# PEDIATRIC AND ADULT NUTRITION IN CHRONIC DISEASES, DEVELOPMENTAL DISABILITIES, AND HEREDITARY METABOLIC DISORDERS

## *Prevention, Assessment, and Treatment*

Third Edition

*Edited by*

Shirley W. Ekvall, Ph.D., FAAMD, FACN, R.D.
Valli K. Ekvall, Ph.D., A.D.D., R.D., L.D.

OXFORD
UNIVERSITY PRESS

OXFORD
UNIVERSITY PRESS

Oxford University Press is a department of the University of Oxford. It furthers the University's objective of excellence in research, scholarship, and education by publishing worldwide. Oxford is a registered trade mark of Oxford University Press in the UK and certain other countries.

Published in the United States of America by Oxford University Press
198 Madison Avenue, New York, NY 10016, United States of America.



First Edition published in 1993
Second Edition published in 2005
Third Edition published in 2017



Library of Congress Cataloging-in-Publication Data
Names: Ekvall, Shirley W., editor. | Ekvall, Valli K., editor.
Title: Pediatric and adult nutrition in chronic diseases, developmental disabilities, and hereditary metabolic disorders
edited by Shirley W. Ekvall, Valli K. Ekvall.
Description: Third edition. | Oxford: Oxford University Press, [2017] | Preceded by Pediatric nutrition in chronic diseases and developmental disorders / edited by Shirley W. Ekvall, Valli K. Ekvall. 2005. | Includes bibliographical references and index.
Identifiers: LCCN 2016006985 (print) | LCCN 2016008795 (ebook) | ISBN 9780199398911 (hardcover : alk. paper) | ISBN 9780199398928 (UPDF) | ISBN 9780199398935 (EPUB)
Subjects: | MESH: Nutritional Physiological Phenomena | Chronic Disease—therapy | Developmental Disabilities—diet therapy | Metabolic Diseases—diet therapy | Nutrition Disorders—prevention & control | Child | Adult Classification: LCC RJ233 (print) | LCC RJ233 (ebook) | NLM QU 145 | DDC 618.92/39—dc23
LC record available at http://lccn.loc.gov/2016006985

9 8 7 6 5 4 3 2 1
Printed by Sheridan Books, Inc., United States of America

*To Ruth and Franklin Rosevear and their daughter, other children with special health care needs, and my late husband, Ray, for their support of this book.*

# Contents

## PART II CHRONIC DISEASES AND DEVELOPMENTAL DISABILITIES

*Shirley W. Ekvall*

### A. Neurological and Developmental



### B. Behavioral and Eating Disorders



### C. Feeding Disorders

### D. Drugs



### E. Miscellaneous Chronic Diseases



## PART III HEREDITARY METABOLIC DISORDERS

*Harvey Levy*

### A. Disorders of Amino Acid Metabolism



### B. Organic Acidemias

# Foreword

The science of Nutrition began in the early part of the 20th century with identification of the essential macronutrients and micronutrients necessary to prevent deficiency diseases and went on to establishing minimal and normal daily requirements of these nutrients. As metabolic pathways were being elucidated, the roles of vitamins, minerals, and trace elements as cofactors or structural components of pathway enzymes were identified.

The unraveling of the genetic code and advances in molecular biology seemed to relegate Nutrition to a secondary role, but that was temporary. The understanding soon evolved that both the genome and its expression are affected by psychosocial as well as biological factors. Of the socioenvironmental factors affecting the genome and its expression, nutrition, beginning in utero and continuing through infancy, childhood, and adulthood, is all-important.

Further, advances in basic and clinical research have enabled children with developmental disorders to survive into adulthood. Because of these advances, nutrition intervention strategies for children with developmental disorders or chronic diseases must have both short- and long-term goals. The short-term goals involve support of growth and development while avoiding deficiencies in both calories and specific nutrients. Long-term goals are equally or even more important. For example, because many children for whom these modern strategies have been successful have reduced physical activity, it is of utmost importance to tailor the diet to match caloric expenditure and avoid the complicating factor of obesity. For children with chronic disorders such as myelomeningocele, obesity can be a devastating management problem. As treatment for developmental disorders and chronic diseases has improved, so has longevity. Therefore, long-term goals must also take into account the avoidance of nutritional risk factors for chronic adult diseases such as hypertension, coronary artery disease, and cancer.

Each child needs an individualized program, depending on the severity of the disorder and his or her personal nature. The family must participate fully in the planning process and act as a full partner with health professionals in the implementation of the nutrition program if the goals are to be achieved and the child is to become as independent as possible. Health care professionals with varied experience and backgrounds should be assembled into a team to provide appropriate guidance and follow-up.

*Pediatric and Adult Nutrition in Chronic Diseases, Developmental Disabilities, and Hereditary Metabolic Disorders*, although directed particularly toward children with special health care needs, provides a wealth of information on current issues in preventive nutrition and normal growth for all ages. As noted in the Contents, the diseases and disorders of children that necessitate nutritional intervention are extremely varied. The diverse topics include acquired disorders such as pica, obesity, and anorexia nervosa; inherited metabolic diseases; and other genetic diseases such as cystic fibrosis, diabetes, and chromosomal defects, as well as the specific nutritional considerations associated with heart diseases, cancer, normal prenatal and postnatal growth, and prematurity.

The first editor, Shirley Walberg Ekvall, is a nationally recognized expert in the field of pediatric nutrition with more than 40 years' experience and numerous publications as well as national and international presentations. She has served as director of a national nutrition workshop for children with special health care needs and as a federal research grant reviewer and editorial consultant for the Surgeon General's Report on Nutrition and Health, several nutrition journals, and various publishers. Valli K. Ekvall has more than 15 years' experience and several publications related to nutrition for both children and adults with developmental disabilities or special health care needs. She also brings the added dimension of knowledge of psychology as it relates to nutrition.

The editors have assembled a knowledgeable and experienced group of respected experts in the fields of nutrition, medicine, and biochemistry to bridge the gap from research to practice in nutrition for each of the chapters in this book. The authors provide a careful analysis and clear guidelines for proper nutrition for children and adults with special health needs. This book is well organized and user-friendly, with consistent headings in each chapter. It is a completely rewritten volume that offers health professionals greater understanding of the nutritional implications of various disease states, how nutrition can affect brain development and learning behavior, and approaches to improving the health status of each person.

Richard Bozian, MD
Professor Emeritus
University of Cincinnati
Department of Internal Medicine
Director
Division of Nutrition
Cincinnati, Ohio
Third Edition

Alvin Mauer, MD
Former Professor of Medicine/Pediatrics
University of Tennessee
Memphis, Tennessee
Former Chairman of the Nutrition Committee/American Academy of Pediatrics
Second Edition

# Preface

Nutrition is a focus of government action. The Healthy People 2020 National Health Promotion and Disease Prevention Objectives provided 10 new topics and policy and action strategies to improve nutrition for the nation. The Surgeon General's Report on Nutrition and Health and the Surgeon General's Report: Children with Special Health Care Needs Campaign both verified the need for better nutrition through early intervention, particularly for children with special health care needs. They are based on Public Law 99-457, which underscores the importance of early intervention and identifies the need for family-centered care and community-based care to reduce nutrition problems and their related costs in our society. Several interdisciplinary national workshops and short courses have been convened to make other disciplines aware of the impact of nutrition on chronic diseases and developmental disorders. The growing recognition of the importance of nutrition has been enhanced by the development of growth charts by the Centers for Disease Control and Prevention based on data from the National Health and Nutrition Examination Surveys (NHANES).

The third edition of this book spans the void between nutrition research and its practical application to children with standard needs, chronic diseases, and intellectual and developmental disabilities. It is completely rewritten, systematically organized, and user-friendly. All chapters are written by MDs and PhDs. The book covers nutrition for numerous chronic diseases and intellectual and developmental disabilities, including inborn errors of metabolism and inherited metabolic disorders. Topics such as botanicals, probiotics, sports nutrition, genetics, and vegetarianism are included in this edition.

Each chapter describes the current status of research on the role of nutrition in intellectual and developmental disorders and chronic diseases of children and helps translate this research into clinical practice. The main focus is on treatment, with the goal of helping children and adults who have special health care needs to develop their potential. Techniques of assessment (including behavior) and prevention for persons of all ages are addressed. In the past 10 years, the help of nutritionists has increasingly been sought to address many behavioral problems such as autism, attention-deficit hypersensitivity disorder, and obesity disorders. Teamwork is required for these very complex problems and is emphasized in this book.

All the disease chapters are consistently organized to cover biochemical and clinical abnormalities, techniques in nutrition evaluation or diagnosis, nutritional treatment or management, and follow-up procedures. Part I stresses preventive techniques in assessing and averting diseases and other high-risk problems. Resource materials and quality assurance standards in nutrition also are addressed. Part II deals with nutrition in people with chronic diseases and intellectual and developmental disabilities. Part III describes inherited metabolic disorders or inborn errors of metabolism and provides methods of diagnosis and nutrition therapy.

This book should continue to be a valuable reference for pediatricians, internists, nutritionists, dietitians, psychologists, family practitioners, pediatric residents, occupational and physical therapists, speech therapists, medical students, nutrition students, nursing students, and other allied health personnel. We hope that its use will help improve the nutrition status of children with special health care needs and will stimulate more research in this field.

*Shirley Walberg Ekvall*
*Cincinnati, Ohio*

# Acknowledgments

We wish to acknowledge Richard Bozian, Harvey Levy, Terri Wallace, Diane Spear, Russell Carroll, Bradley Ekvall, Julia Wahoff, Robert Smith, Carol Henderson, Tina Lu, Alvin Wulfekuhl, Meade Johnson Nutritionals, Abbott Laboratories,Nutricia Co.and Vitaflo for their assistance with this book.

# Contributors

Amal H. Assa'ad, MD
*Professor*
*Director, Allergy and Immunology Fellowship*
*Director, Food Allergy and Eosinophilia Clinic*
*Division of Allergy and Immunology*
*Cincinnati Children's Hospital Medical Center*
*Cincinnati, Ohio*

Keith-Thomas Ayoob, PhD
*Associate Clinical Professor*
*Department of Pediatrics*
*Albert Einstein College of Medicine*
*New York, New York*

Vinod Bansal, MD
*Professor of Medicine*
*Division of Nephrology and Hypertension*
*Loyola University Medical Center*
*Maywood, Illinois*

Steven J. Bachrach, MD
*Pediatrician, Cerebral Palsy, General Pediatrics, and Nutrition*
*Children's Hospital of Philadelphia*
*Philadelphia, Pennsylvania*

Rudolf Bauer, MD, PhD
*Professor*
*Head of the Institute of Pharmacognosy*
*Institut fuer Pharmakognosie*
*Karl-Franzens-Universitaet Graz*
*Graz, Austria*

Patricia J. Becker, MS, RDN, CSP, CNSC
*Pediatric Nutrition Specialist*
*Cincinnati Children's Hospital Medical Center*
*Cincinnati, Ohio*

Susan A. Berry, MD
*Professor and Director*
*Division of Genetics and Metabolism*
*Department of Pediatrics*
*University of Minnesota*
*Minneapolis, Minnesota*

Judith Beto, PhD, RD, FADA
*Research Associate*
*Division of Nephrology and Hypertension*
*Loyola University Medical Center*
*Maywood, Illinois*
*Professor, Nutrition Science*
*Dominican University*
*River Forest, Illinois*

Genila Bibat, MD
*Research Associate*
*Department of Pediatrics*
*Johns Hopkins University School of Medicine and the Neurogenetics Unit*
*Kennedy Krieger Institute*
*Baltimore, Maryland*

Richard Boles, MD
*Assistant Professor of Pediatrics*
*Keck School of Medicine*
*University of Southern California*
*Director of Clinical Genetics*
*Children's Hospital Los Angeles*
*Los Angeles, California*

Eric K. Bonsall, MD
*Board Certified Child and Adolescent Psychiatry*
*Medical Director*
*Hoffman Homes for Youth*
*Littlestown, Pennsylvania*
*Psychiatric Consultant*
*Alternative Rehabilitative Communities*
*Harrisburg, Pennsylvania*

Nga Hong Brereton, MS, LDN, IBCLC
*Research Nutritionist*
*Institute for Clinical ad Translational Research*
*Johns Hopkins University School of Medicine*
*Baltimore, Maryland*

Leah Burke, MD
*Professor*
*Department of Pediatrics and Genetics*
*University of Vermont*
*Burlington, Vermont*

Alison Cassin, MS, RD, CSP, LD
*Dietitian, Eosinophilic Disorder*
*Cincinnati Children's Hospital Medical Center*
*Cincinnati, Ohio*

Frank Cerniglia, Jr. MD
*Director of Pediatric Urology*
*Ochsner Clinic*
*New Orleans, Los Angeles*

Harriet Cloud, MS, RD
*Private Practice: Nutrition Matters*
*Birmingham, Alabama*
*Former Director of Nutrition*
*Center for Development and Learning Disabilities*
*Birmingham, Alabama*

Carmen Cuffari, MD
*Associate Professor*
*Division of Pediatric Gastroenterology*
*Johns Hopkins University School of Medicine*
*Baltimore, Maryland*

Paula Cushing, RD
*Registered Dietitian*
*Tennessee Department of Intellectual and Developmental Disabilities*
*Nashville, Tennessee*

Asad Dalia, MD, PhD
*Assistant Professor of Clinical*
*College of Allied Health Sciences Rehabilitation Sciences*
*University of Cincinnati*
*Cincinnati, Ohio*

Karen Reznik Dolins, EdD, RD, CDN
*Adjunct Associate Professor*
*Columbia University*
*New York, New York*

Teresa D. Douglas, PhD
*Department of Human Genetics*
*Emory University Hospital*
*Atlanta, Georgia*

Daniel J. Driscoll, PhD, MD
*Professor of Pediatrics*
*Molecular Genetics and Microbiology*
*Center for Mammalian Genetics*
*University of Florida*
*Gainesville, Florida*

Shirley W. Ekvall, PhD, FAAMD, FACN, RD
*Professor, Adjunct, Online*
*Nova University*
*Ft. Lauderdale, Florida*
*Former Professor*
*University of Cincinnati*
*Cincinnati, Ohio*
*Former Chief of Nutrition Services*
*Division of Developmental Disabilities*
*Cincinnati Children's Hospital Medical Center*
*Cincinnati, Ohio*

Valli K. Ekvall, PhD, ADD, RD, LD
*Assistant Professor, Adjunct, Online*
*Nova University*
*Ft. Lauderdale, Florida*
*Nutrition Community Consultant,*
*Children/Adults with Developmental Disabilities*
*Cincinnati, Ohio*
*Former Nutrition Consultant*
*Division of Developmental Disorders*
*Cincinnati Children's Hospital Medical Center*
*Cincinnati, Ohio*

Craig A. Erickson, MD
*Adolescent Psychologist*
*Cincinnati Children's Hospital Medical Center*
*Cincinnati, Ohio*

Michael Farrell, MD
*Professor of Pediatrics*
*Department of Gastroenterology and Nutrition*
*Chief of Staff*
*Director*
*Pediatric Residency Program*
*Cincinnati Children's Hospital Medical Center*
*Cincinnati, Ohio*

Sharon Feucht, MA, RD
*Pediatric Dietitian*
*University of Washington*
*Seattle, Washington*

Dianne Frazier, PhD, RD
*Professor Emeritus*
*Department of Pediatrics*
*Division of Genetics and Metabolism*
*University of North Carolina*
*Chapel Hill, North Carolina*

Amy Fuller, RD
*Food and Nutrition Services Manager*
*Ridgecrest Regional Hospital*
*Ridgecrest, California*

Carol J. Henderson, PhD, RD, LD
*Pediatric Dietitian*
*Nutricia Company*
*Baltimore, Maryland*

Melanie Gillingham, PhD, RD
*Associate Professor*
*Department of Molecular and Medical Genetics*
*Oregon Health and Science University*
*Portland, Oregon*

Michele Gottschlich, PhD, RD, CSP, CCRP
*Registered Dietitian*
*Shriner's Hospital for Children*
*Associate Professor*
*Department of Surgery*
*University of Cincinnati*
*Cincinnati, Ohio*

Joan Earle Hahn, PhD, RN
*Professor*
*College of Nursing*
*Director of Nursing Program*
*Keene State College*
*Keene, New Hampshire*

Martica Heaner, PhD
*Health and Fitness Journalist*
*Former Fitness Director*
*New York, New York and Houston, Texas*

Linda Hicks, MEd, RD, MOT
*Occupational Therapist Consultant*
*Nutrition Therapist Consultant*
*Ft. Lauderdale, Florida*

Georgia E. Hodgkin, EdD, MS, RD
*Professor, Nutrition and Dietetics*
*Loma Linda University*
*School of Allied Health Professions*
*Pomona, California*

Violet Hsieh, MPH, RD
*Nutritionist*
*Children's Hospital Los Angeles*
*Los Angeles, California*

Agnes M. Huber, PhD, RD, FAAMD
*Professor Emeritus*
*Department of Nutrition*
*Simmons College*
*Boston, Massachusetts*

Malai Holland, RD, MPH, CD
*Metabolic Nutritionist*
*University of Vermont*
*Burlington, Vermont*

Leslie Huffman, RD
*Dietetic Specialist*
*Chapel Hill, North Carolina*

Patricia D. Jackson, MBCHB, FRCPCH
*Honorary Fellow*
*University of Edinburgh*
*Edinburgh, Scotland*

Lisa Kelchner, PhD
*Associate Professor*
*Department of Communication Sciences and Disorders*
*University of Cincinnati*
*College of Allied Health Sciences*
*Cincinnati, Ohio*

Priya Kishnani, MD
*Professor of Pediatrics*
*Division of Medical Genetics*
*Duke University*
*Durham, North Carolina*

Nancy D. Leslie, MD
*Professor and Head of Metabolic Services*
*Division of Human Genetics*
*Cincinnati Children's Hospital Medical Center*
*Cincinnati, Ohio*

Harvey Levy, MD
*Senior Associate in Medicine and Genetics*
*Children's Hospital Boston*
*Professor of Pediatrics*
*Harvard University*
*Boston, Massachusetts*

Alan B. Lewis, MD
*Professor of Pediatrics*
*Division of Cardiology*
*Keck School of Medicine*
*University of Southern California*
*Children's Hospital Los Angeles*
*Los Angeles, California*

Christina C. Lewis, PhD
*Associate Professor*
*Department of Basic Sciences*
*Samuel Merritt University*
*Oakland, California*

Salisa Lewis, RD, MS, LD
*Dietitian Specialist*
*Cincinnati Children's Hospital Medical Center*
*Cincinnati, Ohio*

Daniel Lovell, MD, MPH
*Associate Director*
*Division of Rheumatology*
*Cincinnatti Children's Hospital Medical Center*
*Professor*
*Department of Pediatrics*
*University of Cincinnati*
*Cincinnati, Ohio*

Elisabeth Luder, PhD, RD
*Former Associate Professor*
*Department of Pediatrics*
*Mount Sinai School of Medicine*
*New York, New York*

Gail B. Mahady, PhD
*Associate Professor*
*College of Pharmacy*
*University of Illinois at Chicago*
*UIC/NIH Center for Botanical Dietary Supplements Research*
*Chicago, Illinois*

Yael Shiloh-Malawsky, MD
*Clinical Assistant Professor*
*Department of Neurology, Division of Child Neurology and Epilepsy*
*University of North Carolina School of Medicine*
*Chapel Hill, North Carolina*

Daniel Mallon, MD
*Pediatric Gastroenterologist*
*Division of Gastroenterology, Hepatology, and Nutrition*
*Associate Program Director for Student and Resident Education*
*Division of Gastroenterology, Hepatology and Nutrition*
*Assistant Professor*
*UC Department of Pediatrics*
*Cincinnati, Ohio*

Dorothy Markowitz, RD, LD
*Director*
*Pediatric Nutrition Services*
*University of Minnesota Masonic Children's Hospital*
*University of Minnesota*
*Minneapolis, Minnesota*

Inez Martincevic, MSc, RD
*Clinical Dietitian*
*The Hospital for Sick Children*
*Toronto, Ontario, Canada*

Theresa Mayes, RD, CSP, CCRC
*Registered Dietitian*
*Certified Clinical Research Coordinator*
*Cincinnati Children's Hospital Medical Center*
*Cincinnati, Ohio*

Helen McCune, MS, RD
*Nutritionist*
*Nutrition Department*
*Shands Hospital*
*University of Florida*
*Gainesville, Florida*

Gary McPhail, MD
*Associate Professor*
*Department of Pulmonary Medicine*
*Cincinnati Children's Hospital Medical Center*
*Cincinnati, Ohio*

Robin C. Meyers, MS, RD
*Nutritionist*
*Children's Hospital of Philadelphia*
*Philadelphia, Pennsylvania*

Jennifer Miller, MD
*Assistant Professor*
*Division of Endocrinology*
*University of Florida*
*Gainesville, Florida*

Mari Mori, MD
*Medical Genetics*
*Duke University*
*Durham, North Carolina*

Kathryn Moseley, MS, RD
*Metabolic Dietitian*
*Division of Medical Genetics*
*Children's Hospital Los Angeles*
*Los Angeles, California*

Ann B. Moser, BA
*Research Associate in Neurology*
*Kennedy Krieger Institute*
*Johns Hopkins University*
*Baltimore, Maryland*

Janine Z. Mundorff, MS, RDN, CNSC
*Chief Dietitian*
*Hoffman Homes Residential Treatment Facility*
*Gettysburg, Pennsylvania*

David L. Nelson, PhD
*Professor*
*Department of Molecular and Human Genetics*
*Baylor College of Medicine*
*Editor, American Journal of Human Genetics*
*Houston, Texas*

Barbara Niedbala, MEd, RD, LDN
*Renal Dietitian*
*Fresenius Kidney Care*
*Chicago, Illinois*
*Former Neonatal Nutritionist*
*Children's Mercy Hospital*
*Kansas City, Missouri*

Omar Niss, MD
*Assistant Professor of Pediatrics*
*Division of Hematology*
*Cincinnati Children's Hospital Medical Center*
*Cincinnati, Ohio*

Viviann Nordin, MD, PhD
*Pediatric Neurologist*
*Section of Child Neurology*
*Department of Pediatrics*
*University Hospital of Lund*
*Children's Hospital*
*Lund, Sweden*

William Nyhan, MD
*Professor Emeritus*
*Pediatrics*
*University of California at San Diego School of Medicine*
*San Diego, California*

Ingrid Ora, MD, PhD
*Pediatric Oncologist*
*Section of Oncology*
*Department of Pediatrics*
*University Hospital of Lund*
*Children's Hospital*
*Lund, Sweden*

Scott Pentiuk, MD
*Pediatric Gastroenterologist*
*Division of Gastroenterology, Hepatology, and Nutrition*
*Assistant Professor*
*UC Department of Pediatrics*
*Cincinnati, Ohio*

Gerald V. Raymond, MD
*Professor*
*Department of Neurology*
*University of Minnesota*
*Minneapolis, Minnesota*

Cecilia Rokusek, EdD, RD, MSc
*Assistant Dean of Research and Innovation*
*Professor of Family Medicine, Public Health, and Nutrition*
*College of Osteopathic Medicine*
*Nova Southeastern University*
*Ft. Lauderdale, Florida*
*Distinguished Visiting Professor of Medicine*
*Comenius University*
*Faculty of Medicine*
*Bratislava, Slovakia*

Howard M. Saal, MD
*Professor of Pediatrics*
*Director of Clinical Genetics*
*University of Cincinnati College of Medicine*
*Division of Human Genetics*
*Cincinnati Children's Hospital Medical Center*
*Cincinnati, Ohio*

Stephanie Sanborn, RD
*Nutritionist*
*Middlebury, Vermont*

Tori L. Schaefer, PhD
*Director, Psychiatry*
*Developmental Disabilities Translational Research Lab*
*Cincinnati Children's Hospital Medical Center*
*Cincinnati, Ohio*

Rayfel Schneider, MBBCh, FRCPC
*Staff Rheumatologist*
*The Hospital for Sick Children*
*Professor and Associate Chair*
*Department of Pediatrics*
*University of Toronto*
*Toronto, Ontario, Canada*

Marshal Shlafer, PhD
*Professor*
*Department of Pharmacology*
*University of Michigan Medical School*
*Ann Arbor, Michigan*

Rebecca J. Shlafer, PhD, MPH
*Assistant Professor*
*Division of General Pediatrics and Adolescent Medicine*
*University of Minnesota*
*Minneapolis, Minnesota*

Rani H. Singh, PhD
*Professor*
*Human Genetics*
*Emory University*
*Atlanta, Georgia*

Wendy Smith, MD
*Director*
*Division of Genetics*
*Maine Pediatric Specialty Group*
*Barbara Bush Children's Hospital*
*Portland, Maine*

Diane Spear, RD, MS
*Nutririon Therapist*
*Division of Developmental Disabilities*
*Registered Dietitian/Nutritionist*
*Oklahoma Department of Health*
*Mannford, Oklahoma*

Virginia A. Stallings, MD
*Professor of Pediatrics*
*University of Pennsylvania School of Medicine*
*Director of Nutrition Center*
*Children's Hospital of Philadelphia*
*Philadelphia, Pennsylvania*

Cynthia Stegeman, ED, RD
*Professor of Dental Hygiene*
*Department of Dental Hygiene*
*University of Cincinnati*
*Cincinnati, Ohio*

Florence Stevens, MS, RD, LD
*Former Developmental Nutritionist*
*Division of Developmental Disabilities*
*Cincinnati Children's Hospital Medical Center*
*Cincinnati, Ohio*

Sandy van Calcar, PhD, RD
*Metabolic Dietitian*
*Molecular and Metabolic Genetics*
*Oregon Health and Science University*
*Portland, Oregon*

Margreet van Rijn, PhD
*Research Specialist*
*Beatrix Children's Hospital*
*University Medical Center of Groningen*
*Groningen, the Netherlands*

Francjan van Spronsen, MD, PhD
*Associate Professor in Metabolic Diseases*
*Division of Metabolic Diseases*
*Beatrix Children's Hospital*
*University Medical Center of Groningen*
*Groningen, the Netherlands*

Julia Wahoff, COTA/L
*Occupational Therapy Consultant*
*Private Practice*
*Cincinnati, Ohio*

Jennifer Walberg-Wolfe, MS
*Exercise Physiologist Consultant*
*Private Practice*
*Bluffton, South Carolina*

Russell E. Ware, MD, PhD
*Director, Division of Hematology*
*Co-Executive Director*
*Cancer and Blood Diseases Institute*
*Cincinnati Children's Hospital Medical Center*
*Cincinnati, Ohio*

Elizabeth Welin, MS, RD, LD
*Pediatric Oncology Dietitian*
*Cincinnati Children's Hospital Medical Center*
*Cincinnati, Ohio*

Melinda Wendland, RD, LD
*Registered Dietitian*
*Division of Nutrition Therapy and the Center for Spina Bifida*
*Cincinnati Children's Hospital Medical Center*
*Cincinnati, Ohio*

Jacqueline Wessel, MEd, RD, CSP, CLE, CNSC
*Registered Dietitian Specialist in the NICU*
*Cincinnati Children's Hospital Medical Center*
*Cincinnati, Ohio*

Tuomas Westermarck, MD, PhD
*Docent in Pediatrics*
*University of Helsinki*
*Former Chief Physician*
*Research Centre Rinnekoti*
*Rinnekoti, Finland*

Sheila M. Wicks, MD
*Professor Biological Sciences*
*Committee Chair for Anatomy and Physiology*
*City Colleges of Chicago*
*Chicago, Illinois*

Rebecca Wilhelm, RD, MS
*Registered Dietitian*
*Division of Nutrition Therapy*
*Cincinnati Children's Hospital Medical Center*
*Cincinnati, Ohio*

Illustrator
Bradley Ekvall, BFA
*Pre-medicine, Fine Arts*
*Co-author/Medical Illustrator, Orthopedics*
*Winners Guide to Pain Relief*
*Former Senior Designer*
*Galerie*
*Cincinnati, Ohio*

# PART I
# PREVENTIVE NUTRITION

*Shirley W. Ekvall*

Preventive nutrition is the focus of Part I.[1] The usual progress of prenatal and postnatal growth and development and the parameters of prematurity are described. The circumstances and behaviors that might interfere with normal growth and the preventive measures and treatments for them are identified. Because the ability to measure nutritional status is key to identifying the possible need for intervention, nutritional status tools and training programs on how to provide nutrition services for children with special health care needs are reviewed. Part I concludes with a discussion of the standards for delivering and evaluating the quality of these nutritional services.

The first three chapters deal with Nutrition and Growth. The effects of early malnutrition on growth reported by Myron Winick are discussed in Chapter 1. The severity, age at onset, and duration of early nutritional deprivation determine the extent of its negative impact on growth and learning capability. The adverse effects of malnutrition on intellectual development are of interest but need further investigation. The interplay of other environmental factors also cannot be ignored.

Adequate maternal nutrients are essential for normal prenatal growth and for development during the first 3 years of life. Ninety percent of brain development and 50% of skeletal growth occur during that period. High-risk factors affecting maternal nutrition and fetal outcome and associated corrective actions are also discussed in Chapter 1. Early prenatal care has increased. Some of the highrisk problems in infancy, such as iron deficiency anemia, hypernatremia, and obesity, are described, along with their treatments, in Chapter 2. Because of the many assessment and treatment factors involved, enteral and parenteral nutrition, fluid balance, increased nutrient needs, and other aspects of nutrition for premature and small-for-gestationalage infants are discussed in Chapter 3. The effects of inadequate nutrition and stress are also presented.

The chapters in Part I relate to early intervention as mandated by Public Law 99-457 (102-119).[2] This law, passed originally in 1986 as an amendment to the Federal Education of the Handicapped Act, focuses on children with special health care needs—that is, children from birth to 3 years of age who have developmental delays or high-risk problems that may result in a developmental delay. Preventive services have now been extended to children ages 3 to 5 years to strengthen the role of the family in their treatment. Children with certain conditions are eligible for early intervention: mental retardation, speech and language impairment, hearing deficit, visual handicap, special learning disability, orthopedic impairment, emotional disturbance, and various other medical conditions categorized as health impairments. Early intervention includes a constellation of physical and cognitive services designed to prevent the need for later special education services.[3] Disciplines involved in early intervention include medicine, nutrition, nursing, special education, speech/language pathology, audiology, psychology, occupational and physical therapy, social work, and dentistry.[4] These services may be interdisciplinary or transdisciplinary in nature.

The US Department of Health and Human Services and the Academy of Nutrition and Dietetics support and encourage nutritional services that are coordinated, interdisciplinary, family centered, and community based for children with special health care needs and advocate the training of students to provide such services.[5–9] The American Academy of Pediatrics and other health care associations also support P.L. 99-457 (102-119). Federal monies are provided to the states to fund early intervention services for children who are developmentally delayed or at high risk from birth. At the state level, these services are administered by departments of education, health, or mental health and developmental disabilities. Nutrition education is a major component of P.L. 99-457 (102-119). Education related to nutrition may not only alleviate the problems of these children with special health care needs (e.g., feeding problems in children with cerebral palsy), so that they can attain their full growth and development, but may also prevent the delay from developing.[9,10]

The techniques used to screen, assess, diagnose, and correct high-risk nutritional problems in children with chronic diseases and developmental disorders, such as those seen in children eligible for services mandated by P.L. 99-457 (102-119), are presented in the second section of Part I, entitled Nutrition Evaluation. The five-point nutritional assessment includes dietary and nutrient intake and physical activity, biochemical values, anthropometric measurements, physical signs, and feeding. Several assessment methodologies are described comprehensively in Chapter 4, including anthropometric illustrations of measurement techniques for developmental disorders in people of all ages. Assessment forms, grids, tables, and illustrations covering the period from infancy to adulthood and beyond are provided in the appendices. Three levels of nutritional status assessment—minilevel (community), mid-level (clinics), and in-depth (physical examination)—are discussed in this chapter.[4]

Without the necessary nutritional resources and training materials at clinics and other community-based programs, nutritional intervention would not be possible. Program-planning tools for implementing community and family-centered care are presented in Chapter 5. One such resource is an interdisciplinary short course for developmental disorders and chronic diseases sponsored annually by Maternal and Child Health clinics in various cities. This course also is available with training manuals[11,12] and videotapes from the University of Cincinnati and other sites.[13]

Detailed quality assurance standards of care for developmental disorders, myelomeningocele, and other topics, as well as several pyramids and Choose My Plate models related to nutrition, physical activity, and ethnicity, are given in the appendices.[14] The 2015 Guidelines for Americans also are shown in the appendices.[15] Quality assurance standards for specific diseases or disorders are discussed throughout the book. The impact of stress and injury, as well as nutrition, is presented in Chapter 6. Other preventive measures are also discussed, including sports nutrition in Chapter 7 and vegetarian diets in Chapter 8.

## References

1. U.S. Department of Health and Human Services, Maternal and Child Health Bureau. *Child Health USA 2014*. http://mchb.hrsa.gov/chusa14/. Accessed May 23, 2016.
2. Individuals with Disabilities Education Act. Early Intervention Program for Infants and Toddlers with Handicaps: Final Regulations. Public Law 99-457 (102-119). *Federal Register*, June 22, 1989.
3. Campbell MK, Kelsey KS. The PEACH survey: a nutrition screening for use in early intervention programs. *J Diet Assoc.* 1994; 94:1156.
4. Ekvall S, Ekvall V. Early intervention and nutrition. In: Stevens F, Ekvall S, eds. *Empowering Children Through Early Intervention with Good Nutrition: Focusing on Culturally Diverse Children with Special Health Care Needs.* Manual #4 MCHB and HRSA. Cincinnati, OH: University of Cincinnati Publications; 2002.
5. U.S. Department of Health and Human Services. *Healthy People 2020*. Office of Disease Prevention and Health Promotion. http://www.healthypeople.gov. Accessed May 23, 2016.
6. Lucas B, Feucht S. *The Benefits of Nutrition Services for a Case Series of Children with Special Health Care Needs in Washington State.* DOH Publication No. 970-212. Olympia, WA: Washington State Department of Health; 1998.
7. Herman D, Baer M. *Cost-Effectiveness of Nutrition Services· for Children with Special Health Care Needs:1.* Los Angeles, CA: University Affiliated Center for Child Development and Developmental Disabilities; 1999.
8. Nardella M, Campo L, Ogata U, eds. *Nutrition Interventions for Children with Special Health Care Needs Manual.* DOH Publication No. 961-158. Olympia, WA: Washington State Department of Health; 2003.
9. Ptomey LT, Wittenbrook W. Position of the Academy of Nutrition and Dietetics: nutrition services for individuals with intellectual and developmental disabilities and special health care needs. *J Acad Nutr Diet.* 2015; 115:593.
10. Position of the Academy of Nutrition and Dietetics: the role of nutrition in health promotion and chronic disease prevention. *J Acad Nutr Diet.* 2013; 113:972.
11. Garvin J, Ekvall S. *Nutrition for Children with Special Health Care Needs: Second Tier Training Kit in Developmental Disorders and Managed Care.* Manual #5 MCHB and HRSA. Cincinnati, OH: University of Cincinnati Publications; 2002.
12. Yang Y, Lucas B, Feucht S, eds. *Nutrition Interventions for Children with Special Health Care Needs*, 3rd ed. DOH Publication No. 961-158. Olympia, WA: Washington State Department of Health; 2010. http://here.doh.wa.gov/materials/nutrition-interventions/15_CSHCN-NI_E10L.pdf. Accessed May 23, 2016.
13. Story M, Holt K., Sofka D. *Bright Future in Practice: Nutrition*, 2nd ed. Arlington, VA; National Center for Education in Maternal and Child Health; 2002.
14. U.S. Department of Agriculture. *My Plate, My Wins: Healthy Eating Solutions for Everyday Life.* http://www.ChooseMyPlate.gov. Accessed May 23, 2016.
15. U.S. Department of Health and Human Services and U.S. Department of Agriculture. *2015–2020 Dietary Guidelines for Americans.* 8th ed. December 2015. http://health.gov/dietaryguidelines/2015/. Accessed May 23, 2016.

# A.

# NUTRITION AND GROWTH

## 1 Prenatal Growth in Pregnancy

SHIRLEY W. EKVALL, VALLI K. EKVALL, AND BARBARA NIEDBALA

The two major sources of developmental disabilities in prenatal growth are genetic inheritance and the intrauterine environment. The genetic disorders include single-gene disorders such as cystic fibrosis, maple syrup urine disease, galactosemia, phenylketonuria, and sickle cell anemia and chromosomal disorders such as trisomy 13, trisomy 18, and trisomy 21 or Down syndrome (see Chapter 60). Conditions affecting the intrauterine environment that give rise to developmental disorders include maternal infection (e.g., herpes simplex type II), maternal diseases, and maternal lifestyle factors (e.g., exposure to toxic substances in the workplace or home, drug abuse, malnutrition, smoking).

### MATERNAL NUTRITION AND FETAL OUTCOME

Improved nutrition during pregnancy, especially beginning in the first trimester, is associated with improved pregnancy outcomes.[1,2] In a systematic review of food subsidy programs in high-income countries, Black et al.[3] found that pregnant food subsidy program participants had a 10% to 20% increased intake of nutrients. This was associated with a small but clinically relevant increase in mean birth weight. In the United States, the Special Supplemental Nutrition Program for Women, Infants and Children (WIC) has been proven to have favorable outcomes.[4] It provides nutrition education and foods, promotes breast-feeding, and provides referrals to health care and social service systems. WIC has been found to produce improved birth outcomes (i.e., reduced rates of premature birth and infant mortality), improved nutrient density in the maternal diet, and improved rates of initiation of breast-feeding.

Barker's hypothesis,[5] that undernutrition in utero permanently changes the body's structure, function, and metabolism in ways that lead to coronary heart disease in later life, has expanded the research field. Some of the ideas and progress in research were reviewed by Wadhwa et al.[6] They examined studies looking at the timing of fetal undernutrition and its effect on types of chronic diseases developing later in life (e.g., insulin resistance, coronary artery disease); the fetal origins of obesity; in utero exposure to maternal stress and its effect on both birth weight and the development of chronic diseases; and epigenetic mechanisms that may account for some of the observations in studies of the developmental origins of health and disease. Offspring born either small for gestational age (SGA) or large for gestational age (LGA) share common risks for a number of behavioral disorders and are at higher risk for obesity later in life.[7] See Chapter 3 for information on the SGA infant.

### TRENDS IN MATERNAL AND INFANT MORTALITY

Global maternal mortality rates have steadily declined over the years. The cause of death varies by region. The four most prevalent causes of maternal death in high-income regions in 2013 were abortion, hypertension, sepsis, and hemorrhage, although all of these decreased significantly between 1990 and 2013. By contrast, the most important causes of maternal death in low-income countries, abortion and hemorrhage, did not change between 1990 and 2013.[8]

According to the World Health Organization, the number of neonatal deaths and stillbirths in developed countries is falling as a result

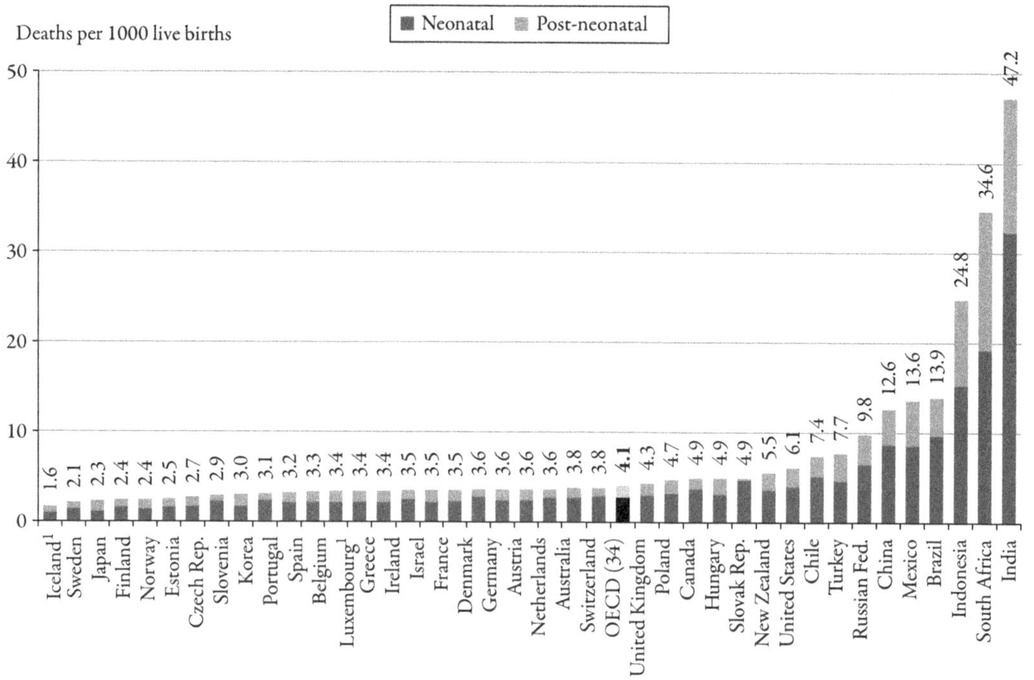


**Figure 1–1.** Infant Mortality Data. Part of the explanation for the relatively high infant mortality rate in the United States is due to a more complete registration of very premature or low birth weight babies than in other countries. From OECD (2013), Health at a Glance 2013: OECD Indicators, OECD Publishing. Used with permission.

of "changing patterns in reproductive health, socioeconomic progress and the quality of obstetric and neonatal facilities."[9] Figure 1–1 illustrates infant mortality rates among industrialized nations. In the United States, the highest fetal mortality occurs at lower gestational ages (<23 weeks), and much of the early fetal mortality is related to congenital anomalies, intrauterine growth restriction, or an underlying maternal medical condition or infection.[10] In the southeastern United States, where fetal mortality is highest, the infant death rate for mothers with prenatal care beginning from the first month was one-fifth of the rate for mothers with no prenatal care.[11]

## BIOCHEMICAL, PATHOLOGICAL, CLINICAL, AND NUTRIENT ABNORMALITIES

The effects of malnutrition are determined by its severity, timing, and duration.[12] When undernourished, the liver, heart, kidney, and skeletal muscle work harder and remain small to spare the brain and lung from damage (Fig. 1–2). The last trimester of pregnancy and the first 6 months after birth are important for brain development. By age 3 years, 90% of brain development has occurred, but the child has increased only 50% in height. The number of brain cells found in Chilean infants who were dying from malnutrition was less than 40% of the number in normal infants (Fig. 1–3). Studies in Mexico by Winick[12] demonstrated that if malnourished infants were rehabilitated, 10% had a total recovery in IQ, 52% were educable, 33% were trainable, and 5% were institutionalized (Fig. 1–4). In the United States and Europe, problems caused by malnutrition include more subtle changes in perceptual thinking, abstract thinking, and verbalization, as well as maladaptive behavior. The incidence of

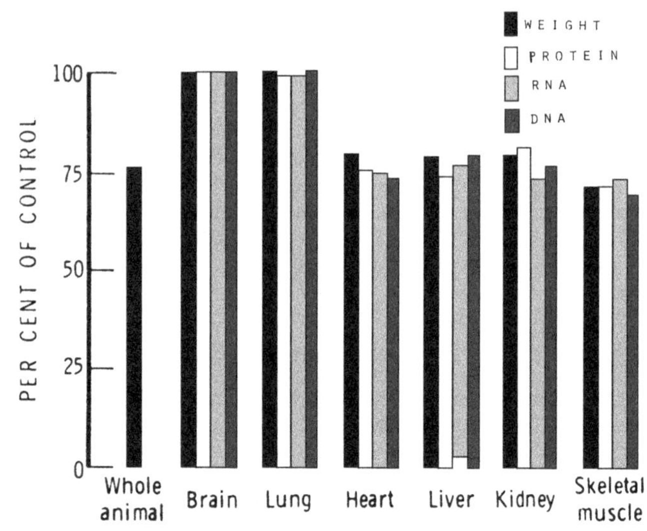


**Figure 1–2.** End of refeeding, period II. (From Winnick M. Cellular changes during early malnutrition. *Currents in Maternal and Child Health.* Columbus, OH: Ross Laboratories; 1971. Used with permission.)

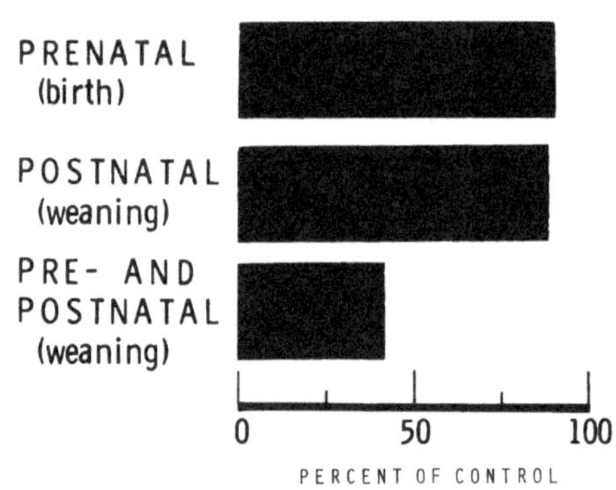


**Figure 1–3.** Malnutrition: total brain cell number. (From Winnick M. Cellular changes during early malnutrition. *Currents in Maternal and Child Health.* Columbus, OH: Ross Laboratories; 1971. Used with permission.)

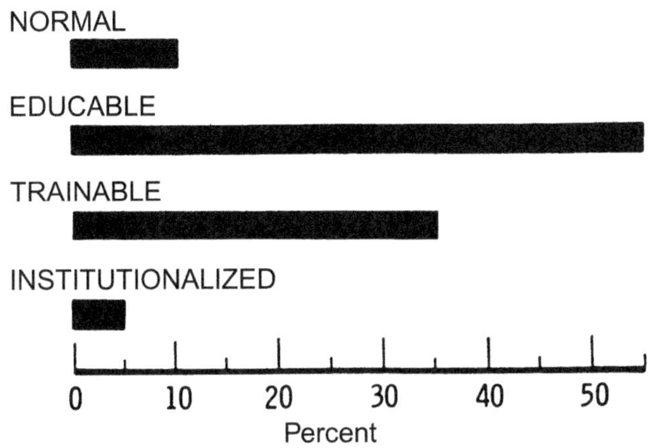


**Figure 1–4.** Infantile marasmus. (From Winnick M. Cellular changes during early malnutrition. *Currents in Maternal and Child Health.* Columbus, OH: Ross Laboratories; 1971. Used with permission.)

**Table 1–1.** Environmental Factors Suspected of Causing Congenital Malformation in Human Beings (Teratogenic)

| *Contaminants and Additives* | *Product Use* |
|---|---|
| Cadmium | Alcohol |
| Cyclamates | Cigarettes |
| Dioxin | Coffee |
| Dichlorodiphenyl trichloroethane (DDT) | Gasoline |
| Food colorings | Lysergic acid diethylamide (LSD) |
| Hair dyes | Marijuana |
| Lead | Methadone |
| Mercury* | Phencyclidine |
| Monosodium glutamate | Tea |
| Nitrates | Tobacco chewing |
| Nitrites | Toluene sniffing |
| Polyhalogenated biphenyls | |
| Saccharin | *Occupational Exposure* |
| Sodium fluoride | Anesthetic gases |
| 2,4,5-T herbicide | Fat solvents |
| | Hair spray |
| *Natural Substances* | Hexachlorophene |
| Blighted potatoes | Hydrocarbons |
| Cyanide in cassava | Organic solvents |
| Goitrogens in brassicae | Printing trades |
| | Smelters |
| | University laboratories |

*Of all the substances listed, only mercury is today considered a proven human teratogen. From Kalter H, Warkany J. Congenital malformations: etiologic factors and their role in prevention (first of two parts). *N Engl J Med.* 1983; 308:424; and Kalter H. Teratology in the 20th century: environmental causes of congenital malformations in humans and how they were established. *Neurotoxicol Teratol.* 2003; 25:131.

fetal malnutrition is estimated to range from 3% to 10% of live births in developed countries and from 15% to 20% in developing countries.[13,14]

A major risk factor for developmental disabilities is the mother herself. Pregnancy during adolescence, short interpregnancy intervals, and too little or too much weight gain in the mother are associated with poor outcomes.[15,16] Multiple dietary factors influence outcome. Protein-energy malnutrition and deficiencies of iron, zinc, folate, vitamin $B_{12}$, and vitamin A are well known to cause infant morbidities.[17] The risk of spina bifida, a neural tube defect (see Chapter 11), can be significantly reduced by supplemental folic acid, particularly for low-income women with reduced absorption of folic acid.[18] Excessive ingestion of vitamins A and D, calcium, and iodine also may result in prenatal damage to the infant. Variations of vegetarian diets (e.g., vegan, plant-based) can be healthful but also may put the fetus at risk for nutrient deficiencies.[19,20] Pica leading to lead intoxication or nutrient deficiencies and excessive ingestion of alcohol (>5 oz of whiskey or equivalent per day) directly affect fetal development (see Chapters 14 and 23).

Drug use by the mother, either therapeutic or recreational, may affect the fetus. The use of antiepileptic drugs, more than 30 of which are in common use, has expanded to treat other types of disorders in the mother, such as depression, migraine headaches, and panic disorder.[21] Use of antiepileptic drugs, especially valproic acid, is implicated in raising the risk of embryonic malformations including microcephaly, growth retardation, hypoplasia of the midface and fingers, cardiac malformations, hypospadias, facial clefts, and neural tube defects. Oral contraceptive users present with consistently lower serum vitamin $B_{12}$ concentrations independent of their dietary intake.[22] Diuretics reduce oxygen to the fetal brain. Tetracycline produces abnormalities in bone development, including decalcification of dentition. Thalidomide, diethylstilbestrol, lysergic acid diethylamide (LSD), warfarin, antihistamines, cortisone, some antibiotics and tranquilizers, and Accutane (isotretinoin, a vitamin A analog) have caused major problems in prenatal growth,[23,24] although other environmental substances and drugs have been accepted as nonteratogenic with customary use (Tables 1–1 and 1–2). Drugs such as heroin and barbiturates can produce withdrawal in the infant.[25] Heroin (which causes hyperkalemia), morphine (which results in calcium inhibition), and cocaine (which depresses appetite) are more damaging; their use results in lower birth weight than is seen with barbiturate addiction, and their ingestion is a form of abuse.[26] Cigarette smoking is linked with low birth weight, pregnancy complications, more physiological stress symptoms in the newborn at birth, and lower IQ throughout life.[27,28] In utero marijuana exposure has not been implicated in any major fetal growth or physical abnormalities,[29] but there is some evidence that marijuana causes problems with neurological development resulting in hyperactivity or poor cognitive function.[30]

Other high-risk maternal indicators include chronic disease; a prior child with birth defects; 15% underweight or 20% overweight[31]; a poor obstetric or fetal history; hemoglobin lower than 11 g/dL or hematocrit lower than 33% in the second trimester; proteinuria; and glucosuria. Environmental substances at first suspected of causing congenital malformation in humans are shown in Table 1–1; of these, only mercury has been proven to be a human teratogen. The critical periods in human development are presented in Figure 1–5.

Some maternal diseases can affect prenatal growth, including epilepsy, diabetes, heart disease, phenylketonuria, Rh blood factor, hypertension (related to toxemia), and anemia. In such cases, laboratory values for hemoglobin, hematocrit, serum transferrin, transferrin saturation, thiamine, riboflavin, and urinary *n*-methyl nicotinamide (mg/g of creatinine) differ from the acceptable adult values.

**Table 1–2.** Presumably Nonteratogenic Drugs and Drug Classes in Customary Use

| | |
|---|---|
| Adrenocorticoids | Lithium* |
| Amphetamines | Meclizine |
| Nonquinine antimalarials | Nalidixic acid |
| Aspirin | Oral hypoglycemics |
| Bendectin | D-Penicillamine* |
| Captopril | Phenothiazines |
| Clomiphene | Podophyllum |
| Diazepam | Propoxyphene |
| Ergonovine | Sulfonamides |
| Imipramine | Tuberculostatics |

*Since 1983, it has been questioned whether lithium and D-penicillamine may be teratogenic. From Kalter H, Warhany J. Congenital malformations: etiologic factors and their role in prevention (first of two parts). *N Engl J Med.* 1983; 308:424 (see Chapter 27); and Kalter H. Teratology in the 20th century: environmental causes of congenital malformations in humans and how they were established. *Neurotoxicol Teratol.* 2003; 25:131.

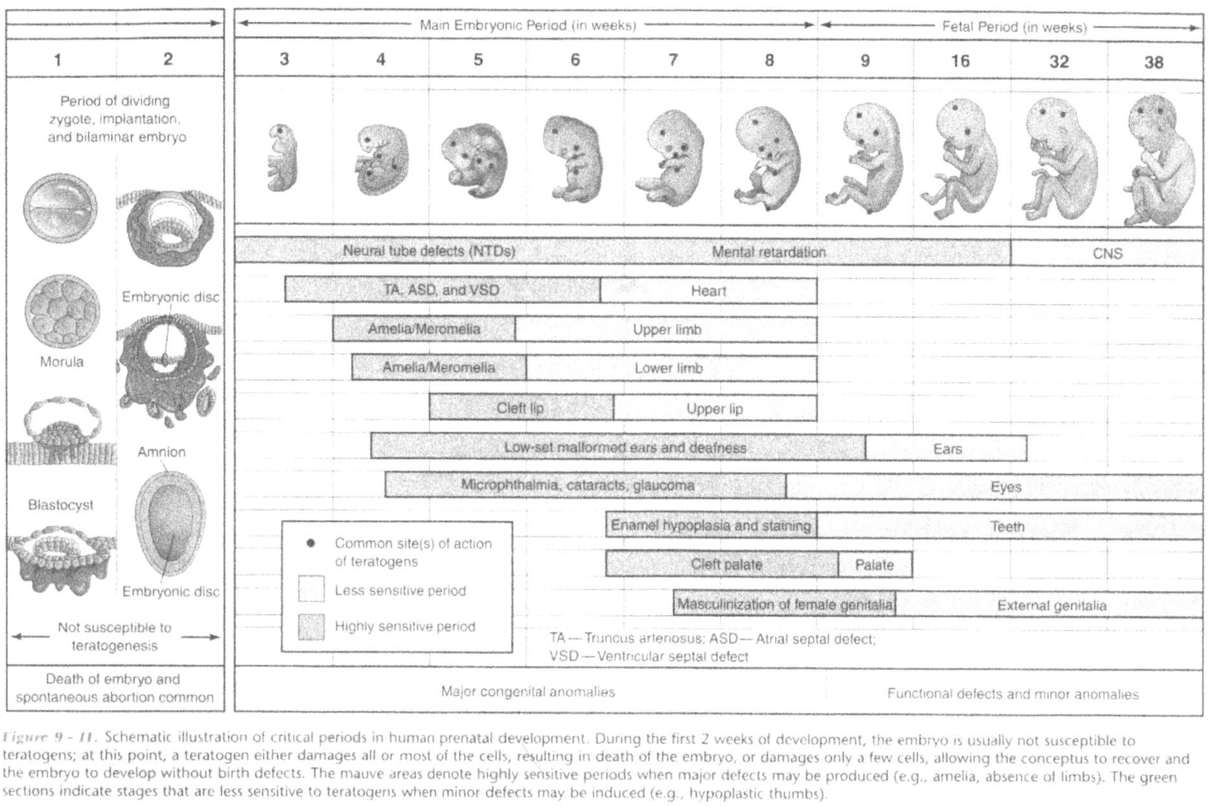


**Figure 1–5.** Schematic illustration of critical periods in human prenatal development. During the first 2 weeks of development, the embryo is usually not susceptible to teratogens. After that point, a teratogen either damages all or most of the cells, resulting in death of the embryo, or damages only a few cells, allowing the conceptus to recover and the embryo to develop without birth defects. (From Moore KL. *Before We Are Born: Essentials of Embryology and Birth Defects,* 6th ed. Philadelphia: Saunders; 2003. Used with permission.)

## FACTORS TO BE CONSIDERED IN NUTRITIONAL EVALUATION AND DIETARY MANAGEMENT

A suggested assessment of the mother includes her medical history and physical screening of four parameters: dietary history and food frequency; anthropometric measures of the mother's fatfold, height, and weight; physical activity of the mother; and laboratory test results (see the WIC nutritional assessment form and computerized perinatal nutrition assessment form in Appendix 5.) The mother should be asked about the quantities of various foods eaten and any unusual food habits, such as pica during pregnancy, in the dietary history. Women who are malnourished before pregnancy and during early pregnancy require additional nutrients[32] and dietary counseling, especially teenagers whose bodies are still growing. The recommended daily food intakes for pregnant adolescents, pregnant adults, and lactating women are shown in Table 1–4. Because this daily food plan may be low in some nutrients, such as folate and other B vitamins (depending on

**Table 1–3.** Embryopathology Reported in Animal Models with Specific Nutritional Imbalances

| | | |
|---|---|---|
| Water | Deficiency | — |
| Food | Deficiency | — |
| Food and water | Deficiency | — |
| Vitamin A | Deficiency | Excess |
| Vitamin D | Deficiency | Excess |
| Vitamin K | Deficiency | — |
| Vitamin E | Deficiency | — |
| Vitamin C | Deficiency | Excess |
| Riboflavin | Deficiency | — |
| Thiamine | Deficiency | — |
| Niacin | Deficiency | — |
| Pyridoxine | Deficiency | — |
| Folic acid | Deficiency | — |
| Pantothenic acid | Deficiency | — |
| Vitamin $B_{12}$ | Deficiency | — |
| Calcium | Deficiency | Excess |
| Magnesium | Deficiency | — |
| Iodine | Deficiency | Excess |
| Copper | Deficiency | — |
| Manganese | Deficiency | — |
| Zinc | Deficiency | — |
| Iron | Deficiency | — |

From Brent RL. Maternal nutrition and congenital malformations. In: Young BK, ed. *The Patient Within the Patient: Problems in Perinatal Medicine.* Vol. 21. March of Dimes Birth Defects Foundation. New York: Alan Liss; 1985:1. (See also http://www.modimes.org).

**Table 1–4.** Daily Food Plan

| Food Group | Adolescent Pregnancy | Adult Pregnancy | Lactation |
|---|---|---|---|
| *Milk* (milk products may be used) | 5 c | 4 c | 6 c |
| Meat, liver, poultry, eggs, or beans | 2 servings (4 oz ea.) | 2 servings (3 oz ea.) | 4 servings ($2^1/_2$ oz ea.) |
| *Fruit* (vitamin C food source) | 2 servings | 2 servings | 2 servings |
| Other fruits | 2 servings | 2 servings | 2 servings |
| *Vegetables* as a source of vitamin A | 1 serving | 1 serving | 1 serving |
| Other vegetables (including raw vegetables) | 2 servings | 2 servings | 2 servings |
| *Bread and cereal* (whole grain preferred) | 5–6 servings | 4 servings | 5 servings |
| *Other* foods | Foods to meet caloric needs may be selected from above groups, or fats and sweets may be added in moderation (about 200 calories) | | |
| *Liquids* | 8–12 c | 8–12 c | 12 c |

**Table 1–5.** Dietary Reference Intake (DRI) During Pregnancy and Lactation for Women Ages 19 to 30 Years

| | Nonpregnant, Nonlactating Adult | Pregnancy | Lactation |
|---|---|---|---|
| Energy* (kcal) | 1791 | 1986 | 2138 |
| Protein* (g) | 63.3 | 78.2 | 79.7 |
| Vitamin A (μg/d)† | 700 | 770 | 1300 |
| Zinc (mg/d)† | 8 | 11 | 12 |
| Copper (μg/d)† | 900 | 1000 | 1300 |
| Calcium (mg/d) | 1000 | 1000 | 1000 |
| Phosphorus (mg/d) | 700 | 700 | 700 |
| Magnesium (mg/d) | 310 | 350 | 310 |
| Vitamin D (μg/d) | 5 | 5 | 5 |
| Fluoride (mg/d) | 3 | 3 | 3 |
| Thiamine (mg/d) | 1.1 | 1.4 | 1.4 |
| Riboflavin (mg/d) | 1.1 | 1.4 | 1.6 |
| Niacin (mg/d) | 14 | 18 | 17 |
| Vitamin $B_6$ (mg/d) | 1.3 | 1.9 | 2.0 |
| Folate (μg/d) | 400 | 600 | 500 |
| Vitamin $B_{12}$ (μg/d) | 2.4 | 2.6 | 2.8 |
| Panthothenic acid (mg/d) | 5 | 6 | 7 |
| Biotin (μg/d) | 30 | 30 | 35 |
| Choline (mg/d) | 425 | 450 | 550 |
| Vitamin C (mg/d) | 75 | 85 | 120 |
| Vitamin E (mg/d) | 15 | 15 | 19 |
| Selenium (μg/d) | 55 | 60 | 70 |

From Food and Nutrition Board, Institute of Medicine. *Dietary Reference Intakes: Applications in Dietary Assessment.* Washington, DC: National Academies Press; 2000. (See Appendix 1.)

*From the Food and Nutrition Board, Institute of Medicine. *Dietary Reference Intakes for Energy, Carbohydrate, Fiber, Fat, Fatty Acids, Cholesterol, Protein and Amino Acids (Macronutrients).* Washington, DC: National Academies Press; 2002.

†From the Food and Nutrition Board, Institute of Medicine. *Dietary Reference Intakes for Vitamin A, Vitamin K, Arsenic, Boron, Chromium, Copper, Iodine, Iron, Manganese, Molybdenum, Nickel, Silicon, Vanadium and Zinc.* Washington, DC: National Academies Press; 2002.

the foods selected), a prenatal vitamin supplement is typically recommended by the physician during both pregnancy and lactation.[18] The daily diet during pregnancy should include approximately 14 extra grams of protein, 300 extra calories, and increased quantities of most vitamins and minerals, except for vitamin D, calcium, and phosphorus, as noted in Table 1–5. (See the Dietary Reference Intakes in Appendix 1.) The Institute of Medicine of the National Academy of Sciences recommends three meals and two snacks per day.[33]

## VITAMIN AND MINERAL DEFICIENCIES AND EXCESSES

The micronutrients most likely to be important for maternal, infant, and child outcomes are iron, iodine, folate, vitamin $B_{12}$, vitamin D, calcium, selenium, and zinc.[34] Without iron supplementation, most women exhaust their iron stores and are iron deficient, as manifested by low ferritin levels.[35] Iron supplementation appears to be needed until about 20 to 24 weeks' gestation. If no iron supplementation is given, it takes about 2 years after delivery to attain prepregnancy ferritin levels.[36] Consumption of ascorbic acid and meat, fish, or poultry may increase nonheme iron bioavailability fourfold.[37] Iodine deficiency in the mother leads to lower IQ in the infant due to hypothyroxinemia; it also is associated with higher rates of spontaneous abortion, reduced birth weight, and increased infant mortality.[38] An adequate intake of folic acid content is essential to prevent megaloblastic anemia and to decrease the risk of a neural tube defect. However, there is some controversy about the effect of folate supplementation on birth outcomes, particularly the development of wheezing and asthma.[39] Vitamin $B_{12}$ deficiency (<148 pmol/L) is associated with adverse maternal and neonatal outcomes, including developmental anomalies, spontaneous abortion, preeclampsia, and low birth weight (<2500 g).[40]

The intake of vitamin D is often too low to sustain healthy circulating levels of the prehormone 25(OH)D. Low serum 25(OH)D levels have been linked to altered brain development.[41] Low maternal intake of vitamin C has been associated with a twofold increase in the risk of preeclampsia.[35] Villar and Belizan[42] reported that individuals with high calcium intake have lower blood pressure and that rats with restricted calcium intake develop hypertension, which is reversible by calcium supplementation. Moreover, the eclampsia syndrome is similar to tetany caused by hypocalcemia, a finding that requires more research; the symptomatology has also shown a correlation with diet.[42,43] Zinc deficiency results in impaired synthesis of nucleic acids. According to one study, addition of zinc to prenatal iron and folate supplements can improve maternal and neonatal zinc status.[44] Adequate zinc intake is critical to cognition and to the electrophysiology and behavioral activity of the brain. However, zinc supplementation does not lead to increased birth weight or a reduction in the incidence of low birth weight.[45] Vitamin A is needed for the transport of protein, a carrier of zinc into the blood. Low manganese levels, as measured in the mother's hair (which may be an inaccurate technique), have been found in mothers of infants with congenital malformations[46]; high manganese levels have also caused congenital problems. Magnesium deficiency may be responsible for spasms of the umbilical and placental vasculature.[47,48] Magnesium supplementation may be useful in reducing the risk for gestational-age babies.[49]

Problems resulting from excess minerals due to vitamin/mineral supplementation can include excessive calcium and iodine, as noted in animal models. Problems caused by iodine deficiency still occur in some parts of the world, however.[43,50] Guidelines for supplementation safety exist.[50] For example, beta-carotene (chemically one-half of vitamin A) is much safer than supplemental vitamin A to reduce the retinol intake.[51] Preelampsia symptoms can be eased by reducing the number of calories and/or the amounts of proteins, lipids, simple sugars, and sodium, but particularly proteins and sodium.[50]

## LEAD CONTAMINANTS AND FOOD FADDISM

It is critical to evaluate malnutrition with poor dietary habits or pica[52] and the presence of a risky maternal environment in the home (e.g., presence of organic or fat solvents such as oven cleaners or degreasers). Many substances, such as organic mercury compounds and benzene, are of particular concern. Not only environmental lead but also arsenic and other heavy metals that enter the food chain may seriously deplete body stores of vitamin C, iron, and other essential nutrients (e.g., zinc, magnesium, calcium), leading to intrauterine growth retardation, decreased immune defenses, impaired psychosocial faculties, and other disabilities associated with malnutrition.[53] Maternal hobbies or workplace environments involving lead-based or organic solvents also need to be considered and evaluated.[54,55] These contaminants can cause even more problems when superimposed on malnutrition (see Chapter 23).

Leakage of lead from zinc-lined soldering seams in old cans of vegetables and fruits needs to be evaluated by public health workers and nutritionists. The calcium in evaporated or canned milk is less of a problem because the calcium in milk chelates with the lead, which is then excreted (skeletal calcium is the dominant contributor to blood lead during pregnancy and in the postpartum period).[56] Hot water running through lead pipes can also contribute significant amounts of lead, half of which is absorbed.[56] Deficiencies in body calcium, zinc, iron, and protein are associated with increased uptake of lead.[56] Lead can also produce alterations in vitamin D, calcium, and phosphorus homeostasis.[57] When mothers smoke, the birth weight of the infant is smaller. The lead in the tobacco plant that the child inhales as smoke is even more damaging for a child with low birth weight because of the increased oxygen requirement. High dietary sodium intake produces greater loss of calcium in the urine because sodium and calcium compete for the same recovery mechanism in the kidney (see DASH Diet Appendix 1 for Healthy Eating).[58] High sodium intake thus has a negative effect on the protective action of calcium to prevent lead toxicity.

The consumption of foods such as unpasteurized milk and juice, imported cheeses, partially cooked eggs, raw and smoked seafood, and meat spreads and pâtés exposes the mother to potentially harmful bacteria,[59–61] and eating large amounts of certain fish exposes the fetus to mercury.[62]

## AGE

The incidence of low birth weight is increased by one-third in infants born to adolescent mothers. Early prenatal care promotes better pregnancy outcomes for younger teenagers than for older teens or adults.[63] Encouraging young adolescents to gain larger amounts of weight during pregnancy may be one way to decrease the risk of low-birth-weight deliveries.[64–66] Infants born to mothers younger than 15 or older than 40 years of age have lower birth weight and a higher incidence of Down syndrome (see Chapter 15).[67]

## WEIGHT GAIN

Body mass and weight gain of approximately 12.5 kg significantly influence birth weight.[60,63] Each kilogram of maternal weight gain in underweight, ideal weight, and moderately overweight women increases the infant birth weight by 25.9, 28.3, and 17.8 g, respectively.[68,69] When assessing the nutritional requirements of pregnant women, weight gain related to the changes due to the pregnancy itself must be considered.[70] As shown in Table 1–6, a prenatal weight gain of 25 to 35 lb produces an optimal pregnancy outcome for a single infant; 35 to 45 lb is optimal for twins.[71,72] The caloric cost of pregnancy is about 70,000 calories. The pregnant woman who does not gain sufficient weight must catabolize maternal tissue; this may produce ketosis and thus may impair the neurological development of the fetus.[73] The Institute of Medicine reexamined its recommendations for gestational weight gain in 2009 and summarized the findings in "Weight Gain During Pregnancy: Reexamining the Guidelines."[74] Brown et al.[75] found that more than 50% of underweight women failed to gain more than 9 kg in pregnancy, and their infants weighed less than 2501 g; therefore, weight gain is of critical importance to underweight women who become pregnant. Siega-Riz et al.[76] found a significant relationship between weight gain at 20 weeks' gestation and infant birth weight. Nutritionists have developed a prenatal weight gain intervention program using social marketing methods to encourage early weight gain.[77,78]

Muscati et al.[79] and Hruba and Kachlik[80] found that smoking is significantly associated with reduced prenatal weight gain. Smoking during pregnancy has a negative influence on birth weight.[80] The resting metabolic rate increased more during pregnancy than previous estimates on well-nourished women would indicate, and the increase was significantly correlated with the birth weight of the baby.[81] Increased incidences of hypertension (43%), hyperglycemia (16.9%), and subnormal urinary estriol excretion (18.6%) were found in obese pregnant women.[81] The complications of labor also are much greater with obesity. Although obese pregnant women are at greater risk for complications, weight gain is recommended at the amount listed in Figure 1–6 to ensure optimal birth outcomes. The figure shows recommended weight gain as related to prepregnancy weight and weight gain for selected subsets.

The fetus is fed initially by the trophoblast (via secretion of uterine milk from the uterine glands), then by the syncytium (formed between maternal and fetal tissues) after the blastocyst is implanted in the uterine epithelium, and finally by the placenta (through placental circulation). The velocity of weight gain peaks at 33 to 34 weeks' gestation at about 220 g/wk[82] (Fig. 1–7; see Chapters 2 and 3). Carbohydrates reach the fetus as glucose, which is used to synthesize fat. The essential lipids and phospholipids in the cell walls and nervous system are transferred to the fetus from the maternal circulation. The lipid content is 1% at 20 weeks, 2.8% at 34 weeks, and 15% at term. The nitrogen (as polypeptides, proteins, and immunoglobulins) that is required for the synthesis of many different proteins reaches the fetus mainly by active transport of amino acids. The proportion of protein increases with gestational age and is greater than that of fat until 35 weeks' gestation[82] (Fig. 1–8). The rate of calcium increases from 0.3 g/wk at 18 weeks to 2.6 g/wk at 40 weeks (Fig. 1–9).

**Table 1–6.** Weight Gain Related to Pregnancy

| | Weight (lb) |
|---|---|
| Baby | 7.0–8.5 |
| Placenta | 2.0–2.5 |
| Increase in weight of uterus | 2.0 |
| Amniotic fluid | 2.0 |
| Increase in weight of breasts | 1.0–4.0 |
| Increase in blood volume and extracellular fluid | 8.0–10 |
| Mother's stores* | 3.0–6.0 |
| Total | 25.0–35.0 |

*Extra stores of fat and a little protein are required to support the energy needed for pregnancy, labor, delivery, and milk production.

Trace elements enter the fetus early in gestation, probably in the plasma attached to specific proteins, whereas water-soluble vitamins cross the placenta by active transport because their concentration is higher in fetal than in maternal blood. Fat-soluble vitamins are found in lower concentrations in the fetus than in maternal plasma, but the method of transfer is unknown. The oxygen consumption of the fetus is 30 kcal/kg/24 hr in utero, 32 kcal/kg/24 hr at birth, and 43 kcal/kg/24 hr by the first day of life.[81]

## EXERCISE

The literature on physical activity and pregnancy has evolved over the last 50 years, and there is currently sufficient empirical evidence to support the promotion of moderate to vigorous prenatal physical activity for maternal health benefits.[83] Moderate to vigorous physical activity during pregnancy has been linked to better health outcomes for mothers and their children. The American College of Obstetricians and Gynecologists (ACOG) released guidelines in 2002 advising pregnant women to engage in at least 150 minutes of moderate-intensity physical activity each week.[84]

## DISEASES OR DISORDERS

Infants born to smokers weigh up to 300 g less at birth owing to a chronic decrease in placental blood flow.[79,80] Alcohol and drugs should be avoided during pregnancy (see Chapters 14 and 27). Data from human studies regarding caffeine use are inconsistent. Caffeine should be used minimally, or intake should be lower than 150 mg/day; late spontaneous abortions are more likely with higher levels.[33] A 5-oz cup of coffee has approximately 128 mg of caffeine; a 5-oz cup of black tea, 46 mg; a 5-oz cup of green tea, 32 mg; and 12 oz of cola, 53 mg.

In the United States, geophagia, pagophagia, and anylophagia are the most commonly reported practices of pica during pregnancy. Anemia (iron deficiency) and zinc deficiency are common problems with pica (see Chapter 23). Clay and starch are the most commonly ingested substances. Pregnant women need to be questioned about food cravings and pica in particular (especially because of the harmful effects of lead toxicity).

Mothers with diabetes have a higher incidence of congenital malformations in their infants. In rats, these malformations are caused by reduced arachidonic acid during organogenesis. Acute administration of zinc and arachidonic acid significantly increased glucose disposition in diabetic (ob/ob) mice; the study authors recommended these two compounds as a dietary supplement to control hyperglycemia[85] in patients with type 2 diabetes.[86] Women who are obese are more likely to develop gestational diabetes during pregnancy. In addition, women who are diabetic tend to deliver infants who weigh more than 9 lb, and some of these infants may develop gross motor impairment and inattention.[87] Frequently, these infants are delivered by cesarean section before they reach full term. Eating a well-balanced diet and exercising regularly are particularly important for the mother with diabetes. Reviewing foods eaten in historical times can be of benefit.[88]

In recent years, toxemia in pregnancy has become less life-threatening because blood pressure has come to be controlled more effectively, reducing the incidence of intracranial hemorrhage. Prompt use of blood transfusion and broad-spectrum antibiotics for complications is needed.[89] The mean serum level of placental isoferritin was found to be low in women with preeclamptic toxemia compared with

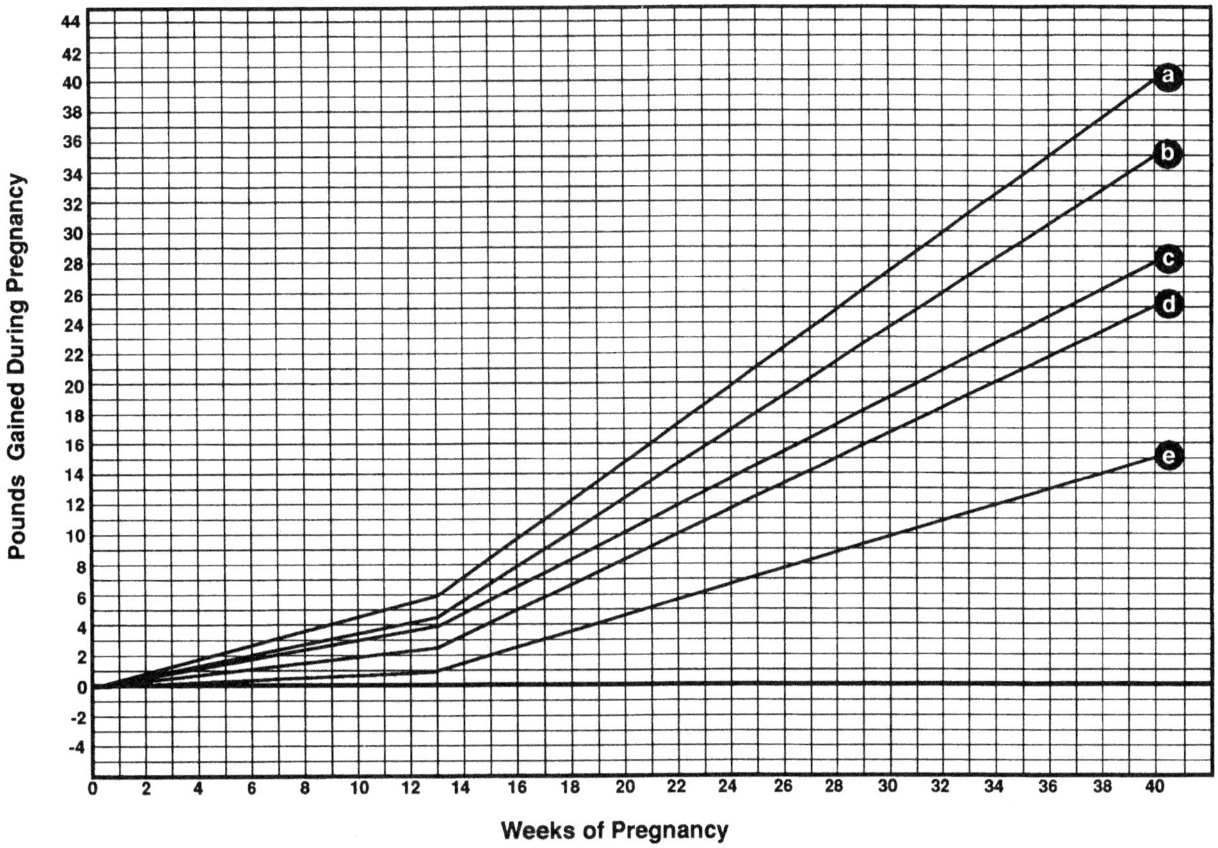


| Weight Before Pregnant | Keep Pregnant Weight in this Range |
|---|---|
| Normal | b - d |
| Underweight | a - c |
| Overweight | d - e |

**Figure 1–6.** Recommended weight gain during pregnancy. (Adapted from National Academy of Science. *Nutrition During Pregnancy.* Rosemount, IL: National Dairy Council; 1991. Used with permission.)

women experiencing a normal pregnancy. For this reason, placental isoferritin may be a useful marker for preeclamptic toxemia during pregnancy.[90] It appears that the fetus whose mother has toxemia is unlikely to be thrombocytopenic during labor and delivery; therefore, scalp blood counts and cesarean delivery to avoid labor probably are not required.[89] The Doppler ultrasound measurement of cardiac output in the fetus has been validated.[90] Treatment of hypertension with medication during pregnancy may not be needed unless blood pressure is higher than 170/100 mm Hg because diuretics can decrease the fetal oxygen supply.[91,92] If medication is needed, calcium channel blockers cause less low fetal weight than atenolol in the first trimester.[92] Antioxidants may reduce the risk of hypertension,[92] as may calcium

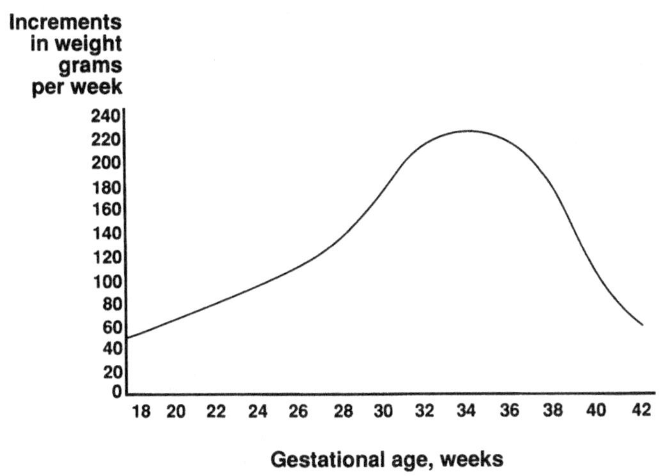


**Figure 1–7.** Velocity of weekly weight gain in utero. (From Widdowson EM. Fetal and neonatal nutrition. *Nutr Today*. 1987; 22:16. Used with permission.)

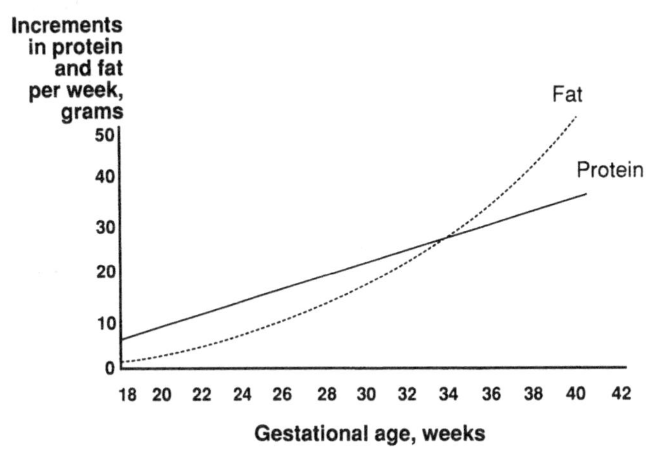


**Figure 1–8.** Increments of fat and protein in the fetal body per week. (From Widdowson EM. Fetal and neonatal nutrition. *Nutr Today*. 1987; 22:16. Used with permission.)

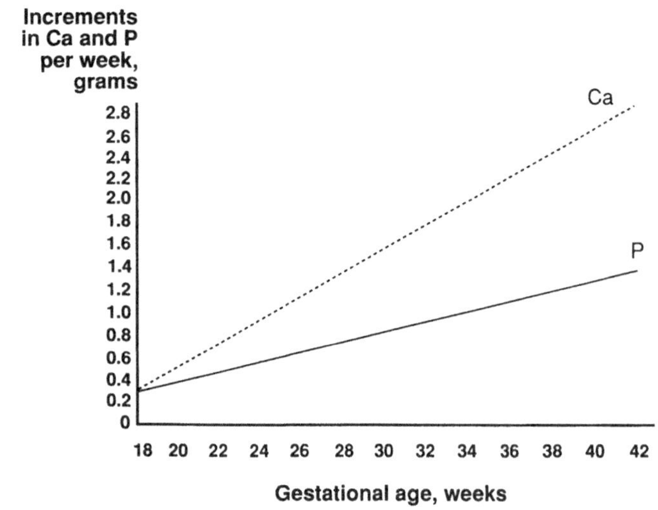


**Figure 1–9.** Increments of calcium (Ca) and phosphorus (P) in the fetal body per week. (From Widdowson EM. Fetal and neonatal nutrition. *Nutr Today*. 1987; 22:16. Used with permission.)

supplementation.[93] A diet that contains less than 1 g sodium and 2 g calcium per day may be helpful. Prevention should be the goal.[94] Proteinuria should be evaluated for its cause if it occurs at 1+, 2+, or 3+ levels. Among women requiring parenteral nutrition, the frequency of complications secondary to centrally inserted venous catheters is greater in pregnant women than in nonpregnant women.[95] Peripherally inserted catheters may be preferable.

## PREVENTION MANAGEMENT

An annotated resource list may be found in a training module of the Prevention Strategies for Developmental Disabilities program, *The Impact of Nutritional Status Before Conception, During Pregnancy, and in Early Childhood.*[96,97] Nutrition resources on prenatal growth are also readily available from the following sources: Food, Dairy and Nutrition Councils; selected federal information clearinghouses and national resource centers; Planned Parenthood affiliates; Maternal and Child Health projects; WIC projects; March of Dimes chapters (Maternal Nutrition Modules 1–10 and *Inside My Mom*); the American Dietetic Association (e.g., position papers for healthy pregnancy outcome); and dietary departments in hospitals. By contracts between the National Academy of Sciences and the U.S. Department of Health and Human Services Health Resources and Services Administration; the Centers for Disease Control and Prevention Division of Nutrition, Physical Activity and Obesity; the National Institutes of Health Eunice Kennedy Shriver National Institute of Child Health and Human Development; the National Institutes of Health National Institute of Diabetes and Digestive and Kidney Diseases; the U.S. Department of Health and Human Services Office on Women's Health; the U.S. Department of Health and Human Services Office of Disease Prevention and Health Promotion; and the March of Dimes, the Institute of Medicine has produced a valuable resource with information on weight gain and nutrient supplementation during pregnancy entitled *Weight Gain During Pregnancy: Reexamining the Guidelines*.[74] The Institute of Medicine has also provided dietary references for vitamins and minerals.[98]

Because the need to assess nutrition parameters in prenatal growth is so critical, dietitians and nutritionists should be employed in obstetric and pediatric offices. Likewise, because homeless women have higher pregnancy rates (11.4% versus 5% for American women overall) and lower-birth-weight infants (16.3%) than low-income women at 11.4%, as well as overall birth rates in New York City (7.4%),[99] dietitians and nutritionists should be used as consultants to homeless shelters.[100,101] This is very cost-effective, eliminating the need for subsequent costly health care in the United States. Third-party reimbursement for nutrition services also is cost-effective.

Preventive measures are important in reducing infant mortality. Because lower net weight gains in pregnancy are associated with an increased risk for the infant, young adolescent, Asian-American, and African-American mothers should strive for higher weight gains based on prepregnancy weight for height or body mass index (BMI) (weight/height$^2$) (see Fig. 1–5). The recommended weight gain is as follows:

- Low BMI (<19.8) = 28–40 lb
- Normal BMI (19.8–26.0) = 25–35 lb
- High BMI (26.0–29.0) = 15–25 lb

Adolescents and underweight women tend to report prepregnancy weight and height more accurately than overweight women do. Using pictures to show stages of growth and development of the fetus and plotting the weight change on a grid (see Fig. 1–5) can reinforce the importance of weight gain, particularly for adolescents.[102]

In Guatemala, a study examined women who became pregnant with a second child and continued to breast-feed into the second trimester of pregnancy. The stress of lactation depleted maternal nutrient stores but did not affect fetal growth significantly.[103] Intake of certain nutrients (i.e., iron, zinc, calcium, copper, magnesium, vitamins D and $B_{12}$, and folate) and caloric intake should be further studied to relate maternal and fetal nutritional status to pregnancy outcome.[104] If a daily multivitamin/mineral preparation is recommended at the beginning of the second trimester, it should contain iron (27 mg), zinc (11 mg), copper (1000 µg), calcium (1000 Cityase clarify this sentence; it is hard to understand which figures are being compared. Are you repeating the 11.4% figure for pregnancy in homeless women, or is this the rate of LBW infants in low-income women? Also, is the 7.4% figure for New York City a pregnancy rate or the rate of LBW Please verify all dosages.mg), vitamin $B_6$ (2 mg), folate (600 µg), vitamin C (85 mg), and vitamin D (5 µg); it should be taken between meals or at bedtime[74] (see Table 1–5). In addition, a mixture of docosahexanoic acid and arachidonic acid may benefit both the maternal and neonatal long-chain polyene status.[105] The Dietary Reference Intakes from the Institute of Medicine are listed in Appendix 1.

It is important to understand the physiology of pregnancy and nutritional metabolism.[106] Susser and Stein[107] found that to enhance infant birth weight, the maternal diet appears to deserve more attention than weight gain. However, nutritional intervention is important in both single and twin pregnancies because of the risk of obesity.[108] Because many people patronize fast-food establishments and other restaurants, dietitians and nutritionists should encourage the reduction of sodium, sugar, and fat content in foods and the increased use of whole-grain products, nuts, vegetables, and fruits. The evidence of reduced intake of folate, iron, and calcium (i.e., more soft drinks and less milk) in the United States and other countries is alarming.[109,110] The original position paper on vegetarian diets by the American Dietetic Association and Dietitians of Canada[111] and the updated practice paper on healthy pregnancy outcomes,[112] as well as Chapter 8 in this text (on vegetarian diets), should be reviewed. Restaurants also would benefit from input by nutritionists and dietitians, particularly through the National Restaurant Association.

## LACTATION

A 2015 position paper on breast-feeding by the Academy of Nutrition and Dietetics[113] stated:

> It is the position of the Academy of Nutrition and Dietetics that exclusive breastfeeding provides optimal nutrition and health protection for the first 6 months of life, and that breastfeeding with complementary foods from 6 months until at least 12 months of age is the ideal feeding pattern for infants. Breastfeeding is an important public health strategy for improving infant and child morbidity and mortality, improving maternal morbidity, and helping to control health care costs. Research continues to support the positive effects of human milk on infant and maternal health, as it is a living biological fluid with many qualities not replicable by human milk substitutes. Recent research advancements include a

greater understanding of the human gut microbiome, the protective effect of human milk for premature infants and those born to women experiencing gestational diabetes mellitus, the relationship of breastfeeding with human immunodeficiency virus, and the increased ability to characterize cellular components of human milk.

Breast-feeding has the advantage of reducing allergens if there is a history of allergies in the family and of increasing immunoglobulin. In order to reduce the risk of atopic disease in the infant, mothers with a family history of atopic disease should breast-feed for longer than 15 weeks.[114] Breast-feeding may protect against clinical symptoms of some diseases (e.g., celiac disease, Crohn's disease) and may bestow psychological benefits.[113] These advantages are particularly important for children with developmental disorders or chronic illness who are prone to upper respiratory infections. Benefits to the mother include more rapid loss of weight gained during pregnancy, enhanced maternal-infant bonding, amenorrhea, and more rapid uterine involution. However, the mother who does not choose to breast-feed should not be made to feel guilty, because infant formulas are nutritious. Another benefit of breast-feeding is its association with lower blood pressure later on for children born prematurely. Weight gain in breast-fed infants is usually 1 to 2 lb less at the end of the first, but adequate growth in length occurs, as was noted in a 1-year study by Diaz et al. (Figs. 1–10 and 1–11).[115] In a study in the United Kingdom of children born preterm, the long-term benefit of breast-milk feeding to reduce atherosclerosis was evidenced by a lower C-reactive protein level and a lower ratio of low-density to high-density lipids.[116]

Breast-feeding practices among various cultures in the United States are changing. In 1998, about 68% of white infants, 45% of African-American infants, and 66% of Hispanic infants were breast-fed. Southeast Asian infants had the lowest rate.[117] Morbid obesity (BMI >40) led to risk of an early termination of breast-feeding.[118] Some situations, such as multifetal pregnancy, need special consideration.[119] For preterm infants, breast milk provides less protein, calcium, and phosphorus and fewer trace elements than are available in the uterus; therefore, a supplemental formula is needed as well (see Chapter 3). However, extended breast-feeding should be encouraged for the premature infant.[120,121] Although most medications are excreted into breast milk at concentrations that are not harmful to the infant, some may be harmful, so all medications should be investigated.[114] To breast-feed successfully, working mothers need extra support and guidance; part-time employment, flexible schedules, and partial breast-feeding may be helpful. Teaching the mother to drink a lot of fluids, get plenty of rest, and know that adequate infant weight gain (0.5–1 oz per day after the fifth day) can be achieved by 8 to 12 feedings every 24 hours, producing five to seven soaking wet diapers and five to seven dirty diapers, gives the mother confidence that the infant is receiving adequate nourishment. Swallowing should be heard; there should be no rooting after feeding; and the breast should feel empty after feeding.

During lactation, at least 16 g more protein and 340 calories more than the adult DRIs should be consumed, and the intake of vitamins and minerals (except for vitamin D, iron, calcium, and phosphorus) should be increased as well (see Table 1–5). The daily food plan for lactation is shown in Table 1–4. A study of maternal nutrition during lactation was undertaken at the request of the Maternal and Child Health Program for lactating women. The following nutrients should not be consumed above the recommended daily allowance for lactation because they are secreted into human milk: iodine, vitamins $B_6$, vitamin D, and selenium. Major minerals (i.e., calcium, phosphorus, sodium, and potassium) in human milk are not affected by the mother's diet. The stores of vitamin C, thiamine, biotin, folate, and vitamins $B_{12}$, A, and E, as well as the composition of fatty acids in the mother's diet, may influence the nutrients in human milk; however, the influence of other vitamins and trace minerals is unknown. Omega-3 and omega-6 fatty acids, as in Canadian requirements, and choline[122] have been added to the list of increased nutrients needed in pregnancy. (Table 1–7 shows choline food sources.)

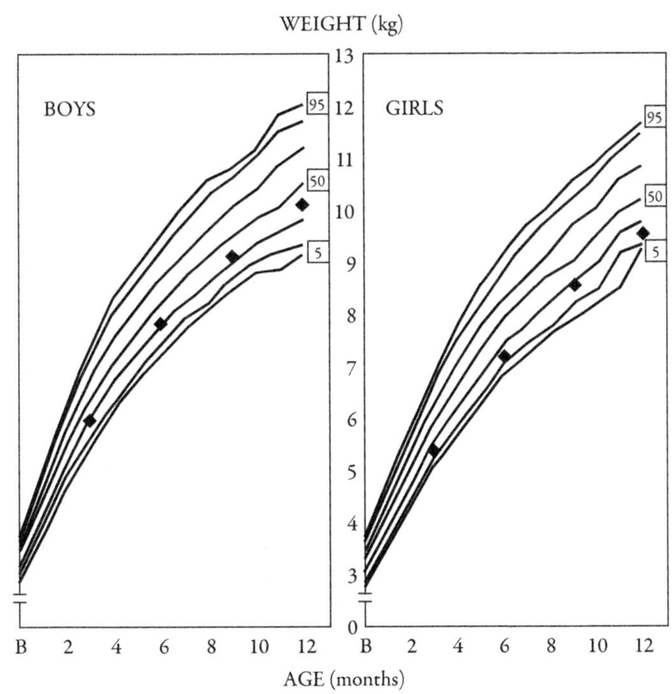


**Figure 1–10.** Weight percentile curves for exclusively breast-fed boys ($n = 628$ at birth) and girls ($n = 589$ at birth) compared with the 50th percentile values of the World Health Organization (WHO)/National Center for Health Statistics (NCHS) reference. (From Diaz S. Herreros C, Aravena R, et al. Breast-feeding duration and growth of fully breast-fed infants in a poor urban Chilean population. *Am J Clin Nutr.* 1995; 62:371. Used with permission.)

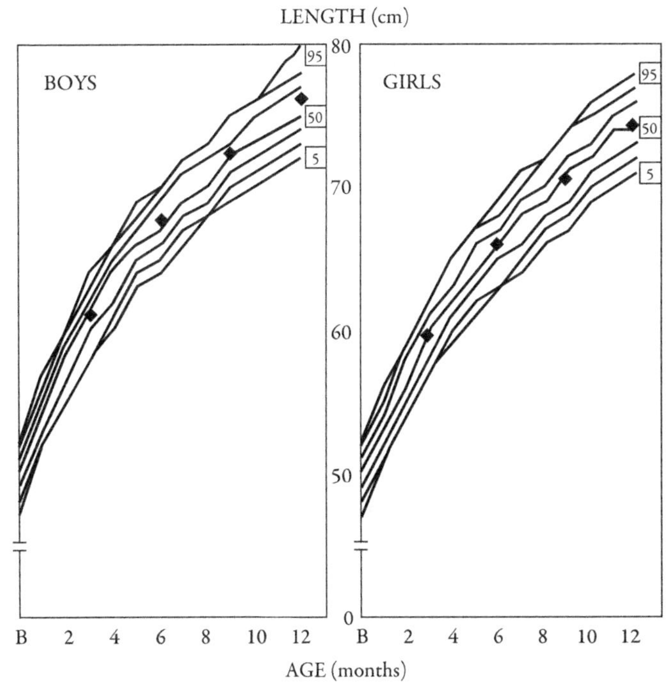


**Figure 1–11.** Length percentile curves for exclusively breast-fed boys ($n = 628$ at birth) and girls ($n = 589$ at birth) compared with the 50th percentile values of the World Health Organization (WHO)/National Center for Health Statistics (NCHS) reference. (From Diaz S. Herreros C, Aravena R, et al. Breast-feeding duration and growth of fully breast-fed infants in a poor urban Chilean population. *Am J Clin Nutr.* 1995; 62:371. Used with permission.)

**Table 1–7.** Choline Content of Some Common Foods[*,†]

| | | Choline | GPCho | PCHo | PtdCho | SM | Total Choline |
|---|---|---|---|---|---|---|---|
| Dairy products/eggs | Cheese | 1.59 | 2.30 | 0.64 | 7.37 | 4.59 | 16.50 |
| | Eggs | 0.62 | 0.60 | 0.61 | 238.43 | 10.74 | 251.00 |
| | Whole milk | 3.67 | 7.52 | 1.85 | 0.61 | 0.65 | 14.29 |
| | Skim milk | 2.81 | 9.70 | 1.66 | 0.75 | 0.71 | 15.63 |
| Meat | Beef | 3.57 | 3.86 | 0.53 | 62.43 | 7.77 | 78.15 |
| | Chicken | 5.27 | 1.20 | 3.45 | 44.44 | 11.48 | 65.83 |
| | Bacon | 12.06 | 14.52 | 2.68 | 85.58 | 10.05 | 124.89 |
| | Pork | 2.19 | 22.51 | 1.18 | 70.45 | 6.42 | 102.76 |
| | Atlantic cod | 17.73 | 30.04 | 1.57 | 32.90 | 1.38 | 83.63 |
| | Salmon | 8.62 | 5.89 | 1.07 | 48.02 | 1.84 | 65.45 |
| Cereals/grains | Wheat germ, toasted | 69.19 | 33.78 | 4.19 | 44.92 | ND | 152.08 |
| | Wheat bran | 50.89 | 4.36 | 2.06 | 17.77 | ND | 74.39 |
| | Wheat bread | 17.98 | 4.93 | 0.29 | 3.33 | ND | 26.53 |
| | White bread | 6.04 | 3.33 | 0.24 | 2.56 | ND | 12.17 |
| | Oat bran | 4.41 | 33.25 | 0.68 | 20.23 | ND | 58.57 |
| | Oats | 1.25 | 1.64 | ND | 4.53 | ND | 7.42 |
| | Rice | 0.72 | 0.95 | ND | 0.42 | ND | 2.08 |
| Fruits/fruit products | Apples | 0.33 | ND | ND | 3.11 | ND | 3.44 |
| | Bananas | 3.20 | 5.60 | 0.51 | 0.44 | ND | 9.76 |
| | Grapefruit | 3.56 | 1.16 | 0.25 | 2.55 | ND | 7.53 |
| | Grapes | 4.80 | ND | 0.62 | 0.21 | ND | 5.63 |
| | Oranges | 4.68 | 1.10 | 0.51 | 2.09 | ND | 8.38 |
| Vegetables | Broccoli | 8.45 | 1.32 | 9.30 | 20.98 | ND | 40.06 |
| | Carrots | 6.82 | ND | 1.13 | 0.84 | ND | 8.79 |
| | Cucumber | 3.99 | 0.48 | 0.91 | 0.58 | ND | 5.95 |
| | Peppers | 3.62 | ND | 1.19 | 0.74 | ND | 5.54 |
| | Spinach | 1.69 | ND | 1.13 | 21.97 | ND | 24.78 |
| | Tomatoes | 4.40 | ND | 1.83 | 0.50 | ND | 6.74 |
| | Yellow corn | 8.93 | 0.64 | 1.68 | 10.70 | ND | 21.95 |
| | Peas | 2.16 | 0.79 | 0.68 | 23.88 | ND | 27.51 |
| Beverages | White wine | 3.56 | 1.59 | ND | ND | ND | 5.15 |
| | Brewed tea | 0.37 | ND | ND | ND | ND | 0.37 |
| | Coffee | 1.89 | 0.67 | ND | 0.03 | 0.03 | 2.62 |
| Legumes/legume products | Peanuts | 17.59 | 1.27 | 1.79 | 31.81 | ND | 52.47 |
| | Peanut butter | 25.04 | 1.25 | 1.64 | 35.09 | ND | 63.02 |
| | Beans, navy | 14.02 | 0.78 | 0.56 | 11.57 | ND | 26.93 |
| | Soybeans | 47.27 | 2.92 | 1.12 | 64.56 | ND | 115.87 |
| Fast food | Cheese pizza | 6.68 | 1.42 | 0.81 | 4.17 | 0.90 | 13.98 |
| | French fries | 12.14 | 3.94 | 0.81 | 5.18 | ND | 22.06 |
| | Fast food hamburger | 5.66 | 4.50 | 0.88 | 20.34 | 2.85 | 34.23 |
| | Hot dog and bun | 4.51 | 1.88 | 0.81 | 20.72 | 2.14 | 30.06 |

[*]From Allen LH. Anemia and iron deficiency: effects on pregnancy outcome. *Am J Clin Nutr.* 202; 130:443S Foods were stored in a glass container at −20°C overnight and then stored at −80°C until analyzed using LC-ESI-IDMS.

[†]Data (mean of duplicate determinations) are presented for choline compounds (mg choline moiety/100 g food). Total choline is the sum of choline, phosphocholine (PCho), glycerophosphocholine (GPCho), phosphatidylcholine (PtdCho), and sphingomyelin (SM) in the food. ND = not detected.

Increased fluids as well as increased nutrients are recommended for the mother's diet during lactation. Problems appear to occur in the following types of mothers[102] (see Appendix 1):

- High-risk mothers who consume less than 1800 calories per day (supplement daily with large amounts of nutrient-dense foods and a multivitamin/mineral supplement)
- Vegetarian mothers who avoid animal foods (take a daily supplement of 2.6 μg vitamin $B_{12}$)
- Mothers who have low calcium intake or lactose intolerance, although lactose tolerance may improve during pregnancy (take a 600-mg elemental calcium supplement with meals)
- Mothers who have limited exposure to sunlight and consume few vitamin D–fortified foods (take a daily supplement of 10 μg vitamin D).

Mothers should not breast-feed if they have human immunodeficiency virus (HIV) infection or are using drugs, alcohol, or large amounts of tobacco and caffeine (with abstinence after birth, they may breast-feed).[114,117] Regional poison control centers and university pharmacies are excellent sources for drug nutrition information.

Colostrum provides only 18 kcal/kg/24 hr, but it provides 12.5 g immunoglobulin (12–15% protein) on day 1 and 1% to 2% by day 5, which limits bacterial and viral antigens in the intestinal tract. Colostrum also binds iron and makes it unavailable to *Escherichia coli* in the intestine, thereby inhibiting bacterial growth. Colostrum has two times as much vitamin A, eight times as much carotenoids, and five times as much vitamin $B_{12}$ per 100 mL as mature milk. Because nutrition after birth is less efficient than during pregnancy, 120 kcal/kg/24 hr is needed during the first month and 100 kcal/kg/24 hr during the second month. Breast milk provides about 100 kcal/kg/24 hr or less, but some nutrients are better absorbed in breast milk.

The newborn infant should be given the following: 7.5 μg vitamin D daily if sunlight exposure is limited, a fluoride supplement daily if the water source contains less than 0.3 ppm fluoride, and 1 to 2 mg vitamin K immediately after birth (once only).[123] At 6 months, the infant should be given foods rich in bioavailable iron or a daily low-dose iron supplement.[114] Research is needed on the relationship between maternal diet during lactation and maternal nutritional status and milk volume. The urinary ratio of lactose to creatinine has been investigated as a research and clinical tool for estimating lactation performance.[124] It is now considered a gross (imprecise) measure. Improving growth in very-low-birth-weight infants during the first 28 days is a major research challenge.[125]

Some additional concerns to be addressed by pediatric nutritionists are the premature introduction of solid foods and the thickening of formula with cereal in the bottle for infants younger than 4 months of age. These are common practices, especially in rural areas. Mothers and grandmothers also need education on the selection of solid foods (i.e., how to select higher-nutrient, lower-fat weaning foods) and on the limitation of high-calorie drinks.

It is the responsibility of the dietitian and nurse to provide education and training about breast-feeding and lactation to other health care professionals and to the public. Cultural sensitivity, less formula distribution, supportive workplaces, and reduced language barriers also are necessary to better coordinate services for minority groups.[126–128]

## SUMMARY AND FOLLOW-UP

In high-risk pregnancies, prenatal care is particularly important. Fetal malnutrition may lead to adult disease.[5,6] Dietary and physical examinations, anthropometric measures, biochemical data, and medical histories are needed at each clinic visit. Mothers who breast-feed need education about food selection because a poorly balanced diet may increase the risk of atopic sensitization of the infant.

Another area of concern is the interaction of nutrition and infection (e.g., HIV), which influences the health status of children. Disease, age, feeding patterns, and diet all interact to affect the child's health. Problems can occur in two ways. The infant or child may have a poor nutritional status that leads to a compromised immune system and reduced resistance to infection. The problem may also begin with an infectious disease accompanied by appetite loss, anorexia, elevated metabolism, and malabsorption (one example is diarrhea). For HIV-infected newborns, disease is one of the most potent factors in the undernutrition and infection cycle (see Chapter 29).

### References

1. Wrottesley SV, Lamper C, Pisa PT. Review of the importance of nutrition during the first 1000 days: maternal nutritional status and its associations with fetal growth and birth, neonatal and infant outcomes among African women. *J Dev Orig Health Dis.* 2015; 7:144.
2. Nnam NM. Improving maternal nutrition for better pregnancy outcomes. *Proc Nutr Soc.* 2015; 74:454.
3. Black AP, Brimblecombe J, Eyles H, Morris P, Vally H, O'Dea K. Food subsidy programs and the health and nutritional status of disadvantaged families in high income countries: a systematic review. *BMC Public Health.* 2012; 12:1099.
4. Chock LR, Hayes DK, Tomiyasu DW. Insights in public health. The Special Supplemental Nutrition Program for Women, Infants and Children: strengthening families for 40 years. Maddock J, Hayes D, St John TL, Starr R, eds. *Hawaii J Med Public Health.* 2014; 73:295.
5. Barker DJ. The origins of the developmental origins theory. *J Intern Med.* 2007; 261:412.
6. Wadhwa PD, Buss C, Entringer S, Swanson JM. Developmental origins of health and disease: brief history of the approach and current focus on epigenetic mechanisms. *Semin Reprod Med.* 2009; 27:358.
7. Grissom NM, Reyes TM. Gestational overgrowth and undergrowth affect neurodevelopment: similarities and differences from behavior to epigenetics. *Int J Dev Neurosci.* 2013; 31:406.
8. Kassebaum NJ, Bertozzi-Villa A, Coggeshall MS, et al. Global, regional, and national levels and causes of maternal mortality during 1990–2013: a systematic analysis for the Global Burden of Disease Study 2013. *Lancet.* 2014; 384(9947):980.
9. World Health Organization. *Neonatal and Perinatal Mortality: Country, Regional and Global Estimates.* Geneva: WHO; 2006.
10. MacDorman MF, Gregory ECW. Fetal and perinatal mortality: United States, 2013. *Natl Vital Stat Rep.* 2015; 64:1.
11. He X, Akil L, Aker WG, Hwang H-M, Ahmad HA. Trends in infant mortality in United States: a brief study of the southeastern states from 2005–2009. Scott J, ed. *Int J Environ Res Public Health.* 2015; 12:4908.
12. Winick M. Nutrition education in medical schools and residency training. In: Lifshitz, F., ed. *Childhood Nutrition.* Boca Raton, FL: CRC Press; 1995.
13. Ramacharndran P. Maternal nutrition—effect on fetal growth and outcome of pregnancy. *Nutr Rev.* 2002; 60:S26.
14. Hamaoui E, Hamaoui M. Nutritional assessment and support during pregnancy. *Gastroenterol Clin North Am.* 2003; 32:59.
15. Ramakrishnan U, Imhoff-Kunsch B, Mortorell R. Maternal nutrition interventions to improve maternal, newborn, and child health outcomes. *Nestle Nutr Inst Workshop Ser.* 2014; 78:71.
16. van der Berg JW, Sen S, Chomitz VR, et al. The role of systemic inflammation linking maternal BMI to neurodevelopment in children. *Pediatr Res.* 2016; 79:3.
17. Haider BA, Yakoob MY, Bhutta ZA. Effect of multiple micronutrient supplementation during pregnancy on maternal and birth outcomes. *BMC Public Health.* 2011; 11(Suppl 3):S19.
18. Wilson RD, Genetics committee, Wilson RD, Audibert F, et al. Pre-conception folic acid and multivitamin supplementation for the primary and secondary prevention of neural tube defects and other folic acid-sensitive congenital anomalies. *J Obstet Gynaecol Can.* 2015; 37:534.
19. Piccoli GB, Clari R, Vigotti FN, et al. Vegan-vegetarian diets in pregnancy: danger or panacea? A systematic narrative review. *BJOG.* 2015; 122:623.
20. Pistollato F, Sumalla Cano S, Elio I, et al. Plant-based and plant-rich diet patterns during gestation: beneficial effects and possible shortcomings. *Adv Nutr.* 2015; 6:581.
21. Wlodarczyk BJ, Palacios AM, George TM, Finnell RH. Antiepileptic drugs and pregnancy outcomes. *Am J Med Genet A.* 2012; 158A:2071.
22. McArthur JO, Tang H, Petocz P, Samman S. Biological variability and impact of oral contraceptives on vitamins $B_6$, $B_{12}$ and folate status in women of reproductive age. *Nutrients.* 2013; 5:3634.
23. Bigby M, Stern RS. Adverse reactions to isotretinoin. *J Am Acad Dermatol.* 1988; 18:543.
24. Rothman KJ, Moore L, Singe MR, et al. Teratogenicity of high vitamin A intake. *N Engl J Med.* 1995; 333:1369.
25. Jacobson S, Chiodo LM, Sokol R., Jacobson JL. Validity of maternal report of prenatal alcohol, cocaine, and smoking in relation to neurobehavioral outcome. *Pediatrics.* 2002; 109:815.
26. Hannigan JH, Armant DR. Alcohol in pregnancy and neonatal outcome. *Semin Neonatal.* 2000; 5:243.
27. Minnes S, Lang A, Singer L. Prenatal tobacco, marijuana, stimulant, and opiate exposure: outcomes and practice implications. *Addict Sci Clin Pract.* 2011; 6:57.
28. Moylan S, Gustavson K, Øverland S, et al. The impact of maternal smoking during pregnancy on depressive and anxiety behaviors in children: the Norwegian Mother and Child Cohort Study. *BMC Med.* 2015; 13:24.
29. Hall W, Degenhardt L Adverse health effects of non-medical cannabis use. *Lancet.* 2009; 374:1383.
30. Metz TD, Stickrath EH. Marijuana use in pregnancy and lactation: a review of the evidence. *Am J Obstet Gynecol.* 2015; 213:761.
31. Abrams B, Altman SL, Pickett KE. Pregnancy weight gain: still controversial. *Am J Clin Nutr.* 2000; 71(Suppl 5):1233S.
32. Georgieff MK. Nutrition and the developing brain: nutrient priorities and measurement. *Am J Clin Nutr.* 2007; 85:614S.
33. Institute of Medicine. *Dietary Reference Intakes for Vitamin A, Vitamin K, Arsenic, Boron, Chromium, Copper, Iodine, Manganese, Molybdenum, Nickel, Silicon, Vanadium, and Zinc.* Washington, DC: National Academy Press; 2001.
34. Darnton-Hill I, Mkparu UC. Micronutrients in pregnancy in low- and middle-income countries. *Nutrients.* 2015; 7:1744.
35. Zhang C, Williams M, King I, et al. Vitamin C and the risk of anemia—results from dietary questionnaire and plasma assay. *Epidemiology.* 2002; 13:409.
36. Mahomed K. Iron supplementation in pregnancy. *Cochrane Database Syst Rev.* 2000; (2):CD000117.
37. Monsen E. Iron nutrition and absorption: dietary factors which impact iron bioavailability. *J Am Diet Assoc.* 1998; 88:786.
38. Morse NL. Benefits of docosahexaenoic acid, folic acid, vitamin D and iodine on foetal and infant brain development and function following maternal supplementation during pregnancy and lactation. *Nutrients.* 2012; 4:799.
39. Wang T, Zhang HP. Is folate status a risk factor for asthma or other allergic diseases? *Allergy Asthma Immunol Res.* 2015; 7:538.
40. Finkelstein JL, Layden AJ, Stover PJ. Vitamin B-12 and perinatal health. *Adv Nutr.* 2015; 6:552.
41. Calvo MS, Whiting SJ, Barton CN. Vitamin D intake: a global perspective of current status. *J Nutr.* 2005; 135:310.
42. Villar J, Belizan JM. Same nutrient, different hypothesis: disparities in trials of calcium supplementation during pregnancy. *Am J Clin Nutr.* 2000; 71:1375S.
43. Lauro V, Pisani,C, Zacche G. Correlation between changes in symptomatology and changes in diet. *Acta Biomed Aleneo Parmense.* 1997; 68(Suppl 1):95.
44. Caulfield LE, Zavaketa N, Figueroa A. Adding zinc to prenatal iron and folate supplements improves maternal and neonatal zinc status in a Peruvian population. *Am J Clin Nutr.* 1999; 69:1257.
45. Zahiri Sorouri Z, Sadeghi H, Pourmarzi D. The effect of zinc supplementation on pregnancy outcome: a randomized controlled trial. *J Matern Fetal Neonatal Med.* 2015; Sept 12 [Epub ahead of print].
46. Moro R, Gialanella G, Zhang YX, Perrone L, DiToro R. Trace elements in full-term neonate hair. *J Trace Elem Electrolytes Health Dis.* 1992; 6:27.
47. Handwerker SM, Altura BT, Royo B, Altura BM. Ionized serum magnesium levels in umbilical cord blood of normal pregnant women at delivery: relationship to calcium, demographics and birth weight. *Am J Perinatol.* 1993; 1:392.
48. Sibai BM., Villar MA, Bray E. Magnesium supplementation during pregnancy: a double-blind randomized controlled clinical trial. *Am J Obstet Gynecol.* 1989; 161:115.
49. Merialdi M, Garoroli G, Villar J, et al. Nutritional interventions during pregnancy for the prevention or treatment of impaired fetal growth: an overview of randomized controlled trials. *J Nutr.* 2003; 133(5 Suppl 2):1626S.
50. Tiwari BD, Godbole MM, Chattopadhyay N, Mandal A, Mithal A. Learning disabilities and poor motivation to achieve due to prolonged iodine deficiency. *Am J Clin Nutr.* 1996; 63:782.

51. Voyles LM, Turner RE, Lukowski MJ, Langkamp-Henken B. High levels of retinol intake during the first trimester of pregnancy result from use of over-the-counter vitamin supplements. *J Am Diet Assoc.* 2000; 100:1068.
52. Pathak P, Singh P, Kapil U, Raghuvanshi RS. Prevalence of iron, vitamin A, and iodine deficiencies amongst adolescent pregnant mothers. *Indian J Pediatr.* 2003; 70:299.
53. Hamilton S, Rothenberg SJ, Khan FA, Manalo M, Norris KC. Neonatal lead poisoning from maternal pica behavior during pregnancy. *J Natl Med Assoc.* 2001; 93:317.
54. Graff JC, Murphy L, Ekvall S, Gagnon M. In-home toxic chemical exposures and children with intellectual and developmental disabilities. *Pediatr Nurs.* 2006; 32:596.
55. Tyler C, White-Scott S, Ekvall S, Abulafia L. Environmental health and disabilities: a life span approach. *Family Community Health.* 2008; 31:287.
56. Rye JE, Ziegler EE, Nelson SE, Fomon SJ. Dietary intake of lead and blood lead concentration in early infancy. *Am J Dis Child.* 1983; 137:886.
57. Keen CL, Hanna LA, Lanoue L, et al. Developmental consequences of trace mineral deficiencies in rodents: acute and long-term effects. *J Nutr.* 2003; 133(5 Suppl 1):1477S.
58. Martini LA, Cuppari L, Colugnati FA, et al. High sodium chloride is associated with low bone density in calcium stone–forming patients. *Clin Nephrol.* 2000; 54:85.
59. Heiman KE, Garalde VB, Gronostaj M, et al. Multistate outbreak of listeriosis caused by imported cheese and evidence of cross-contamination of other cheeses, USA, 2012. *Epidemiol Infect.* 2015; Jun 30 [Epub ahead of print].
60. Goldberg G. Nutrition in pregnancy: the facts and fallacies. *Nursing Standard.* 2002; 17:39.
61. Committee on Infectious Diseases; Committee on Nutrition; American Academy of Pediatrics. Consumption of raw or unpasteurized milk and milk products by pregnant women and children. *Pediatrics.* 2014; 133:175.
62. U.S. Department of Health and Human Services. *Food Safety for Pregnant Women.* http://www.FoodSafety.gov. Accessed May 17, 2016.
63. Lenders CM, McElrath TF, Scholl TO. Nutrition in adolescent pregnancy. *Curr Opin Pediatr.* 2000; 12:291.
64. Pathak P, Singh P, Kapil U, Raghuvanshi RS. Prevalence of iron, vitamin A and iodine deficiencies amongst adolescent pregnant mothers. *Indian J Pediatr.* 2003; 70:299.
65. Combs-Orme T. Health effects of adolescent pregnancy: implications for social workers. *Fam Soc.* 1993; 74:344.
66. Chauliac M, Raimbault AM. Adolescent pregnancy. *Dev Sante.* 1992; (98):23.
67. Reichman NE, Pagnini DL. Maternal age and birth outcomes: data from New Jersey. *Fam Plan Perspect.* 1997; 29:268.
68. Hediger ML, Scholl TO, Belsky DH, et al. Patterns of weight gain in adolescent pregnancy: effects on birth weight and preterm deliveries. *Obstet Gynecol.* 1989; 74:6.
69. Ekblad U, Grenman S. Maternal weight gain during pregnancy and pregnancy outcome. *Int J Gynaecol Obstet.* 1992; 39:277.
70. Segel JS, McAnarney ER. Adolescent pregnancy and subsequent obesity in African-American girls. *J Adolesc Health.* 1994; 15:491.
71. Luke B, Hediger ML, Nugent C, et al. Body mass index: specific weight gains associated with optimal birth weights in twin pregnancies. *J Reprod Med.* 2003; 48:217.
72. Ayustawati, Matsubara S, Minakami H, Ohkuchi A, Izumi A, Sato I. Symphysis-fundus height and weight gain pattern in Japanese women with twin pregnancies. *J Reprod Med.* 2003; 48:277.
73. Sebire NJ, Jolly M, Harris J, Regan L, Robinson S. Is maternal underweight really a risk factor for adverse pregnancy outcome? A population-based study in London. *BJOG.* 2001; 108:61.
74. Institute of Medicine (IOM) and National Research Council (NRC). *Weight Gain During Pregnancy: Reexamining the Guidelines.* Washington, DC: The National Academies Press; 2009.
75. Brown JE, Murtaugh MA, Jacobs DRJr, Margellos HC. Variation in newborn size according to pregnancy weight change by trimester. *Am J Clin Nutr.* 2002; 76:205.
76. Siega-Riz AM, Adair LS, Hobel CJ. Maternal underweight status and inadequate rate of weight gain during the third trimester of pregnancy increases the risk of preterm pregnancy. *J Nutr.* 1996; 126:146.
77. Hickey CA. Sociocultural and behavioral influences on weight gain during pregnancy. *Am J Clin Nutr.* 2000; 71:1364S.
78. Olson CM, Strawderman MS. Modifiable behavioral factors in a biopsychosocial model predict inadequate and excessive gestational weight gain. *J Am Diet Assoc.* 2003; 103:48.
79. Muscati SK, Koski KG, Gray-Donald K. Increased energy intake in pregnant smokers does not prevent human fetal growth retardation. *J Nutr.* 1996; 126:2984.
80. Hruba D, Kachlik P. Influence of maternal active and passive smoking during pregnancy on birth weight in newborns. *Cent Eur J Public Health.* 2000; 8:249.
81. Spaaij CJ, van Raaif JM, de Groot LC, van der Heijden LJ, Boekholt HA, Hautvast JG. Effect of lactation on resting metabolic rate and on diet and work-induced thermogenesis. *Am J Clin Nutr.* 1994; 59:42.
82. Widdowson EM. Fetal and neonatal nutrition. *Nutr Today.* 1987; 22:16.
83. Downs DS, Chasan-Taber L, Evenson KR, Leiferman J, Yeo S. Physical activity and pregnancy: past and present evidence and future recommendations. *Res Q Exer Sport.* 2012; 83:485.
84. ACOG Committee opinion number 267, January 2002: exercise during pregnancy and the postpartum period. *Obstet Gynecol.* 2002; 99:171.
85. Hwang IK, Go VL, Harris DM, Yip I, Song MK. Effects of arachidonic acid plus zinc on glucose disposal in genetically diabetic (ob/ob) mice. *Diabetes Obes Metab.* 2002; 4:124.
86. Petry C, Eaton M, Wobken JD, Mills MM, Johnson D, Georgieff MK. Iron deficiency of liver, heart, and brain in newborn infants of diabetic mother. *Pediatrics.* 1992; 121:109.
87. Orno, A, Ratzon N, Greenbaum C, Wolf A, Dulitzky M. School-age children born to diabetic mothers and to mothers with gestational diabetes exhibit a high rate of inattention and fine and gross motor impairment. *J Pediatr Endocrinol Metab.* 2001; 14(Suppl 1):681.
88. Rosevear R. *Nutrition in Biblical Times.* Cincinnati, OH: Clifton Hills Press; 1996.
89. George JN. The association of pregnancy with thrombotic thrombocytopenic purpura—hemolytic uremic syndrome. *Curr Opin Hematol.* 2003; 10:339.
90. Harman CR, Baschat AA. Comprehensive assessment of fetal wellbeing: which Doppler tests should be performed? *Curr Opin Obstet Gynecol.* 2003; 15:147.
91. Churchill D, Perry IJ, Beevers DG. Ambulatory blood pressure in pregnancy and fetal growth. *Lancet.* 1997; 349:7.
92. Bayliss H, Churchill D, Beevers M, Beevers DG. Anti-hypertensive drugs in pregnancy and fetal growth: evidence for pharmacological programming in the first trimester. *Hypertens Pregnancy.* 2002; 21:161.
93. Buchner HC, Cook RJ, Gyat FH, Lang JD, Cook DJ, Hatala R, Hunt I. Effects of dietary calcium supplementation on blood pressure: a metanalysis of randomized controlled trials. *JAMA.* 1996; 275:1016.
94. Dekke G, Sibai B. Primary, secondary and tertiary prevention of pre-eclampsia. *Lancet.* 2001; 357:209.
95. Strevens H, Wide-Swensson D, Hansen A, et al. Glomerular endotheliosis in normal pregnancy and pre-eclampsia. *BJOG.* 2003; 110:831.
96. Ekvall S, Hedrick B. *The Impact of Nutritional Status Before Conception, During Pregnancy, and in Early Childhood.* Training Module IV: Prevention Continuing Education in Rural Areas Project (84–1). Ohio Developmental Disabilities Council and Ohio Department of Mental Retardation and Developmental Disabilities (funded by P.L. 50-602), 1992.
97. Ekvall SM, Ekvall VK. The importance of nutrition in the prevention of intellectual disabilities. 10th World Congress of the International Association for the Scientific Study of Intellectual Disabilities (IASSID) and the Finnish Society for Biological Medicine. *Trends Biomed Finland.* 1996; 7:22.
98. National Academy of Science; Institute of Medicine; Food and Nutrition Board. *Dietary Reference Intakes: The Essential Guide to Nutrient Requirements.* Washington, DC: National Academies Press; 2006.
99. Luder E, Cupens-Okado E, Karen-Roth A, Martinez-Weber C. Health and nutrition survey in a group of urban homeless adults. *J Am Dietetic Assoc.* 1990; 90:1387.
100. Han B, Wells BL, Taylor AM. Use of health care for the homeless program services and other health care services by homeless adults. *J Health Care Poor Underserved.* 2003; 14:87.
101. Langnase K, Muller MJ. Nutrition and health in an adult urban homeless population in Germany. *Public Health Nutr.* 2001; 4:805.
102. American Dietetic Association. Position of the American Dietetic Association: nutrition intervention in the treatment of anorexia nervosa, bulimia nervosa, and eating disorder not otherwise specified (EDNOS). *J Am Diet Assoc.* 2001; 101:810.
103. Villar J, Rivera J. Nutritional supplementation during two consecutive pregnancies and the interim lactation period: effect on birth weight. *Pediatrics.* 1988; 81:51.
104. Picciano MF. Pregnancy and lactation: physiological adjustments, nutritional requirements and the role of dietary supplements. *J Nutr.* 2003; 133:1997S.
105. DeGroo, R, Hornstra G, Van Houweligen A, Roumen F. Effect of α-linoleic acid supplementation during pregnancy on maternal and neonatal polyunsaturated fatty acid status and pregnancy outcome. *Am J Clin Nutr.* 2004; 79:251.
106. King JC. Physiology of pregnancy and nutrient metabolism. *Am J Clin Nutr.* 2000; 71:1218S.
107. Susser M, Stein Z. Timing in prenatal nutrition: a reprise of the Dutch Famine Study. *Nutr Rev.* 1994; 52:84.
108. Leese B, Jomeen J, Denton J. Appropriate maternal weight gain in singleton and twin pregnancies: what is the evidence? *Hum Fertil (Camb).* 2012; 15:194.
109. Wang DD, Leung CW, Li Y, et al. Trends in dietary quality among adults in the United States, 1999 through 2010. *JAMA Intern Med.* 2014;174(10):1587.
110. Louie JC, Tapsell LC. Intake of total and added sugars and nutrient dilution in Australian children and adolescents. *Br J Nutr.* 2015; 114:1875.
111. American Dietetic Association; Dietitians of Canada. Position of the American Dietetic Association and Dietitians of Canada: vegetarian diets. *Can J Diet Pract Res.* 2003; 64:62.
112. Kaiser LL, Campbell CG, Academy Positions Committee Workgroup. Practice paper of the Academy of Nutrition and Dietetics abstract: nutrition and lifestyle for a healthy pregnancy outcome. *J Acad Nutr Diet.* 2014; 114:1447.
113. Lessen R, Kavanagu K. Position of the academy of nutrition and dietetics: promotion and supporting breastfeeding. *J Acad Nutr Diet.* 2015; 115:444.
114. Peddleston J. Canadian Pharmaceutical Association position paper on breastfeeding and infant nutrition. *J Hum Lact.* 1997; 13:99.
115. Diaz S, Herreros C, Aravena R, Eugenia M, Reyes M, Schiappacasse V. Breast-feeding duration and growth of fully breastfed infants in a poor urban Chilean population. *Am J Clin Nutr.* 1995; 62:371.
116. Singhal A, Cole T, Fewell M, Lucas A. Breastmilk feeding and lipoprotein profile in adolescents born preterm: follow up of a prospective randomized study. *Lancet.* 2004; 363:1571.
117. Position of the American Dietetic Association: breaking the barriers to breast feeding. *J Am Diet Assoc.* 2001; 101:1213.
118. Baker JL, Michaelsen KF, Sorensen TI, Rasmussen KM. High prepregnancy body mass index is associated with early termination of full and any breastfeeding in Danish women. *Am J Clin Nutr.* 2012; 86:404.
119. Brown JE., Carlson M. Nutrition and multifetal pregnancy. *J Am Diet Assoc.* 2000; 100:343.
120. Morton JA. Strategies to support extended breastfeeding of the premature infant. *Adv Neonatal Care.* 2002; 2:267.
121. Morton JA. Breastfeeding the premature infant. *Pediatr Ann.* 2003; 32:290.
122. Zeisel SH., Niculescu MD. Choline and phosphatidylcholine. In: Shils ME, Shike M, Ross AC, et al., eds. *Modern Nutrition in Health and Disease*, 10th ed. Baltimore: Lippincott Williams & Wilkins; 2006.
123. Ziegler EE., Fomon SJ. Strategies for the prevention of iron deficiency: iron in infant formula and baby foods. *Nutr Rev.* 1996; 54(11 pt 1):348.

124. Kalkwalf HJ, Kalis M. Urinary lactose: changes postpartum and relation with breast milk production. *Am J Clin Nutr.* 1997; 65:744.
125. Bloom BT, Mulligan J, Arnold C et al. Improving growth of very low birth weight infants in the first 28 days. *Pediatrics.* 2003; 112:8.
126. Loiselle CG, Semenic SE., Cote B, Lapointe M, Gendron R. Impressions of breast-feeding information and support among first-time mothers within a multi-ethnic community. *Can J Nurs Res.* 2001; 33:31.
127. Stevens F, Ekvall S. eds. *Empowering Children Through Early Intervention with Good Nutrition: Focusing on Culturally Diverse Children with Special Health Care Needs.* Manual IV. Cincinnati, OH: University of Cincinnati Publications; 2002.
128. Ptomey LT, Wittenbrook W. Position of the Academy of Nutrition and Dietetics: nutrition services for individuals with intellectual and developmental disabilities and special health care needs. *J Acad Nutr Diet.* 2015; 115:1347.

# 2 Postnatal Growth in Infancy

JACQUELINE WESSEL, BARBARA NIEDBALA, AND SHIRLEY W. EKVALL

Nutritional intake, from birth on, must be adequate for proper growth and development. Nutrition should be provided to the infant in a way that is appropriate for his or her developing motor skills and that enhances nurturing between infant and caregiver. The American Academy of Pediatrics (AAP), the World Health Organization (WHO), and other groups identify breast-feeding as the ideal method of feeding and nurturing infants and the use of human milk as ideal to achieve optimal infant and child health.[1–4] The nursing relationship confers many benefits to both the mother and the infant. Human milk is considered the gold standard for nutrition and immune protection for the term infant.[4] Human milk supports the optimal growth of term infants, providing essential substances, nutrients, and bioactive and immunologic constituents; it also promotes a favorable microbial colonization, which leads to priming and maturation of the gut.[5]

The bioactive and immunologic elements of human milk protect babies against infection and inflammation and contribute to immune maturation.[6] Part of the immune protection may be attributed to the establishment of beneficial bacteria in the gastrointestinal tract of the infant fed with human milk.[6] Human milk contains probiotics, including *Bifidobacterium bifidum* and *Lactobacillus*,[5] as well as prebiotic oligosaccharides that promote the growth of these bacteria.[6] The bifidus flora of the human milk–fed infant is thought to activate the immune system and defend against pathogens.[7–10] Breast-feeding protects against respiratory infections,[7] diarrhea,[7,8] and otitis media[9] and reduces infant morbidity worldwide.[10] Infants who are not fed human milk have a twofold greater risk of morbidity.[10] The use of human milk has also has been associated with higher developmental scores.[11] However, because of their clinical condition, not all infants can be breast-fed, and human milk may need to be given by other methods, such as a specialized bottle or a nasogastric, nasojejunal, gastric, or gastrojejunal tube. There is loss of human milk fat when given in a continuous feeding. Strategies to address this problem are discussed elsewhere.[12]

Unfortunately, the use of recreational drugs is not uncommon in pregnant and lactating women. The Academy of Breastfeeding Medicine has useful practical guidelines.[13] In general, adequately nourished mothers who are narcotic dependent but enrolled and participating in a drug treatment program and who have had consistent prenatal care with no other contraindications (e.g., human immunodeficiency virus [HIV] infection) are supported in their decision to breast-feed their infants.[13]

Infant formula composition is based on human milk and is continually being modified to replicate the substances in human milk more closely. The bacterial colonization pattern of the human milk–fed infant is different from that of formula-fed infants.[14] Some term infant formulas now have added prebiotics, and some have added probiotics. Although the AAP recommends breast-feeding as the ideal way to nourish infants,[15] sometimes it is not an option. In such cases, iron-fortified infant formula is the best choice.[15]

## FACTORS TO BE CONSIDERED IN NUTRITIONAL EVALUATION

Problems in infant nutrition often center on birth weight and the baby's functional abilities. The Apgar score at birth and the Ballard scoring system are important indices of the maturity and functional abilities of the infant.[16,17] The percentage of acceptable weight loss after birth for a term breast-fed infant has often been quoted as 5% to 7%. A recent systematic review of the literature found a range of 3.79% to 8.6%; however, the studies that were reviewed often did not meet the methodological criteria.[18] More research needs to be done to more clearly answer this fundamental question.

### Growth Assessment

For term infants, the WHO growth charts are now recommended for use during the first 24 months of life; after that, the Centers for Disease Control and Prevention (CDC) charts are used to 19 years (see Appendices 3–2 to 3–5, related to WHO Growth Grids).[19] The CDC charts are based on data from primarily formula-fed infants in Ohio obtained between 1929 and 1975.[19] The WHO charts, released in 2006, are based on the growth of breast-fed infants of well-nourished mothers in Brazil, Ghana, India, Norway, Oman, and the United States, using data collected from 1997 to 2003.[20] Infants were followed longitudinally from birth to 24 months, and a cross-sectional component was used from 18 to 71 months.[20] A comparison of the two charts is available; breast-fed infants, who would have appeared to falter from 2 months onward, track along the WHO mean Z score and weight for age.[19] Because the WHO charts are based on healthy, breast-fed infants, they are deemed prescriptive rather than descriptive and demonstrate that healthy infants and children from around the world who are raised in healthy environments and follow recommended feeding practices (i.e., breast-feeding by well-nourished mothers) have strikingly similar patterns of growth.[19] Because a healthy, breast-fed infant is the model for growth, it makes sense to use a growth curve based on those infants. WHO has educational materials that provide instructions on how to plot and interpret growth measurements.[21]

The assessment of pediatric malnutrition has been a focus of nutrition professionals.[22–27] Identifying malnourished patients is key to the work in pediatric malnutrition. The Academy of Nutrition and Dietetics and the American Society of Parenteral and Enteral Nutrition recommend that a standardized set of indicators be used to identify malnutrition, as follows:

1. When a single data point is available, indicators are the Z score for weight for length/height, the body mass index (BMI) for age or length/height for age, or the mid-upper arm circumference (MUAC).
2. When two or more data points are available, indicators may also include weight gain velocity for ages up to 2 years, weight loss for ages 2 to 20 years, deceleration in the weight-for-length/height Z score, and inadequate nutrient intake. The goal is to use as many data points as possible.[21]

It is hoped that the use of standardized parameters will lead to a more accurate identification of malnutrition, so that interventions can occur and improve outcomes.[22,23] In adults, malnutrition has been seen as a precursor to the development of pressure ulcers.[28] If this is also true in the pediatric population, the recognition and treatment of malnutrition could avoid painful pressure ulcers. These parameters are designed to be used in both inpatient and outpatient settings.[22,23]

Malnutrition in the first year is an especially troubling problem. In Egypt, health care providers, using similar tools, evaluated the common causes in their area for stunted growth.[29] Experts are now working on tools for the assessment of neonatal malnutrition because the current tools can be used only from 6 months onward. Z scores and

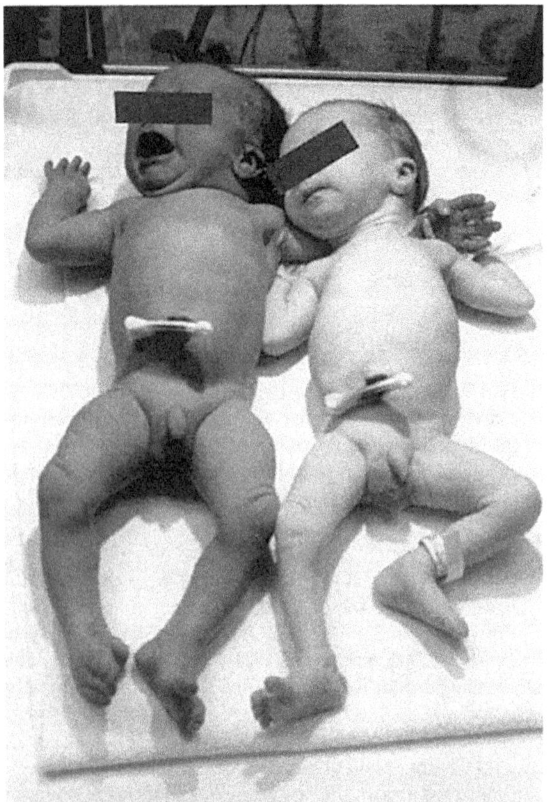

**Figure 2–1.** Comparative size of a normal infant *(left)* and a small-for-gestational age infant *(right)*, both born at full term. (Courtesy of F. Hall, D.O., Section of Neonatal/Perinatal Medicine, the Children's Mercy Hospital of Kansas City. Used with permission.)

standard deviation scores measure departure from the median. They are calculated from normal distributions (for length) and non-normal distributions (for weight).[21] Along with the educational materials on how to plot and interpret growth measurements, WHO offers a Z score calculator.[21] Z score use is recommended because it can be a more accurate descriptor of where the infant is on the growth curve, especially when the infant is either below the 3rd percentile or above the 97th percentile. Z scores can accurately describe the growth as either a negative number (below the median), such as −1.17, or a positive number (above the median), such as +2.25. Changes within a percentile band can be better expressed by the use of Z scores; with traditional charting, a measurement just above the 3rd percentile and one just below the 15th percentile would both be reported as "3rd to 15th percentile."

Measurement of the MUAC is recommended as a tool to identify and track malnutrition.[21] Again, the standards are for infants 6 months and older, although a newer study reported use of the technique with infants aged 1 to 6 months and provided guidelines for the cut-off score to determine severe malnutrition.[30] Another study reviewed various methods to examine overweight in preterm and term infants measured at hospital discharge. MUAC was found to be an inexpensive method to evaluate increased fat deposition in preterm and term infants.[31] Although further research needs to be done to establish neonatal standards, a single MUAC measurement at 6 to 14 weeks has been shown to have predictive value.[21] The MUAC measurement technique is explained in United Nations Children's Fund (UNICEF) training videos.[32] Measuring tapes are also available from UNICEF and are color coded for infants and children from 6 months to 5 years of age.[33]

The WHO growth chart can be used to determine whether term infants are born severely small (<3rd percentile), small for gestational age (SGA, <10th percentile), appropriate for gestational age (AGA), or large for gestational age (LGA, >90th percentile)[7,8] (Figs. 2–1 and 2–2). The prenatal history and the parents' heights should be evaluated for infants who measure either SGA or LGA because such infants can present with significant postnatal sequelae. The normally growing infant follows his or her own percentile rank from 6 weeks after birth, and deviations from the individual trajectory of a baby's growth should be investigated.

## Intrauterine Growth Restriction

Although infants with intrauterine growth restriction (IUGR) are traditionally thought of as also being SGA, this is not always the case. IUGR or fetal growth restriction (FGR) is a diagnosis based on at least two fetal measurements taken 3 weeks apart.[34] Growth restriction is the result of arrested growth or a shift in growth rate measured longitudinally.[34] In utero, a fetus could have faltering growth and a drop in percentiles but still be born at or even above the 10th percentile, thus differentiating between IUGR from SGA.

## Small-for-Gestational-Age Infants

Babies who are born SGA (i.e., <10th percentile) or extremely SGA (<3rd percentile)[34] could be just small infants born appropriately sized

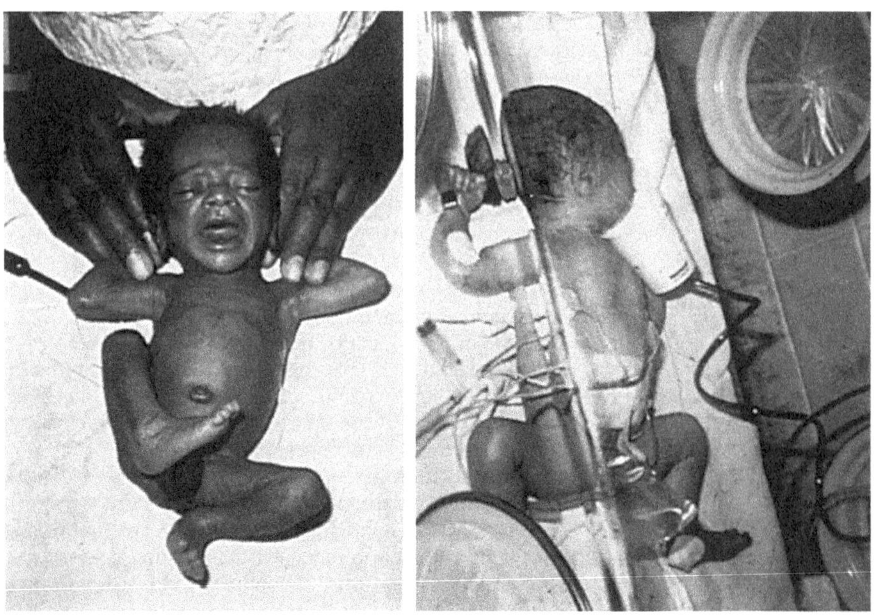

**Figure 2–2.** Comparative size and posturing behavior of a term small-for-gestational-age infant *(left)* and a preterm appropriate-for-gestational-age infant *(right)*. (Courtesy of the Perinatal Research Institute, Cincinnati OH. Used with permission.)

for their small parents. However, that is not the case for most SGA infants. Children who are born SGA or with FGR are at risk for minor cognitive deficits leading to school difficulties and for metabolic syndrome.[34] In the newborn period, morbidity and mortality are higher than in appropriately sized newborns of the same gestational age. The initial management of an SGA newborn includes avoidance of hypothermia and close monitoring of blood glucose.

In mothers at risk for having an SGA infant, serial ultrasound assessments have shown that maternal weight gain is associated with fetal growth throughout pregnancy but has a differential relationship across gestation.[35] Among women with an SGA infant identified in mid-gestation, increased maternal weight gain was associated with a decreased probability of fetal SGA 7 weeks later.[35] Maternal overweight and obesity have been associated with increased risks of macrosomia and IUGR.[36] Maternal anemia has been associated with lower-birth-weight infants.[36]

There has been considerable concern about infants who are initially SGA. The "developmental origins of adult health and disease" hypothesis indicates that environmental factors, particularly maternal undernutrition, act in early life to program the baby to be at risk for adverse health outcomes such as cardiovascular disease, obesity, and the metabolic syndrome in adult life.[37] This programming results from early physiological tradeoffs to promote fetal survival. Restriction of placental growth and function appears to result in an increased dependence of maintenance of arterial blood pressure on the sequential recruitment of the sympathetic nervous system and the fetal hypothalamic-pituitary-adrenal (HPA) axis. These adaptive changes appear to set up the infant for the later problems.[37] Because of this potential, there has been a great deal of controversy about what the growth trajectory should be for term SGA infants after birth.

A study from the US Collaborative Perinatal Project[38] examined five different growth trajectories for term SGA infants and compared their outcomes with those of term AGA infants. Of the SGA babies, those who exhibited no catch-up growth (22%) had a higher risk of infection in infancy, showed growth restriction, and had low IQ scores at 7 years. A smaller group (8.9%) had excessive catch-up growth leading to higher risk of overweight or obesity and elevated blood pressure at 7 years. Babies with slow catch-up growth (17%) or with regression in growth after 4 months (15%) had higher risks of growth restriction and low IQ score. However, those babies with appropriate catch-up growth (37%) did not have increased risk of adverse outcomes. Linear growth trajectories showed similar findings. The conclusion was that the optimal growth trajectory for term SGA infants may be fast catch-up growth to about the 30th percentile during the first several months, with modest catch-up growth thereafter to about the 50th percentile by 7 years of age.[38] Another study showed that infants with early catch-up growth (before 4 months of age) had slightly higher IQ scores at 4 years.[39] Early rapid growth in infants not born SGA appears to produce no difference in IQ score.[40]

The long-term survival of SGA infants is less than that of AGA or LGA infants, particularly in the first year of life, and they remain at a higher risk of dying early until age 30 years.[41]

### Large-for-Gestational-Age Infants

The risk factors for having an LGA infant include diabetes, maternal age, parity, prepregnancy BMI, ethnicity, weight gain during pregnancy, gender of fetus, and gestational age at birth.[42] It is important to identify infants who are LGA; for example, an infant of a diabetic mother could present with hypoglycemia after birth and should be monitored appropriately.[42] A further concern for LGA infants is that there may be central adipose tissue which could lead to the development of metabolic syndrome in childhood.[43] LGA infants also have been shown to have an increased risk of developing childhood acute lymphoblastic leukemia (relative risk [RR], 1.66; 95% confidence interval [CI], 1.32–2.10).[44,45]

Not all LGA infants are the same, however. The LGA infants of normoglycemic mothers were shown to have a higher proportion of lean body mass than those infants whose mothers who had gestational diabetes mellitus (GDM). Even among AGA infants, there was a higher proportion of fat mass in those infants whose mothers were diabetic.[46]

Research is ongoing about the specific effects of elevated glucose levels and glycemic control on infant outcomes. There is some evidence that hyperglycemia in the second trimester (rather than earlier or later) may lead to a greater risk for a diabetic woman to have an infant who is LGA.[47] The Hyperglycemia and Adverse Pregnancy Outcome (HAPO) study was conducted to determine the associations of GDM and obesity with adverse pregnancy outcomes. Both maternal GDM and obesity were independently associated with adverse pregnancy outcomes, and their combination had a greater impact than either one alone.[48] Prepregnancy obesity and severe obesity are also related to stillbirth, with placental disease, umbilical abnormalities, hypertension, and fetal anomalies being the leading causes.[49]

### Body Composition

In the past, weight gain was a focus in the assessment of neonatal growth. Then came the concept of proportional growth, which acknowledged that growth of all parameters (i.e., weight, length, and head circumference) is very important.[50] Weight for length became an important metric. A new BMI chart for premature infants, based on the Olsen growth curve, is now available.[51] The next step in nutrition assessment is to measure lean body mass. A thorough review of techniques was published in 2014.[52] Methods used for measurement of lean body mass in infants were described by Rice and Valentine.[53] A correlation of the differences between old and new software for bone density measurement (dual-energy absorptiometry, or DXA) and the relationship of DXA measurements to skin fold measurements and air displacement plethysmography (the PEA POD Infant Body Composition System) has been published.[54] A study by Hediger et al.[55] indicated why this information is important. In the third National Health and Nutrition Examination Survey (NHANES) study, SGA infants were found to have a deficit in muscularity based on measurements of MUAC and mid-upper arm muscle area from 2 months to 4 years. LGA infants were found to have a surfeit of muscularity but less of a surfeit of fatness.[55] Whether these findings will be validated with the use of newer techniques remains to be seen.

## OTHER NUTRITIONAL CONSIDERATIONS

### Hypoxic Ischemic Encephalopathy

The Apgar score at birth is an important index of the maturity and functional abilities of the infant. Infants with very low Apgar scores may present with hypoxic ischemic encephalopathy (HIE) and may have varying degrees of morbidity, including low IQ score and cerebral palsy.[56] Therapeutic hypothermia is now a standard of care for infants with HIE and has been associated with higher developmental scores.[56,57] These infants may develop some metabolic alterations such as hypomagnesemia,[58] hypocalcemia,[59] hypoglycemia,[60,61] and hyperglycemia.[60,61]

Because their calorie needs can be very different from those of the average infant, infants with HIE may have abnormal growth in the postnatal period.[62] Some have lower calorie needs over time, probably related to the reduction that is seen in head circumference growth, which is a marker of brain growth. For these infants, it is important not to just continue to decrease calories by "watering down" the formula or human milk. This could lead to inadequate nutrients and, at the extreme end, inadequate electrolytes. It is essential to work with a dietitian to reduce calories if growth is excessive while keeping nutrient and electrolyte levels adequate. Other infants with HIE have high calorie needs and may fail to thrive.[62] This may be related to the higher tone they exhibit, which contributes to higher calorie needs. Some infants have failure to thrive due to difficulty feeding once the obligatory suck reflex is gone, or they may never have had a good suck at all. Some infants require more calories to perform simple movements, especially if their tone is high; they may need more calories for adequate growth. The use of higher protein intake during the first year of life has been studied as a means to combat failure to thrive in these infants.[63]

Because these infants may have an inefficient or abnormal suck, well-meaning practitioners sometimes add cereal to their feedings. This creates a higher-calorie feed with increased carbohydrate, potentially creating an allergy, and increased calories (from 19–20 to ≥30 kcal/oz). The result may be greater problems with overweight and obesity. A guideline for follow-up of infants with HIE has been published.[64]

Coordination of the suck-swallow reflex is dependent on postconception age and usually is not developed fully until 34 to 36 weeks' gestation. In addition, inappropriate foods or methods of feeding can lead to poor nutritional status and poor feeding skill development or aggravate already existing problems. Common feeding practices that should be discouraged are (1) early introduction of solid foods (before 6 months of age); (2) thickening of formula with infant cereal; (3) giving liquids other than breast milk or formula (e.g., juice) in the first 6 months; (4) "propping" bottles for feeding before the infant is able to hold a bottle; and (5) use of an infant feeder to push strained foods into the infant's mouth.

## Malnutrition

Nutritional adequacy of the diet relates to health concerns other than growth, and postnatal development, in turn, can influence nutritional status. Malnutrition during critical periods of both intrauterine and postnatal development can have irreversible effects on intellectual potential and behavior,[65] and early severe undernutrition can have deleterious effects on basic cognitive functions.[66] Certain substances not normally regarded as essential may become essential if their precursors are limited in the diet or if the processes of conversion are reduced in activity due to abnormal gene function or developmental immaturity.[67,68] Bone modeling and skeletal effects probably result from a complex sequence of hormonal changes in interaction with nutritional factors.[67] Positive manipulation of the diet, through emphasis on particular food groups or the addition of supplements, is being studied more frequently.

Docosahexaenoic acid (DHA) and arachidonic acid (ARA) are long-chain omega-6 fatty acids normally found in human milk. These substances are now being added to infant formulas and human milk fortifiers based on research on the association of DHA and ARA intake, forms, and ratios with brain levels, visual function, and cognitive ability in healthy breast-fed infants.[69] In some areas of the world, mothers produce breast milk with higher DHA and ARA content than in other areas. In central Europe, fortification with 200 mg/day of DHA from midpregnancy to lactation improved the DHA status of infants and babies.[70] The initial DHA content of breast milk in this region was similar to that seen in the US state of Missouri.[71] The relationship of these nutrients to growth was shown in a study linking formula fortified with DHA and ARA with improved weight and length/height for age but not with higher BMI from birth to 6 years.[72] Another study showed that preterm infants fed supplemented formulas had increased lean body mass and reduced fat mass by 1 year of age.[73]

## Obesity

Obesity is an increasingly significant health problem in industrialized countries, and its accompanying morbidities include hypertension, diabetes, cardiovascular and respiratory diseases, orthopedic disorders, and psychosocial dysfunction.[74] Prenatal undernutrition has been linked with greater obesity. In a study of women who were pregnant during the Dutch famine in World War II (1944–1945) and their offspring, researchers observed an increase of more than 120% in weight for height (based on the 1948 WHO standards) among 19-year-old military recruits whose mothers were malnourished only during the first trimester of pregnancy.[75] Those whose mothers were malnourished in the second or third trimester had a lower mean birth weight and lower adult BMI but a higher incidence of type 2 diabetes than those whose mothers had only first-trimester malnutrition.[76] Also, there was a decrease in obesity among recruits whose mothers were malnourished in the immediate postnatal period.[75] These findings led to the idea that early intrauterine malnutrition affects the hypothalamic development and early postnatal malnutrition affects the number of adipocytes.[75]

Some have speculated that there is an interaction between the prenatal environment and the function of pancreatic beta cells, hypothalamus, liver, and other organs in the regulation of adult homeostasis including energy and cardiovascular function. Barker hypothesized that the fetus has to adapt to malnutrition in utero and makes changes that later affect metabolic, cardiovascular, and endocrine functions in the adult.[77–79]

The relative contributions of socioeconomic and behavioral factors operating in fetal and infant life, childhood, and adulthood to these obesity-associated diseases is an important research area.[79,80] It has been commonly thought that bottle-feeding and the early introduction of solid foods in infancy lead to infantile obesity because of the caregiver's tendency to encourage the infant to finish all of each feeding. Some studies suggest that breast-feeding is protective against obesity[82–86]; others do not provide any conclusive evidence pertaining to the method of feeding as a causative agent in the development of obesity.[87,88] Predominant breast-feeding during the first 6 months of life was shown in one study to protect against a higher BMI in adolescence.[89] No link has been shown between the age at which solid foods are introduced and obesity.[90] Although nutrition and dietary habits learned early in life have effects on health status and disease well into adulthood,[91] no association has been shown between the relative proportions of dietary carbohydrate, protein, and fat in early childhood and obesity.[92]

Although it is possible to document a direct relationship between increased caloric intake and obesity on the societal level, it has been difficult to do so on the individual level. Most studies have reported no correlation between individual caloric intake and degree of adiposity.[93,94] After a child becomes overweight or obese, a steady state with little weight change may occur, explaining in part the average or below-average reported caloric intake of these individuals. Another theory is that the overweight child has lowered energy output.[95,96]

From the time solid foods are introduced, the infant learns valuable lessons about the role of food. Individual differences in control of food intake are determined to a large extent by childhood feeding practices.[97,98] Infants should triple their birth weight by 12 months, but many infants in the United States are doing so by 6 months. Poor eating behaviors practiced by family members that have led to their obesity are likely to be learned and practiced by the growing infant and toddler. These behaviors include eating past the point of satiety, "cleaning the plate," and using food as a method of showing affection or relieving emotional stress. Although children can have a genetic and epigenetic tendency toward obesity,[99–101] the environment clearly plays a greater role in its development.

Caution must be used when interpreting research studies aimed at preventing obesity. The primary physiological function of adipose tissue is energy storage; it is a means of modifying mortality risk during the nutritionally turbulent period of infancy.[102] Secondary functions of adipose tissue include thermoregulation, cushiony protection for organs, and storage of fat-soluble vitamins and essential fatty acids. Emphasis is being placed on early nutritional intake in the hope of preventing adult obesity.[103] Results may not be applicable to different cultures, however, because what prevents a public health problem in a developed country may afford the best level of nutritional protection in an underdeveloped one.

The BMI (based on weight/height$^2$) correlates well with the percentage of body weight as fat.[104] The BMI is recommended as the most suitable index for ascertaining the degree of adiposity in children.[105] Using this measurement alone, overweight is commonly defined as a BMI greater than the 85th percentile for age and sex, and obesity as a BMI greater than the 95th percentile. Percentile graphs are shown in Appendix 3. Children with atrophy of the lower extremities or abnormal growth of the limbs usually need separate growth charts because the height is squared in BMI and is not appropriate.

Prevention of excess weight is the best protection against the complications of obesity. Increasing the proportion of adults, adolescents, and children who practice healthy dietary habits and increasing the proportion who maintain adequate physical activity are goals of Healthy People 2020 (see Appendix 1–4).[104]

Treatment of obesity requires simultaneously increasing energy expenditure and decreasing caloric intake. In growing children, weight maintenance is the objective because stature will continue to increase. Although treatment appears simple and straightforward, in practice it is a challenge for the family to modify the environment that contributed to the abnormal rate of weight gain. Dietz[107] suggested the following basic practices: promoting breast-feeding, implementing regular family meals, restoring to parents the responsibility for what children are offered and restoring to children the choice of whether to eat what is offered, and reducing the amount of time that children are allowed to watch television. Dietitians may assist family members in determining the nutritional adequacy of the current diet and realistic caloric needs; the requirements of individuals vary in relation to a wide variety of factors.[108] The measurement of energy intake in infants is far from straightforward, and the possibility of significant error is great.[109] As children mature and become more independent, nutrition education is naturally adapted to the needs of adolescents. The use of school health programs is increasing and may be valuable in preventing obesity.[110] Physical education should be included in all school programs. Be sure that children in infant day care and preschool programs are getting adequate movement and exercise. Mothers should be taught during pregnancy about infant feeding. They should be cautioned not to put cereal in bottles and not to give milk at bedtime (i.e., to put only water in the bottle at bedtime if a bottle is needed). Only 1 to 2 tablespoons of food should be given, not the whole jar at one time, even though the label states that one jar equals one serving; it is important to control portion size (see Table 4–6 in Chapter 4).

## BIOCHEMICAL AND CLINICAL ABNORMALITIES

### Iron Deficiency Anemia

Simple methods of preventing iron deficiency (ID) and iron deficiency anemia (IDA) have existed for more than 70 years, yet they remain a significant health problem. Globally, the incidence in preschool children is estimated at 47%.[111] In the United States, the incidence of ID in toddlers (12–36 months) is 7%, and the incidence of IDA in toddlers is 2%.[112,113] Anemia in the first year of life is an important warning sign of potential nutritional deficiencies. Prompt diagnosis and treatment are important not only to correct the anemia but also to prevent any long-term problems associated with deficiencies.[114] Because of the widespread use of iron-fortified infant formulas and cereal products, there has been a decline in the incidence of IDA during the first year of life, but it becomes a significant issue in children between 1 and 2 years of age.[115]

Common symptoms associated with ID are nonspecific and include fatigue, irritability, and restlessness. Adverse effects of anemia include decreased energy, reduced tolerance to heat and cold stress, and cellular immunoincompetence due to the decreased hemoglobin level and the body's compensatory mechanisms to improve oxygen transport. Iron-dependent tissue enzymes are affected, causing health impairment even before the anemia occurs.[116,117] ID also affects mental and motor development. Developmental test scores of iron-deficient children are significantly lower than those of children with sufficient iron stores.[118] However, correction of the ID may not result in improvement in test scores due to various factors such as the timing of the ID, other nutrient deficiencies, limitations of the developmental test, and poor social background.[119]

Full-term, healthy infants are born with sufficient iron stores to provide for rapid tissue growth during the first 4 to 6 months of life. Requirements then gradually increase, from approximately 2 mg/day (the recommendation for infants <6 mo of age) to approximately 11 mg/day (recommended for infants 7–12 mo of age).[120] Risk factors for ID include the size of the infant and the gestational age (infants with IUGR or premature birth have smaller reserves of iron), as well as the time at which the umbilical cord was clamped (immediate clamping of the cord deprives the infant of a substantial portion of birth body iron).[121] Regardless of birth weight or gestational age, all infants need a reliable exogenous source of iron during the second period of rapid growth, between 4 months and 2 years of life.

The laboratory indices used in the diagnosis of ID and IDA correspond to the overlapping stages of iron depletion. The first stage, loss of storage iron, is reflected by a fall in serum ferritin concentration. A decline in circulating iron occurs next and may be measured by serum iron or transferrin saturation. At that point, iron-dependent enzymes are impaired, and some of the deleterious effects of ID are seen, even before the circulating hemoglobin concentration drops. Free erythrocyte protoporphyrin also increases at that stage and is often used in the differential diagnosis. The final stage is a decrease in hemoglobin concentration, indicating anemia. IDA is microcytic; therefore, a decrease in the mean corpuscular volume is also seen.[116,117]

No single laboratory value definitively indicates the presence of ID or IDA. Rather, diagnosis of these states depends on the results of three or more indices. Accepted laboratory values for ID, used in the NHANES 2003–2006 study, are as follows: serum ferritin, <14 μg/dL; transferrin saturation, <12%; and erythrocyte protoporphyrin, >1.24 nmol/L RBCs.[120] Anemia is defined as a hemoglobin concentration of less than 11 g/dL.[122] In cases of mild anemia, infection, or chronic disease, ID may be difficult to diagnose correctly. A therapeutic trial of iron is often given in such cases.

### Factors To Be Considered in the Evaluation, Prevention, and Management of Anemia

Breast milk contains 0.3 mg/L of a highly absorbable form of iron; approximately 50% this iron is available to the infant.[123] However, ID may occur if the infant is exclusively breast-fed for longer than 6 months. The AAP has recommended that breast-fed term infants receive iron supplementation of 1 mg/kg/day, starting at 4 months of age (earlier for premature and SGA infants) and continuing until appropriate iron-containing complementary foods have been introduced.[115] Despite controversy regarding gastrointestinal intolerance and the possibility of increased infections, the AAP concluded that infant formulas containing 12 mg/L of iron are safe to use in those infants who are not breast-feeding.[115] Weaning from breast milk or iron-fortified formula to whole cow's milk before 12 months of age is associated with a significantly higher incidence of ID, allergy to milk protein, and type 1 diabetes.[124]

When beicost is introduced, the risk of an iron-deficient diet begins. The iron present in foods commonly given to infants is primarily nonheme iron, a poorly absorbable form. Iron-fortified infant cereal, vegetables, and fruits contain iron in this form. The addition of ascorbic acid (from fruit juice or added to food) and small amounts of heme iron (from meat, fish, or poultry) can greatly increase the iron absorption from typical infant foods.[125]

The iron requirement for children older than 1 year of age is 7 mg/day.[115] Supplements may be necessary for those toddlers not consuming adequate iron-rich foods. The AAP recommends general screening for anemia at 1 year of age.[115] Treatment of established ID or IDA consists of providing supplemental oral iron at a dosage of 3 to 6 mg/kg/day.[126] Treatment should continue for 3 to 4 months, with iron levels verified in the laboratory before treatment is ended. The iron supplement is best absorbed when it is given between meals and with an ascorbic acid–containing food source such as 2 to 4 oz of orange juice. The diet should be reviewed for reliable sources of iron, particularly as the child's milk source changes from breast milk or iron-fortified formula to whole cow's milk after 1 year of age.

### Hypernatremic Dehydration

Breast-feeding–associated neonatal hypernatremia occurs in up to 2% of neonates.[127] It is characterized by excessive weight loss (>10%) and is significantly associated with cesarean delivery, primiparity, breast anomalies or breast-feeding problems, excessive prepregnancy maternal weight, delayed first breast-feeding, lack of previous breast-feeding experience, and low maternal education level.[128] The infant's weight should be monitored closely during the first 2 weeks after delivery.

Hypernatremic dehydration also occurs in older infants and toddlers, but most often it is the result of an infectious diarrheal disease in combination with inappropriate fluid therapy.[129] Other cases occur in relation to disease states such as diabetes insipidus, diabetes mellitus, renal disease, underlying neurological disorders, and salt poisoning. Dietary errors could potentially cause severe dehydration; for example, skim milk, which has a high renal solute load, can overburden the infant kidney, especially if inadequate water is consumed. This is an

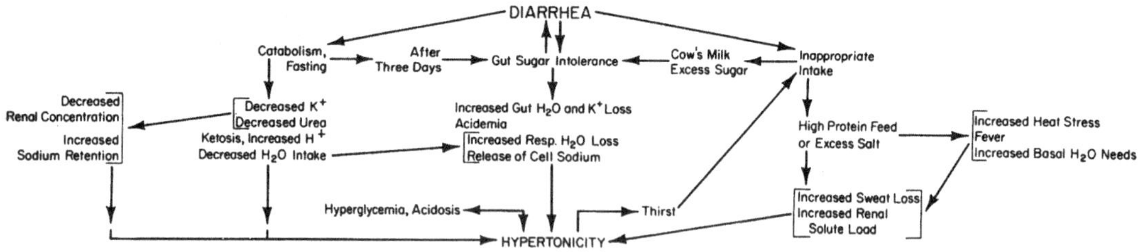


**Figure 2–3.** Events leading to the development of hypernatremic dehydration after diarrheal losses. (From Hirschorn N[130]. The treatment of acute diarrhea in children: a historical and physiological perspective. *Am J Clin Nutr.* 1980; 33:637.)

impetus for the constant education by health care professionals regarding breast-feeding and/or formula-feeding of infants, the appropriate age at which to introduce solid foods, and the types of solid foods. Infants and children are more susceptible to dehydration because of (1) their large ratio of body surface area to weight, which causes more evaporative water losses; (2) their susceptibility to metabolic water loss during febrile periods[130]; and (3) a normally higher metabolic rate in children weighing less than 15 kg[131] (Fig. 2–3).

In a small child with diarrhea, increased gastrointestinal water and potassium losses induce further respiratory water loss and a release of non-extracellular sodium that may result in hypernatremia.[132] Inappropriate fluid therapy (see Chapter 4 for adequate fluid requirement based on age) can aggravate the existing water deficit and sodium retention when a fluid that is too high in sodium is given. Figure 2–3 illustrates the events in hypernatremia.

Hypernatremic dehydration is defined as dehydration associated with an elevated serum sodium concentration of 150 mEq/L or higher; the normal range is 136 to 145 mEq/L.[132] It reflects a body water deficit relative to sodium. Severe dehydration does not have to occur for the infant to become hypernatremic; one study documented that 50% of infants with hypernatremic dehydration were less than 10% dehydrated.[133] Infants presenting with hypernatremic dehydration may show few of the usual signs of dehydration (e.g., dry shrunken tongue, diminished skin turgor, lack of tears). More often, signs of central nervous system dysfunction (e.g., lethargy, irritability, seizures) are apparent. These signs may occur in as many as 70% of infants when the serum sodium concentration rises above 158 mEq/L.[134] In developed countries, it is relatively easy to diagnose and treat dehydration with either intravenous solutions or oral rehydration solutions (ORS). In developing countries, resources are scarce and it is important to determine which children with diarrhea are at risk for severe disease and require hospital admission and intravenous fluids; a WHO dehydration scale[135] is in widespread use, but more accurate methods are still needed.[136]

## Factors To Be Considered in the Management of Diarrhea-Related Hypernatremia

Correct management of mild, moderate, or severe diarrhea-related dehydration is necessary to prevent the majority of cases of hypernatremic dehydration. Bouts of infectious diarrhea may be treated successfully at home, thereby avoiding the costs and complications associated with hospitalization. The usual symptoms of this acute illness are increased frequency of loose or watery stools, vomiting, and a decreased intake of food and fluid. ORS such as Pedialyte and Enfalyte have been designed specifically for use in developed countries for treatment of these symptoms in otherwise healthy children. These solutions contain 30 to 60 mEq/L of sodium together with small amounts of glucose to facilitate sodium absorption; they also contain potassium, chloride, zinc, and an anionic base.[137] Table 2–1 gives examples of branded solutions.

**Table 2–1.** Composition of Oral Electrolyte Solutions

| Oral Rehydration Solution | $Na^+$ (mEq/L) | $K^+$ (mEq/L) | Osmolality |
|---|---|---|---|
| Pedialyte | 45 | 20 | 250 |
| Enfalyte | 50 | 25 | 160 |

**Table 2–2.** Sodium Content and Osmolality of Clear Liquids

| Product | $Na^+$ (mEq/L) | Osmolality (mOsm/kg $H_2O$) |
|---|---|---|
| Chicken broth | 251–357 | 501 |
| 7-Up | 5–7 | 548 |
| Cola drinks | 1.3–6.5 | 750 |
| Kool-Aid | 0.9–1.1 | 251–509 |
| Jell-O | 22–27 | 644 |
| Sports drinks | 20 | 330 |
| Apple juice | 5 | 730 |
| Ginger ale | 0.8–2.7 | 557 |
| Popsicles | 4.7–5.6 | 719 |

Adapted from Wendland, BE, Arbus GS. Oral fluid therapy: sodium and potassium content and osmolality of some commercial "clear" soups, juices, and beverages. *Can Med Assoc J.* 1979; 21:564; and Snyder J. The continuing evolution of oral therapy for diarrhea. *Semin Pediatr Infect Dis.* 1994; 5:231.

Different ORS are available for use in developing countries, and more research and education is being directed at prevention of gastroenteritis through the continuation of breast-feeding for longer periods and the use of probiotics, antiemetics, and antidiarrheal agents.[138]

Vomiting is not a contraindication to the use of ORS. When fluid is administered by spoon in 5-mL amounts, rather than through a nipple or cup, retention is usually successful (Table 2–2; see Table 2–1). When the clinician recommends an ORS, guidelines should be given as to the amount to be offered per day and whether any other fluids may be offered. To ensure the correct dilution and final electrolyte content, ready-to-feed solutions are preferred to powders that must be mixed with water.

Cases of hypernatremic dehydration caused by dietary errors alone do not constitute a large percentage of cases in the United States; however, it is important to address this problem and its prevention. All infants, as well as any small children who have severe psychomotor retardation or are comatose, are unable to communicate thirst and therefore are the most susceptible to hypernatremic dehydration caused by a faulty diet. A diet that is excessive in sodium, together with inadequate free water, is likely to cause hypernatremic dehydration in the absence of increased water loss. If hyperosmolar feedings are given in addition to inadequate water and excessive sodium, vomiting and diarrhea may result, causing hypernatremia and dehydration to occur more rapidly.

## Vitamin D Deficiency

Breast milk contains low amounts of vitamin D, and infants traditionally have been exposed to sunlight to prevent rickets. Since the early 1900s, milk has been fortified with 400 IU vitamin D per quart, and

**Table 2–3.** Categories of Vitamin D Status

| | Serum 25-Hydroxyvitamin D Level | |
|---|---|---|
| Category | nmol/L | ng/mL |
| Risk of deficiency | <30 | <12 |
| Risk of inadequacy | 30–49 | 12–19 |
| Sufficiency | 50–125 | 20–50 |
| Above which there may be reason for concern | >125 | >50 |

infant formulas have been similarly fortified. It is now well known that vitamin D crosses the placenta, and term infants are generally protected from vitamin D deficiency for the first 2 to 3 months of life.[139] However, vitamin D–deficiency rickets is still a global problem, and the incidence is highest in countries where children are unable to be outside owing to religious or cultural customs or climatic conditions.[140] Increasing the vitamin D concentration of breast milk to adequate levels can be done by supplementation of the breast-feeding mothers.[141] In countries where routine health care is available, vitamin D–deficiency rickets is easily prevented.

Four categories of vitamin D status are defined by the Institute of Medicine based on serum levels of the prehormone, 25-hydroxyvitamin D[142] (Table 2-3). The prevalence of serum vitamin D deficiency in children aged 1 to 8 years was 1% in the United States in 2001–2006,[143] although there is evidence that the incidence is rising dramatically.[144] Vitamin D deficiency (hypovitaminosis D), as defined by serum level, is associated with obesity; high levels of adipose tissue sequester the vitamin and make it less available to the body.[145] Hypovitaminosis D leads to increased risk of multiple adverse health effects, including lower respiratory tract infections and type 1 diabetes in children.[141]

## SUMMARY

Evaluation of postnatal growth is an essential component of primary pediatric care. Breast-feeding confers a wide range of benefits to both infant and mother. In cases in which breast-feeding is not possible, other methods to convey human milk to the baby are needed. If the mother is unable to express human milk, iron-fortified infant formula is indicated.

Deviation of an infant from his or her previous Z score or growth curve channel on the WHO growth curve should be promptly investigated. Dietitians are an important part of that investigation; they work in concert with lactation consultants if the infant is breast-feeding or the mother is expressing human milk.

Evaluation of family dietary practices and nutrition education are essential components of primary pediatric care; they are a worthwhile long-range investment for the child.[146] In nutritional evaluation and counseling with families, the pediatrician, nurse, or dietitian should be aware of and investigate abnormal growth patterns. Z scores should be used to help keep track of growth. For infants with a developmental disorder, use of a combination of the WHO growth curve and the particular chart can be helpful in evaluating growth. It is important to be aware of the risk factors for vitamin and mineral deficiencies. Hyperlipidemia in infancy is addressed in Chapter 32 of this text, and elevated lead levels in infancy are discussed in Chapter 23.

### References


1. American Academy of Pediatrics, Work Group on Breastfeeding. Breastfeeding and the use of human milk (RE9729). *Pediatrics.* 1997; 100:1035.
2. World Health Organization. Global targets 2025: breastfeeding policy brief. 2014. http://www.who.int/nutrition/publications/globaltargets2025_policybrief_breastfeeding/en/. Accessed May 19, 2016.
3. United Nations Children's Fund, *World Health Organization. Breastfeeding Advocacy Initiative: For the Best Start in Life.* Geneva: WHO; 2015.
4. World Health Organization. *Infant and Young Child Feeding: Model Chapter.* Geneva: WHO; 2009.
5. Andreas NJ, Kampmann B, Mehring Le-Doare K. Human breast milk: a review on its composition and bioactivity. *Early Hum Dev.* 2015; 91:629.
6. Civardi E, Garofoli F, Mazzucchelli I, et al. Enteral nutrition and infections: the role of human milk. *Early Hum Dev.* 2014; 90(Suppl 1):S57.
7. Beaudry M, Dufour R, Marcoux S. Relation between infant feeding and infections during the first six months of life. *J Pediatr.* 1995; 126:191.
8. Dewey KG, Heinig MJ, Nommsen-Rivers LA. Differences in morbidity between breast-fed and formula-fed infants. *Pediatrics.* 1995; 126:696.
9. Duncan B, Ey J, Holberg CJ, et al. Exclusive breastfeeding for at least 4 months protects against otitis media. *Pediatrics.* 1993; 91:867.
10. Yang YS, Yu SY. The effect of exclusive breastfeeding on development and incidence of infection in infants. *J Hum Lact.* 1996; 12:27.
11. Mortensen EL, Michaelsen KF, Sanders SA, et al. The association between duration of breastfeeding and adult intelligence. *JAMA.* 2002; 287:2365.
12. Wessel J. Human milk. In Corkins MR, ed. *The A.S.P.E.N. Pediatric Nutrition Support Core Curriculum*, 2nd ed. The American Society for Parenteral and Enteral Nutrition. Silver Spring, MD: ASPEN Publications; 2014.
13. Reece-Stremtan S, Marinelli KA, Academy of Breastfeeding Medicine. ABM clinical protocol #21: guidelines for breastfeeding and substance abuse disorder, revised 2015. *Breastfeeding Med.* 2015; 10:135.
14. Voreades N, Kozil A, Weir TL. Diet and the development of the human intestinal microbiome. *Front Microbiol.* 2014; 5:494.
15. American Academy of Pediatrics, Committee on Nutrition. *Pediatric Nutrition Handbook*, 6th ed. Elk Grove Village, IL: AAP; 2008.
16. American Congress of Obstetricians and Gynecologists. The Apgar Score. Committee Opinion Number 644, October 2015. http://www.acog.org/Resources-And-Publications/Committee-Opinions/Committee-on-Obstetric-Practice/The-Apgar-Score. Accessed May 19, 2016.
17. The New Ballard Score. http://www.ballardscore.com/Pages/ScoreSheet.aspx. Accessed May 19, 2016.
18. Thulier D. Weighing the facts: a systematic review of expected patterns of weight loss in full-term, breastfed infants. *J Hum Lact.* 2016; 32:28.
19. Grummer-Strawn L, Reinold C, Krebs N; Centers for Disease Control and Prevention. Use of World Health Organization and CDC growth charts for children aged 0-59 months in the United States. *MMWR Recomm Rep.* 2010; 59(RR09):1.
20. de Onis M, Garza C, Onyango AW, et al. WHO growth standards for infants and young children. *Arch Pediatr.* 2009; 16:47.
21. World Health Organization. *Training Course for Child Growth Assessment WHO Growth Standards.* Geneva: WHO; 2008.
22. Becker PJ, Nieman Carney L, Corkins MR, et al. Consensus statement of the Academy of Nutrition and Dietetics/American Society for Parenteral and Enteral Nutrition: indicators recommended for the identification and documentation of pediatric malnutrition (undernutrition). *J Acad Nutr Diet.* 2014; 114:1988.
23. Becker PJ, Nieman Carney L, Corkins MR, et al. Consensus statement of the Academy of Nutrition and Dietetics/American Society for Parenteral and Enteral Nutrition: indicators recommended for the identification and documentation of pediatric malnutrition (undernutrition). *Nutr Clin Pract.* 2015; 30:147.
24. Joosten KF, Hulst JM. Malnutrition in pediatric hospital patients: current issues. *Nutrition.* 2011; 27:133.
25. Hulst JM, Zwart H, Hop WC, Joosten KF. Dutch national survey to test the STRONGkids nutrition al risk screening tools in hospitalized children. *Clin Nutr.* 2010; 29:106.
26. Durakbasa ÇU, Fettahoglu S, Bayar A, et al. The prevalence of malnutrition and effectiveness of STRONGkids tool in the identification of malnutrition risks among pediatric surgical patients. *Balkan Med J.* 2014; 31:313.
27. Beer SS, Juarez MD, Vega MW, Canada NL. Pediatric malnutrition: putting the new definition and standards into practice. *Nutr Clin Pract.* 2015;30:609.
28. Litchford MD, Dorner B, Posthauer ME. Malnutrition as a precursor of pressure ulcers. *Adv Wound Care (New Rochelle).* 2014; 3:54.
29. Kavle JA, Flax VL, Abdelmgeid A, et al. Factors associated with early growth in Egyptian infants: implications for addressing the dual burden of malnutrition. *Matern Child Nutr.* 2016; 12:139.
30. Chand S, Shah, D. Mid-upper arm circumference for detection of severe acute malnutrition in infants aged between one and six months. *Indian Pediatr.* 2015; 52:528.
31. Daly-Wolfe KM, Jordan KC, Slater H, et al. Mid-arm circumference is a reliable method to estimate adiposity in preterm and term infants. *Pediatr Res.* 2015; 78:336.
32. United Nations Children's Fund. *Measuring MUAC Training Video.* http://www.unicef.org. Accessed May 20, 2016.
33. United Nations Children's Fund. *Mid-Upper Arm Circumference Measuring Tapes.* UNICEF Technical Bulletin No. 13, revision 2. New York: UNICEF Supply Division; 2014.
34. Vayssiere C, Sentilhes I, Ego A, et al. Fetal growth restriction and intra-uterine growth restriction: guidelines for clinical practice from the French College of Gynecologists and Obstetricians. *Eur J Gynecol Reprod Biol.* 2015; 193:10.
35. Hinkle SN, Johns AM, Albert PS, et al. Longitudinal changes in gestational weight gain and the association with intrauterine fetal growth. *Eur J Obstet Gynecol Reprod Biol.* 2015; 190:41.
36. Wrottesley SH, Lamper C, Pisa PT. Review of the importance of nutrition during the first 1000 days: maternal nutritional status and its associations with fetal growth and birth, neonatal and infant outcomes among African women. *J Dev Orig Health Dis.* 2016; 7:144.
37. McMillen IC, MacLaughlin SM, Muhlhausler BS, et al. Developmental origins of adult health and disease: the role of periconceptional and foetal nutrition. *Basic Clin Pharmacol Toxicol.* 2008; 102:82.
38. Lei X, Chen Y, Ye J, et al. The optimal postnatal growth trajectory for term small for gestational age babies: a prospective cohort study. *J Pediatr.* 2015; 166:54.
39. Varella MH, Moss WJ. Early growth patterns are associated with intelligence quotient scores in children born small-for-gestational age. *Early Hum Dev.* 2015; 91:491.
40. Beyerlein A, Ness AR, Streuling I. Early rapid growth: no association with later cognitive functions in children born not small for gestational age. *Am J Clin Nutr.* 2010; 92:585.
41. Wennerstrom EC, Simonsen J, Melbye M. Long term survival of individuals born small and large for gestational age. *PLoS One.* 2015; 10:e0138594.
42. Lawrence EJ. A matter of size: part 2. Evaluating the large-for-gestational-age neonate. *Adv Neonatal Care.* 2007; 7:187.
43. Boney CM, Verma A, Tucker R, Vohr BR. Metabolic syndrome in childhood: association with birth weight, maternal obesity, and gestational diabetes. *Pediatrics.* 2005; 115:e290.
44. Sprehe MR, Barahmani N, Cao Y, et al. Comparison of birth weight corrected for gestational age and birth weight alone in prediction of development of childhood leukemia and central nervous system tumors. *Pediatr Blood Cancer.* 2010; 54:242.
45. Oksuzyan S, Crespi CM, Cockburn M, et al. Birth weight and other perinatal characteristics and childhood leukemia in California. *Cancer Epidemiol.* 2012; 36:e359.
46. Uebel K, Pusch K, Gedrich K, et al. Effect of maternal obesity with and without gestational diabetes on offspring subcutaneous and preperitoneal adipose tissue development from birth up to year-1. *BMC Pregnancy Childbirth.* 2014; 14:138.

47. Kerssen A, de Valk HW, Visser GH. Increased second trimester maternal glucose levels are related to extremely large-for-gestational-age infants in women with type I diabetes. *Diabetes Care.* 2007; 30:1069.
48. Catalano PM, McIntyre HD, Cruickshank JK. The Hyperglycemia and Adverse Pregnancy Outcome study: associations of GDM and obesity with pregnancy outcomes. *Diabetes Care.* 2012; 35:780.
49. Bodnar LM, Parks WT, Perkins K, et al. Maternal prepregnancy obesity and cause-specific stillbirth. *Am J Clin Nutr.* 2015; 102:858.
50. Olsen I, Lawson ML, Meinzen-Derr J, et al. Use of a body proportionality index for growth assessment of preterm infants. *J Pediatr.* 2009; 154:496.
51. Olsen I, Lawson ML, Ferguson AN, et al. BMI curves for preterm infants. *Pediatrics.* 2015; 135:e572.
52. Prado CM, Heymsfield SB. Lean tissue imaging: a new era for nutritional assessment and imaging. *JPEN J Parenter Enteral Nutr.* 2014; 38;940.
53. Rice MS, Valentine CJ. Neonatal body composition: measuring lean mass as a tool to guide nutrition management in the neonate. *Nutr Clin Pract.* 2015; 30:625.
54. Barbour LA, Hernandez TL, Reynolds RM, et al. Striking differences in estimates of infant adiposity by new and old DXA software, PEAPOD and skin-folds at 2 weeks and 1 year of life. *Pediatr Obes.* 2015; Jul 22 [Epub ahead of print]. doi: 10.1111/ijpo.12055.
55. Hediger ML, Overpeck MD, Kuczmarski RJ, et al. Muscularity and fatness of infants and young children born small- or large-for-gestational-age. *Pediatrics.* 1998; 102:e60.
56. Rei M, Ayres-de-Campos D, Bernardes J. Neurological damage arising from intrapartum hypoxia/acidosis. *Best Pract Res Clin Obstet Gynaecol.* 2016; 30:79.
57. Jacobs SE, Berg M, Hunt R, et al. Cooling for newborns with hypoxic ischemic encephalopathy. *Cochrane Database Syst Rev.* 2013; (1):CD003311.
58. Tocco NM, Hodge AE, Jones AA, et al. Neonatal therapeutic hypothermia-associated hypomagnesemia during parenteral nutrition therapy. *Nutr Clin Pract.* 2014; 29:246.
59. Prempunpong C, Efanov I, Sant'Anna G. Serum calcium concentrations and incidence of hypocalcemia in infants with moderate or severe hypoxic-ischemic encephalopathy: effect of therapeutic hypothermia. *Early Hum Dev.* 2015; 91:535.
60. Basu SK, Kaiser JR, Guffey D, et al. Hypoglycemia and hyperglycemia are associated with unfavourable outcome in infants with hypoxic ischemic encephalopathy: a post hoc analysis of the CoolCap Study. *Arch Dis Child Fetal Neonatal Ed.* 2016; 101:F149.
61. Nadeem M, Murray DM, Boylan GB, et al. Early blood glucose profile and neurodevelopmental outcome at two years in neonatal hypoxic-ischemic encephalopathy. *BMC Pediatr.* 2011; 11:10.
62. Vohr BR, Stephens BE, McDonald SA, et al. Cerebral palsy and growth failure at 6 to 7 years. *Pediatrics.* 2013; 132:e905.
63. Merhar SL, Meinzen-Derr J, Sprague J, et al. Safety and tolerability of enteral protein supplementation for infants with brain injury. *Nutr Clin Pract.* 2015; 30:546.
64. Robertson CM, Perlman M. Follow-up of the term infant after hypoxic-ischemic encephalopathy. *Paediatr Child Health.* 2006; 11:278.
65. Skull A, Ruben A, Walker AC. Malnutrition and microcephaly in Australian aboriginal children. *Med J Aust.* 1997; 166:412.
66. Perales CG, Heresi E, Pizarro F, Colombo M. Cognitive functions of school children with normal IQ and histories of severe and early malnutrition. *Arch Latinoam Nutr.* 1996; 46:282.
67. Wharton BA, Scott PH. Distinctive aspects of metabolism and nutrition during infancy. *Clin Biochem.* 1996; 29:419.
68. Matokovic V. Nutrition, genetics and skeletal development. *J Am Coll Nutr.* 1996; 15:556.
69. Ryan AS, Astwood JD, Gautier S, et al. Effects of long chain polyunsaturated fatty acid supplementation on neurodevelopment in childhood: a review of human studies. *Prostaglandins Leukot Essent Fatty Acids.* 2010; 82:305.
70. Bergmann RL, Haschke-Becher E, Klassen-Wigger P, et al. Supplementation with 200 mg/day docosahexaenoic acid from mid-pregnancy through lactation improves the docosahexaenoic acid status of mothers with a habitually low fish intake and of their infants. *Ann Nutr Metab.* 2008; 52:157.
71. Otto SJ, Houwelingen AC, Antal M, et al. Maternal and neonatal essential fatty acid status in phospholipids: an international comparison study. *Eur J Clin Nutr.* 1997; 51:232.
72. Currie LM, Tolley EA, Thodosoff JM, et al. Long chain polyunsaturated fatty acid supplementation in infancy increases length- and weight-for-age but not BMI to 6 years when controlling for effects of maternal smoking. *Prostaglandins Leukot Essent Fatty Acids.* 2015: 98:1.
73. Groh-Wargo S, Jacobs J, Auestad N, et al. Body composition in preterm infants who are fed long-chain polyunsaturated fatty acids: a prospective, randomized, controlled trial. *Pediatr Res.* 2005; 57:712.
74. Gortmaker S, Dietz WH, Sobel AM, Whehler CA. Increasing pediatric obesity in the United States. *Am J Dis Child.* 1987; 151:535.
75. Ravelli AC, Stein ZA, Susser MW. Obesity in young men after famine exposure in utero and early infancy. *N Engl J Med.* 1976; 295:349.
76. Ravelli AC, van der Meulen JH, Michels RP, et al. Glucose tolerance in adults after prenatal exposure to famine. *Lancet.* 1998: 351:173.
77. Barker DJ. Maternal nutrition, fetal nutrition, and diseases later in life. *Nutrition.* 1997; 13:807.
78. Barker DJ, Clark PM. Fetal undernutrition and disease in later life. *Rev Reprod.* 1997; 2:105.
79. Barker DJ. Fetal origins of cardiovascular disease. *Ann Med.* 1999: 31(Suppl 1):3.
80. Lamont DW, Parker L, Cohen MA, et al. Early life and later determinants of adult disease: a 50 year follow-up study of the Newcastle Thousands Families cohort. *Public Health.* 1998; 112:85.
81. Lucas A. Programming by early nutrition: an experimental approach. *J Nutr.* 1998; 128(Suppl 2):401S.
82. Overfeeding in the first year of life. *Nutr Rev.* 1973; 31:116.
83. Crow RA, Fawcet JN, Wright P. Maternal behavior during breast- and bottle-feeding. *J Behav Med* 1980; 3:259.
84. Liese AD, Hirsch T, vonMutius E, et al. Inverse association of overweight and breast feeding in 9- to 10-year-old children in Germany. *Int J Obes Relat Metab Disord.* 2001; 25:1644.
85. Hediger ML, Overpeck MD, Kuczmarshi RJ, Ruan NJ. Association between breast feeding and overweight in young children. *JAMA.* 2001; 285:2453.
86. von Kries R, Koletzko B, Sauerwald T, et al. Breastfeeding and obesity: cross sectional study. *BMJ.* 1999; 319:147.
87. Fawzi WW, Forman MR, Levy A, et al. Maternal anthropometry and infant feeding practices in Israel in relation to growth in infancy: the North African Infant Feeding Study. *Am J Clin Nutr.* 1997; 65:1731.
88. Stettler M, Zemel BS, Kumanyika S, Stallings VA. Infant weight gain and childhood overweight status in a multicenter cohort study. *Pediatrics.* 2002; 109:194.
89. Gillman MW, Rifas-Shiman SL, Camargo CAJr, et al. Risk of overweight among adolescents who were breastfed as infants. *JAMA.* 2001; 285:2461.
90. Agras WS, Kraemer HC, Berkowitz RI, et al. Influence of early feeding style on adiposity at 6 years of age. *J Pediatr.* 1990; 116:805.
91. Strauss RS. Childhood obesity. *Pediatr Clin North Am.* 2002; 49:175.
92. Wolman PG. Feeding practices and prevalence of obesity in preschool children. *J Am Diet Assoc.* 1984; 84:436.
93. Rolland-Cachera MF, Bellisle F. No correlation between adiposity and food intake: why are working class children fatter? Am J Clin Nutr. 1986; 44:779.
94. Martorell R, Stein AD, Shroeder DG. Early nutrition and later adiposity. *J Nutr.* 2001; 131:874.
95. Ball EJ, O'Connor J, Abbott R, et al. Total energy expenditure, body fatness, and physical activity in children aged 6–9 years. *Am J Clin Nutr.* 2001; 74:524.
96. Rocandio AM, Ansotegui L, Arroyo M. Comparison of dietary intake among overweight and nonoverweight schoolchildren. *Int J Obes Rel Metab Disord.* 2001; 25:1651.
97. Birch LL. Development of food acceptance patterns in the first years of life. *Proc Nutr Soc.* 1998; 57:617.
98. Spruijt-Metz D, Lindquis CH, Birch LL, Fisher JO, Goran MI. Relation between mothers' child-feeding practices and children's adiposity. *Am J Clin Nutr.* 2002; 75:581.
99. Rolland-Cachera MF, Deheeger M, Bellisle F. Early adiposity rebound is not associated with energy or fat intake in infancy. *Pediatrics.* 2001; 108:218.
100. Dorosty AR, Emmett PM, Reilly JJ, ALSPAC Study Team. Factors associated with early adiposity rebound. *Pediatrics.* 2000; 105:1115.
101. Heerwagen MJ, Miller MR, Barbour LA, et al. Maternal obesity and fetal metabolic programming: a fertile epigenetic soil. *Am J Physiol Regul Integr Comp Physiol.* 2010; 299:R711.
102. Kuzawa CW. Adipose tissue in human infancy and childhood: an evolutionary perspective. *Am J Phys Anthropol.* 1998; 27(Suppl):177.
103. Whitaker RC, Pepe MS, Wright JA, et al. Early adiposity rebound and the risk of adult obesity. *Pediatrics.* 1998; 101:e5.
104. Roche AF, Siervogel RM, Chumlea WC, Webb P. Grading fatness from limited anthropometric data. *Am J Clin Nutr.* 1981; 34:2831.
105. Rolland-Cachera MF, Sempe M, Guilloud-Bataille M, et al. Adiposity indices in children. *Am J Clin Nutr.* 1982; 36:178.
106. U.S. Department of Health and Human Services, Washington, DC: Healthy People 2020: *2020 Topics and Objectives.* http://www.healthypeople.gov/2020/topics-objectives. Accessed May 19, 2016.
107. Dietz WH. The obesity epidemic in young children. *BMJ.* 2001; 322:313.
108. Wells JC. Energy metabolism in infants and children. *Nutrition.* 1998; 14:817.
109. Davies PS. Energy requirements for growth and development in infancy. *Am J Clin Nutr.* 1998; 68:939S.
110. Illuzzi S, Cinelli B. A coordinated school health program approach to adolescent obesity. *J School Nurs.* 2000; 16:12.
111. McLean E, Cogswell M, Egli I, et al. Worldwide prevalence of anaemia, WHO Vitamin and Mineral Nutrition Information System, 1993–2005. *Public Health Nutr.* 2009; 12:444.
112. Centers for Disease Control and Prevention. Iron deficiency—United States 1999–2000. *MMWR Morb Mortal Wkly Rep.* 2002; 51:897.
113. Centers for Disease Control and Prevention. *2nd National Report on Biochemical Indicators of Diet and Nutrition in the U.S. Population. 3: Trace Elements.* http://www.cdc.gov/nutritionreport/pdf/Trace.pdf. Accessed May 19, 2016.
114. Gallagher PG, Ehrenkranz RA. Nutritional anemias in infancy. *Clin Perinatol.* 1995; 22:671.
115. Baker RD, Greer FR, The Committee on Nutrition. Clinical report—diagnosis and prevention of iron: deficiency and iron-deficiency anemia in infants and young children (0–3 years of age). *Pediatrics.* 2010; 126:1.
116. Finch CA, Cook JD. Iron deficiency. *Am J Clin Nutr.* 1984; 39:471.
117. Scrimshaw NS. Iron deficiency and its functional consequences. *Compr Ther.* 1985; 40:40.
118. Grantham-McGregor S, Ani C. A review of studies on the effect of iron deficiency on cognitive development in children. *J Nutr.* 2001; 131:649S.
119. Pollitt E. The developmental and probabilistic nature of the functional consequences of iron-deficiency anemia in children. *J Nutr.* 2001; 131:669S.
120. Burke RM, Leon JS, Suchdev PS. Identification, prevention and treatment of iron deficiency during the first 1000 days. *Nutrients.* 2014; 6:4093.
121. Chapparo CM. Setting the stage for child health and development: prevention of iron deficiency in early infancy. *J Nutr.* 2008; 138:2529.
122. Cogswell ME, Looker AC, Pfeiffer CM, et al. Assessment of iron deficiency in US preschool children and nonpregnant females of childbearing age: National Health and Nutrition Examination Survey 2003–2006. *Am J Clin Nutr.* 2009; 89:1334.

123. Saarinen UM. Need for iron supplementation in infants on prolonged breast-feeding. *J Pediatr.* 1978; 93:177.
124. Leung AK, Sauve RS. Whole cow's milk in infancy. *Paediatr Child Health.* 2003; 8:419.
125. Engelmann MD, Sandstrom B, Michaelson KF. Meat intake and iron status in late infancy: an intervention study. *J Pediatr Gastroenterol Nutr.* 1998; 26:36.
126. Özdemir N. Iron deficiency anemia from diagnosis to treatment in children. *Turk Pediatri Ars.* 2015; 50:11.
127. Bolat F, Oflaz MB, Guven AS, et al. What is the safe approach for neonatal hypernatremic dehydration? A retrospective study from a neonatal intensive care unit. *Pediatr Emerg Care.* 2013; 29:808.
128. Lavagno C, Camozzi P, Renzi S, et al. Breastfeeding-associated hypernatremia: a systematic review of the literature. *J Hum Lact.* 2016; 32:67.
129. Forman S, Crofton P, Huang H, et al. The epidemiology of hypernatraemia in hospitalised children in Lothian: a 10-year study showing differences between dehydration, osmoregulatory dysfunction and salt poisoning. *Arch Dis Child.* 2012; 97:502.
130. Hirschorn N. The treatment of acute diarrhea in children: a historical and physiological perspective. *Am J Clin Nutr.* 1980; 33:637.
131. Ahmed I, Agusto-Odutola TB. Hypernatremia in diarrheal infants in Lagos. *Arch Dis Child.* 1970; 45:97.
132. McCauley D, Blackhall MI. Hypernatremic dehydration in infantile gastroenteritis. *Arch Dis Child.* 1961; 36:543.
133. Habel AH, Simpson H. Osmolar relation between cerebrospinal fluid and serum in hyperosmolar hypernatremic dehydration. *Arch Dis Child.* 1976; 51:660.
134. Rosenbloom L, Sills JA. Hypernatremic dehydration and infant mortality. *Arch Dis Child.* 1975; 50:750.
135. World Health Organization. *The Treatment of Diarrhoea: A Manual for Physicians and Other Senior Health Workers.* 4th ed. Geneva: WHO; 2005.
136. Hoxha T, Xhelili L, Azemi M, et al. Comparing the accuracy of the three dehydration scales in children with acute diarrhea in a developing country of Kosovo. *Mater Sociomed.* 2015; 27:140.
137. King CK, Glass R, Bresee JS, Duggan C; Centers for Disease Control and Prevention. Managing acute gastroenteritis among children: oral rehydration, maintenance, and nutritional therapy. *MMWR Recomm Rep.* 2003; 52:1.
138. Ciccarrelli S, Stolfi I, Caramia G. Management strategies in the treatment of neonatal and pediatric gastroenteritis. *Infect Drug Resist.* 2013; 29:133.
139. Hillman LS, Haddad JG. Human perinatal vitamin D metabolism: I. 25-hydroxyvitamin D in maternal and cord blood. *J Pediatr.* 1974; 84:742.
140. Pettifor JM. Nutritional rickets: deficiency of vitamin D, calcium, or both? *Am J Clin Nutr.* 2004; 80:1725S.
141. Dawodu A, Wagner CL. Prevention of vitamin D deficiency in mothers and infants worldwide: a paradigm shift. *Paediatr Int Child Health.* 2012; 32:3.
142. Institute of Medicine. *Dietary Reference Intakes for Calcium and Vitamin D.* Washington, DC: National Academies Press; 2010.
143. Looker AC, Johnson CL, Lacher DA, et al. *Vitamin D Status: United States 2001–2006.* NCHS Data Brief, no. 59. Hyattsville, MD: National Center for Health Statistics; 2011.
144. Williams R. Prevalence of hypovitaminosis D and its association with comorbidities of childhood obesity. *Perm J.* 2014; 18:32.
145. Harel Z, Flanagan P, Forcier M, Harel D. Low vitamin D status among obese adolescents: prevalence and response to treatment. *J Adolesc Health.* 2011; 48:448.
146. Kleinman RE, ed. Committee on Nutrition, American Academy of Pediatrics. *Pediatric Nutrition Handbook.* 5th ed. Elk Grove Village, IL: AAP; 2004.

# 3 Problems of Prematurity

JACQUELINE WESSEL, BARBARA NIEDBALA, AND SHIRLEY W. EKVALL

Prematurity is defined as birth before 37 weeks of gestation. Although most infants born prematurely have low birth weights, the terms *prematurity* and *low birth weight* are not synonymous. A widely accepted classification of infants by birth weight is shown in Table 3–1.

In 2012, there were more than 450,000 preterm births in the United States, or approximately 1 of every 9 births.[1] Causes include premature rupture of the membranes, maternal hypertensive disorders, preterm spontaneous labor, and antepartum hemorrhage. Also associated with premature delivery are low maternal weight, low socioeconomic status, diabetes, nephritis, anemia, fetal anomalies, infection, and multiple pregnancy. Mortality and morbidity are related to birth weight, gestational age, and etiology. Survival rates for extremely low-birth-weight (ELBW) infants and infants at the limits of viability (22–25 weeks' gestation) have improved dramatically over time.[2] There has not, however, been an accompanying drop in the incidence of disability.[2] The rates of impaired neurodevelopmental outcomes in the moderate to severe category, which include mental disability, cerebral palsy, epilepsy, blindness, and moderate to severe hearing impairment, have not changed much in the last 20 years.[2–6] Rates of disability generally increase with decreasing gestational age and birth weight. There are numerous reports on the incidence of disabilities, not only for the ELBW infants[2–6] but also for moderately preterm and late preterm infants.[7]

## PHYSIOLOGICAL, FUNCTIONAL, AND IATROGENIC PROBLEMS

The premature infant must adapt to extrauterine life despite having immature organ systems. Nutrition plays a primary role: Adequate substrate material must be present for growth and development to continue outside the uterus. The premature infant's immature renal and gastrointestinal systems require a lower renal solute load and smaller-volume feedings; respiratory distress syndrome and patent ductus

Symbols: X - 1st Exam O - 2nd Exam

NEUROMUSCULAR MATURITY

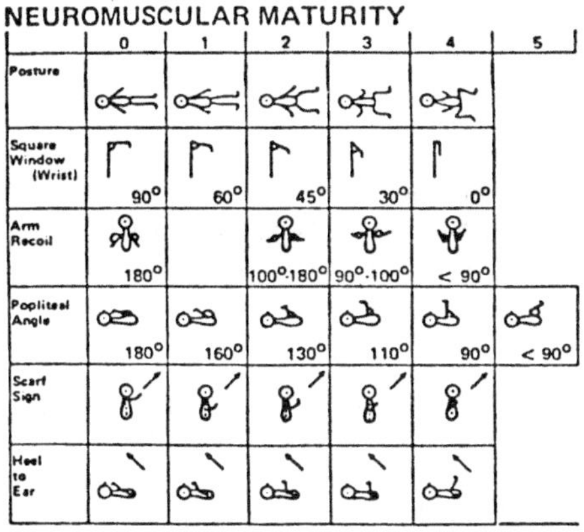


PHYSICAL MATURITY

| | 0 | 1 | 2 | 3 | 4 | 5 |
|---|---|---|---|---|---|---|
| SKIN | gelatinous red, transparent | smooth pink, visible veins | superficial peeling &/or rash, few veins | cracking pale area, rare veins | parchment, deep cracking, no vessels | leathery, cracked, wrinkled |
| LANUGO | none | abundant | thinning | bald areas | mostly bald | |
| PLANTAR CREASES | no crease | faint red marks | anterior transverse crease only | creases ant. 2/3 | creases cover entire sole | |
| BREAST | barely percept. | flat areola, no bud | stippled areola, 1–2 mm bud | raised areola, 3–4 mm bud | full areola, 5–10 mm bud | |
| EAR | pinna flat, stays folded | sl. curved pinna, soft with slow recoil | well-curv. pinna, soft but ready recoil | formed & firm with instant recoil | thick cartilage, ear stiff | |
| GENITALS Male | scrotum empty, no rugae | | testes descending, few rugae | testes down, good rugae | testes pendulous, deep rugae | |
| GENITALS Female | prominent clitoris & labia minora | | majora & minora equally prominent | majora large, minora small | clitoris & minora completely covered | |

Gestation by Dates ________ wks

Birth Date ________ Hour ________ am pm

APGAR ________ 1 min ________ 5 min

MATURITY RATING

| Score | Wks |
|---|---|
| 5 | 26 |
| 10 | 28 |
| 15 | 30 |
| 20 | 32 |
| 25 | 34 |
| 30 | 36 |
| 35 | 38 |
| 40 | 40 |
| 45 | 42 |
| 50 | 44 |

SCORING SECTION

| | 1st Exam=X | 2nd Exam=0 |
|---|---|---|
| Estimating Gest Age by Maturity Rating | ______Weeks | ______Weeks |
| Time of Exam | Date ______ Hour ______ am pm | Date ______ Hour ______ am pm |
| Age at Exam | ______Hours | ______Hours |
| Signature of Examiner | ______ M.D. | ______ M.D. |

**Figure 3–1.** Postnatal growth in infancy: estimation of gestational age by maturity rating. This is a newborn maturity rating and classification. The scoring system is from Ballard, J.L., et al. A simplified assessment of gestational age. *Pediatr. Res.* 1977; 11:374. Figures adapted from Sweet, A.Y. Classification of the low birth weight infant. In: Klaus, M.H., Fararoff, A.A., eds. *Care of the High-Risk Infant.* Philadelphia: W.B. Saunders; 1977; 47. Used with permission.

**Table 3–1.** Classification of Infants by Birth Weight

| Classification | Weight (g) |
|---|---|
| Low birth weight (LBW) | 1500–2500 |
| Very low birth weight (VLBW) | 1000–1499 |
| Extremely low birth weight (ELBW) | <999 |
| Micropremie | <750 |

arteriosus may necessitate further fluid restriction. Many aspects of the gastrointestinal system are immature, including the forward propulsion of enteral nutrients.[8] Advanced medical technologies such as temperature regulation, total parenteral nutrition (TPN), and surfactant therapy enable infants with inefficiently functioning organs to survive but may induce other clinical problems. Assisted ventilation requires the infant to be tube-fed or parenterally supplied with nutrients; it may also result in palatal groove formation, tooth enamel hypoplasia, and acquired cleft palate. Frequent phlebotomy may lead to iatrogenic anemia. The infant has an extremely high mineral accretion rate; because current parenteral and enteral formulas cannot provide for the infant's ideal needs, the result is metabolic bone disease.

## FACTORS TO BE CONSIDERED IN NUTRITIONAL EVALUATION

### Anthropometric Data

Baseline measurements of birth weight, length, and head circumference are performed according to standard procedures. Loss of 5% to 10% of the birth weight occurs during the first week of life due to a physiological diuresis. Thereafter, weight gain is dependent on nutritional intake. Healthy, enterally fed premature infants usually regain their birth weight by the second postnatal week. Once the birth weight is regained, average daily weight gain can approximate intrauterine rates. Because of complicating morbidities, however, most premature infants do not achieve the median birth weight of the reference fetus at the same postmenstrual age.[9] Growth curves specific to preterm infants are used; the two most commonly used charts are the Fenton-WHO[9,10] and the Olsen[11] premature growth curves. When an infant reaches the gestational age of 40 weeks, the WHO growth curve can be used. When the WHO growth curve is used in an electronic health record (EHR), an adjustment can be made to view the corrected age on the growth curve. Infant ages are corrected until 2 or 3 years using these curves. Z score calculations are available for both of these curves, and some of them will appear on the EHR; if not, they can be calculated through use of a website such as Peditools (http://www.Peditools.org) or an iPhone app such as Neonatal Growth Chart 2013 (https://itunes.apple.com/us/app/neonatal-growth-chart-2013/id670834784?mt=8). Gender-specific BMI curves are also now available.[12] See Appendix 3 for various growth charts.

### Biochemical Assessment

Infants receiving parenteral nutrition should be monitored routinely for electrolytes, blood urea nitrogen, calcium, phosphorus, magnesium, alkaline phosphatase, total protein, albumin, triglycerides, and liver function. In all premature infants, clinical signs of specific nutrient deficiencies and documentation of dietary inadequacy should be sought before laboratory assessments are made. Zinc, folate, vitamin A, and essential fatty acid deficiencies may occur in individual infants who have exceptionally low prenatal stores or dietary deficiencies. Serum prealbumin or retinal-binding protein (RBP) concentrations may be better markers of nutritional status and nitrogen balance in premature infants because of their shorter half-life; however. RBP is sometimes thought to be too sensitive to be helpful, and prealbumin may be the better marker. A more thorough discussion is available elsewhere.[13] Premature infants with inadequate protein and energy intake have significantly low prealbumin and RBP concentrations.

### Clinical Assessment

The infant should be routinely inspected for signs of nutritional deficiencies, such as edema, dermatitis, and changes in hair color. Late-occurring peripheral edema and/or pulmonary edema may be signs of overhydration, vitamin E deficiency, or hypoalbuminemia. Dry skin or flaky dermatitis suggests essential fatty acid or zinc deficiency. Overall evaluation of the adipose tissue and musculature is crucial.

There are no good predictive signs of enteral feeding intolerance. Increased gastric residues, abdominal distention, and emesis were previously used.[14–16] However, a small amount of gastric residue is normal. Gastric residuals are no longer measured in many nurseries because the numbers were most often a sign of a normal premature infant's disorganized motility rather than a warning sign for the development of necrotizing enterocolitis.[14,15] In a study by Shulman et al., there was no correlation between achievement of full feedings and gastric residual volume; small bowel, colonic, or whole bowel permeability; fecal calprotectin (a measure of gastrointestinal inflammation); gastric emptying; or abdominal distention.[17]

### Nutritional Intake

Intakes of energy, protein, fat, vitamins, and minerals from parenteral and enteral formulas are calculated from nursing records of the infant's actual intake and output. Intravenous (IV) solutions other than parenteral nutrition solutions (e.g., dextrose used for medication administration, calcium gluconate), oral vitamin/mineral supplements, human milk fortifiers, and other intakes should be duly recorded. Emesis should be subtracted from the total enteral intake. The caloric density and osmolality of the enteral formula must be considered when assessing the infant's gastrointestinal tolerance. High caloric density may be associated with decreased gastric emptying. There is no significant difference in emptying time between formulas with 20 versus 24 kcal/oz, but a density greater than 24 kcal/oz may cause delayed gastric emptying.[18] Gastric emptying in preterm infants does not seem to be affected by osmolality, volume, or energy density individually, but reducing the osmolality and increasing the feeding volume increased gastric emptying.[19] When various vitamin, mineral, and oral medication preparations are mixed together with infant formula, the osmolality may be calculated by the method of Ernst et al.[20] Spreading out medications instead of clustering them improves the tolerance and decreases the osmolar load. Other drug-nutrient interactions should be considered when assessing nutritional intake and the causes of formula intolerance. Diuretic therapy, specifically furosemide, causes hypercalciuria and hypokalemic hypochloremic alkalosis. Potassium chloride supplementation is typically warranted. Long-term antibiotic treatment is a well-known causative factor in diarrhea because it destroys the gut flora necessary for carbohydrate digestion. Amphotericin use is associated with renal tubular dysfunction and hypokalemia.

### Feeding Ability

Coordination of the suck-swallow reflex is dependent on postconceptional age and is not usually fully developed until 34 to 36 weeks of gestation. Other developmental disorders affecting the central nervous system or musculature may further delay the development of suck-swallow coordination. Gagging, choking, spitting, apnea, severe bradycardia, and cyanosis are indications that the infant is not yet ready for nipple feeding. An evaluation of feeding readiness by assessment of behavior and other cues during a feeding is often done by nurses and therapists.[21,22] The use of cue-based feeding techniques has decreased the length of time most infants need to attain full oral feeding.[23] Breast-feeding should be started in the neonatal intensive care unit (NICU) before discharge. Some infants breast-feed better than they bottle-feed. Test weights, a technique in which the infant is weighed before and after breast-feeding, can give an estimate of the milk volume taken in by the infant. Lactation consultants are an invaluable resource to an NICU.

## NUTRITIONAL MANAGEMENT

The goal of nutritional care for the premature infant is a well-grown infant with a body composition and chemical balance matching those of, first, the fetus in utero and then the term infant who is nourished postnatally by mother's milk. The preterm infant inevitably accumulates a significant nutrient deficit during the first few weeks of life.[24] It takes time to establish recommended intakes, and the intake is rarely maintained. Energy and protein intakes are notably short of goals.[25] More aggressive nutritional management is recommended, particularly for ELBW infants for whom acute respiratory illness has taken precedence in clinical care.[26–33] Two key strategies have been proposed: (1) earlier administration of parenteral amino acids and (2) integration with enteral feedings in the first few days of life.[29] These strategies are aimed at decreasing postnatal weight loss, obtaining an earlier return to birth weight, and promoting early positive nitrogen retention and energy balance.

## Parenteral Nutrition

In the first days of life, the infant's fluid therapy is monitored carefully to allow for slow diuresis and to keep the sodium, glucose, and acid-base balance stable. Higher fluid intakes in the second to fourth day of life and in the first 10 days of life have been associated with an increased risk of developing severe bronchopulmonary dysplasia.[34,35] Parenteral nutrition is now started with amino acids as the first IV feeding. In healthy very low-birth-weight (VLBW) infants, both stable isotope and nitrogen balance studies have shown that most plasma amino acid concentrations decline significantly after birth if the infant has no protein intake. The degree of protein loss is approximately 1.2 to 1.4 g/kg/day and can be ameliorated by providing that amount of protein. However, because the daily in utero protein accretion is 2.1 g/kg/day, a total protein intake of at least 3.5 g/kg/day is needed to keep the preterm infant on track with expected in utero accretion rates.[36] Thureen et al.[37] demonstrated no evidence of protein intolerance during the first week of life in ventilated neonates who received amino acid intakes of up to 2.9 g/kg/day. Therefore, sufficient protein delivery to achieve positive nitrogen balance can be attained by providing at least 1.5 g/kg/day. Many clinicians routinely start with 3 g/kg protein and increase the intake to 4.0 g/kg/day. Studies suggest that it may not be necessary to increase protein administration incrementally; infants can be started at or near the maximal recommended protein intake.[38]

A balanced delivery of energy from glucose and lipid (rather than exclusively from one or the other) is recommended. The goals are to meet the resting energy expenditure (60 kcal/kg/day), so as to prevent or reduce catabolism, and to promote weight gain by further increasing the energy intake. Initial IV glucose infusion rates of approximately 6 mg/kg/min are usually well tolerated, and as long as hyperglycemia does not develop, the infusion rate can be advanced over a period of several days to 10 to 12 mg/kg/min.[39] If hyperglycemia occurs at glucose infusion rates of less than 4 mg/kg/min, insulin can be infused at 0.05 to 0.1 U/kg/hr. The infusion rate then is adjusted based on frequent measurements of the plasma glucose concentration. Insulin infusion has been shown to be safe, with infrequent episodes of hypoglycemia and no adverse effect on long-term neurodevelopmental outcome.[40] The addition of protein to IV fluids helps to decrease hyperglycemia.[41]

Lipid administration of 0.5 to 1.0 g/kg/day prevents essential fatty deficiency, which could develop within 72 hours in premature infants because of their limited fat stores. Lipid also provides a concentrated source of energy while minimizing overall fluid intake and lowering total solution osmolality. Lipid emulsion can be started at 1 g/kg/day beginning on the first day of life and advanced to a maximum of 3.0 g/kg/day, depending on serum triglyceride clearance.[42] Addition of carnitine (2–5 mg/kg) to parenteral nutrition promotes fatty acid oxidation and prevents carnitine deficiency.[43] Complications of lipid infusion include hypertriglyceridemia and hyperglycemia, because premature infants have a reduced ability to clear lipids from their blood. Twenty percent rather than 10% lipid emulsions are used because the 10% emulsions have a higher phospholipid content that interferes with plasma triglyceride clearance, resulting in higher triglyceride and plasma cholesterol concentrations. The total daily lipid dose should be spread out over 24 hours. For surgical neonates and those likely to be receiving parenteral nutrition for an extended period with a minimum amount of enteral nutrition, a lipid restriction to 1 g/kg/day might be warranted.[44,45] A higher glucose infusion rate is then needed for growth.

Vitamin, mineral, and trace element requirements for parenteral nutrition are summarized in Table 3–2. It is difficult to provide calcium and phosphorus in amounts large enough to prevent metabolic bone disease. In-depth research of the vitamin and mineral needs of preterm infants was discussed by Tsang et al.[46]

**Table 3–2.** Suggested Parenteral Intakes of Vitamins and Trace Elements

| Vitamin | Amount per Kilogram per Day |
|---|---|
| Vitamin A (µg) | 280–500 |
| Vitamin E (mg) | 2.8 |
| Vitamin K (µg) | 100 |
| *Vitamin D (IU) | 60–400 |
| Ascorbic acid (mg) | 25 |
| Thiamine (µg) | 350 |
| Riboflavin (µg) | 150 |
| Pyridoxine (µg) | 180 |
| Niacin (mg) | 6.8 |
| Pantothenate (mg) | 2.0 |
| Biotin (µg) | 6.0 |
| Folate (µg) | 56 |
| Vitamin $B_{12}$ | 0.3 |
| **Trace Element** | **Amount per Kilogram per Day** |
| *Calcium (mg) | 60–80 |
| *Magnesium (mg) | 4.3–7.2 |
| Zinc (µg) | 400 |
| Iron (µg) | 200 |
| Copper (µg) | 15–20 |
| Selenium (µg) | 1.5–2 |
| Manganese (µg) | 1.0 |
| Iodide (µg) | 1.0 |
| Molybdenum (µg) | 0.25 |
| Chromium (µg) | 0.20 |
| *Phosphorus (mg) | 48–60 |

Adapted from Green HL, Hambidge KM, Schanler R, et al. Guidelines for the use of vitamins, trace elements, calcium, magnesium, and phosphorus in infants and children receiving total parenteral nutrition: report of the Subcommittee on Pediatric Parenteral Nutrient Requirements from the Committee on Clinical Practice Issues of the American Society for Clinical Nutrition. *Am J Clin Nutr.* 1988; 48:1324; and Tsang Uauy R, Koletzko B, Zlotkin S, eds. *Nutrient Requirements in Preterm Infants.* Cincinnati: Digital Education Publishing; 2004.
*Note in mg or IU.

*Minimal enteral nutrition* (MEN) refers to the enteral feeding of formula, human milk, or both.[47] Advantages of MEN are thought to be a shorter time to full enteral feeds and increased feeding tolerance. The role of parenteral nutrition is to provide rapid, maximal nutrition, and the role of MEN is to "prime" the gut and stimulate normal gastrointestinal activity. The documented benefits include fewer days on parenteral nutrition, less interruption of feedings, and fewer infants with sepsis.[48,49]

Typically, trophic or minimal enteral feedings are started if an infant is hemodynamically stable within the first 24 to 48 hours of life. If there is a period of minimal or trophic feeding, then advancements are started at 20 to 160 mL/kg/day. Fortification of human milk over time ranges from a total of 25 mL/day to 100 mL/day. It is important to fortify while TPN is still in place to avoid the drop in nutrition that occurs when human milk is given alone without fortification. If human milk from the mother is not available, many centers use donor human milk. It is obtained from a milk bank under the auspices of the Human Milk Banking Association of North America (HMBANA), which maintains strict guidelines for the testing of donor mothers and pasteurization methods. Although there is some loss of immune protection, donor human milk still conveys some protection. However, this milk may be from a different stage of lactation because many women donate when their infants are 6 to 10 months old. This mature milk, which is perfectly suited to their own infant, has a lower content of protein and zinc, nutrients that naturally decline over time and are highest in preterm milk during the early part of milk production. Additional fortification may be needed for growth.[31–33] Sodium supplementation may also be helpful and can be monitored by serial urine sodium assays.[50]

## Enteral Nutrition

Preterm infants fed enterally in the hospital should be given a calcium:phosphorus ratio between 1.7 and 2.0 (Table 3–3) and a range of intakes as follows: calcium, 120–200 mg/kg/day; phosphorus, 60–140 mg/kg/day; magnesium 8–15 mg/kg/day; vitamin D,

**Table 3–3.** Required Calcium (Ca) and Phosphorus (P) Intakes to Meet the Fetal Accretion Rate

| Gestational Age (wk) | Weight (g) | Fetal Accretion Rate (mg/kg/day) | | Required Intake (mg/kg/day) Human Milk* | | Preterm Formula† | |
|---|---|---|---|---|---|---|---|
| | | Ca | P | Ca | P | Ca | P |
| 28 | 1150 | 120 | 71 | 240 | 79 | 185 | 100 |
| 32 | 1715 | 125 | 72 | 250 | 81 | 190 | 101 |
| 36 | 2710 | 130 | 80 | 260 | 90 | 200 | 113 |

*Retention of calcium is 50% of intake; retention of phosphorus is 89% of intake.
†Retention of calcium from US commercial premature formulas is 65% of intake; retention of phosphorus from these formulas is 71% of intake.
From Tsang R, Uauy R, Koletzko B, Zlotkin S, eds. *Nutrient Requirements in Preterm Infants*. Cincinnati, OH: Digital Education Publishing; 2004.

400–1000 IU/day. These are new recommendations from Koletzko, Poindexter, and Uauy.[51] Enteral nutrition is provided by various methods, depending on the infant's condition. Oral tube placement is preferable in those with respiratory distress because infants are usually nose breathers. Intermittent bolus gavage feeding appears to be the most physiological feeding method. The gallbladder contracts better after bolus rather than continuous feedings, apparently related to a decreased release of cholecystokinin with continuous feedings.[52] Continuous feedings may be used in those infants whose respiratory status is compromised during bolus feedings and in those who exhibit delayed gastric emptying without ileus. Nonnutritive sucking on a pacifier is associated with earlier tolerance of nipple feeding and earlier hospital discharge.[53] Breast-feeding or bottle-feeding may be attempted in infants who have reached a postconceptional age of 32 to 34 weeks. The transition from gavage to nipple feeding is gradual and depends on the infant's suck-swallow coordination and tolerance. Signs of respiratory distress, gagging, or choking may be present during some, but not all, feedings. Experimentation with nipple types and sizes may be helpful. Enlarging the hole in nipples is not recommended because it affects the infant's ability to learn to integrate the muscle activity involved in oral control.

Preterm human milk contains higher concentrations of fat, protein, sodium, chloride, magnesium, and iron on a gram-per-liter basis than mature human milk.[54,55] Despite these higher concentrations, however, lowered growth rate and inadequate bone mineralization are common in preterm infants fed their own mother's milk because of insufficient volume or a variable concentration of nutrients relative to the infant's extreme needs. However, the ease of digestion and the presence of host defense mechanisms and growth factors in human milk cannot be reproduced technologically in formula. The feeding of human milk is thought to provide significant protection from infection and necrotizing enterocolitis.[56] Human milk fortifiers are used to increase the calcium, phosphorus, magnesium, protein, energy, and vitamin A and D levels, as well as the levels of other vitamins and minerals. Liquid high-protein fortifiers are now available.

Premature infant formula, in comparison to standard formula, provides a higher modified protein content; modified fat and carbohydrate; and significantly higher calcium and phosphorus contents. Formulas containing 67, 81, and 100 kcal/dL are available, although many protocols now start with the high-protein 81 kcal/dL rather than the 67 kcal/dL formula. There are now 30 kcal/oz ready-to-feed premature infant formulas, and they can be diluted to make formulas with 25 through 29 kcal/oz. This is typically more desired than the use of additives, which may skew the ratios of carbohydrate, protein, and fat. Breast milk or formula used for enteral feeding may begin at full strength,[33,57] with the volume dependent on the infant's size. Energy needs are estimated at 110 to 130 kcal/kg/day in VLBW infants, and protein needs at 3.5 to 4.5 g/kg/day.[51] Use of these intakes in uncomplicated infants should result in weight gain of approximately 30 g/day. If it does not, the dietitian should investigate the reasons for poor growth. In some instances, the answer is simple (e.g., the baby never gets the volume that is prescribed). Many centers have found that infants were more likely to achieve the desired intake and fewer feedings were held after they stopped checking gastric aspirates.

Postnatal iron needs are high, and iron supplementation may begin at 2 weeks of age as long as plasma vitamin E is normal. Otherwise, supplementation of iron should begin at least by the eighth postnatal week. Supplements of 2 to 4 mg/kg/day are given to human milk–fed infants. The infant on an iron-containing premature formula may receive 2 mg/kg/day elemental iron. If the birth weight is less than 1000 g, 4 mg/kg/day is given; if it is 1000 to 1500 g, 3 mg/kg/day is given; and if it is 1501 to 2500 g, 2 mg/kg/day is given.[58]

Vitamin E supplementation is often necessary because of poor placental transfer, inadequate stores, and postnatal malabsorption. Vitamin E requirements are increased by high intakes of both iron and polyunsaturated fatty acids. The recommended intake is 2.2 to 11 mg/kg/day of α-tocopherol.[51] Infants receiving premature formula may not need additional vitamin E supplementation unless iron supplements are given concurrently. Studies suggest that infants who are at high risk for bronchopulmonary dysplasia (BPD) and have low serum α-tocopherol levels may benefit from vitamin A supplementation during the acute stage of respiratory distress. To achieve a serum retinol level greater than 20 μg/dL, doses of 2000 U intramuscularly every other day may be used.[59] Selenium supplementation may also have an effect because lowered selenium levels are documented in these infants.[60] Daily enteral docosahexaenoic acid (DHA) supplementation alternatives also may be needed for the premature infant.[61]

Calcium, phosphorus, and vitamin D supplements are usually necessary for both human milk–fed and formula-fed infants (see Table 3–3). Although the minimum requirement for these minerals is unknown, if hypophosphatemia occurs, the calcium:phosphorus ratio should be manipulated to obtain a ratio between 1.4 and 2.0.[57] Metabolic bone disease occurs in relation to calcium and phosphorus deficiency but may not be amenable to dietary therapy.[62] However, premature infants may still develop vitamin D–deficiency rickets if not provided with a minimum of 400 IU/day; some require more, with a range of 400 to 1000 IU/day recommended.[51] A general pediatric multivitamin is usually provided daily to premature infants, although the requirements of these infants are still unclear.

## Prognosis and Follow-up

Slow growth and behavioral eating difficulties are common nutritional problems in premature infants after hospital discharge. There are many challenges, even though there is a preterm discharge formula class that has a nutrient profile between those of premature infant formula and term infant formula.[63] The neurodevelopmental outcome is consistently reported as improved in preterm breast-fed infants,[64–66] and mothers perceive specific advantages.[67] Therefore, more evaluation and support should be given to the family to continue breast-feeding when growth parameters fall below recommended levels. Table 3–4 presents the parameters that indicate nutritional deficiencies in infants up to 34 weeks' gestation or 1800 g birth weight.[68]

Early weaning to solid food should be firmly discouraged; the use of human milk fortifier for home use or the use of premature formula after discharge should be carefully evaluated for individual infants. Improving postdischarge nutrition in preterm infants is a primary goal, with research being directed to human milk fortifiers and infant formulas.[69,70] Metabolic bone disease persists throughout childhood in children born prematurely[68] and is the probable cause of the persistent short stature seen in these children. However, VLBW females reportedly catch up in growth by age 20 years, whereas VLBW males remain significantly shorter and lighter than their term counterparts.[71]

**Table 3–4.** Parameters That Indicate Nutritional Deficiencies in Infants up to 34 Weeks' Gestation or 1800 g Birth Weight

| | |
|---|---|
| Gain in weight | <25 g/day |
| Gain in length | <1 cm/wk |
| Gain in head circumference | <0.5 cm/wk |
| Phosphorous | <4.5 mg/dL |
| Alkaline phosphatase | >450 IU/L |
| Urea nitrogen | <5 mg/dL |
| Prealbumin | <10 mg/dL |
| Retinol-binding protein | <2.5 mg/dL |

In this new era in premature infant nutrition, nutrition is provided immediately[72] and sustained throughout the NICU stay[33]; in many circumstances, it is then continued throughout the first year of life,[51] with monitoring in a High-Risk Infant Follow-up clinic. Current outcomes may be better. It is known that early nutrition (in the first week of life) with increased intakes of protein and energy is associated with higher Mental Development Index scores and lower likelihood of length/growth restrictions at 18 months in ELBW infants.[73] The first week may be pivotal, but there must be a concerted effort to provide excellent nutrition throughout the NICU stay and beyond to maximize neurodevelopment and prevent nutritional stunting.

## References


1. Centers for Disease Control and Prevention. Reproductive Health. http://www.cdc.gov. Accessed May 23, 2016.
2. Stephens BE, Vohr BR. Neurodevelopmental outcome of the premature infant. *Pediatr Clin North Am.* 2009; 56:631.
3. Hintz SR, Kendrick DE, Wilson-Costello DE, et al. Early childhood developmental outcomes are not improving for infants born at <25 weeks gestational age. *Pediatrics.* 2011; 127:62.
4. Gargus RA, Vohr BR, Tyson JE, et al. Unimpaired outcomes for extremely low birth weight infants at 18 to 22 months. *Pediatrics.* 2009; 124:112.
5. Keir A, McPhee A, Wilkinson D. Beyond the borderline: outcomes for inborn infants born at ≤500 gm. *J Paediatr Child Health.* 2014; 50:146.
6. Jarjour IT. Neurodevelopmental outcome after extreme prematurity: a review of the literature. *Pediatr Neurol.* 2015; 52:143.
7. Johnson S, Evans TA, Draper ES, et al. Neurodevelopmental outcomes following late and moderate prematurity: a population-based cohort study. *Arch Dis Child Fetal Neonatal Ed.* 2015; 100:F301.
8. Berseth CI. Feeding methods for the preterm infant. *Semin Neonatol.* 2001; 6:417.
9. Fenton TR, Kim JH. A systematic review and meta-analysis to revise the Fenton growth chart for preterm infants. *BMC Pediatr.* 2013; 13:59.
10. Fenton TR, Nasser R, Eliasziw M, et al. Validating the weight gain of preterm infants between the reference growth curve of the fetus and the term infant. *BMC Pediatrics.* 2013; 13:92.
11. Olsen IE, Groveman SA, Lawson ML, et al. New intrauterine growth curves based on United States data. *Pediatrics.* 2010; 125:e214.
12. Olsen IE, Lawson ML, Ferguson AN, et al. BMI curves for preterm infants. *Pediatrics.* 2015; 135:e572.
13. Banh L. Serum proteins as markers of nutrition: what are we treating? Nutrition Issues in Gastroenterology, Series #43. *Practical Gastroenterol.* 2006; 30:46.
14. Fanaro S. Feeding intolerance in the preterm infant. *Early Hum Dev.* 2013; 89:S13.
15. Lucchini R, Bizzarri B, Giampietro S, et al. Feeding intolerance in preterm infants: how to understand the warning signs. *J Matern Fetal Neonat Med.* 2011; 24(Suppl 1):72.
16. Hair AB, Peluso AM, Hawthorne KM, et al. Beyond necrotizing enterocolitis prevention: comparing outcomes with an exclusive human milk-based diet. *Breastfeed Med.* 2016; 1:70.
17. Shulman RJ, Ou CN, Smith EO. Evaluation of potential factors predicting attainment of full gavage feedings in preterm infants. *Neonatology.* 2011; 99:38.
18. Siegel M, Lebenthal E, Krantz B. Effect of caloric density of gastric emptying in premature infants. *J. Pediatr.* 1984; 104:118.
19. Ramirez A, Wong WW, Shulman RJ. Factors regulating gastric emptying in preterm infants. *J Pediatr.* 2006; 149:475.
20. Ernst IA, Williams JM, Glick M., Lemons IA. Osmolality of substances used in the intensive care nursery. *Pediatrics.* 1983; 72:347.
21. McCain GC. An evidence-based guideline for introducing oral feeding to healthy preterm infants. *Neonatal Netw.* 2003; 22:45.
22. Thoyre S, Park J, Pados B, et al. Developing a co-regulated, cue-based feeding practice: the critical role of assessment and reflection. *J Neonatal Nurs.* 2013; 19:139.
23. Wellington A, Perlman JM. Infant-driven feeding in premature infants: a quality improvement project. *Arch Dis Child Fetal Neonatal Ed.* 2015; 100:F495.
24. Embleton NE, Pang N, Cooke RJ. Postnatal malnutrition and growth retardation: an inevitable consequence of current recommendations in preterm infants? *Pediatrics.* 2001; 107:270.
25. Carlson SJ, Ziegler EE. Nutrient intakes and growth of very low birth weight infants. *J Perinatol.* 1998; 18:252.
26. Adamkin DH. Issues in the nutritional support of the ventilated baby. *Clin Perinatol.* 1998; 25:79.
27. Thureen PJ, Hay WWJr. Intravenous nutrition and postnatal growth of the micropremie. *Clin Perinatol.* 2000; 27:197.
28. Ziegler EE, Thureen PJ, Carlson SJ. Aggressive nutrition of the very low birthweight infant. *Clin Perinatol.* 2002; 29:225.
29. Adamkin DH. Two key strategies in the nutritional management of the extremely low birth weight infant. *Przegl Lek.* 2002; 59(Suppl 1):14.
30. Hay WWJr. Aggressive nutrition of the preterm infant. *Curr Pediatr Rep.* 2013; 1:229.
31. Hanson C, Sundermeier KJ, Dugick L, et al. Implementation, process, and outcomes of nutrition best practices for infants <1500 g. *Nutr Clin Pract.* 2011; 26:614.
32. Donovan R, Puppala B, Angst D, Coyle BW. Outcomes of early nutrition support in extremely low-birth-weight infants. *Nutr Clin Pract.* 2006; 21:395.
33. Prince A, Groh-Wargo S. Nutrition management for the promotion of growth in very low birthweight premature infants. *Nutr Clin Pract.* 2013; 28:659.
34. Guo MM, Chung CH, Chen FS, et al. Severe bronchopulmonary dysplasia is associated with higher fluid intake in very low birthweight infants: a retrospective study. *Am J Perinatol.* 2015; 30:155.
35. Oh W, Poindexter BB, Perritt R, et al. Association between fluid intake and weight loss during the first ten days of life and risk of bronchopulmonary dysplasia in extremely low birth weight infants. *J Pediatr.* 2005; 147: 786.
36. Evans RA, Thureen P. Early feeding strategies in preterm and critically ill neonates. *Neonatal Netw.* 2001; 20:7.
37. Thureen P, Anderson A, Baron K, et al. Protein balance in the first week of life in ventilated neonates receiving parenteral nutrition. *Am J Clin Nutr.* 1998; 68:1128.
38. Thureen PJ, Melara D, Fennessey PV, Hay WWJr. Effect of low versus high intravenous amino acid intake on very low birth weight infants in the early neonatal period. *Pediatr. Res.* 2003; 53:24.
39. Dweck HS, Cassady G. Glucose intolerance in infants of very low birth weight: I. Incidence of hyperglycemia in infants of birth weight 1,110 grams or less. *Pediatrics.* 1974; 53:189.
40. Heald A, Abdel-Latif ME, Kent AL. Insulin infusion for hyperglycaemia in very preterm infants appears safe with no effect on morbidity, mortality, and long term neurodevelopmental outcome. *J Matern Fetal Neonatal Med.* 2012; 25:2415.
41. Mahaveer A, Grime C, Morgan C. Increasing early protein intake is associated with a reduction in insulin-treated hyperglycemia in very preterm infants. *Nutr Clin Pract.* 2012; 27:399.
42. American Academy of Pediatrics. Use of intravenous fat emulsions in pediatrics. *Pediatrics.* 1981; 68:738.
43. Borum PR. Carnitine in parenteral nutrition. *Gastroenterology.* 2009; 137:S129.
44. Sanchez SE, Braun LP, Mercer LD, et al. The effect of lipid restriction on the prevention of parenteral nutrition associated cholestasis in surgical infants. *J Pediatr Surg.* 2013; 48:573.
45. Cober MP, Teitelbaum DH. Prevention of parenteral nutrition associated liver disease: lipid minimization. *Curr Opin Organ Transplant.* 2010; 15:330.
46. Tsang R, Uauy R, Koletzko B, Zlotkin S, eds. *Nutrient Requirements in Preterm Infants.* Cincinnati, OH: Digital Education Publishing; 2004.
47. Berseth CL. Minimal enteral feedings. *Clin Perinatol.* 1995; 22:195.
48. Tyson JE, Kennedy KA. Minimal enteral nutrition for promoting feeding tolerance and preventing morbidity in parenterally fed infants. *Cochrane Database Syst. Rev.* 2000; (2):CD000504.
49. Kennedy KA, Tyson JE, Chamnanvanikij S. Early versus delayed initiation of progressive enteral feedings for parenterally fed low birth weight or preterm infants. *Cochrane Database Syst. Rev.* 2000; (2):CD001970.
50. Isemann B, Mueller EW, Narendran V, Akinbi H. Impact of early sodium supplementation on hyponatremia and growth in premature infants: a randomized controlled trial. *JPEN J Parenter Enteral Nutr.* 2016; 40:342.
51. Koletzko B, Poindexter BB, Uauy R, eds. *Nutritional Care of Preterm Infants.* Basel, Switzerland: Karger Publishing, 2014.
52. Jawaheer G, Shaw NJ, Pierro A. Continuous enteral feeding impairs gallbladder emptying in infants. *J Pediatr.* 2001; 138:822.
53. Pinelli J, Symington A, Ciliska D. Nonnutritive sucking in high-risk infants: benign intervention or legitimate therapy? *J Obstet Gynecol Neonatal Nurs.* 2002; 31:582.
54. Anderson GH. Human milk feeding. *Pediatr Clin North Am.* 1985; 32:335.
55. Assad M, Elliott MJ, Abraham JH. Decreased cost and improved feeding tolerance in VLBW infants fed an exclusive human milk diet. *J Perinatol.* 2016; 36:216.
56. Schanler RJ. The use of human milk for premature infants. *Pediatr Clin North Am.* 2001; 48:207.
57. Hay WWJr, Lucas A, Heird WC, et al. Workshop summary: nutrition of the extremely low birth weight infant. *Pediatrics.* 1999; 104:1360.
58. Dallman PR. Iron deficiency in the weanling: a nutritional problem on the way to resolution. *Acta Paediatr Scand.* 1986; 323:59.
59. Atkinson SA. Special nutritional needs of infants for prevention of and recovery from bronchopulmonary dysplasia. *J Nutr.* 2001; 131:942S.
60. Falciglia H, Johnson JR, Sullivan J, et al. Role of antioxidant nutrients and lipid peroxidase in premature infants with respiration distress syndrome and bronchopulmonary dysplasia. *Am J Perinatol.* 2003; 20:97.
61. Baack M, Puumala SE, Messier SC, et al. Daily enteral DHA supplementation alleviates deficiency in premature infants. *Lipids.* 2016; 51: 423.
62. Faerk J, Petersen S, Peitersen B, Michaelsen KF. Diet and bone mineral content at term in premature infants. *Pediatr Res.* 2000; 47:148.
63. Carver JD, Wu PY, Hall RT, et al. Growth of preterm infants fed nutrient enriched or term formula after hospital discharge. *Pediatrics.* 2001; 107:683.
64. Horwood LJ, Fergusson DM. Breastfeeding and later cognitive and academic outcomes. *Pediatrics.* 1998; 101:e9.
65. Temboury MC, Otero A, Polanco I, et al. Influence of breastfeeding on the infant's intellectual development. *J Pediatr Gastroenterol Nutr.* 1994; 18:32.
66. Vohr BR, Poindexter BB, Dusick AM, et al. Persistent beneficial effects of breast milk ingested in the neonatal intensive care unit on outcomes of extremely low birth weight infants at 30 months of age. *Pediatrics.* 2007; 120:e953.

67. Kavanaugh K, Meier P, Zimmermann B, Mead L. The rewards outweigh the efforts: breastfeeding outcomes for mothers of preterm infants. *J Hum Lact.* 1997; 13:15.
68. Hall RT. Nutritional follow-up of the breastfeeding premature infant after hospital discharge. *Pediatr Clin North Am.* 2001; 48:453.
69. Lucas A, Fewtrell MS, Morley R, et al. Randomized trial of nutrient-enriched formula versus standard formula for postdischarge preterm infants. *Pediatrics.* 2001; 108:703.
70. Reis BB, Hall RT, Schanler RJ, et al. Enhanced growth of preterm infants fed a new powdered human milk fortifier: a randomized, controlled trial. *Pediatrics.* 2000; 106:581.
71. Hack M, Schluchter M, Cartar L, et al. Growth of very low birth weight infants to age 20 years. *Pediatrics.* 2003; 112:e30.
72. Valentine CJ, Fernandez S, Rogers LK, et al. Early amino acid administration improves preterm infant weight. *J Perinatol.* 2009; 29:428.
73. Stephens BE, Walden RV, Gargus RA, et al. First week protein and energy intakes are associated with 18 month developmental outcomes in extremely low birth weight infants. *Pediatrics.* 2009; 123:1337.

# B.

# NUTRITION EVALUATION

## 4 Nutritional Assessment

SHIRLEY W. EKVALL, DIANE SPEAR, VALLI K. EKVALL, JENNIFER WALBERG-WOLFE, AND PAULA CUSHING

Nutritional assessment is defined by the Academy of Nutrition and Dietetics (Academy) as a systematic approach to collect, record, and interpret relevant data from patients, clients, family members, caregivers, and other individuals and groups.[1,2] After data are collected, the practitioner uses past experience and reference standards to assimilate the information into an assessment that provides an understanding of the individual's nutritional status. The Academy's four-step Nutrition Care Process (NCP) is a problem-solving method used to address nutrition-related problems and provide safe and effective quality nutrition care. The NCP supports nutrition screening as the first step to identify people at nutritional risk who would benefit from an assessment by a registered dietitian/nutritionist.[3] Similarly, the American Society for Parenteral and Enteral Nutrition (A.S.P.E.N.) defines nutrition screening as "a process to identify an individual who is malnourished or who is at risk for malnutrition to determine if a detailed nutritional assessment is indicated."[4]

Nutritional evaluation at the Cincinnati Children's Hospital Medical Center, Division of Developmental Disabilities (CCDDD) uses a multidisciplinary approach: (1) screening and/or referral; (2) nutritional assessment; (3) interpretation of assessment; (4) an intervention or treatment plan; and (5) a follow-up plan.[5] There are three levels of nutritional assessment: an *in-depth assessment* performed as part of a complete physical examination; a *mid-level assessment* performed in a specialty clinic, such as a myelomeningocele, cerebral palsy, or high-risk infant clinic; and a *mini-level assessment* performed in the home or community. The choice of assessment depends on the expertise and amount of time available, the age of the child or adult, and the identified problem. This chapter focuses primarily on the in-depth nutritional assessment.

### MALNUTRITION

Malnutrition is a commonly identified risk factor that triggers the need for nutritional assessment. Malnutrition is generally described as any disorder of nutrition, including overnutrition and undernutrition. Malnutrition occurs when an individual has inadequate intake of protein or energy (or both) over a prolonged period resulting in loss of fat stores and/or muscle wasting.[6] Economically, socially, and educationally deprived populations are at risk for malnutrition. Some of the people at highest risk for nutritional and oral health problems include children born prematurely, children with failure to thrive, special needs children with developmental delays, adults with developmental disabilities, people taking multiple medications, and people with gastrointestinal problems such as lactose intolerance, gastroesophageal reflux, or dysphagia.

The Academy and A.S.P.E.N. have published consensus statements on the characteristics[6] and indicators[7] recommended for the identification and documentation of pediatric malnutrition (undernutrition). These recommendations differ from traditional and historical definitions of malnutrition in that they are based on etiology, consider multiple manifestations of undernutrition, and differentiate between nonsevere and severe malnutrition in the adult population and between mild, moderate, and severe malnutrition in the pediatric population. Clinical characteristics of adult malnutrition are inadequate food and nutrient intake, weight loss, loss of subcutaneous fat, muscle loss, fluid accumulation, and reduced grip strength; identification of two of these six characteristics is recommended for the diagnosis of either severe or nonsevere malnutrition.[6] Recommended indicators for pediatric malnutrition if only one data point is available include the Z score for weight for height/length, body mass index (BMI) for age, length/height for age, and mid-upper arm circumference (MUAC). If two or more data points are available, indicators of weight-gain velocity, weight loss, deceleration in the weight-for-length/height Z score, and inadequate nutrient intake apply.[7]

The International Statistical Classification of Diseases and Related Health Problems, 10th revision (ICD-10) code assignments for malnutrition depend on the type and severity, as well as physician documentation. The ICD-10 classifications are described as follows:

1. *Kwashiorkor* (E40) is a severe type of malnutrition characterized by skin and hair pigment changes, edema, slow growth, and pathological changes in the liver, including fatty infiltration, necrosis, and fibrosis.
2. *Nutritional marasmus* (E41) is characterized by severe tissue wasting, loss of subcutaneous fat, and often dehydration.
3. *Marasmic kwashiorkor* (E42) includes both diagnoses with severe protein-calorie malnutrition.
4. *Unspecified severe protein-calorie malnutrition* (E43) includes signs and symptoms of malnutrition with starvation edema.
5. *Protein-calorie malnutrition of moderate and mild degree* (E44).
6. *Retarded development following protein-calorie malnutrition* (E45) includes short stature, stunting, and slow growth due to malnutrition.
7. *Unspecified protein-calorie malnutrition* (E46) due to unbalanced or insufficient diet or to defective assimilation or utilization of nutrients.

Early malnutrition (in the cerebellum) causes a reduction in the number of cells in the cerebrum and brain stem (see Figs. 1–2 and 1–3 in Chapter 1). In an underdeveloped country, 19 children experiencing malnutrition in the first year of life were followed for 4 years after rehabilitation. Only 10% achieved normal intelligence; 52% were educable, 33% were trainable, and 5% were institutionalized.[8,9] In the United States, subtle changes in development, such as delays in language or cognitive development, may be related to malnutrition, especially if it occurred before 6 months of age[9] (see Fig. 1–4 in Chapter 1). Long-term effects have also been reported in children from Chili.[10]

Malnutrition can be produced by disease or disability, such as fever, cardiovascular disease, diabetes mellitus, cystic fibrosis, and cerebral palsy. Some disease-related problems are malabsorption, anorexia, hypermetabolic and metabolic dysfunction, organ failure, and treatment-induced causes (Table 4–1).[11] Obesity also may be a form of malnutrition, either *primary* and *secondary*, particularly in people who are immobile. Obesity is a pathological condition in which there is an accumulation of fat in excess of what is needed for body functioning. For both primary and secondary malnutrition, the grade of malnutrition may be evaluated according to Waterlow's classification (Table 4–2).[12] An initial nutritional medical screening for clients at risk of malnutrition is often obtained before referral for an in-depth nutritional assessment (Table 4–3). Health care providers should be well informed about these criteria so that they can make appropriate referrals for the in-depth assessment (Table 4–4).

**Table 4–1.** Conditions That Affect Nutritional Status

| Condition | Increased Nutrient Needs |
|---|---|
| Infections | Vit A, Vit C, Fe, N, Calories, $H_2O$, Na, K |
| Drugs | Vit C, N, Na, K, Vit $B_{12}$, folic acid |
| Emotion | Iodine, Vit C, Vit B complex, Ca, N |
| Malnutrition | Vit C, Vit A, N, Chol, K, P |
| Obesity | Calories, macronutrients and micronutrients |
| Immobilization | Ca, Na, K, N, $H_2O$ |
| Malabsorption | Vit C, Vit B complex, Vit A, Vit D, Vit E, Vit $B_{12}$, fat, calories, $H_2O$, N, Ca, P, Na, K |
| Physical activity | Vit C, Vit B complex, N |
| Pregnancy and lactation | Ca, N, Fe, folic acid |
| Surgery | Vit C, Vit $B_{12}$, K, N, $H_2O$ |
| Burns or injury | Vit C, Vit B complex, K, N |
| Environment (heat) | Ca, Cu, Mg, P, K, Fe, N, Na |

Ca = calcium; Chol = choline; Cu = copper; Fe = iron; $H_2O$ = water; K = potassium; N = nitrogen; Na = sodium; P = phosphorus; Vit = vitamin.

**Table 4–2.** Assessment of Malnutrition: Waterlow Classification

| Grade of Malnutrition | Weight for Height, % of Standard | Height for Age, % of Standard |
|---|---|---|
| 0 | >90 | >95 |
| 1 | 81–90 | 90–95 |
| 2 | 70–80 | 85–89 |
| 3 | <70 | <85 |

From Waterlow JC. *Protein-Energy Malnutrition*. London: Edward Arnold; 1992, with permission.

## IN-DEPTH NUTRITIONAL ASSESSMENT

A comprehensive evaluation is needed when assessing nutritional status in the child or adult with intellectual and developmental disabilities (IDD).[13] Evaluation of nutrition status encompasses a five step approach using key elements of an in-depth nutritional assessment: dietary, anthropometric, physical and clinical, biochemical, and feeding/behavioral (Table 4–5). A problem identified in the assessment of dietary intake often manifests physiologically in the biochemical assessment, later on in the anthropometric assessment, and finally in the physical signs and symptoms. For this reason, the problem should be addressed at the dietary state—the first level of assessment.

The NCP nutrition-related assessment data include the pertinent food and nutrition history, anthropometric and biochemical measurements, nutrition-focused physical examination and clinical findings, physiological and disease conditions, and functional and behavioral status, including social and cognitive function, psychological and emotional factors, quality-of-life measures, and change readiness.[1,2]

Specific to the child or adult with IDD, the nutritional assessment should include the impact of disability on nutritional status, current therapies and daily living supports, social skills, mealtime assistance and dining skills, mobility, sensory processing needs, social and communication skills, level of independence, and cognitive level.[14]

Frequently encountered issues in nutritional assessment of children are specialty measuring techniques or equipment, specialized growth charts, and sensory processing or food selectivity issues.[15] Two frequently encountered issues in nutritional assessment for adults are collecting valid dietary intake data and determining energy needs. Assessment of nutrition and energy requirements is challenging because they vary depending on the disability diagnosis, severity of the disability, mobility status, age, medications, and feeding problems.[15]

## DIETARY HISTORY

In this part of the assessment, information on both the developmental and the current dietary history is obtained. Food and nutrition intakes are calculated, and conditioning factors, such as problems of malabsorption and medication use, are evaluated. For the person with a developmental delay or chronic illness, it is particularly important to know what is actually being consumed; a large amount of the food may be spilled during the feeding or eating process. Socioeconomic information is also reviewed in the dietary assessment. Three methods for collecting dietary data are available: (1) a food list—the quantity of food eaten over time; (2) a food record—inventory of the food on hand at the beginning and end of a study or plate waste record; and (3) a family food account—description of the food purchased. Food intake patterns based on the food groups for different ages are shown in Table 4–6.

The food list method that is used most frequently is a list or diary (1–3 days or 7 days) of food consumed. Food lists are useful in obtaining

**Table 4–3.** Initial Nutritional Screening Data

The presence of one or more of the following conditions should alert the health care professional that the patient has the potential of developing malnutrition or has had a condition in the past requiring special nutritional care. Incorporation of the following questions and observations into a routine history and physical examination can facilitate identification of patients who are at risk for malnutrition.

*General*
Does the patient have any conditions that cause nutrient loss, such as malabsorption syndromes, draining abscesses, wounds, fistulas, or protracted diarrhea?
Does the patient have any conditions that increase the need for nutrients, such as fever, burn, injury, sepsis, or antineoplastic therapies?
Has the patient been NPO for 3 days or more?
Is the patient receiving a modified diet or diet restricted in one or more nutrients?
Is the patient on a diet that is modified in texture or consistency of liquids due to choking/aspiration risk?
Is the patient being enterally or parenterally fed?
Does the patient describe food allergies, lactose intolerance, or limited food preferences?
Is the patient on a diet that is modified in texture or consistency of liquids due to choking/aspiration risk?
Has the patient experienced recent unexplained weight loss?

*Gastrointestinal*
Does the patient complain of nausea, indigestion, vomiting, diarrhea, or constipation?
Does the patient exhibit glossitis, stomatitis, or esophagitis?
Does the patient have difficulty chewing or swallowing?
Does the patient have a partial or total gastrointestinal obstruction?
What is the patient's state of dentition?

*Cardiovascular*
Does the patient have ascites or edema?
Is the patient able to perform activities of daily living?
Does the patient have congestive heart failure?

*Genitourinary*
Does fluid input approximately equal fluid output?
Does the patient have an ostomy?
Is the patient undergoing hemodialysis or peritoneal dialysis?

*Respiratory*
Is the patient receiving mechanical ventilatory support?
Is the patient receiving oxygen via nasal prongs?
Does the patient have chronic obstructive pulmonary disease?

*Skin*
Does the patient describe nail or hair changes?
Does the patient have rashes or dermatitis?
Does the patient have dry or pale mucous membranes or decreased skin turgor?
Does the patient have pressure areas on the sacrum, hips, or ankles?

*Extremities*
Does the patient have pedal edema?
Does the patient exhibit cachexia?

Modified from *Nutritional Assessment: What Is It? How Is It Used?* Columbus, OH: Ross Laboratories; G593. Used with permission.

presumptive evidence of dietary inadequacies but not the absolute values consumed. In general, a deficiency in one nutrient is a good indicator of other nutritional problems. Figure II-2 in the introduction for Part II of this book shows the deficiencies of nutrients found in children with developmental disabilities over a 10-year period.

The dietary history is based on the 24-hour recall of foods eaten and the food summary, which is a frequency cross-check of the 24-hour recall. The food summary is evaluated according to a 16-point system. Points are subtracted for the intake of large quantities of sugar, salt, soft drinks, sweet desserts, and foods high in saturated fat and cholesterol or if the diet contains inadequate amounts of fiber and water. If the score is lower than 10, the parent or caregiver is given a 3-day dietary diary to complete, and a follow-up visit is scheduled. The nutrient content of the 3-day diet diary is then analyzed using food composition tables and compared with the Dietary Reference Intakes (see Appendix 1). At CCDDD, 56 nutrients are calculated from the 3-day diet diary and the 24-hour recall. Daily fluid needs are calculated according to the following requirements based on the child's weight:

- For 1 to 10 kg, 100 mL/kg
- For 10 to 20 kg, 1000 mL plus 50 mL/kg
- For each kilogram over 10 kg and for weights through 20 kg, 1500 mL plus 20 mL/kg
- For each kilogram over 20 kg, 1500 to 1800 $mL/m^2$ based on body surface area[16–18]

Fiber requirements are 5 g plus 1 g per year of age for children (see Chapter 36 for more details).

**Table 4–4.** Referral Criteria for an In-Depth Nutritional Assessment

*Specialty Clinic**
Younger than 3 years of age
Height or weight <10th or >75th percentile or a large discrepancy in weight for height
Mechanical feeding problems
Conditions such as allergies, chronic diarrhea, excessive use of vitamins, food faddism
Family income <$25,808 for four people
Mother younger than 20 years of age at time of child's birth
Postmenarcheal adolescent girl

*Hospital*
Height <85% of standard (stunted)
Weight for height <90% of standard (underweight) or >120% of standard (obese)
Weight loss ≥5% of usual body weight
Serum albumin <3 g/dL (<2.5 g/dL in an infant)
Lymphocyte count <1500 cells/µL
Sustained fever, major organ failure, etc.
Nothing passed orally for ≥2 days without parenteral nutrition
On clear full-liquid diet for ≥2 days
Referred by other disciplines

*From the Cincinnati Children's Hospital Medical Center, Division of Developmental Disabilities, Cincinnati, OH.

## ANTHROPOMETRY ASSESSMENT

The National Health and Nutrition Examination Survey (NHANES) and the Centers for Disease Control and Prevention (CDC) provide the basis for anthropometric measurements. Accumulated data were used to develop age- and sex-specific percentile distributions for the various anthropometric measurements.[19] Normal growth and developmental changes are presented in Table 4–7. Adjustment for parental stature is shown in Table 4–8.

Standard procedures are used in the measurement of *height* (recumbent length if <2 years of age and <1 m in length; otherwise, standing stature or upper-to-lower body ratio); *weight; body mass index; head circumference* (≤6 years); *triceps* skinfold (TSF), subscapular skinfold (SSF), and thorax and other skinfolds; *arm circumference* (after infancy); *chest circumference* (in infancy to age 5, particularly in underdeveloped countries); upper and lower *arm length* (in atrophy of lower extremities); *arm span* (in atrophy of lower extremities); *other* circumferential measurements; and *bone* or *skeletal age*.[20–22]

Accurately measured height and weight are essential for a determination of nutrition status. Height combined with weight is used to calculate ideal body weight (IBW), body surface area (BSA), and BMI. These measurements have implications for epidemiologic research, obesity assessment, and nutrition status as well as for screening and interventions for disorders such as osteoporosis.[14] They can be used to calculate doses of chemotherapy drugs, anesthetic agents, other medications, and mechanical ventilation settings. Height and weight are

**Table 4–5.** Guidelines for Nutritional Status Assessment

| Dietary Assessment (Minimal) | Biochemical Assessment (Minimal) | Anthropometric Assessment (Minimal) | Physical or Clinical Signs (Minimal) | Feeding and Behavioral Assessment (Minimal) |
|---|---|---|---|---|
| Feeding history questionnaire<br>24-Hour recall<br>Food frequency recall<br>Observation of food purchased in the home (if visit made to home) | Hemoglobin or complete blood count<br>Hematocrit<br>Routine urinalysis | Head circumference<br>Weight—beam scale<br>Height:<br>Recumbent<br>Standing<br>Upper and lower ratio (if needed) | Medical and dental records<br>Clinical signs of malnutrition<br>Skin<br>Lips-tongue-gums<br>Teeth<br>Eyes | Parental/staff perception<br>Professional perception |
| (Midlevel) Minimal | (Midlevel) Minimal | (Midlevel) Minimal Plus | (Midlevel) Minimal Plus | (Midlevel) Minimal Plus |
| Parental/staff knowledge:<br>Nutrition-drug interaction<br>Basic nutrition<br>Fiber and fluid<br>Caloric expenditure | | Plot growth curve<br>Special growth grids | Physical limitations score<br>Allergies<br>Infections | Gross motor<br>Fine motor<br>Reinforcers |
| (In-Depth) Midlevel Plus | (In-Depth) Midlevel Plus | (In-Depth) Midlevel Plus | (In-Depth) Midlevel Plus | (In-Depth) Midlevel Plus |
| 3-Day diet diary<br>Quantitative<br>Supplements<br>Special diet<br>Physical activity record<br>Caloric expenditure<br>Mobility | Transferrin saturation<br>Total serum protein and albumin<br>Fasting glucose<br>Serum urea nitrogen<br>Quantitative urinary plasma amino acid screen<br>Organic acids | Skinfold or fatfold:<br>Triceps<br>Subscapular<br>Abdominal (obese)<br>Arm circumference<br>Waist circumference (obese)<br>Bone age or density (as needed) | Clinical signs of malnutrition:<br>Hair<br>Posture<br>Abdomen<br>Skeletal development<br>General appearance—behavior, speech<br>Prenatal history—maternal weight gain and diet<br>Postnatal history of chronic illness or disease<br>Blood pressure | Physical:<br>Oral reflexes (suck, swallow, chew)<br>Neuromuscular development (fine and gross motor)<br>Behavioral:<br>Parent-child interaction<br>Reinforcers<br>Environmental influences |
| (Special Conditions) | | | | |
| Anticonvulsant | Folic acid and vitamin C<br>Vitamin D and calcium<br>Alkaline phosphates<br>Pyridoxine | | | |
| Prader-Willi | Glucose tolerance test | | | |
| Pica | Lead, hemoglobin | | | |

Adapted from Smith MA, ed. *Guides for Nutritional Assessment of the Mentally Retarded and Developmentally Disabled.* Memphis, TN: University of Tennessee Child Development Center for Health Services; 1976.

**Table 4–6.** Food Intake Patterns for Optimal Nutrition at Various Age Levels

| Food Group* | Servings per Day | Average Size of Servings | | | | | | | | | |
|---|---|---|---|---|---|---|---|---|---|---|---|
| | | 0–2 Mo | 3–4 Mo | 5–7 Mo | 8–12 Mo | 1 Yr | 2–3 Yr | 4–5 Yr | 6–9 Yr | 10–12 Yr | 13–16 Yr |
| *Milk and Cheese* | 4 | | | | | | | | | | |
| 1.5 oz cheese = 1 c (8 oz) milk | | ~1 c† formula with iron | ~1¼ c† formula with iron | ~1 c† formula with iron | ¾ c formula with iron | ¾ c whole milk | ½ c | ½ c | ¾–1 c | 1 c | 1 c |
| *Meat Group* | 2 | | | | | | | | | | |
| Lean meat, fish | | — | — | — | 1 T egg yolk | 1 egg | 1 egg | 1 egg | 1 egg | 1 egg | 1 egg |
| Egg, poultry | | — | — | 1 T | 3 T | 3 T | 3–4 T | 4 T | 4–6 T | 6–8 T | 8 T |
| Peanut butter | | — | — | — | — | — | 1 T | 2 T | 2–3 T | 3 T | 3 T |
| Dried beans, peas | | — | — | — | — | ¼ c | ¼ c | ½ c | ½ c | ¾ c | ¾ c |
| *Fruits and Vegetables* | 4‡ including | | | | | | | | | | |
| Vitamin C source (citrus fruits, berries, tomato, cabbage, cantaloupe) | 1 | — | — | ¼ c | ¼ c | ½ c | ½ c | ½ c | ½ c or 1 medium orange | ½ c or 1 medium orange | ½ c or 1 medium orange |
| Vitamin A source (green or yellow fruits and vegetables) | 1 | — | — | 1 T | 2 T | 2 T | 3 T | 4 T | 4 T | ⅓ c | ½ c |
| Other fruits and vegetables | 2 | — | — | 1 T | 2 T | 2 T | 3 T | 4 T | 4 T | ⅓ c | ½ c |
| *Bread or Grains*† | 4 | | | | | | | | | | |
| Bread | | — | — | — | ½ sl | ½ sl | 1 sl | 1–1½ sl | 1–2 sl | 2 sl | 2 sl |
| Cooked cereal | | — | — | 1 T | 2 T | ¼ c | ⅓ c | ½ c | ½ c | ¾ c | 1 c or more |
| Dry cereal | | — | — | — | — | 6 T | ½ c | ¾ c | ¾ c | 1 c | 1 c or more |
| Macaroni, spaghetti, rice | | — | — | — | — | ¼ c | ⅓ c | ½ c | ½ c | ¾ c | 1 c or more |

Adapted by Marjorie Michell and Shirley Ekvall from Bennet MJ, Hansen AJ. *Four Groups of the Daily Food Guide.* USDA Publication No. 30. Washington, DC: Institute of Home Economics.

*Fats added only if needed to meet caloric needs after 1 year of age.

†Breast-feeding or quantity of formula according to physician prescription.

‡Add more if needed for calories or other nutrients (particularly antioxidants).

**Table 4–7.** Normal Increases in Weight and Length from Birth to Adolescence

| Weight | Change | Normal Weight (lb [kg]) |
|---|---|---|
| Birth | | 7.7 (3.5) |
| 6 mo | Doubles | 15.4 (7.0) |
| 1 yr | Triples | 23.1 (10.5) |
| 2 yr | Quadruples | 28.0 (13.0) |
| 2 yr to adolescence | About 5.0 lb/yr | |
| Adolescence | About 10.0 lb/yr | |
| **Length** | **Change** | **Normal Length (in. [cm])** |
| Birth | | 19.5 (50.0) |
| 1 yr | | 30.0 (74.0) |
| 4 yr | Doubles | 41.0 (100.0) |
| 13 yr (girls) | Triples | 60.0 (150.0) |
| ≥13 yr (boys) | Rapid linear growth | |

From Cincinnati Children's Hospital Medical Center, Division of Developmental Disabilities, Nutrition Department (extrapolated from Growth Grids, Appendix 3).

also used to calculate energy, protein, and fluid needs. Inaccuracies in these measurements can result in inaccurate IBW, BSA, and BMI values as well as inaccurate calculation of nutrient needs, with profound effects on outcomes. Often, it is essential to use two or more anthropometric measurements and compare them or take an average. Skinfold measurements may be useful when height or weight is difficult to obtain or more measurements are needed.

Height, weight, and skinfold measurements in adults need to be obtained at least annually or more often based on health status or health care prevention and monitoring procedures.[14] Measurement variations may affect the course of care, such as initiation of weight-based medications or dosage changes, new medical diagnoses, and diagnostic studies or procedures requiring medications.

Height, weight, and head circumference should be plotted on standard growth grids developed from the NHANES data to determine the child's height-for-age, weight-for-age, and weight-for-height ratios. A deviation of 15% or one standard deviation above or below the mean is abnormal. Special grids have been developed for children with Down syndrome, myelomeningocele, Prader-Willi syndrome, sickle cell anemia, and other conditions. Children with special health care needs may be at special growth risk because of their disability. Specialized charts can be used for children with various disabilities, but the National Center for Health Statistics (NCHS)/CDC charts should be used in conjunction with the specialized growth charts for the recommended measurements and plotting procedures.[22] The height-to-weight ratio should be used for children with other special health care needs. At birth, length is related to maternal height, but by age 2 years, length correlates best with mean parental height. A 1-month-old infant gains 30 g and grows 1.5 mm each day. A 3-year-old child gains 5 g and grows 0.2 mm per day.[23]

Heights and weights of both biological and adoptive parents and siblings should be documented to determine the relationship of growth to the child's genetic potential and to identify growth retardation caused by nutritional and other factors. The impact of nutrition on anthropometric measures was illustrated by a study of parent-child pairs in which Garn found the dimensions of adoptive parents and children to be similar.[24] They were genetically unrelated, but after living together they began to resemble each other in growth and stature, fatness, and even urinary analysis values and serum vitamin levels.

**Table 4–8.** Adjustments for Parental Stature (in Centimeters) To Be Made to Measured Length (≤2 Years) or Stature (>2 Years)

| | Short Parents | | Tall Parents | |
|---|---|---|---|---|
| Age (yr) | Boys | Girls | Boys | Girls |
| Birth | +1 | 0 | −1 | −1 |
| 2 | +3 | +3 | −4 | −4 |
| 4 | +4 | +4 | −6 | −6 |
| 6 | +6 | +6 | −7 | −7 |
| 8 | +7 | +6 | −9 | −8 |
| 10 | +8 | +6 | −10 | −8 |
| 12 | +8 | +7 | −10 | −9 |
| 14 | +8 | 7+ | −10 | −8 |
| 16 | +11 | +8 | −15 | −10 |
| 18 | +13 | +7 | −17 | −9 |

## Measurement of Height

Accurate height measurement is an important part of nutritional assessment and intervention. Height should be measured directly whenever possible, rather than relying on memories of clients or families. Height measurement alone is an important indicator of nutritional status, bone health, and various health problems.[14]

Standing height is the most accurate method for obtaining a height measurement. A number of common disabilities and disease processes can make it difficult to measure standing height because of structural anomalies (e.g., kyphosis, scoliosis), neuromuscular issues (e.g., atrophy, contractures), or sensory and compliance issues. Other methods of measuring height may need to be considered. Recumbent or supine height and arm span measurements are used for people who are unable to stand or have lower limb dysfunction. Knee height and forearm length are additional methods of height measurement. In some cases, it may be helpful to use more than one method of measurement and compare the results.

Height measurements are recorded to the nearest quarter inch or centimeter. Many studies have shown recumbent height to be longer than standing height by about 2 cm and thus to be a more accurate measure of length. (This difference is 1.8 cm by age 2 years, gradually decreases to 1.1 cm by age 9, then gradually increases to 1.9 cm by age 16 in boys and age 14 in girls; the 1.9 cm difference then remains until age 28 for both sexes.[21]) Refer to Tables/Figures/Appendix for guidelines on obtaining height measurements, giving the actual numbers and titles of the items you are referencing when specifics are needed.

### Height Measurement in Children

Height or stature and length should be measured to the nearest 0.5 cm and repeated twice for increased reliability.

*Standing height.* Use a dermographic pencil, a measuring tape, and a leveler, clipboard, or block. Height is measured with a flexible steel or plastic-coated measuring tape attached to the wall or door frame. The child stands against the tape or stadiometer with the shoes removed and the heels, lower back, and shoulders touching the wall or door frame; a block of wood or slipboard is lowered to make firm contact with the child's scalp (Figs. 4–1 and 4–2).

*Recumbent height.* Use a rigid measuring board or head board and two people; if the child is younger than 2 years of age or less than 1 m in length, a head board should be used. The child lies on his or her back in the center of the measuring board. One person holds the crown of the child's head against the head board; the other person grips both of the child's ankles with one hand and places the child's heel firmly against the foot board, which is manipulated with the other hand. If the infant's knees are flexed, they should be firmly but gently pressed down on the table with the lateral edge of the hand. The head board is turned upright to measure an older child (Fig. 4–3).

*Sitting height.* Sitting height from crown to rump is used to determine the length of children whose legs are severely deformed or shorter than normal. Use an anthropometer, and place the child in an erect, sitting position with the head oriented; measure the vertical distance from the sitting surface to the vertex (top of the head).

*Arm length and arm span.* Measure each distance twice to the nearest 0.1 cm. Upper arm length, when multiplied by a factor, can be used to determine height. Use a plastic-coated tape measure; place the child in an erect standing position, with the upper arms hanging at the sides and arms flexed 90 degrees. For upper arm length, measure the distance from the acromion process to the radiale. Arm span is often measured, and it should equal the height. Stretch both arms maximally with the child's back against the wall; measure from the tip of one middle finger to the tip of the other middle finger.

*Knee height.* To measure knee height, use a knee height caliper. The child should be lying on his or her back with the left knee and ankle bent to 90 degrees. Place the caliper down against the thigh, about 2 inches behind the patella (kneecap), and measure twice to the nearest 0.1 cm.

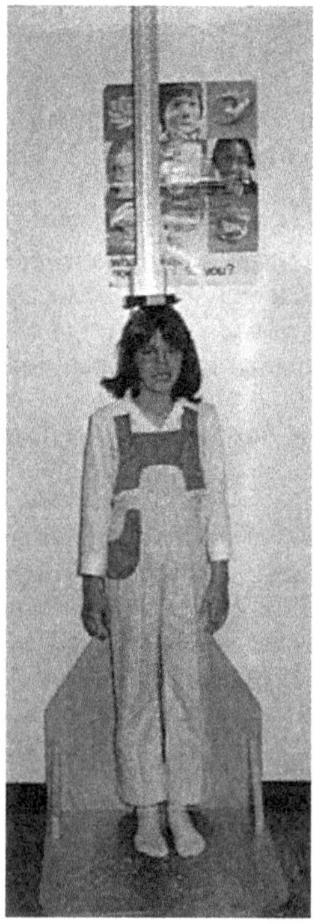

**Figure 4–1.** Measuring stature. (From the Cincinnati Children's Hospital Medical Center, Division of Developmental Disabilities, Nutrition Department, Cincinnati, OH. Used with permission.)

### Height Measurement in Adults

*Standing height.* Use a wall-mounted stadiometer, a measuring rod on a platform scale, rafter's square, or other flat object resting on top of the head. Ensure that the floor surface is even and firm. The person removes his or her shoes and stands erect, looking straight ahead with shoulders relaxed, arms at sides, legs straight, and heels together and flat on the floor; the shoulder blades, buttocks, and heels should touch the wall. Mark at the bottom of the stadiometer, measuring rod, rafter's square, or other object and measure the length.

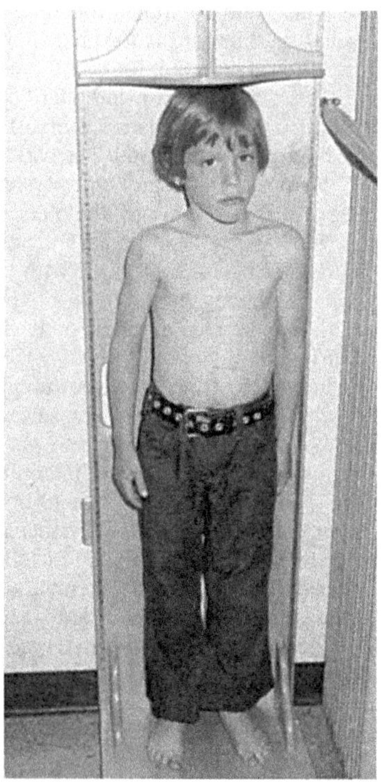

**Figure 4–2.** Upright measurement with the head board. (From the Cincinnati Children's Hospital Medical Center, Division of Developmental Disabilities, Nutrition Department, Cincinnati, OH. Used with permission.)

*Supine measurement.* Position the person on a bed without pillows or wedges, lying as flat as possible with the body and limbs straight. Mark the surface at the tip of the head and at the base of the heels. Move the person, and measure the length of the flat surface. This method may be contraindicated if the person has gastroesophageal reflux disease, a feeding tube, or another condition that prevents him or her from lying flat. Adjustments or precautions in using this method may be needed.

*Demi-span measurement.* Extend one of the person's arms out as straight as possible. Using a flexible measuring tape, measure the length from the notch in the sternum to the tip of the middle fingertip. Doubling this measurement provides an *estimate* of height. This may be the only method available to obtaining a height for some people.

*Knee height.* The method of measuring knee height for adults is the same as described for children.

It is often necessary to use two or more anthropometric measurements for comparison and/or to use an average of the measurements for nutrition calculations.

## Measurement of Weight

Weight measurement is an essential indicator of overall nutrition status as well as an important parameter in determining energy needs. Accurate body weight measurement is crucial in assessing nutritional health status and monitoring weight change over time. Whenever possible, the dietitian should observe and record how a person is weighed in order to assess the procedure for accuracy and consistency.

Accurate and reliable weights are frequently used to monitor the effectiveness of nutrition intervention and progress toward the person's goals. An individual may have a nutrition plan for weight loss, or to gain weight, that requires periodic weight measurements to assess progress. People receiving enteral nutrition also need regular weight monitoring to evaluate response to the prescribed formula regimen and to achieve or maintain healthy weight status. Physicians and nursing personnel may use weight information to assess health risk and monitor the impact of medications or other treatments prescribed.

Regular weights assist dietitians and health professionals to be proactive in identifying weight stability, unintentional weight loss, or undesirable weight gain and to help reduce health risks. It is important that weights be taken accurately every time. Any weight change, whether gain or loss, should be reviewed. Any significant change in weight could be a "red flag" and may indicate a serious medical problem.

Information for estimating body weights of patients with amputations is shown in Figure 4-4. For limbs, the segmental weight averages are for left and right. These figures are helpful in estimating desired body weight and making adjustments for people with paraplegia or quadriplegia and those with reduced muscle mass.

### Weight Measurement in Children

Weight should be measured with the use of a beam scale[22] unless the child weighs less than 13.6 kg or 30 lb, in which case an infant scale should be used. The scale should be checked weekly. To weigh an infant or small child, remove all of the child's clothing and shoes, balance the infant scale and place the child on it, and weigh twice to the nearest 30 g. For a child weighing more than 13.6 kg (30 lb), use a beam scale with a capacity of 220 to 350 lb and a support pillar. Have the child remove his or her shoes and all clothing except underwear; balance the scale and place the child in a standing position on the scale, facing the beam with hands on hips or on a support pillar. Weigh twice to the nearest 100 g; the child steps off the scale after each measurement (Fig. 4–5).

### Weight Measurement in Adults

A reliable method of weighing and accurate weights are not always available, especially in a community home setting. Weight measurement can be particularly challenging for people in wheelchairs and

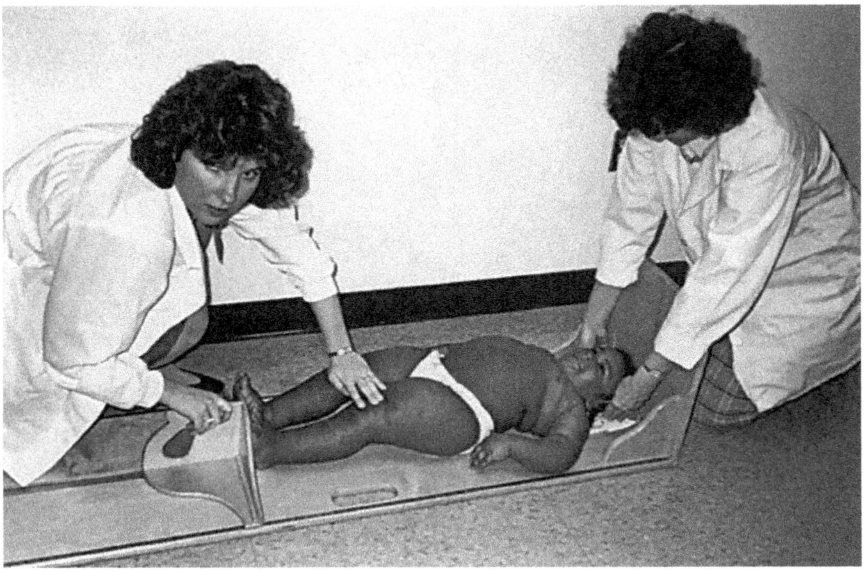

Figure 4–3. Head board measurement in a supine or recumbent position. (From the Cincinnati Children's Hospital Medical Center, Division of Developmental Disabilities, Nutrition Department, Cincinnati, OH. Used with permission.)

people who are unable to stand unassisted on floor scales. These individuals benefit from a scale that allows the person to sit in a chair or roll a wheelchair onto the scale.

Additional issues with obtaining weights involve those individuals who have limited or no access to a scale, have a scale that is broken or malfunctioning, or have a scale that does not allow them to stand on it easily. When issues related to weights and scales are identified, dietitians are encouraged to communicate with agency management and work toward a resolution.

If facilities and residential agencies are not consistently obtaining weights because of unavailability of a wheelchair scale, the following are possible suggestions:

- Consider contacting local resources for permission to use their scale, such as a doctor's office, hospital, nursing home or assisted living center, Coop, local gym, fire station, dialysis clinic, facility or business with a loading dock scale, local recycling center, or urgent care/walk-in clinic.
- Consider purchasing a scale; an agency may want to purchase a scale for use with individuals they support who live or work in close proximity.
- Agencies and homes who have a wheelchair scale may be willing to allow others to use it.
- Go to and search for mobility or wheelchair clinics in nearby locations for scale availability.
- If a person has or needs a Hoyer lift for transfers, consider purchasing a scale attachment.
- Contact local medical equipment vendors or agencies with equipment retrieval programs for scales to place in a home, vocation worksite, or agency location.

When weights are taken with the individual in a wheelchair, a variety of factors can affect weight measurement, including pieces of the wheelchair that may be removed or left on at the time of weighing (e.g., foot rests, head rest, lap tray) and extra items such as backpacks, coats, or blankets, which should be removed.

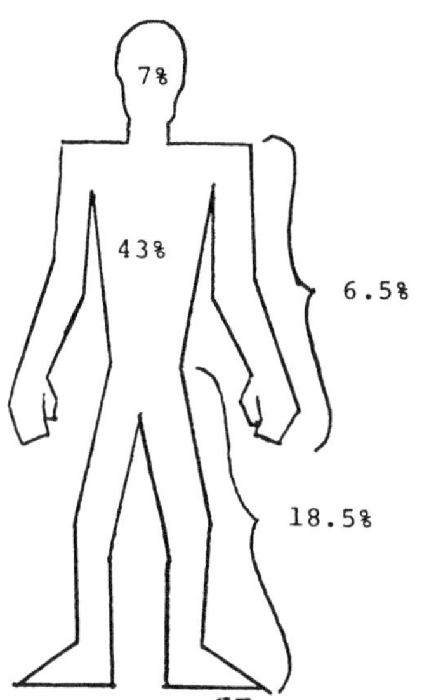


Figure 4–4. Segmental weights for limbs. (Modified from Brunnstrom S. *Clinical Kinesiology.* Philadelphia: F.A. Davis; 1972.)

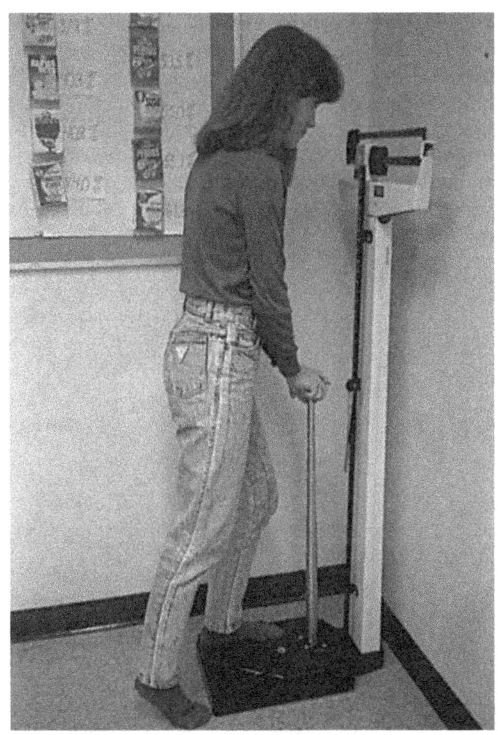

Figure 4–5. Person being weighed using a support pillar. (From the Cincinnati Children's Hospital Medical Center, Division of Developmental Disabilities, Nutrition Department, Cincinnati, OH. Used with permission.)

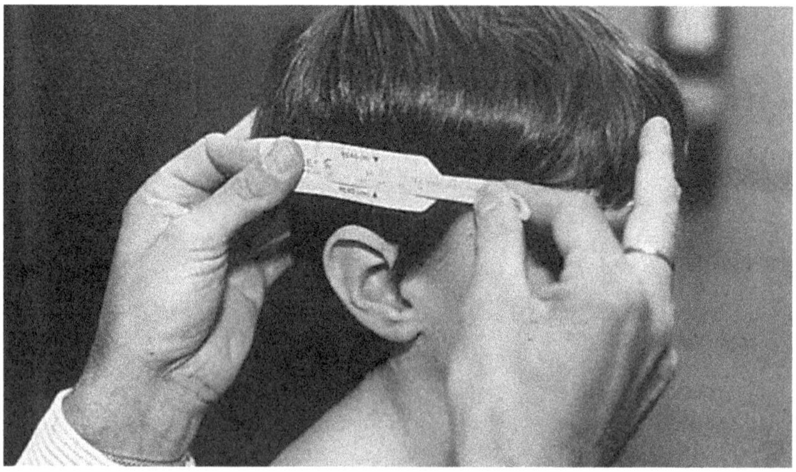

**Figure 4–6.** Head circumference measurement. (From Chumlea WC. Assessing growth and nutritional status of children who are chronically ill or handicapped. In: Ekvall S, Stevens F, eds. *Nutritional Needs of the Handicapped/Chronically Ill Child.* Manual III. Cincinnati, OH: Children's Hospital Medical Center, Division of Developmental Disabilities; 1989, with permission.)

## Circumferential and Skinfold Measurements

*Head circumference.* The head circumference is an important measure in young children because it reflects brain growth. The rate of brain growth is greatest during the last trimester of pregnancy and the first 6 months after birth. However, it is important to take head circumference measurements through age 6 years in a child who is developmentally delayed. Head circumference should be measured with a nonstretchable tape; use a flexible, narrow (7-mm wide), steel or plastic-coated tape. Apply the tape firmly around the head, above the supraorbital ridges or the most prominent part of the frontal bulge anteriorly and over that part of the occiput that yields the maximal frontal-occipital circumference. Measure twice to the nearest 0.1 cm (Fig. 4–6).

*Skinfold thickness.* The most commonly measured skinfold thickness in nutritional assessment is the TSF. However, other measurements may be more accurate indicators of body fat. The sum of multiple skinfold thickness measurements, including triceps, biceps, chin, subscapular, midaxillary, paraumbilical, suprailiac, thigh, and medial calf skinfolds, may be more accurate (see Appendix 8). However, in routine clinical practice, adequate accuracy and reproducibility can be obtained from measurement and summation of just the TSF and SSF thicknesses.[25] TSF and SSF grids have been developed for boys and girls aged 0 to 6 years, 6 to 12 years (TSF), and 12 to 18 years (SSF). These grids correlate well with total fat and percent body fat in children. Other measurement techniques can be found in Appendix 8. Use Lange or Holtain calipers and a tape measure; measure twice to the nearest 0.2 mm on all skinfolds.

*Triceps skinfold.* The distribution of subcutaneous fat varies from individual to individual and changes with aging, but alterations caused by dietary changes appear to occur proportionately throughout the body. Therefore, changes in subcutaneous fat are assumed to reflect changes in total body fat. TSF is a good general index of growth and nutritional status. TSF thickness provides an estimate of body fat, and the arm muscle circumference or area that is calculated from the TSF thickness and upper arm circumference provides an indication of body muscle, skeletal mass, lean body mass (LBM), or the somatic proteins (see "Biochemical Assessment"). Because caloric needs and perhaps nutrient needs are based on LBM or fat-free mass, which is active tissue (rather than the more inactive fat tissue), it is essential to determine LBM. A 24-hour urinary creatinine measurement also provides an indication of skeletal muscle or somatic proteins (Fig. 4–7).

*Subscapular skinfold thickness.* Place the person in a standing, erect position with the shoulders and arms relaxed; measure by grasping the skin and subcutaneous tissues 1 cm below the tip of the right scapula, with the forefinger at the lower tip of the scapula.[25] The skinfold forms a line about 45 degrees below the horizontal, extending diagonally toward the right elbow. Place the calipers perpendicular to the length of the fold about 1 cm over the inferior angle of the scapula, directly lateral to the finger at the mark (Fig. 4–8).

*Medial calf skinfold.* Place the person in a standing position. Measure the medial calf circumference at the most prominent part of the lower leg first, and mark the point. Grasp the skin and subcutaneous fat 1 cm above the marked point at the medial calf muscle, and apply the calipers at the marked point to measure calf skinfold (CSF); for the lateral CSF, use the side instead of the medial calf muscle.

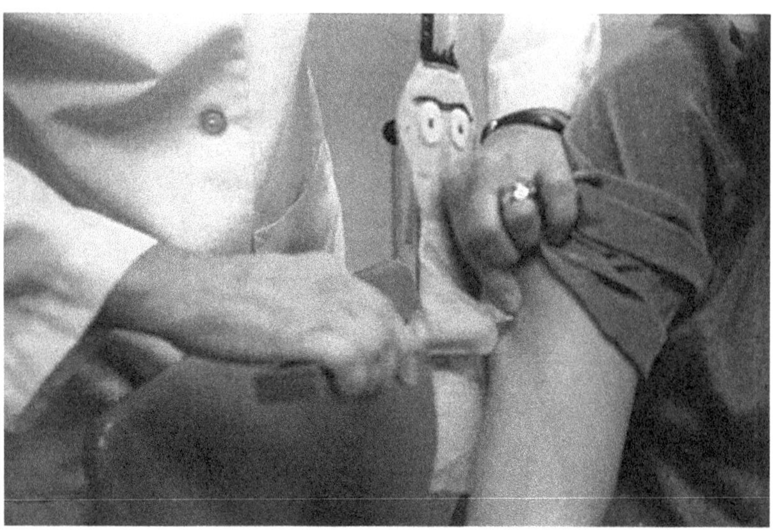

**Figure 4–7.** Triceps skinfold measurement using a puppet. (From the Cincinnati Children's Hospital Medical Center, Division of Developmental Disabilities, Nutrition Department, Cincinnati, OH. Used with permission.)

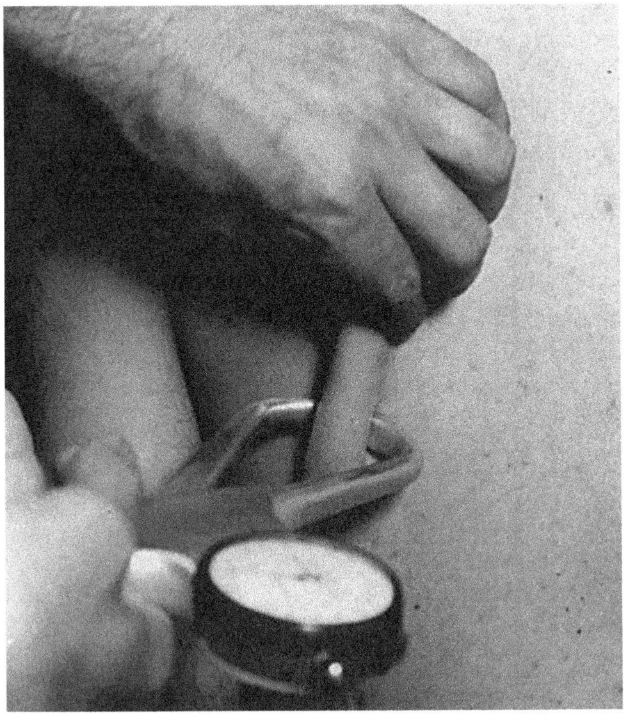

**Figure 4–8.** Subscapular skinfold measurement. (From Chumlea WC. Assessing growth and nutritional status of children who are chronically ill or handicapped. In: Ekvall S, Stevens F, eds. *Nutritional Needs of the Handicapped/Chronically Ill Child.* Manual III. Cincinnati, OH: Children's Hospital Medical Center, Division of Developmental Disabilities; 1989, with permission.)

*Midarm muscle circumference (MAMC).* The MAMC is derived from the following formula:

$$\text{MAMC or (cm)} = \text{midarm circumference (cm)}: 3.14 \times \frac{\text{triceps skinfold (TSF) in mm}}{10}$$

MAMC (in centimeters) estimates somatic protein, and TSF (in millimeters) estimates subcutaneous fat, but variability in size of the bone is not determined. The midarm muscle area (MAMA) is calculated by the following equation:

$$\frac{\text{midarm circumference (cm)} - \left(3.14 \times \frac{\text{TSF mm}}{10}\right)}{12.56}$$

A combination of TSF and upper arm circumference is used to compute the upper arm muscle area in children using the nomogram developed by Gurney and Jelliffe[25] (Fig. 4–9). The *corrected MAMA* (cMAMA) by Heymsfield et al.[26] uses the same equation but subtracts 20% for bone (−6.5 for females, −10 for males); a nomogram using this correction factor is not available. The MAMA prediction equations are not recommended for persons having a relative weight of 125% or greater or a TSF thickness greater than the 85th percentile. The MAMA appears to be a useful index for body muscle in young children; it is significantly correlated with creatinine excretion in this population.[27] For all of the techniques described here, circumferences are measured with the use of plastic-coated, nonstretchable tape; measurements are determined twice to the nearest 0.1 cm.

Arm muscle area is a more physiological parameter than arm muscle circumference and skinfold or fatfold measures. Changes in the arm muscle area result in larger changes in the arm muscle area values as a function of the formula used to calculate it. The mid-upper arm muscle area can be calculated from the TSF and the upper arm circumference by using the arm anthropometry nomogram for the appropriate age.

*Medial calf circumference.* Place the person in a sitting position with the feet flat on the floor; apply tape to the most prominent area of the calf.

*Waist, abdomen, and hip circumferences.* Place the person in a standing position with the feet together, weight evenly distributed, and arms hanging at the sides (place infants on their backs). Measure the horizontal circumference at the waist, at the largest part of the abdomen, and at the hip (largest part of the buttocks area) during normal breathing.

Circumferential and skinfold measurements may best be utilized as a means of determining physiological change over time, particularly when evaluating body composition and weight change.

## Application of Anthropometric Measures in a Nutritional Assessment

Anthropometric measurements are useful in completing a nutritional assessment (Table 4–9). The more measurements one can obtain, the more precisely the person's body composition can be interpreted and the more accurate the nutritional assessment. However, clinical measurements must be both reliable (two measurement samples) and accurate (using adequate equipment and proper technique), or wrong conclusions regarding nutritional status, growth, and intervention may be drawn. Incremental growth charts showing the velocity, slope of the curve, or rate of growth per unit of time allow comparison of a child's growth rate with that of American children in the general population. Thus, the amount of change or increment from one visit to the next can be quantified.

BMI compares weight to height but is not useful in children with unusual body composition (e.g., increased LBM). It is calculated by the following equation:

$$\text{BMI} = \frac{\text{weight (kg)}}{\text{height (m}^2\text{)}}$$

The BMI may correlate better with body fat than body weight.[28] Increased central adiposity combined with dyslipidemia, hypertension, hyperglycemia, and abnormal glucose tolerance ultimately produces the metabolic syndrome, leading to excessive lower and upper body fat stores.[28] A BMI of 25 to 29.9 is an indication of overweight, and a BMI of 30 or greater indicates obesity in adults.[29] However, this figure cannot be translated into recommendations of how much weight to lose. Mei et al. compared the BMI with other methods for measuring body fatness.[30] The BMI in adolescence is correlated more closely with percent body fat in girls, whereas TSF is correlated more closely with body fat in boys.[31] A TSF thickness of 60% to 80% indicates a moderate deficit; less than 60%, a severe deficit; and more than 85%, an excess of body fat.

The weight-for-height ratio is the most widely used index for measurement of adipose tissue, but it does not differentiate muscle and soft tissue from fat, especially in young children. Two skinfold measurements (TSF with SSF or CSF) can be used to determine body fat. An arm muscle circumference of 75% to 85% represents a moderate to mild deficit; less than 75% is a severe deficit. Skeletal muscle, like fat, can be used as an energy source if calories are not sufficient, although it is not intended for that purpose. Muscle can be estimated by MAMA, MAMC, and CHI.

The relationship of head circumference to recumbent length is a useful indicator; length should not exceed head circumference by more than 40 percentile points, or vice versa. For example, a 6-month-old boy with a height of 70 cm (80th percentile) and a head circumference of 41.5 cm (5th percentile) should be evaluated further. The gestational age of the child must be assessed properly in the first 2 or 3 years of life. If the child is determined to be at 32 weeks' gestation or later, correction must be made until he or she reaches 24 months of age, whereas for an infant born at 28 weeks' gestation or earlier, correction must be made until 36 months of age. Usually, by age 4 years, corrections for gestational age are no longer needed. Scores used

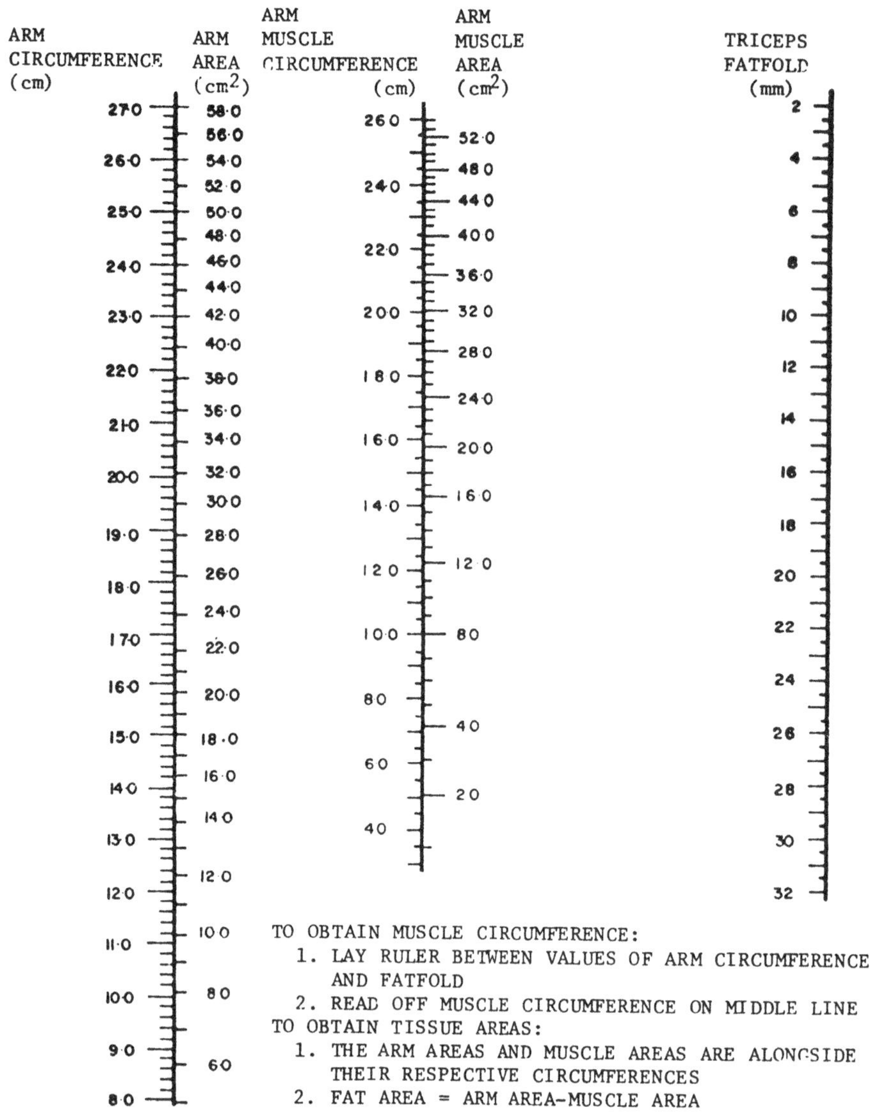


**Figure 4–9.** Arm anthropometry nomogram for children. (From Gurney JM, Jelliffe DB. Arm anthropometry in nutritional assessment: a nomogram for rapid calculation of muscle circumference and cross-sectional muscle and fat areas. Am J Clin Nutr. 1973; 26:912, with permission.)

to categorize data are calculated according to the formula shown in Table 4–10.

## Anthropometric Assessment of Children with Special Needs

Anthropometric assessments of children with special needs must employ alternative measurement techniques[32] and special growth grids or charts for certain disorders or diseases. The grid should be used to plot longitudinal data on the child to determine whether he or she is improving, deteriorating, or remaining the same. Parental stature or weight is rarely the cause of weight or length above the 95th or below the 5th percentile. Abnormal growth may be related to weight-tallness; obesity; edema; length or stature (e.g., tall parents, accelerated maturation, Marfan syndrome, pituitary gigantism); weight for length or weight for stature (e.g., obesity, edema, achondroplasia); head circumference (hydrocephaly); and TSF thickness (obesity).

Causes for growth below the 5th percentile may be indicated by

- *Weight*—shortness, malnutrition, chronic renal disease, psychosocial deprivation, infectious disease, iron deficiency anemia
- *Length or stature*—short parents, malnutrition, psychosocial deprivation, delayed maturation, and endocrinopathies, especially hypothyroidism and hypopituitarism
- *Chromosomal and genetic abnormalities* (e.g., Turner syndrome)
- *Chronic renal disease*
- *Weight for length or weight for stature*—dehydration, recent febrile illness, recent malnutrition, Marfan syndrome
- *Head circumference*—microcephaly (e.g., fetal alcohol syndrome, craniostenosis, genetic disorders
- *Triceps skinfold thickness*—malnutrition, chronic illness such as cystic fibrosis

Accurate measures of height and weight can still be obtained in children who cannot stand. The TSF and arm circumference measurements obtained in the upright position correlate significantly with those obtained in the supine position (Figs. 4–10 and 4–11). Arm span or arm length can be multiplied by a factor to measure length. Upper arm length (rather than lower arm length or total arm length), multiplied by a factor, correlates most significantly when evaluating children with myelomeningocele. Leg length plus a factor can be used to measure length or weight if the child has normal leg development and is older than 6 years of age. Weight can be measured by a movable wheelchair beam scale or by weighing the caregiver and child together and then subtracting the caregiver's weight.

Each recumbent position measurement is taken in the same body location as the corresponding standing measurement. Recumbent measurement techniques for TSF, SSF, and MAMC can be used with a few exceptions. The arm being measured for MAMC is placed alongside the body with the palm up and raised slightly by placing a sandbag under the elbow (see Fig. 4–10). Measurement of TSF and SSF is made with the child lying on the side with one arm extending from the front of the body at a 45-degree angle, the trunk in a straight line, and the legs bent and tucked up slightly. The arm being measured rests along the trunk, palm down. An imaginary line connecting the

**Table 4–9.** Some Anthropometric Measurements Applied in Nutritional Assessment

| Measurement | Age Groups | Nutritional Indication | Reproducibility | Advantages | Disadvantages | Observer Error | Interpretation |
|---|---|---|---|---|---|---|---|
| Weight | All groups | Present nutritional status, undernutrition and overnutrition | Good | Common in use | Difficult in field<br>Cannot determine body composition<br>Need accurate age<br>Height related (insensitive) | <100 g in children<br><250 g in adults | <60% severe<br>60–80% moderate<br>80–90% mild<br>90–100% normal<br>110–120% overweight<br>>120% obese |
| Height | All groups | Chronic nutritional status (undernutrition) | Good | Common in use<br>Simple to do in field | Other factors play a role | <0.5 cm in children<br><3.0 cm in adults | <80% dwarf<br>80–93% short<br>93–105% normal<br>>105% giant |
| | Age 7 yr | Chronic undernutrition in early childhood | Good | | | | |
| Head circumference | Age 0–4 yr | Intrauterine and childhood nutrition (chronic undernutrition) | Good | Simple | Other factors play a role (e.g., brain development) | <0.5 cm | |
| Midarm circumference | All groups | Present undernutrition and overnutrition | Fair | Simple<br>Age independent<br>Child need not be stripped<br>Suitable for rapid survey | No limits for overnutrition<br>No standard for adults | <0.5 cm | <75% severe<br>75–80% moderate<br>80–85% mild<br>>85% normal |
| Skinfold thickness (subscapular or triceps) | All groups | Present undernutrition and overnutrition | Fair | Measures body composition<br>Detects obesity in adults | Needs expensive caliper<br>Difficult with children and in the field<br>? Ethnic differences | 1.0–1.5 mm | Similar to item (1) |
| Weight/height/ age ratio | All groups | Present undernutrition and overnutrition | Good | Index of body build<br>Age independent (1–4 yr and adult) | Need proper scales, need trained personnel | | <75% severe<br>75–85% moderate<br>85–90% mild<br>90–110% normal<br>110–120% overweight<br>>120% obese |
| Ratio of midarm circumference to head circumference | Age 3–48 mo | Present undernutrition | Good | Simple<br>Age independent<br>Sex independent<br>Any person can do it in field | No standard for adults | | <0.25 severe<br>0.25–0.28 moderate<br>0.28–0.31 mild<br>0.31–0.35 normal<br>>0.35 obese |
| Ratio of chest circumference to head circumference | Age 1–2 yr | Present undernutrition | Fair or poor | Simple, age independent | For limited ages<br>No classification method | | <1 malnourished<br>>1 normal |

From McLaren DS. Nutritional assessment. In: McLaren DS, Burman D, eds. *Textbook of Pediatric Nutrition,* 2nd ed. New York: Churchill-Livingstone; 1982. Used with permission.

acromion processes should be perpendicular to the surface of the bed and the spine (see Fig. 4–11). Standards for measurement of standing

**Table 4–10.** Adjusted Ages at Which Growth Measurements Should Be Plotted for Infants of Various Gestational Ages (GA) at Birth

| | Adjusted Age (mo) for Plotting | | |
|---|---|---|---|
| Actual Age (mo) | 28 wk GA | 32 wk GA | 36 wk GA |
| 3 | 0 | 1 | 2 |
| 6 | 3 | 4 | 5 |
| 9 | 6 | 7 | 8 |
| 12 | 9 | 10 | 11 |
| 15 | 12 | 13 | 14 |
| 18 | 15 | 16 | 17 |
| 21 | 18 | 19 | 20 |
| 24 | 21 | 22 | 23 |
| 27 | 24 | 25 | 26 |
| 30 | 27 | 28 | 29 |
| 33 | 30 | 31 | 32 |
| 36 | 33 | 34 | 35 |

From Moore W, Roche A, eds. *Pediatric Anthropometry,* 3rd ed. Columbus, OH: Ross Laboratories; 1987. Used with permission.

height (stature), recumbent length, head circumference, skinfold thickness, and arm circumference for chronically ill and handicapped children are adapted from Chumlea and Roche.[21] Growth charts for the general population can be seen in Appendix 3, and those for children with specific developmental disorders in Appendix 2. Body compartment assessments are shown in Table 4–11.

## Body Composition

LBM has been measured mainly by the doubly labeled water method or by whole body potassium 40 ($^{40}$K) count. Most techniques measure the whole body average, such as the 24-hour excretion of creatinine as a measure of muscle mass, dilution of oxygen-labeled water as a measure of total body water, and the radioactive $^{40}$K count as a measure of body cell mass. Other advanced technologies are becoming available that evaluate the four compartments (water, protein, mineral, and fat) and are particularly useful in disease states. The distribution of fat and muscle at selected sites, which can predict the risk of certain metabolic diseases, requires imaging techniques such as magnetic resonance imaging (MRI),[33] dual-energy X-ray absorptiometry (DEXA),[34,35] or computed tomography (CT). These are expensive techniques and are used mainly for research (Table 4–12).

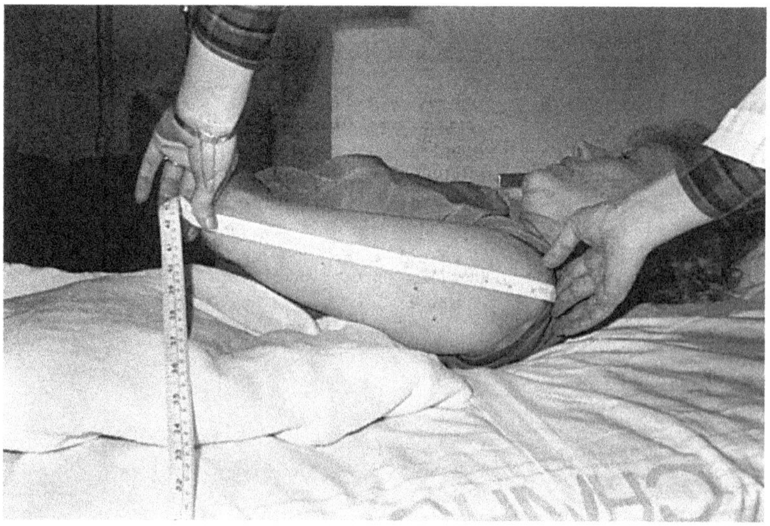

**Figure 4–10.** Recumbent upper arm measurement technique. (From the Cincinnati Children's Hospital Medical Center, Division of Developmental Disabilities, Nutrition Department, Cincinnati, OH. Used with permission.)

Bioelectrical impedance (BIA) is another method of determining total body water and fat as well as fat-free mass (FFM) or LBM composition in human subjects. The method is based on the nature of electrical conduction, which is influenced by water and electrolyte distribution. Because the FFM or LBM contains almost all of the water and conducting electrolytes in the body, electrical conductivity is far greater in FFM than in fat mass. The equation developed by Lukaski and Bolonchuk[36] to measure FFM is

$$\text{FFM}(\text{LBM}) = [(0.734\,\text{Ht})/\text{R}] \times 0.116\,\text{Wt} + 0.096\,\text{X} + 0.878 \times \text{gender} - 4.03$$

where Ht = height in centimeters, Wt = body weight in kilograms, R = resistance, X = reactance, and gender = 1 (male) or 0 (female).

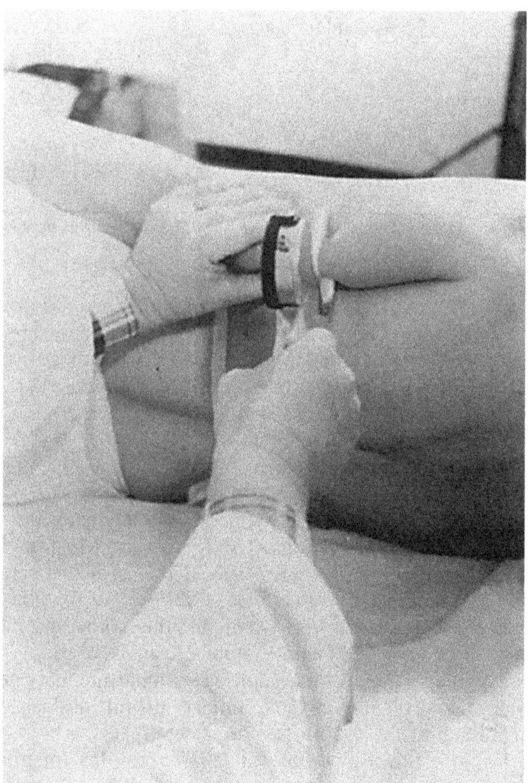

**Figure 4–11.** Recumbent triceps skinfold measurement technique. (From Chumlea WC, Roche AF. Nutritional anthropometric assessment of non-ambulatory persons using recumbent techniques. *Am J Anthrop.* 1984; 63:1.)

Five independent variables seemed adequate for predicting FFM in a study conducted by Guo et al.[37] For men, the selected variables were weight, lateral and midaxillary skinfolds, arm circumference, and BIA; for women, they were weight, lateral CSF and TSF, SSF, and BIA.

The multicomponent model of Slaughter et al.[38] is based on the following equation:

$$\%\,\text{body fat} = \frac{(2.74 - 0.71\,\text{body water}) + 1.27\,\text{bone mineral} - 2.045) \times 100}{\text{body density}}$$

This model reflects the concentrations of water, protein, and mineral and thus appears to be more accurate than the Siri two-component model, which includes only percent body fat and body density from underwater weighing:

$$\%\,\text{body fat} = \left(\frac{4.95 - 4.5}{\text{body density}}\right) \times 100$$

Body density may be measured by $^{40}K$, underwater weighing, and skinfold measurement; bone mineral may be measured by photon absorption (see "Biochemical Assessment"). The most accurate prediction equation for children 8 years and older is based on a multicomponent system for determining percent body fat that includes density, water, and bone and uses the sum of the TSF and CSF measurements[38]:

**Table 4–11.** Body Compartments and Common Methods of Assessment

| Body Compartment | Assessed By | Interpretation Affected By |
|---|---|---|
| Adipose | Skinfold measurements, body weight | Presence of clothing and dressings, technician error, patient age, hydration status, frame size |
| Somatic proteins—skeletal muscle | Body weight, arm muscle circumference, creatinine height index (CHI) | Same as above, plus completeness of sample collection, stress, injury, patient age, body build, renal function |
| Visceral proteins | Serum albumin, serum transferrin | Nephrotic syndrome, albumin infusion, stress, injury, blood products, patient hydration status, liver function |
| Plasma proteins—extracellular skeleton | | |

From Nutritional Assessment: *What Is It? How Is It used?* Columbus, OH: Ross Laboratories. Used with permission.

**Table 4–12.** Limitations of Methods of Determining Human Body Composition*

| Method | Cost | Technical Difficulty | Precision: Fat-Free Mass | Precision: % Fat |
|---|---|---|---|---|
| Water | | | | |
| Deuterium | 2 | 3 | 3 | 3 |
| Oxygen 18 | 5 | 5 | 4 | 4 |
| Tritium | 3 | 3 | 3 | 3 |
| Potassium | 4 | 4 | 4 | 3 |
| Creatinine | 2 | 3 | 2 | 1 |
| Densitometry | | | | |
| Immersion | 3 | 4 | 5 | 5 |
| Plethysmography | 4 | 3 | 5 | 5 |
| Skinfold thickness | 1 | 2 | 2 | 2 |
| Arm circumference | 1 | 3 | 2 | 2 |
| Neuron activation | 5 | 5 | 5 | 5 |
| Photon absorptiometry | 4 | 4 | 4 | 4 |
| 3-Methylhistidine | 2 | 3 | 3 | ?† |
| Electrical conductivity | 5 | 1 | 4 | 4 |
| Impedance | 2 | 1 | 4 | 4 |
| Computed tomography | 5 | 5 | ? | ? |
| Ultrasound | 3 | 3 | 3 | 3 |
| Infrared interactance | 4 | 3 | 3 | 3 |
| Magnetic resonance | 5 | 5 | ? | ? |

*The ranking system of limitations is an ascending scale, from 1 (least) to 5 (greatest).
†Unknown at this time.
From Lukaski H. Methods for assessment of human body compostion: traditional and new. *J Am Clin Nutr*. 1987; 46:537. Used with permission.

$$\text{Male \% body fat} = 0.735(\text{TSF} + \text{CSF}) + 1.0$$

$$\text{Female \% body fat} = 0.610(\text{TSF} + \text{CSF}) + 5.1$$

The sum of TSF and SSF may also be used to determine percent body fat, but these values must be calculated separately for various age groups and therefore are much more complicated to use than TSF and CSF measurements[38] (see Appendix 8 for nomograms for percent body fat based on TSF+SSF and TSF+CSF.)

Guo et al.[37] developed a prediction equation to estimate the body composition (FFM) of children from 10 to 18 years of age and, indirectly, the percent body fat using only BIA, height, and weight, without the need for any other anthropometric measures by cross-validation. Methods to determine body fat based on BIA are useful but require expensive BIA equipment ($4000–$5000) rather than the inexpensive caliper ($200) used in the TSF and CSF equation of Lohman. Body composition based on skinfold measurements can be as accurate as BIA if the measurements are taken accurately. Both are better predictors than BMI, particularly in men.[38] Hydration may also affect BIA measurements. However, skinfolds may not be as good a predictor as circumferential measures if body fat is greater than 35%.

Fat patterning differences related to age, ethnic group, fatness, physical activity, and areas of the body can be evaluated with the use of skinfold equations. Likewise, basic equations are being modified for calculation of adult obesity. A target weight for adults can be used to achieve a certain percent body fat and is accurate as long as the percent body fat is determined correctly. The target weight formulas are as follows:

$$\text{Fat weight} = \text{total body weight} \times \text{\% body fat}$$

$$\text{FFM} = \text{total body weight} - \text{fat weight}$$

$$\text{Target weight} = \text{\%FFM} / (100 - \text{desired body fat})$$

Segmental measures can be useful in children who cannot stand.

## Physical Activity Assessment

Physical activity is universally recommended for maintenance of good health. For children and adults with disabilities, however, options for exercise may be limited by the nature of the disability, by the built environment, and by inaccessibility of programs, equipment, and services offered in community recreation facilities.[39,40] Children and adults with intellectual, physical, and sensory disabilities need and should have access to programs in which they can learn and participate in team and individual sports. Most of all, they should be given the opportunity to interact with peers, both with and without disabilities, while being physically active.[41]

Information about physical activity is obtained either from the 24-hour recall of physical activity or from the 3-day diet/activity diary. It is necessary to evaluate the level of physical activity to determine the person's caloric needs from muscle mass or LBM. Caregivers should also know that caloric requirements and the need for physical activity vary with activity level. To condition the cardiovascular system, one should engage in 20- to 30-minute periods of exercise at least three times per week in target heart rate (THR). The THR range for an individual is determined by subtracting the age in years from 220 and then multiplying that figure by 55% (for a low-end THR) or by 75% or 85% (for a high-end THR). Swimming and fast walking are two excellent forms of aerobic exercise that involve large muscle groups and are recommended for children and adults with special health needs. Other aerobic exercises are bicycling, aerobic dancing, rowing, biking, skating, skiing, and jogging. Anaerobic exercises include sprinting, weight lifting, and calisthenics. Physical activity should focus on fun and enjoyment while promoting increases in strength and endurance, skill development, improved self-esteem, enhanced bone formation, reduced stress, weight management, and decreases in heart disease risk factors.

Parents and family members of people with developmental disorders or chronic illnesses have developed innovative exercise games and equipment to meet their special needs, such as a body-sized skateboard that is moved by the arms or an exercise bike that provides necessary physical supports. Studies in physical activity for individuals with intellectual disabilities have revealed moderate to strong evidence that physical activity positively affects balance, muscle strength, and quality of life.[42–45] Research in this area needs to be translated into practice, specifically the development of physical activity programs that are adaptable to the needs of individuals with intellectual disability. Consultation with an occupational therapist and/or a physical therapist may be needed to ensure that the physical activity is safe and appropriate for the individual.

## Energy Expenditure: Calorie Needs

The *basal metabolic rate* (BMR), or resting metabolic rate (RMR), is measured in a post-malabsorptive state and at complete rest in a thermoneutral environment, which is an artificial condition. In practice, BMR is reflective only of the resting state and is called the *resting energy expenditure* (REE). These terms are interchangeable. The REE is the largest component of total energy expenditure (TEE). The REE correlates well with LBM and differs from the BMR by less than 10%. The thermic effect of food varies with the food content and is only 5% to 10% of the energy ingested. (Methods for calculating REE related to activities are noted in Table 4–13.) The differences in LBM account for about 80% of the variability when measuring the REE for individuals of the same sex and similar height, weight, and age.

Changes in body composition at different ages are affected by disease; these changes, in turn, markedly affect energy needs. The LBM of infants (1.7–2.0 × REE) is higher than that of adults (1.45–1.50 × REE). Sex differences in body composition are small until children reach adolescence, when young men have greater LBM and young women have more fat. When calculating energy needs, requirements may be determined by actual weight or by median weight according to sex, age, and height. The weight of undernourished or obese individuals should be adjusted to normal height and weight. People with large body frames require more energy per unit of time than those with small frames. Yet, when individuals of the same weight vary in height and thus in BMI, height or stature variations have little effect on energy needs, except in the elderly and perhaps in African-Americans with a lower REE. Weight is thus the influencing factor in BMR, RMR, and REE. Pregnant and lactating women need additional calories. For children

**Table 4–13.** Approximate Energy Expenditure for Various Activities in Relation to Resting Needs for Men and Women of Average Size

| Active Category* | Representative Value for Activity Factor per Unit Time of Activity |
|---|---|
| Resting | REE × 1.0 |
| Sleeping, reclining | |
| Very light | REE × 1.5 |
| Seated and standing activities, painting trades, driving, laboratory work, typing, sewing, ironing, cooking, playing cards, playing a musical instrument | |
| Light | REE × 2.5 |
| Walking on a level surface at 2.5 to 3 mph, garage work, electrical trades, carpentry, restaurant trades, housecleaning, child care, golf, sailing, table tennis | |
| Moderate | REE × 5.0 |
| Walking 3.5 to 4 mph, weeding and hoeing, carrying a load, cycling, skiing, tennis, dancing | |
| Heavy | REE × 7.0 |
| Walking with load uphill, tree felling, heavy manual digging, basketball, climbing, football, soccer | |

*When repeated as multiples of basal needs, the expenditures of men and women are similar. From the National Research Council REE, resting energy expenditure.

younger than 10 years of age, caloric needs are based on normal growth patterns; after age 10, the caloric needs of boys and girls differ.

*Physical activity* is the second largest component of TEE. For sedentary people, increasing physical activity during their leisure time is essential to increasing their LBM and ultimately their nutrient needs. The activity factor is multiplied by the REE to determine energy needs or estimated energy requirement (EER). The total energy factor for digestion of food is small but may necessitate an additional 7% of TEE in research compared with clinical situations. Conventional formulas for estimating TEE are inaccurate and generally overestimate energy expenditure for nonambulatory patients with severe developmental disabilities. An example of conditions that can alter energy needs is cerebral palsy—type (athetoid, spasticity, or mixed), hyperactivity, and low muscle tone.

Another method of assessing energy needs is based on the *basal energy expenditure* (BEE), or basal energy requirement, which is the measure of energy needs when at complete rest. The BEE does not account for activity level, stress factors, temperature, specific dynamic action of food, or other conditioning factors. It can be estimated in three ways: (1) multiply the metabolic rate (kcal/hr) by 24; (2) for children weighing more than 15 kg and measuring greater than 85 cm in height and who are near ideal body weight (IBW), use the Mayo Clinic nomogram to determine surface area. Then use this equation: (m) × (kcal/m/hr × 24 hr/day = kcal/day); (3) for persons 18 years and older who are close to IBW, use the Harris-Benedict equations:[46] BEE (men) = 66 + (13.75 × W) + (5.0 × H) − (6.8 × A); BEE (women) = 655 + (9.6 × W) + 1.70 × H) − (4.7 × A), where W = weight in kilograms, H = height in centimeters, and A = age in years; and (4) The BEE is then multiplied by a factor for activity level and for stress (e.g., head trauma). However, a revised Harris-Benedict equation[46] is needed for the malnourished person because of increased resting oxygen consumption: female REE = 447,593 = 3098 S + 9.247 Wt − 4.330 A, and male REE = 88.362 + 4700 S + 13.397 Wt − 5677 A. Many methods are given because it is very difficult to evaluate energy needs in children with developmental disabilities.

**Table 4–14.** Energy Needs of Nutritional Therapy

| Type of Therapy | Protein Requirement (g/24 hr) | Energy Requirement (kcal/24 hr) |
|---|---|---|
| Parenteral anabolic therapy | | 1.75 × BEE |
| Oral anabolic therapy | | 1.50 × BEE |
| Oral maintenance therapy | | 1.20 × BEE |
| Prescriptions for anabolism* | | |
| Oral protein-sparing therapy | 1.5 × Weight | |
| Total parenteral nutrition | (1.2 to 1.5) × Weight | 40 × Weight |
| Oral hyperalimentation | (1.2 to 1.5) × Weight | 40 × Weight |

*Levels of protein intake are to be adjusted according to blood urea nitrogen values and nitrogen balance.
BEE = basal energy expenditure; Weight = actual weight in kilograms.
From Blackburn GL, Bistrian BR, Maini BS, Schlamm HT, Smith MF. Nutritional and metabolic assessment of the hospitalized patient. *JPEN J Parenter Enteral Nutr.* 1977; 1:11. Used with permission.

**Table 4–15.** Nutritional Needs of Children Receiving Enteral Feeding (Birth to Age 15 Yr)

| Energy Needs | Protein Needs (g/kg) | |
|---|---|---|
| Basal = (55 − 2 × age) × kg | 0–6 mo | 2.2 |
| Maintenance = 20% × basal | 6 mo–1 yr | 1.6 |
| Growth = 50% × basal | 1–3 yr | 1.2 |
| *Activity = 0 − 25% × basal | 4–6 yr | 1.1 |
| Sepsis − 13%/1 degree C × basal | 7–14 yr | 1.0 |
| Simple trauma = 20% × basal | | |
| Multiple injuries = 40% × basal | | |
| Burns = 50 − 100% × basal | | |

*50% × basal in very active children.
Adapted from Seashore J. Nutrition support of children. *Yale J Biol Med.* 1984; 51:111. Used with permission.

The TEE can be determined in several ways, depending on the problem, the age of the client, and the expertise available. The most exact methods are a doubly labeled water method of indirect calorimetry[47,48] and measurement of $^{40}$K in the whole body counter.[49] These methods have been evaluated in persons with developmental disorders as well. A less precise method is to multiply BEE by factors for activity, stress, and fever. Several procedures can be used to determine caloric needs based on energy expenditure. The following method is used by McCardle et al.[50]

1. BMR cal/24 hr × surface area;
2. Physical activity cal = BMR × 5 × a physical activity factor (i.e., sedentary, 20%; light, 30%; moderate, 40%; very active, 50%)
3. Food digestion cal = (BMR cal + physical activity cal) × 10%
4. Total energy needs = BMR cal + physical activity cal + food digestion cal

Energy needs of those requiring enteral and parenteral feeding are noted in Tables 4–14[51] and 4–15.[52]

Box 4–1 shows a quick method to determine the caloric needs of adults, which can be useful in a mini-assessment. It is adapted from the *Official Pocket Guide to Diabetic Exchanges* published by the American Diabetes Association.[53]

Another simple method of determining caloric needs is based on weight and activity level (sedentary, moderate, or active). For an overweight individual, the range of adjustment for activity level is 20 to 30 cal/kg; for a person of normal weight, it is 30 to 40 cal/kg; and for an underweight individual, it is 30 to 50 cal/kg.[50] It is recommended that standard formula calculations be compared in addition to clinical judgment.

## ASSESSMENT OF PHYSICAL AND CLINICAL SIGNS

In malnutrition, physical and clinical signs are often the last to appear, usually after a prolonged inadequate intake of nutrients. Therefore, dietary depletion should be evaluated carefully and corrected when it first appears so that the potential for the child's growth is not reduced by inadequate nutrition. Many signs of malnutrition are subclinical, however. It is necessary to evaluate frequently to become a good clinician who is knowledgeable about the clinical and physical signs of malnutrition[54,55] (Table 4–16).

According to the World Health Organizations, the physical signs are classified as (1) those associated with nutritional deficiency; (2) those that need further investigation (e.g., malnutrition due to chronic problems or poverty); and (3) those not related to malnutrition. A physical signs assessment should evaluate the oral musculature and its possible

**Box 4–1.** Method to Determine Caloric Needs of Adults

1. Determine body build by dividing height (in centimeters) by wrist measurement (in centimeters). Measure the wrist from the styloid process, which is above the radius (outer bone of the forearm, thumb side) to the ulna (large inner bone of the forearm, opposite the thumb side). Determining the frame size by elbow breadth may be even more accurate.

| Build | Men | Women |
|---|---|---|
| Small | 10.4 | 11.1 |
| Medium | 9.6–10.4 | 10.1–11.0 |
| Large | 9.6 | 10.1 |

2. Calculate the desirable body weight (DBW):

| Build | Men | Women |
|---|---|---|
| Small | Allow 106 lb for first 5 ft of height, plus 6 lb for each additional inch | Allow 100 lb for first 5 plus 5 lb for each additional inch |
| Medium | Subtract 10% | Subtract 10% |
| Large | Add 10% | Add 10% |

3. Determine caloric needs based on activity level. Basal level equals DBW activity level in pounds: (a)Sedentary = DBW × 3; (b) Moderate = DBW × 5; and (c) Strenuous = DBW × 10.
4. Add calories for indicated weight gain, growth (pregnant women), and lactation: *Pregnancy*—add 195 cal/day to gain 22–27 lb in 9 months *Lactation*—add 347 cal/day
5. Subtract calories for indicated weight loss (to lose 1 lb/wk, subtract 500 cal/day).

**Table 4–16.** Clinical Nutrition Examination

| Clinical Findings | Possible Deficiency | Possible Excess |
|---|---|---|
| *Hair, Nails* | | |
| Flag sign (transverse dyspigmentation of hair | Protein, copper | |
| Hair easily pluckable | Protein | |
| Hair thin, sparse | Protein, biotin, zinc | Vitamin A |
| Nails spoon-shaped | Iron | |
| Nails lackluster, transverse ridging | Protein, calories | |
| *Skin* | | |
| Dry, scaling | Vitamin A, zinc, essential fatty acids | Vitamin A |
| Erythematous eruption (sunburn-like) | | Vitamin A |
| "Flaky paint" dermatosis | Protein | |
| Follicular hyperkeratosis | Vitamin A, vitamin C; essential fatty acids | |
| Nasolabial seborrhea | Niacin, pyridoxine, riboflavin | |
| Petechiae, purpura | Ascorbic acid, vitamin K | |
| Pigmentation, desquamation (sun-exposed areas) | Niacin (pellagra) | |
| Subcutaneous fat loss | Calories | |
| Yellow pigmentation sparing sclerae (benign) | | Carotene |
| *Eyes* | | |
| Angular blepharitis | Riboflavin | |
| Band keratitis | | Vitamin D |
| Corneal vascularization | Riboflavin | |
| Dull, dry conjunctiva | Vitamin A | |
| Fundal capillary microaneurysms | Ascorbic acid | |
| Papilledema | | Vitamin A |
| Scleral icterus (mild) | Pyridoxine | |
| *Perioral Area* | | |
| Angular stomatitis | Riboflavin | |
| Cheilosis | Riboflavin | |
| *Oral Area* | | |
| Atrophic lingual papillae | Niacin, iron, riboflavin, folate, vitamin $B_{12}$ | |
| Glossitis (scarlet, raw) | Niacin, pyridoxine, riboflavin, vitamin $B_{12}$, folate | |
| Hypogeusesthesia (also hyposmia) | Zinc, vitamin A | |
| Magenta tongue | Riboflavin | |
| Swollen, bleeding gums (if teeth are present) | Ascorbic acid | |
| Tongue fissuring, edema | Niacin | |
| *Glands* | | |
| Parotid enlargement | Protein | |
| Sjögren syndrome | Ascorbic acid | |
| Thyroid enlargement | Iodine | |

(*continued*)

**Table 4–16.** Continued

| Clinical Findings | Possible Deficiency | Possible Excess |
|---|---|---|
| *Heart* | | |
| Enlargement, tachycardia, high-output failure | Thiamine (wet beriberi) | |
| Small size, decreased output | Calories | |
| Sudden failure, death | Ascorbic acid | |
| *Abdomen* | | |
| Hepatomegaly | Protein | Vitamin A |
| *Muscles, Extremities* | | |
| Calf tenderness | Thiamine, ascorbic acid (hemorrhage into muscle) | |
| Edema | Protein, thiamine | |
| Muscle wastage (especially temporal area, dorsum of hand, spine) | Calories | |
| *Bones, Joints* | | |
| Beading of ribs (child) | Vitamin C, vitamin D | |
| Bone and joint tenderness (child) | Ascorbic acid (subperiosteal hemorrhage) | Vitamin A |
| Bone tenderness (adult) | Vitamin D, calcium, phosphorus (osteomalacia) | |
| Bulging fontanelle (child) | | Vitamin A |
| Craniotabes, bosselation (child) | | Vitamin D |
| *Neurologic Considerations* | | |
| Confabulaton, disorientation | Thiamine (Korsakoff psychosis) | |
| Decreased position and vibratory senses, ataxia | Vitamin $B_{12}$, thiamine | |
| Decreased tendon reflexes, slowed relaxation phase | Thiamine | |
| Drowsiness, lethargy | | Vitamin A, vitamin D |
| Ophthalmoplegia | Thiamine, phosphorus | |
| Weakness, paresthesias, decreased fine tactile sensation | Vitamin $B_{12}$, pyridoxine, thiamine | |
| *Other* | | |
| Delayed healing and tissue repair (e.g., wound, infarct, abscess) | Ascorbic acid, zinc, protein | |
| Fever (low-grade) | | Vitamin A |

From Weinsier RE, Butterworth CE Jr. *Handbook of Clinical Nutrition*. St. Louis: Mosby; 1981. Used with permission.

**Table 4–17.** Normal Blood Pressure at Various Ages

| Ages | Mean Systolic Pressure ± 2 SD | Mean Diastolic Pressure ± 2 SD |
|---|---|---|
| Newborn | 80 ± 16 | 46 ± 16 |
| 6–12 mo | 80 ± 29 | 60 ± 10* |
| 1 yr | 96 ± 30 | 66 ± 25* |
| 2 yr | 99 ± 25 | 64 ± 25* |
| 3 yr | 100 ± 25 | 67 ± 23* |
| 4 yr | 99 ± 20 | 65 ± 20* |
| 5–6 yr | 94 ± 14 | 55 ± 9 |
| 6–7 yr | 100 ± 15 | 56 ± 8 |
| 7–8 yr | 102 ± 15 | 56 ± 8 |
| 8–9 yr | 105 ± 16 | 57 ± 9 |
| 9–10 yr | 107 ± 16 | 57 ± 9 |
| 10–11 yr | 111 ± 17 | 58 ± 10 |
| 11–12 yr | 113 ± 18 | 59 ± 10 |
| 12–13 yr | 115 ± 19 | 59 ± 10 |
| 13–14 yr | 118 ± 19 | 60 ± 10 |

*In this study, the point of muffling was taken as the diastolic pressure.
From Nadas AS, Fyler DC, eds. *Pediatric Cardiology*, 3rd ed. Philadelphia: Saunders; 1972. Used with permission.

relationship to feeding problems; use of drugs (e.g., anticonvulsants); general appearance; and behavioral characteristics. Blood pressure should be measured in all children older than 3 years of age (Table 4–17). Physical signs of excessive weight change need to be investigated thoroughly. Severe weight loss is loss greater than 2% in 1 week, 5% in 1 month, 7.5% in 3 months, or 10% in 6 months.[56,57]

## BEHAVIORAL HEALTH AND PSYCHOSOCIAL EVALUATION

Social and psychological components are increasingly important parts of the nutritional assessment and must be considered when planning the proper nutrition intervention. It is estimated that 35% to 40% of people with IDD also live with psychiatric disorders.[58] A longitudinal study found that more than 40% of a cohort of 1318 adults with IDD were diagnosed with four or more comorbidities, including 18% diagnosed with anxiety disorder and 17.8% with depression.[59]

Evaluation of behavioral health status is particularly crucial if the child, family, adult, or caregivers are in a stressful state. Calorie and protein needs may need adjustment during times of stress (Table 4–18). The degree of stress is often related to the magnitude of change brought about by various life situations. The Holmes Social Readjustment Rating Scale[60] assigns numerical values to a number of stressful situations (Tables 4–19 and 4–20). Standardized instruments are available to measure the following conditions:

- Anxiety state: 40-item STAI[61]
- Depression: Beck Depression Inventory Index[62]
- Functional status: Karnofsky Performing Status Assessment[63]
- Quality of life: Quality of Life Index[64] (designed by a sociologist) or Spitzer Quality of Life Index[65] (designed by a physician) (see Appendix 9)
- Mood states, Profile of Mood States[66] (measuring tension-anxiety, digression-dejection, anger-hostility, fatigue-inertia, and confusion-bewilderment).

Adolescence is a time of change and stress in Western society. There are three stages of adolescence, each involving significant psychosocial changes: (1) ages 10 to 14 years—early puberty, with changes in body image; (2) ages 14–18 years—peer groups, with cognitive awakening and much risk taking; and (3) ages 18–21 years—separation from family, less peer involvement, and increased self-sufficiency. Changes taking place in adolescence are related to the needs for autonomy, independence, assumption of adult sexual and work roles, and economic independence.[67] Adulthood can be seen as an extension of development that starts in childhood and continues through adolescence (Fig. 4–12).

In adolescence, stress is caused by changes in body image, sexuality conflicts, academic and athletic pressures, and relationships

**Table 4–18.** Calorie and Protein Needs in Stress

| Stress Level | Clinical Setting | Estimated Total Need (kcal/kg/day) | NPC:N | AA (g/kg/day) | AA | % Total kcal as CHO | Fat |
|---|---|---|---|---|---|---|---|
| 0 | Simple starvation | 28 | 150:1 | 1.0 | 15 | 60 | 25 |
| 1 | Elective surgery | 32 | 100:1 | 1.5 | 20 | 50 | 30 |
| 2 | Polytrauma | 40 | 100:1 | 2.0 | 25 | 40 | 35 |
| 3 | Sepsis | 50 | 80:1 | 2.5 | 30 | 70 | 0 |

From Cerra FB, ed. Open forum: Branched chain amino acids. I: stress nutrition. *Nutr Support Services.* 1985;5:8. Used with permission.

with peers and others.[67] Adolescence can be much less stressful if the child has a good self-image, has been treated well by parents consistently, and has healthy eating patterns.[67] The peak period of growth occurs in adolescence, beginning at age 13.5 years for boys and 11.5 years for girls.[68] A boy may gain 9.5 cm and a girl 8.3 cm in height during a single year. The nutritional status of a North American adolescent is assessed better by the Tanner and Davis maturational charts than by standard growth grids because nutrient needs in adolescence are related to maturity, not age. Boys tend to have a weight/fat gain early in puberty and then become leaner, whereas girls tend to have a constant rise in adipose tissue. Men may not reach maximum adult height until the third decade of life.[68] The body composition of adolescents is shown in Appendix 9. Women

**Table 4–19.** Stress Caused by Changes in Life Situation

| Life Event | Mean Value |
|---|---|
| Death of spouse | 100 |
| Divorce | 73 |
| Marital separation | 65 |
| Jail term | 63 |
| Death of close family member | 63 |
| Personal injury or illness | 53 |
| Marriage | 50 |
| Fired at work | 47 |
| Marital reconciliation | 45 |
| Retirement | 45 |
| Change in health of family member | 44 |
| Pregnancy | 40 |
| Sex difficulties | 39 |
| New family member | 39 |
| Business readjustment | 39 |
| Change in financial state | 38 |
| Death of close friend | 37 |
| Change to different line of work | 36 |
| Change in number of arguments with spouse | 35 |
| Mortgage over $10,000 | 31 |
| Foreclosure of mortgage or loan | 30 |
| Change in responsibilities at work | 29 |
| Son or daughter leaving home | 29 |
| Trouble with in-laws | 29 |
| Outstanding personal achievement | 28 |
| Wife begins or stops work | 26 |
| Beginning or ending school | 26 |
| Change in living conditions | 25 |
| Revision of personal habits | 24 |
| Trouble with boss | 23 |
| Change in work hours or conditions | 20 |
| Change in residence | 20 |
| Change in school | 20 |
| Change in recreation | 19 |
| Change in church activities | 19 |
| Change in social activities | 18 |
| Mortgage or loan less than $10,000 | 17 |
| Change in sleeping habits | 16 |
| Change in number of family get-togethers | 15 |
| Change in eating habits | 15 |
| Vacation | 13 |
| Christmas | 12 |
| Minor violations of the law | 11 |

Adapted from Holmes TH. The social readjustment rating scale. *J Psychosom Res.* 1967; 11:213.

**Table 4–20.** Ways to Cope More Effectively with Stress

| | |
|---|---|
| *Strengthen your body* | |
| Learn to relax. | Control all your input. |
| Eat a nutritionally balanced diet. | Have medical check-ups. |
| Get proper rest. | Dress in a way that feels right. |
| Get regular exercise. | Practice good posture. |
| Lose weight. | |
| *Develop self-understanding* | |
| List your goals. | Keep track of your stress level. |
| Listen to the rhythm of your body. | Make use of the helping professions. |
| Write a diary or journal. | Be honest with yourself. |
| Get feedback from others on how they perceive you. | Find out what is controllable in your life and what isn't. |
| Analyze your strengths and weaknesses. | |
| *Improve your mind* | |
| Read about stress and human growth. | Clear your mind. |
| Be sensitive to all dimensions of life. | Take a course. |
| Do light reading. | Go to the public library. |
| Think about great ideas. | |
| *Develop healthy attitudes* | |
| Think positively. | Practice living in the present. |
| Develop the attitude of gratitude. | Don't be afraid of failure. |
| Learn to accept what you cannot change. | Get friendly with leisure. |
| Learn to love yourself. | |
| *Control your emotions* | |
| Admit to yourself how you feel. | Face your fears. |
| Practice self-expression. | Experiment with new feelings. |
| Work off your anger. | |
| *Improve your personal relationships* | |
| Seek out friendships. | Listen to others. |
| Share yourself with significant others. | Don't criticize and blame others. |
| Contact new people. | Give in occasionally. |
| Do something for others. | Make clear choices. |
| Take charge of getting involved. | Face painful questions directly. |
| *Control your job* | |
| Focus on one thing at a time. | Redefine your job. |
| Manage your time. | Take some time off. |
| Define the purpose of work. | Be assertive. |
| Don't try to be perfect. | |
| *Lift your spirit* | |
| Keep things in proper perspective. | Encourage your gentleness. |
| Work toward deepening your life. | Engage in organized religious activity. |
| Allot time for daily meditation. | Laugh. |
| Learn to let go. | Learn to play. |
| *Improve your environment* | |
| Spend time in a new environment. | Reduce excessive noise. |
| Find security. | Rearrange and redecorate your home. |
| Change residences. | Control the television set. |
| *Live a healthy lifestyle* | |
| Be yourself. | Set up desirable futures. |
| Arrange to have variety in your life. | Take time to be alone. |
| Take one thing at a time. | Plan relaxed vacations. |
| Don't let things drift. | Practice relaxed driving. |
| Learn to vary your pace. | Develop your own list of coping devices. |
| Plan for maximum comfort. | Develop a hobby. |

Adapted from Holmes TH. The social readjustment rating scale. *J Psychosom Res.* 1967; 11:213.

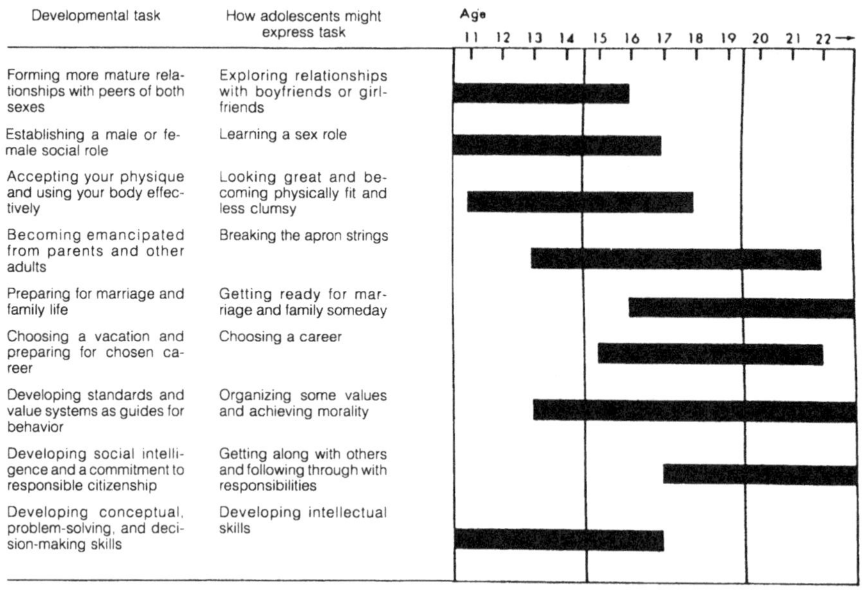


**Figure 4–12.** Developmental tasks in adolescents. (From Eggert LL. Psychological development in adolescence. In: Mahan LK, Rees Z, eds. Nutrition in Adolescence. St. Louis, MO: Mosby; 1984, with permission.)

on diets, athletes, ballet dancers, and others may have delayed menarche until age 19 years due to reduced fatness (hormones are stored in fat tissue). Hemoglobin values should be 13 g/dL or more for boys and 12 g/dL or more for girls.

Adolescent boys and girls are at risk for iron deficiency anemia, particularly because of boys' increased muscle mass, menses in girls, and marginal intakes of calcium, riboflavin, and vitamin A.[69] Teenage girls and boys often skip breakfast and snack frequently.[70] Likewise, teenagers eat many meals away from home. Many adolescent girls are overweight or obese (especially members of minority ethnic groups), and may be on diets.[71] Pregnancy at 15 to 17 years of age or younger is a high-risk problem in that increased nutrients are needed for the adolescent and the growing fetus.[72–74]

Adolescents usually respond well to invitations to both participate in and solve problems in nutrition planning. Therefore, they should be interviewed separately from their parents or caregivers. The interview also must be nonjudgmental. Dietitians and nutritionists working with adolescents need to be knowledgeable about sports nutrition, eating disorders (anorexia nervosa, bulimia, and obesity), alcohol and drug abuse, nutrient-drug interactions, and affective mood disorders, psychiatric illnesses, behavioral therapies, and psychotherapies, particularly those related to eating, mood, and developmental disorders.[75] They also need extensive listening and counseling skills[75] and must be able to provide nutrition education, both to the adolescent alone and to the family as a whole. Core areas of nutritional assessment for an adolescent are weight history, height, sexual maturity, reproductive history, food beliefs, dietary behaviors, fluid balance and hydration, iron status, medications, exercise patterns, and elimination patterns. Specialized training for working with this population is available at 8 adolescent health centers and 22 university-affiliated programs for developmental disorders in the United States.

The nutritionist should be aware of the special concerns of adolescent participation in athletic events and should encourage physical activity. For example, a complex carbohydrate diet and reduced exercise for a few days before an athletic event may be useful for some high-endurance sports.[76–78] Typically, a well-balanced diet with adequate protein, iron, and fluid that meets the Dietary Reference Intakes (DRIs) for age is recommended. Added calories (preferably supplied by complex carbohydrates) may be needed, depending on the calories expended in competition, and increased fluids should be given to replace those lost in perspiration. Special psychic-type foods, such as concentrated sweets and unusual diets, are of no benefit and should be evaluated individually. Alcohol use can lead to obesity; protein-energy malnutrition; deficiencies in thiamine, folate, and other vitamins; and depletion of magnesium and zinc. The second most commonly used drug, cocaine, as well as other stimulants, such as amphetamines, result in weight loss, abnormal dietary patterns, and nutrient deficiencies.[79] Most patients with mood disorders show weight loss, but increased appetite, particularly in the winter, occurs in a few patients. Schizophrenia may produce delusions in relation to certain foods or fluids, which may result in nutrient deficiencies, protein-energy malnutrition, and dehydration.

The nutritionist must become knowledgeable about psychiatric illnesses and their treatment, including their neurobiochemistry and neurophysiology. Diet and psychotropic medications can produce dry mouth, riboflavin deficiency, constipation, weight gain, nausea, and loose stools. When used in combination with alcohol, they can produce further sedation; caffeine can reduce their effectiveness. Large amounts of ascorbic acid may decrease the absorption of antipsychotics, and exercise may eliminate the effect of antidepressants. Increased sodium can eliminate lithium's activity, but a low-sodium diet can cause lithium retention and toxicity. Drug-induced malnutrition is covered in more detail in Chapter 27. With chemical dependency, the biological, psychological, and social factors must be investigated.[79] It is essential for the dietitian to become a member of the treatment team for both assessment and rehabilitation. Likewise, drug abuse, inadequate nutrition, and lack of prenatal care are problems in homeless pregnant girls that must be addressed by dietitians because the average infant mortality rate is double in this population (24.9/1000)[80] (see Chapter 1). Problems of anemia, diarrhea, nutritional deficiencies, and lead poisoning are common among the homeless.[81,82] In addition to the problems of the general population, children with special needs may have more challenges and may require separate growth charts, such as those for cerebral palsy and myelomeningocele.[53,82–85]

## FEEDING AND EATING ASSESSMENT

In performing a feeding assessment, one must know the normal milestones of feeding skill development, such as grasping the cup with both hands by age 15 months.[83] Ideally, a feeding assessment is conducted in conjunction with a speech and language pathologist or an occupational therapist. The person must be observed while eating. The child must be able to chew before he or she is able to speak; simulating this problem requires trying to speak without moving the tongue. Simulating swallowing problems requires tilting the neck toward the cervical spine and trying to swallow. A menu developed at CCDDD to help with the mechanics of feeding includes the following:

- Thin, peeled apple slices or orange sections with tough membranes removed
- Cereals cooked in milk with raisins or fruit added to increase texture

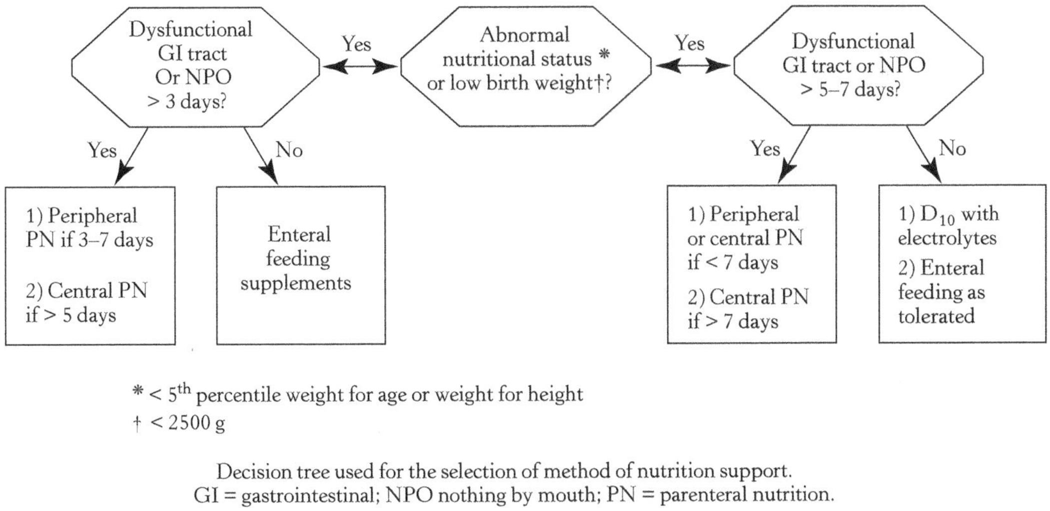


**Figure 4–13.** Decision tree used for the selection of method of nutrition support. $D_{10}$ = dextrose 10%; *GI* = gastrointestinal; *NPO* = nothing by mouth; *PN* = parenteral nutrition. (From Hendricks K, Duggan C, Walker W. Manual of Pediatric Nutrition. Hamilton, Ontario: B.C. Decker; 2000, with permission.)

- Graham cracker bits or animal crackers sprinkled on pudding
- Toast sticks, enriched animal crackers, zwieback, and dry cereals (preferably not sugar-coated) that may be used to encourage finger feeding
- Cooked vegetables and fruits, gradually advanced to raw ones, such as carrots
- Cottage cheese in varying degrees of lumpiness, combined with fruits, such as applesauce, to encourage acceptance
- Cheeses with varying degrees of hardness, used by themselves or combined with whole-grain crackers
- Hamburger, meatballs, tender chicken, meat cubes, and, finally, more chewy meats.

Until feeding milestones are accomplished, a combination of cottage cheese, yogurt, ice cream, pureed fruit, citrotein jello, and formula may be used to increase protein and calories. Feeding the child with disabilities is a challenge for many disciplines.[86–92] These disciplines, particularly occupational therapy, dentistry, and speech and hearing, also provide information related to feeding problems. A psychologist may assist in the area of motivation. The feeding assessment sections of the forms used by CCDDD are shown in Appendices 4 and 5. The feeding skill assessment chart can be used to observe changes over several visits. The Mueller Prespeech and Feeding evaluation can be an important interdisciplinary assessment tool (see Appendix 4). Feeding assessment is described in more detail in Chapter 24, and enteral and parenteral nutrition in Chapter 35. Tube feedings may be needed if the child is not obtaining 75% of the needed calories and nutrients (DRIs) and 90% of the fluid requirements[93,94] (see Fig. 4–13).

The treatment or intervention plan is designed to achieve a behavioral objective. It specifies the goal, time frame for completion, and measurement of accomplishment. The interpretation of the findings of the in-depth nutritional assessment includes a summary of the pertinent nutritional history, current nutritional status, anthropometry data, biochemistry, clinical or physical signs, presenting nutritional problem, impression or diagnosis, and recommendations. Evaluation points for the CCDDD summary are shown in Appendix 4.

Adults with developmental disabilities experience an array of eating problems and require a range of mealtime assistance strategies. As individuals with IDD age, the levels of support at mealtime greatly increase, from needing a small amount of support such as adaptive equipment to needing moderate to full support in order to eat an adequate amount of food and liquid in a safe manner.[12] The nutritionist should work with the team or circle of support to address all aspects of mealtime. Eating assistance is described in more detail in Chapter 24.

## BIOCHEMICAL ASSESSMENT

Laboratory or biochemical tests provide the most precise and most quantitative method of evaluating nutritional status. Biochemical data are used to detect marginal deficiencies before any overt clinical or physical signs appear or to corroborate questionable dietary histories. The laboratory test is the most expensive method of evaluation. The interpretation of the data is sometimes difficult because it may be correlated with dietary or other assessment parameters.

Large intakes of some nutrients, such as fat, or an imbalance of nutrients can produce biochemical abnormalities.[96] Likewise, a deficiency of one nutrient may indicate other nutrient abnormalities. A nutrient deficiency may be caused not only by decreased intake but also by *inhibiting factors*, such as excessive excretion or loss, increased requirements for the nutrient, or the presence of analogs. Progressive depletion of a nutrient results in the following sequential changes in nutrition status: lowered plasma concentration; lowered intercellular fluid concentration; lowered concentrations of red and white blood cells; lowered intracellular concentration; biochemical and physiological abnormalities in pyruvate, kynurenic acid, phosphatase, *p*-hydroxyphenyl acids, electrocardiographic findings, electroencephalographic findings, and dark adaptation; morphological change; and, ultimately, death of the cell.

The four most important biochemical measures in nutritional assessment are urinary excretion of nitrogen and creatinine, serum protein level, skin testing of cellular immunity, and determination of the percentage of lymphocytes. The choice of laboratory tests depends on the expertise required, the cost of the tests, and the child's problem.[97] Laboratory equipment is required for calorimetry, fluorometry, spectrophotometry, chromatography, and microbiological assay (Table 4–21). Consent of the person, parent, or guardian is required to perform biochemical tests for research studies. To minimize the trauma and cost of repeated tests, one should always consult the person's chart to see if a recent blood chemistry value is available.

### Creatinine

Somatic proteins are found in skeletal muscle, whereas visceral proteins are found in other body compartments.[98] The urinary excretion of creatinine correlates well with the status of skeletal muscle. However, it is difficult to collect a 24-hour urine sample from children, which is needed to calculate the creatinine height index (CHI):

$$\text{CHI} = \frac{\text{measured urinary creatinine}}{\text{ideal urinary creatinine}} \times 100$$

where ideal creatinine excretion is IBW × 23 mg for men and IBW × 18 mg for women. A value 60% to 80% lower than that level is considered moderate depletion, and a value more than 60% lower indicates severe depletion.

### Serum Protein Level

Albumin is a better measure of protein nutrition than the globulins, as it has a shorter biologic half-life.[99,100] The visceral proteins in the

**Table 4–21.** Biochemical Chart

| Test | Specimen (Method)* | Normal Range or Mean Value in Children† | Amount of Specimen‡ (mL) |
|---|---|---|---|
| Hemoglobin | Whole blood (cyanmethemoglobin) | 12.5 g/dL (100 mL) | 0.1 |
| Hematocrit | Whole blood (micro-centrifuge) | 35–37% | 0.1 |
| Iron | Serum (chromogenic complex) | 50–60 μg/dL | 2.0 |
| Transferrin saturation | Serum (Fe saturation) | ≥20% | 2.0 |
| Copper | Serum (chromogenic complex, atomic absorption) | 70–140 μg/dL | 3.0 |
| Magnesium | Serum (chromogenic complex, atomic absorption) | 1.5–2.1 mEq/L | 3.0 |
| Zinc | Serum (atomic absorption) | 80–120 μg/dL | 2.0 |
| Calcium | Serum (chromogenic complex, atomic absorption) | 9–10 mg/dL | 0.5 |
| Phosphorus | Serum (chromogenic complex) | 3.5–5.5 mg/dL | 0.5 |
| Vitamin A | Serum (chromogenic complex, fluorometric) | 30–65 μg/dL | 2.0 |
| Carotene | Serum (optical density) | 80–200 μg/dL | 1.0 |
| Vitamin D | Serum (25OH-cholecalciferol) | 15–40 ng/mL | 5.0 |
| Ascorbic acid | Plasma (chromogenic complex, fluorometric) | 0.5–1.5 mg/dL | 1.0 |
| Folic acid | Serum, erythrocytes (radioimmunoassay, microbiological) | 5–6 ng/mL | 1.0 |
| Vitamin $B_{12}$ | Serum (radioimmunoassay, microbiological) | 200–1000 pg/mL | 1.0 |
| Vitamin $B_6$ | Erythrocytes (AST-ALT index) | 1.5 | 1.0 |
| Pyridoxic acid | Urine (chromogenic complex) | ≥0.8 mg/24 hr | 5.0 |
| Thiamine | Erythrocytes, serum, urine (transketolase, TPP effect, fluorometric) | 0–14% TPP effect | 2.0 |
| Riboflavin | Erythrocytes, serum, urine (glutathione reductase fluorometric) | Activation coefficient <1.20 | 2.0 |
| Protein (total) | Serum (chromogenic complex, biuret) | 6–8 g/dL | 0.2 |
| Albumin | Serum (chromogenic complex, bromcresol green) | 3.5–5.0 g/dL | 0.2 |
| Blood urea nitrogen | Serum (chromogenic complex, enzymatic) | 10–20 mg/dL | 0.5 |
| Glucose | Serum (chromogenic, enzymatic) | 70–90 mg/dL | 0.5 |
| Essential amino acids | Serum (amino acid analyzer) | Varies for amino acid | 0.5–5.0 |
| Alkaline phosphatase | Serum (chromogenic, enzymatic) | Infants, 100–150 mU/mL<br>Children, 50–125 mU/mL | 0.1 |

Modified from H. V. Nino, Ph.D., Christ Hospital, Cincinnati, OH.
*Use of serum or plasma is adequate in most cases; however, the type of specimen is determined by the analytical method. Determinations of micronutrients in serum, plasma, or urine can be used to establish correlations among them and with other metabolites and functional tests (e.g., TPP activation) to assist in the biochemical evaluation.
†Variability of values dependent on age. Values indicated are guidelines for the interpretation of results.
‡Volume of specimen is determined by the analytical method.
ALT = alanine aminotransferase; AST = aspartate aminotransferase; Fe = iron; TPP = thiamine pyrophosphate.

liver, such as retinol-binding protein, prealbumin, and transferrin, have even shorter half-lives than albumin and therefore are even more sensitive in detecting early nutritional changes. However, the serum transferrin assay is not routinely available in clinical laboratories. Transferrin can be calculated from the total iron-binding capacity (TIBC) by use of the following equation[31]: calculated transferrin = (0.68 × TIBC) + 21. Ranges of serum transferrin and serum albumin levels give some indication of malnutrition severity[25] (Table 4–22).

## Immune Competence

Immunological abnormalities, such as a reduction in lymphocyte count, are indicators of poor nutritional status. The *total lymphocyte count*, an indication of immune reserves, is calculated according to the following equation:

$$\frac{\%\,\text{lymphocytes} \times \text{WBC}}{100}$$

where WBC = white blood cell count. Mild depletion is indicated by a value of 1200 to 2000 cells/mm³, moderate depletion by 800 to 1199/mm³, and severe depletion by less than 800/mm³. Cell-mediated immunity is determined by intradermal testing with such antigens as streptokinase, streptodornase, *Candida* and *Trichopyton* species, mumps, and the purified protein derivative of tuberculin (PPD). Intact

**Table 4–22.** Visceral Protein and Immune Competence Studies That Are Useful in Nutritional Assessment of Malnutrition

| | Half-Life | Normal | Malnutrition Values: Mild | Moderate | Severe |
|---|---|---|---|---|---|
| *A Protein* | | | | | |
| Albumin | 21 days | 3.5–5.5 g/dL | 3.0–3.5 g/dL | 2.1–3.0 g/dL | <2.1 g/dL |
| Transferrin | 10 days | 200–400 mg/dL | 150–175 mg/dL | 100–150 mg/dL | <100 mg/dL |
| Thyroxine-binding protein | 2 days | 15.7–29.6 mg/dL | | | |
| Retinol-binding protein | 12 hr | 2.6–7.6 mg/dL | | | |
| Somatomedin C | 2 hr | 0.4–2 U/mL | | | |
| *B Immunity* | | | | | |
| Total lymphocyte count (% lymphocytes × WBC) | | | 1200–2000/m³ | 800–1199/m³ | <800/m³ |
| Cell-mediated immunity (immune function): antigen analysis, including streptokinase, streptodornase, *Candida* spp., mumps, PPD | | | | | |

Modified from Long CR. Historic review of nutritional assessment techniques in applying new technology to nutritional assessment. In: Gussler JD, ed. *Report of the Ninth Ross Roundtable on Medical Issues*. Columbus, OH: Ross Laboratories; 1989. Used with permission.
PPD = purified protein derivative of tuberculin; WBC = white blood count.

immunity is indicated by one or more positive responses (i.e., a wheal measuring at least 5 × 5 mm). Anergy, or diminished reactivity to specific antigens, is frequently associated with increased sepsis and higher mortality rates.

Nutrients that are important in maintaining immunocompetence include nucleotides (found mainly in meat, poultry, fish, eggs, milk, nuts, and legumes); a balance of omega-6 fatty acids or linoleic acid (vegetable seed oils, meat, and milk) with omega-3 fatty acids (fish oils, canola oil, walnut or soybean oils, and plant leaves); zinc (meat, eggs, milk, poultry, whole grain, and oysters); iron (liver, beef, poultry, eggs, and raisins); and vitamin A (leafy green or dark yellow vegetables, liver, and cheese). However, some of these nutrients—iron, zinc, fat, omega-6 fatty acids, and linoleic acid—can suppress immunity when administered in high amounts.

A Prognostic Nutritional Index (PNI) with four parameters, developed by Mullen et al., provides a quantitative estimate of the risk of anergy, sepsis, and death[101]:

$$\mathrm{PNI} = 158\% - \begin{bmatrix} (16.6 \times \mathrm{ALB}) + (0.78 \times \mathrm{TSF}) + \\ (0.2 \times \mathrm{TFN}) + (5.8 \times \mathrm{DH}) \end{bmatrix}$$

where ALB = serum albumin concentration (g/dL); TSF = triceps skinfold (mm); TFN = transferrin (g/dL); and DH = delayed hypersensitivity in interdermal cellular immunity testing—the grade of reactivity to any of three antigens (*Candida,* mumps, or streptokinase/streptodornase) is indicated by a score of 0 (nonreactive), 1 (<5 mm induration), or 2 (>5 mm induration). The higher the percentage, the higher the mortality rate. For example, if ALB = 3.0 g/dL, TSF = 10.1 mm, and TFN = 155 g/dL, then PNI = 63.5%. The 63.5% risk of anergy, sepsis, or death is high in this malnourished person. A PNI of less than 30% indicates mild risk; 30% to 59% indicates moderate risk; and greater than 60% indicates high risk.[101]

### Bone Mineralization and Bone Age

For the child younger than 10 years of age who is immobile, is taking an anticonvulsant, or is growth retarded, a *bone mineralization* measurement using the left forearm is useful to determine the loss of minerals. The photon absorption method using a bone mineral analyzer is preferred.[102–104]

For bone age, radiography of the hand and wrist is an accurate method to assess skeletal age with minimal skin radiation. The procedure is modified for children older than 3 years of age and requires an X-ray machine and a plastic paddle to obtain a left hand and wrist posteroanterior radiograph. In the clinical estimate, maturation of skeletal age should be correlated with other findings, such as motor performance, mental age, race, height, weight, and nutrition status. DEXA also can be used to determine bone age, but it results in more radiation exposure.[105,106]

## IN-DEPTH NUTRITIONAL ASSESSMENT OF AGING ADULTS

As the child with developmental disorders and chronic diseases passes through adolescence into adulthood, other biochemical, dietary, anthropometric, and physical signs are manifested. Aging may occur more rapidly than in the general population. The BMR, TEE, and BEE decrease approximately 20% between 30 and 90 years of age; the calcium content of the skeleton decreases; collagen and elastin become more polymerized; and connective tissue becomes brittle.[107] The female hormones estrogen and progesterone decline more than do male hormones, leading to greater osteoporosis in women. Estrogen is found in most foods of plant or animal origin. It is particularly high in soybean oil, palm kernel oil, cabbage, wheat germ, clover, and eggs, but its estrogenic biological activity is only about 1% to 0.1%. Women with high calcium and estrogen levels have significantly greater bone density than women with lower calcium and estrogen levels.

Levels of high-density lipoproteins (HDL) and low-density lipoproteins (LDL) may change with age. The LDL is calculated as follows:

$$\frac{\text{cholesterol} - \text{triglycerides}}{5} - \text{HDL} = \text{LDL}$$

Normal desirable adult values are as follows: LDL, 62 to 130 mg/dL; HDL, 32 to 72 mg/dL; cholesterol, 120 to 200 mg/dL; triglycerides, 15 to 200 mg/dL; LDL/HDL ratio, 1.0 to 4.0; and cholesterol/HDL ratio, 1.9 to 4.2. Values for children can be found in Chapter 54; body weight and saturated fat intake appear to be important indicators of cholesterol in children. HDL is composed of 50% protein, 18% cholesterol, 30% phospholipids, and 2% triglycerides; LDL contains 25% protein, 43% cholesterol, 23% phospholipids, and 9% triglycerides; and very-low-density lipoprotein (VLDL) contains 13% protein, 15% cholesterol, 12% phospholipids, and 60% triglycerides. Diets supplemented with eicosapentaenoic acid (EPA) and docasahexaenoic acid (DHA) from fish oil significantly lower systolic blood pressure (by 4.5 mm Hg) but produce a 4% increase in LDL cholesterol.[108]

The stroke-reducing effect of the blood pressure reduction would be expected to outweigh the effect of the rise in cholesterol. Therefore, blood pressure levels should be checked frequently with supplementation. Because obesity is a major problem in the United States, research has focused on the use of drug therapy to treat obesity in adults. Anorectic drugs are being developed, such as centrally acting drugs (those that utilize opioid receptors, peptide antagonists), thermogenic drugs (adrenergic antagonists), and gastrointestinal drugs (enzyme inhibitors, absorption inhibitors, and synthetic foods).[109–111] Serotoninergic drugs, such as fluoxetine, have been used for weight control and depression. Adrenergic agents, such as amphetamines, have been used to suppress appetite. (Serious side effects and death have occurred related to the use of ephedra.) Gut peptides increase satiety.[112] However, all of these drugs should be carefully studied before they are used in children with morbid obesity.

In older persons of both sexes, the kidneys, liver, and pancreas function less efficiently. Overloading the body with sweets may result in insulin deficiency and may influence the development of diabetes and the metabolic syndrome. Sodium intake is typically 10,000 to 25,000 mg/day and needs to be reduced because the requirement of the daily U.S. diet is only 200 to 500 mg.[113] Chloride measurement may be available to check the compliance of the patient on a low-sodium diet. Medications may stay in the body longer because of less efficient kidney function. The need for protein and calcium is increased.[114] Likewise, folic acid and vitamin $B_{12}$ frequently become deficient. Problems of adolescents such as alcohol abuse, overmedication, depression or mood disorders, and anorexia also plague the elderly (see Appendix 9 for a Depression Inventory). In addition, lactose intolerance, poor hydration or constipation, and poor oral health may occur, particularly in the disabled older adult. Social ills and institutionalization that affect the one-fourth of elderly people who live near the poverty line and the one-third who live alone compound the nutritional problems of this population. Arthritis and osteoporosis may also bring about changes in physical activity and meal preparation. Inappropriate food intake (one-third of elderly individuals skip meals), reduced midarm circumference or TSF, and multiple medications (taken by almost one-half of this population) must be evaluated.

Adults with developmental disorders who are living in group homes or supported environments need to obtain at least one-third of their DRIs in the evening meal, especially when working outside the home.[115] At least 64% of meals were found in one study to contain only two food groups, and snacks mainly added calories rather than other nutrients.[114,115] Carbohydrate overeating has been reported among adults with intellectual disability who were depressed.[116] A classification related to behavior has been developed.[103]

Serum albumin appears to be the simplest and best single predictor of mortality and can provide early identification of increased risk of death in the elderly population. However, changes in serum albumin do not become apparent for 3 to 4 weeks. Serum transferrin is more sensitive and has a shorter half-life, but iron deficiency can elevate the transferrin level, so the test must be interpreted carefully. Serum transferrin measurement should be repeated every 7 to 10 days, and serum albumin every 3 to 4 weeks. Electrolytes, calcium, and phosphorus should be checked regularly. If serum albumin and transferrin are normal, it is assumed that there is no loss of organ mass or functional impairment. If malnutrition is identified, protein and calorie assessments are essential. For the hospitalized patient, determination of the nitrogen balance may be important and should be repeated every 3 to 4 weeks. If the nitrogen balance is positive, 1 g means a gain of 1 oz of protoplasm; a negative nitrogen balance of 16 g means a loss of 1 lb of muscle, cardiac muscle, or organ tissue.

If there is a loss of one-third of LBM, a diagnosis of malnutrition is made, which often is associated with death.[118] The total lymphocyte count should be 20% to 40% of WBCs; however, an infection can elevate WBCs and result in a misdiagnosis of nutritional inadequacy.[118] Energy expenditure is determined indirectly by measuring oxygen consumption. By also determining carbon dioxide production, the substrate (or substrates) being oxidized can be assessed and the respiratory quotient (RQ) calculated. A caloric equivalent for 1 L of oxygen is assigned based on this RQ, resulting in a more accurate measure of energy requirements.

A nutritional assessment for this population includes evaluation of anthropometry, biochemical measurements, nutritional diagnosis, energy-protein requirements, and nutritional therapies (see Appendix 10 for details). Anthropometry, biochemical, and dietary tests provide information on body fat stores, muscle mass, visceral proteins, and immunocompetence. Assigning the adult the proper classification or nutritional diagnosis is important. If visceral proteins, lymphocyte count, and cellular immunity are moderate or severely depleted, a kwashiorkor state is noted (weight may be normal). If weight, creatinine, and cellular immunity are moderately depleted, a marasmus or starvation state is noted (albumin may be normal). If both are depleted, it is a mixed state. Because the nutrition status at the time of admission in the elderly population correlates with the risk of subsequent complications, even when selected non-nutritional factors are controlled, protein and caloric intake and weight must be determined when making a diagnosis. Albumin and weight loss are essential parameters. The nutrition diagnosis should be documented.[119]

**Table 4–23.** Criteria for Nutrition Referral to Specialty Clinics

| |
|---|
| *High-Risk Infant Clinic* |
| Seizure disorder |
| Hydrocephalus |
| Multiple congenital anomalies |
| Chromosomal anomalies |
| Condition requiring neurosurgical intervention |
| Metabolic disorders |
| Fetal drug and alcohol syndromes |
| Congenital infectious diseases: STORCH (syphilis, toxoplasmosis, rubella, cytomegalovirus, herpes) |
| Any question of developmental disorder |
| *Myelomeningocele Clinic* |
| Age <5 yr |
| Weight >50th or <5th percentile or discrepancy in height and weight |
| Mobility loss >25% |
| Mechanical feeding problems |
| Premenarchal adolescent girls |
| Certain conditions such as allergy, diarrhea, excessive use of vitamins or medications, food faddism |
| *Cerebral Palsy Clinic* |
| Height <10th percentile and weight >75th percentile |
| Mobility loss <25% |
| Sudden weight loss or gain |
| Mechanical or behavioral feeding problems |
| Gastrointestinal problems (especially diarrhea or constipation) |
| Conditions that affect food intake, such as allergy, vegetarianism, low income, food faddism, excessive use of vitamins or medications, family problems |
| Parents' request for nutrition consultation |

## MID-LEVEL ASSESSMENT

The mid-level nutritional assessment is performed in outpatient clinics, such as the high-risk infant (Early Intervention), myelomeningocele, and cerebral palsy clinics at CCDDD. The criteria for referral to these clinics are shown in Table 4–23. The CCDDD nutritionist participates in assessing the nutritional status of children referred for nutrition problems to the clinic. This evaluation requires about 20 minutes per child as part of the interdisciplinary team assessment or involving only the nutrition discipline. Nutrition record forms used for mid-level assessment in these clinics are shown in Appendix 4.

The child's calorie, protein, fluid, and basic nutrient needs are determined, as well as the caregiver's knowledge of calorie expenditure, nutrition, fiber, and fluid needs. Developmental milestones, drug interactions, anthropometric measurements, physical activity, biochemical signs, physical signs, and socioeconomic condition should also be assessed. The interpretation or summary is structured as subjective, objective, assessment, and plan (SOAP), with specified recommendations, follow-up, and goals including a timetable and measurement methods. A 3-day diet/physical activity diary is collected if the child is determined to be at high nutritional risk (food summary score <10; see "Dietary History").

Children with feeding problems often require additional nutrition follow-up.[120–130] The BEE equation multiplied by a 1.3 stress factor (with weight adjusted by 50%) gave the best energy expenditure value for mechanically ventilated patients.[131] African-American children appear to have a lower REE, which should be used in determining energy needs.[132] Fruit and vegetable intake has been correlated with increased bone mass in girls in early puberty and may require follow-up.[133] Weight management is a major concern in follow-up for children with disabilities[134]; guidelines for exercise testing provides some assistance in this area.[135]

## MINI-LEVEL ASSESSMENT

The mini-level nutritional assessment is an interdisciplinary evaluation that frequently is performed in the community (see Table 4–1). The nurse or teacher may evaluate the physical and behavioral conditions of the child (see the Screening/Mini-Evaluation in Appendix 4), which are often closely related to the nutritional status. The nutritionist may obtain information on height and weight and some other physical signs (e.g., mouth, eyes, hair, skin, nails). A 100-point food frequency list based on the USDA MyPlate model, with emphasis on whole grains, increased fiber, and high-density nutrients, may be useful in the mini- and mid-level assessments (see Appendix 4). The social worker may obtain information on food purchasing or preparation while making the home visit. The occupational therapist, dentist, or physician may obtain information on feeding problems. The mini-assessment may also function as a screening device for nutrition problems.

Family-centered care for children with special health care needs is of special importance in the interdisciplinary mini-level evaluation.[136] Public Law 99-457 authorizes early intervention programs for infants and toddlers with potential developmental delays. Development of individualized family service plans requires specialized education in pediatric nutrition for children with developmental disorders (behavioral and feeding skills), cultural diversity, community nutrition, and interdisciplinary teams (see Chapter 5 on community programs). When preschool children appear cognitively ready to learn about food, nutrition, and health, greater effort must be made to educate them about vegetables and fruits[137] and early increased physical activity.[138] Nutrition education programs for parents of children in the Head Start program have had a positive effect on the quality of the diet for their children. Reliable tools are being developed to assess hunger and food insecurity.[139] These tools need to be culturally sensitive.[140] Ideas of health promotion/prevention[141] as primary nutrition, and nutrition services for the special health care needs of children as secondary nutrition, are essential.

## SUMMARY

Individuals with IDD can be at an increased nutritional risk because of problems associated with eating and swallowing, food medication interactions, metabolic disorders, decreased mobility, psychosocial aspects, and environmental issues. Nutritional assessment of the child or adult with a developmental disability or chronic illness uses five parameters: diet and physical activity, biochemical signs, anthropometric measurements, physical signs, and feeding or eating. Physical and clinical signs are often the last to appear when nutrients are deficient. Assessment of dietary intake is often the initial indicator that deficiencies or excesses are occurring. The level of assessment employed—in-depth, mid-level, or mini-level—depends on the problem, the age of the person, and the time and expertise available.

For persons with nutritional and developmental disorders, it is important to assess the level of support and assistance needed to carry out the nutrition plan as well as the participation and education of family members, caregivers, and the individual. The dietitian needs to consider effective approaches to communication and education with regard to the person's cognitive, intellectual, and physical abilities as well as those of the family or care providers. Behavioral responses or actions, both positive and negative, in individuals with IDD communicate wants, needs, and emotions.[13] Determining what the person is trying to communicate helps to identify appropriate supports and interventions needed to achieve outcomes.

When evaluating a person who has a syndrome or condition with which one are unfamiliar, it is important to take the time to research whether the condition has unique nutritional implications. Interpretation of the assessment findings or diagnosis and the follow-up or treatment plan by the nutritionist/dietitian is essential. Assessment often requires multiple measures or parameters in addition to use of clinical judgment.[13] The nutritionist/dietitian is the key in reducing health care costs by preventing nutrition problems or correcting these problems early so that the person can develop to his or her full potential.

Family-centered care for children with special health care needs is of special importance in the interdisciplinary mini-level evaluation.[136] P.L. 99-457 authorizes early intervention programs for infants and toddlers with potential developmental delays. Specialized education in pediatric nutrition with developmental disorders (behavioral and feeding skills), cultural diversity, community nutrition, and interdisciplinary teams is needed to develop the individualized family service plans. When preschool children appear cognitively ready to learn about food, nutrition, and health, greater effort must be made to educate them about vegetables and fruits[137] and early increased physical activity.[138] Nutrition education programs for parents of children in the Head Start program have had a positive effect on the quality of the diet for their children. Reliable tools are being developed to assess hunger and food insecurity.[139] These tools need to be culturally sensitive.[140] Ideas of health promotion/prevention[141] as primary nutrition, and nutrition services for adults with developmental disabilities as well as the special health-care needs of children as secondary nutrition, are essential.

Successful development of the individual's nutrition care plan requires an interdisciplinary approach to person-centered planning involving the person, family, care providers, and other health care professionals. Nutritional assessment recommendations should address implementation of the nutrition plan, including education and training, monitoring, and documentation of progress in achieving nutrition outcomes; these are essential elements for an effective plan and team process. The interdisciplinary approach to nutrition care can be the most effective way to assist individuals to achieve desired nutrition outcomes.

### References


1. Lacey K, Pritchett E. Nutrition care process and model: ADA adopts road map to quality care and outcomes management. *J Am Diet Assoc.* 2003; 103:1061.
2. Writing Group of the Nutrition Care Process/Standardized Language Committee. Nutrition care process and model part 1: the 2008 update. *J Am Diet Assoc.* 2008; 108:1113.
3. Academy of Nutrition and Dietetics Evidence Analysis Library. Nutrition screening: definitions and criteria. 2014. http://andevidencelibrary.com/topic.cfm?cat=3958. Accessed May 23, 2016.
4. Cober MP, Robinson D, Adams S, et al. *American Society for Parenteral and Enteral Nutrition (A.S.P.E.N.): Definitions of Terms, Styles, and Conventions Used in A.S.P.E.N. Board of Directors–Approved Documents.* May 2015. http://www.nutritioncare.org/Clinical_practice_Library/. Accessed May 26, 2016.
5. S. Ekvall and Staff, Cincinnati Center of the Division of Developmental Disabilities. *xxx*. Cincinnati, OH: Children's Hospital Medical Center.
6. White JV, Guenter P, Jensen G, et al. Consensus statement of the Academy of Nutrition and Dietetics/American Society for Parenteral and Enteral Nutrition: characteristics recommended for the identification and documentation of adult malnutrition (undernutrition). *J Acad Nutr Diet.* 2012; 112:730.
7. Becker PJ, Carney LN, Corkins MR, et al. Consensus statement of the Academy of Nutrition and Dietetics/American Society for Parenteral and Enteral Nutrition: indicators recommended for the identification and documentation of pediatric malnutrition (undernutrition). *J Acad Nutr Diet.* 2014; 114:1988.
8. Winick M, ed. *Nutrition, Pre- and Postnatal Development.* New York: Kluwer Academic/Plenum; 1979.
9. DeLong GR. Effects of nutrition on brain development in humans. *Am J Clin Nutr.* 1993; 57(Suppl):286S.
10. Ivanovic DM, Leiva BP, Perez HT, et al. Nutritional status, brain development and scholastic achievement of Chilean high-school graduates from high and low intellectual quotient and socio-economic status. *Br J Nutr.* 2002; 87:81.
11. Simko M, Cowell C, Gilbride J. *Nutrition Assessment: A Guide for Planning Intervention*, 2nd ed. Burlington, MA: Jones & Bartlett; 1995.
12. Waterlow JC. *Protein-Energy Malnutrition.* London: Edward Arnold; 1992.
13. Cushing P, Spear D, Novak P, et al. Academy of Nutrition and Dietetics: standards of practice and standards of professional performance for Registered Dietitians (Competent, Proficient, and Expert) in intellectual and developmental disabilities. *J Acad Nutr Diet.* 2012; 112;1454.
14. Cushing P, Spear D, Geerts S, et al. *The Adult with Intellectual and Developmental Disabilities: A Resource Tool for Nutritional Professionals.* Behavioral Health Nutrition Dietetic Practice Group of the Academy of Nutrition and Dietetics. Chicago: Academy of Nutrition and Dietetics; 2008.
15. Position of the Academy of Nutrition and Dietetics: nutrition services for individuals with intellectual and developmental disabilities and special health care needs. *J Nutr Diet.* 2015; 115;593.
16. Twin Cities District Dietetic Association. Enteral and parenteral nutrition support. In: *Manual of Pediatric Nutrition.* Minneapolis, MN: Turner Publishing Company; 1998.
17. Heller KE, Sohn W, Burt BA, Feigal RJ. Water consumption and nursing characteristics of infants by race and ethnicity. *J. Public Health Dent.* 2000; 60:140.
18. Kleiner SM. Water: an essential but overlooked nutrient. *J. Am. Diet Assoc.* 1999; 99:200.
19. Life Sciences Research Office, Federation of American Societies for Experimental Biology. *Nutrition Monitoring in the United States: An Update Report on Nutrition Monitoring.* Prepared for the U.S. Department of Agriculture and the U.S. Department of Health and Human Services. USDHHS Publication No. (PHS) 89-1255. Public Health Service, Washington, DC: U.S. Government Printing Office; 1989.
20. Lohman TG, Roche AF, Martorell M. *Anthropometric Standardization Reference Manual.* Champaign, IL: Human Kinetics Books; 1988.
21. Chumlea WC, Roche AF. Nutritional anthropometric assessment of non-ambulatory persons using recumbent techniques. *Am J Anthrop.* 1984; 63:1.
22. Ogden CL, Kuczmarski RJ, Flegal KM, et al. Centers for Disease Control and Prevention 2000 growth charts for the United States: improvements to the 1977 National Center for Health Statistics version. *Pediatrics.* 2002; 109:45.
23. Roche AF, Davila GH. Differences between recumbent length and stature within individuals. *Growth.* 1974; 38:313.
24. Garn S. The anthropometric assessment of nutritional status. In: Smith MA, ed. *Guides for Nutritional Assessment of the Mentally Retarded and the Developmentally Disabled.* Proceedings of the Third National Nutrition Workshop for Nutritionists from University Affiliated Facilities, sponsored by the Bureau of Community Health Services. Memphis, TN: The Child Development Center, University of Tennessee Center for Health Services.
25. Gurney JM, Jelliffe DB. Arm anthropometry in nutritional assessment: a nomogram for rapid calculation of muscle circumference and cross-sectional muscle and fat areas. *Am J Clin Nutr.* 1973; 26:912.
26. Heymsfield S, McManus C, Smith J, Stevens V, Nikon D. Anthropometric measurement of muscle mass: revised equations for calculating bone-free arm muscle area. *Am J Clin Nutr.* 1982; 36:680.
27. Trowbridge F, Hiner C, Robertson A. Arm muscle indicators and creatinine excretion in children. *Am J Clin Nutr.* 1982; 36:691.
28. Bray GA, Champagne CM. Obesity and the metabolic syndrome: implications for dietetics practitioners. *J Am Diet Assoc.* 2004; 104:86.
29. Centers for Disease Control and Prevention. Division of Nutrition, Physical Activity, and Obesity, National Center for Chronic Disease Prevention and Health Promotion. *About Child and Teen BMI.* Last updated May 15, 2015. http://www.cdc.gov/healthyweight/assessing/bmi/childrens_bmi/about_childrens_bmi.html.
30. Mei Z, Grummer-Strawn LM, Pietrobelli A, Goulding A, Goran MI, Dietz WH. Validity of body mass index compared with other body-composition screening indexes for the assessment of body fatness in children and adolescents. *Am J Clin Nutr.* 2002; 75:978.
31. Johnston FE. Validity of triceps skinfold and relative weight as measures of adolescent obesity. *J Adolesc Health Care.* 1985; 6:185.
32. Belt-Niebala B, Ekvall S, Mai Cook C, Oppenheimer S, Wessel J. Linear growth measurement: a comparison of single arm-lengths and arm-span. *Dev Med Child Neurol.* 1986; 28:319.
33. Taicher GZ, Tinsley FC, Reiderman A, Heiman ML. Quantitative magnetic resonance (QMR) method for bone and whole-body composition analysis. *Anal Bioanal Chem.* 2003; 377:990.

34. Steiner MC, Barton RL, Singh SJ, Morgan MD. Bedside methods versus dual energy X-ray absorptiometry for body composition measurement in COPD. *Eur Respir J.* 2002; 19: 626.
35. Salvatoni A, Brambilla P, Deiana M, Nespoli L. Application of DEXA in body composition assessment in children. *Ann Diagn Paediatr Pathol* 1998; 2:49.
36. Lukaski HC, Bolonchuk WW, Siders WA, et al. Chromium supplementation and resistance training: effects of body composition, strength, and trace element status of men. *Am J Clin Nutr.* 1996; 63:954.
37. Guo SM, Roche AF, Houtkooper L. Fat-free mass in children and young adults predicted from bioelectric impedance and anthropometric variables. *Am J Clin Nutr.* 1989; 50:435.
38. Slaughter MW, Lohman TG, Boileau RA, et al. Skinfold equations for estimations of body fatness in children and youth. *Human Biol.* 1988; 60:709.
39. Rimmer J, Riley B, Wang E, Rauworth A, Jurkowski J. Physical activity participation among persons with disabilities: Barriers and facilitators. *Am J Prev Med.* 2004; 26:419.
40. Mitchell L, Zivianni J, Boyd R. Characteristics associated with physical activity among independently ambulant children and adolescents with unilateral cerebral palsy. *Dev Med Child Neur.* 2014; 57:;167.
41. Heller T, McCubbin J, Drum C, Peterson J. Physical activity and nutrition health promotion interventions: what is working for people with intellectual disabilities? *Intellect Dev Disabil.* 2011; 49:26.
42. Bartlo P, Klein P. Physical activity benefits and needs in adults with intellectual disabilities: systematic review of the literature. *Am J Intellect Dev Disabil.* 2011; 116:220.
43. Hsieh K, Heller T, Bershadsky J, Taub S. Impact of adulthood stage and social-environmental context on body mass index and physical activity of individuals with intellectual disability. *Intellect Dev Disabil.* 2015; 53:100.
44. Schijndel-Speet M, Evenhuis H, Wijck R, Empelen P, Echteld M. Facilitators and barriers to physical activity as perceived by older adults with intellectual disability. *Intellect Dev Disabil.* 2014; 52:175.
45. Pett M, Clark L, Eldredge A, et al. Effecting healthy lifestyle changes in overweight and obese young adults with intellectual disability. *Am J Intellect Dev Disabil.* 2013; 118:224.
46. Roza A, Shizgal H. The Harris-Benedict equation reevaluated: resting energy requirements and body cell mass. *Am J Clin Nutr.* 1984; 40:168.
47. Black AE, Cole TJ. Within- and between-subject variation in energy expenditure measured by the doubly-labelled water technique: implications for validating reported dietary energy intake. *Eur J Clin Nutr.* 2000; 54:386.
48. Bandini LG, Schoeller DA, Fukagawa NK, Wykes LJ, Dietz WH. Body composition and energy expenditure in adolescents with cerebral palsy or myelodysplasia. *Pediatr Res.* 1991; 29:70.
49. Grogan CB, Ekvall SM. Body composition of children with myelomeningocele, determined by $^{40}$K, urinary creatinine and anthropometric measures. *J Am Coll Nutr.* 1999; 18:316.
50. McCardle WD, Katch FI, Katch VI. *Exercise Physiology: Energy, Nutrition, and Human Performance.* Philadelphia: Lippincott, Williams & Wilkins; 2001.
51. Blackburn GL, Bistrian BR, Maini BS, Schlamm HT, Smith MF. Nutritional and metabolic assessment of the hospitalized patient. *JPEN J Parenter Enteral Nutr.* 1977; 1:11.
52. Seashore J. Nutrition support of children. *Yale J Biol Med.* 1984; 51:111.
53. American Diabetes Association. *The Official Pocket Guide to Diabetic Exchanges: Choose Your Foods,* 3rd ed. Alexandria, VA: American Diabetes Association; 2011.
54. McLaren DS. Nutritional assessment. In: McLaren DS, Burman D, eds. *Textbook of Pediatric Nutrition*, 2nd ed. New York: Churchill-Livingstone; 1982.
55. Moore W, Roche A, eds. *Pediatric Anthropometry*, 3rd ed. Columbus, OH: Ross Laboratories; 1987.
56. Lukaski H. Methods for assessment of human body composition: traditional and new. *J Am Clin Nutr.* 1987; 46:537.
57. Weinsier RL, Butterworth CEJr. *Handbook of Clinical Nutrition.* St. Louis: Mosby; 1981.
58. Ervin D, Williams A, Merrick J. Primary care: mental and behavioral health and persons with intellectual and developmental disabilities. Pediatric Faculty Publications, Paper 158. *Front Public Health.* 2014;2:76.
59. Rimmer JH, Hsieh K. Longitudinal health and intellectual disability study on obesity and health risk behaviors. Presented at the State of Science Conference on Lifespan Health and Function of Adults with Intellectual Disabilities: Translating Research into Practice, Bethesda, MD; May 26, 2011: 57. http://www.aucd.org/docs/ncbddd/May%20 2011%20ID%20Surveillance/Health%20Frontier%20meeting%20proceedings.pdf
60. Holmes TH. The social readjustment rating scale. *J Psychosom Res.* 1967; 11:213.
61. Spielberger CD, Gorsuch RL, Lushene RE. *STAI Manual for the State-Trait Anxiety Inventory: Self-Evaluation Questionnaire.* Palo Alto, CA: Consulting Psychologists Press; 1970.
62. Beck A, Ward C, Mendelson M, Mock J, Erbaugh J. An inventory for measuring depression. *Arch Gen Psychiatry.* 1961; 4:561.
63. Liem BJ, Holland JM, Kang MY, Hoffelt SC, Marquez CM. Karnofsky Performance Status Assessment: resident versus attending. *J Cancer Educ* 2002; 17:138.
64. Padilla GV, Presant C, Grant MM, Metter G, Lipsett J, Heide F. Quality of life index for patients with cancer. *Res Nurs Health.* 1983; 6:117.
65. Spitzer WO, Dobson AJ, Hall J, Measuring the quality of life of cancer patients: a concise QL-index for use by physicians. *J Chronic Dis.* 1981; 34:585.
66. McNair D, Lorr M, Droppleman L. *EITS Manual for the Profile of Mood States.* San Diego, CA: Educational and Industrial Testing Service; 1981.
67. Elkind D. *The Hurried Child: Growing Up Too Fast Too Soon*, 3rd ed. Cambridge, MA: Perseus; 2001.
68. Hulanecha B, Korlarg F. The final phase of growth in height. *Ann Human Biol.* 1983; 1:429.
69. Harnack L, Stang J, Story M. Soft drink consumption among U.S. children and adolescents: nutritional consequences. *J Am Diet Assoc.* 1999; 99:436.
70. Stang J, Bayer CT. Position of the American Dietetic Association: child and adolescent food and nutrition programs. *J Am Diet Assoc.* 2003; 103:887.
71. Roberston R, Williams A, Sward K, et al. A comparison of skinfolds and leg-to-leg bioelectrical impedance for the assessment of body composition in children. *Dyn Med.* 2003; 26:5.
72. Stang J, Story MT, Harnack L, Neumark-Sztainer D. Relationships between vitamin and mineral supplement use, dietary intake and dietary adequacy among adolescents. *J Am Diet Assoc.* 2000; 100:905.
73. Dwyer JT, Stone EJ, Yang M, et al. Prevalence of marked overweight and obesity in a multiethnic pediatric population: findings from the Child and Adolescent Trial for Cardiovascular Health (CATCH) study. *J Am Diet Assoc.* 2000; 100:1149.
74. Neutzling MB, Taddei JA, Gigante DP. Risk factors of obesity among Brazilian adolescents: a case-control study. *Public Health Nutr.* 2003; 6:743.
75. Jensen DV, Noerholm V, Martiny K, Bech P. The internal and external validity of the Major Depression Inventory in measuring severity of depressive states. *Psychol Med.* 2003; 33:351.
76. Golding L, Meyers C, Sinning W. *The Y's Way to Physical Fitness*, 3rd ed. Champaign, IL: Human Kinetics Books; 1989.
77. Rogol A, Clark R, Roemmich JN. Growth and pubertal development in children and adolescents: effects of diet and physical activity. *Am J Clin Nutr.* 2000; 72(Suppl):521S.
78. Maynard LM, Wisemandle E, Roche AF, Chumlea WC, Guo SS, Siervogel RM. Childhood body composition in relation to body mass index. *Pediatrics.* 2001; 107:334.
79. American Dietetic Association. Position of the American Dietetic Association: integration of medical nutrition therapy and pharmacotherapy. *J Am Diet Assoc.* 2010; 110:950.
80. Wiecha JL, Dwyer JT, Dunn-Strohecker M. Nutrition and health services needs among the homeless. *Public Health Rep.* 1991; 106:364.
81. Luder E, Cupens-Okado E, Karen-Roth A, Martinez-Weber C. Health and nutrition survey in a group of urban homeless adults. *J Am Diet Assoc.* 1990; 90:1387.
82. Johnson LJ, McCool AC. Dietary intake and nutritional status of older adult homeless women: a pilot study. *J Nutr Elder.* 2003; 23:1.
83. American Academy of Pediatrics (AAP) Committee on Children with Disabilities. Care coordination: integrating health and related systems of care for children with special health care needs. *Pediatrics.* 1999; 104:978.
84. Krick J, Murphy-Miller P, Zeger S, Wright E. Pattern of growth in children with cerebral palsy. *J Am Diet Assoc.* 1996; 97:680.
85. LaFollette P, Ekvall S, Oppenheimer S. Effect of level of lesion and quality of ambulation on growth chart measurements in children with myelomeningocele: a pilot study. *J Am Diet Assoc.* 1992; 92:7.
86. Stevenson R. Feeding and nutrition in children with developmental disabilities. *Pediatr Ann.* 1995; 24:255.
87. Tolia V, Ventimiglia J, Kuhns L. Gastrointestinal tolerance of a pediatric fiber formula in developmentally disabled children. *J Am Coll Nutr.* 1997; 16:224.
88. Smit E, Crespo CJ. Dietary intake and nutritional status of U.S. adult marijuana users: results from the Third National Health and Nutrition Examination Survey. *Public Health Nutr.* 2001; 4:781.
89. Thomas AG, Akobeng AK. Technical aspects of feeding the disabled child. *Clin Nutr Metab Care.* 2000; 3:221.
90. Stacy M, Holt K, Sopha D. *Bright Futures in Practice: Nutrition.* Washington, DC: Georgetown University, National Center for Education, Maternal and Child Health; 2000.
91. Morris SE, Klein MD. *Pre-Feeding Skills: Comprehensive Resources for Mealtime Development,* 2nd ed. Tucson, AZ: Communication Skills Builders; 2003.
92. Nadas AS, Fyler DC, eds. *Pediatric Cardiology*, 3rd ed. Philadelphia: Saunders; 1972.
93. Lewis G, Ekvall S, Ekvall V. Neurologic handicapping conditions. In: *The A.S.P.E.N. Nutrition Support Practice Manual.* Silver Spring, MD: American Society for Parenteral and Enteral Nutrition; 1998.
94. Marra MV, Boyer AP. Position of the American Dietetic Association: nutrient supplementation *J Am Diet Assoc.* 2009; 109:2073.
95. Ekvall S, Ekvall V. Nutrition support for children with developmental delays. In: Baker S, Baker R, Davis A, eds. *Pediatric Nutrition Support.* Sudbury, MA: Jones and Bartlett Publishers; 2005.
96. Van Horn L. Nutritional assessment and treatment strategies. Buehler Center on Aging, McGaw Medical Center, Northwestern University. Chicago: Galter Health Sciences Library. Last updated June 9, 1999. http://www.galter.northwestern.edu/geriatrics/chapters/nutritional_assessment.cfm.
97. Kleinmann RE, Committee on Nutrition. *Pediatric Nutrition Handbook*, 5th ed. Elk Grove Village, IL: American Academy of Pediatrics; 2004.
98 Keshaviah PR, Nolph KD, Moore HL, et al. Lean body mass estimation by creatinine kinetics. *J Am Soc Nephrol.* 1994; 4:1475.
99. Beck FK, Rosenthal TC. Prealbumin: a marker for nutritional evaluation. *Am Family Physician.* 2002; 65:1575.
100. Kasvosve I, Delanghe J. Total iron binding capacity and transferrin concentration in the assessment of iron status. *Clin Chem Lab Med.* 2000; 40:1014.
101. Mullen JL, Buzby GP, Waldman MT, Gertner MH, Hobbs CL, Rosato EF. Prediction of operative morbidity and mortality by preoperative nutritional assessment. *Surg Forum.* 1979; 30:80.
102. Wong JC, Lewindon P, Mortimer R, Shepherd R. Bone mineral density in adolescent females with recently diagnosed anorexia nervosa. *Int J Eat Disord.* 2001; 29:11.
103. Cameron JR, Mazess RB, Sorenson JA. Precision and accuracy of bone mineral determination by direct photon absorptiometry. *Invest Radiol.* 1968; 3:141.
104. Namsung R, Tsang RC. Factors affecting newborn bone mineral content: in utero effects on newborn bone mineralization. *Proc Nutr Soc.* 2000; 59:55.

105. San Roman P, Palma JC, Otec MD, Nevado E. Skeletal maturation determined by cervical vertebrae development. *Eur J Orthod.* 2002; 24:303.
106. Steiner MC, Barton RL, Singh SJ, Morgan MD. Bedside methods versus dual energy X-ray absorptiometry for body composition measurement in COPD. *Eur Respir J.* 2002; 19: 626.
107. Anderson J. Dietary calcium and bone mass through the life cycle. *Nutr Today* 1990; 2:9.
108. Kestin M, Clifton P, Belling GB, Nestel PJ. n-3 fatty acids of marine origin lower systolic blood pressure and triglycerides but raise LDL cholesterol compared with n-3 and n-6 fatty acids from plants. *Am J Clin Nutr.* 1990; 51:1028.
109. Halpern A, Mancini MC. Treatment of obesity: an update on anti-obesity medications. *Obes Rev.* 2003; 4:25.
110. Gillum RF. Indices of adipose tissue distribution, apolipoproteins B and A1, lipoprotein (a), and triglyceride concentration in children aged 4–11 years. The Third National Health and Nutrition Examination Survey. *J Clin Epidemiol.* 2001; 54:367.
111. Shenkin A, Cederblad G, Elia M, Isaksson B, International Federation of Clinical Chemistry. Laboratory assessment of protein-energy status. *Clin Chim Acta* 1996; 253(1–2):S5.
112. Batterham RL, Bloom SR. The gut hormone peptide YY regulates appetite. *Ann N Y Acad Sci.* 2003; 994:162.
113. Schroder H, Schmelz E, Marrugat J. Relationship between diet and blood pressure in a representative Mediterranean population. *Eur J Nutr.* 2002; 41:161.
114. Bartali B, Salvini S, Turrini A, et al. Age and disability affect dietary intake. *J Nutr.* 2003; 133:2868.
115. Mercer KC, Ekvall SW. Comparing the diets of adults with mental retardation who live in intermediate care facilities and in group homes. *J Am Diet Assoc.* 1992; 92:356.
116. O'Brien G, Whitehouse A. A psychiatric study of deviant eating behavior among multiply handicapped adults. *Br J Psychiatry.* 1990; 157:281.
117. O'Brien G. The classification of problem behaviour in Diagnostic Criteria for Psychiatric Disorders for Use with Adults with Learning Disabilities/Mental Retardation (DC-LD). *J Intellect Disabil Res.* 2003; 47(Suppl 1):32.
118. Shuran M, Nelson R. Updated nutritional assessment and support of the elderly. *Geriatrics.* 1986; 41:48.
119. Sullivan D, Patch G, Walls R, Lipschitz D. Impact of nutrition status on morbidity and mortality in a select population of geriatric rehabilitation patients. *Am J Clin Nutr.* 1990; 51:749.
120. Okosun IS, Liao Y, Rotimi CN, Dever GE, Cooper RS. Impact of birth weight on ethnic variations in subcutaneous and central adiposity in American children aged 5–11 years. A study from the Third National Health and Nutrition Examination Survey. *Int J Obes Relat Metab Disord.* 2000; 24:479.
121. Throughton KE, Hill AE. Relation between objectively measured feeding competence and nutrition in children with cerebral palsy. *Dev Med Child Neurol.* 2001; 43:187.
122. Cunningham JJ. Body composition and nutrition support in pediatrics: what to defend and how soon to begin. *Nutr Clin Pract.* 1995; 10:177.
123. Littlewood RA, Wotten M, Trocki O, Shepherd RW, Shepherd K. Reduced body cell mass following severe head injury in children: implications for rehabilitation. *Pediatr Rehabil.* 1999; 3:95.
124. Tse P, Leung S, Chan T, Sien A, Chan A. Dietary fiber intake and constipation in children with severe developmental disabilities. *J Paediatr Child Health.* 2000; 36:236.
125. Spender Q, Stein A, Dennis J, Reilly S, Percy E, Cave D. An exploration of feeding difficulties in children with Down syndrome. *Dev Med Child Neurol.* 1996; 38:681.
126. Tawfik R, Dickson A, Clarke M, Thomas AG. Caregivers' perceptions following gastrostomy in severely disabled children with feeding problems. *Dev Med Child Neurol.* 1997; 39:746.
127. Trier E, Thomas AG. Feeding the disabled child. *Nutrition.* 1998; 14:801.
128. Hawdon JM, Beauregard N, Slattery J, Kennedy G. Identification of neonates at risk of developing feeding problems in infancy. *Dev Med Child Neurol.* 2000; 42:235.
129. Ekvall B, Ekvall V. High sodium and low calcium, vitamin D, magnesium and physical activity in children with developmental disorders and the general population. In: Elmadfa I, Konig J, eds. 17th International Congress of Nutrition, Vienna, Austria, Aug 2001. *Ann Nutr Metab* 2001; 45(Suppl 1):A231.
130. Manikam R, Perman J. Pediatric feeding disorders. *J Clin Gastroenterol.* 2000; 30:34.
131. Barak N. Assessment of resting energy expenditure in mechanically ventilated patients. *Am J Clin Nutr.* 2004; 79:341.
132. DeLang J, Bray G, Harsha D, Volaufova J. Energy expenditure in African-American and white boys and girls in a 2-year follow-up of the Baton Rouge Children's Study. *Am J Clin Nutr.* 2004; 79:268.
133. Tylavsky FA, Holliday K, Danish R, Womack C, Norwood J, Carbone L. Fruit and vegetable intakes are an independent predictor of bone size in early pubertal children. *Am J Clin Nutr.* 2004; 79:311.
134. Ekvall S, Ekvall V. Obesity in myelomeningocele: dietetics in physical medicine and rehabilitation network. *Am Diet Assoc.* 1997; 17:2.
135. *Guidelines for Exercise Testing and Prescription*, 6th ed. Philadelphia: Lippincott, Williams & Wilkins; 2000.
136. Ekvall S. Obesity in children. *Exceptional Parent.* 2003; 33(6):102.
137. Griebble L, Falciglia G, Davis A, Couch S. A curriculum based on social learning theory emphasizing food exposure and positive parent-child feeding strategies: a pilot study. *J Am Diet Assoc.* 2003; 103:100.
138. Wells JC, Ritz P. Physical activity at 9–12 months and fatness at 2 years of age. *Am J Human Biol.* 2001; 13:384.
139. Holben DH, American Dietetic Association. Position of the American Dietetic Association: food insecurity in the United States. *J Am Diet Assoc.* 2010; 110:1368.
140. Ekvall S, Stevens F, eds. *Empowering Children Through Early Intervention with Good Nutrition: Focusing on Culturally Diverse Children with Special Health Care Needs.* Manual IV. Cincinnati: University of Cincinnati Publications; 2002.
141. Slawson DL Fitzgerald N, Morgan KT. Position of the Academy of Nutrition and Dietetics: the role of nutrition in health promotion and chronic disease prevention. *J Acad Nutr Diet.* 2013; 113:972.

# 5 Community-Based Nutrition Services and Resources

CECILIA ROKUSEK, SHARON FEUCHT, LISA KELCHNER, AND JOAN EARLE HAHN

This chapter provides an overview of resources for individuals with special needs, including physical or intellectual disabilities and chronic disease impacting persons throughout the lifespan. Resources for infants, children, adolescents, adults, and older adults are discussed. As the number of persons with intellectual and developmental disabilities (IDD) living to age 55 years and older increases, focused attention is being given to this growing older adult population (see Chapter 61).

## INTRODUCTION

Significant advances in research and practice over the past 25 years have advanced understanding of the importance of nutritional care for persons with IDD and challenging chronic diseases. As a result, knowledge and resources have expanded at the local, state, national, and international levels. The American Academy of Nutrition and Dietetics reaffirms the importance of nutrition for persons with IDD throughout the lifespan.[1] Nutrition is essential to life, development, longevity, and overall quality of life for everyone. This chapter provides a guide for dietitians, nutritionists, and interprofessional practitioners to identify the nutrition resources available to them as they work to provide nutrition planning for persons with IDD throughout the lifespan. Resources include training, funding, and replicable materials for use and dissemination to persons with IDD, their families, and carepartners.

Even though understanding of the importance of good nutrition for individuals with IDD has increased significantly over the past 20 years, the connection between nutrition and the overall wellness of persons with IDD has still not been achieved. There continues to be a lack of access to high-quality interprofessional practice and ongoing intervention that should include nutrition. Further, there is an inadequate preparation of health care providers to meet the interprofessional needs of persons with IDD.[2] Overall, individuals with IDD and their families are not involved enough in public health and prevention activities focused on nutrition, exercise, and overall wellness. This paucity of attention to prevention activities has led to an increased incidence of chronic diseases among individuals of all ages with IDD.[3] When examining the overall community response and identification of resources, one must look at all of the programs available to the entire community that focus on prevention and healthy lifestyles, and persons of all ages with IDD should be included.[4] These individuals should be connected to the entire primary health care system, which should be focused on individual patient-centered, coordinated, and collaborative care that emphasizes health and wellness throughout the lifespan.

When identifying resources in the community related to the nutritional well-being of individuals with IDD, no matter what the age, one must examine all of the interprofessionally related resources that interact with nutrition. Most commonly, these include dentistry, occupational therapy, physical therapy, medicine, nursing, and speech and language pathology.

## SERVICES AND RESOURCES FOR CHILDREN

The need for nutrition services for children with special health care needs (CSHCN) has increased significantly in communities throughout the country. Deinstitutionalization, integrated community living programs, supported employment options, least-restrictive learning environments, worksites for adolescents, full integration in the school systems, and a philosophy of inclusion or normalcy continue as the mandates of community-based systems to serve the education, social, and health care needs of all persons with special needs. These directives challenge nutrition professionals to focus more efforts on the community setting, which can include the home, the clinic, early intervention services, and the school.

Because the nutrition needs of those with developmental disabilities vary, as do the skills required to meet those needs, the interprofessional role of the nutrition professional has become increasingly important as a key member of the health care team. It is essential that the nutritionist focusing on developmental disabilities work closely with the parents or primary caregivers, allied health professionals and nurses (e.g., speech clinicians, physical therapists), physicians, food service personnel (in a school setting), teachers, and health care financing agencies (i.e., insurance companies and federal and state entitlement programs).[5]

The interprofessional team approach enhances a sense of cooperation among all professionals united by a common goal of achieving optional medical and nutritional support for all individuals. More interprofessional training is needed to inform health care administrators and other team members about the impact of good nutrition for CSHCN including needs related to developmental disabilities and chronic illnesses. Training materials and programs are available, including information on cultural diversity.[6,7] The Maternal and Child Health Bureau (MCHB) also provides interprofessional training opportunities around the United States, including opportunities for nutrition training.[8]

Nutrition intervention for persons with developmental disabilities can be both preventive and restorative. The community environment may pose a challenge for persons seeking either preventive or restorative intervention. Registered dietitians (RDs) may not be available on a daily basis in the health care delivery system or in the community setting. These settings depend most on nutrition consultants to provide the direction and clinical expertise for persons with special needs. The consultant, whether in the health care setting, in the home, or elsewhere, must ensure that the individuals ongoing nutrition needs are met and that there is close collaboration with parents, teachers, and related health care professionals including nurses, speech therapists, physical therapists, occupational therapists, and social workers (Box 5–1). Unfortunately, many early intervention sites and schools do not employ a qualified nutrition professional, despite the need for services and the implied mandate in the Individuals with Disabilities Education Act (IDEA), discussed later.

Although the model for provision of services at the community level—in Head Start/Early Head Start programs, early intervention for infants and toddlers, schools, and adult service agencies—is primarily that of consultation, the enhanced role of nutrition services in the community delivery system will require more registered dietitians and nutritionists (RDNs) in the future. In general, nutrition professionals within community settings should strive to:

- Be advocates for nutrition services and funding and their incorporation throughout the interprofessional planning process for individuals requiring special nutrition and feeding interventions.
- Develop nutritional care that is family centered and coordinated with all other services provided.

**Box 5–1.** Nutrition Services for Children with Special Needs

The competencies listed in this document describe assessment, intervention, and follow-up services provided by nutritionists skilled in the delivery of nutrition services to high-risk children. Such individuals will have been credentialed by the Commission on Dietetic Registration of the American Dietetic Association and will be registered dietitians (RDs). They will have received specialized training and will be involved in continuing education addressing the needs of children at risk.

## *DIRECT CARE SERVICES*

I. *Perform Assessment*
  A. Nutrition Status
    1. Collect and interpret anthropometric and growth data.
    2. Assess clinical status with special attention to problems affecting nutritional status; define the need to refer.
    3. Assess dietary intake.
    4. If appropriate, collect feeding history, which may affect current food intake.
    5. Collect and/or assess the need to collect biochemical data.
    6. Collect medication information, which may affect nutrient needs.
    7. Collect data regarding mobility status and physical activity.
  B. Feeding Skills
    1. Assess feeding skill development, considering present level of function to determine normal versus delayed feeding skills.
    2. Assess oral motor development to determine normal, delayed, or pathological development and the need for referral to appropriate therapy.
    3. Evaluate appropriateness of food textures offered, based on feeding development.
  C. Feeding Behavior
    1. Collect information on caregiver-child interactions; if appropriate, observe feeding.
    2. Define non-eating behaviors (e.g., throwing food, refusing to eat, gagging), which affect nutrient intake.
    3. Define eating behaviors (e.g., pica, using fingers/utensils appropriately, stuffing food into the mouth), which affect feeding skill development.
  D. Feeding Environment
    1. Evaluate the feeding environment (i.e., equipment, timing of meals and snacks, sanitation, and safety).
    2. Assess caregiver's knowledge of food sources and appropriate foods for the child.
    3. Assess caregiver's economic ability to provide food for the child and use of available resources.
  E. Caregiver's Expectations
    1. Evaluate appropriateness of caregiver's expectations for feeding skills.
    2. Evaluate appropriateness of caregiver's expectations for quantity of food the child should consume.

II. *Develop Nutrition Care Plan*

III. *Provide Counseling and Consultation*
  A. Counsel caregiver regarding
    1. Improving nutrient deficiencies/excesses through food sources and/or supplements.
    2. Feeding skills and appropriate foods to support developmental progress.
    3. Management of feeding behaviors.
    4. Improvement of feeding environment within the framework of the individual's need, socioeconomic status, and lifestyle.
  B. Provide consultation to health care professionals (e.g., therapists, physician, public health nurse) in these methods for improving the child's nutrient and energy intake.
  C. Make referrals to appropriate health professionals and health care agencies.
  D. Participate in interagency and interprofessional team conferences to determine priorities for therapy, follow-up, and referral.

IV. *Monitor Effectiveness of Nutrition Care Plan and Counseling and Follow Up as Needed*

## *AGENCY AND CONSULTATIVE SERVICES*

I. *Nutrition Education*
  A. Collect and evaluate materials on nutrition and feeding for use by families, caregivers, and health professionals.
  B. Develop, arrange, conduct, and evaluate nutrition education programs for health professionals and the public.

II. *Policy Making and Program Planning*
  A. Identify individuals at nutritional risk by soliciting consumer and professional input.
  B. Assess nutrition and diet-related health problems in the community.
  C. Plan or participate in planning, developing, implementing, and evaluating the nutrition components of community programs.
  D. Consult with group centers or health agencies regarding nutrition standards and nutrition care criteria.

This document was prepared by the participants of the first short-term Nutrition and Handicapped Children Training Program of the Child Development and Mental Retardation Center, University of Washington. These activities were supported by the State of Washington Department of Social and Health Sciences, Bureau of Parent-Child Health Services (sponsoring number 1640-67510).

- Provide leadership in the development, implementation, and ongoing evaluation of an integrated nutrition services component.
- Work to develop an agency-specific nutrition program and manual outlining program requirements and policy standards.
- Provide ongoing technical assistance and in-service training in nutrition to other interprofessional staff.
- Work closely with state and private accreditation agencies on quality assurance.

Community nutrition programs at all levels must include the following components[5]:

- Screening
- Complete assessment
- Development of nutrition care plans through an individualized family service plan (IFSP), individualized education plan (IEP) or an individualized habilitation plan (IHP)
- Implementation of a nutrition care plan by an interprofessional team, including parents/guardians when appropriate
- Nutrition counseling focusing on the individual with special needs and his or her ability to follow through on the recommendations made
- Follow-up and referral to other community agencies when appropriate.

## RESOURCES THROUGHOUT THE LIFESPAN

The key to independent living and an enhanced quality of life is education and support that promotes inclusion and fosters a healthy lifestyle throughout the lifespan.[4] For example, overweight adults with Down syndrome most appropriately should join local weight loss groups rather than be put in a segregated, one-on-one weight loss program or a group program only for persons with developmental disabilities. Individuals with Down syndrome have a higher tendency toward overweight and obesity throughout life.[9]

Adults with intellectual disability have a higher prevalence of obesity and overweight compared with the general population.[10] In addition, individuals with IDD who are living in community settings have a higher prevalence of obesity and more elevated risk factors for cardiovascular disease and other chronic diseases than do other adults.[11–13]

As one assesses community resources to help reduce the problems associated with overweight and obesity, it is important to note that adults with intellectual disability who reside in community settings likely have adopted health behaviors similar to those of the general public.[14,15] Adults with IDD residing in community settings typically have elevated dietary fat intake and low fruit and vegetable intake, similar to the general public, and this is of growing serious concern. These dietary habits lead to an elevated body mass index and increased risk for development of adverse health conditions.[3,16]

In fact, nurse practitioners conducting an in-home preventive intervention with 84 adults ages 29 to 68 years with IDD in the community reported using nursing interventions to address nutritional health for at least two-thirds of the participants in the study. The majority (85%) received nursing intervention for health education, and four nursing interventions were most likely to occur together: weight management, nutrition management, health screening, and behavior management.[17] These findings support the need for follow-up with registered dietitians/nutritionists.

Promotion of health and prevention of secondary or other disabling conditions are essential. To address the need for education about health promotion, training programs for staff and health promotion interventions have been designed and adapted for individuals with developmental disabilities to include nutrition-specific interventions or combined interventions (e.g., physical activity and healthy eating). These programmatic interventions have shown effectiveness in a number of health outcomes.[8] All community resources should be identified carefully so that the most appropriate school or agency can deliver a comprehensive and fully integrated nutrition program.

The impact of nutrition services for persons with developmental disabilities is ongoing and lifelong. Nutrition services for the infant, child, adolescent, or adult with special needs should be integrated fully through the IEP and/or IHP. The age of the individual will determine the agency or school that can assist in the provision of appropriate nutrition services. Specific services and resources are described later.

## INDIVIDUALS WITH DISABILITIES ACT

The IDEA.[18] provides funds to states for the education of students with disabilities under a detailed service mandate. This law ensures that all children ages 3 through 21 years who are enrolled in public schools and need special education and related services receive a free, appropriate public education regardless of the level or severity of their disability. Because of the increasing number of medically fragile and technology-dependent children who are being fully integrated into the public schools, the role of the RD in the school system must be expanded.

The IDEA requires that states ensure that these children receive an IEP based on their specific needs in the least restrictive environment possible. The law also provides guidelines for determining what related services (e.g., transportation, augmentative or assistive devices, medical services) are needed and outlines a due process procedure to make sure that the rights of children with disabilities are fully protected.

School-age children and adolescents with special needs may also require specialized nutrition services. As part of the required services, and with emphasis on the least restrictive environment, children can participate in the National School Lunch and School Breakfast Programs.[19] Therefore, school lunch programs must provide special-needs children and adolescents with the assistance they need to meet their dietary requirements so that they can participate fully in the educational process.[20]

### Section 504 of the Rehabilitation Act and Education

Section 504 of the federal Rehabilitation Act of 1973 applies to elementary, secondary, and postsecondary schools and prohibits discrimination on the basis of disability in programs or activities that receive federal financial assistance. This law is enforced by the Office of Civil Rights and prohibits specific discriminatory activities, including the assignment of students with special disabilities to segregated classes or facilities. In elementary and secondary schools, children with disabilities may be assigned separate facilities or courses of special education only when such placement is necessary to provide them equal educational opportunities and when these facilities or services are comparable to the others. For more information on student placement under Section 504, visit the website of the US Department of Education Office of Civil Rights (http://www2.ed.gov/about/offices/list/ocr/docs/placpub.html).

### Early Intervention

In 1986, IDEA expanded to provide statewide early intervention services designed to help infants and toddlers with developmental delays or diagnosed disabilities. Federal assistance is provided to states to establish early intervention services for infants and toddlers with disabilities from birth to 3 years of age and their families.[21] The early intervention program is available in every state and is coordinated by a state's lead agency. This agency must ensure that all infants and toddlers with disabilities in the state who may have a developmental delay or a diagnosed disability are identified and evaluated. This agency conducts public awareness and child find activities throughout the state to let residents know that early intervention services are available to help eligible infants and toddlers with disabilities. Early intervention programs provide another opportunity for the involvement of RDNs in meeting the challenging nutrition needs of the population from birth through 3 years of age using a family-centered, coordinated team approach.[22] Parents and caregivers must be informed of all the interprofessional services available, and each child is provided an Individual Family Service Plan (IFSP).

## OTHER COMMUNITY PROGRAMS

Nutrition professionals may be called on to work in schools and hospitals; Head Start/Early Head Start programs; child care settings; Early and Periodic Screening, Diagnostic, and Treatment (EPSDT) programs; and state interagency councils, which provide direction and a coordinated plan for the state's future work with the preschool population.[19,22] While working in these community settings, nutritionists may interact with programs such as the Special Supplemental Nutrition Program for Women, Infants, and Children (WIC), the Supplemental Nutrition Assistance Program (SNAP), child health specialty clinics, and university training programs.[23]

Community-based care means that community services are available and accessible, financial support is coordinated, and a coordinated system of care has been established to facilitate delivery of services. The role of the dietitian/nutritionist in a community setting is to connect families with these systems and services by identifying needs,[23,24] coordinating and providing care, advocating for services, and supporting families. The remaining sections of this chapter provide information that will assist in identifying services to provide community-based care.

### Medical Insurance and Services

With the advent of the Patient Protection and Affordable Care Act (PPACA), or just the Accountable Care Act (ACA), CSHCN may benefit from the emphasis on improved delivery of quality care and the promotion of medical homes, patient- and/or family -centered care, and use of electronic medical records. In addition, health plans can no longer limit or deny coverage for preexisting conditions in children younger than 19 years of age.[25] Federal programs and assistance to states to provide health programs to those with disabilities and the poor are available. The programs described here vary in focus and from state to state.

### Medicaid

Medicaid is a federal program (Title XIX of the Social Security Act) that pays for health services for selected individuals who are poor, elderly, blind, or disabled or who are enrolled in certain programs including Medicaid waivers. Medicaid covers children whose families receive assistance and is financed with both federal and state funds. The amount varies by state. Medicaid waivers are state-run programs that use federal funding to pay for health care for individuals with certain health conditions. Medicaid waivers allow CSHCN to receive health care without being institutionalized. They give states the flexibility to design publicly financed health care programs outside of the Medicaid statute and regulations. Each state has different waivers with specific eligibility requirements and services. More information about Medicaid is provided online.[26]

### State Child Health Insurance Program

The State Child Health Insurance Program (Title XXI of the Social Security Act), also known as the Children's Health Insurance Program (CHIP), provides comprehensive benefits to children in low-income families. States determine whether they will participate and design their own program within federal guidelines. States have the ability to design their CHIP program to stand alone and provide assistance to children from uninsured, low-income families; to use the funds to expand Medicaid eligibility; or to use federal funding to expand both Medicaid and a separate CHIP. Medicaid expansion CHIP programs provide the standard Medicaid benefit package, including EPSDT services, which includes all medically necessary services including mental health and dental services.[27]

### Early and Periodic Screening, Diagnostic, and Treatment Programs

EPSDT programs provide comprehensive and preventive health care services for children younger than 21 years of age who are enrolled in their state's Medicaid program. EPSDT is key to ensuring that children and adolescents receive appropriate preventive, dental, mental health, developmental, and specialty services. States must inform Medicaid-eligible individuals of EPSDT services and age-appropriate immunizations. States must provide or arrange for screening services for all children and arrange (directly or through referral) for corrective treatments needed after the screenings.[28] Services can include assistive communication devices, durable medical goods, nutritional supplements, personal assistance, speech therapy, physical therapy, and occupational therapy.

### Title V Maternal and Child Health Services Block Grant Program

The Title V Maternal and Child Health Services Block Grant Program—the nation's oldest federal-state partnership—aims to improve the health and well-being of women, particularly mothers, and children.[29–31] Funding is available to every state and jurisdiction. Using federal guidelines, states provide matching funds to the federal block grant. These funds are used for programs including health assessments and interventions; provision of quality care for pregnant women, mothers, and children; reductions in infant mortality; and family-centered and community-based systems of coordinated care for CSHCN.

These services are available to all children who have or are at increased risk for chronic physical, developmental, behavioral, or emotional conditions and who also require health and related services of a type or amount beyond those required by children generally. State programs include child health specialty clinics. Each state develops and submits its own yearly Title V application. State plans can be accessed online.[32]

Programs of the United States Department of Agriculture (USDA) Food and Nutrition Service (FNS) provide funding for a variety of food assistance programs to individuals and groups. This includes food distribution programs, child nutrition programs, and SNAP (formerly known as the Food Stamp program). FNS works with public, private, and non-profit partners to increase food security and reduce hunger by providing children and low-income people access to food, a healthful diet, and nutrition education. Several of the programs are described here. Additional information about these programs can be accessed on the USDA website.[33]

### Supplemental Nutrition Assistance Program

SNAP, a federal program funded through the USDA FNS, serves as the first line of defense against hunger. SNAP offers nutrition assistance to millions of eligible, low-income individuals and families and provides economic benefits to communities. The FNS works with state agencies, nutrition educators, and neighborhood and faith-based organizations to ensure that those eligible for nutrition assistance can make informed decisions about applying for the program and can access benefits.

### Special Supplemental Nutrition Program for Women, Infants and Children

WIC is a federal program that provides supplemental foods, nutrition education, and referrals to health care for income-eligible pregnant, breast-feeding, and postpartum women and infants and children up to the age of 5 years. Medical or nutritional risk factors are determined by qualified health care professionals, including RDNs.

### National School Lunch Program

The National School Lunch Program (NSLP) is a federally assisted meal program with specific requirements that operates in public and nonprofit private schools and residential child care institutions. It provides nutritionally balanced, low-cost or free lunches and snacks to children and adolescents. Schools receive cash subsidies and donated commodities from the USDA for each meal served. Reduced-price or free lunches are available based on the family's income relative to the federal poverty level. Schools may also provide the School Breakfast Program, which operates similarly to the NSLP. Schools also receive funds for serving half-pints of milk.

### Supplemental Security Income

The Supplemental Security Income (SSI) program pays monthly benefits to income-eligible individuals who are 65 years of age or older, blind, or disabled. Children may qualify if they meet the Social Security Administration's definition of disability and if their income and assets fall within the guidelines. It is important to know that once a child is determined to be disabled and is eligible for SSI, referrals for health care services are made through the CSHCN provisions of the Social Security Act. These are state-administered programs and may have a different name at the state level. Local public health departments, community health centers, social services offices, and hospitals can provide information on these services. To learn more about this program visit the SSI website.[34]

### Head Start and Early Head Start

Head Start and Early Head Start programs support the comprehensive development of children from birth to age 5 years in centers, in child care partner locations, and in their own homes. Head Start services are delivered by public and private nonprofit and for-profit community agencies. Head Start promotes the school readiness of young children from low-income families, and services include early learning, health, and family well-being. Programs include developmental screenings as well as connecting families with health related services.[35]

### Family Voices

Family Voices is a national, nonprofit, family-led organization that promotes quality health care for all children and youth, especially those with special needs. The work occurs at local, state, regional, and national levels. The Family Voices website provides information and education regarding CSHCN and networking and support for families.[36]

### Healthy Start

Healthy Start is a federal program that works to prevent infant mortality by targeting communities with rates at least 1.5 times the national average. It also focuses on reduction of low birth weight, preterm birth, and maternal mortality and maternal morbidity. The program helps the nation's most disadvantaged children survive infancy and live longer, more productive lives. Funds are provided to community-based organizations, universities, and local health departments to develop Healthy Start programs.[37]

### National Healthy Start Association

The National Healthy Start Association (NHSA) is an organization committed to improving birth outcomes and health disparities that exist within communities of color throughout the United States. As the membership association for the federal Healthy Start program, NHSA promotes the development of community-based maternal and child health programs, particularly those addressing the issues of infant mortality, low birth weight, and racial disparities in perinatal outcomes, and care for newborns, mothers and families.[38]

### Association of University Centers on Disabilities Research and Education Services

The Association of University Centers on Disabilities (AUCD) is a network of University Centers for Excellence in Developmental Disabilities (UCEDDs). These interprofessional centers help to advance policy and practice for and with individuals who have IDD, their families, and communities. There are 67 UCEDDs—at least one in every US state and territory. UCEDDs help the movement of information from research to the community for people with disabilities, members of their families, state and local government agencies, and community providers. Projects include those that provide training, technical assistance, service, research, and information sharing, with a focus on building the capacity of communities to sustain all their citizens.[39]

### Leadership Education in Neurodevelopmental and Related Disabilities

AUCD programs on Leadership Education in Neurodevelopmental and Related Disabilities (LEND) provide long-term, graduate-level interprofessional training as well as interprofessional services and care to improve the health of infants, children, and adolescents with disabilities. Trainees from diverse professional disciplines, including nutrition, are prepared to assume leadership roles in their respective fields and ensure high levels of interprofessional clinical competence. LEND programs are federally funded through the Maternal and Child Health Bureau of the Health Resources and Services Administration (HRSA).

LEND programs operate within a university system, usually as part of a UCEDD or other larger entity, and in collaboration with local university hospitals and/or health care centers. There are currently 43 LENDs in 37 states. Although each LEND program is unique, with its own focus and expertise, they all provide interprofessional training, have faculty and trainees in a wide range of disciplines, and include parents or family members as paid program participants.[40]

### Elderly Nutrition Program

The Elderly Nutrition Program (ENP), funded by the Department of Health and Human Services (DHHS), provides meals and nutrition education to the elderly (persons older than 60 years of age) and to individuals younger than 60 years with disabilities who reside in housing occupied primarily by elderly persons. It was established in 1968 as a 3-year demonstration and research program of nutrition for the elderly funded by the Administration on Aging (AOA) under Title IV of the Older Americans Act (OAA). Amendments to the reauthorized OAA in 1992 strengthened requirements for targeting services to those in greatest economic or social need, with special attention to low-income minorities. Elderly individuals can receive low-cost, nutritious meals in community settings where they can also receive social and rehabilitative services. This program, also known as the Congregate Meal Program, provides an excellent opportunity for elderly persons with developmental disabilities to be integrated more fully into the community with other elderly persons. For current information on these sites, visit the AOA website (http://www.aoa.gov/nutrition/default.htm).

### Special Projects of Regional and National Significance

To meet the intent of the various programs and laws, nutrition professionals will be called on to work in a variety of community settings, including schools, hospitals, public health departments, Head Start agencies, WIC programs, and community health centers. Training is essential in working with children, adolescents, and adults with a disability or chronic illness. The HRSA, through the MCHB, is a key resource in providing training through Title V, Special Projects of Regional and National Significance (SPRANS). Nutrition training is one of the many opportunities available through this training source. These training programs promote the healthy nutrition of children, adolescents, women, and families by providing graduate training to nutritionists and RDNs. Trainees are prepared for leadership roles in public health nutrition. In addition, short-term training is provided to individuals from a variety of disciplines focused on both clinical and public health approaches to maternal and child nutrition.

## FUNDING

Funding for nutrition services in community agencies is a complex issue. The need for third-party reimbursement and adequate funding for nutrition services must be addressed on an ongoing basis. Resources should be available for nutrition services, both personnel and materials, such as feeding equipment and special-formula diets. The American Academy of Pediatrics publication, *Bright Futures in Practice: Nutrition*, addresses many of the issues for children.[8] These resources are readily available for RDNs working in the community. Ongoing training for nutrition professionals should be provided at the pre-service and in-service levels several times throughout a calendar year.

RDs can provide ongoing consultation. Dietitians and graduate-level nutritionists can make a significant contribution to the success and overall productivity, independence, and integration of persons with IDD into the community (Box 5–2). Achievement of this goal in any community environment is dependent on interagency interprofessional collaboration, individual, and family involvement at the preschool, elementary, and adult levels. Nutrition professionals must be advocates for their services in the educational setting, especially for CSHCN.

## SUMMARY

Nutrition practice in the field of developmental disabilities has offered and continues to offer services within multiple modalities to improve the nutrition status of these children and their families. Each local community is dependent on federal and state funding for cutting-edge projects, as well as on philanthropic endeavors to address in particular the cycle of childhood and family hunger and the increased dynamics of societal homelessness, which increase the risk that children will be identified as developmentally delayed. Increased numbers of collaborative endeavors are evident in local communities, including food pantries and food banks, specialized ethnic and faith-based initiatives that focus on improving the health and nutrition of poor children from minorities and their families, nutrition counseling efforts to teach children and parents about healthy foods and lifestyles, efforts of United Way and Community Chest resulting in the development of a "Dial a Dietitian Hotline," and local newsletters, flyers, brochures, and videos that are available in community libraries.

**Box 5–2.** Financing Structure for Nutrition Services

*I. Title XIX Medicaid*

Authorized through the Social Security Act; administered by the Health Care Financing Administration (HCFA)

For all ages

Immediate Care Facilities for the Mentally Retarded (ICF-MR) (may or may not be institution based)

Home and Community-Based Waiver (HCBS); must be noninstitutional (food cannot be purchased with this money)

Eligibility includes all those who are eligible and receiving Supplemental Security Income (SSI)—aged, blind, and disabled. Also can include others as determined by individual states with approval of federal governmental regulation agency (HCFA).

*II. Education Dollars*

Through P.L. 99-457 (Education of the Handicapped Act Amendments, 1986), nutrition services may be identified as a needed, reimbursable service.

Through P.L. 94-142 (Education for All Handicapped Students Act, 1976), the provision of a free and appropriate education for all students may include nutrition services when needed.

Head Start programs provide nutrition services.
School lunch should be provided to all students, including those with special needs.

*III. Social Services Block Grant Money*

For all ages

Individual states determine what services can be purchased for special needs (nutrition may not be included; only "non-institutional" types of services).

*IV. Maternal and Child Health*

Funded through Title V of the Social Security Act

Through the provision of nutrition services at the state level and at specialty clinics such as those for individuals with phenylketonuria (PKU), spina bifida, or Down syndrome, people gain access to specialized nutrition services and resources.

*V. Entitlement Programs**

Income dependent

Special Supplemental Nutrition Program for Women, Infants, and Children (WIC) —should contain nutrition education provided by a qualified nutrition professional.

Supplemental Nutrition Assistance Program (SNAP)—should contain nutrition education provided by a qualified nutrition professional.

*These programs are administered through various agencies from state to state.
From Rokusek C. Vermillion, SD: South Dakota University Affiliate Program, USD School of Medicine; 1989.

RDNs and licensed graduate level nutritionists need to be involved in community-based services to provide families with financing options and resources in the community for training as well as research.[41] Incorporating components of nutrition assessment and quality nutrition services is important for all persons. Targeting outcomes and measuring food intake/energy output of persons with IDD is important throughout the lifespan (Fig. 5–1). As resources expand, it is important to monitor research in the field. In addition, to developing best practices, it is critical that results of innovative feeding and nutrition programs are documented and tracked over time.

In developing and identifying ongoing resources, an integrated and interprofessional approach to examining all needed and relevant services needs to be taken. This includes active involvement of the family members and persons with IDD. In examining comprehensive and integrated services for persons with IDD throughout the lifespan, it is important to examine the overall health of the individual with IDD and the relationship of the health status to overall dietary intake and exercise (energy output) potential. Prevention of disease and health promotion must always be taken into consideration. It is well established that individuals with IDD have a higher incidence of obesity than those in the overall general population. Severe obesity has been related to a lifespan reduction of 5 to 20 years.[2] Concurrent with the higher incidence of obesity, as in the overall population, there is a higher rate of type 2 diabetes, cardiovascular disease, and metabolic syndrome.[17]

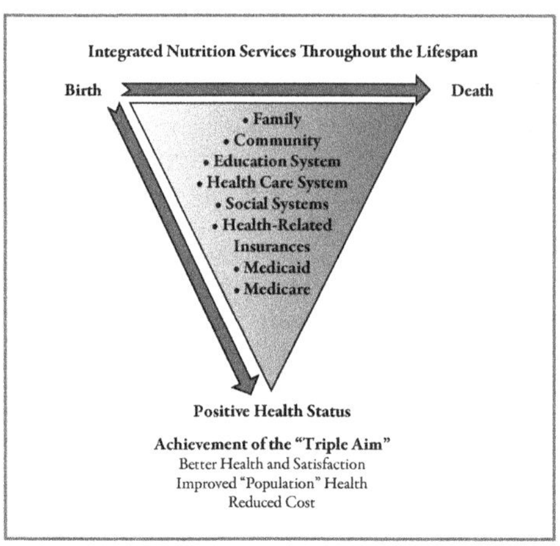


**Figure 5–1.** Integrated nutrition services throughout the lifespan. C. Rokusek, 2016

Many times the onset of overweight and obesity in the IDD population begins early, with family members giving food as a reward or enabling children with IDD to eat whatever they want and however much they want.[42] Good nutrition for everyone starts at birth (and even earlier, during pregnancy). The Healthy People 2020 initiative emphasizes the importance of "health promotion and reduction of chronic disease through the consumption of healthful diets and achievement and maintenance of healthy body weight for everyone."[43] It is important for the family and all members of the medical and social interprofessional team to prevent overweight and obesity in the IDD population. There are many reasons for increased obesity in this population other than overeating, including genetic conditions, behavioral issues, use of atypical antipsychotics, use of tricyclic antidepressants, inability to make food choices, use of food as a coping mechanism, and use of food by parents or staff to control individual behavior.[43]

Utilizing resources in the community through local extension services, universities, libraries, and weight loss programs such as Weight Watchers can be effective. In addition, maintaining an appropriate and reasonable level of exercise or movement is critically important. All persons with IDD need to be involved in planning and selecting good food choices. Starting early is the key. In the home, school setting, and community-based living environment, good nutrition should be emphasized with individual choices. In community living, staff should receive training on nutrition and exercise. Persons with IDD of all ages should be involved whenever possible in making good choices and in preparing their own foods. Nutrition education should be ongoing, focusing on food variety and healthy food choices. Menu planning is important for everyone. Often, local grocery stores and grocery chains offer healthy menu options and even week-long menu plans. These resources can often be accessed online.

Good nutrition information and resources for families, care partners, and professionals can be accessed anytime using technology for providers and families. For example, portion control is a critical component in nutrition, and the "Choose My Plate" model can be a guide in this area. It provides an easy to understand, visual approach to both portion control and food groupings.[44]

The term "telehealth" has several operational definitions, and multiple terms (e.g., e-health, telemedicine, telerehab) are used to describe a similar scope of service. Broadly, telehealth is a model of health care that uses medical information exchanged from one site to another via electronic communications as a means to improve a patient's health status.[45] It can involve connected care across a spectrum of electronically enabled, consultative, direct patient care, educational, and self-management services. The Academy of Nutrition and Dietetics refers to "telepractice" and describes it as interactive use, by any health care providers (including RDs), of "electronic information and telecommunications technologies to engage in the diagnosis, evaluation, and treatment of patients or clients at a remote location through means such as teleconferencing."[46] Further designation is made for services that require engaging in real-time direct patient interactions at a distance (synchronous), indirect or store-and-forward patient interactions (asynchronous), and dissemination of nutrition information that is not personalized but general in nature. Telehealth can be used as a primary, adjunct, or hybrid approach to individual care and information exchange.

In the field of nutrition science and dietetics, use of telehealth is both feasible and effective for supporting individuals of all ages in their homes as they manage chronic conditions such as diabetes and obesity or as they pursue wellness through nutrition. Studies examining the feasibility of telehealth or mobile health technology report high levels of satisfaction with the convenience, increased access to care, and personal support it provides.[47] At this time, constraints related to use of telehealth do exist and in some instances can be significant. Successful use depends on adequate connectivity, appropriate technology to support Web- or software-based teleconferencing platforms, appropriate patient selection, and compliance with all federal, state, and discipline-specific policies regarding security, privacy, standards of care, scope of practice, and reimbursement. This is a growing area of service for individuals with IDD and their families in rural or isolated areas.

## References


1. Ptomey LT, Wittenbrook W. Position of the Academy of Nutrition and Dietetics: nutrition services for individuals with intellectual and developmental disabilities and special health care needs. *J Acad Nutr Diet.* 2015; 115:593.
2. Gronhuis S, Aman M. Overweight and obesity in youth with developmental disabilities: a call to action. *J Intellect Dis Res.* 2014; 58:787.
3. Draheim CC, Stanish HI, Williams DP, McCubbin JA. Dietary intake of adults with mental retardation who reside in community settings. *Am J Ment Retard.* 2007; 112:392.
4. US Department of Health and Human Services, Office of the Surgeon General, Office on Disability. *The 2005 Surgeon General's Call to Action to Improve the Health and Wellness of Persons with Disabilities: Calling You to Action.* Rockville, MD: US Department of Health and Human Services, Office of the Surgeon General; 2005. http://www.ncbi.nlm.nih.gov/books/NBK44667/. Accessed June 3, 2016.
5. Yang Y, Lucas B, Feucht S, eds. *Nutrition Interventions for Children with Special Health Care Needs Manual*, 3rd ed. Publication No. 961-158. Olympia, WA: Washington State Department of Health; 2010. http://here.doh.wa.gov/materials/nutrition-interventions. Accessed June 3, 2016.
6. Garvin J, Ekvall S. *Nutrition for Children with Special Health Care Needs: Second Tier Training Kit in Developmental Disorders and Managed Care.* Manual #5. Cincinnati, OH: Maternal and Child Health Bureau and Health Resources Services Administration and University of Cincinnati Publications; 2002.
7. Stevens F, Ekvall S. Cultural diversity and developmental disabilities. In: Stevens F, Ekvall S, eds. *Empowering Children through Early Intervention with Good Nutrition: Focusing on Culturally Diverse Children with Special Health Care Needs.* Manual #4. Cincinnati, OH: University of Cincinnati Publications; 2002.
8. Bright Futures in Practice: Nutrition Pocket Guide. https://brightfutures.aap.org/Bright%20Futures%20Documents/BFNutrition3rdEdPocketGuide.pdf. Accessed June 3, 2016.Bright Futures in Practice: Nutrition Pocket Guide. https://brightfutures.aap.org/Bright%20Futures%20Documents/BFNutrition3rdEdPocketGuide.pdf
9. Rubin SS, Rimmer JH, Chicoine B, Braddock D, McGuire DE. Overweight prevalence in persons with Down syndrome. *Am J Ment Retard.* 1998; 36:175.
10. Yamaki K. Body weight status among adults with intellectual disability in the community. *Am J Ment Retard.* 2005; 43:1.
11. Rimmer JH, Braddock D, Fujiura G. Prevalence of obesity in adults with mental retardation: implications for health promotion and disease prevention. *Am J Ment Retard.* 1993; 31:105.
12. Rimmer JH, Braddock D, Fujiura G. Cardiovascular risk factor levels in adults with mental retardation. *Am J Ment Retard.* 1994; 98:510.
13. Rimmer JH, Braddock D, Marks B. Health characteristics and behaviors of adults with mental retardation residing in three living arrangements. *Res Dev Disabil.* 1995; 16:489.
14. Crespo CJ, Keteyian SJ, Heath GW, Sempos CT. Leisure-time physical activity among US adults. Results from the Third National Health and Nutrition Examination Survey. *Arch Intern Med.* 1996; 156:93.
15. Ernst ND, Sempos CT, Briefel RR, Clark MB. Consistency between US dietary fat intake and serum total cholesterol concentrations: the National Health and Nutrition Examination Surveys. *Am J Clin Nutr.* 1997; 66:9655.
16. Anderson LL, Humphries K, McDermott S, et al. The state of the science of health and wellness for adults with intellectual and developmental disabilities. *Intellect Dev Disabil.* 2013; 51:385.
17. Hahn JE. Using NIC in an APRN-led preventive model for adults aging with developmental disabilities. *J Nurs Sch.* 2014; 46:304.
18. US Department of Education. *Building the Legacy: IDEA 2004.* Individuals with Disabilities Act. http://idea.ed.gov/. Accessed June 3, 2016.
19. Axtman CD, Davis J, Rokusek C. *A Survey on Nutrition Attitudes, Knowledge, and Needs of School Lunch Directors in Relation to Special Needs Populations.* Pierre, SD: South Dakota Department of Education; 1983.
20. Dwyer J, Egan MC, eds. *The Right to Grow: Putting Nutrition Services for Children with Special Long-Term Development and Health Needs into Action.* Boston: Frances Stern Nutrition Center, New England Medical Center Hospital; 1986.
21. US Health and Human Services. *IDEA 2004: Building the Legacy—Part C (birth–2 years old).* Individuals with Disabilities ACT (IDEA), http://idea.ed.gov/part-c/search/new. Accessed June 3, 2016.
22. Campbell MK, Kelsey KS. The Peach Survey: a nutrition screening to use in early intervention programs. *J Am Diet Assoc.* 1994; 94:1156.
23. Cloud HH. Update on nutrition for children with special needs. *Top Clin Nutr.* 1997; 13:21.
24. Stang J, Bayerl CT; American Dietetic Association. Position of the American Dietetic Association: child and adolescent food and nutrition programs. *J Am Diet Assoc.* 2010; 110:791.
25. Patient Protection and Affordable Care Act (PPACA): child and adolescent food and nutrition assistance programs. *J Am Diet Assoc.* 2010; 110:791.
26. Medicaid.gov: Keeping America Healthy. Website. http://www.medicaid.gov/index/html. Accessed June 3, 2016.
27. Medicaid.gov: Keeping America Healthy. *Children's Health Insurance Program (CHIP).* http://www.medicaid.gov/chip/chip-program-information.html. Accessed June 3, 2016.
28. Medicaid.gov. *Benefits: Early and Periodic Screening, Diagnostic, and Treatment.* http://www.medicaid.gov/Medicaid-CHIP-Program-Information/By-Topics/Benefits/Early-and-Periodic-Screening-Diagnostic-and-Treatment.html. Accessed June 3, 2016.
29. Division of Services for Children with Special Health Needs (DSCSHN). Fact Sheet http://mchb.hrsa.gov/about/factsheets/dschcnfacts.pdf. Accessed June 3, 2016.
30. US Department of Health and Human Services, Health Resources and Services Administration. *Maternal and Child Health Bureau: fact sheet.* http://www.hrsa.gov/about/pdf/mchb.PDF. Accessed June 3, 2016.
31. US Department of Health and Human Services, Health Resources and Services Administration, Maternal and Child Health Bureau. *Division of State and Community Health: fact sheet.* http://mchb.hrsa.gov/about/factsheets/dschfacts.pdf. Accessed June 3, 2016.
32. US Department of Health and Human Services, Health Resources and Services Administration, Maternal and Child Health Bureau. *Title V State Action Plans.* http://mchb.hrsa.gov/programs/titlevgrants/stateactionplans.html. Accessed June 3, 2016.
33. United States Department of Agriculture, Food and Nutrition Service Programs. *About FNS.* http://www.fns.usda.gov/about-fns. Accessed June 3, 2016.
34. Social Security Administration. *Supplemental Security Income (SSI) Benefits.* https://www.ssa.gov/disabilityssi/ssi.html. Accessed June 3, 2016.
35. US Department of Health and Human Services, Administration for Children and Families, Office of Head Start. Website. http://www.acf.hhs.gov/programs/ohs. Accessed June 3, 2016.
36. Family Voices. Website. http://familyvoices.org. Accessed June 3, 2016.
37. US Department of Health and Human Services, Health Resources and Services Administration, Maternal and Child Health. *Healthy Start.* http://mchb.hrsa.gov/programs/healthystart/index.html. Accessed June 3, 2016.
38. National Healthy Start Association. Website. http://www.nationalhealthystart.org/. Accessed June 3, 2016.
39. Association of University Centers on Disabilities. *About UCEDD.* https://www.aucd.org/template/page.cfm?id=667. Accessed June 3, 2016.
40. Association of University Centers on Disabilities. *About LEND.* https://www.aucd.org/template/page.cfm?id=473. Accessed June 3, 2016.
41. Bradley-Davalos C. *Staff Education: Nutrition Education in the Intellectually/Developmentally Disabled Community.* Master's Project, School of Nursing and

Health Professions, University of San Francisco, California; 2015. http://repository.usfca.edu/capstone/224. Accessed June 3, 2016.
42. Mulrooney H. Weight management and learning disabilities. *Practice Nurs.* 2014; 25:81.
43. US Office of Disease Prevention and Health Promotion. *HealthyPeople.gov: Nutrition and Weight Status.* Site last updated 06/03/2016. http://www.healthypeople.gov/2020/topics-objectives/topic/nutrition-and-weight-status. Accessed June 3, 2016.
44. US Department of Agriculture. ChooseMyPlate.gov. Website. www.choosemyplate.gov. Accessed June 3, 2016.
45. American Telemedicine Association. *Core Operational Guidelines for Telehealth Services Involving Provider-Patient Interactions.* May 2014. http://www.americantelemed.org/docs/default-source/standards/core-operational-guidelines-for-telehealth-services.pdf?sfvrsn=6. Accessed June 3, 2016.
46. Bussey C, Michael P. Telehealth: opportunities and pitfalls. *J Am Diet Assoc.* 2008; 108:1296.
47. Shigaki CL, Koopman RJ, Kabel A, Canfield S. Successful weight loss: how information technology is used to lose. *Telemedicine and e-Health.* 2014; 20:144.

# 6 Nutritional Support After Injury

THERESA MAYES AND MICHELE GOTTSCHLICH

The stress of trauma invokes a multitude of physiological events that affect an individual's nutrition status by altering substrate production and utilization and thereby impacting dietary requirements. In addition, the hypermetabolism and hypercatabolism that accompany critical injury result in rapid weight loss and erosion of muscle mass and bone in association with depletion of nitrogen and visceral protein. Untoward outcomes such as poor wound healing, depressed lung function, increased risk of infection, extended hospital stay, and higher mortality may characterize the posttrauma state. Appropriate provision of nutrients after injury promotes anabolic adaptation and improves these outcomes.

## BIOCHEMICAL ABNORMALITIES

Cuthbertson and Tilstone[1] described a biphasic pattern of events that occur in trauma or stress (Table 6–1). The two distinct periods of ebb and flow are increasingly pronounced, depending on the severity of the injury. The initial ebb phase is characterized by depressed metabolism, whereas the subsequent flow phase is defined by a number of factors that mediate hypermetabolism and hypercatabolism.

Hormonal alterations that follow stress appear to drive the response to injury. Heightened secretion of catecholamines, glucocorticoids, and glucagon contributes to increased energy needs and the proteolytic state.[2–5] These catabolic hormones also stimulate gluconeogenesis and glycogenolysis, producing the hyperglycemia that is characteristic of the posttraumatic period. In addition, in response to stress, serum insulin levels are disproportionate to the rise in glucagon, which fosters tissue insulin resistance and hyperglycemia as well. As a result, glucose protocols have increasingly been applied in the critical care setting,[6,7] although controversy exists regarding its efficacy in all intensive care populations.[8] In order for the host to survive, appropriate nutrition support—primarily adequate calories, protein, fluid and electrolytes—must be provided to minimize the breakdown of lean body mass and maximize the synthesis of sufficient protein to transition to anabolism.

### Nutrition Support

The enteral route is the preferred method of nutrient delivery in the critical care population. Increased intestinal blood flow, preserved gastrointestinal function, decreased mucosal atrophy, and reduced bacterial translocation have been proven with enteral alimentation.[9,10] Questions remain regarding the most safe and efficacious time at which to initiate enteral support after trauma. There has been concern that enteral feeds delivered to patients who are receiving inotropic agents or during periods of poor perfusion may decrease blood flow to the splanchnic bed, resulting in gut ischemia. However, there is evidence suggesting that enteral nutrition may exert a protective effect on the gastrointestinal tract.[10–16] An algorithm has been developed to assist the clinician during fluid resuscitation and pressor dependence (Fig. 6.1). It is important to consider trophic enteral feeds during times of poor perfusion as a means to sustain gut integrity. Glutamine also appears to have a protective effect in preventing intestinal mucosal damage.[17,18] Once hemodynamic stability is achieved, the enteral regimen may be advanced to goal rate.

The preferred route for enteral access to the critically ill patient depends on the duration of access, alertness of the patient, and gastrointestinal function. These patients often have an increased potential for aspiration pneumonia secondary to gastric paresis. Transpyloric feeding tube placement can overcome this problem. In patients with short-term enteral access needs presenting with an intact gag reflex and normal gastric function, successful placement of a gastric feeding tube is possible; however, diligent monitoring of residual is required. To choose the most appropriate enteral product for the patient, one must match the nutritional requirements of the clinical condition with the composition of the formula. The enteral choice must take into account digestive and absorptive capacity, organ dysfunction, fluid requirement, and degree of hypermetabolism and hypercatabolism.

Parenteral nutrition is associated with depressed immune response, heightened incidence of bacterial translocation, increased number of infectious episodes, and access issues. As a result, intravenous support is primarily reserved for patients with a nonfunctioning gastrointestinal tract. The American Society for Parenteral and Enteral Nutrition and the American College of Critical Care Medicine have published guidelines distinguishing conditions in which nutrition support via the enteral versus the parenteral route is appropriate.[19] When parenteral nutrition is indicated, simultaneous trophic enteral feeds are recommended, if possible, to promote gut mucosal integrity.

## FACTORS TO BE CONSIDERED IN NUTRITIONAL EVALUATION

### Energy Assessment

A plethora of energy assessment equations exist in critical care. Basal energy expenditure (BEE) as predicted by the Harris-Benedict[20] and Schofield[21] equations, with alterations for activity and injury factors,[22] has been reliably used by clinicians for decades (Box 6–1; Tables 6–2 and 6–3). The recommendation for energy needs during the ebb phase of injury generally falls below normal. As the patient transitions to the flow response, caloric needs increase exponentially. As the individual progresses to the adaptive phase, energy requirements return to normal.

In general, the resting energy expenditure (REE) derived from indirect calorimetry is more accurate than estimates provided by equations. Indirect calorimetry allows the nutrition support regimen to be tailored to meet the individual energy needs of the patient. Energy requirements are frequently skewed by predictive equations for conditions such as head injury, inflammatory bowel disease, ventilator failure, chronic pulmonary disease, trauma, obesity, burns, and sepsis. As a result, indirect calorimetry is of particular importance during these conditions. Typically, REE is adjusted by 20% to 40% to allow for stress factors that are not inherent in the measurement. The respiratory quotient is available from indirect calorimetry testing and provides an additional assessment of the adequacy of substrate provision.

### Protein Requirements

Based on age, the normal pediatric population requires approximately 0.8 to 2.2 g of protein per kilogram body weight per day. Conditions of critical illness increase protein demands to as high as 4 to 5 g/kg/day, depending on age, fluid status, renal function, and the extent of injury, which determine the severity of protein loss or turnover. These values should be based on preinjury weight or ideal body weight in an obese individual. Determination of nitrogen balance is also a helpful guide to protein provision. Critically ill patients with complicating kidney or liver disease may require further alterations in the daily protein recommendation.

**Table 6–1.** Metabolic Alterations Produced by Stress

| | Ebb Response | Flow Response | |
|---|---|---|---|
| | | Acute Phase | Adaptive Phase |
| Dominant Factors | Loss of plasma volume<br>Poor tissue perfusion<br>Shock<br>Low plasma insulin levels | Increased total body blood flow<br>Elevated catecholamines<br>Elevated glucagon<br>Elevated glucocorticoids<br>Normal or elevated serum insulin<br>High glucagon:insulin ratio | Stress hormone response subsiding<br>Convalescence |
| Metabolic and Clinical Characteristics | Decreased oxygen consumption<br>Depressed resting energy expenditure (REE)<br>Decreased blood pressure<br>Cardiac output below normal<br>Decreased body temperature | Catabolism<br>Hyperglycemia<br>Increased respiratory rate<br>Increased oxygen consumption and hypermetabolism<br>Increased carbon dioxide production<br>Increased body temperature<br>Redistribution of polyvalent cations such as zinc and iron<br>Increased urinary excretion of nitrogen, sulfur, magnesium, phosphorus, potassium, and creatinine<br>Accelerated gluconeogenesis<br>Fat mobilization<br>Increased use of amino acids as oxidative fuels | Anabolism<br>Normoglycemia<br>Energy expenditure diminished<br>Nutrient requirements approaching preinjury needs |

Adapted with permission from Gottschlich MM, Alexander JW, Bower RH. Enteral nutrition in patients with burns or trauma. In: Rombeau JL, Caldwell MD, eds., *Enteral and Tube Feeding*, vol 1. Philadelphia: Saunders; 1990: 307.

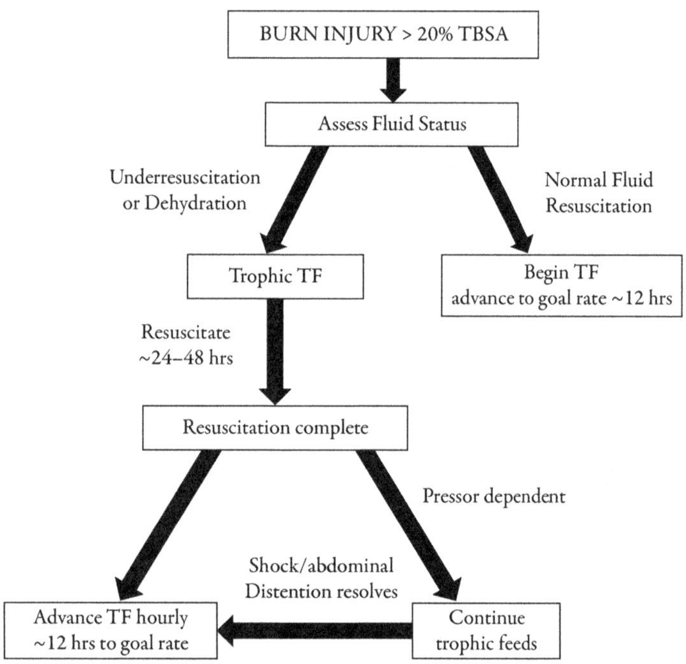


**Figure 6–1.** Enteral nutrition support clinical decision algorithm for patients with burns. TBSA = total body surface area; TF = feeds.

**Box 6–1.** Harris-Benedict Equation*

***Total Energy Expenditure (TEE) = Basal Energy Expenditure (BEE) × Activity Factor (AF) × Injury Factor (IF)***

***For Males:***

*BEE = 66.5 + (13.8 × weight in kg) + (5 × height in cm) − (6.8 × age in years)*

***For Females:***

*BEE = 655.1 + (9.6 × weight in kg) + (1.8 × height in cm) − (4.7 × age in years)*

From Harris J, Benedict FA. Biometric study of basal metabolism in man. *Proc Natl Acad Sci U S A*. 1918; 4:370.[20]

*BEE is calculated by the Schofield equation[21]; activity and injury factors were presented by Long et al.[22]

**Table 6–2.** Shofield Equation

| Age | Basal Energy Expenditure (kcal per day) |
|---|---|
| Males <3 yr | (0.17 × weight in kg) + (1.517 × height in cm) − 617.6 |
| Males 3–10 yr | (19.6 × weight in kg) + (0.1303 × height in cm) + 414.9 |
| Males 10–18 yr | (16.3 × weight in kg) + (0.1372 × height in cm) + 515.5 |
| Females <3 yr | (16.25 × weight in kg) +(1.0232 × height in cm) − 413.5 |
| Females 3–10 yr | (16.97 × weight in kg) + (1.618 × height in cm) + 371.2 |
| Females 10–18 yr | (8.365 × weight in kg) + (4.65 × height in cm) + 200 |

From Schofield WN. Predicting basal metabolic rate: new standards and review of previous work. *Hum Nutr Clin Nutr*. 1985; 39:5.

## Fluid and Electrolyte Requirements

Adequate fluid provision is important to maintain acid-base balance and hemodynamic stability. In addition, routine monitoring and replacement of electrolytes is necessary in the critical care setting. Electrolytes serve a vital role in cellular metabolism and function, and intracellular electrolytes such as potassium, phosphorus, and magnesium are needed to promote anabolism.

## Clinical and Laboratory Tests

### Anthropometry

Fluctuations in weight, independent of fluid shifts, represent an important indicator of the adequacy of nutrition support. It is important to obtain an admission or preinjury weight and to monitor the adequacy of calorie provision with biweekly weight assessments. A goal of 90% to 110% of the admission or preinjury weight indicates optimal nutrition intervention. Triceps skinfold thickness and midarm muscle circumference measurements are inexpensive ways of determining changes in body composition. Fat and somatic stores can be easily depleted after stress. Measurement of both on admission and at weekly intervals thereafter indicates the adequacy of the calorie and protein regimens.

**Table 6–3.** Long's Activity and Injury Factors

| Activity Factors | Injury Factors |
|---|---|
| Bedrest: 1.2 | Minor Surgery: 1.2 |
| Ambulatory: 1.3 | Skeletal Trauma: 1.35 |
| | Major Sepsis: 1.6 |
| | Severe Burns: 2.1 |

From Long C, Schaffel N, Geiger C, Schiller WR, Blakemore WS. Metabolic response to injury and illness: estimation of energy and protein needs from indirect calorimetry and nitrogen balance. *J Parenter Enteral Nutr*. 1979; 3:452.

### Laboratory Tests

Serum albumin and prealbumin are the most common biochemical elements used to assess the adequacy of nutrition support. Albumin is a known prognostic indicator correlating with clinical outcome. Changes in albumin over short periods are most likely the result of fluid shifts, wound exudation, blood loss, albumin infusion, overhydration, or underhydration. Because of its long half-life (approximately 3 weeks), trending albumin is a better predictor of nutrition status over time. Prealbumin has a much shorter half-life and is therefore more often used to monitor the nutrition status of a stress or trauma patient on a weekly basis. Trends are also plotted, taking into account the impact of impaired renal function and inflammation[23,24] which can increase levels, as well as liver disease, which is known to decrease levels.

In addition to monitoring of hepatic transport proteins, nitrogen balance studies are performed to assess the adequacy of protein provision. Most often, nitrogen balance is calculated as follows:

$$\text{Nitrogen balance} = \text{nitrogen intake} - (\text{nitrogen output} + 4)$$

where nitrogen output (24 hour urinary urea nitrogen in grams) is subtracted from nitrogen intake (protein intake in grams in 24 hours divided by 6.25). An additional 4 g of nitrogen is added to nitrogen output to account for insensible losses, as in sweat and stool. A negative nitrogen balance indicates insufficient protein intake; therefore, an increase in protein intake is warranted. A positive nitrogen balance in the range of +1 to +3 indicates adequate protein intake during periods when protein is needed to replenish depleted stores. After visceral protein stores are adequately repleted, a goal of zero nitrogen balance is in order. The validity of nitrogen balance can be skewed in patients with renal insufficiency or excess fluid or nitrogen loss from wounds.

## SUMMARY

The stress of critical illness leads to multiple pathophysiological events that affect nutrition status. Initiation of a nutrition support plan that combats the debilitating hypermetabolic and hypercatabolic cascades of injury and includes a care plan with ongoing assessment of the regimen's adequacy is essential to reduce morbidity and improve survival.

### References


1. Cuthbertson D, Tilstone WJ. Metabolism during the postinjury period. *Adv Clin Chem.* 1969; 12:1.
2. Hepner KM, Hebbeger KM, Day J., et al. Glucagon regulation of energy metabolism. *Physiol Behav.* 2010; 100:545.
3. Fryberg DA, Glefand RA, Jahn LA, et al. Effects of epinephrine on human muscle glucose and protein metabolism. *Am J Physiol Endocrinol Metab.* 1995; 268:E55.
4. Matthews DE, Pesola G, Campbell RG. Effect of epinephrine on amino acid and energy metabolism in humans. *Am J Physiol Endocrinol Metab.* 1990; 258:E948.
5. Ballian N, Rabiee A, Andersen DK, Elahi D, Gibson BR. Glucose metabolism in burn patients: the role of insulin and other endocrine hormones. *Burns* 2010; 36:599.
6. Jeschke MG, Klein D, Herndon DN. Insulin treatment improves the systemic inflammatory reaction to severe trauma. *Ann Surg.* 2004; 239:553.
7. Cochran A, Davis L, Morris S, Saffle JR. Safety and efficacy of an intensive insulin protocol in a burn-trauma intensive care unit. *J Burn Care Res.* 2008; 29:187.
8. Griesdale DEG, de Souza RJ, van Dam RM, et al. Intensive insulin therapy and mortality among critically ill patients: a meta-analysis including NICE-SUGAR study data. *Can Med Assoc J.* 2009; 180:821.
9. Hadfield RJ, Sinclair DG, Houldsworth PE, Evans TW. Effects of enteral and parenteral nutrition on gut mucosal permeability in the critically ill. *Am J Respir Crit Care Med.* 1995; 152:1545.
10. Goldberg RF, Austen WG, Zhang X, et al. Intestinal alkaline phosphatase is a gut mucosal defense factor maintained by enteral nutrition. *Proc Natl Acad Sci U S A.* 2007; 105:3551.
11. Panchal AK, Manzi J, Connolly S, et al. Safety of enteral feedings in critically ill children receiving vasoactive agents. *J Parenter Enteral Nutr.* 2016; 40:236.
12. Flordeli Lasierra JL, Pérez-Vela JL, Umezawa Makikado LD, et al. Early enteral nutrition in patients with hemodynamic failure following cardiac surgery. *J Parenter Enteral Nutr.* 2015; 39:154.
13. Yang S, Wu X, Yu W, Li J. Early enteral nutrition in critically ill patients with hemodynamic instability: an evidence-based review and practical advice. *Nutr Clin Pract.* 2014; 29:90.
14. Gottschlich MM, Jenkins ME, Mayes T, Kagan RJ, Warden GD. An evaluation of the safety of early vs. delayed enteral support and effects on clinical, nutritional and endocrine outcomes after severe burns. *J Burn Care Rehabil.* 2002; 23:401.
15. McClave SA, Wei-Kuo C. Feeding the hypotensive patient: does enteral feeding precipitate or protect against ischemic bowel? *Nutr Clin Pract.* 2003; 18:279.
16. Zaloga GP, Roberts PR, Marik P. Feeding the hemodynamically unstable patient: a critical evaluation of the evidence. *Nutr Clin Pract.* 2003; 18:285.
17. Windle M. Glutamine supplementation in critical illness: evidence, recommendations and implications for clinical practice in burn care. *J Burn Care Res.* 2006; 27:764.
18. Garcia de Lorenxo A, Zarazaga A, Garcia Luna P. Clinical evidence for enteral nutritional support with glutamine: a systemic review. *Crit Care Med.* 2002; 30:2022.
19. McClave SA, Martindale RG, Vanek VW, et al. Guidelines for the provision and assessment of nutrition support therapy in the adult critically ill patient: Society of Critical Care Medicine (SCCM) and American Society for Parenteral and Enteral Nutrition (A.S.P.E.N.). *J Parent Enteral Nutr.* 2009; 33:277.
20. Harris J, Benedict FA. Biometric study of basal metabolism in man. *Proc Natl Acad Sci U S A.* 1918; 4:370.
21. Schofield WN. Predicting basal metabolic rate: new standards and review of previous work. *Hum Nutr Clin Nutr.* 1985; 39:5.
22. Long C, Schaffel N, Geiger C, Schiller WR, Blakemore WS. Metabolic response to injury and illness: estimation of energy and protein needs from indirect calorimetry and nitrogen balance. *J Parenter Enteral Nutr.* 1979; 3:452.
23. Yang HT, Yim H, Cho YS, et al. Serum transthyretin level is associated with clinical severity rather than nutrition status in massively burned patients. *J Parenter Enteral Nutr.* 2014; 38:966.
24. Shields BA, Pidcoke HF, Chung KK, et al. Are visceral proteins valid markers of nutritional status in the burn intensive care unit? *J Burn Care Res.* 2014; 36:375.

# 7 Sports Nutrition

KAREN REZNIK DOLINS AND MARTICA HEANER

Nutrition and physical activity play a dual role in good health. Because the two are inextricably linked, it is important to avoid focusing on one area while neglecting the other. Both regular exercise and good nutrition can provide a wide array of physiological, psychological, and functional health benefits to all children, especially those with chronic illnesses or developmental disorders. When implementing physical activity regimens, one should follow established exercise guidelines and make any necessary modifications as dictated by the child's specific medical condition. Nutritional intake should meet the child's basic nutrition needs to optimize health as well as to enhance the child's physical performance.

Sports nutrition is a relatively new area of research. Little is known about the best protocols for physical activity and sports nutrition in many special populations, including ill children and those with disabilities. Exercise plans and nutrition regimens should be tailored to the specific needs of the child whenever possible.

## HEALTH BENEFITS OF PHYSICAL ACTIVITY

Regular physical activity conditions the growing body in a variety of ways.[1] It is essential for the development of strong, healthy bones and muscles; aids in weight control; and appears to have mental health benefits as well, resulting in a heightened sense of well-being. The fitness benefits of exercise lead to functional improvements in everyday life, including improved energy levels, stamina, posture, coordination, and stability. Physical activity also plays a role in disease management and prevention, helping children to optimize blood lipid and blood pressure levels, improve lung capacity and cardiovascular function, and maintain glucose tolerance.

Children with a chronic disease or developmental disorder will obtain the same benefits from regular physical activity as healthy children do. Exercise can help improve their quality of life. Sometimes a child with a chronic illness is discouraged from exercising. Unless there are disease or health condition–specific contraindications to certain types of exercise, physical activity should be encouraged to optimize the many physiological systems it affects, including the skeletal, muscular, and cardiovascular systems. Because all children can benefit from physical activity, it is important to allow them to be active, within individually determined limitations, and to teach them how do so safely.

Special Olympics is an international nonprofit organization that provides athletic training and competition to individuals with mental retardation. More than 4 million athletes in 170 countries and millions of volunteers participate in Special Olympics games every year. The programs include 30 summer and winter sports, such as swimming, cycling, golf, soccer, bowling, basketball, gymnastics, roller skating, running, and tennis. The association strives to help participants "develop improved physical fitness and motor skills, greater self-confidence, and a more positive self-image."[2]

Not all physical activities are equivalent in the physiological changes they induce. Fitness training is highly specific. An exercise that is cardiovascular based, such as walking or running, may increase a child's muscle mass to a lesser degree than what might be possible with a resistance activity such as weight training, calisthenics, or gymnastics. Conversely, many resistance activities may not provide significant cardiovascular improvements or the same rise in caloric expenditure as that provided by a traditional aerobic pursuit. Participating in a solitary fitness activity such as cycling will not produce the same neuromuscular and coordination benefits as performing a more skill-based activity. For that reason, it is important to *cross-train*—that is, to include a variety of different sports and activities in an overall program. Children who are encouraged to move not only will have fun but will be empowered by a sense of their own physical strength. The Centers for Disease Control calls for parents, schools, and communities to create opportunities for physical activities that are enjoyable and promote confidence in children's and teens' ability to be physically active.

## YOUNG ATHLETES' BILL OF RIGHTS

The Young Athletes' Bill of Rights[3] includes the following:

1. The right to have the opportunity to participate in sports regardless of ability level.
2. The right to participate at a level commensurate with each child's developmental level.
3. The right to have qualified adult leadership.
4. The right to participate in a safe and healthy environment
5. The right of each child to share leadership and decision making.
6. The right to play as a child and not as an adult.
7. The right to proper preparation for participation in sports.
8. The right to equal opportunity to strive for success.
9. The right to be treated with dignity by all involved.
10. The right to have fun through sports.

Benefits of regular exercise include cardiovascular fitness, muscular strength and stamina, flexibility and mobility, improved gross motor skills, improved agility and stability, hormonal regulation, and an improved sense of well-being and self-confidence.

## HEALTH RISKS OF INACTIVITY

Almost half of Americans aged 12 to 21 years are not vigorously active on a regular basis.[4] Factors that play a role include increased time spent watching television and using computers, removal of physical activity from two-thirds of the schools, and fewer outdoor play opportunities for many children. Inactivity and poor nutrition go hand in hand. A child who is trapped in an increasingly inactive life may be inclined to eat more and to make poor food choices—especially if excess television watching subjects the child to the massive marketing campaigns that junk-food manufacturers aim at children. Survey data show that 41.3% of children spend 3 or more hours playing video or computer games and 32.5% watch television for 3 or more hours on school days.[5] An underused, poorly fed body will suffer a decline in health status that may place the child at greater risk for a variety of health disorders and diseases.

### Obesity

Obesity rates have been rising dramatically among America's youth, although recent evidence suggests a leveling off at about 17%.[6] Epidemiologic data reveal that a child who is obese at 12 years of age has approximately a 75% chance of being obese as an adult.[7] Children with special health care needs may be especially prone to obesity in later years. As obesity increases, so does the risk for chronic diseases, including type 2 diabetes mellitus, dyslipidemia, and hypertension in both children and adults. Tracking a child's height, weight, and body composition throughout childhood can reliably indicate whether these parameters are within the recommended range.[7] Because successful treatment of obesity in adults is rare, it has been suggested that aggressive treatment should start with the emergence of overweight in a children.[8] Exercise, along with dietary and behavior modification, is an essential component of a treatment program for childhood obesity (see Chapter 18). The American Academy of Pediatrics (AAP) has urged pediatricians to take a proactive stance, advocating for physical education programs that promote fitness.[9]

### Diabetes

The National Institutes of Health reported that the percentage of children diagnosed with type 2 diabetes rose from less than 5% before 1994 to between 30% and 50%.[9] One of every 433 children younger than 20 years of age is affected.[10] Type 2 diabetes is more prevalent in youth with a body mass index (BMI) greater than the 85th percentile in the United States and Europe.[11] Impaired glucose tolerance was found in one study to affect 25% of obese children between 4 and 10 years of age and 21% of obese adolescents between 11 and 18 years of age.[12] Clinicians must be on the lookout for undiagnosed symptoms of type 2 diabetes in overweight or inactive children. These symptoms include polyuria, polydipsia, polyphagia, blurred vision, fatigue, headache, poor wound healing, and weight loss (see Chapter 48).

### Osteopenia

Bone density increases to approximately 90% of its peak level during the adolescent years. Weight-bearing physical activity (e.g., jumping), along with adequate calcium, magnesium, fluoride, and vitamin D intake, especially during growth periods, is essential to optimize peak bone density. Participation in weight-bearing physical activity throughout childhood and adolescence contributes to lifelong bone health.[13]

Certain types of activity are more weight-bearing than others and may result in greater bone mass increases due to greater force production or impact stimulus. Exercise stimulus is site specific. Jumping and high-impact movements with the lower body tend to affect the hip and lumbar spine. Forceful muscular action with the upper body, such as ball throwing, racket hitting, resistance training, and maneuvers with body weights (e.g., propulsive hand stands, swinging on rails), affect the wrist. Gymnasts, for example, have been found to have greater bone mineral density than age-matched controls. The magnitude of the force applied to the muscles and bones is more important in producing bone changes than the number of times that stress is applied. Gymnasts who perform high-impact movements sporadically exhibit better bone density than runners who experience moderate impact over an extended period.

Increased bone mineral density established during childhood has been found to be maintained in adults, even when they are no longer engaging in high levels of physical activity.[14] Therefore, exercise in childhood may help reduce the risk of fractures in postmenopausal women. Young girls who undereat or are underweight may remain in a prepubertal state for many years, especially if they participate in sports in which weight control is emphasized. The delay in the onset of estrogen action can result in undermineralized bone.[15] Young girls and women who are extremely active may also be susceptible to the cluster of conditions known as the female athletic triad: disordered eating, amenorrhea, and osteoporosis.

### Hyperlipidemia and Hypercholesterolemia

Hyperlipidemia and hypercholesterolemia were recognized by the 1985 Panel for the National Institutes of Health Consensus Development Conference on the Health Implications of Obesity as two of the adverse effects of obesity. Dietary therapy, weight loss, and regular physical activity have been recommended as effective methods to lower elevated levels of total cholesterol, low-density lipoprotein (LDL) cholesterol and triglycerides and to raise low levels of high-density lipoprotein (HDL) cholesterol in overweight and obese persons with dyslipidemia.[16] Aerobic fitness, as measured by peak oxygen uptake, is inversely related to blood cholesterol levels and fat mass.[17] It has been demonstrated that aerobic training results in an increase in peak oxygen uptake when performed at intensities greater than 80% of maximal heart rate (see Chapter 32).

## FACTORS TO BE CONSIDERED IN NUTRITIONAL EVALUATION

### Growth

A primary concern of the school-age child is the achievement of normal growth. Height and weight should be evaluated using National Center for Health Statistics growth charts, and BMI should be calculated (http://pediatrics.aappublications.org/content/pediatrics/125/2/361.full.pdf). Height and weight should be plotted routinely to allow for the identification of either overnutrition or undernutrition. When height and weight fall into markedly different percentiles, weight-for-height may be a more sensitive index of appropriate growth than weight-for-age because body weight is related more closely to size than to age. However, children may have atrophy of the extremities, making this calculation less useful. Growth charts have been developed for these disorders (see Appendix 2).

### Weight

A healthy body weight is one that is in proportion to height. Although underweight or overweight (BMI >95th percentile) may have a detrimental effect on physical performance, altering the body weight will not necessarily improve performance. Any attempts to change the body weight of a child who is clearly underweight or overweight should be made with the aid of a physician or nutritionist to ensure adequate nutritional intake. Excessive weight loss may affect a child's growth rate, nutrition status, hormone levels, and bone mineral content and may contribute to psychological stress preliminary to an eating disorder. It is also important to emphasize good nutrition through nutrition education so that the child, parent, or coach will avoid improper weight management, fluid restriction, and misuse of dietary supplements.[8]

### Body Composition

Physiological changes in bone density and in the proportion of body water in adolescents going through puberty make it difficult to use body fat and weight measurements as rigid evaluation criteria.[8] Because there are currently no standards of comparison for young athletes that are specific for sport and gender, the clinician must use sound clinical judgment and growth charts to assess optimal weight. Evaluation of body composition should take into account the fact that children have higher body water content and lower bone mineral content than adults, and therefore their body density is lower. Equations using conversion constants from adult samples may overestimate body fat by 3% to 6%. The chemical composition of fat-free mass (i.e., water, minerals, protein) changes with passage through puberty; therefore, use of skinfolds, body widths, and circumferences may not accurately assess changes in body fat. Estimates of body fat must use a multicomponent approach. Changes may be tracked using skinfold thickness without calculation of percent body fat. Use of body composition assessments to manipulate body fat for sports performance should be avoided because this practice may adversely affect growth and development.

### Dietary Habits

Nutritional adequacy can be assessed with the use of a food frequency questionnaire and a 24-hour dietary recall. For the best assessment, both the parents and the child should be interviewed, and the child should be questioned away from the parents to avoid answers that are based on parental expectations.[8] To facilitate recall of meal patterns, it is useful to ask not just what was consumed but details on dietary behaviors: Is breakfast normally eaten? Is lunch consumed at home or at school? What are the favorite snacks, and how often does snacking occur? Are dinners spent eating in front of the television or with the family? When are fluids consumed? Questions about the type, duration, and intensity of regular physical activities should be included to better assess energy expenditure.

## GUIDELINES FOR PHYSICAL ACTIVITY

Children, as well as adults, are advised to engage in moderate-intensity physical activity for 30 minutes on most days of the week.[4] It is crucial to start young in order to instill familiarity and a positive association with fitness activities. A physical fitness program should include strength, flexibility, and aerobic components (see Appendix 7, Children's Pyramid Physical Activity).

### Resistance Training

Strength or resistance training using free weights or weight machines has been found to increase strength in children and adolescents. The AAP has confirmed that strength training programs for preadolescents and adolescents can prevent injuries and impact long-term health. Strength training can be safe and effective if proper resistance training techniques and safety precautions are followed. In 2008, the AAP issued the following recommendations for strength training[18]:

- Before the individual begins a formal strength training program, a medical evaluation should be performed by a pediatrician. If indicated, a referral may be made to a sports medicine physician who is familiar with the various strength training methods as well as their risks and benefits for preadolescents and adolescents.
- Preadolescents and adolescents should avoid competitive weight lifting, power lifting, body building, and maximal lifts until they reach physical and skeletal maturity.
- Aerobic conditioning should be coupled with resistance training if general health benefits are the goal.
- Strength training programs should include warm-up and cool-down components.
- A general strengthening program should address all major muscle groups and exercise through the complete range of motion.
- Specific strength training exercises should be learned initially with no load (resistance). Once the exercise skill has been mastered, incremental loads may be added.
- Progressive resistance exercise requires successful completion of 8 to 15 repetitions in good form before the weight or resistance is increased. It is generally recommended that resistance training be performed 2 to 3 days a week.[18,19]
- Any sign of injury or illness from strength training should be evaluated before the exercise in question is continued.

Other forms of resistance training use body weight and/or impact forces. Physical activity that places a load on the bone will stimulate bone growth and optimize bone mineral density. Jumping exercises such as jumping rope or jumping jacks are particularly effective. When modifying resistance exercise for a child's special limitations, it is important to search for tools that may enhance performance. A variety of differently shaped weights and resistance-band products can make holding a weight easier. Many exercises can be performed by a person in a wheelchair.

### Cardiovascular Exercise

The American College of Sports Medicine defines cardiorespiratory fitness as the ability to perform large-muscle, dynamic, moderate- to high-intensity exercise for prolonged periods. The following guidelines are recommended[19]:

- An exercise session should include a warm-up period of approximately 10 minutes, an endurance phase of 20 to 60 minutes, and a cool-down period of 5 to 10 minutes.
- The duration of the activity depends on its intensity. Easier movements can be performed for longer periods. Vigorous exercise should be performed in intervals, interspersing periods of work and rest, or for a shorter overall duration.
- If recreational games are included along with bona fide fitness training, the experience of successful participation, as opposed to winning or losing, should be emphasized. Because the skill level and perception of effort are not always the same as the intensity level, monitoring of the heart rate and perceived exertion is recommended. Whenever possible, requirements should be modified to cope with the limitations of an ill or handicapped child.
- Both the intensity and the duration of exercise determine the total caloric expenditure. Clinical and low-fit populations can improve the fitness with lower-intensity, longer-duration sessions. Intensity can be estimated by monitoring the heart rate, breathing rate, and/or perceived exertion. Looking for physical signs of fatigue, such as reduced ability or slack posture, can also be helpful.
- Medications that may influence heart rate or fatigue should be considered when determining the amount and intensity of activity.
- The recommended rate of progression in an exercise conditioning program depends on the functional capacity, medical and health status, age, individual activity preferences and goals, and the individual's tolerance of the current level of training. Deconditioned individuals should be allowed more time to adapt to each stage of conditioning before progressing further.
- Cardiorespiratory exercise should be performed on most days of the week. An ill or deconditioned individual can benefit from breaking up longer sessions. For example, three 10-minute sessions can be used instead of one 30-minute session.
- If a child has limited mobility or is confined to a wheelchair, an aerobic effect can be elicited by rhythmic, continuous movements of the arms.

### Flexibility

According to the American College of Sports Medicine, flexibility is the ability to move a joint through its complete range of motion. The following recommendations should be considered when performing range-of-motion exercises[19]:

- Avoid stretching "cold." An active warm-up period that includes mobility and temperature-raising movements should precede vigorous stretching. Alternatively, stretching can be performed after physical activity, rather than before it. However, an active warm-up should be included before vigorous activity.
- Several types of stretching can improve range of motion, including static, ballistic, and proprioceptive neuromuscular facilitation. Static stretching, in which a position is held for 10 to 30 seconds to the point of mild discomfort but never pain, is the most commonly recommended method.
- Yoga, Pilates, and other flexibility-based disciplines can improve flexibility. One should be careful to avoid extreme positioning, uncomfortable joint angles, and progressing faster than is comfortable.
- Three to four repetitions of a stretch that is held for 10 to 30 seconds are performed on at least 2 to 3 days per week. Daily stretching is most effective.
- Children with limited mobility can be assisted with their stretching exercises.

## DIETARY MANAGEMENT

The nutritional requirements for active children are similar to those for sedentary children, allowing for the additional energy needs of activity. Calories consumed must be adequate to provide for physical activity as well as normal growth. It can be difficult to assess energy expenditure in children because of variations in age, gender, stage of development, and body composition. A compendium has been developed to assign energy costs to various activities in children, but practitioners should use caution because this remains a work in progress.[20,21] It also should be recognized that children whose movements are less efficient require more kilocalories per unit of body weight.

A variety of foods should be included from each of the food groups in the Choose MyPlate guidelines (http://www.choosemyplate.gov/). To achieve the health benefits of physical activity, active youth should be encouraged to minimize their intake of saturated fats and cholesterol, consume sweets in amounts that will allow for the maintenance of energy balance, and consume adequate dietary calcium and vitamin K, along with physical activity, to allow for optimal bone mineralization. These nutrients are ideally obtained through whole foods rather than supplements. A child can be educated as to appropriate types of snacks and times of snacking to enhance energy levels. The child should be taught how to make nutritious choices, such as selecting a healthier item from a vending machine or a fast-food restaurant. Breakfast helps replenish glycogen stores that are depleted overnight.

**Table 7–1.** Caloric Equivalents of a Child's Activities (in Kilocalories per 10 Minutes of Activity)

| | Body Weight (kg) | | | | | | | | | |
|---|---|---|---|---|---|---|---|---|---|---|
| Activity | 20 | 25 | 30 | 35 | 40 | 45 | 50 | 55 | 60 | 65 |
| Basketball | 34 | 43 | 51 | 60 | 68 | 77 | 85 | 94 | 102 | 110 |
| Calisthenics | 13 | 17 | 20 | 23 | 26 | 30 | 33 | 36 | 40 | 43 |
| Cycling | | | | | | | | | | |
| 10 km/hr | 15 | 17 | 20 | 23 | 26 | 29 | 33 | 36 | 39 | 42 |
| 15 km/hr | 22 | 27 | 32 | 36 | 41 | 46 | 50 | 55 | 60 | 65 |
| Figure skating | 40 | 50 | 60 | 70 | 80 | 90 | 100 | 110 | 120 | 130 |
| Ice hockey (on-ice time) | 52 | 65 | 78 | 91 | 104 | 117 | 130 | 143 | 156 | 168 |
| Running | | | | | | | | | | |
| 8 km/hr | 37 | 45 | 52 | 60 | 66 | 72 | 78 | 84 | 90 | 95 |
| 10 km/hr | 48 | 55 | 64 | 73 | 79 | 85 | 92 | 100 | 107 | 113 |
| Soccer (game) | 36 | 45 | 54 | 63 | 72 | 81 | 90 | 99 | 108 | 117 |
| Swimming | | | | | | | | | | |
| Breast stroke 30 m/min | 19 | 24 | 29 | 34 | 38 | 43 | 48 | 53 | 58 | 62 |
| Front crawl | 25 | 31 | 37 | 43 | 49 | 56 | 62 | 68 | 74 | 80 |
| Back stroke | 17 | 21 | 25 | 30 | 34 | 38 | 42 | 47 | 51 | 55 |
| Tennis | 22 | 28 | 33 | 39 | 44 | 50 | 55 | 61 | 66 | 72 |
| Walking | | | | | | | | | | |
| 4 km/hr | 17 | 19 | 21 | 23 | 26 | 28 | 30 | 32 | 34 | 36 |
| 6 km/hr | 24 | 26 | 28 | 30 | 32 | 34 | 37 | 40 | 43 | 48 |

Adapted with permission from Bar-Or O. *Pediatric Sports Medicine for the Practitioner*. New York: Springer; 1983.

If a child feels too excited or nervous to eat before an event, rather than pressuring the child to eat, one should encourage the consumption of liquids such as sports drinks or juices.

Excessive consumption of protein, calories, or other nutrients will not improve athletic performance. The use of protein supplementation is not recommended and has not been shown to improve athletic performance, muscle development, or strength. Research on the safety and efficacy of other nutritional supplements in enhancing exercise performance is unavailable in children. Of concern, young athletes using such supplements may develop a false sense of security and may be less likely to attribute progress to their training and diet. Some coaches may encourage a child to overeat or supplement or may deny regular fluids as part of the training discipline. Efforts should be made to educate coaches and parents on the special needs of a child with a medical condition (Table 7–1). Guidelines on snacks and their timing are as follows:

- One to 2 hours before exercise: fruit or vegetable juice, sports drink, fresh fruit
- Two to 3 hours before exercise: fruit or vegetable juice, sports drink, fresh fruit, breads, bagels, crackers
- Three or more hours before exercise: fruit or vegetable juice, sports drink, fresh fruit, breads, bagels, crackers, low-fat yogurt, pasta with tomato sauce, cereal with low-fat milk
- Within 2 hours after exercise: fresh fruit, sports drink, bread, bagels, crackers

## FLUID NEEDS OF ACTIVE CHILDREN

Dehydration can dramatically affect a child's ability to perform well. As little as a 2% decrease in body weight from fluid loss (e.g., a 1.2-lb loss for a 60-lb child) can lead to a significant decrease in muscular strength and stamina.[22] Adequate hydration is essential to regulate body temperature. Additional factors contributing to reduced performance and heat illness include extreme exertion in the heat and the wearing of uniforms and equipment that act to retain heat. Research shows that children are able to safely exercise in the heat as long as they maintain adequate hydration, avoid clothing that may result in heat retention, and rest sufficiently.[22]

Challenges to maintaining adequate hydration include children's diminished sense of thirst; a child may be quite dehydrated before he or she feels thirsty. Fluid should be readily available, and fluid breaks should be scheduled regularly. Children should be advised to drink on a schedule rather than relying on thirst.

One must be alert for signs of dehydration or underfeeding, including early fatigue, irritability, or a sudden drop in performance. Those supervising exercise for children with special needs should be aware that certain conditions will increase the likelihood of heat illness. For example, children with mental retardation may not recognize the need to replace fluid losses. Those with diabetes mellitus, diabetes insipidus, or gastrointestinal infection may experience greater than normal fluid losses. Certain congenital heart defects may result in excessive sweating, whereas cystic fibrosis may result in diminished thirst. Certain medications have diuretic effects. Finally, anorexia or obesity also affects thermoregulation.

Based on these consideration, the AAP has issued the following recommendations for exercising in cold or hot weather or for prolonged periods[22]:

- The intensity of activities that last 15 minutes or longer should be reduced whenever relative humidity, solar radiation, and air temperature are above critical levels. One way of increasing rest periods on a hot day is to substitute players on a team frequently.
- At the beginning of a strenuous exercise program or after traveling to a warmer climate, the intensity and duration of exercise should be limited initially and then gradually increased over a period of 10 to 14 days to ensure acclimatization to the heat. If such a period is not available, practice and competition periods should be curtailed.
- Before prolonged physical activity, the child should be well hydrated. During the activity, periodic drinking should be enforced. For example, every 20 minutes, a child weighing 40 kg should drink 150 mL of cold tap water or a flavored carbohydrate-electrolyte beverage (250 mL for an adolescent weighing 60 kg), even if the child does not feel thirsty. Weighing before and after a training session can verify hydration status if the child is weighed wearing little or no clothing.
- Clothing should be light-colored, lightweight, and limited to one layer of absorbent material to facilitate evaporation of sweat. Sweat-saturated garments should be replaced by dry garments. Rubberized sweatsuits should never be used to produce loss of weight.

Children and adolescents with medical conditions have special issues with respect to participation in athletic activities. The pediatrician can play an important role in determining whether a child with a health condition should participate in certain sports by assessing the child's health status, suggesting appropriate equipment or modifications to decrease the risk of injury, and educating the athlete and parents on the risks of injury in relation to the child's condition.[23]

## References


1. Centers for Disease Control and Prevention. *Health benefits of physical exercise.* http://www.cdc.gov/physicalactivity/basics/pa-health/. Accessed June 6, 2016.
2. Special Olympics. Website. www.specialolympics.org. Accessed June 6, 2016.
3. Martens R, Seefeldt V, eds. *Guidelines for Children's Sports.* Washington, DC: American Alliance for Health, Physical Education, Recreation and Dance; 1979.
4. US Department of Health and Human Services. *2008 Physical Activity Guidelines for Americans.* ODPHP Publication No. U0036; October 2008. Washington, DC: US DHHS, Office of Disease Prevention and Health Promotion. http://www.health.gov/paguidelines/pdf/paguide.pdf. Accessed June 6, 2016.
5. Centers for Disease Control and Prevention, Youth Risk Behavior Survey. Trends in the Prevalence of Physical Activity and Sedentary Behaviors: National YRBS, 1991–2013. http://www.cdc.gov/healthyyouth/data/yrbs/results.htm. Accessed June 6, 2016.
6. Ogden CL, Carroll MD, Kit BK, Flegal KM. Prevalence of childhood and adult obesity in the United States, 2011–2012. *JAMA.* 2014; 311:806.
7. Klish WJ. Childhood obesity. *Pediatr Rev.* 1998; 19:312.
8. Hoelscher DM, Kirk S, Ritchie L, Cunningham-Sabo L; Academy Positions Committee. Position of the Academy of Nutrition and Dietetics: interventions for the prevention and treatment of pediatric overweight and obesity. *J Acad Nutr Diet.* 2013; 113:1375.
9. US Preventive Services Task Force. Screening for obesity in children and adolescents: US Preventive Services Task Force recommendation statement. *Pediatrics.* 2010; 125:361.
10. Pettitt DJ, Talton J, Dabelea D, et al. Prevalence of Diabetes in U.S. Youth in 2009: the SEARCH for Diabetes in Youth Study. *Diab Care.* 2014; 37:402.
11. Rosenbloom, AL, Silverstein JH, Amemiya S, Zeitler P, Klingensmith GJ. Type 2 diabetes in children and adolescents. *Pediatr Diabetes.* 2009; 10(suppl 12):17.
12. Sinha R, Fisch G, Teague B, et al. Prevalence of impaired glucose tolerance among children and adolescents with marked obesity. *N Engl J Med.* 2002; 346:802.
13. Gunter KB, Almstedt HC, Janz KF. Physical activity in childhood may be the key to optimizing lifespan skeletal health. *Exerc Sport Sci Rev.* 2012; 40:13.
14. Bass S, Pearce G, Bradney M, et al. Exercise before puberty may confer residual benefits in bone density in adulthood: studies in active prepubertal and retired female gymnasts. *J Bone Miner Res.* 1998; 13:500.
15. Roemmich JN, Richmond RJ, Rogol AD. Consequences of sport training during puberty. *J Endocrinol Invest.* 2001; 24:708.
16. Stefanick ML. Physical activity for preventing and treating obesity-related dyslipoproteinemias. *Med Sci Sports Exerc.* 1999; 31(11 suppl):S609.
17. Baquet G, VanPraagh E, Berthoin S. Endurance training and aerobic fitness in young people. *Sports Med.* 2003; 33:1127.
18. American Academy of Pediatrics Council on Sports Medicine and Fitness, McCambridge TM, Stricker PR. Strength training by children and adolescents. *Pediatrics.* 2008; 121:835.
19. American College of Sports Medicine. *ACSM's Guidelines for Exercise Testing and Prescription*, 9th ed. Philadelphia: Lippincott Williams & Wilkins; 2014.
20. Ridley K, Olds T. Assigning energy costs to activities in children: a review and synthesis. *Med Sci Sports Exerc.* 2008; 40:1439.
21. Lyden K, Keadle SK, Staudenmayer J, Freedson P, Alhassan S. Energy cost of common activities in children and adolescents. *J Phys Act Health.* 2013;10:62.
22. Council on Sports Medicine and Fitness and Council on School Health, Bergeron MF, Devore C, Rice SG; American Academy of Pediatrics. Climatic heat stress and exercising children and adolescents. *Pediatrics.* 2011; 128:e741.
23. Rice SG. Medical conditions affecting sports participation. *Pediatrics.* 2008; 121:841.

# 8 Vegetarian Diets Across the Lifespan

GEORGIA E. HODGKIN

Increasing numbers of people in the United States are choosing vegetarian diets. A Roper poll in 2000 estimated that 2% of the adult population was vegetarian, and 2% of children aged 6 to 17 years said they never ate meat, fish, or poultry.[1] A Harris poll in 2015 indicated that 3.4% of the adult population was vegetarian. Of the 2015 subgroups, 6% of the 18- to 34-year-olds never ate meat, fish, or poultry, and 7% of those households earning less than $50,000 were vegetarian. The 2015 poll suggested that the younger population and those with lower incomes chose vegetarian diets more frequently than the general population. The reason that young people were choosing vegetarian diets was not determined to be related to beliefs, length of time on the job, or other factors.[2]

Vegetarian diets usually differ from carnivorous diets only in the source of the protein consumed, yet quite a variety of vegetarian diets have been defined. The label often is descriptive of the protein foods excluded or included. Typically, meat, fish, and poultry are excluded. When dairy milk is included, the diet is referred to as a lacto-vegetarian diet. Likewise, adding eggs changes the name to ovo-vegetarian, with both milk and eggs added, the diet is referred to as lacto-ovo-vegetarian. A total vegetarian diet, commonly referred to as vegan, excludes all animal products, including honey. Table 8–1 summarizes the various vegetarian diets.

Some persons choose to use the phrase "plant-based" diet. This diet is based in plants but uses meat as a condiment.[3–6] Therefore, it is not strictly a vegetarian diet. The term "semivegetarian" also refers to a diet that includes meat on an infrequent basis.

Vegetarian diets are preferred by the public for a number of reasons, including health, religious, economic, and environmental concerns. The environmental concern relates to the disparity in resources used to produce nutrients for humans from plants compared with those needed to produce nutrients from animals for human consumption. An example is water use. It requires 4 gallons of water to produce 1 g of protein from beef, whereas 1 g of protein from soybeans requires 0.5 gallons.[8] Such comparisons would seem to recommend vegetarian diets.

## HEALTH BENEFITS OF VEGETARIAN DIETS

A cohort of the Adventist Health Study-2 (AHS-2) included 15,200 men and 26,187 women in the United States and Canada. Data showed that vegetarians had a lower risk for developing diabetes than nonvegetarians.[9] A lower incidence of colorectal cancer was shown for the 96,354 in the AHS-2 data set, and there was also a much lower risk among the pesco-vegetarians compared with nonvegetarians.[10] Health benefits have been shown for vegetarian diets in regard to cardiovascular disease,[11] hypertension,[12] and metabolic syndrome.[13] Even mood benefits from vegetarian meals, in spite of vegetarians' lower intakes of eicosapentaenoic acid (EPA) and docosahexaenoic acid (DHA), which are important in the regulation of brain function and structure.[14] Of a cohort of 73,308 participants in AHS-2, 2570 deaths occurred over 5.79 years, suggesting that vegetarian diets lead to reduced all-cause mortality.[11]

## IMPLEMENTING A VEGETARIAN DIET

It is the position of the American Dietetic Association (now known as the Academy of Nutrition and Dietetics)[7] that:

> Appropriately planned vegetarian diets, including total vegetarian or vegan diets, are healthful, nutritionally adequate, and may provide health benefits in the prevention and treatment of certain diseases. Well-planned vegetarian diets are appropriate for individuals during all stages of the lifecycle, including pregnancy, lactation, infancy, childhood, and adolescence, and for athletes.

Tools for meal planning have been developed by the US Food and Drug Administration (FDA), Department of Agriculture (USDA), and Department of Health and Human Services (DHHS) and are available to the public. Three are particularly helpful. The *food label* shows the serving size and nutrients in the food. A *food graphic*, currently known as MyPlate, displays the food groups and the portion of each meal suggested to come from that group. The third tool is the *Dietary Guidelines for Americans,* which gives recommendations for choices in all food groups. My Vegetarian Plate[15] is a food graphic that displays balanced nutrition meeting nutrient needs for healthy groups of people (see Appendix 7–7, *My Vegetarian Plate*). The proportion of food from each group is represented on the graphic.

Appendix 7–8, *My Vegetarian Plate Food Guide*, includes three commonly recommended calorie levels. The number of servings needed to reach each calorie level is given, as is the amount of various foods that equals one serving. Nutrients provided generally by each food group are listed, as well as foods that are the better sources of those nutrients. Foods are divided into groups because they provide a common set of nutrients; therefore, it is unwise to skip any of the groups.

To determine the recommended calorie level for an individual, go to http://www.choosemyplate.gov and click on SuperTracker. The site determines a Daily Food Plan based on four points of information: age, gender, weight, and height. The Daily Food Plan states the number of servings needed to meet the recommended calorie level. Consult Appendix 7–8 for the size of the portions served at a meal.

When foods are chosen from a wide variety within in each food group, nutrient needs will be met as well as calorie needs supplied. The graphic provides the Dietary Reference Intake for all nutrients when appropriately planned.

## NORMAL GROWTH IN CHILDREN

Well-planned vegetarian diets support normal growth and development in children. Both lacto-ovo-vegetarian diets and vegan diets meet nutrient needs throughout the lifespan.[7] Table 8–2 gives the recommended number of servings for children in each age group by gender.[16]

## NUTRIENTS OF CONCERN WITH VEGETARIAN DIETS

Vegetarian diets can provide all the amino acids necessary for metabolism. Improved methods of processing and preparation have increased the digestibility of plant proteins.[16] The combining of plant proteins to achieve "complete" protein at each meal is not necessary. The full complement of amino acids can be provided from a diet composed of a variety of plant proteins consumed throughout the day. Typical meal planning includes a variety of foods in a day's menu that will provide all of the amino acids needed for protein synthesis. A mixed and varied diet of sufficient calories ensures adequate protein for growth and maintenance throughout the lifespan.[17]

**Table 8–1.** Foods Included and Excluded from Vegetarian Diets

| Type of Vegetarian Diet | Foods Included | Foods Excluded |
|---|---|---|
| Lacto-vegetarian | Milk | Meat, fish, poultry, and eggs |
| Ovo-vegetarian | Eggs | Meat, fish, poultry, and milk |
| Lacto-ovo-vegetarian | Milk and eggs | Meat, fish, poultry |
| Pesco-vegetarian | Fish | Meat and poultry |
| Pollo-vegetarian | Chicken | Meat and fish |
| Total vegetarian or vegan | No animal products of any kind | Meat, fish, poultry, milk, eggs; some do not use honey |
| Macrobiotic[7] | Grains, legumes, vegetables; lesser amounts of fruit, nuts, seeds; some add fish | Meat, poultry, sometimes fish, milk, eggs, some vegetables, some fruits |
| Fruitarian[7] | Fruits and vegetables that are botanically fruits; nuts and seeds | All others |

From Craig WJ, Mangels AR. Position of the American Dietetic Association: vegetarian diets. *J Am Diet Assoc.* 2009; 109:1266.

Beyond the protein content of vegetarian diets are concerns for iron and zinc intake. Rational assumptions regarding vegetarian diets would lead to an expected compromised iron and zinc status because fiber and other substances in plant foods interfere with the absorption of those minerals. However, vegetarian diets provide an abundance of nonheme iron along with enhancers of absorption, most notably vitamin C. The net result is that vegetarians are no more at risk of iron deficiency anemia than are omnivores.[18] With modern food processing procedures, such as soaking, heating, sprouting, fermenting, and leavening, the reduced absorption of nutrients may be lessened. Adequate zinc absorption is more likely assured if leavened or sourdough breads, sprouts, and soaked legumes are included in the menu. Hence, the conclusion is the same for zinc as for iron: Vegetarians are no more at risk for deficiency than those who do not subscribe to vegetarian diets.[19,20] Foods that provide zinc and nonheme iron are listed in Table 8–3.

Like omnivorous diets, vegetarian diets that include milk may be adequate in calcium. Total vegetarian or vegan diets, however, must be carefully planned to meet the calcium requirements of children. See Table 8–3 for dietary sources of calcium. Soy milk may be fortified with calcium if a calcium salt is used in the processing of the soybean. The label on the product indicates whether a serving contains 20% to 30% of the Daily Value (DV) for calcium, which is comparable to cow's milk. The bioavailability of calcium in soy milk is approximately 75% of that in cow's milk. The methods used to measure absorption of calcium may be overestimated by as much as 50% in soy milks.[21]

Vitamin D sources include sunshine and fortified foods. The principal fortified food in the US diet is cow's milk. If cow's milk is eliminated from the diet, care must be taken to ensure that another source is provided. Vitamin $B_{12}$ is found only in animal products. The milk and eggs in lacto-ovo-vegetarian diets may supply the daily requirement, but total vegetarian diets must be supplemented, either through foods that are fortified or by a synthetic supplement. Omega-3 fatty acids may come from vegetarian sources. With planning, a vegetarian diet can meet all of these nutrient needs. Fortification of foods and supplements help to provide a variety of approaches to vegetarian meal planning.[22]

## DIETARY MANAGEMENT

Parameters have been developed for the application of vegetarian diets to a number of disease processes.[23] Recommendations for multiple diets are available. Diets across the lifespan for a number of pathologies have been published, for children as well as adults.[23]

Children exhibiting failure to thrive show significant growth delays, most often from nutritional deprivation due to psychosocial factors. In this instance, both protein and calories are lacking, and when these are provided, catch-up growth will be seen. Infants should receive formulas that are no more calorically dense than 24 kcal/oz; additional calories may come from rice cereal, vegetable oils, or medium-chain triglyceride oils. Older children may be offered more calorie-dense

**Table 8–2.** Servings for Vegetarian Children*

| | Age Range, Gender, and Calories (with Age Used for the Stated Calorie Level[16]) | | | | | | | |
|---|---|---|---|---|---|---|---|---|
| | 1–2 yr | | 3–8 yr | | 9–13 yr | | 14–18 yr | |
| Food Group | M (1046 cal at NAS) | F (992 cal) | M (1742 cal at 6 yr) | F (1642 cal at 6 yr) | M (2279 cal at 11 yr) | F (2071 cal at 11 yr) | M (3152 cal at 16 yr) | F (2368 cal at 16 yr) |
| Breads/cereals (80 cal) | 3.5 | 3 | 6 | 5.5 | 10.5 | 9 | 14 | 10 |
| Vegetables (25 cal) | 1 | 1 | 3 | 2 | 3 | 3 | 5 | 4 |
| Fruits (60 cal) | 2 | 2 | 3 | 3 | 3.5 | 3.5 | 4.5 | 4 |
| Milk/dairy (Whole, 160 cal; LF, 120 cal; 100 cal) | 2.5 Whole | 2.5 Whole | 3 LF | 3 LF | 3 NF | 3 NF | 4 NF | 3.5 NF |
| Protein foods (medium-fat, 75 cal) | 2 | 2 | 5 | 5 | 6.5 | 6.5 | 8 | 6 |
| Fats and oils (45 cal) | 1 | 1 | 4 | 3 | 5.5 | 4 | 10 | 6 |
| Desserts (with 1 tsp sugar and 2 g fat, 45 cal) | 1 | 1 | 2 | 2 | 2 | 2 | 4 | 3 |
| Total calories | 1040 | 1000 | 1740 | 1630 | 2250 | 2063 | 3145 | 2345 |
| % Fat | 32 | 33 | 33 | 33 | 28† | 28† | 31† | 29† |
| % Protein | 16 | 17 | 18 | 18 | 17 | 18 | 16 | 16 |

*Amounts per serving:
Breads/cereals = 1 slice bread (30 g), ¾ c cold unsweetened cereal, ½ c hot cereal, ⅓ c pasta/rice, ¼ bagel or muffin (4 oz), ½ English muffin, 3–4 crackers (30 g)
Vegetables = 1 c raw leafy, ½ c chopped raw, ½ c cooked, 6 oz juice
Fruits = 1 medium piece, 1 c berries, ¼ c dried fruit, ½ c unsweetened canned fruit or juice
Milk/dairy = 1 c milk, 1 c yogurt, 1¾ oz cheese, 1½ c cottage cheese, 1½ c ice cream
Protein foods = ½ c cooked beans, ½ c tofu, ¼ c nuts/seeds, 2 T nut butter, ¼ c meat alternative, 1 egg
Fats and oils = 1 tsp oil, margarine, mayonnaise, or nut butter; ⅛ avocado, 1½ tsp tahini
Desserts = 1 small cookie, 1 small piece of candy (e.g., 1/5 of a 1.9-oz chocolate bar, 11 Gummi Savers, 1 LifeSaver lollipop, 13 M&Ms, 5 M&Ms with peanuts or small turtle candy), 5 animal crackers, ¼ small piece of cake, ⅓ cupcake, 1/6 small piece of pie
†Calculations are based on medium-fat protein choices. Children's menus could include high-fat protein foods such as cheeses or nut butters for these age groups, raising the % fat.
LF, low-fat; NF, nonfat.

**Table 8–3.** Calcium, Iron, and Zinc Content of Selected Foods

| Food | Amount | Content (mg) |
|---|---|---|
| *Calcium* | | |
| Milk, cow's | 1 cup | 300 |
| Milk, soy, calcium fortified | 1 cup | 350–299 |
| Yogurt | 1 cup | 300–150 |
| Milk, almond, fortified | 1 cup | 200 |
| Cheese, cheddar | 1 oz | 204 |
| Collards, cooked | ½ c | 133 |
| Orange juice, calcium fortified | ½ c | 175 |
| Cottage cheese, 2% fat | ½ c | 103 |
| Kale, frozen, boiled | ½ c | 90 |
| Soybeans, cooked | ½ c | 87 |
| Almonds | ¼ c | 74 |
| Molasses, blackstrap | 1 T | 41 |
| Tortilla, corn or flour | 1 (6-in. diameter) | 40–19 |
| Bread, white | 1 slice | 38 |
| Broccoli, cooked | ½ c | 36 |
| Bread, whole wheat | 1 slice | 30 |
| Meat alternative products | 1 serving | 15–4 |
| Margarine, oil, or butter | 1 tsp | 2–0 |
| *Iron* | | |
| Total cereal (General Mills) | ¾ c | 18 |
| Cream of Wheat, instant, cooked | ¾ c | 11.9 |
| Cheerios or Wheaties | 1 c | 9.5–4.5 |
| Meat alternatives | 1 serving | 7.2–0.36 |
| Great Northern or pinto beans, cooked | 1 c | 3.77–3.57 |
| Bagel, plain | 3.7 oz | 3.23 |
| Prune juice, canned | 1 c | 3.02 |
| Spaghetti, cooked | 1 c | 1.79 |
| Apricots, dried | ½ c (halves) | 1.73 |
| Raisins | ½ cup | 1.31 |
| Almonds, dried | 1 oz (24 nuts) | 1.26 |
| Pistachios, dried | 1 oz (47nuts) | 1.16 |
| Tomato juice | 8 oz | 1.04 |
| Bread, white | 1 slice | 0.94 |
| Walnuts, English or Persian, dried | 1 oz (14 halves) | 0.81 |
| Bread, whole wheat | 1 slice | 0.68 |
| Egg, boiled | 1 | 0.60 |
| Butter, margarine, and oils | | 0.0–0.02 |
| *Zinc* | | |
| Total cereal (General Mills) | ¾ c | 15.0 |
| Meat alternatives | 1 serving | 4.79–0.03 |
| Oatmeal, cooked | 1 c | 2.34 |
| Tofu, raw firm | 3 oz | 1.33 |
| Garbanzo beans or lentils, cooked | 1/2 c | 1.27 |
| Brown rice, cooked | 1 c | 1.23 |
| Milk, cow's, nonfat | 1 c | 1.03 |
| Lima, kidney, pinto beans, cooked | ½ c | 0.93 |
| Peanut butter | 2 T | 0.93 |
| Cheddar cheese | 1 oz | 0.87 |
| Bagel, 3.7 oz, 1 | 1 (3.7 oz) | 0.81 |
| Potato, baked with skin | 21/4 | 173 |
| Green peas, frozen, boiled | ½ c | 0.53 |
| Egg, boiled | 1 | 0.52 |
| Broccoli, boiled | 1 c | 0.52 |
| Whole wheat bread | 1 slice | 0.50 |
| White bread | 1 slice | 0.18 |
| Carrots, sliced, boiled | ½ c | 0.16 |

Data from Pennington JS, Spungen J. *Bowes and Church's Food Values of Portions Commonly Used*, 19th ed. Philadelphia: WoltersKluwer/Lippincott Williams & Wilkens; 2010.

foods, such as whole milk, cheese, dried fruits, avocado, or peanut butter, in a pleasant environment interacting with others, free of electronics but with untidiness tolerated. Low-calorie liquids (e.g., water, soda, juice) are limited at meal-time to increase the consumption of high-calorie solids.[23] Ketogenic diets may be used for children with epilepsy. These diets are very high in fat to produce the ketones β-hydroxybutyrate and/or acetone, which may be the cause of their anticonvulsant effect. Although these diets are high in fat (85–95% of calories), protein is moderate and carbohydrate is very low. Plant protein sources that are very low in carbohydrate have been identified.[23] Children who need to follow a kidney-protective diet may be accommodated by a vegetarian diet; exchange lists are available to plan for plant proteins in their meal patterns.[23] This is also true for children diagnosed with diabetes mellitus. Serving sizes of vegetarian meat alternative products have been calculated to fit within the exchange lists for diabetes. Vegetarian approaches to diets for persons with inborn errors of metabolism (e.g., maple syrup urine disease, phenylketonuria, galactosemia, fructosemia, cystic fibrosis) have also been described.[23]

Adults with a wide spectrum of pathologies may be prescribed a diet that can be based on a vegetarian meal plan. The renal exchange lists for plant proteins apply to adults and children who must follow a kidney-protective diet. The adult diabetic may use the plant protein exchange lists for diabetics. For the majority of the US population who are overweight, following the serving sizes and number of servings provided in the *My Vegetarian Plate Food Guide* will optimize the potential of achieving and maintaining a healthful weight. For the few who are underweight, increasing the number of servings of the nutritious foods in the *My Vegetarian Plate Food Guide* will maximize the potential of reaching a suitable weight goal.

A vegetarian meal plan may address a myriad of disorders, such as cancers, cardiovascular diseases, gastrointestinal complaints, mineral imbalances, neurological disorders, pulmonary diseases, and trauma.[23] The foods to avoid and those to encourage remain similar to recommendations for people who choose carnivorous diets. The difference for the vegetarian is the protein source; it is from plants rather than from the animal kingdom. To reiterate, all the amino acids the body needs for its multitude of varied proteins may be synthesized from the amino acids found in vegetarian meals that provide sufficient calories from a variety of foods.[17]

## SUMMARY

Appropriately planned vegetarian diets will support growth and maintenance across the lifespan. Total vegetarians or vegans must ensure that adequate calcium, vitamin D, zinc, iron, vitamin $B_{12}$, and omega-3 fatty acid sources are provided in their menus. Food choices throughout the day from a variety of sources that meet caloric needs will provide the complete complement of amino acids needed for protein synthesis. Those who require modified diets may continue to follow vegetarian meal plans. References are available to assist in meeting the needs of those wishing to implement vegetarian diets.

### References


1. Wasserman D, ed. How many teens are vegetarian? How many kids don't eat meat? Results from a Vegetarian Resource Group Roper poll. *Vegetarian J.* 2001; 20(1):10.
2. Stahler C. How often do Americans eat vegetarian meals? And how many adults in the U.S. are vegetarian? The Vegetarian Resource Group, May 2015. http://www.vrg.org/journal/vj2011issue4/vj2011issue4poll.php. Accessed June 6, 2016.
3. American Institute for Cancer Research. *10 Ways to Reduce Your Cancer Risk.* Washington, DC: American Institute for Cancer Research; 2000.
4. American Institute for Cancer Research. *The New American Plate*. Washington, DC American Institute for Cancer Research; 2000.
5. US Department of Agriculture. MyPlate, MyWins: Healthy Eating Solutions for Everyday Life. Website. www.choosemyplate.gov/. Accessed June 6, 2016.
6. US Department of Agriculture, Center for Nutrition Policy and Promotion. *Dietary Guidelines for Americans, 2010–2015*, 8th ed. Prepared for the Committee by the Agricultural Research Service, US Department of Agriculture, US Department of Health and Human Services. May 2010. http://www.cnpp.usda.gov/sites/default/files/dietary_guidelines_for_americans/2010DGACReport-camera-ready-Jan11-11.pdf. Accessed June 6, 2016.
7. Craig WJ, Mangels AR. Position of the American Dietetic Association: vegetarian diets. *J Am Diet Assoc.* 2009; 109:1266.
8. Mekonnen MM, Hoekstra AY. The green, blue and grey water footprint of crops and derived crop products. *Hydrol Earth Syst Sci.* 2011; 15:1577. Available at http://waterfootprint.org. Accessed June 6, 2016.

9. Tonstad S, Stewart K, Oda K, Batech M, Herring RP, Fraser GE. Vegetarian diets and incidence of diabetes in the Adventist Health Study-2. *Nutr Metab Cardiovasc Dis.* 2013; 23:292.
10. Orlich MJ, Singh PN, Sabate J, et al. Vegetarian dietary patterns and the risk of colorectal cancers. *JAMA Intern Med.* 2015; 175:767.
11. Orlich MJ, Singh PN, Sabate J, et al. Vegetarian dietary patterns and mortality in the Adventist Health Study-2. *JAMA Intern Med.* 2013; 173:1230.
12. Pettersen BJ, Anousheh R, Fan J, Jaceldo-Siegl K, Fraser GE. Vegetarian diets and blood pressure among white subjects: results from the Adventist Health Study-2. *Public Health Nutr.* 2012; 15(10):1909.
13. Rizzo M, Sabate J, Jaceldo-Siegl K, Fraser GE. Vegetarian dietary patterns are associated with a lower risk of metabolic syndrome: the Adventist Health Study-2. *Diabetes Care.* 2011; 34:1225.
14. Beezhold BL, Johnston CS, Daigle DR. Vegetarian diets are associated with healthy mood states: a cross-sectional study in Seventh-day Adventist adults. *Nutr J.* 2010; 9:26.
15. Hardinge F. *My Vegetarian Plate.* General Conference of Seventh-day Adventists Nutrition Council. 2013. Silver Springs, MD: Health Ministries, North American Division of Seventh-day Adventists.
16. Institute of Medicine of the National Academies. *Dietary Reference Intakes for Energy, Carbohydrate, Fiber, Fat, Fatty Acids, Cholesterol, Protein, and Amino Acids (Macronutrients).* 2005. Washington, DC: The National Academies Press.
17. Young VR, Pellett PL. Plant proteins in relation to human protein and amino acid nutrition. *Am J Clin Nutr.* 1994; 59(suppl):1203S.
18. Craig WJ. Iron status of vegetarians. *Am J Clin Nutr.* 1994; 59(suppl):1233S.
19. Saunders AV, Craig WJ, Baines SK. Zinc and vegetarian diets. *Med J Aust.* 2013; 199(4 suppl):S17.
20. Gibson RS, Heath AL, Szymlek-Gay EA. Is iron and zinc nutrition a concern for vegetarian infants and young children in industrialized countries? *Am J Clin Nutr.* 2014; 100(suppl 1):459S.
21. Heaney RP, Dowell MS, Rafferty K, Bierman J. Bioavailability of the calcium in fortified soy imitation milk, with some observations on method. *Am J Clin Nutr.* 2000; 71:1166.
22. Craig WJ. Nutrition concerns and health effects of vegetarian diets. *Nutr Clin Pract.* 2010; 25:613.
23. Hodgkin G, Maloney S, eds. *The Loma Linda University Diet Manual: A Handbook Supporting Vegetarian Nutrition.* Loma Linda, CA: Loma Linda University Press; 2003.

# PART II

# CHRONIC DISEASES AND DEVELOPMENTAL DISABILITIES

*Shirley W. Ekvall*

Two studies, conducted in 1990–1991 and 2000–2001,[1] each included 83 children with chronic diseases and/or developmental disorders who had been referred to the Nutrition Department of the Cincinnati Children's Hospital Medical Center, Division of Developmental Disabilities (CCDDD), for in-depth comprehensive office assessment. The survey sample did not include children receiving nutrition in midlevel (specialty clinics) or mini-level (community settings) assessments. Some perspective was provided on the global experience with nutrition for children with special health care needs.[2]

In Figure II–1, the 2001 study is compared to the one from 10 years earlier with the same distribution categories of nutritional disorders: overweight, underweight, feeding problems, nutritional deficiency, bizarre food habits, metabolic disorders, and no problems. In both surveys, 13% of the children were referred because of major nutritional deficiency. A significant percentage of children in most of the other referral categories also had nutritional deficiencies (i.e., <67% of the Recommended Daily Allowance). The CCDDD nutrition assessment surveys revealed a decrease in feeding problems over the intervening decade (13% in 2001 vs 23% in 1991), as well as a decrease in underweight problems (13% in 2001, vs 27% in 1991, a significant change). However, there was a significant increase in overweight problems (35% in 2001 vs 24% in 1991, a significant change), and the prevalence of bizarre food habits almost doubled (15% in 2001 vs 8% in 1991, a significant change).

There was a higher percentage of males in the 2001 compared with the 1991 study. The 2001 study had a smaller percentage of African-American children and higher percentages of Caucasians and other ethnic groups (Table II–1).

One dietary assessment study has reported a deficiency of iron, calories, calcium, niacin, and vitamins A, C, and D in this population.[3] Iron and vitamin C deficiencies correlated with feeding problems.[4] These nutrient deficiencies, as well as others, were found in 4% to 63% of the children in the 2001 CCDDD survey, compared with 8% to 45% of those in the 1991 survey.[1]

Children in the general population suffer from some of the same deficiencies. According to an earlier survey from the Nutritional Monitoring Division of the US Department of Agriculture (USDA), diets of children aged 1 to 5 years were deficient in calcium, zinc, magnesium, vitamin E, and vitamin B6 (in descending order). In addition, adolescents in their late teens in both the USDA and CCDDD surveys and women in the USDA survey were deficient in folate.[5] Folate was the nutrient most often found to be deficient in adolescents, and this was most concerning for pregnant females in their late teens or at older ages because of the increased need for this nutrient during pregnancy.[1] The folate status of adolescents had improved significantly with supplementation by the time of the 2001 study (2%, vs 12% in 1991), but it was still low in some teenagers and adult women.[6] Genetics also plays a role in folate metabolism.[7] Supplementation does not appear to have affected zinc absorption.[8]

Vitamin D was the nutrient most likely to be deficient in 2001, and vitamin E was most often deficient in 1991[9] (Fig. II–2). Other nutrients for which 40% or more children were deficient were zinc (45% in 2001 vs 46% in 1991) and pantothenic acid (42% in 2001 vs 27% in 1991). There were significant changes in the percentages of children with deficiency of fluids (40% in 2001 vs 37% in 1991) and fiber (65% in 2001 vs 60% in 1991). There were also significant reductions in the prevalence of iron deficiency (21% in 2001 vs 52% in 1991) and vitamin C deficiency (7% in 2001 vs 13% in 1991) but an increase in vitamin A deficiency (25% in 2001 vs 16% in 1991). Iron and vitamin C intake improved significantly between 1991 and 2001. Vitamin and mineral supplements were consumed by 47% of the evaluated children in 2001, compared with 36% in 1991.

The CCDDD surveys also showed evidence of excessive intake of some nutrients (i.e., more than 133% of the Dietary Reference Intake [DRI]). The very high percentages of children with excessive intake of specific nutrients considered to be harmful to the body are shown in Figure II–3. Most remarkable is the fact that 95% of the children evaluated in 2001, and 94% in 1991, had an excessive intake of sodium (628% and 621% of DRI, respectively). Daily or more frequent consumption of soft drinks (41%) and candy or sugar items (71%) was noted for children in the 2001 survey, a significant change from the 1991 figures (34% and 30%, respectively).[10] Fat and sodium excess has been shown in other studies of children as well.[11] The CCDDD studies showed intakes of fat and sodium, as well as kilocalories and protein, to be significantly greater than their requirements. Kilocalories significantly increased over the decade (20% in 2001 vs 7% in 1991), although fat intake decreased (29% in 2001 vs 63% in 1991).

A Food Summary Score based on the food groups was calculated (see the in-depth nutrition record in Appendix 4) and was found to be less than 10 points in 54% of the children evaluated in 2001, compared with 40% of those surveyed in 1991, a significant change. This low score reflects an increased intake of energy-dense foods such as soft

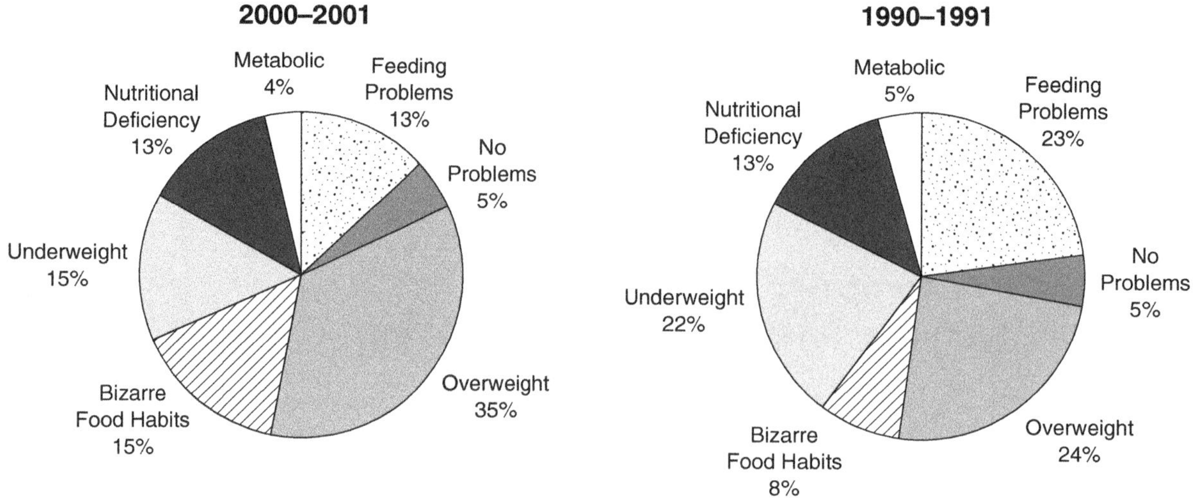


**Figure II–1.** Distribution of nutritional disorders among children referred to the Cincinnati Children's Hospital Medical Center, Division of Developmental Disabilities Nutrition in 2000–2001 and 1990–1991.

drinks, as opposed to nutrient-dense foods. As a result, these children required more treatment sessions to improve their nutrition. The fruit and vegetable groups provide the protective action of antioxidants such as retinoids and beta-carotene, vitamin E, and vitamin A; 56% of the children in 2001 were found to have a low intake of fruits (vs 63% in 1991), and 56% had a low intake of vegetables (vs 57% in 1991). The percentage of children who had a deficient number of servings in the bread group was 76% in 2001, compared with 52% in 1991, representing a significant change to less intake of whole grains. In 2001, 49% of the children had deficient intake in the meat group (vs 45% in 1991), and 56% were deficient in the milk group (vs 24% in 1991; the latter represents a significant decrease in dairy consumption).

A great deal of nutrition education is needed to encourage intake of more nutrient-dense foods, especially for children whose diets are restricted or limited in calories, such as children with the chronic diseases and developmental disorders discussed in Part II.[12] Reduction in the consumption of sugar and sodium in all age groups, and of calories and fat in children older than 2 years of age, is essential. For example, milk or milk products should replace excessive consumption of soft drinks to increase calcium and vitamin D intake. Of the 83 children in each survey, calcium was deficient in 24% of younger children and 66% of adolescents in 2001 (vs 27% and 40%, respectively, in 1991), whereas vitamin D was deficient in 24% of younger children and 66% of adolescents in 2001 (vs 46% and 60%, respectively) in 1991; both findings are of significant concern. The low intake of dietary calcium (54% in 2001 vs 24% in 1991), low vitamin D intake (24% in 2001 vs 46% in 1991), and low physical activity (27% in 2001 vs 59% in 1991) all represent significant changes over the decade and can result in reduced bone mass for children who are developmentally delayed or chronically ill.[13,14] The need for calcium to enhance bone mass is particularly acute during adolescence. Overweight problems require reduced caloric intake, which may further decrease bone mass.[15] Children who are using anticonvulsant medications and who are dark skinned have a superimposed problem of reduced vitamin D absorption (see discussion in Chapter 10). Yet, the use of calcium supplements in children without adequate fluid (40% of the children in 2001 vs 37% in 1991) or with little physical activity and high sodium intake can be harmful to the kidneys. Therefore, calcium intake from the diet is preferred. Increased sodium competes with calcium and creates further calcium loss.[15] This problem illustrates the complexities of nutritional diagnosis and treatment in children with special health care needs.

**Table II–1.** Composition of Study Groups in CCDDD Nutrition Surveys

| | Survey I (1990–1991) | Survey II (2000–2001) |
|---|---|---|
| No. of children | 83 | 83 |
| Mean age (yr) | 5.4 | 5.6 |
| % Male | 69 | 76 |
| % Female | 31 | 24 |
| Race (%) | | |
| Caucasian | 65.1 | 67.5 |
| African American | 32.5 | 27.75 |
| Other | 2.4 | 3.6 |
| Not available | 0 | 1.2 |

CCDDD = Cincinnati Children's Hospital Medical Center, Division of Developmental Disabilities.

Many nutrients may be deficient because of the effects of medications (e.g., anticonvulsants) taken by children with chronic diseases and developmental disorders. For example, in one study, lower thyroxin and higher retinol-binding protein levels were found among children who received diphenylhydantoin, phenobarbital, or other anticonvulsant combinations; however, vitamin A was higher in those taking phenylhydantoin.[13] The effect of medication in nutrition is addressed in Chapter 27. Feeding was a problem in only 13% of the children evaluated in 2001, compared with 23% in 1991 (see Fig. II–1). This topic is presented in Chapter 24 and discussed in Chapters 9, 25, and 35.

In the CCDDD surveys, underweight occurred in 15% of the children evaluated in 2001 and 35% in 1991 (see Fig. II–1), often related to feeding problems. Among children with developmental disorders such as myelomeningocele,[16] Down syndrome, or Prader-Willi syndrome, the prevalence of overweight was 35% in 2001 and 24% in 1991, representing a significant change. In a study in Norway of children with disabilities, the prevalence of feeding disorders was 23% to 43% for those who were had cognitive impairment, 26% to 52% for those with cerebral palsy, and 10% to 49% for those with congenital heart disease.[17] Height was subnormal in 50%, and weight was subnormal in 25% of children with feeding problems. Height-for-age was most deficient in those children with cerebral palsy and cognitive impairment and least deficient in the children with epilepsy.[17] Dysphagia, or difficulty in swallowing, creates one of the greatest risks for malnutrition and severe feeding problems.[18]

Interestingly, in the CCDDD 2001 survey, only 8% of the children in 2001 (vs 20% in 1991) were below the 5th percentile for height; in 2001, 22% (vs 23% in 1991) had a weight-to-height ratio above the 95% percentile, and 2% (vs 11% in 1991) were below the 5th percentile in weight-to-height. Children weighed more in the 2001 survey. Physical activity was low in 27% of the children in 2001, compared

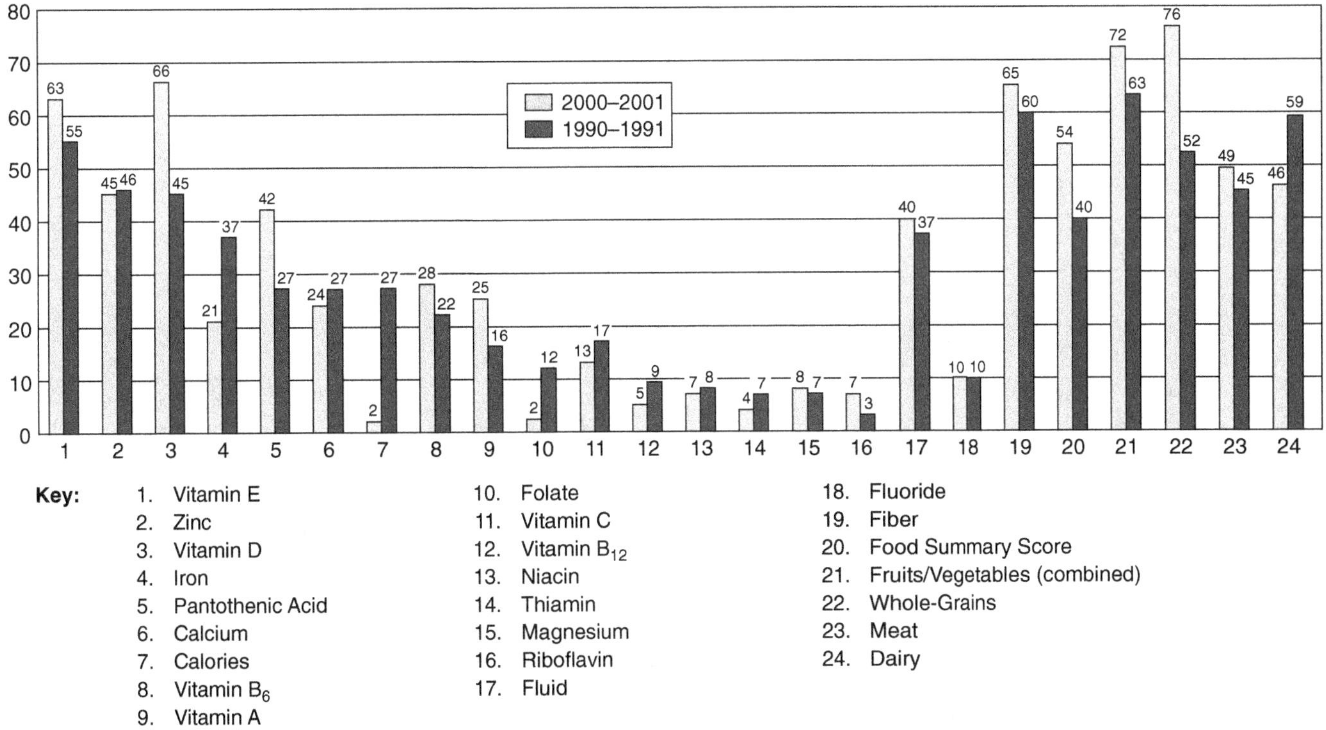


**Figure II–2.** Nutrient deficiencies (percentage of children with less than two-thirds of the required amounts of 24 different nutrients and food groups) in the 2001 and 1991 Cincinnati Children's Hospital Medical Center, Division of Developmental Disabilities Nutrition surveys.

with 59% in 1991, and was high in 1% of the children in 2001, compared with 20% in 1991 (Fig. II–4). This indicates a critical need to continue to address low physical activity, especially for children who have a developmental disorder (see Chapters 4 and 18). A special weight and height growth grid for myelomeningocele is being developed at CCDDD using the national data, and other special growth grids for Down syndrome, sickle cell anemia, Prader-Willi syndrome, Rubenstein-Taybi syndrome, Turner syndrome, Williams syndrome, and other disorders have been created (see Appendix 2). The energy assessment needs are difficult to determine for this population and must be ascertained on an individual basis. The assessment should always include the physical activity level as well as a caloric intake computation because of the effect of physical activity in increasing lean body mass.[16] This problem is addressed in Part II—in Chapter 18 on obesity, Chapter 20 on failure to thrive, and the chapters on other specific diseases—as well as in the discussion of nutritional assessment in Part I.

Psychological, eating, and behavioral disorders such as failure to thrive, anorexia nervosa, and obesity are receiving widespread attention today. Bizarre food habits were noted in 15% of the children evaluated in 2001, compared with 8% of those in 1991. Some of these problems may be neurologically based (e.g., attention-deficit hyperactivity disorder). Children with neurological disorders such as epilepsy, muscular dystrophy, and autism have nutrition and other related problems that require interdisciplinary intervention. For example, the effect of nutrients and neurotransmitters on brain dysfunction is

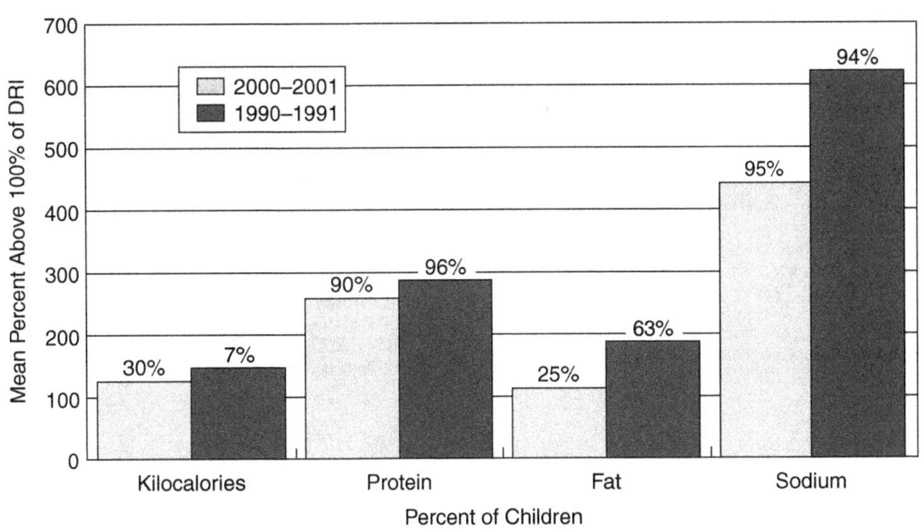


**Figure II–3.** Percentage of children with excess nutrients (mean percent above the Daily Recommended Intake), CCDDD, 2000–2001 and 1990–1991 surveys.

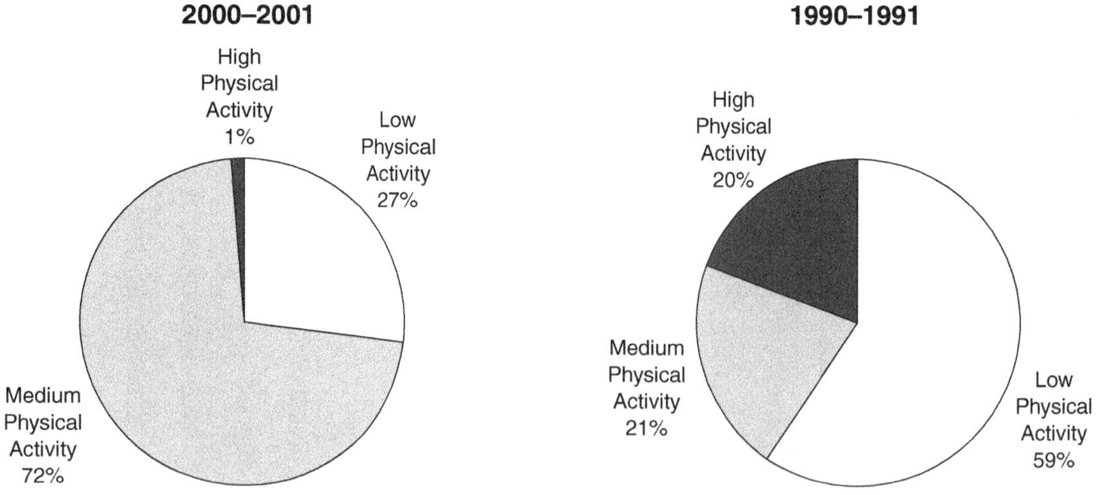


**Figure II–4.** Distribution of physical activity among children referred to the Cincinnati Children's Hospital Medical Center, Division of Developmental Disabilities Nutrition, Nutrition Department for in-depth assessment in 1990–1991 and in 2000–2001.

a promising research area. Some of these topics have been addressed in collaboration by a nutritionist, gastroenterologist, psychologist, and psychiatrist. Children with diseases such as congenital heart disease, cancer, or renal disease require special nutritional management with specific standards of care. In many instances, developmental disorders and chronic diseases overlap; both require long-term, consistent, and preventive care.

Nutrition is the key to open the door to better health. During the past decade, several position papers of the American Academy of Pediatrics Committee on Nutrition have addressed the nutritional health of children in the general population.[19] Position papers on children in the general population (referenced throughout this book) and children with developmental disorders have also been developed by the Academy of Nutrition and Dietetics[20] (www.eatright.org). In addition, the Academy and Nutrition and Dietetics Pediatric Nutrition Practice Group (PNPG), with input from the Behavioral Health and Nutrition Practice Group (BHN) has published quality assurance criteria for several diseases and disorders and has developed other protocols on chronic diseases in draft form (see Appendix 7). Children from low-income families are in particular need of adequate nutrients for proper growth and development.[21] Proper nutrition is cost-effective because it reduces the incidence of infections, anemia, stunted growth, and hospitalization, thereby providing these children with enough energy to develop and learn to their full potential.[22] As Part II demonstrates, the interdisciplinary team approach based on coordination of services and family-centered input provides the best means for improving the health and potential of children with special health care needs, whether the developmental disorders are neurological, behavioral, feeding-related, medication-related, or caused by chronic diseases.

## References

1. Ekvall S. Part II: chronic diseases and developmental disorders. In: Ekvall SW. *Pediatric Nutrition in Chronic Disorders and Developmental Disorders*. 2nd ed, New York: Oxford University Press;2005.
2. Hals J, Ek J, Svalastog AG, Nilsen H. Studies on nutrition in severely neurologically disabled children in an institution. *Acta Pediatr*. 1996; 85:1469.
3. Smith M, Connolly B, McFadden S, et al. *Feeding Management of a Child with a Handicap: A Guide for Professionals*. Memphis: University of Tennessee Center for the Health Sciences, Child Development Center; 1982.
4. Gouge AL, Ekvall SW. Diets of handicapped children: physical, psychological and socioeconomic correlations. *Am J Ment Defic*. 1975; 80:149.
5. Giddens JB, Krug SK, Tsang RC, Guo S, Miodovnik M, Prada JA. Pregnant adolescent and adult women have similarly low intake of selected nutrients. *J Am Diet Assoc*. 2000; 100:1334.
6. Moore LL, Bradlee ML, Singer MR, Rothman KJ, Milunsky A. Folate intake and the risk of neural tube defects: an estimation of dose-response. *Epidemiology*. 2003; 14:200.
7. Shaw GM, Lammer EJ, Zhu H, Baker MW, Neri E, Finnell RH. Maternal periconceptional vitamin use, genetic variation of infant reduced folate carrier (A8OG), and risk of spina bifida. *Am J Genet*. 2002; 108:1.
8. Hansen M, Samman S, Madsen LT, Jensen M, Sorenson S, Sandstrom B. Folic acid enrichment of bread does not appear to affect zinc absorption in young women. *Am J Clin Nutr*. 2001; 74:125.
9. Nesby-O'Dell S, Scanlon KS, Cogswell ME, et al. Hypovitaminosis D prevalence and determinants among African-American and white women of reproductive age: Third National Health and Nutrition Examination Survey, 1998–1994. *Am J Clin Nutr*. 2002; 76:187.
10. Burri BJ, Neidlinger TR. Dietary intakes and serum concentration of vitamin E and total carotenoids of healthy adults with severe physical disabilities are lower than matched controls. *J Am Diet Assoc*. 2002; 102:1804.
11. Laria CM, Oborzanek E, Ernest ND. Choose and prepare foods with less salt: advice for all Americans. *J Nutr*. 2001; 131:536S.
12. Levedahl JW, Oliveira V. Dietary impacts of food assistance programs. In: Frazão E, ed. *America's Eating Habits: Changes and Consequences*. Agriculture Information Bulletin No. AIB-750. May 1999. Washington, DC: US Department of Agriculture, Economic Research Service.
13. Baer MT, Kozlowski BW, Blyler EM, Trahms CM, Taylor ML, Hogan MP. Vitamin D, calcium and bone status in children with developmental delay in relation to anticonvulsant use and ambulatory status. *Am J Clin Nutr*. 1997; 65:1042.
14. Namsung R, Tsang RC. Factors affecting newborn bone mineral content: in utero effects on newborn bone mineralization. *Proc Nutr Soc*. 2000; 59:55.
15. Llama M, Susic D, Frohlich ED. Prevention of hypertension. *Cardiology*. 2002; 17:531.
16. Grayan C, Ekvall S. Body composition of children with myelomeningocele determined by K40, urinary creatinine and anthropometric measures. *J Am Coll Nutr* 1999; 18:316.
17. Thommessen M, Heiberg A, Kase BF, Larsen S, Riis G. Feeding problems, height and weight in different groups of disabled children. *Acta Pediatr Scand*. 1991; 80:527.
18. McCallum SL. The National Dysphagia Diet: implementation at a regional rehabilitation center and hospital system. *J Am Diet Assoc*. 2003; 103:381.
19. American Academy of Pediatrics, Committee on Genetics. Folic acid for the prevention of neural tube defects. *Pediatrics*. 1999; 104:325.
20. Pomey L.T.Wittenbrook W., Position of the Academy of Nutrition and Dietetics. Providing nutrition services for individual intellectual and developmental disabilities and special health care needsl J Acad Nutr Diet. 2015;115:593.
21. US Department of Health and Human Services Maternal and Child Health Bureau. *Child Health USA 2014*. http://mchb.hrsa.gov/chusa14 Accessed May 23, 2016.
22. U.S. Department of Health and Human Services and US Department of Agriculture 2015-2020 Dietary Guidelines for Americans. 8th ed December 2015. http://healtu.gov/dietaryguidelines/2015. Accessed May 23, 2016.

# A. NEUROLOGICAL AND DEVELOPMENTAL

## 9 Cerebral Palsy

ROBIN C. MEYERS, STEVEN J. BACHRACH, AND VIRGINIA A. STALLINGS

Cerebral palsy (CP) is a chronic, nonprogressive motor disability that results from an injury to the developing brain early in life.[1] Dysfunction in motor coordination and muscle tone characterizes CP. Anything that can cause damage to the developing brain can cause CP. Modern imaging techniques[1,2] have shown that in most children with CP, the brain damage occurs before birth. There are three broad categories of etiology, each related to a different time during fetal life: (1) cerebral malformations originating in early fetal life (first 20 weeks of gestation), which include such conditions as lissencephaly and schizencephaly; (2) periventricular lesions or periventricular leucomalacia arising between 24 and 34 weeks of gestation (in utero or after premature birth); and (3) cortical infarction or hemorrhage occurring around the time of a term birth (vascular infarctions or hypoxic-ischemic lesions). Other causes include congenital infections (e.g., cytomegalovirus infection, toxoplasmosis, herpes); injuries occurring after birth (e.g., traumatic brain injury from child abuse or accidents); bacterial meningitis; severe jaundice; and exposure to toxins such as lead or mercury.

CP is the most common childhood disability.[3] Studies from different parts of the United States and the world have yielded rates ranging from 2.0 to 2.8 per 1000 live births during the 1990s.[3] In the United States, there are about 500,000 children younger than 18 years of age with CP, and 10,000 babies are diagnosed with the condition each year. Although full-term infants still comprise most of those with CP (approximately 60–65%), premature infants have a much higher risk of being diagnosed with CP. Compared with the risk of 0.25% for a full-term infant, a baby born weighing less then 1500 g has a 5% risk, and one weighing less than 1000 g has a 10% risk of developing CP.[3]

### TYPES OF CEREBRAL PALSY

CP is classified according to the predominant tone abnormality and the affected region of the body. Muscle tone can be either increased (hypertonic, spastic) or decreased (hypotonic, floppy). Other tone or movement abnormalities include athetosis due to damage to the basal ganglia and ataxia due to cerebellar damage. Spastic CP is by far the most common type. In a classic study published in 1959, spasticity was said to affect 65% to 70% of children with CP, whereas 5% to 10% had ataxic CP, and 10% to 20% had athetoid or dyskinetic CP. It is also not unusual for patients to have a mixed tone picture including both spasticity and athetosis.[4] Over the past 50 years, with changes in medical care, we see fewer cases of athetosis and more of spasticity (70–80%).[5]

If all four limbs are affected in a child with decreased tone, the disorder is described as hypotonic quadriplegia. A child with increased tone affecting primarily the legs is said to have spastic diplegia. There are also classification systems that describe children with CP based on their level of disability. The Gross Motor Function Classification System (GMFCS) scale is based on the gross motor function, with level ranging from 1 (walks without limitations) to 5 (transported by others in a wheelchair).[6] Similar scales exist for fine motor function and oral-motor function.

## SYMPTOMS AND PRESENTATION

The more severe the disability, the earlier the child is likely to present with symptoms and be diagnosed. The main early symptoms of CP fall into three broad categories: abnormality of muscle tone, delayed motor development, and persistence of primitive neurological reflexes. These primitive reflexes are developmental reflexes that are normal in infants up to a certain age (3–6 months) but then fade and are replaced by voluntary motion.[7] These primitive reflexes include the tonic neck reflex , grasp, Moro, tongue thrust, and rooting reflexes. Many of these early infant reflexes persist in children with CP. Normally, organized voluntary motion is delayed, decreased, absent, or erratic in children with CP while abnormal posture and reflexes persist.

Even though the most common tone abnormality is spasticity, infants during the first year of life can be initially hypotonic, developing hypertonicity later. This pattern may include increased tone in arms and legs but low tone in the trunk, making it difficult to sit or stand. By 6 months of age, in a severely affected child in whom all four limbs are affected, parents may notice an increase or decrease in general body tone and failure to achieve such developmental milestones as rolling over, reaching for a toy, or sitting up.

In children with less severe CP, the signs are more subtle; these children often are not diagnosed until 1 to 2 years of age. The most common presenting signs are poor muscle coordination when performing voluntary movements (ataxia); stiff or tight muscles and exaggerated reflexes (spasticity); walking with one foot or leg dragging; walking on the toes, a crouched gait, or a "scissored" gait; and stiff or floppy muscle tone.

Almost all children with hemiplegia will eventually walk (although some will need a cane or braces), whereas approximately 90% of those with diplegia and 30% of those with quadriplegia will be able to walk with the help of assistive devices.[8]

Signs of CP differ from person to person and may change over time. Symptoms may include difficulty with fine motor tasks (e.g., writing, feeding oneself, dressing), gross motor tasks (e.g., sitting, walking, balance), oral-motor function (e.g., swallowing, speaking), and involuntary movements.

Children during the first year of life may show the following:

- Dissociated pattern of development, with gross motor skills lagging far behind language, adaptive, and social skills (if the child has more global problems, all areas of development will lag)
- Excessive fussiness or irritability
- Poor feeding skills
- Stiffness (spasticity) with diapering, feeding, handling, or bathing
- An easily evoked and pronounced startle reflex with sensory stimulation

Different types of CP are usually diagnosed at different ages. *Spastic CP* involves increased muscle tone of the "clasp knife" variety, persistent infant reflexes, and increased deep tendon reflexes in one of the three characteristic patterns: *hemiplegia*, involving the arm and leg on one side of the body; *diplegia,* involving predominantly the lower extremities, although upper extremities may have less severe deficits; and *quadriplegia*, involving all four extremities and possibly including the trunk, head, and neck muscles.

Various combinations of these patterns also occur.[9] *Spastic hemiplegia* is often difficult to diagnose in the first few months of life, and asymmetry may not be noted by the parent or physician until the child is 12 months of age or older. In *spastic diplegia*, the gait is often more affected than hand skills, and the diagnosis is often not made until the child begins to ambulate at about 12 to 15 months of age. Children with *spastic quadriplegia* (SQCP) frequently are severely involved, and the diagnosis may be made early in infancy. These children present with difficulties in positioning, handling, and feeding due to diffusely increased tone, tongue thrusting, and swallowing problems.[7] Except for the most severe cases, the definitive diagnosis is often delayed until 2 years of age to increase the certainty.

*Dyskinetic CP* is associated with abnormalities in muscle tone that affect the entire body. One type of dyskinetic CP is athetoid, in which the child has uncontrolled and continuous involuntary movements; characteristically, these are slow, worm-like, writhing movements usually involving all four extremities as well as the muscles of the neck, face, and trunk. Historically, the common cause of athetoid CP was moderate to severe neonatal jaundice (kernicterus). The ability to treat jaundice has resulted in a significant decline in kernicterus and thus in athetoid CP.[10] The term *mixed CP* refers to the condition in which both athetosis and spasticity are present. *Ataxia* is a type of CP characterized by abnormalities of voluntary movement and balance, such as an unsteady gait.

Although CP is primarily a motor disability, it is often accompanied by developmental problems such as cognitive impairment, learning disabilities, attention-deficit hyperactivity disorder, speech and language disorders, visual or hearing impairments, seizure disorder, and growth retardation.[5] Health care for children with the more complex types of CP (i.e., those with GMFCS level from 3 to 5) is best managed by a multidisciplinary team that includes a developmental pediatrician, registered dietitian, physical therapist, speech therapist, occupational therapist, and other specialists the child may need, such as a neurologist, an orthopedic surgeon, or a gastroenterologist. Growth in children with CP is different from growth in typically developing children.[11–13] The cause is multifactorial but is largely related to oral motor dysfunction, inadequate energy intake, changes in hormones, central nervous system damage, and impaired mobility.[14,15] Growth is an indicator of overall health and well-being. Studies have shown that children with CP who grow better and weigh more miss fewer days of school and use less health care.[11] Brooks et al. showed that children with weights above the 20th percentile on CP-specific growth charts had lower rates of morbidity and mortality.[12] Children with CP are often shorter and lighter than typically developing children. Children with more severe oral motor dysfunction have lower body fat and decreased rates of weight gain and linear growth.[15] This faltering growth can be caused by a combination of factors, including central nervous system damage, lack of weight bearing, and chronic undernutrition.[7,9]

In several studies, a correlation has been observed between the severity of motor involvement, degree of feeding dysfunction, and growth faltering in children with CP.[11,16–18] Because growth can affect health in these children, the proper assessment of growth becomes very important. Nutrition and growth assessment for children with CP is difficult because the standards used are based on typically developing children and are not suitable for children with CP. Assessment is also difficult because of the physical limitations of the children themselves.

## NUTRITION ASSESSMENT

### Anthropometic Measurement

Weight, length/height, and head circumference measurements are essential for all children to assess growth and general health. The triceps skinfold (TSF) is a reliable indicator of fat stores and nutritional status in children with CP.[19] Bioelectrical impedance analysis and dual-energy x-ray absorptiometry (DXA) have been used as tools to assess body composition of these children.[20,21] Because of physical and cooperation limitations of some of the children, certain measurements may be difficult to obtain, and more time may be required for adequate assessment. Changes in weight, skinfold thickness, and knee height for stature and comparison to reference data are all methods for assessing nutritional interventions on an individual patient basis.

### Weight

Weight should be obtained at each visit using standard equipment and techniques. An infant scale is used for infants and small children who cannot stand. Older children who cannot stand should not be weighed on an infant scale; they can be weighed on a bed scale, table scale, chair scale, or wheelchair scale. If none of these methods is available, a caregiver can stand on the scale and have his or her weight "zeroed" out. The child is then given to the caregiver to hold on the scale, and the resulting weight will be that of the child. Weight should be measured with a minimum amount of clothing and without braces.

### Stature

A measurement of stature should be obtained at each visit using standard equipment and techniques. Children younger than 2 years of age and those who cannot stand without crouching or standing on their toes should be measured on a recumbent length board. Standing height should be obtained in children older than age 2 who can stand without crouching or standing on their toes. Both of these measurements are made without shoes or braces.

For children with muscle contracture, who cannot be measured on a recumbent length board, segmental measures are an alternative to standard measurements of stature.[11,14,22] Stevenson et al. found that knee height, tibia length, and upper-arm length are reliable indices of stature in children with CP and derived regression equations from these measures to estimate height in children younger than 12 years of age.[23] These measurements are easily performed in a clinic setting with standard equipment.

### Triceps Skinfold

TSF is a measurement of subcutaneous fat stores and is easy to obtain in a clinic setting. Samson-Fang and Stevenson found that a TSF thickness below the 10th percentile identified 96% of malnourished children with CP. They found it to be a better indicator of malnutrition than weight for length.[24]

### Growth Charts

When properly measured, height or length, weight, head circumference, body mass index, and weight-for-length can be plotted on gender- and age-appropriate growth charts (http://www.cdc.gov/growthcharts) and compared with the child's previous measures and data from reference populations (i.e., typically developing children).

A recumbent length should be plotted on the World Health Organization (WHO) chart for length from birth to 24 months. Standing height should be plotted on the Centers for Disease Control and Prevention (CDC) chart for ages 2 to 20 years. Recumbent lengths obtained on an older child and lengths calculated from segmental measurements should be plotted on the CDC chart for 2- to 20-year-olds. Anthropometric measurements may also be plotted on condition-specific growth charts. However, these may be of limited use because they are descriptive in nature and may be based on a small number of children. The specialty charts are plotted along with the CDC charts for ages 2 to 20 years (see Appendix 2–7 and Appendix 2–8).

### Cerebral Palsy Growth Charts

Several versions of growth charts for children with CP have been published, starting with Krick et al. in 1996.[12,13,25] The Krick charts were a step forward but were limited in scope. In 2007, Day et al. published charts for children with CP that were derived from a large population of children and adolescents who received services from the state of California.[13] These charts were the first to include children up to the age of 20 years and the first to separate children according to their GMFCS level. They allow children's growth data to be plotted on charts based on a population with similar functional disabilities. However, they are still descriptive in nature and do not represent optimal growth in children with CP, so they should be used with caution.

In 2011, Brooks et al. published a set of CP growth charts based on the charts first published in 2007. These charts have a prescriptive component. Knowing that children who grow better and are better nourished use less health care and miss fewer day of social activity, Brooks et al. reexamined the data from the first set of growth charts and found that children with GMFCS level of 1 or 2 had lower rates of morbidity and mortality when their weights were above the 5th percentile on the CP charts. Children in GMFCS levels 3 or 4 who were not being tube fed had lower rates of morbidity and mortality when their weight was above the 20th percentile on the corresponding CP growth chart. The results for GMFCS level 5 children who were tube fed were not as clearcut as for the other groups. There was less morbidity when the level 5 tube-fed children had weights below the 20th percentile but higher rates of mortality. The authors suggested using the 20th percentile as an indicator for the need for closer monitoring of nutrition and growth.[12] These charts have been published in a format similar to that of the CDC charts and can be useful in determining the direction of care and nutritional support for children with CP[12]; they are available at (http://www.lifeexpectancy.org/articles/NewGrowthCharts.shtml)

### Energy Requirements

Estimates of energy requirements for children with CP must take into consideration the degree of neurological impairment, mobility, feeding difficulties, and altered body composition as well as the need for weight gain or weight loss.[15,26] Limited physical activity due to impairments in mobility, muscle strength, and muscle tone might be expected to decrease energy expenditure; however, the energy required for physical activity may actually be greater in persons with disabilities because of low efficiency and the increased work needed to perform the activity. Rose et al. demonstrated higher heart rates and slower walking speeds in children with CP who were ambulatory, suggesting a higher workload.[27] However, although children with CP expend more energy to walk, their total energy expenditure (TEE) is lower because of their lower overall physical activity level and lower fat-free mass (FFM) compared with typically developing children.[28] The reduced TEE in nonambulatory groups can also be attributed to a decrease in physical activity and decreased FFM.[28,29] There are no studies of the protein requirements of children with CP. Whether requirements are altered because of decreased muscle mass is unclear.

Several studies have been conducted to determine daily energy expenditure in children and adolescents with CP. Bandini et al. found that the resting metabolic rate and FFM in a group of nine adolescents with CP (six spastic, one athetoid, and two mixed) were significantly lower than in a group of typically developing adolescents.[30] TEE was also significantly lower than in typically developing adolescents of the same age. Stallings et al. measured energy expenditure in 61 nonambulatory children and adolescents with SQCP and 37 controls.[31] Resting energy expenditure (REE) adjusted for body composition was found to be significantly lower in SQCP subjects with malnutrition, as indicated by low fat stores (TSF <25th percentile for age), when compared with controls, but REE was not different from controls in those children with SQCP who had adequate fat stores. TEE was significantly lower in the SQCP group than in controls. These findings were similar to those of Bandini et al.[30] and suggested that individuals with SQCP have a lower energy requirement—not a higher one, as has often been suggested. The authors suggested that the low REE seen in individuals with low body fat stores was caused by adaptation to chronically low energy intake and resulting malnutrition.[31]

Several options exist for estimating dietary energy needs as a starting point for nutrition management in the setting of CP. Most methods for estimating energy needs are based on typically developing children. These include the Daily Recommended Intakes (DRI) for basal energy expenditure, indirect calorimetry,[31–33] and the WHO equation[34]. Height has been used, but this is not recommended because of the difficulty in obtaining an accurate height measurement in this population, which may lead to underestimation of energy needs. Other equations also include a measurement of height, body composition, and/or body surface area and may result in an inaccurate estimate of energy needs. Each of these methods may overestimate or underestimate energy needs in children with CP, so regardless of the method used, it is critical to monitor weight and linear growth to determine the adequacy of nutritional intake.

### Vitamin and Mineral Status

Vitamin and mineral requirements specific for children with CP are not available. It is assumed that in children with CP who have no complicating factors, vitamin and mineral requirements are comparable to those of typically developing children.

Children with CP are at risk of developing micronutrient deficiencies. Studies have documented low intake of several micronutrients, such as iron, folate, vitamin D, and zinc, in some orally or enterally fed children with CP.[35,36] Others have demonstrated biochemical evidence of deficiency of several micronutrients, including iron, selenium, and essential fatty acids, as well as vitamins C, D, and E.[37–39] Deficiencies may develop because enteral formulas provide adequate amounts of micronutrients based on the age-related DRIs for energy and fluid intake, and this is often more volume than a child with CP receives if his or her energy needs are extremely low.[15,39] Children with CP need their nutrition status evaluated to determine sufficient, but not excessive, intake levels for micronutrients. Tailored nutrient supplementation should be initiated if deficiencies are present, and excessive intakes should be corrected if necessary.

## FEEDING

Poor motor skills contribute to feeding problems in children with CP. Lack of sitting balance; lack of head, mouth, and trunk control; inability to bend the hips sufficiently to enable stretching of the arms forward to grasp or to maintain grasp; and lack of eye-hand coordination enabling food to be brought by the hand to the mouth make the feeding process difficult for children with CP.[18,40] Common feeding problems include difficulties in sucking; poor coordination of swallowing or chewing; abnormal reflexes such as tongue thrust; and poor lip and tongue control. Children with CP have difficulty manipulating food once it is in the mouth, placing them at risk for choking and aspiration. They may become exhausted before finishing a meal. These problems may contribute to poor dietary intake and poor growth.

A study of feeding efficiency in children with severe CP and growth failure found that these children required 2 to 12 times longer to chew and swallow pureed food and 1 to 15 times longer to consume solid food than weight-matched controls.[41] The time required to feed a child with CP is often lengthy, and inadequate time for feeding may compromise the child's nutrient intake. In addition to poor chewing and swallowing, Dahlseng et al. found an association between feeding problems and poor communication skills; they suggested that the inability of children with CP to effectively communicate their need for food or beverages to the caregiver, in addition to poor feeding skills, increases the risk of inadequate dietary intake and poor nutritional status. Children with CP who have oral, pharyngeal, or esophageal dysphagia or gastroesophageal reflux are also at risk for feeding problems.[16]

## DIETARY MANAGEMENT OF COMMON NUTRITIONAL PROBLEMS

### Inadequate Nutrient Intake

As discussed previously, oral-motor dysfunction is often associated with poor intake, poor growth, and undernutrition. Several experts have reported reduced food intake in children with CP.[14,42,43] These findings, along with other reports, highlight the importance of nutritional assessment and a feeding evaluation as essential parts of the clinical assessment of all children with moderate to severe neurodevelopmental disorders.[15,16,26,31,44]

The RD should determine what foods and how much of the foods offered to the child is actually eaten. The child may have spillage or may not have the ability to swallow the foods or liquids offered. The RD should estimate the child's energy and protein needs and take into consideration the appropriate textures and consistencies of foods that the child can tolerate when making recommendations. If fat stores are low, increased caloric intake is warranted. It is important that the RD gather information from caregivers on the child's feeding patterns and tolerated textures.

### Feeding Skills

Feeding is often a long and tiring process for a child with disabilities. Mealtimes, quantities consumed, and the endurance of the child are important factors to consider in the assessment. Finally, the influence of the environment must be considered. Too much environmental stimulation during mealtime is distracting. Management of feeding problems often requires the expertise of an occupational, physical, and/or speech therapist as well as an RD.

Proper positioning and the use of appropriate seating are important for successful feeding. A physical or occupational therapist can help with specialized equipment such as a feeding chair, standing table, or proper alignment in a wheelchair to optimize feeding. Adapted utensils also enhance feeding success. A feeding or occupational therapist can assist with correct positioning and use of such utensils and with improving oral skills, particularly in children younger than 5 years of age.[15] Enhancing oral-motor function may not always result in improved feeding efficiency or weight gain. Because of this and the fact that the child's abilities may decline over time, it is important to evaluate oral feeding skills as part of ongoing follow-up.[15] Also, recurrent pneumonia or wheezing may be an indication of the development or worsening of aspiration. Another approach to improving oral intake is behavioral therapy with a child psychologist trained in CP-specific therapy. This therapy can potentially impact several components of oral feeding in a positive way. The amount of food, the duration of mealtimes, the variety of textures, and mealtime interactions between caregiver and child may all be affected in a positive way.[45]

Although it is important to promote a child's independent feeding skills, it is essential that nutrition status not be compromised for the sake of independence. For some children with CP, feeding difficulties are so severe as to prevent adequate nutrient intake, and a gastrostomy tube (GT) is indicated. Placement of a GT has been shown to improve health in these children (as measured by hospitalizations) as well as parents' worries about their child's health. Improvements in caregiver quality-of-life measures have been demonstrated at 6 and 12 months after GT placement.[46]

Enteral tube feedings should be considered if the child with CP cannot routinely take in enough orally for adequate weight gain, linear growth, and hydration.[15,47] Additional indications for enteral feedings include risk of aspiration with oral feeding and long mealtimes caused by chewing and swallowing dysfunction.[15] Nasogastric or nasojejunal tube feeding is used for short-term nutrition support or in children who are awaiting GT placement. A GT or low-profile device (button) is preferable for those who need long-term enteral nutrition. Children who receive GT support early in the course of their growth faltering have better growth and nutrition outcomes. Children who receive GT feeding at older ages may gain weight, but linear growth deficits may persist.[48] GTs may be placed surgically, by interventional radiology, or by percutaneous endoscopic gastrostomy (PEG) placement.

### Enteral Feeding Regimen

There are many ways to administer tube feedings to a child with CP. Regimens typically include a combination of bolus and continuous feeds. Bolus feedings provide a physiological response similar to oral feeding of meals and snacks, are more convenient, and allow for more flexibility. If the child cannot tolerate the required volume of formula as bolus feeds, the volume can be divided into daytime bolus feeds and nighttime continuous feedings.[15,26] For those who do not tolerate bolus feeds or who receive jejunal feeds, continuous formula infusions are needed for the entire volume of feeding. Formula choice for enteral feedings should take into account the child's age, medical conditions, allergies, estimated caloric requirements, and tolerance.[15,44]

Unless otherwise indicated, a standard, age-appropriate, casein- or whey-based formula is used. With evidence of milk protein allergy or sensitivity, a protein hydrolysate or amino acid formula is used. For children with very low energy needs, special attention should be given to the macronutrient and micronutrient content of the formula. Supplemental vitamins, minerals, or electrolytes can help avoid or treat deficiencies. Formula with added fiber may help prevent constipation but can cause gas and bloating.[44]

### Home-Prepared Tube Feedings

Home-prepared tube feeding (HPTF) is food that has been home cooked, pureed, and bolus-fed through a GT. HPTF was used for many years before the development of commercially prepared, standardized enteral formulas. Some families continue to express an interest in HPTF to replace enteral formulas.[49] HPTF use is also increasing because it is helpful in treating gagging and retching associated with fundoplication. The mechanism leading to the improvement in gagging and retching is unclear. One reason for better tolerance may be the higher viscosity of the HPTF.[50] Regardless of the reason, the support of an RD is essential to plan the components and analyze the composition of the mixture for adequacy of all macronutrients and micronutrients. A nutrient analysis of the HPTF is recommended, especially if HPTF is used as the sole source of nutrition. Close monitoring for gastrointestinal tolerance and growth response is needed. Special care and clean technique are essential for all tube feedings but even more important with HPTF.

### Overweight

In some children with SQCP who do not have oral-motor problems or who are fed by tube, overweight may be a concern. Limited physical activity and reduced FFM both contribute to decreased energy needs. Care must be taken to ensure adequate intake of water, protein, and micronutrients on low-energy diets. Management of overweight in children who have developmental disabilities is discussed in Chapter 18.

### Constipation

Children with CP, especially those with quadriplegic CP who are limited in oral-motor skills and ability to ambulate, are at high risk for constipation. Many of these children have poor intake of fluids and fiber, and many sit in a wheelchair for almost the entire day, with little chance for exercise. High-fiber foods, such as fruits and vegetables, whole-grain breads and cereals, and prune juice, may alleviate constipation. It is essential that adequate fluids be consumed in addition to high-fiber foods. Often, because of swallowing difficulties, children with CP eat pureed foods and limit their fluids severely to reduce the risk of aspiration. Thickening of fluids may support greater fluid intake, although the thickening agents themselves may contribute to constipation.

A number of medications taken by children with CP can also contribute to constipation, including anticholinergics to control drooling (e.g., glycopyrrolate, scopolamine) and the baclofen pump. In turn, chronic constipation can be so uncomfortable as to cause the child to stop eating. Some children with CP have poor gut motility, leading to slow transit of food through the gut and resulting constipation. These children may need more medical treatment for constipation. Beyond diet and fluids, there are a number of laxatives that stimulate the gut to evacuate stool as well as osmotic-type laxatives that work by pulling water into the gut, thus softening the stool and making it easier to pass. Chronic use of laxatives containing mineral oil should be avoided because of interference with absorption of fat-soluble vitamins.

### Gastroesophageal Reflux

Another medical issue that is common to many children, and especially children with CP, is gastroesophageal reflux (GER). Reflux is common in healthy infants and often resolves by 1 year of age. Children with CP are at higher risk for GER that persists with age. The primary symptom is "spitting up" or vomiting shortly after meals, but many children have reflux without these obvious symptoms. Significant vomiting after meals can cause weight loss in a child whose intake may already be barely adequate. Some children with GER develop esophagitis, which in the nonverbal child can be challenging to diagnose. Esophagitis can cause such severe discomfort at mealtimes that a previously good oral eater clamps his teeth shut and turn his head away when offered food. Other children may develop anemia from a low-volume continuous blood loss that is too small to discolor the stools. Others with GER may be obviously in distress for no apparent reason, and not necessarily only at mealtime.

If GER is documented, treatment will likely begin with medications; if these fail to alleviate the symptoms, surgery is an option. Fundoplication involves creation of a valve at the junction of the esophagus and stomach that allows food into the stomach but prevents it from coming back up into the esophagus. An alternative for a child being fed through a GT is to advance the tube into the jejunum and feed directly into the small intestine rather than into the stomach.

## DENTAL PROBLEMS

Dental problems are common in children with CP and may contribute to feeding difficulties. Poor oral hygiene and dentition, dental caries, enamel hypoplasia, bruxism, and malocclusion are encountered frequently. Hyperplasia of the gums may occur with long-term use of phenytoin and phenobarbital, two anticonvulsant drugs. Poor dental hygiene may contribute to poor chewing, hyperplasia of gums, or hypersensitivity in the mouth.

Unresolved dental problems often have a negative impact on food intake as well as the child's health and quality of life. Tooth brushing twice a day is the most important daily activity to maintain good oral hygiene and prevent future dental decay and gum problems. For the infant and young child, effective oral hygiene can be accomplished by wiping the teeth with a moist washcloth or gauze. If the child has problems with head and neck control, he or she can be positioned in a wheelchair, in a parent's lap, or lying down. If the child can tolerate a toothbrush and not gag, a soft brush may be used with circular motions. If the child cannot tolerate a toothbrush, one can brush with toothpaste on a cotton-tipped swab or soft washcloth. If the child is able to brush on her own, the parent still needs to monitor technique and go over areas that may have been missed.

Fluoride is important for reducing the risk of dental decay. It is available as a flavored liquid, chewable tablet, or mouth rinse. Topical fluoride can be applied at dental visits every 6 months. The need for fluoride depends on the amount of fluoride in the local water supply. Cavities also can be reduced by improving the diet, for example by consuming whole fruits rather than soft drinks, sticky snacks, cookies, or sugary fruit drinks.

## BONE HEALTH

Many factors, including nutritional factors, predispose the child with CP to poor bone health. However, the most profound factor is the lack of weight-bearing, which affects children with the most severe forms of CP, usually SQCP. Bone is very sensitive to musculoskeletal stress, and the lack of stress in nonambulatory people results in a form of osteoporosis known as *disuse osteoporosis*. Fractures without trauma (called *fragility fractures*) are common among children who are nonambulatory because of their CP. As many as 25% of children older than age 10 with SQCP have had a fragility fracture,[51] and once a child has had one such fracture, the risk for additional fractures increases.[52,53]

Calcium and phosphorus are the principal minerals that make up bone. Vitamin D plays a major role in the absorption of these minerals in the gut and their incorporation into bone matrix. In children with CP, poor food intake, and particularly deficiencies in intake of calcium and vitamin D and lack of sunlight exposure, also contribute to poor bone health. Other factors include delayed puberty and medications that can lower bone density, such as certain anticonvulsants, proton pump inhibitors used to treat reflux, and the injectable birth control drug Depo-Provera. Often, the only factors that can be addressed are the nutritional factors. Improved intake of minerals and vitamins can at least slow the progression of osteoporosis, if not actually reverse it. Sometimes, alternative medications with less effect on bone density can help, as can encouragement of standing or walking as often as tolerated. If, despite these measures, the child has fragility fractures, bisphosphonates are often prescribed to improve bone density.

## SUMMARY

Children with the complex forms of CP (GMFCS score 3–5) should be managed by a multidisciplinary team that includes a physician, nurse, RD, speech therapist, occupational therapist, and physical therapist. The nutrition management of a child with CP includes short-and long-term goals for growth, evaluation of nutrition status, assessment of dietary intake, and behavioral objectives. Routine clinical care should include anthropometric and dietary assessments as well as an assessment of feeding skills and progress in the treatment of nutrition-related problems. Health professionals working with care providers must recognize the significant role of each member of the team and work together with professionals and caregivers to promote the overall health and well-being of the child.

## ACKNOWLEDGMENTS

The authors would like to acknowledge Melanie Beach, MS, RD, and Chelsea Ale for their help with the preparation of this chapter, and Linda Bandini, PhD, and Shirley W. Ekvall, PhD, RD, for their contributions to this chapter in the previous edition.

### References

1. Sugimoto T, Woo M, Nishida N, et al. When do brain abnormalities in cerebral palsy occur?: an MRI study. *Dev Med Child Neurol.* 1995; 37:285.
2. Truwit CL, Barkovich AJ, Koch TK, Ferriero DM. Cerebral palsy: MR findings in 40 patients. *AJNR Am J Neuroradiol.* 1992; 13:67.
3. Blair E, Watson L. Epidemiology of cerebral palsy. *Semin Fetal Neonatal Med.* 2006; 11:117.
4. Crothers B, Paine R. *The Natural History of Cerebral Palsy.* Cambridge, MA: Harvard University Press; 1959.
5. Johnson M, Hoon A, Kaufmann W. Neurobiology, diagnosis and management of cerebral palsy. In: Accardo P, ed. *Capute and Accarodo's Neurodevelopmental Disabilities in Infancy and Childhood,* vol 1, 3rd ed. Baltimore, MD: Brookes Publishing; 2008.
6. Palisano R, Rosenbaum P, Walter S, Russell D, Wood E, Galuppi B. Development and reliability of a system to classify gross motor function in children with cerebral palsy. *Dev Med Child Neurol.* 1997; 39:214.
7. Menkes J. Perinatal asphyxia and trauma. In: Menkes J, ed. *Textbook of Child Neurology,* 3rd ed. Philadelphia: Lea & Febiger; 1985.
8. da Paz A, Burnett S, Brga L. Walking prognosis in cerebral palsy: a 22 year retrospective analysis. *Dev Med Child Neurol.* 1994; 36:130.
9. Lord J. Cerebral palsy: a clinical approach. *Arch Phys Med Rehabil.* 1984; 65:542.
10. Bhutani V, Johnson L, Gourley G. Hyperbilirubinemia and kernicterus: epidemiology, etiology and therapy. *Pediatr Acad Soc Abstr.* 2003; (May):398A.
11. Stevenson RD, Conaway M, Chumlea WC, et al. Growth and health in children with moderate-to-severe cerebral palsy. *Pediatrics.* 2006; 118:1010.
12. Brooks J, Day S, Shavelle R, Strauss D. Low weight, morbidity, and mortality in children with cerebral palsy: new clinical growth charts. *Pediatrics.* 2011; 128:e299.
13. Day SM, Strauss DJ, Vachon PJ, Rosenbloom L, Shavelle RM, Wu YW. Growth patterns in a population of children and adolescents with cerebral palsy. *Dev Med Child Neurol.* 2007; 49:167.
14. Kuperminc MN, Stevenson RD. Growth and nutrition disorders in children with cerebral palsy. *Dev Disabil Res Rev.* 2008; 14:137.
15. Marchand V, Motil KJ. Nutrition support for neurologically impaired children: a clinical report of the North American Society for Pediatric Gastroenterology, Hepatology, and Nutrition. *J Pediatr Gastroenterol Nutr.* 2006; 43:123.
16. Arvedson JC. Feeding children with cerebral palsy and swallowing difficulties. *Eur J Clin Nutr.* 2013; 67(suppl 2):S9.
17. Fung EB, Samson-Fang L, Stallings VA, et al. Feeding dysfunction is associated with poor growth and health status in children with cerebral palsy. *J Am Diet Assoc.* 2002; 102:361.
18. Dahlseng MO, Finbraten AK, Juliusson PB, Skranes J, Andersen G, Vik T. Feeding problems, growth and nutritional status in children with cerebral palsy. *Acta Paediatr.* 2012; 101:92.
19. Samson-Fang L, Fung E, Stallings VA, et al. Relationship of nutritional status to health and societal participation in children with cerebral palsy. *J Pediatr.* 2002; 141:637.
20. Henderson RC, Lark RK, Renner JB, et al. Dual X-ray absorptiometry assessment of body composition in children with altered body posture. *J Clin Densitom.* 2001; 4:325.
21. Bell K, Boyd R, Walker J, Stevenson R, Daves P. The use of bioelectrical impedance analysis to estimate total body water in young children with cerebral palsy. *Clin Nutr.* 2013; 32:579.
22. Samson-Fang L, Bell KL. Assessment of growth and nutrition in children with cerebral palsy. *Eur J Clin Nutr.* 2013; 67(suppl 2):S5.
23. Stevenson RD. Use of segmental measures to estimate stature in children with cerebral palsy. *Arch Pediatr Adolesc Med.* 1995; 149:658.
24. Samson-Fang LJ, Stevenson RD. Identification of malnutrition in children with cerebral palsy: poor performance of weight-for-height centiles. *Dev Med Child Neurol.* 2000; 42:162.
25. Krick J, Murphy-Miller P, Zeger S, Wright E. Pattern of growth in children with cerebral palsy. *J Am Diet Assoc.* 1996; 96:680.
26. Mascarenhas MR, Meyers R, Konek S. Outpatient nutrition management of the neurologically impaired child. *Nutr Clin Pract.* 2009; 23:597.
27. Rose J, Medeiros JM, Parker R. Energy cost index as an estimate of energy expenditure of cerebral-palsied children during assisted ambulation. *Dev Med Child Neurol.* 1985; 27:485.
28. Bell KL, Davies PS. Energy expenditure and physical activity of ambulatory children with cerebral palsy and of typically developing children. *Am J Clin Nutr.* 2010; 92:313.
29. Walker JL, Bell KL, Boyd RN, Davies PS. Energy requirements in preschool-age children with cerebral palsy. *Am J Clin Nutr.* 2012; 96:1309.
30. Bandini LG, Schoeller DA, Fukagawa NK, Wykes LJ, Dietz WH. Body composition and energy expenditure in adolescents with cerebral palsy or myelodysplasia. *Pediatr Res.* 1991; 29:70.
31. Stallings VA, Zemel BS, Davies JC, Cronk CE, Charney EB. Energy expenditure of children and adolescents with severe disabilities: a cerebral palsy model. *Am J Clin Nutr.* 1996; 64:627.
32. Krick J, Murphy PE, Markham JF, Shapiro BK. A proposed formula for calculating energy needs of children with cerebral palsy. *Dev Med Child Neurol.* 1992; 34:481.
33. Otten JJ, Hellwig JP, Meyers LD, eds; Food and Nutrition Board; Institute of Medicine. *Dietary Reference Intakes: The Essential Guide to Nutrient Requirements.* Washington, DC: The National Academies Press; 2006:92.
34. Food and Agriculture Organization, World Health Organization, United Nations University. *Expert Consultation: Human Energy Requirements.* Food and Nutrition Technical Report Series I. Rome: FAO; October 2001.
35. Hillesund E, Skranes J, Trygg KU, Bohmer T. Micronutrient status in children with cerebral palsy. *Acta Paediatr.* 2007; 96:1195.
36. Kilpinen-Loisa P, Pihko H, Vesander U, Paganus A, Ritanen U, Makitie O. Insufficient energy and nutrient intake in children with motor disability. *Acta Paediatr.* 2009; 98:1329.
37. Jones M, Campbell KA, Duggan C, et al. Multiple micronutrient deficiencies in a child fed an elemental formula. *J Pediatr Gastroenterol Nutr.* 2001; 33:602.
38. Hals J, Bjerve KS, Nilsen H, Svalastog AG, Ek J. Essential fatty acids in the nutrition of severely neurologically disabled children. *Br J Nutr.* 2000; 83:219.
39. Piccoli R, Gelio S, Fratucello A, Valletta E. Risk of low micronutrient intake in neurologically disabled children artificially fed. *J Pediatr Gastroenterol Nutr.* 2002; 35:583.
40. Bell KL, Samson-Fang L. Nutritional management of children with cerebral palsy. *Eur J Clin Nutr.* 2013; 67(suppl 2):S13.
41. Gisel EG, Patrick J. Identification of children with cerebral palsy unable to maintain a normal nutritional state. *Lancet.* 1988; 1:283.
42. Sullivan PB, Juszczak E, Lambert BR, Rose M, Ford-Adams ME, Johnson A. Impact of feeding problems on nutritional intake and growth: Oxford Feeding Study II. *Dev Med Child Neurol.* 2002; 44:461.
43. Stallings VA, Charney EB, Davies JC, Cronk CE. Nutrition-related growth failure of children with quadriplegic cerebral palsy. *Dev Med Child Neurol.* 1993; 35:126.
44. Shaikhkhalil A, Meyers R. Neurological Impairment. In: Corkins MR, ed. *The A.S.P.E.N. Pediatric Nutrition Support Core Curriculum.* Silver Spring, MD: A.S.P.E.N. Publishing; 2015:261.
45. Linscheid T. Behavioral treatments for pediatric feeding disorders. *Behav Modif.* 2006; 30:6.
46. Sullivan PB, Juszczak E, Bachlet AM, et al. Impact of gastrostomy tube feeding on the quality of life of carers of children with cerebral palsy. *Dev Med Child Neurol.* 2004; 46:796.
47. Kuperminc MN, Gottrand F, Samson-Fang L, et al. Nutritional management of children with cerebral palsy: a practical guide. *Eur J Clin Nutr.* 2013; 67(suppl 2):S21.
48. Sanders KD, Cox K, Cannon R, et al. Growth response to enteral feeding by children with cerebral palsy. *JPEN J Parenter Enteral Nutr.* 1990; 14:23.
49. Mortensen M. Blenderized tube feeding: clinical perspectives on homemade tube feeding. *PNPG Post: A Publication of the Pediatric Practice Group of the American Dietetic Association.* 2006; 17(Fall):104.
50. Pentiuk S, O'Flaherty T, Santoro K, Willging P, Kaul A. Pureed by gastrostomy tube diet improves gagging and retching in children with fundoplication. *JPEN J Parenter Enteral Nutr.* 2011; 35:375.
51. Henderson RC, Lark RK, Gurka MJ, et al. Bone density and metabolism in children and adolescents with moderate to severe cerebral palsy. *Pediatrics.* 2002; 110(1 Pt 1):e5.
52. Stevenson RD, Conaway M, Barrington JW, Cuthill SL, Worley G, Henderson RC. Fracture rate in children with cerebral palsy. *Pediatr Rehabil.* 2006; 9:396–403.
53. King W, Levin R, Schmidt. Prevalence of reduced bone mass in children and adults with spastic quadriplegia. *Dev Med Child Neurol.* 2003; 45:12.

# 10 Seizures and Epilepsy

YAEL SHILOH-MALAWSKY, LESLIE HUFFMAN, TUOMAS WESTERMARCK, AND SHIRLEY W. EKVALL

Seizures occur in approximately 10% of all people at some time during their lives. An epileptic seizure is a transient occurrence of signs and/or symptoms caused by abnormal excessive or synchronous neuronal activity in the brain.[1] An acute provoked seizure is a seizure that occurs in the context of an acute brain insult or systemic disorder; examples are acute stroke, hypoglycemia, and alcohol withdrawal. Seizures are classified as *generalized*, when they rapidly engage both hemispheres, or as *focal* (previously *partial*), when they originate within an area in one hemisphere.[2] Commonly recognized generalized seizure types include generalized tonic-clonic seizures (formerly called *grand mal*) and absence seizures (formerly called *petit mal*). Other types of generalized seizures are tonic, clonic, atonic, and myoclonic seizures. Some seizures are not clearly define as generalized or focal; an example is infantile spasms.[2] Anyone can have a seizure if the appropriate metabolic conditions are present. Relevant conditions include numerous metabolic and nutritional abnormalities.

About 0.5% to 1% of people have epilepsy, a disorder of the brain characterized by an enduring predisposition to generate epileptic seizures. The definition of epilepsy requires the occurrence of at least one unprovoked epileptic seizure.[1,3] Epilepsy is a family of disorders; it comprises many different diseases and conditions. The 2010 revised classification of seizures and epilepsy[2] defines the cause of epilepsy as either *genetic*, when epilepsy is the direct result of known genetic defects, or *structural/metabolic* (previously *symptomatic*), when there is a known underlying brain abnormality (e.g., remote stroke, brain tumor) or a metabolic disorder known to be associated with epilepsy. At times, the etiology is described as *unknown* (previously *cryptogenic*).

Epilepsy most commonly develops during the first year of life, and more than half of epilepsy cases manifest before age 21. Another peak in epilepsy onset occurs in older age, related to the accumulation of brain insults from such conditions as remote stroke, trauma, or tumors.[4] Potential causes of epilepsy in infants and children include acute brain-injuring insults such as perinatal asphyxia, sepsis, and hypoglycemia and chronic causes such as brain malformations and genetic disorders.

## BIOCHEMICAL ABNORMALITIES

Common metabolic causes of acute provoked seizures are hypoxia, hypoglycemia, and electrolyte abnormalities. Hypoglycemia is more likely than hyperglycemia to cause seizures. Typical causes of hypoglycemia include hyperinsulinemic states such as insulinomas, nesideoblastosis, and excess insulin administration. It is important to recognize hypoglycemia early because antiepileptic drugs (AEDs) are unlikely to abort an ongoing seizure if the hypoglycemia is not corrected. Hypoglycemia is particularly important to recognize because there is an increased risk of permanent brain injury if this condition is prolonged.

As with hypoglycemia, seizures due to electrolyte imbalances need to be treated with appropriate correction of the underlying abnormalities; mere administration of AEDs is ineffective. The electrolyte abnormalities most commonly associated with seizures are hyponatremia and hypocalcemia.[5,6] Less frequently seen in clinical practice are hypomagnesemia, hypophosphatemia, and hypokalemia.[7–9] A common cause of hyponatremia is diarrhea when the fluid loss is replaced by a hypotonic solution. Another cause is hyponatremia due to use of the medication desmopressin, which is often administered to children with nocturnal enuresis. Hypocalcemia may be seen in vitamin D deficiency, renal disease, parathyroid disease, and pseudohypoparathyroidism (target organ resistance to parathyroid hormone).

## FACTORS TO BE CONSIDERED IN NUTRITIONAL EVALUATION

Nutritional deficiencies and genetic/metabolic disorders can cause or contribute to seizures, and some epilepsy syndromes respond to specific treatments based on diet or supplementation of cofactors (vitamin-responsive epilepsies). These include, among others, disorders of pyridoxine (vitamin $B_6$), folinic acid, and glucose transporter 1 (GLUT1) deficiency.[10]

Abnormalities of pyridoxine metabolism due to genetic/metabolic disorders or decreased intake (pyridoxine deficiency) result in inadequate levels in the brain of pyridoxal phosphate (PLP), the active form of vitamin $B_6$, leading to an hyperexcitable state that provokes seizures. Two genetic epilepsies cause PLP deficiency: pyridoxine-dependent seizures and PLP-dependent epilepsy.

Pyridoxine-dependent seizures result from an autosomal recessive disorder caused by mutations in the *ALDH7A1* gene, which encodes the protein antiquitin.[11] Seizures usually manifest in neonates but can appear later in infancy. These seizures are refractory to antiseizure medications, and the electroencephalogram (EEG) activity is very abnormal. Treatment with intravenous bolus of pyridoxine (50–100 mg) has a dramatic effect. In typical cases, the seizures stop within minutes and the EEG normalizes. There is a small risk of respiratory arrest associated with acute pyridoxine administration. Lifelong therapy with a daily dose of 50 to 200 mg of pyridoxine is effective in preventing seizures in most patients. PLP-dependent epilepsy is an autosomal recessive disorder caused by mutation in the *PNPO* gene, which is involved in the conversion of vitamin $B_6$ derived from food to PLP. It is characterized by neonatal seizures that are refractory both to conventional AEDs and pyridoxine administration.[12] Seizures are responsive to large daily doses of pyridoxal 5′-phosphate, 10 to 80 mg/kg/day in three or four divided doses enterally.

Dietary deficiency of pyridoxine is fairly uncommon. Isoniazid can interfere with pyridoxine metabolism and cause seizures.[13] High intake of gingko has also been reported to cause seizures because it acts as an antagonist of pyridoxine.[14]

Another group of vitamin B–responsive epileptic disorders are the cerebral folate deficiency seizures and folinic acid–responsive seizures. Cerebral folate deficiency is characterized by low folates in the cerebrospinal fluid. The syndrome has been associated with both genetic and acquired conditions; the underlying etiology is not always well understood. In some cases, cerebral folate deficiency has been shown to be related to blocking of folate receptors by autoantibodies. It has also been shown to be associated with specific genetic mutations, such as *ALDH7A1* and folate receptor 1 (*FOLR1*) gene mutations, as well as diverse metabolic and genetic disorders. Folinic acid–responsive seizures are characterized by cessation of seizures after oral administration of folinic acid (3–5 mg/kg/day).[15,16]

The GLUT1 deficiency syndrome causes low glucose concentration in the cerebrospinal fluid; it is a genetic disorder caused by mutation of *SLC2A1*, the gene that encodes GLUT1.[17] The classic patient with GLUT1 deficiency syndrome has drug-resistant seizures beginning in the first year of life; however, the phenotype is highly variable. Lumbar puncture should be performed with the patient in a fasting state to establish the diagnosis. Ketogenic diet (KD) is the treatment of choice of patients with GLUT1 deficiency; it has been shown to be highly effective in controlling the seizures and improving developmental outcome, although neurobehavioral and motor deficits persist in most cases.[18]

Other metabolic abnormalities are associated with seizures or epilepsy and respond to specific diets or nutritional supplementation. Among these are biotin deficiency, biotinidase deficiency (an enzyme abnormality), creatine deficiency, aminoacidopathies (e.g., maple syrup urine disease, phenylketonuria [PKU]), urea cycle defects (associated with hyperammonemia), Menke disease (associated with decreased serum copper and ceruloplasmin), galactosemia, hyperglycinemia, and porphyria.[10]

## NUTRITIONAL CONSIDERATIONS AND ANTIEPILEPTIC DRUGS

There are a few anecdotal reports suggesting that some foods and dietary contents might influence the occurrence of seizures, but there is little evidence that avoidance of certain foods will decrease seizure occurrence in children with epilepsy.[19] Caffeine is a psychostimulant, but despite theoretical concerns, there is insufficient evidence to support pro-seizure effects of caffeine in animals or humans.[20] Anecdotal reports have suggested that the high-intensity sweetener aspartame can cause seizures in some vulnerable individuals, but systematic investigations of this possibility have not supported these reports.[21] Grapefruit juice can cause an increase in the serum concentration of carbamazepine (and therefore toxicity) as a result of inhibition of enzymes in the liver and gut wall.[22]

Women treated with AEDs are at increased risk for fetal malformations.[23] There are numerous possible mechanisms for the teratogenicity, including folate deficiency. Carbamazepine, phenobarbital, and phenytoin interfere with folate absorption and may induce a folate deficiency. Supplementation with at least 0.4 mg/day folate (as recommended for all women of child-bearing potential), and up to 4 mg/day (recommended for women with a previously affected child), is recommended for women of child-bearing age with epilepsy who are at risk of becoming pregnant.[24]

Virtually all AEDs are excreted in breast milk. The concentration of these drugs is usually small enough that the effect on the nursing infant is negligible, although sedation has been reported with some AEDs (e.g., phenobarbital, primidone, ethosuximide). Although the data are limited, it has been shown that valproic acid, phenobarbital, phenytoin, and carbamazepine do not penetrate into breast milk in amounts that might be clinically important.[24] Overall, the benefits of breast-feeding outweigh the risk of infant exposure to the low concentration of AEDs in breast milk, and breast-feeding should be encouraged unless symptoms emerge.[25]

The effect of AEDs on bone health and vitamin D metabolism raises important nutritional considerations. The risk for skeletal fractures in patients with epilepsy is two to five times greater than in the general population. Multiple factors contribute to this risk, including seizures, falls, and comorbidities. In addition, the use of AEDs alone is associated with an increased risk of fractures.[26] AEDs were shown to have clinical effects on bone health by multiple mechanisms, including effect on vitamin D metabolism. Optimization of calcium and vitamin D intake and routine screening for calcium and vitamin D metabolites are recommended for all persons with epilepsy treated with AEDs.[19,27]

## DIETARY MANAGEMENT

### Ketogenic Diet

For centuries, it has been observed that fasting and starvation are associated with a reduction in seizures. The KD, initially described by Wilder in 1921, was formulated to mimic the biochemical effects of starvation—that is, to induce ketosis.[28] The KD was used extensively in the early to middle 20th century as a treatment for epilepsy. Its use waned as a greater variety of more conveniently administered AEDs became available. However, despite an ever-increasing number of AEDs, a significant proportion of patients remain refractory to drug treatment. In 1992, neurologists at the Johns Hopkins School of Medicine reported surprisingly high efficacy using the KD to treat medically refractory epilepsy in children, and it has remained an important option for epilepsy treatment. It is usually considered for children who have multiple seizures every week and for whom at least two (and usually more) AEDs have proved ineffective. It is also considered if surgical intervention has either failed or is not an option.[29,30] When considering the KD, it is important to evaluate for metabolic conditions that may contraindicate a very-high-fat diet. Such conditions include carnitine deficiencies, beta-oxidation defects, porphyria, and pyruvate carboxylase deficiency.[31]

The underlying biochemical mechanism of the KD antiseizure effect is still unclear. Achieving a state of ketosis seems critical, and caloric restriction alone may have some antiseizure effect.[31,32] There is experimental evidence for four distinct molecular mechanisms that could contribute to the antiseizure effect of these diets. These mechanisms include carbohydrate reduction, activation of adenosine triphosphate (ATP)–sensitive potassium channels by mitochondrial metabolism, inhibition of the mammalian target of rapamycin (mTOR) pathway, and inhibition of glutamatergic excitatory synaptic transmission.[33]

To achieve a state of ketosis, the KD comprises a strictly monitored number of calories, a high proportion of fat, and a combination of low-protein and low-carbohydrate foods. In the past, fluid was restricted in these patients. This is no longer practiced according to Wirrell, who stated that there is little evidence that fluid restriction is needed or beneficial.[31,32] In addition, there are some reports that fluid restriction as part of the KD increases the incidence of constipation and kidney stones. The "dose" of the KD is expressed as a ratio of fat to combined protein and carbohydrate (by weight) and most commonly ranges from 3:1 to 4:1. Meal size, calories, and timing are strictly controlled. Patients started on the KD become ketotic, and parents monitor urine ketones daily with the use of urine chemsticks. Serum ketones are also elevated and can be monitored by measuring the serum concentration of beta-hydroxybutyrate. With these metabolic changes, a patient's breath may smell sweet or may smell of acetone.

Over the past few decades, multiple versions of the KD have been established. These include the classic KD, the modified Atkins diet (MAD), the medium-chain triglyceride (MCT) oil diet, and low glycemic index diet.

The classic KD maintains a 3:1 or 4:1 ratio of fat to combined protein and carbohydrate, with 80% to 90% of calories in the diet from fat. In the past, the diet had to be calculated by hand, and foods were labeled as ketogenic or antiketogenic:

$$\frac{\text{Ketogenic}}{\text{Antiketogenic}} = \frac{0.90\text{ fat} + 0.46\text{ protein} + 0.0\text{ carbohydrate}}{0.10\text{ fat} + 0.58\text{ protein} + 1.0\text{ carbohydrate}}$$

Today, the classic KD meals are calculated with the use of a computerized nutrient database program such as KetoDietCalculator (ketodietcalculator.org), with all food weighed on a digital gram scale. Many creative ketogenic recipes are now widely available through the efforts of dedicated dietitians and parent networks, and the increased variety has made the classic KD more palatable. There are also commercially available products that permit easier administration of the KD via gastrostomy tube feedings. In several studies, the classic KD resulted in a greater than 50% decrease in seizures in about half of treated children and complete seizure control in 10% to 15%.[34] Table 10–1 shows a sample paradigm for calculating the initial KD composition.

The MAD has become popular as an alternative to the KD. It is a less restrictive option because it limits carbohydrate intake without requiring protein and calorie restriction, weighing of foods, or hospitalization when starting the diet.[35] This version is most often used for adult patients who do not respond to medication and are not candidates

**Table 10–1.** Calculation of a Typical Ketogenic Diet (KD) Composition

| Steps in Calculation | Example Calculation |
|---|---|
| 1. Determine caloric recommendation based on RDA; the KD should supply 75% and 100% of this amount, depending on activity level. | Assume a 6-year-old child with an ideal weight of 20 kg; the KD should supply 68 kcal/kg. |
| 2. Calculate total calories per day. | 20 kg × 68 kcal/kg = 1360 kcal/day |
| 3. Choose the starting ratio, usually 3:1 or 4:1. | 4:1 ratio = 36 kcal F for every 4 kcal combined (P + C); 36 kcal + 4 kcal = 40 kcal per "unit" of food |
| 4. Calculate total "units" of food per day. | 1360 kcal/day ÷ 40 kcal/unit = 34 units/day |
| 5. Calculate F using the determined ratio. | 4 × 34 units = 136 g F per day |
| 6. Total of P + C will usually be 1 × units/day. | 1 × 34 units = 34 g (P + C) |
| 7. Calculate P requirement using RDA. | At 1 g P per 1 kg body weight, 1 g/kg × 20 kg = 20 g P |
| 8. The allotment of C is the (P + C) total from step 6 minus the P requirement from step 7. | 34 g − 20 g = 14 g C |
| 9. The total daily diet is divided equally into three or four meals. | Intake of 136 g F, 20 g P, and 14 g C in three meals daily = 45 g F, 7 g P, and 5 g C per meal |
| 10. Fluids should be calculated at 0.7–1.0 of the daily maintenance requirements and divided throughout day. | For a 20-kg child, 1050–1500 mL/day should be consumed, or 70–100 mL/hr over 15 waking hours |

C = carbohydrate; F = fat; P = protein; RDA = recommended daily allowance.

for surgical intervention, but it is becoming more common for pediatric patients as well. The average adult patient begins the MAD by restricting carbohydrates to 15 to 20 g/day, and pediatric patients begin at 10 to 15 g/day.[36] MAD outcomes are comparable to those of the KD. In a retrospective review, about 48% of patients (adults and children combined) had a greater than 50% reduction, 26% had a greater than 90% reduction, and 13% became seizure free over a period of 3 to 6 months when MAD was used before the KD.[36]

The last two alternatives to the KD most used in the United States are the MCT oil diet and the Low Glycemic Index Treatment (LGIT). The MCT oil variation was traditionally considered more palatable than the classic KD. MCT oil is used as the primary source of fat calories, thereby decreasing the "volume" of fat the patient receives (Table 10–2). As improvements have been made to the classic KD, the MCT oil diet is less readily used. The LGIT limits the amount of carbohydrate, similar to MAD, but emphasizes carbohydrates that are lower on the glycemic index. Table 48–1 in Chapter 48 provides a glycemic index list. For additional information, visit the website of the Charlie Foundation for Ketogenic Therapies (www.charliefoundation.org).

The average duration of therapy with the KD and its alternatives ranges from 2 to 3 years. In some reported cases, the KD has been continued as long as 20 years.[31] Supplementation with a multivitamin, calcium, and vitamin D are very important while on the KD or a KD alternative. Both medications and supplements should be taken in tablet form (i.e., a nonchewable, non-orodispersible tablet) or compounded in a sugar-free solution because of the carbohydrate content in these products.

Selecting those patients most likely to benefit from the KD remains a challenge. Because starting the KD involves hospitalization (in most cases), extensive education, and a commitment of at least 3 months, it is desirable to be able to predict with greater precision which patients are most likely to sustain a reduction in seizures.[34] Age is a frequently cited component: The average patient ranges from 1 to 12 years of age, although there are reports of effective treatment in adults, adolescents, and infants.[34–36]

The type of seizure and epilepsy syndrome should be considered when screening candidates for a trial of the KD. Multiple published case series have shown the KD and its alternatives to be an effective antiseizure treatment.[31,32,36–39] Success has also been reported for children with infantile spasms, Lennox-Gastaut syndrome, Rett syndrome, and Landau-Kleffner syndrome. KD is the recommended treatment for GLUT1 deficiency.[18,40–42]

Like other epilepsy treatments, the KD involves some risks. Common adverse effects can be short or long term. Short-term side effects may include lethargy, constipation, dehydration, hypoglycemia, emesis, weight change, increased hypercholesterolemia, and dyslipidemia. Long-term effects may include growth retardation, gastrointestinal disturbances, changes in bone metabolism, pancreatitis, increased bruising, and renal stones.[31,43] To improve initial tolerance of the diet, the meals are often started at one-third of the target size (calories), given as a liquid (shake) or as regular food. Input from a dietitian is essential in implementing and fine-tuning the diet. Detrimental effects of the KD have been reported; these include heart disease and death, although they occur very rarely.[31]

## Follow-up

Children prescribed the KD need to be followed closely by their physician and dietitian. Monitoring of weight and height is important for adjusting the calorie intake and ensuring that adequate growth continues. Parents should check urine ketones daily; a review of their values

**Table 10–2.** Calculation of the Medium-Chain Triglyceride (MCT) Diet

| Steps in Calculation | Example Calculation |
|---|---|
| 1. Establish caloric needs according to the RDA. | Assume a value of 1900 kcal/day. |
| 2. Determine the amount of MCT oil to be given (50–70% of total kcal); 1 g MCT = 8.3 kcal, and 1 tbsp (15 mL) MCT = 14 g | 60% × 1900 kcal = 1140 kcal from MCT<br>1140 kcal ÷ 8.3 kcal/g= 137 g MCT<br>137 g ÷ 14 g/tbsp = 9.8 tbsp (147 mL) MCT |
| 3. Determine the calories to be provided by foods exclusive of MCT. | 1900 − 1140 = 760 kcal |
| 4. Establish P intake according to RDA (at least 36 g of P for a 5- to 7-year-old child weighing 28 kg) | Assume 41 g of protein is needed.<br>41 g x 4 kcal/g = at least 164 kcal P |
| 5. Estimate maximum calories (19% of total) to be given in form of C. | 19% × 1900 = no more than 361 kcal from C<br>361 kcal ÷ 4 kcal/g = no more than 90 g of C |
| 6. Estimate maximum calories for P + C (29% of total) | 29% × 1900 = no more than 551 kcal from (P + C) |
| 7. Estimate minimum calories to be given in the form of F exclusive of MCT (11% of total) | 11% × 1900 = at least 209 kcal from other F<br>209 kcal ÷ 9 kcal/g = 23 g F other than MCT |
| 8. After determining all of these dietary requirements, calculate the dietary pattern using exchange lists. | The dietary requirements can be met by consumption of 9.8 tbsp MCT, 23 g other F, 41 g P, and 90 g C, plus 26 additional kcal to total 1900 kcal/day |

[a]See Chapter 48.
C = carbohydrate; F = fat; P = protein; RDA = recommended daily allowance; tbsp = tablespoon.

will help determine whether the KD ratio needs to be increased or calories adjusted. Poor ketosis and excessive weight gain can indicate too many calories, too low a ketogenic ratio, or compliance problems. Careful assessment of the child for hair loss, lethargy, poor wound healing, abnormal bruising or bleeding, and behavior changes is also important. Laboratory values commonly checked at clinic visits are electrolytes (including calcium and phosphorus), glucose, complete blood count, total protein, albumin, amylase, blood urea nitrogen, beta-hydroxybutyrate, and creatinine. Urine is checked for blood and crystals, which could be early signs of renal stones. Also, follow-up visits are a good time to determine whether to decrease or discontinue concomitant AEDs if seizure control has improved since the introduction of the KD.

## References


1. Fisher RS, van Emde Boas W, Blume W, et al. Epileptic seizures and epilepsy: definitions proposed by the International League Against Epilepsy (ILAE) and the International Bureau for Epilepsy (IBE). *Epilepsia.* 2005; 46:470.
2. Berg AT, Berkovic SF, Brodie MJ, et al. Revised terminology and concepts for organization of seizures and epilepsies: report of the ILAE Commission on Classification and Terminology, 2005–2009. *Epilepsia.* 2010; 51:676.
3. Fisher RS, Acevedo C, Arzimanoglou A, et al. ILAE official report: a practical clinical definition of epilepsy. *Epilepsia.* 2014; 55:475.
4. Annegers JF, Hauser WA, Lee JR, Rocca WA. Incidence of acute symptomatic seizures in Rochester, Minnesota, 1935–1984. *Epilepsia.* 1995; 36:327.
5. Bhalla P, Eaton FE, Coulter JBS, Amegavie FL, Sills JA, Abernethy LJ. Lesson of the week: hyponatraemic seizures and excessive intake of hypotonic fluids in young children. *BMJ.* 1999; 319:1554.
6. Sheth DP. Hypocalcemic seizures in neonates. *Am J Emerg Med.* 1997; 15:638.
7. Vanpee D, Dive A, Ossemann M, Gillet JB. Refractory seizure with hypokalaemia: seizures related to theophylline intoxication. *Postgrad Med J.* 2001; 77:209.
8. Paul VK, Vaswami M, Singh M, Sekhar C, Deorari AK. Seizures in neonates and young infants due to hypomagnesemia. *Indian J Pediatr.* 1997; 64:725.
9. Miller DW, Slovis CM. Hypophosphatemia in the emergency department therapeutics. *Am J Emerg Med.* 2000; 18:457.
10. Papetti L, Parisi P, Leuzzi V, et al. Metabolic epilepsy: an update. *Brain Dev.* 2013; 35:827.
11. Scharer G, Brocker C, Vasiliou V, et al. The genotypic and phenotypic spectrum of pyridoxine-dependent epilepsy due to mutations in ALDH7A1. *J Inherit Metab Dis.* 2010; 33:571.
12. Kuo MF, Wang HS. Pyridoxal phosphate-responsive epilepsy with resistance to pyridoxine. *Pediatr Neurol.* 2002; 26:146.
13. Pellock JM, Howell J, Kendig EL, Baker H. Pyridoxine-deficiency in children treated with isoniazid. *Chest.*1985; 7:658.
14. Kajiyama Y, Fujii K, Takeuchi H, Manabe Y. Ginkgo seed poisoning. *Pediatrics.* 2002; 109:325.
15. Gallagher RC, Van Hove JLK, Scharer G, et al. Folinic acid-responsive seizures are identical to pyridoxine-dependent epilepsy. *Ann Neurol.* 2009; 65:550.
16. Aylett SB, Varadkar S, Fassone E, et al. Cerebral folate deficiency associated with a novel homozygous nonsense mutation in FOLR1. *J Inherit Metab Dis.* 2012; 35:S138.
17. Seidner G, Alvarez MG, Yeh JI, et al. GLUT-1 deficiency syndrome caused by haploinsufficiency of the blood-brain barrier hexose carrier. *Nat Genet.* 1998; 18:188.
18. Klepper J. Glucose transporter deficiency syndrome (GLUT1DS) and the ketogenic diet. *Epilepsia.* 2008; 49(suppl 8):46.
19. Asadi-Pooya AA, Mintzer S, Sperling MR. Nutritional supplements, foods, and epilepsy: is there a relationship? *Epilepsia.* 2008; 49:1819.
20. Zagnoni PG, Albano C. Psychostimulants and epilepsy. *Epilepsia.* 2002; 43(suppl 2):28.
21. Butchko HH, Stargel WW, Comer CP, et al. Aspartame: review of safety. *Regul Toxicol Pharmacol.* 2002 ;35:S1.
22. Garg SK, Kumar N, Bhargava VK, Prabhakar SK. Effect of grapefruit juice on carbamazepine bioavailability in patients with epilepsy. *Clin Pharmacol Ther.* 1998; 64:286.
23. Pennell PB. Antiepileptic drugs during pregnancy: what is known and which AEDs seem to be safest? *Epilepsia.* 2008; 49(suppl 9):43.
24. Harden CL, Pennell PB, Koppel BS, et al. Practice parameter update: management issues for women with epilepsy. Focus on pregnancy (an evidence-based review): vitamin K, folic acid, blood levels, and breastfeeding. Report of the Quality Standards Subcommittee and Therapeutics and Technology Assessment Subcommittee of the American Academy of Neurology and American Epilepsy Society. *Neurology.* 2009; 73:142.
25. Meador KJ. Breastfeeding and antiepileptic drugs. *JAMA.* 2014; 311:1797.
26. Shen C, Chen F, Zhang Y, Guo Y, Ding M. Association between use of antiepileptic drugs and fracture risk: a systematic review and meta-analysis. *Bone.* 2014; 64:246.
27. Sheth RD, Pack A.Wyllie E, Pennell PB. Bone health and fractures in epilepsy. In: Wyllie E, Cascino GD, Gidal BE, Goodkin HP, eds. *Wyllie's Treatment of Epilepsy: Principles and Practice,* 5th ed: chapter 46. Philadelphia: Wolters Kluwer Health/Lippincott Williams & Wilkins; 2011.
28. Wilder RM, Winter MD. The threshold of ketogenesis. *J Biol Chem.* 1922; 52:393.
29. Vining EP. The ketogenic diet. *Adv Exp Med Biol.* 2002; 497:225.
30. Ekvall S. *Nutrition for Special Health Care Needs, Children to Adults.* A self study course based on the book, *Pediatric and Adult Nutrition in Standard, Chronic Diseases and Intellectual and Developmental Disabilities: Prevention, Assessment, and Treatment*, edited by S. Ekvall and V. Ekvall (Oxford University Press, 3rd ed., 2016).
31. Kossoff E, Freeman J, Turner Z, Rubenstein JE. *Ketogenic Diets: Treatments for Epilepsy and Other Disorders.* New York: Demos Medical Publishing; 2011.
32. Wirrell EC. Ketogenic ratio, calories, and fluids: do they matter? *Epilepsia.* 2008; 49(suppl 8):17.
33. Danial NN, Hartman AL, Stafstrom CE, Thio LL. How does the ketogenic diet work?: four potential mechanisms. *J Child Neurol.* 2013; 28:1027.
34. Zupec-Kania B, Neal E, Schultz R, Roan ME, Turner Z, Welborn M. An update on diets in clinical practice. *J Child Neurol.* 2013; 28:1015.
35. Kossoff EH, Rowley H, Sinha SR, Vining EP. A prospective study of the modified Atkins diet for intractable epilepsy in adults. *Epilepsia.* 2008; 49:316.
36. Kossoff EH, Cervenka MC, Henry BJ, Haney CA, Turner Z. A decade of the modified Atkins diet (2003–2013): results, insights, and future directions. *Epilepsy Behav.* 2013; 29:437.
37. Tolaymat A, Nayak A, Geyer JD, Geyer SK, Carney PR. Diagnosis and management of childhood epilepsy. *Curr Probl Pediatr Adolesc Health Care.* 2015; 45:3.
38. Levy RG, Cooper PN, Giri P. Ketogenic diet and other dietary treatments for epilepsy. *Cochrane Database Syst Rev.* 2012; 3:CD001903.
39. Neal EG, Chaffe H, Schwartz RH, et al. The ketogenic diet for the treatment of childhood epilepsy: a randomised controlled trial. *Lancet Neurol.* 2008; 7:500.
40. Freeman JM, Vining EP. Seizures decrease rapidly after fasting: preliminary studies of the ketogenic diet. *Arch Pediatr Adolesc Med.* 1999; 153:946.
41. Shafrir Y, Prensky AL. Acquired epileptiform opercular syndrome: a second case report, review of the literature, and comparison to the Landau-Kleffner syndrome. *Epilepsia.* 1995; 36:1050.
42. Liebhaber GM, Riemann E, Baumeister FA. Ketogenic diet in Rett syndrome. *J Child Neurol.* 2003; 18:74.
43. Plonka-Póltorak E, Westermarck T, Kaipainen P, Kaski M, Atroshi F, eds. Trace elements, antioxidant enzymes and free carnitine levels among epileptic patients treated with valproate monotherapy. In: Atroshi F, ed. *Pharmacology and Nutritional Intervention in the Treatment of Disease.* Croatia: InTech; 2014.

# 11 Myelomeningocele

FRANK CERNIGLIA JR. MD. AND SHIRLEY W. EKVALL

Myelomeningocele (MM), the most serious type of the neural tube defect (NTD), is also known as spina bifida. It arises embryonically during the transformation of the neuroectoderm into a neural tube as it detaches from the cutaneous ectoderm. It is the most common malformation resulting from a disturbance in neurotation and occurs when a child is born with a protruding lesion along the midline of the spinal cord that blocks closure of the neural tube[1] (Fig. 11–1).

The defect takes form between 26 and 30 days' gestation; the later its development, the lower the lesion.[2] Removal of the sac and closure of the neural defect usually are performed within 24 to 48 hours after birth to avoid infection. The sac contains meninges, dura, cerebral spinal fluid, and other neural elements. The effects of spina bifida depend on the level of the sac or lesion and the type of lesion and contents of the sac. The higher the sac and the more neural elements it contains, the greater the extent of impairment. Manifestations range from weakness in the lower extremities to complete paralysis of the legs, loss of sensation, incontinence of urine and feces, and abnormalities of the hips, knees, and feet. Approximately 90% of children with MM have hydrocephalus, which is not fatal if treated promptly, before brain tissue is destroyed. A ventriculoatrial or ventriculoperitoneal shunt is used to relieve the pressure[3] (Fig. 11–2).

The median IQ of children with MM is 88.[4] Even with normal intelligence, many children with MM have a learning disability. Trophic ulcers, spontaneous fractures, and deformities of the lower extremities occur because of decreased ambulation. Obesity follows and usually is related to the level of the lesion; higher lesions produce the greatest amount of obesity.[5]

The incidence of MM was about 5 per 10,000 births in the United States and 6.7 per 10,000 births in Ireland before the late 1990s.[6] In the United States, the prevalence of NTDs declined significantly after mandatory folic acid fortification of foods. The incidence of having a child affected by spina bifida in the United States is highest for Hispanic women (4.17 per 10,000), compared with non-Hispanic White women (3.22 per 10,000) and non-Hispanic Black or African-American women (2.64 per 10,000).[7]

Recurrence in families in which one child has spina bifida is 2.5 times greater than the incidence in the general population.[8] However, first-born children are at greatest risk for MM.[9] With surgical correction of hydrocephalus, removal of the lesion, prevention of renal damage, and provision of aggressive nutrition, orthopedic therapy, and other multidisciplinary therapies, survival has improved to 80% to 95% compared with earlier levels of 50% to 70%.[3]

## BIOCHEMICAL ABNORMALITIES

Among the proposed causal factors are amphetamines, oral contraceptives, potato glycoalkaloids, nitrites, salicylates, geography, maternal age (especially >35 years), maternal illness, socioeconomic status, migration, ethnicity, and hyperthermia.[10] Watkins et al.[11] found that a woman's risk increases with high body mass index (BMI). Drugs such as valproic acid also have been investigated, but currently the most promising area of research involves nutritional deficiencies.[12] Several studies have shown that insulin-dependent diabetic women have more infants with congenital abnormalities, including neural defects. Aminopterin, a powerful folic acid antagonist, has produced NTDs in humans.[13] Maternal alcohol ingestion during neurotation also may lead to NTDs.[13]

Although the etiology of MM is unknown and may involve both genetic and environmental factors, prenatal screening is available that can detect raised alpha-fetoprotein levels in amniotic fluid associated with spina bifida and other NTDs.[14] One study found that maternal dieting behaviors involving restricted food intake during the first trimester were associated with increased risk of NTDs.[15] Ultrasound monitoring is frequently performed prenatally for women and can show head malformations before 20 weeks' gestation.

High levels of urinary excretion of *p*-hydroxyphenylacetic acid (pHPAA), 4-hydroxy-3-methoxymandelic acid (HMMA), and homovanillic acid (HVA) found in children with MM may be caused by a disorder in the metabolism of ascorbic acid.[16] Ekvall et al.[17] reported low levels of ascorbic acid and zinc in children with MM; however, these children were able to become ascorbic acid saturated with ascorbic acid supplementation. In the Ekvall study, 40 children with MM were matched for age, sex, race, and physical activity and divided evenly into a group receiving ascorbic acid supplementation and a control group. Dietary intake of ascorbic acid was measured to rule out any influence on serum levels. Over an average period of 3.2 years, the experimental group with supplementary ascorbic acid had significantly higher ascorbic acid and vitamin $B_{12}$ levels than the control group and did not show deficiency in serum vitamin $B_{12}$ levels, anemia, or an elevated mean corpuscular volume.[17] It can be concluded that the demethylation/remethylation cycle of methionine, being folate and vitamin $B_{12}$ dependent, is crucial for embryonic and fetal growth, probably through generation of DNA, proteins, and polyamines.[12,18]

Maternal periconceptual vitamin usage and genetic variation in reduced folate carrier (A8OG polymorphism) in the infant produce a risk of spina bifida.[19] An increased dietary intake of methionine, as well as folate and vitamin $B_{12}$, reduced the risk of MM.[20] Up to 80% of children with spina bifida also have a latex allergy resulting from increased exposure to latex products.[21] Patients with MM have decreased bone mineral density and are at risk for pathological bone fractures.[22]

## FACTORS TO BE CONSIDERED IN NUTRITIONAL EVALUATION

### Nutritional Deficiency

Most research has focused on deficiencies of folic acid, zinc, the multivitamin supplement methionine, and genetic variants. Based on an early small study, Laurence et al.[23] recommended that 0.4 mg of folic acid be administered with the first dose beginning 28 days before conception to decrease the incidence of NTD. In a double-blind study, they investigated the effect of folic acid supplementation in early pregnancy and before conception in women who previously had given birth to a child with an NTD. There was no recurrence in 10 women who received folic acid but six recurrences in 17 women who had no folate supplementation. The authors concluded that a good diet and folate supplementation were beneficial[23] (Table 11–1). Boddie et al.[24] found that the risk of spina bifida could be significantly reduced by supplemental folic acid; however, absorption of polyglutamyl folate may vary among women. Both interventional and observational studies suggest than folic acid supplementation may reduce the incidence of neural tube defects by and average of about 70%.

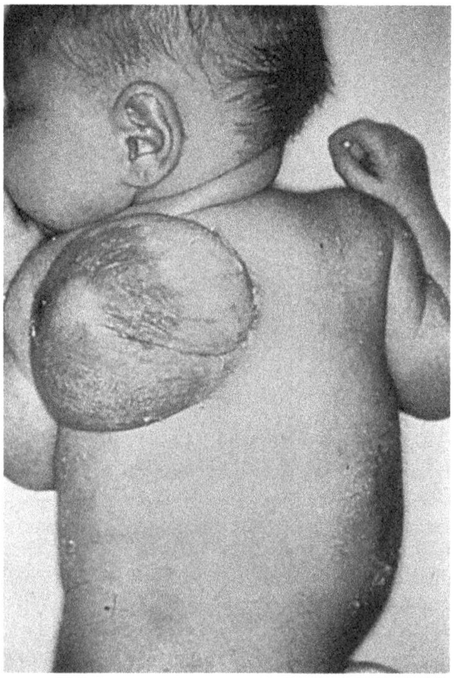

**Figure 11–1.** Protruding sac along the midline of the spinal cord, which produces nonclosure of the neural tube. (From the Cincinnati Children's Hospital Medical Center, Division of Developmental Disabilities, Cincinnati, OH. Used with permission.)

Smithells et al.[9] compared 234 mothers in England who took a supplemental Pregnavite Forte F vitamin preparation every day 28 days before conception with 219 mothers in the United States who did not receive that vitamin preparation. The supplemented mothers had only a 0.9% occurrence of NTD, compared with 5.1% in the unsupplemented mothers. This vitamin preparation contained slightly fewer vitamins and minerals than the current US Dietary Reference Intakes (DRIs), except for increased iron sulfate. The researchers' choice of controls was questionable, but the finding called for further research in this area. Molloy et al.[25] suggested the need for better maternal nutritional status evaluation, and particularly for increased folic acid and vitamin $B_{12}$ early in pregnancy.

A study by Butterworth and Bendich[26] indicated that consuming multivitamin supplements containing folic acid during the periconceptional period reduces the number of children born with serious malformations. Multivitamin supplementation also has been associated with a reduced incidence of other congenital malformations. An earlier study[27] showing the relation of NTD risk to multivitamin intake in general, and to folic acid in particular, involved 23,491 women who had alpha-fetoprotein screening or amniocentesis at approximately 16 weeks' gestation; 49 of these women (3.5 per 1000), evaluated at delivery, gave birth to infants with an NTD. The prevalence of NTDs among infants of women who used folic acid with multivitamins during the first 6 weeks of pregnancy was only 0.09 per 1000, compared with a prevalence of 0.12 to 0.59 per 1000 among those whose mothers used multivitamins without folic acid.

Scholl et al.[28] found that women with a low mean daily folate intake had an approximately twofold greater risk of preterm delivery and infant low birth weight after maternal characteristics, energy intake, and other correlated nutrients were controlled. The inclusion of folic acid in the multivitamin during the first 6 weeks of pregnancy was most significant in reducing the incidence of NTD. A study in seven countries[29] firmly concluded that supplementation with 4 mg folic acid (10 times the US DRI) significantly lowered the recurrence of fetal NTD and recommended increased folic acid for women with a previous NTD-affected pregnancy. Folic acid supplementation was also recommended for all pregnant women, but the quantity was not given.

An objective was added to the Healthy People 2000 initiative from the US Department of Health and Human Services to promote the use of folic acid in reducing NTDs.[30] Multivitamins reduce the risk of nonsyndromic NTD cases associated with other birth defects. All females of child-bearing age should be taking a folic acid supplement of 0.4 mg/day and consuming a diet rich in folate.[31] The estimated annual number of NTD-affected pregnancies in the United States declined from 4000 in 1995–1996 to 3000 in 1999–2000, possibly because of the folic acid fortification program.[32] Because many pregnancies are unplanned, supplementation should not await plans for pregnancy.[31] For all women, synthetic folic acid, consumed as supplements or in fortified foods, may be the best way to increase folate blood levels.[31]

In 1999, Kloeblen[33] assessed the folate-related knowledge and behaviors of pregnant women and found that populations of low-income pregnant women were likely to benefit from the folate fortification of grain products. Since that time, 0.1 mg (100 μg) folic acid per 100 g of product has been added to many flour and other cereal and grain products. The fortification of grain products with folic acid has not been found to decrease absorption of zinc, a concern during fortification discussions.[34] Yet in one of the most advanced countries in the world, this new recommendation has had little effect on patients' folate intake.[35] Consumption of more than 1000 μg of folic acid per day may require further study of zinc and vitamin $B_{12}$ as genetic markers. Most people consume only 200 μg of folic acid per day in their diet. The synthetic form of folic acid is better absorbed than that in food. Studies in other countries have also found low levels of folate in women of child-bearing age.[36–38]

In earlier research, Bergmann et al.[39] found increased zinc concentrations in hair samples from pregnant women who had already produced one child with NTD. The plasma zinc level in maternal blood also was significantly lower in 54 women delivering infants with congenital abnormalities. Nevin[40] found significantly higher amounts of zinc and copper in the amniotic fluid of mothers in the NTD group. In the study by Smithells et al.,[9] supplementation did not include zinc and copper, but zinc as a catalyst could have been spared by increased iron

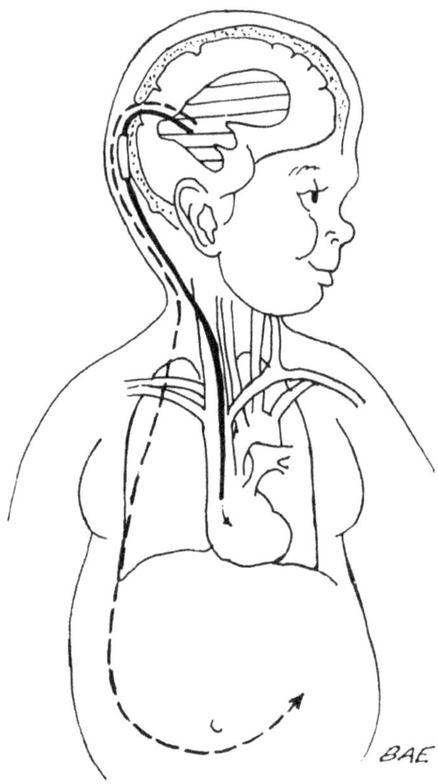

**Figure 11–2.** A ventriculoatrial shunt or ventriculoperitoneal shunt is used to relieve pressure.

**Table 11–1.** Statistically Significant Results of Studies on Neural Tube Defects (NTDs) and Folic Acid Supplementation

| Study | Design | Subjects | Results | Relative Risk | Comments |
|---|---|---|---|---|---|
| *Interventional Studies* | | | | | |
| Smithells et al.[9] | United Kingdom Nonrandomized, controlled, multicenter trial | • Pregnant women with a prior NTD-affected pregnancy<br>• Supplemented mothers took 0.36 mg folic acid plus a multivitamin daily; unsupplemented mothers took placebo from at least 1 mo before conception through first trimester | • 3 NTD pregnancies among 454 supplemented women<br>• 24 NTD | 0.14 | 86% risk reduction |
| UK MRC Study[29] | United Kingdom Randomized, controlled, multicenter trial | • Pregnant women with a prior NTD-affected pregnancy<br>• Supplemented mothers took 0.36 mg folic acid plus a multivitamin daily; unsupplemented mothers took placebo from at least 1 mo before conception through the first trimester | • 6 NTD pregnancies among 593 supplemented women<br>• 21 NTD pregnancies among 602 unsupplemented women | 0.28 | 72% risk reduction |
| *Observational Studies* | | | | | |
| Bower and Stanley | Western Australia Case-control study | • Pregnant women without a prior NTD-affected pregnancy<br>• Spina bifida case babies and normal control babies<br>• Highest folate quartile compared with the lowest<br>• History of taking a multivitamin supplement containing folic acid from at least 1 mo before conception through the first trimester | • 77 cases; 154 controls<br>• Highest folate quartile compared with lowest<br>• Increasing protective effect observed from lowest to highest quartile | 0.25 | 75% risk reduction |
| Mulinare et al. | Atlanta, Georgia Case-control study | • Pregnant women without a prior NTD-affected pregnancy<br>• NTD case babies and normal control babies<br>• History of taking a multivitamin supplement containing 0–0.8 mg folic acid from at least 1 mo before conception through the first trimester | • 24 supplemented NTD cases<br>• 157 unsupplemented NTD cases<br>• 1075 unsupplemented controls | 0.40 | 60% risk reduction |
| Milursky et al.[27] | New England Prospective cohort study | • Pregnant women without a prior NTD-affected pregnancy<br>• NTD case babies and normal control babies<br>• History of taking a multivitamin supplement with or without 0.1–1.0 mg folic acid from at least 1 mo before conception through the first trimester | • 10 NTD pregnancies among 10,713 women who took a multivitamin with folate<br>• 39 NTD pregnancies among 11,944 women who took a multivitamin without folate | 0.28 | 72% risk reduction |

supplementation. Ekvall et al.[17] also showed a reduction in serum zinc, as well as ascorbic acid, in children with MM. The synergistic effect of ascorbic acid and folic acid must be considered. Favier et al.[41] also asked whether zinc deficiency might be responsible for NTDs. The island of Puerto Rico has combined the efforts of media, pharmacy, and health agencies in promoting folic acid supplementation as a good model. Future research may include

- Testing of multivitamin preparations
- Examining the effects of other environmental factors including vitamin $B_{12}$ and folic acid,[42] methionine (which converts homocysteine to methionine),[43] riboflavin, and zinc
- Looking at genetic factors such as polymorphic genes,[44] particularly the folate metabolism and the N(5)N(10)-methylenetetrahydrofolate reductase (MTHFR) genotype in mothers of offspring with NTD[45]
- Identifying women and siblings at risk with one affected child
- Improving the diets of women during child-bearing ages.

## Height

The mean birth length of children with NTDs is significantly lower than that of other infants. Reduced length and atrophy of the lower extremities seem to produce the reduced height of children with NTDs, although other problems, such as hydrocephalus, renal disease, and malnutrition, may contribute to it. Few data exist on anthropometric measures or the stages of puberty in children with MM. In a study by Rosenblum et al.,[46] children with MM who had a lower lesion showed no reduction in stature, whereas 43% of those with midlevel lesions and 80% of those with high lesions were below the 3rd percentile in height. LaFollette-Atencio et al.[47] determined that lesions in general resulted in a significant reduction in stature but identified no specificity related to the level of the lesion. Yet, in several studies, the level of the lesion significantly affected ambulation. Asher and Olson[48] also found that the most important variable affecting ambulation was the level of the lesion. LaFollette-Atencio et al.[47] showed that the linear growth rate of children with a high lesion who were wheelchair bound began to decline over time and increased weight ensued, whereas children with high lesions who were ambulatory showed more normal growth curves in both height and weight. Keeping the child walking or physically active and out of the wheelchair is essential to avoid weight gain, regardless of the level of the lesion.

There are two methods of determining stature, using arm span or single arm length multiplied by a factor.[49] An arm span-to-height ratio has been developed. The measured arm span is multiplied by 1.0 if there is no leg muscle mass loss (sacral lesion), by 0.95 if there is partial leg muscle loss (midlevel and lower lumbar lesions), or by 0.9 if there is complete leg muscle loss (high lumbar or thoracic lesion).[50] However, children who have a high lesion or who are bedridden or wheelchair bound cannot be measured in this manner, and the procedure requires two observers. Belt et al.[51] found that upper arm length was less affected by a high lesion than arm span in 48 children with MM. In the 9.5- to 10.5-year age group, for example, the upper arm length multiplied by 5.3 could be used to determine stature, thereby allowing the identification of pathological factors affecting growth. This procedure requires only one observer. Structural anthropometric measurements have been determined for male and female wheelchair-mobile adults. Industrial workstations for wheelchair-mobile adults should be developed.

## Weight

Overweight is the most frequent nutritional disease in patients affected by MM. It can be speculated that childhood and adolescent obesity in patients with MM occurs as a result of complex interactive factors and is not strictly related to energy intake and degree of motor impairment.[52] Children with MM give the impression of being overnourished despite seemingly low energy intake, according to Dahl and Gebre-Medhin.[53] LaFollette-Atencio et al.[47] observed that children with MM started to gain weight by age 4, when bracing or walking began. In their study of 100 children with MM, the weight-to-height index was above the 95th percentile for both girls and boys, suggesting obesity. Because of shortness of stature, conventional methods for nutrition assessment may underestimate obesity in children with MM. The purpose of this study was to provide a reliable growth chart for determining body proportion in children with MM rather than using BMI, which squares stature.

Further investigations with more children are now being conducted by the Cincinnati Children's Hospital Medical Center, Division of Developmental Disabilities (CCDDD). In a growth chart with data from several different centers, children with MM tended to follow their own growth curve from 4 to 10 years, with girls reaching peak growth at 8 to 9 years and boys at 10 to 12 years (earlier than children without MM).

## Skinfolds

In a study of body composition, Grogan and Ekvall[54] found that the abdominal and thoracic skinfolds and the waist and abdominal circumferences were correlated significantly with percent body fat measured in the whole body counter. Fat appeared to accumulate around the hips and lower areas of the body below the neurological lesion. Hayes-Allen[5] found a significant correlation between weight and subscapular skinfold thickness in children with MM. Shepherd et al.[55] found decreased body cell mass and total body water (with increased extracellular fluid and decreased intercellular fluid) as well as increased percent body fat after age 3 to 4 years, particularly in children with high lesions. Physical maturation occurs earlier in children with MM (11.4 years, compared with 12.5–12.7 years for children without MM), possibly related to increased adipose tissue or obesity. Green et al.[56] also found that growth in weight influences sexual maturation in children with MM.

## Caloric Needs

Children with MM often do not appear overweight on age-based growth charts; therefore, weight-for-height or calories per centimeter of height must be used to determine caloric needs. In one study of minimally active children with MM who were older than 8 years of age, the caloric level was only 7 kcal per centimeter of height, yet weight loss was slight; only 9 to 11 kcal/cm was required to maintain weight.[54] The purpose of this study was to find a way to prevent obesity in children with MM by investigating the effects of growth, calories, and physical activity on body composition in these children. This information can be applied to clinical practice to determine caloric needs and to correlate body fatness with anthropometry measures. Based on lean body mass (LBM), caloric needs for these children are about 50% of the DRI, or approximately 9 cal/cm for maintenance or 7 cal/cm for weight loss after 6 years of age. Grogan and Ekvall[54] found that physical activity increased LBM (and thereby caloric needs) better than diet restriction.

Braune and Fischer[57] determined that loss of one limb in children without MM resulted in a 15% reduction in the caloric requirement. Perhaps a reduction of weight and caloric needs due to limb reduction or atrophy should be considered in MM: Should a 30% or greater reduction in calories occur with atrophy of both limbs? Because there is decreased LBM and increased adipose tissue in paralyzed lower extremities, fat comprises a higher proportion of the body mass, and available standards tend to underestimate the extent of obesity. In a study of eight adolescent girls with MM using the doubly labeled water method, Bandini et al.[58] measured energy needs of 10.2 kcal/cm (range, 8.4–12.8 kcal/cm) in four nonambulatory girls and 12.6 kcal/cm (range, 11.9–13.2 kcal/cm) in four ambulatory girls. All subjects appeared to have developed their upper torso LBM. Caloric restrictions may need to begin at 3 to 4 years of age, when the child should be walking. By that age, the limbs are failing to grow adequately, and stature is starting to decrease on the growth chart.[47,59]

## Physical Activity

Overweight and obesity can impair ambulation potential to such a degree that children must spend their lives in a wheelchair if physical activity is not started early in life. In a study of 14 children with MM, increasing physical activity had more effect than reducing caloric intake for increasing LBM and reducing adipose tissue.[54] Because increasing the LBM increases caloric needs, physical activities such as swimming are crucial and should begin in infancy. Waist circumference correlates well with weight and may possibly be used as a surrogate measurement for weight. School-age children with MM should be able to monitor their weight independently. Further study of waist circumference and other anthropometric measures is being conducted at the CCDDD. Groups such as Wheelies Clubs for those in wheelchairs have helped increase LBM and reduce weight.

## Physical Signs, Constipation, and Feeding Skills

Physical signs of malnutrition or dental problems should be noted during each clinic visit. Poor skin condition due to pressure sores, increased weight, and lack of sensation in the lower extremities must be evaluated at each clinic visit by the nurse and nutritionist and corrected. Constipation may be caused by the neurogenic bowel (without adequate system control), inactivity, a diet low in fiber and fluid, or the use of anticholinergic drugs to treat the neurogenic bladder. Feeding skills should be reviewed as needed in relation to the bulbar palsy produced by the Arnold-Chiari brain malformation.

## Urinary Tract Infections

Urinary tract infections (UTIs) produce significant health problems. Acidification of the urine by dietary means helps decrease bacterial growth. For this application, the acid-ash diet, which is high in meats, poultry, seafood, eggs, fats, and cereals and low in vegetables and fruits, has been promoted. The acid-ash foods include all foods from the meat and bread groups; a few from the vegetable group (corn, hominy, lentils) and the fruit group (cranberries, plums, prunes); and cakes, cookies, and plain gelatin. Most fats are neutral, except for bacon and high-sodium foods. Candy, coffee, and tea also are neutral. Milk and milk products (except for cheese) are alkaline-ash, as are all fruits and vegetables except those few mentioned previously, carbonated beverages, chocolate, and items prepared with baking powder or soda. However, the lack of adequate fruits and vegetables, especially over a long period of time, makes this diet controversial.

Synthetic vitamin C also may be used to acidify the urine to maintain a pH between 5.5 and 6.[17] Bacterial adherence to the uroepithelium is recognized as an important mechanism in the initiation and pathogenesis of UTIs. The anti-adhesive property of cranberries probably helps to prevent UTIs in two ways: first, it directly prevents *E. coli* from adhering to uroepithelial cells, and second, it selects for less adherent bacterial strains in the stool.[60] Blueberries have been shown to contain similar anti-adherence compounds.

## Drug-Nutrient Interactions

Epilepsy occurs in approximately 20% of patients with MM. The following medications frequently are used: anticonvulsants for seizures, anticholinergics for bladder control, and antibiotics for frequent infections of the upper urinary tract.

# DIETARY MANAGEMENT

Criteria for nutrition referral to the Myelomeningocele Clinic at the CCDDD are age less than 5 years; weight above the 35th or below the 5th percentile or a discrepancy in height and weight; mobility loss greater than 25%; mechanical feeding problems; premenarchal adolescent girl; and certain conditions, such as allergy, diarrhea, excessive use of vitamins, or food faddism. Prevention of health problems through the use of low-calorie, high-nutrient-dense foods is emphasized when the child is very young, because it is hard to change eating patterns after 3 years of age (Table 11–2). It is important to emphasize the introduction of solid foods after 6 months of age, using only 1 tbsp initially. Parents and caregivers must understand how much food is enough, limit intake to the amount adequate for growth, and not use food as a reward or a substitute for love. They must be models for their children with MM by eating low-calorie, nutrient-dense foods themselves to help the child establish good food patterns.

At a CCDDD Summer Preschool Program, children with MM were educated in the use of low-calorie, high-nutrient-dense foods while their caregivers watched through a one-way mirror. This nutrition education is as important as teaching the diabetic exchange system to the parents of children with diabetes. Foods with a high fiber content, particularly prunes, juice, and plenty of water (8 c/day) help relieve constipation and facilitate weight control. Adequate nutrients—especially zinc, ascorbic acid, vitamin $B_{12}$, and folic acid[61]—must be maintained in the diet of the child and also that of the mother, who is at risk of producing a second child with MM. The child with MM may already have low serum levels of ascorbic acid and zinc. Lead levels should also be monitored in pregnancy and in the child with MM.[62] Lowered weight gain in pregnancy also may be a risk factor.[63]

**Table 11–2.** Nutritional Assessment for Myelomeningocele: University-Affiliated Cincinnati Center for Developmental Disorders Clinic*

I. Dietary intake (based on 3-day annual food record or 24-hr recall with food frequency)
   A. Nutrients (calories, vitamins, minerals, protein)
   B. Fluids, fiber/bulk with bowel function
   C. Energy expenditure/ambulation
   D. Dietary modifications and compliance
   E. Client caregiver understanding
      1. Solid food after 6 mo
      2. Increased texture
      3. Good feeding skills
      4. Low-calorie, high-nutrient-dense foods and high-calorie, low-nutrient- dense foods
      5. Demonstrate 1-day meal plan
         a. Number and size of servings
         b. Weight control/calorie expenditure
         c. Fluid and fiber
         d. Reward nonfood items
         e. Drug and nutrient interactions
         f. Modification, if needed
II. Anthropometry
   A. Weight for height
      1. 2–10 yr: keep between 10th and 75th percentile†
      2. 10–17 yr: keep between 10th and 90th percentile†
   B. Fatfold thickness (for children >1 yr, keep between 10th and 90th percentile for age and sex)
      1. Triceps
      2. Abdominal
      3. Waist circumference
   C. Upper arm length
III. Biochemical
   A. Iron status
   B. Nutrient supplementation
   C. Drugs affecting nutrient use/need
IV. Physical signs—clinical and dental
V. Feeding—skills and behaviors
VI. Care plan
   A. Behavioral objective
      1. Problem
      2. Goal
      3. Timetable and how measured
      4. Subjective-objective assessment plan (SOAP) notes
   B. Intervention—within 2 wk of assessment

From Ekvall S. Myelomeningocele: nutrition implications. *Top Clin Nutr.* 1988; 3(3):44. Used with permission.

*Follows quality assurance guidelines.

†Keep in 25th percentile for age if possible.

School-age children should be allowed to select and determine their physical activity and to measure their own waist circumference (having been prepared for this independence during the preschool years). The parents or siblings and the child with MM should plan, prepare, and shop for food together. By this time, the child should have developed good dental care practices and be able to plan a 1-day menu.

By the preteen period, children with MM should be in charge of their weight control and exercise programs, including setting appropriate goals, keeping food records, taking their own measurements, and making decisions about follow-up care. Because weight affects self-image, parents or siblings and the interdisciplinary team (i.e., physician, nutritionist, social worker, nurse, physical therapists, psychologist) need to teach the young child with MM self-motivation techniques and the importance of the diet (e.g., using the waist circumference tool) and activities such as the Wheelies Club.

Dietary restrictions are imposed when weight is above the 25th percentile for age or the 10th percentile for height on standard National Center for Health Statistics growth charts. The multidisciplinary approach to weight control has been described by Hanson and Graves.[64] Killiam et al.[65] discussed other rehabilitation measures related to weight for the child with MM. A wheelchair, bed, or chair scale can be used to measure weight; infants can be held by their mothers. A gross measurement of weight can be obtained by using a tape measure to gauge the change in waist circumference over time if no other method is available. This method has the advantage of giving children a feeling of control over their weight. Obesity produces significant health problems.

Exercise should be started in infancy because it increases LBM and thus increases caloric needs. Because the child should be kept below the 25th percentile of weight for age, increased exercise should be stressed by all members of the interdisciplinary team.[66] The physical therapist and nutritionist must plan exercise goals together beginning when the child is in infancy. Because all children may not be seen by a nutritionist, criteria for screening or referral should be developed, and the Complete Quality Assurance Standards for Myelomeningocele and Developmental Disorders[67] should be used. Nutrients related to drug interaction must be evaluated.

The association of spina bifida and eating disorders must be considered; some children with MM use weight loss as a source of power that can somehow compensate for their losses and neurological limitations.[68] Clinicians caring for patients with spina bifida need to understand that these children may be at risk for development of an eating disorder. Such awareness should influence the quality of nutrition counseling (prevention aspect) and the clinical assessment of sudden weight loss.

The March of Dimes Resource Center[69] has very useful information to encourage folic acid consumption by all women of child-bearing age, as do the American Academy of Pediatrics[70] and the Centers for Disease Control and Prevention.[71] Scientists and physicians also need to better understand which cases occur due to inadequate folic acid consumption or other causes unrelated to folic acid and the biological mechanisms to prevent NTDs.[68,71,72] The dose-response relationship of folic acid has been estimated.[73] The interference of too much folic acid masking vitamin $B_{12}$ deficiency[74] or reducing zinc absorption must be researched further.

## Follow-up

Physical activity, caloric intake, anthropometric factors, and biochemical factors must be monitored and measurable goals specified in the follow-up care plan. The 3-day diet and physical activity diary or a 24-hour dietary recall and frequency cross-check must be obtained weekly in infancy, monthly after 1 month of age, and every 3 months after 1 year of age until the child reaches school age, after which it is obtained approximately every 6 months. The diet diaries may extend to the high-risk mother, because preconception diet counseling is essential for her.[75] The 24-hour dietary recall (including high-fiber foods, fluids, and nutrient-dense snacks[76]), a food frequency record, and a physical activity score are necessary for all MM children who are immobilized or taking anticonvulsant medications.

Awareness of the importance of folate to prevent MM and NTDs is needed in all MM clinics, with the dietitian or nutritionist as the educator. Three ways to increase folic acid intake are stressed: (1) increase your intake of folate-rich foods; (2) take a vitamin supplement with folic acid; (3) increase your intake of foods fortified with folic acid.[77] Anthropometric measures (weight, height, skinfolds, circumferences) should be performed each time the child is seen by the nutrition department. At the same time, biochemical information, physical signs, and any feeding problems should be evaluated. Bone mineralization measurements also should be taken as needed. A case study approach can be used to evaluate some of these follow-up procedures.[78] As the child grows into adulthood, weight management,[79] developmental concerns,[80] pressure ulcers,[81] and anxiety often become greater issues and need to be addressed and followed.[82]

## References


1. Seller MJ. Sex, neural tube defects, and multisite closure of the human neural tube. *Am J Med Genet.* 1995; 58:332.
2. McLaurin RL, Warkany J. Management of spina bifida and associated anomalies. *Comp Ther.* 1986; 12:60.
3. Oppenheimer S. Twenty-year review: Cincinnati experience. In: McLaurin R, Oppenheimer S, Dias L, Kaplan WE, eds. *Spina Bifida: A Multidisciplinary Approach.* New York: Praeger; 1986.
4. Raimondi AJ. Intellectual development in shunted hydrocephalic children. *Am J Dis Child.* 1974; 127:664.
5. Hayes-Allen MC. Obesity and short stature in children with myelomeningocele. *Dev Med Child Neurol Suppl.* 1972; 27:59.
6. Lorber J. Where have all the spina bifida gone? *Midwife Health Visit Community Nurse* 1986; 22(3):94.
7. Boulet SL, Yang Q, Mai C, et al. Trends in postfortification prevalence of spina bifida and anencephaly in the United States. *Birth Defects Res A Clin Mol Teratol.* 2008; 82:527.
8. Laurence KM. The natural history of spina bifida cystica: detailed analysis of 407 cases. *Arch. Dis. Child.* 1964; 39:41.
9. Smithells RW, Nevin NC, Seller MJ, et al. Further experience of vitamin supplementation for prevention of neural tube defect recurrences. *Lancet.* 1983; 1:1027.
10. Lemire RJ. Causes of neural tube defects. In: McLaurin RL, Oppenheimer S, Dias L, Kaplan, WE, eds. *Spina Bifida: A Multidisciplinary Approach.* New York: Praeger; 1986.
11. Watkins ML, Scanlon KS, Mulinare J, Khoury MJ. Is maternal obesity a risk factor for anencephaly and spina bifida? *Epidemiology.* 1996; 7:507.
12. Hernandez-Diaz S, Werler MM, Walker AM, Mitchell AA. Neural tube defects in relation to use of folic acid antagonists during pregnancy. *Am J Epidemiol.* 2001; 153:961.
13. Friedman JM. Can maternal alcohol ingestion causes neural tube defects? *J Pediatr.* 1982; 101:232.
14. Brock DJ, Bolton AE, Scrimgeour JB. Prenatal diagnosis of spina bifida and anencephaly through maternal plasma-alpha-fetoprotein measurement. *Lancet.* 1974; 1:767.
15. Carmichael SL, Shaw GM, Schaffer DM, Laurent C, Selvin S. Dieting behaviors and risk of neural tube defects. *Am J Epidemiol.* 2003; 158:1127.
16. McKiben B, Toseland PA, Duckworth T. Abnormalities in vitamin C metabolism in spina bifida. *Dev Med Child Neurol.* 1968; 10(suppl s15):55.
17. Ekvall S, Chen IW, Bozian R. The effect of supplemental ascorbic acid on serum vitamin $B_{12}$ levels in myelomeningocele patients. *Am J Clin Nutr.* 1981; 34:1356.
18. Eskes TK. Neural tube defects, vitamins and homocysteine. *Eur J Pediatr.* 1998; 157(suppl 2):S139.
19. Shaw GM, Lammer EJ, Zhu H, Baker MW, Neri E, Finnell RH. Maternal periconceptional vitamin use, genetic variation of infant reduced folate carrier (A8OG), and risk of spina bifida. *Am J Med Genet.* 2002; 108:1.
20. Shaw GM, Velie EM, Schaffer DM. Is dietary intake of methionine associated with a reduction in risk for neural tube defect–affected pregnancies? *Teratology.* 1997; 56:295.
21. Szepfalusi A, Rainer S, Bernert G, Dietrick W, Spitzauer S, Urbanek R. Latex sensitization in spina bifida appears disease associated. *J Pediatr.* 1999; 134:344.
22. Quan A, Adams R, Ekmark E, Baum M. Bone mineral density in children with myelomeningocele. *Pediatrics.* 1998; 102(3):E34.
23. Laurence KM, Nanci J, Miller M, Campbell H. Increased risk of recurrence of pregnancies complicated by fetal neural tube defects in mothers receiving poor diets, and possible benefit of dietary counseling. *Br Med J.* 1980; 281:1592.
24. Boddie A, Delow R, Nackashi J, et al. Folate absorption in women with a history of neural tube defect–affected pregnancy. *Am J Clin Nutr.* 2000; 72:154.
25. Molloy AM, Kirke P, Hillary I, Weir DG, Scott JM. Maternal serum folate and vitamin B-12 concentrations in pregnancies associated with neural tube defects. *Arch Dis Child.* 1985; 60:660.
26. Butterworth CE Jr, Bendich A. Folic acid and the prevention of birth defects. *Annu Rev Nutr.* 1996; 16:73.
27. Milursky A, Jick H, Jick SS, et al. Multivitamin/folic acid supplementation in early pregnancy reduces the prevalence of neural tube defects. *JAMA.* 1989; 262:2847.
28. Scholl TO, Hediger ML, Schall JI, Khoo CS, Fischer RL. Dietary and serum folate and their influence on the outcome of pregnancy. *Am J Clin Nutr.* 1996; 63:520.
29. MRC Vitamin Study Research Group. Prevention of neural tube defects: results of the Medical Research Council Vitamin Study. *Lancet.* 1991; 338:131.
30. Centers for Disease Control and Prevention, National Center for Health Statistics. *Healthy People 2000 Review, 1995–96.* Hyattsville, MD: Public Health Service, 1996.
31. Neuhouser ML, Beresford SA, Hickock DE, Monsen ER. Absorption of dietary and supplemental folate in women with prior pregnancies with neural tube defects and controls. *J Am Coll Nutr.* 1998; 17:625.
32. Centers for Disease Control and Prevention. Spina bifida and anencephaly before and after folic acid mandate—United States 1995–1996, and 1999–2000. *MMWR Morb Mortal Wkly Rep.* 2004; 53(17):362.
33. Kloeblen A. Folate knowledge, intake from fortified grain products, and periconceptional supplementation patterns of a sample of low-income pregnant women according to the Health Belief Model. *J Am Diet Assoc.* 1999; 99:33.
34. Hansen M, Samman S, Madsen LT, Jensen M, Sorenson S, Sandstrom B. Folic acid enrichment of bread does not appear to affect zinc absorption in young women. *Am J Clin Nutr.* 2001; 74:125.
35. Berg MJ, Van Dyke DC, Chenard C, et al. Folate, zinc, and vitamin B-12 intake during pregnancy and postpartum. *J Am Diet Assoc.* 2001; 101:242.
36. Wartanowicz M, Ziemlanski S, Bulhak-Jachymczyk B, Konopka L. Assessment of nutritional folate status and selected vitamin status of women of childbearing age. *Eur J Clin Nutr.* 2001; 55:743.
37. Iqbal MM. Prevention of neural tube defects by periconceptual use of folic acid. *Pediatr Rev.* 2000; 21:58.
38. Kihlberg R, Bui TH, Jorgensen C, Soderhjelm L. Folic acid protects against neural tube defects—but how many women of reproductive age have been informed about this fact? *Lakartidningen.* 1999; 96:1961.
39. Bergmann KE, Makosh G, Tews KH. Abnormalities of hair zinc concentration in mothers of newborn infants with spina bifida. *Am J Clin Nutr.* 1980; 33:2145.
40. Nevin N. Prevention of neural tube defects in an area of high incidence. In: Dobbing J, ed. *Prevention of Spina Bifida and Other Neural Tube Defects.* New York: Academic Press; 1983.
41. Favier M, Favier A, Robert E, Guignier M, Malinas Y. Can zinc deficiency in the mother be responsible for the occurrence of spina bifida aperta in the fetus? [in French]. *Rev Fr Gynecol Obstet.* 1987; 82(10):575.
42. Martinez de Villarrea LE, Delgado-Enciso L, Valdez-Leal R, et al. Folate levels and N(5),N(10)-methylenetetrahydrofolate reductase genotype (MTHFR) in mothers of offspring with neural tube defects: a case-control study. *Arch Med Res.* 2001; 32:277.
43. Wilson A, Platt R, Wu Q, et al. A common variant in methionine synthase reductase combined with low cobalamin (vitamin $B_{12}$) increases risk for spina bifida. *Mol Genet Metab.* 1999; 67:317.
44. Christensen B, Arbour L, Tran P, et al. Genetic polymorphisms in methylenetetrahydrofolate reductase and methionine synthase, folate levels in red blood cells, and risk of neural tube defects. *Am J Med Genet.* 1999; 84:151.
45. Van der Put NM, van den Heuvel IP, Steegerss-Theunissen RP, et al. Decreased methylene tetrahydrofolate reductase activity due to the 677→T mutation in families with spina bifida offspring. *J Mol Med (Berl).* 1996; 74:691.
46. Rosenblum MF, Finegold DN, Charney EB. Assessment of stature of children with myelomeningocele, and usefulness of arm-span measurement. *Dev Med Child Neurol.* 1983; 25:338.
47. LaFollette-Atencio P, Ekvall-Walberg S, Oppenheimer S, Grace E. The effect of level of lesion and ambulation on growth chart measurements in children with myelomeningocele—a pilot study. *J Am Diet Assoc.* 1992; 94:858.
48. Asher M, Olson J. Factors affecting the ambulatory status of patients with spina bifida cystica. *J Bone Joint Surg.* 1983; 65:350.
49. Engstrom FM, Roche AF, Mukherjee D. Differences between arm-span and stature in white children. *J Adolesc Heath Care.* 1981; 2:19.
50. Shurtleff D, Lamers J, Goiney T, Gordon L. Are myelodysplastic children fat?: anthropometric measures—a preliminary report. *Spina Bifida Ther.* 1982; 4:1.
51. Belt B, Ekvall S, Cook C, Oppenheimer S, Wessel J. Linear growth measurement: a comparison of single arm-lengths and arm span. *Dev Med Child Neurol.* 1986; 28:319.
52. Fiore P, Picco P, Castagnola E, et al. Nutritional survey of children and adolescents with myelomeningocele (MMC) overweight associated with reduced energy intake. *Eur J Pediatr Surg.* 1998; 8(suppl 1):34.
53. Dahl M, Gebre-Medhin M. Feeding and nutritional problems in children with cerebral palsy and myelomeningocele. *Acta Paediatr.* 1993; 82:816.
54. Grogan C, Ekvall S. Body composition of children with myelomeningocele, determined by $^{40}$K, urinary creatinine and anthropometric measures. *J Am Coll Nutr.* 1999; 8:316.
55. Shepherd K, Roberts D, Golding L, Thomas B, Shepherd R. Body composition in myelomeningocele. *Am J Clin Nutr.* 1991; 53:1.
56. Green S, Frank M, Zackmann M, Prader A. Growth and sexual development in children with myelomeningocele. *Eur Pediatr.* 1985; 144:146.
57. Braune W, Fisher O. In: Brunnstrom S, ed. *Clinical Kinesiology.* Philadelphia: F.A. Davis; 1972.
58. Bandini LG, Schoeller DA, Fukogawa NK, Wyhes L, Dietz WH. Body composition and energy expenditure in adolescents with cerebral palsy and myelodysplasia. *Pediatr Res.* 1991; 29:70.
59. Duval-Beupere G, Kaci M, Lougovoy J, Caponi M, Touzeau C. Growth of trunk and legs of children with myelomeningocele. *Dev Med Child Neurol.* 1987; 29:225.
60. Lowe FC, Fagelman E. Cranberry juice and urinary tract infections: what is the evidence? *Urology.* 2001; 57:407.
61. McDonnell R, Johnson Z, Doyle A, Sayers G. Folic acid knowledge and use among expectant mothers in 1997: a comparison with 1996. *Ir Med J.* 1999; 92:296.

62. Bound JP, Harvey PW, Francis BJ, Awwad F, Anthony CG. Involvement of deprivation and environmental lead in neural tube defects: a matched case-control study. *Arch Dis Child.* 1997; 76:107.
63. Shaw GM, Todoroff K, Carmichael SL, Schaffer DM, Selvin S. Lowered weight gain during pregnancy and risk of neural tube defects among offspring. *Int J Epidemiol.* 2001; 30:60.
64. Hanson R, Graves M. Current concepts: care and habilitation of children with myelomeningocele—a multidisciplinary approach. *J Miss State Med Assoc.* 1987; 28:145.
65. Killiam PE, Apida L, Manilla KJ, Varni JS. Behavioral pediatric weight rehabilitation for children with myelomeningocele. *Am J Matern Child Nurs.* 1983; 8:280.
66. Ekvall S. Myelomeningocele: nutrition implications. *Top Clin Nutr.* 1988; 3(3):44.
67. Ekvall S, Wheby E, eds. *Quality Assurance Standards for Myelodysplasia: Manual II. Clinical Nutrition: Nutritional Needs of the Child with a Handicap or Chronic Illness.* Cincinnati, OH: University of Cincinnati Publications; 1987.
68. Silber TJ, Shaer C, Atkins D. Eating disorders in adolescents and young women with spina bifida. *Int J Eat Disord.* 1999; 25:457.
69. March of Dimes Resource Center, P.O. Box 1657, Wilkes-Barre, PA 18703; telephone 888-MODIMES; website at www.modimes.org. Information on folic acid is available at http://www.marchofdimes.org/pregnancy/take-folic-acid-before-youre-pregnant.aspx. Accessed June 13, 2016.
70. American Academy of Pediatrics, Committee on Genetics. Folic acid for the prevention of neural tube defects. *Pediatrics.* 1999; 104:325.
71. Centers for Disease Control and Prevention. Folic acid and prevention of spina bifida and anencephaly, 10 years after the U.S. Public Health Service recommendation. *MMWR Morb Mortal Wkly Rep.* 2002; 51(RR13):1.
72. Hall JG, Solehdin F. Genetics of neural tube defects. *Ment Retard Dev Disabil.* 1998; 4:269.
73. Moore LL, Bradlee ML, Singer MR, Rothman KJ, Milunsky A. Folate intake and the risk of neural tube defects: an estimation of dose-response. *Epidemiology.* 2003; 14:200.
74. Ray JG, Blom HJ. Vitamin $B_{12}$ insufficiency and the risk of neural tube defects. *QJM.* 2003; 96:289.
75. Distrude A, Prince A. Provision of optimal nutrition care in myelomeningocele. *Top Clin Nutr.* 1990; 5:34.
76. Ekvall S, Hedrick B. *The Impact of Nutritional Status Before Conception, During Pregnancy, and Early Childhood: Training Module VI.* Prevention Continuing Education in Rural Areas Project (84–1). Columbus: Ohio Developmental Disabilities Council and Ohio Department of Mental Retardation and Development Disabilities; 1992.
77. French MR, Barr SI, Levy-Milne R. Folate intake and awareness of folate to prevent neural tube defects: a survey of women living in Vancouver, Canada. *J Am Diet Assoc.* 2003; 103:181.
78. Ekvall S. Appendix C: myelomeningocele case study C. In: Ekvall S. *Nutrition for Special Health Care Needs, Children to Adults.* A self study course based on the book, *Pediatric and Adult Nutrition in Standard, Chronic Diseases and Intellectual and Developmental Disabilities: Prevention, Assessment, and Treatment*, edited by S. Ekvall and V. Ekvall (Oxford University Press, 3rd ed., 2016).
79. Nelson MD, Widman LM, Albresch, RT, Havel PJ, Styne, DM, McDonald CM. Metabolic syndrome in adolescents with spinal cord dysfunction. *J Spinal Cord Med.* 2007; 30(suppl 1):5127.
80. Cushing P. *The Adult with Intellectual and Developmental Disabilities: A Resource Tool for Nutritional Professionals.* Chicago: Academy of Nutrition and Dietetics, 2008.
81. Skipper A. Challenges in pressure ulcers and wound healing. *Nutr Clin Pract.* 2010; 25:13.
82. Lin M, Zabel A, Discanno GE, et al. Correlates of depression and anxiety symptoms in young adults with spina bifida. *J Pediatr Psychol.* 2010; 35:778.

# 12 Nutrients, Neurotransmitters, and Brain Dysfunction

ERIC K. BONSALL, JANINE Z. MUNDORFF, VALLI K. EKVALL, AND SHIRLEY W. EKVALL

As the executive center of the central nervous system (CNS), the brain modulates the complex, dynamically integrated biological network that determines mood, cognition, and behavior and controls physiological homeostasis. The brain comprises only 2% of the adult body weight but requires 15% of the total cardiac output and, remarkably, consumes 20% to 30% of the body's resting metabolic energy. Afferent inputs provide signals to the CNS for control of satiety or food-seeking,[1] and an organism's subsequent nutritional status affects CNS chemistry. The brain does not have large energy stores and therefore depends on a continuous supply of oxygen, glucose, and other nutrients for optimal development and function. In a multifactorial study in Chile, prenatal nutritional indicators were the most important independent variables related to head size.[2] An individual's diet and the subsequent formation of specific precursor compounds greatly impact CNS function by influencing neurotransmitters and neuropeptides. This chapter reviews the current research linking nutritional state with CNS activity and the role of nutrients in the modulation of neurotransmitter synthesis and action related to cognition and maintenance of homeostasis.

## BIOCHEMISTRY AND PHYSIOLOGY

Neurotransmitters are compounds that are found locally within specific neuronal systems and are released on depolarization of the nerve cell.[3] The inside of a nerve cell, or neuron, is maintained approximately 70 mV negative with respect to the outside of the cell by a system of ion pumps and channels involving primarily sodium, potassium, calcium, and chloride. A nerve impulse is propagated down an individual neuron by a decrease in this transmembrane potential, termed *depolarization*, that physically travels down the neuron to the terminal bouton. A small space, the synaptic cleft, separates the presynaptic terminal bouton from the postsynaptic neuron. On depolarization of the terminal portion, a neurotransmitter is secreted into the synapse and subsequently is recognized and bound by a postsynaptic receptor. The further propagation of an impulse down the postsynaptic neuron is a function of the balance between the concentration of the neurotransmitter in the synapse, the affinity of presynaptic (reuptake) and postsynaptic receptors for the neurotransmitter, the density of those presynaptic and postsynaptic receptors, and whether the particular neurotransmitter is excitatory (leading to transmembrane depolarization) or inhibitory (leading to transmembrane hyperpolarization).

A multitude of neurotransmitters have been identified. These substances can be divided broadly into two major classes: (1) the traditional neurotransmitters synthesized in the nerve terminal and (2) the neuropeptide transmitters, which are typically small, protein-like molecules synthesized in the neuron cell body.[4] Traditional neurotransmitters include the catecholamines (norepeinephrine, epinephrine, and dopamine), the biogenic amines (serotonin and histamine), the amino acids (aspartic acid, glutamic acid, glycine, gamma-aminobutyric acid, homocysteine, and taurine), and acetylcholine. The list of putative neuropeptides is lengthy and growing. They include compounds that are found in the gastrointestinal tract, pancreas, pituitary, and even cells of the immune system.[5]

The human genome contains approximately 90 genes related to neuropeptide precursors, and about 100 neuropeptides have been isolated in mammalian brains.[6] A partial listing of neuropeptides with the potential for CNS nutritional status modulation via bidirectional brain-gut communication includes vasoactive intestinal polypeptide (VIP), cholecystokinin octapeptide (CCK-8), substance P, methionine and leucine, enkephalin, insulin, and glucagons.[3] Also important to overall nutritional and health status are CNS neuropeptides involved in the regulation of neuroendocrine pathways. These pathways include hypothalamic control of growth hormone (growth hormone–releasing hormone, somatostatin), adrenal function (corticotropin-releasing hormone, arginine vasopressin), thyroid function (thyrotropin-releasing hormone), and gonadal function (gonadotropin-releasing hormone).[7] Additional neuropeptides of note include angiotensin II, bradykinin, vasopressin, oxytocin, carnosine, bombasin, neurotensin, galanin-like neuropeptide (associated with regulation of appetite), and neuropeptide Y (associated with increased food intake and storage of energy as fat).[3,8]

Studies have shown that traditional neurotransmitters often coexist with neuropeptides in a single neuron, a concept known as *colocalization*.[4] This is contrary to the classical scientific literature, which held that each neuron contains only a single neurotransmitter. For example, it is now known that neurons containing norepinephrine may also contain galanin, encephalin, and neuropeptide Y, whereas those containing acetylcholine may also contain VIP and substance P. Each postsynaptic neuron is regulated by the interplay of excitatory and inhibitory forces from multiple presynaptic neurons or possibly from single presynaptic neurons in which two types of neurons are colocalized. In addition to receptor-mediated presynaptic control of transmitter release, the production of neurotransmitters is also regulated by metabolic events that influence plasma levels of amines depending on voluntary behaviors such as exercise and eating. It is well established that the amounts of amine neurotranmitters are influenced by alterations in blood plasma levels of precursors related to nutritional status and prolonged physical activity.[9,10]

## FACTORS TO BE CONSIDERED IN THE EVALUATION OF NUTRIENTS AND NEUROTRANSMITTER SYNTHESIS AND FUNCTION

The influence of in utero and perinatal nutrition in cognitive and behavioral development, especially for preterm infants, is of particular interest. For example, the importance of adequate choline for acetylcholine synthesis during normal brain development needs to be emphasized, especially in pregnancy.[11]

The nutrient iron also has a key role in the development of the nervous system. According to Beard,[12] 10% to 30% of reproductive-age females and 40% to 70% of pregnant women in Latin America may be iron deficient. The educational level of the mother seems to have an effect on the iron status of the child and the child's psychomotor development.[11] Iron deficiency anemia can be a significant nutritional problem in the first 5 years of life, with alteration in cognition and adverse effects on the development of the CNS.[12] Iron also plays an essential part in the formation and maintenance of myelin and can have an impact on the morphology, physiology, and biochemistry of many organs, even before signs of anemia appear.[12–14] Iron deficiency has been associated with a variety of processes that can affect brain functioning, including mitochondria electron transport, neurotransmitter synthesis and degradation, protein synthesis, and organogenesis.[12]

**Table 12–1.** Some Physiological and Potentially Therapeutic Effects of Nutrients on Brain

| Nutrient | Food Constituent That Increases Brain Levels | Effects | Food Source |
|---|---|---|---|
| Tryptophan | Carbohydrates | *Physiological:* Decreased appetite for carbohydrates; drowsiness; calmness; modulates sensitivity to pain | Beef (broiled), 3.5 oz<br>Skim milk (2% fat), 8 oz<br>Veal, round (cooked), 3.5 oz<br>Cottage cheese, 8 oz |
| | | *Therapeutic:* Depression; insomnia | Chicken (roasted), 3.5 oz<br>Tuna fish (canned), 3 oz |
| Tyrosine | Tyrosine | *Physiological:* Subjective vigor | Cottage cheese (2% fat), 8 oz<br>Skim milk, 8 oz |
| | | *Therapeutic:* Hypertension, shock; hyperprolactinemia; depression; Parkinson's disease | Chicken (roasted), 3.5 oz<br>Cheddar cheese, 4 oz<br>Turkey or ham luncheon meat, 2 oz<br>Evaporated milk, 4 oz |
| Choline | Lecithin | *Therapeutic:* Tardive dyskinesia; memory disorders; mania; ataxias | Chicken egg yolk, 1 large<br>Wheat (cooked), 8 oz<br>Rice, long grain (cooked), 8 oz<br>Lamb leg (raw), 3.5 oz<br>Beef (cooked), 3.5 oz<br>Milk (whole), 8 oz |

Modified from Wurtman RJ, Maher TJ. Strategies for assessing the effects of food additives on the brain and behavior. *Fundam Appl Toxicol.* 1984; 4(3 pt 2):S318.

Fortunately, the brain is resilient and does have some resistance to damage from nutritional deficiencies after birth (e.g., protein-energy malnutrition) as long as there is adequate psychomotor stimulation. Iron status has an active role in a child's sensitivity to infection and his or her ability to become engaged with the surrounding environment and learn from it.[13,14]

With another nutrient, manganese, accidental intoxication during total parenteral nutrition administration has resulted in the onset of parkinsonism with psychiatric symptoms. The patients' symptoms and magnetic resonance imaging abnormalities improved with discontinuation of manganese supplementation and the addition of levadopa treatment.[15] Therefore, careful attention should be given to the long-term intravenous use of this nutrient.

Substantial evidence suggests that specific neurotransmitters are sensitive to relatively mild physiological fluctuations in the quality of foods eaten, even in a single meal.[16–18] Brain neurotransmitter synthesis is affected by specific dietary precursors[19,20] and by more global nutritional status.[21,22] Dietary precursors and their companion neurotransmitters are presented in Table 12–1. The steps in the conversion of these nutrients into neurotransmitters and the regulatory enzymes involved are illustrated in Figure 12–1. Because the brain is separated from the peripheral circulation, these nutrients must pass through the blood–brain barrier, either by diffusion through the capillary endothelial cell membrane or by active transport mechanisms (Fig. 12–2).

Concentrations of amino acids in plasma are affected in two ways. One way is through the exogenous rhythm, which is controlled by the food that is consumed. A high-protein meal increases the level of amino acids in plasma. An internally set, endogenous circadian rhythm also controls amino acid concentration. In humans, the plasma amino acid levels are lowest between 2 A.M. and 4 A.M., but eating continuously or at night can affect these natural internal rhythms. The overall nutritional status of an individual affects neurotransmitter synthesis.[21,22] Foods ingested by malnourished individuals have less competition and therefore can have a more pronounced effect. The rate of synthesis and the amount of neurotransmitter release can result in affective, cognitive, and behavioral changes, thus directly linking nutrient intake with the global functioning of an individual[23] (Table 12–2). Specific neurotransmitters and their relationships to nutrient intake are reviewed in more detail in the following sections.

## Docosahexaenoic Acid

Docosahexaenoic acid (DHA) is essential for the growth and development of the brain in infants and for the maintenance of normal brain function in adults.[24] A diet rich in DHA can help improve learning ability; conversely, its deficiency is associated with deficits in learning. DHA is taken into the brain in preference to other fatty acids.[24] Deficiencies in DHA may be associated with fetal alcohol syndrome, attention-deficit hyperactivity disorder (ADHD), cystic fibrosis, phenylketonuria (PKU), unipolar depression, aggressive hostility, and adrenoleukodystrophy. Decreases of DHA in the brain are associated with cognitive decline during aging and the onset of sporadic Alzheimer's disease.[24] DHA is the active component in fatty fish (e.g., salmon, tuna, mackerel) and in mother's milk. It is found in low levels in both meat and eggs but is not usually present in infant formulas. DHA has been shown to have a positive effect on diseases such as hypertension, arthritis, atherosclerosis, depression, adult-onset diabetes, myocardial infarction, thrombosis, and some cancers.[24] Eicosapentaenoic acid (EPA), another omega-3 fatty acid, is now available in foods such as eggs and infant formula in Europe and Japan.[24]

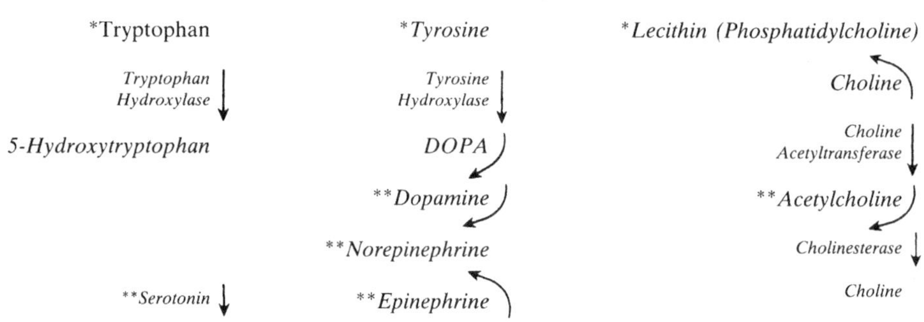


**Figure 12–1.** Steps in the conversion of nutrients into neurotransmitters. * = dietary precursor; ** = neurotransmitter; DOPA = 3,4-dihydroxyphenylalanine.

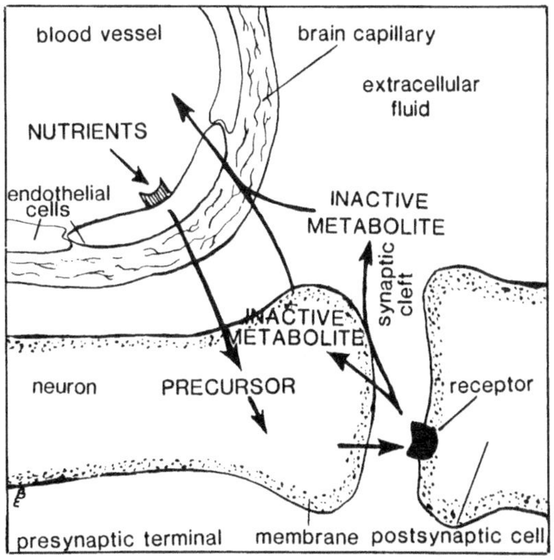


**Figure 12–2.** The pathway of nutrient molecules crossing the blood–brain barrier. (Modified from Wurtman RJ, Wurtman JJ, Regan MM, McDermott JM, Tsay RH, Breu JJ. Effects of normal meals rich in carbohydrates or proteins on plasma tryptophan. *Am J Clin Nutr*. 2003; 77:128.)

## Serotonin

Tryptophan, or 5-hydroxytryptamine, is an amino acid that acts as the primary substrate in the synthesis of serotonin. Tryptophan is first hydroxylated and then decarboxylated to form serotonin. Serotonin is found in platelets, mast cells, and enterochromaffin cells of the gastrointestinal tract. Only 1% to 2% of the serotonin in the body is synthesized in the brain.[25] Because serotonin does not cross the blood–brain barrier, synthesis can occur only if there is an adequate supply of tryptophan from the periphery[26] (see Table 12–1). Tryptophan cannot be synthesized in the blood through protein ingestion or body protein breakdown, and thus it is truly an essential amino acid. Along with tyrosine, it is transported across the blood–brain barrier via a carrier mechanism that is specific for large neutral amino acids.[14,16] Major dietary sources of tryptophan and serving sizes are shown in Table 12–1.[26]

The pathway of nutrient molecules crossing the blood–brain barrier can be seen in Figure 12–2. Because of the competitive nature of amino acid transport, the effect of food ingestion on brain tryptophan is not related to tryptophan content alone. The uptake of an individual amino acid is proportional to the ratio between its concentration and that of its competitors.[11,22,27] For example, protein ingestion causes a greater increase in plasma branched-chain amino acids relative to tryptophan, thereby decreasing the ratio of plasma tryptophan to neutral amino acid (TRP/NAA) and therefore decreasing brain tryptophan uptake. Conversely, carbohydrate ingestion increases the plasma TRP/NAA ratio, thus increasing tryptophan availability to the brain.[14,16] The increase is caused by the carbohydrate-induced insulin release that increases uptake of all amino acids into tissue but has a lesser effect on tryptophan, which is carried in plasma both free and bound to albumin.[16] Because of its competitive advantage in the blood, more tryptophan than other amino acids enters the brain. Thus, protein ingestion decreases the brain serotonin level, whereas tryptophan administration and carbohydrate ingestion increase the concentration of brain tryptophan and, in turn, that of serotonin.[14,16]

The neurobehavioral effects of serotonin are far-ranging and include important effects on mood.[28] Young et al.[29] reported on the effects of tryptophan-free, balanced, and tryptophan-loaded diets on mood in normal volunteers. The tryptophan-free diet produced a mildly depressed mood, which correlated with low plasma tryptophan concentrations. The tryptophan-loaded diet elevated mood in normal volunteers.[30] Serotonin also may affect sexual behavior, impulsiveness and suicide, and the sensation of pain.[31–33] Serotonin is implicated in obsessive-compulsive disorder and other anxiety disorders.[34] Tryptophan has been reported to improve sleep, presumably through serotonergic mechanisms.[35] Suppression of serotonin synthesis can cause insomnia.[36]

Preliminary tests have shown that serotonergic mechanisms likely have a role in the pathophysiology of migraine headaches. Associated with throbbing pain, nausea, photophobia, and paresthesias, migraines are a vascular disorder rather than a problem primarily of the brain. Symptoms of migraine are believed to be related to vasoconstriction followed by vasodilation of the intracranial and extracranial cerebral arteries. Anxiety and fatigue are the best-known predecessors. Stress triggers can include schoolwork, an excess of extracurricular activities, relationship difficulties, disruption of lifestyle, and feeling sad all of the time.[37] For those who are most vulnerable to migraines, certain foods that have a high level of vasoactive compounds (e.g., tyramine, phenylethylamine) may set off an attack. For sensitive individuals, foods containing the following major substances should be avoided: ripened cheeses (cheddar, Gruyere, Stilton, Brie, Camembert), chocolate, and alcoholic drinks (especially red wine). Other food triggers include vinegar (except white vinegar); sauerkraut; sour cream and yogurt; caffeine; nuts and peanut butter; hot fresh breads, raised coffee cakes, and doughnuts; lima beans, navy beans, and pea pods; monosodium glutamate (MSG); canned figs; citrus fruits; bananas; pizza; pork; fermented sausages, bologna, pepperoni, and hot dogs; food dyes; and Nutrasweet.[37] Odor triggers include but are not limited to perfume, gasoline, and various food odors. Other vasoactive substances, such as serotonin and histamine, are also seen as causative agents.

The role of serotonin needs to be further investigated; it has been found to both cause and relieve migraine headaches in conflicting research.[37] Migraines have been treated effectively with a serotonin precursor (5-hydroxytryptophan, or 5-HTP) and with a serotonin antagonist. Tryptophan was also found to be effective in doses of 2 to 4 g/day in 75% of a 20-patient treatment group in preliminary research. Use of tryptophan and 5-HTP is outside the typical pharmacologic treatment, which ranges from sedatives, neuroleptics, antidepressants, and beta-adrenergic antagonists to antiserotonin and antihistaminic agents. These have all worked with varying degrees of success in different individuals.[37] The fact that these drugs have such a wide range of action to treat the same problem demonstrates the difficulty that researchers face in trying to develop a single specific theory on the cause and treatment of migraine. The research on tryptophan and 5-HTP is preliminary and requires closer, more controlled studies.

Hepatic coma may be caused in part by increased serotonin synthesis in the brain.[38] A comatose state may be promoted further by increased uptake of phenylalanine (as a result of increased plasma levels of this amino acid) into the brain. High levels of phenylalanine in the brain inhibit tyrosine hydroxylase and thereby decrease synthesis of the neurotransmitters dopamine and norepinephrine.[39] These catecholamines are thought to be important for normal alertness. Another

**Table 12–2.** Dietary Precursors Affecting Neurotransmitter Function

| Food Source | Blood Amine | Brain Neuron Substrate | Regulatory Enzyme | Neurotransmitter |
|---|---|---|---|---|
| Protein | Tyrosine | Tyrosine | Hydroxylase | Dopamine or norepinephrine |
| | Tryptophan | Tryptophan | Hydroxylase | Serotonin |
| | Histidine | Histidine | Decarboxylase | Histamine |
| | Threonine | Threonine | Serine transhydroxymethylase | Glycine |
| Lecithin | Choline | Choline | Choline acetyltransferase | Acetylcholine |

Modified from Anderson GH, Woodend D. Effect of glycemic carbohydrates on short-term satiety and food intake. *Am J Clin Nutr*. 2002; 76:1023.

factor that may influence hepatic encephalopathy is elevated ammonia levels. Patients with hepatic encephalopathy have been treated with the use of parenteral formulas containing increased amounts of branched-chain amino acids to increase alertness.[40]

The influence of serotonin on carbohydrate appetite has been studied.[41] Increased serotonergic activity selectively decreases carbohydrate intake.[42] Conversely, low brain levels of tryptophan and serotonin have been linked with increased carbohydrate intake.[43]

> The rate of tryptophan's conversion to serotonin is related to the proportion of carbohydrates in the person's diet. Carbohydrates stimulate the release of insulin, which facilitates the uptake of most amino acids into the peripheral tissues. Blood tryptophan levels, however, are unaffected by insulin and so the proportion of tryptophan in the blood and in relation to other amino acids increases when carbohydrates are consumed. Insulin speeds tryptophan's entry into the CNS, where it enters a cluster of neurons known as the raphe nuclei. There it is converted to serotonin. The level of serotonin in turn figures in a feedback mechanism, affecting the amount of carbohydrate an individual subsequently chooses to eat. When the feedback mechanism is disturbed, as we believe happens cyclically in patients with Seasonal Affective Disorder (SAD), carbohydrate-craving obesity and premenstrual dysphoric disorder (PMS), the brain fails to respond when carbohydrates are eaten, and so the desire for them persists longer than it should.[41]

Drugs that selectively facilitate serotonin-mediated neurotransmission cause weight loss, whereas drugs that block serotonin-mediated transmission and antidepressants that interact with neurotransmitters other than serotonin have the opposite effect, often inducing carbohydrate intake and weight gain. The mechanisms behind mood and appetite disorders and their link to serotonin are being elucidated.[44,45] Some therapies, such as phototherapy and medications, are being discovered and refined as the research process continues. The following foods are high in serotonin and tend to increase the feeling of fullness: avocados, bananas, blue-red plums, red plums, dates, eggplant, papayas, passion fruit, pineapple, plantain, bananas, and tomatoes.[46]

SAD, carbohydrate-craving obesity, and PMS have many symptoms in common, including depression, lethargy, inability to concentrate, and episodic bouts of overeating and excessive weight gain. The eating binges often recur in a cyclic pattern. These disorders are affected by biochemical disturbances in two distinct biological systems. One system involves the hormone melatonin, which affects mood and subjective energy levels. The other involves the neurotransmitter serotonin, which regulates the appetite for carbohydrate-rich foods. Both systems are influenced by photoperiodism, the earth's daily dark-light cycle.[41] Persons with SAD experience both depression and carbohydrate craving during seasons of low light, in the fall and winter. Sleep quality is often poor even though the individual sleeps 9 to 10 hours a night. Weight gain often results from overeating of carbohydrates and lessened activity. When spring returns, however, it is as though a switch had been flipped: These individuals become vibrant and full of energy once again. The pounds that were gained are usually lost, and life returns to normal. For SAD sufferers, the craving for carbohydrates occurs in the fall and winter and lasts for several months. For those who experience carbohydrate-craving obesity, the craving is a daily cycle, with the most vulnerable times being the late afternoon and evening. PMS patients' cravings occur during the last week of the luteal phase of the menstrual cycle, begin to remit within a few days after the onset of menstruation, and are usually absent in the week following menses.[41]

Why do these cravings occur? One theory suggests that these foods are consumed to stabilize mood. Persons with carbohydrate-craving obesity have been found to have greater susceptibility to depression. When noncravers consumed carbohydrates, they became sleepy, but for carbohydrate cravers, the consumption of carbohydrates was calming, raising their spirits and clearing their minds—much like a cup of coffee.[41] It has been proposed that these foods are consumed for their perceived psychological benefit, despite the negative cost to the person's health and appearance. Although as many as two-thirds of all obese individuals may be carbohydrate cravers, not all carbohydrate cravers are obese. Some are able to control their weight through exercising and consuming lower-fat carbohydrates such as popcorn or jellybeans.[41] Moreover, some overweight individuals have no special liking for carbohydrates and do their overeating at meals rather than by snacking. Clearly, there is no single pattern that creates and maintains obesity. It is both noteworthy and interesting that SAD sufferers and carbohydrate cravers' symptoms of depression and craving can be eliminated by light therapy.[41]

## Catecholamines

The catecholamines consist of substances involved in the body's fight-or-flight response (i.e., epinephrine and norepinephrine) and dopamine, which is involved in involuntary movement and plays a part in psychosis. Dopamine also has a major role in reward-mediated behaviors. The rate of synthesis of all catecholamines is controlled by the conversion of tyrosine to 3,4-dihydroxyphenylalanine (DOPA) (see Fig. 12–1). Tyrosine hydroxylase, the enzyme that controls this step, is activated whenever nerves are firing rapidly. At these times, the enzyme can handle much more tyrosine than is normally present in the brain. Therefore, whenever tyrosine levels in the brain increase, more catecholamines are synthesized.[47] Fruits with a high dopamine concentration include red and yellow bananas; moderate amounts of dopamine are found in avocado, cocoa bean powder, broccoli, and Brussels sprouts. The dopamine concentration is highest near the skin, and the serotonin concentration is highest near the center of the fruit.[48]

The relationship between diet composition, brain catecholamines, and brain tyrosine metabolism is not well understood. Tyrosine is formed in the liver and, to a limited extent, in the brain from phenylalanine; however, phenylalanine itself is an essential amino acid, and its conversion to tyrosine is probably insufficient to satisfy the body's need for tyrosine. In a study using kittens, the dietary requirement for phenylalanine was reduced by half when tyrosine was substituted for it.[49] Although single meals containing both carbohydrate and protein increase brain tyrosine, with protein having the greater effect, chronic high-protein feeding decreases the tyrosine concentration in the brain.[17,18] A large dose of tyrosine raises brain tyrosine levels and lowers tryptophan levels. Likewise, a large tryptophan or carbohydrate dose can lower brain tyrosine levels and may thereby compromise central catecholaminergic transmission.[17,18] This compromising effect is shown with a 50 mg/kg dose of tryptophan, which produces increased fatigue and decreased pain sensitivity without impairing sensorimotor activity.[50] Protein-containing meals that raise serum tyrosine levels also increase dopamine synthesis in the retina and make humans less depressed.[51] However, patients with depression who are treated with monoamine oxidase inhibitors can be affected adversely by foods high in tyramine, such as aged cheese, undistilled spirits, and mushrooms (see Chapter 27). Tyrosine can also reduce high blood pressure and raise low blood pressure by its effect on norepinephrine-releasing neurons.[52–55] However, tyrosine had no effect on the sympathetic nervous system in young mice.[56] A decarboxylated product of tyrosine—tyramine—can cause norepinephrine release from neurons and may also decrease catecholamine synthesis.[57]

Catecholamine neurotransmitters respond to vitamins and minerals in a wide variety of ways. The effects are much like those of dietary precursors. Vitamin $B_{12}$ and folate affect transmethylation. Folate is the precursor of a necessary cofactor in tyrosine hydroxylase activity. A high percentage of depressed patients have poor folate status.[58] Vitamin $B_6$ deficiency has been linked to a decrease in dopaminergic neuron function in the rat corpus striatum.[59] Vitamin A is involved in the physiology of the retina,[60] and vitamin E acts as an antioxidant in brain tissue. Both ascorbic acid and copper affect the conversion of dopamine to norepinephrine. Magnesium has been shown to influence aggressive behavior in mice while altering the potency of catecholamine-stimulating drugs.[60] Iron, a cofactor of tyrosine hydroxylase activity, is also linked to impaired phenylalanine conversion to tyrosine when it is deficient.[61] Iron-deficient rats have shown inhibition of serotonin and dopamine and a reduction in selective attention and vigilance. Zinc deficiency has caused lethargy and apathy in children and reduced cognition in all age groups.[62–64] Zinc and iron are the most prevalent trace elements in the brain. Essential fatty acid intake has been reported to modulate dopamine activity.[65] The effects of marginal deficiencies of these vitamins and minerals need further exploration.

## Acetylcholine

Acetylcholine is the neurotransmitter at the neuromuscular junction that controls all voluntary movement, and it is also the neurotransmitter of the parasympathetic nervous system. Within the CNS, acetylcholine may be linked to aggression, depression, the stress response, and possibly schizophrenia.[64] Research supports a strong role for this neurotransmitter in memory and the cognitive dysfunction associated with aging.[65] Acetylcholine is synthesized by the action of choline acetyltransferase on choline (see Fig. 12–1). Choline is essential in humans when methionine is not available in excess. Folic acid and vitamin $B_{12}$ also enhance choline metabolism. Dietary intake of choline-lecithin or choline-containing compounds elevates the blood choline concentration. Choline is transported across the blood–brain barrier by a specific carrier that is capable of handling much more choline than is normally present. Therefore, when the blood choline concentration rises, more choline enters the brain. This, in turn, increases the synthesis of acetylcholine. The neurotransmitter is then available for release.

Human milk is rich in choline compounds, particularly in the mammary epithelial cells; those cells concentrate choline from maternal blood, especially during the first 30 days of lactation. Phosphocholine was increased when pregnant rats were fed choline.[66] Bioavailability may differ in breast milk and infant formulas. Human milk has a significantly higher phosphocholine concentration, the same or a lower glycerophosphocholine concentration, and phosphatidylcholine and sphingomyelin concentrations similar to those of bovine milk or bovine-derived infant formulas. Soy-derived infant formulas have lower glycerophosphocholine and sphingomyelin concentrations and higher phosphatidylcholine concentrations than either human milk or bovine milk–derived formulas.

Choline has been used with some success in the treatment of tardive dyskinesia, an involuntary motor movement disorder associated with long-term use of neuroleptics. The usefulness of supplemental choline in the treatment of Alzheimer's disease is questionable, but several studies have suggested possible preventive effects.[67] For example, choline has been shown to enhance memory in rat pups in utero. Choline's availability is key in the development of the brain. Choline specifically affects the rate of creation and destruction of nerve cells in the brains of human infants.[68] Stores of choline can be depleted in the mother during pregnancy and lactation. Eggs and liver are the best dietary sources of choline. Choline has a direct effect on nerve cell signaling and cell signaling as well as lipid transport and metabolism.[69]

## Vitamin D

Vitamin D is a fat-soluble vitamin that is naturally present in foods such as salmon, mackerel, sardines, cod liver oil, liver, organ meats, and egg yolks.[70] Children seldom consistently consume these foods. Dermal synthesis and vitamin D–fortified foods are the major sources of the vitamin.[70]

Vitamin D and its metabolites have a significant clinical role because of their involvement in calcium homeostasis and bone metabolism through endocrine mechanism.[70] In its hormone function, vitamin D modulates gene expression and regulates the immune system.[71] Vitamin D is a neuroactive steroid that may function as a modulator in brain development.[72] Vitamin D receptors are widespread in brain tissue, showing neuroprotective effects.[73]

Groups at risk for vitamin D deficiency include premature infants, exclusively breast-fed infants, dark-skinned children or adults, and those on vegetarian and highly restrictive diets. Others at risk include children or adults living together at higher latitudes or with limited sun exposure; children or adults with conditions of malabsorption; and those who are taking certain medications such as anticonvulsants or antiretroviral drugs.[74]

Vitamin D deficits or vitamin D receptor dysfunction are linked to numerous brain dysfunctions. In both animals and humans, vitamin D serves as an important regulator of neuroprotection, antiepileptic and anticalcification effects, neuroimmunomodulation, interplay with neurotransmitter and hormones, modulation of behaviors, brain aging, and some other, less-explored brain processes.[71] In a large 100-bed residential psychiatric treatment facility, 23.1% of males and 41.3% of females required vitamin D supplementation (unpublished data, Hoffman Homes for Youth, August 2015). Continued research is needed to explore the role of vitamin D in neuropsychiatric disorders.

## Histidine

Histidine, an amino acid, can be taken intraperitoneally or by dietary alteration to increase brain levels of both histidine and histamine, but histamine cannot be produced totally by histidine. Glycine, a nonessential amino acid and a neurotransmitter, can be synthesized in the brain by serine and threonine and needs further investigation. Histamine is involved in allergic and autonomic nervous system responses.[75,76] Weight gain patterns have been associated with the use of antipsychotic medications and have correlated with differential histamine H receptor affinity in adult males.[77] An investigation of children and adolescents taking a variety of second-generation antipsychotic medications found that weight gain patterns also correlated with histamine H receptor affinity.[78] Other possible mechanisms for weight gain associated with second-generation antipsychotic medications include antagonism of 5-HT, A/2A/2C receptors, and effects on alpha$_2$-adrenergic receptors influencing pancreatic beta cells.[79]

## Directions for Further Research and Applications

There is great interest in the impact of nutrition on mood, cognition, and behavior.[80] Future research will involve determining the factors that control the rate at which precursor amino acids are resynthesized into polyproteins and the formation of active peptides that affect behavior.[18] One example of the effect of neuropeptides on behavior is neuropeptide Y (NPY), one of the most plentiful neurotransmitters in the brain. It is now believed that NPY plays an important role in feeding and body weight regulation. NPY-overexpressing mice exhibited significantly increased body weight gain with transiently increased food intake after a 50% sucrose-loaded diet. They later developed both hyperglycemia and hyperinsulinemia with no change in glucose excursion throughout a 1-year observation period.[81] Several peptides produced in the hypothalamus have been isolated from foods.[82] Thyrotropin-releasing hormone has been found in alfalfa and luteinizing hormone–releasing hormone in oat leaves.[17] Monosodium glutamate may damage hypothalamic neurons in young, immature rats.[83] Likewise, erythrosine (red dye FD&C #3) appears to inhibit spermatogenesis in mice and may increase the binding of estrogen receptors to growth-stimulating properties in humans.[84,85]

Broad knowledge of the signs and symptoms of a range of psychiatric disorders and the standard pharmacological and psychotherapeutic treatments is required for the dietitian as a member of a multidisciplinary team working with psychiatrically ill patients. Many psychiatric illnesses manifest with eating disturbances as part of their core symptomatology. Major unipolar depression is an illness that afflicts approximately 10% of women and 5% of men during their lifetime.[79] This illness can develop in early latency and perhaps even in the preschool period. The core feature of this disorder is recurrent episodes of depressed mood that are frequently accompanied by appetite disturbances, sleep disruption, fatigue, feelings of guilt, and suicidal ideation. The etiology is multifactorial, involving the interaction of an inherited vulnerability with environmental stressors. Current treatments include psychotherapy, antidepressant therapy, and electroconvulsive therapy. The potential adjunctive role of dietary manipulation in the treatment of depressed patients and in the maintenance of normal mood in vulnerable individuals is an area in need of investigation.

Comprehensive management of the eating disorders anorexia nervosa and bulimia nervosa clearly requires the input of a skilled nutritionist. Anorexia nervosa is a life-threatening illness of extreme weight loss and distorted body image. Schizophrenia can involve delusions that can result in a greatly increased intake of certain foods or can produce a catatonic state with almost no solid or liquid intake. Homeless people with schizophrenia, a group presumed to be at high risk for malnutrition, have not been studied systematically.

More well-designed studies involving nutrients as part of the treatment of psychiatric illnesses are warranted. Perhaps more importantly, the possible preventive role of good nutritional status needs further research. For additional information, see the chapters in this text on autism (Chapter 13), anorexia nervosa and bulimia (Chapter 22), fetal alcohol syndrome (Chapter 14), drug-induced malnutrition (Chapter 27), and ADHD (Chapter 19).[20]

## References


1. Bray GA. Afferent signals regulating food intake. *Proc Nutr Soc.* 2000; 59:378.
2. Ivanovic DM, Leiva BP, Perez HT, et al. Head size and intelligence, learning, nutritional status and brain development. Head, IQ, learning, nutrition and brain. *Neuropsychologia.* 2004; 42:1118.
3. Synder SH. Forty years of neurotransmitters: a personal account. *Arch Psychiatry.* 2002; 59:983.
4. Steingard RJ, Schmidt C, Coyle JT. Basic neuroscience: critical issues for understanding psychiatric disorders. *Adolesc Med.* 1998; 9:205.
5. Gan X, Zhang L, Solomon GF, Bonavida B. Mechanism of norepinephrine-mediated inhibition of human NK cytotoxic functions: inhibition of cytokine secretion, target binding, and preparation for cytotoxicity. *Brain Behav Immun.* 2002; 16:227.
6. Fricker LD. Neuropeptides and other bioactive peptides: from discovery to function. *Colloquium Series on Neuropeptides* 2012; 1(3):1. doi: 10.4199/C00058EDIVOIY201205NPE003.
7. Molitch ME. Neuroendocrinology and the neuroendocrine system. In: Goldman L, Bennett JC, eds. *Cecil Textbook of Medicine.* Philadelphia: WB Saunders; 2000.
8. Man PS, Lawrence CB. Galanin-like peptide: a role in the homeostatic regulation of energy balance? *Neuropharmacology.* 2008; 55:1.
9. Conlay LA, Wurtman RJ, Blusztajn K, Coviella IL, Maher TJ, Evoniuk GE. Decreased plasma choline concentrations in marathon runners. *N Engl J Med.* 1986; 315:892.
10. Feinstrom JD, Wurtman RJ. Brain serotonin content: physiological dependence on plasma tryptophan levels. *Science.* 1971; 173:149.
11. Zeisel SH. Choline: essential for brain development and function. *Adv Pediatr.* 1997; 44:263.
12. Beard JL. Iron deficiency and neural development: an update. *Arch Latinoam Nutr.* 1999; 49:34S.
13. Guesry P. The role of nutrition in brain development. *Prev Med.* 1998; 27:189.
14. Roncagliolo M, Garrido M, Walter T, Peirano P, Lozoff B. Evidence of altered central nervous system development in infants with iron deficiency anemia at 6 mo: delayed maturation of auditory brainstem responses. *Am J Clin Nutr.* 1998; 68:683.
15. Nagatomo S, Umehara F, Hanada K, et al. Manganese intoxication during total parenteral nutrition: report of two cases and review of the literature. *J Neurol Sci.* 1999; 162:102.
16. Fernstrom JD, Wurtman RJ. Brain serotonin content: physiological regulation by plasma neutral amino acids. *Obes Res.* 1997; 5:377.
17. Anderson GH, Woodend D. Effect of glycemic carbohydrates on short-term satiety and food intake. *Am J Clin Nutr.* 2002; 76:1023.
18. O'Rourke DA, Wurtman JJ, Wurtman RJ, et al. Aberrant snacking patterns and eating disorders in patients with obsessive-compulsive disorder. *J Clin Psychiatry.* 1994; 55:445.
19. Charmandari E, Kino T, Souvatzoglou E, Chrousos GP. Pediatric stress: hormonal mediators and human development. *Horm Res.* 2003; 59:161.
20. Yogman MW, Zeisel SH. Nutrients, neurotransmitters and infant behavior. *Am J Clin Nutr.* 1985; 42:352.
21. Harmer CJ, Rogers RD, Tunbridge E, Cowen PJ, Goodwin GM. Tryptophan depletion decreases the recognition of fear in female volunteers. *Psychopharmacology.* 2003; 167:411.
22. Lawrie SM, MacHale SM, Power MJ, Goodwin GM. Is the chronic fatigue syndrome best understood as a primary disturbance of the sense or effort? *Psychol Med.* 1997; 27:995.
23. Wurtman RJ, Wurtman JJ, Regan MM, McDermott JM, Tsay RH, Breu JJ. Effects of normal meals rich in carbohydrates or proteins on plasma tryptophan. *Am J Clin Nutr.* 2003; 77:128.
24. Horricks JA, Yeo YK. Health benefits of docosahexaenoic acid (DHA). *Pharmacol Res.* 1999; 40:211.
25. Scrimshaw NS. Malnutrition, brain development, learning and behavior. *Nutr Res.* 1998; 18:351.
26. Wurtman RJ, Maher TJ. Strategies for assessing the effects of food additives on the brain and behavior. *Fundam Appl Toxicol.* 1984; 4(3 pt 2):S318.
27. Levitsky DA, Strupp BJ. Malnutrition and the brain: changing concepts, changing concerns. *J Nutr.* 1995; 125(8 suppl):2212S.
28. Blier P, Montigny C, Chaput Y. A role for the serotonin system in the mechanism of action of antidepressant treatments: preclinical evidence. *J Clin Psychiatry.* 1990; 51:14.
29. Young SN, Smith SE, Pihl RO, Ervin FR. Tryptophan depletion causes a rapid lowering of mood in normal males. *Psychopharmacology.* 1985; 87:173.
30. Charney DS, Heninger GR, Reinhard JF. The effect of intravenous L-tryptophan on prolactin and growth hormone and mood in healthy subjects. *Psychopharmacology.* 1982; 77:217.
31. Maher TJ, Ulus IH, Wurtman RJ. Phentermine and other monoamine-oxidase inhibitors may increase plasma serotonin when given with fenfluramines. *Lancet.* 1999; 353:38.
32. Brown G, Linnoila MI. CSF serotonin metabolite (5-HIAA) studies in depression, impulsivity and violence. *J Clin Psychiatry.* 1990; 51:31.
33. Von Knorring L, Perris C, Oreland L, Eisemann M, Eriksson U, Perris H. Pain as a symptom in depressive disorders and its relationship to platelet monamine oxidase activity. *J Neural Transm.* 1984; 60:1.
34. Murphy DL, Pigott TA. A comparative examination of a role for serotonin in obsessive-compulsive disorder, panic disorder and anxiety. *J Clin Psychiatry.* 1990; 51:53.
35. Hartmann E. Effects of L-tryptophan on sleepiness and on sleep. *J Psychiatr Res.* 1983; 17:107.
36. Gross C, Zhang X, Stark K, et al. Serotonin A receptor acts during development to establish normal anxiety-like behavior in the adult. *Nature.* 2002; 416:396.
37. Wasiewski WW. Preventive therapy in pediatric migraine. *J Child Neurol.* 2001; 16:71.
38. Fernstrom JD. Aromatic amino acids and monoamine synthesis in the central nervous system: influence of diet. *J Nutr Biochem.* 1990; 1:508.
39. Dodsworth JM, James JH. Depletion of brain norepinephrine in acute hepatic coma. *Surgery.* 1974; 75:811.
40. Fischer JE, Rosen HM. The effect of normalization of plasma amino acids on hepatic encephalopathy in man. *Surgery.* 1976; 80:77.
41. Wurtman RJ, Wurtman JJ. Carbohydrates and depression: serotonin and seasonal affective disorder. In: Masters RD, ed. *The Neurotransmitter Revolution.* New York: Raven Press; 1994.
42. O'Rourke DA, Wurtman JJ, Wurtman RJ, et al. Aberrant snacking patterns and eating disorders in patients with obsessive-compulsive disorder. *J Clin Psychiatry.* 1994; 55:445.
43. Wurtman RJ, Wurtman JJ. Brain serotonin, carbohydrate-craving, obesity and depression. *Adv Exp Med Biol.* 1996; 398:35.
44. Rausch JL. Treatment of premenstrual mood symptoms. *Psychiatr Clin North Am.* 1993; 16:829.
45. Wallin MS, Rissanen AM. Food and mood: relationship between food, serotonin and affective disorders. *Acta Psychiatr Scand Suppl.* 1994; 377:36.
46. Pawlak L. *Weight Matters: Appetite—the Brain-Body Connection.* Emeryville, CA: Biomedical General Corporation; 1998.
47. Asanuma M, Miyazaki I, Ogawa N. Dopamine- or L-DOPA-induced neurotoxicity: the role of dopamine quinine formation and tyrosinase in a model of Parkinson's disease. *Neurotoxicol Res.* 2003; 5:165.
48. Feldman JM, Lee EM, Castleberry CA. Catecholamine and serotonin content of foods: effect on urinary excretion of homovanillic and 5-hydroxyindoleacetic acid. *J Am Diet Assoc.* 1987; 87:1031.
49. Williams JM, Morris JG, Rogers QR. Phenylalanine requirement of kittens and the sparing effect of tyrosine. *J Nutr.* 1987; 117:1102.
50. Lehnert H, Reinstein DK, Strowbridge BW, Wurtman RJ. Neurochemical and behavioral consequences of acute, uncontrollable stress: effects of dietary tyrosine. *Brain Res.* 1984; 303:215.
51. Delion S, Chalon S, Herault J, et al. Chronic alphalinolenic acid deficiency alters dopaminergic and serotonergic neurotransmission in rats. *J Nutr.* 1994; 24:3466.
52. Gelenberg AJ, Wojick JD. Tyrosine for the treatment of depression. *Am J Psychiatry.* 1980; 137:622.
53. Fernstrom MH, Fernstrom JD. Effects of chronic protein ingestion on rat central nervous systems tyrosine levels and in vivo tyrosine hydroxylation rate. *Brain Res.* 1995; 672:97.
54. Yamauchi A, Shizuka F, Yamamoto T, et al. Amino acids and glucose differently increased extracellular 5-hydroxyindoleacetic acid in the rat brain. *J Nutr Sci Vitaminol.* 1995; 41:325.
55. Leonard BE. Basic aspects of neurotransmitter function. In: Leonard BE, ed. *Fundamentals of Psychopharmacology.* New York: Wiley; 1977.
56. Fernstrom MH, Fernstrom JD. Effects of chronic protein ingestion on rat central nervous system tyrosine levels and in vivo tyrosine hydroxylation rate. *Brain Res.* 1995; 672:97.
57. Fernstrom MH, Fernstrom JD. Acute tyrosine depletion reduces tyrosine hydroxylation rate in rat central nervous system. *Pharmacol Lett.* 1995; 57:97.
58. Fukii A, Matsumoto H, Yamamoto H. Effect of vitamin B complex on neurotransmission and neurite outgrowth. *Gen Pharmacol.* 1996; 27:995.
59. Gospe SMJr, Hecht ST. Longitudinal MRI findings in pyridoxine-dependent seizures. *Neurology.* 1998; 51:74.
60. Conner WE, Neuringer M, Reisbick S. Essential fatty acids: the importance of (n-3) fatty acids in the retina and brain. *Nutr Res.* 1992; 50:21.
61. Gordon N. Iron deficiency and the intellect. *Brain Dev.* 2003; 25:3.
62. Gould MG, Gershwin MD, Hendricks AG. Developmental zinc deficiency and behavior. *J Nutr.* 1995; 125:22:635.
63. Delion S, Chalon S, Guilloteau D, et al. α-Linolenic acid dietary deficiency alters age-related changes of dopaminergic and serotonergic neurotransmission in the rat frontal cortex. *J Neurochem.* 1996; 66:1582.
64. Raedler TJ, Knable MB, Jones DW, et al. In vivo determination of muscarinic acetylcholine receptor availability in schizophrenia. *Am J Psychiatry.* 2003; 160:118.
65. Giacobini E. Cholinesterases: new roles in brain function and in Alzheimer's disease. *Neurochem Res.* 2003; 28:515.
66. Garner SC, Mar M-H, Zeisel SH. Choline distribution and metabolism in pregnant rats and fetuses are influenced by dietary choline content of the maternal diet. *J Nutr.* 1995; 125:2851.
67. Teaktong T, Graham A, Court J, et al. Alzheimer's disease is associated with a selective increase in alpha7 nicotinic acetylcholine receptor immunoreactivity in astrocytes. *Glia.* 2003; 41:207.
68. Beelke M, Sannita WG. Cholinergic function and dysfunction in the visual system. *Methods Find Exp Clin Pharmacol.* 2002; 24(suppl D):113.
69. Zhou FM, Wilson C, Dani JA. Muscarinic and nicotinic cholinergic mechanisms in the mesostriatal dopamine systems. *Neuroscientist.* 2003; 9:23.
70. Ross AC, Taylor CL, Yaktine AL, Del Valle HB. *Dietary Reference Intakes for Calcium and Vitamin D.* Institute of Medicine (US) Committee to Review Dietary Reference Intakes for Vitamin D and Calcium. Washington, DC: National Academies Press; 2011.

71. Kalueff AV, Tuohimaa P. Neurosteroid hormone vitamin D and its utility in clinical nutrition. *Curr Opin Clin Nutr Metab Care.* 2007; 10:9.
72. Harms LR, Burne THJ, Eyles DW, McGrath JJ. Vitamin D and the brain: *Best Pract Res Clin Endocrinol Metab.* 2011; 25,657.
73. Soni M, Kos K, Lang IA, Jones K, Melzer D, Llewellyn DJ. Vitamin D and cognitive function. *Scand J Clin Lab Invest Suppl.* 2012; 243:79.
74. Holick MF, Binkley NC, Bischoff-Ferrari HA, et al. Evaluation, treatment and prevention of vitamin D deficiency: an Endocrine Society clinical practice guideline. *J Clin Endocrinol Metab.* 2011; 96:1911.
75. McLeod JG, Tuck RR. Disorders of the autonomic nervous system: part I. Pathophysiology and clinical features. *Ann Neurol.* 1987; 21:419.
76. McLeod JG, Tuck RR. Disorders of the autonomic nervous system: part II. Investigation and treatment. *Ann Neurol.* 1987; 21:519.
77. Wirshing DA, Wirshing WG, Kysar L, et al. Novel antipsychotics: comparison of weight gain liabilities. *J Clin Psychiatry.* 1999; 60:358.
78. Ibikunle JO, Bonsall EK. Weight changes in children and adolescents on atypical antipsychotics. Presented at the annual meeting of the American Psychiatric Association, New Orleans, May 5–10, 2001. *New Research Abstracts*; 2001: 8.
79. Benazzi F. Is there a link between atypical and early-onset "unipolar" depression and bipolar II disorder? *Compr Psychiatry.* 2003; 44:102.
80. Charmandari E, Kino T, Souvatzoglou E, Chrousos GP. Pediatric stress: hormonal mediators and human development. *Horm Res.* 2003; 59:161.
81. Kaga T, Innui A, Okita M, et al. Modest over-expression of neuropeptide Y in the brain leads to obesity after high-sucrose feeding. *Diabetes.* 2001; 50:1206.
82. Smith SR, de Jonge L, Pellymounter M, et al. Peripheral administration of human corticotrophin-releasing hormone: a novel method to increase energy expenditure and fat oxidation in man. *J Clin Endocrinol Metab.* 2001; 86:1991.
83. Bogdanov MB, Wurtman RJ. Effects of systemic or oral ad libitum monosodium glutamate administration on striatal glutamate release, as measured using microdialysis in freely moving rats. *Brain Res.* 1994; 660:337.
84. Abdel Aziz AH, Shouman SA, Attia AS, Saad SF. A study on the reproductive toxicity of erythrosine in male mice. *Pharmacol Res.* 1997; 35:457.
85. Dees C, Askari M, Garrett S, Gehrs K, Henley D, Ardies CM. Estrogenic and DNA-damaging activity of Red No. 3 in human breast cancer cells. *Environ Health Perspect.* 1997; 105:625.

# 13 Autism Spectrum Disorder

CAROL J. HENDERSON, VIVIANN NORDIN, AND SHIRLEY W. EKVALL

## BACKGROUND AND ORIGINAL DESCRIPTION OF THE DISORDER

Leo Kanner, a pioneer in child psychiatry, first described "infantile autism" in 11 children in 1943 as a rare condition generally defined by its clinical characteristics and core symptoms that included impaired social skills (lack of emotional contact and resistance to change), isolated areas of interest, and delayed and disordered language. Co-occurring symptoms including growth impairment, atypical feeding, and gastrointestinal (GI) problems such as reflux and rumination were documented in 7 of these 11 original cases.[1] Over time, it has become apparent that autism spectrum disorder (ASD) is a heterogeneous disorder with regard to its clinical presentation, etiology, underlying neurobiology, and degree of severity. In 1944, Hans Asperger identified a group of children with often milder symptoms compared to individuals diagnosed with ASD. These children had impairment of social interaction; restricted, repetitive, and stereotyped patterns of behavior; and possibly delayed motor skills.[2] However, in contrast to ASD, there were no clinically significant delays in language or cognitive development.[3]

## DIAGNOSIS: DSM-5 AND ICD-10

ASD is typically diagnosed on the basis of behavioral symptoms, without reference to etiology. However, considerable research has been devoted to investigations of etiological factors. Although no single cause has been identified, the available data suggest that ASD results from different sets of causal factors including genetic and environmental or epigenetic factors.[4] ASD is currently defined by the American Psychiatric Association's *Diagnostic and Statistical Manual of Mental Disorders, Fifth Edition* (DSM-5) as a single disorder that comprises disorders that were previously considered separate: ASD, Asperger's syndrome, childhood disintegrative disorder, and pervasive developmental disorder not otherwise specified.[5] Although the term "Asperger's syndrome" is no longer in the DSM-5, it is still used by some and is generally thought to represent the mild end of the autism spectrum.[5]

The current DSM-5 diagnostic criteria for ASD are listed in Box 13-1. The term "spectrum" in ASD refers to the wide range of symptoms and severity. ASD is a serious neurodevelopmental disorder with symptoms described in two main areas: (1) deficits in social communication and social interaction and (2) restricted, repetitive patterns of behavior, interests, or activities. The latter area includes signs of hyperreactivity or hyporeactivity to sensory input or unusual sensory interests. Specifications are called for if there is any co-occurrence with intellectual impairment, language impairment, medical conditions, or other neurodevelopmental disorders. Individuals who have marked deficits in social communication but whose symptoms do not otherwise meet criteria for ASD should be evaluated for social (pragmatic) communication disorder.[6]

The *International Classification of Diseases* (ICD-10)[3] is published by the World Health Organization; a diagnostic collaboration is currently formulating criteria for the next edition, ICD-11. Currently, for the diagnostic process to be complete, it must include (1) a comparison to ICD-10 criteria in order to find the diagnostic term that best describes the child's problems; (2) penetration of the background neuropsychological, cognitive, and linguistic factors; and (3) consideration of background neurobiological factors.[3]

## EPIDEMIOLOGY AND CONTRIBUTING FACTORS

ASD was originally reported to be a rare condition with a prevalence of 2 to 5 per 10,000 children.[7] However, 2014 data from the Centers for Disease Control and Prevention (CDC) estimated a US prevalence of 1 in 68 children 8 years of age (approximately 1 in 42 boys and 1 in 189 girls).[8] Studies in Asia, Europe, and North America have identified individuals with ASD with an average prevalence of about 1%.[9] The rise in ASD incidence has occurred during a time of diagnostic and legislative changes affecting the definition of ASD and the availability of services for developmental disabilities.[10] The incidence and prevalence of ASD have been rising in recent decades, but the relative contributions from heightened awareness, changes in definitions, more complete ascertainment, improved diagnosis, greater funding for services, and an increased desire on the part of parents to seek services for affected children are difficult to determine, and the potential causes for this trend are not entirely known.[8,10–13]

## EARLY SIGNS AND DETECTION

Subtle signs of ASD may be identified as early as age 2 years or even younger and may be depicted in family videos from the first birthday[14] or in prospective studies of younger siblings of children with ASD. In one prospective study, parents of low-risk controls and high-risk infant siblings recorded any concerns they had regarding their children's development between 6 and 24 months of age. At 3 years of age, an independent, gold-standard diagnostic assessment for ASD was conducted in all participants. Parents of high-risk children who received an ASD diagnosis reported more concerns than parents of low-risk or high-risk children who did not have ASD. Within the high-risk group, the total number of parental concerns predicted a subsequent diagnosis of ASD as early as 12 months of age. Concerns regarding sensory behavior and motor development predicted a subsequent diagnosis of ASD as early as 6 months, whereas concerns about social communication and repetitive behaviors did not predict diagnosis of ASD until after 12 months.[15] By age 2 years, a diagnosis by an experienced professional can be considered very reliable.[16,17] However, on average, children identified with ASD are not diagnosed until after age 4.[8] Often, the diagnosis of ASD is not suspected until the preschool period or later, when problems arise because the child is expected to cooperate in a structured school setting. In some children, the clinical picture is complex and ASD coexists with other disabilities or diseases.

Regression—a loss of previously established skills—can occur. Rates and onset of regression have been debated. A meta-analysis of 85 articles representing 29,035 participants with ASD found an overall prevalence rate for regression of 32.1% (95% confidence interval [CI], 29.5% to 34.8%) occurring at a mean of 1.78 years (95% CI, 1.67 to 1.89 years). Regression prevalence rates differed according to four types: language regression, 24.9%; language/social regression, 38.1%; missed regression, 32.5%; and unspecified regression, 39.1%.[18] Estimates of the prevalence of regression vary depending on the definition used. Requiring loss of language (i.e., defining regression as loss of both language and social skills rather than either one) significantly

**Box 13–1.** Diagnostic Criteria for Autism Spectrum Disorder*

The American Psychiatric Association's *Diagnostic and Statistical Manual, Fifth Edition* (DSM-5) provides standardized criteria to help diagnose Autism Spectrum Disorder 299.00 (comparable to Autistic Disorder F84.0 in the ICD-10); for details, see the DSM-5 manual.

A. Persistent deficits in social communication and social interaction across multiple contexts, as manifested by the following, currently or by history (examples are illustrative, not exhaustive):
   1. Deficits in social-emotional reciprocity, ranging, for example, from abnormal social approach and failure of normal back-and-forth conversation; to reduced sharing of interests, emotions, or affect; to failure to initiate or respond to social interactions.
   2. Deficits in nonverbal communicative behaviors used for social interaction, ranging, for example, from poorly integrated verbal and nonverbal communication; to abnormalities in eye contact and body language or deficits in understanding and use of gestures; to a total lack of facial expressions and nonverbal communication.
   3. Deficits in developing, maintaining, and understanding relationships, ranging, for example, from difficulties adjusting behavior to suit various social contexts; to difficulties in sharing imaginative play or in making friends; to absence of interest in peers.

   *Specify* current severity: Severity is based on social communication impairments and restricted, repetitive patterns of behavior.

B. Restricted, repetitive patterns of behavior, interests, or activities, as manifested by at least two of the following, currently or by history (examples are illustrative, not exhaustive):
   1. Stereotyped or repetitive motor movements, use of objects, or speech (e.g., simple motor stereotypies, lining up toys or flipping objects, echolalia, idiosyncratic phrases).
   2. Insistence on sameness, inflexible adherence to routines, or ritualized patterns of verbal or nonverbal behavior (e.g., extreme distress at small changes, difficulties with transitions, rigid thinking patterns, greeting rituals, need to take same route or eat same food every day).
   3. Highly restricted, fixated interests that are abnormal in intensity or focus (e.g., strong attachment to or preoccupation with unusual objects, excessively circumscribed or perseverative interest).
   4. Hyperreactivity or hyporeactivity to sensory input or unusual interests in sensory aspects of the environment (e.g., apparent indifference to pain/temperature, adverse response to specific sounds or textures, excessive smelling or touching of objects, visual fascination with lights or movement).

   *Specify* current severity: Severity is based on social communication impairments and restricted, repetitive patterns of behavior.

C. Symptoms must be present in the early developmental period (but may not become fully manifest until social demands exceed limited capacities, or may be masked by learned strategies in later life).

D. Symptoms cause clinically significant impairment in social, occupational, or other important areas of current functioning.

E. These disturbances are not better explained by intellectual disability (intellectual developmental disorder) or global developmental delay. Intellectual disability and ASD frequently co-occur; to make comorbid diagnoses of ASD and intellectual disability, social communication should be below that expected for general developmental level.

   *Specify* if:
   With or without accompanying intellectual impairment
   With or without accompanying language impairment
   Associated with a known medical or genetic condition or environmental factor
   Associated with another neurodevelopmental, mental, or behavioral disorder
   With catatonia.

*Note: Individuals with a well-established DSM-IV diagnosis of autistic disorder, Asperger disorder, or pervasive developmental disorder not otherwise specified should be given the diagnosis of ASD. Individuals who have marked deficits in social communication but whose symptoms do not otherwise meet criteria for ASD should be evaluated for social (pragmatic) communication disorder.

underestimates the frequency of developmental regression. The typical age at onset of regression ranges between 15 and 30 months; the average age is approximately 21 months.[18]

## AUTISM RESEARCH

Research on the biology of autism is performed in many areas, ranging from genes and gene products (proteins) to cell function and anatomy to functional integration in networks.[19] Differences are found between ASD children and comparison groups of children with typical development, but often there is an overlap of findings between children with ASD versus other developmental disorders and/or psychiatric conditions. Genetic research has found deletions, multiplications, and mutations in genes regulating synaptogenesis and synaptic function, genes regulating cell migration and apoptotic mechanisms, and neurotransmitters and their receptors. Conditions involving various forms of neuropathology may coexist with ASD (e.g., fragile X syndrome, Rett syndrome). In one neuropathological study, variations ranging from subtle changes in the arrangements of the minicolumns of the cortex to more obvious malformations of the brain were shown.[20] Maldevelopment of the cortex is a finding in many cases of epilepsy, a common comorbid condition in children with ASD.[21]

ASD is a condition that has defined criteria but heterogenic findings in neurobiological investigations. Dysfunction in neural networks and in connectivity between brain areas may be a common factor. In ASD, in social communication is a core finding resulting from impairment in an area that requires the coordination of large networks of cells. Skills that use only limited networks may be spared, allowing some individuals with ASD to have good abilities in restricted areas.[20]

### Genetic Factors

In approximately 10% to 20% of children with ASD, a thorough medical investigation will find some specific neurobiological disorder; yet, each defined condition is an explanation only for small subgroups of ASD cases.[22] In genetic investigations, a range of deviations may be found:

- Chromosomal aberrations (e.g., Down syndrome) may be present. The majority of children with Down syndrome have social communication as a positive part of their development, but some have co-occurring ASD.
- Microdeletions and microduplications (copy number variations) are found with the use of new methods. In one study by Nicholl et al.,[23] copy number variations of clinical significance were found in 5% of all ASD cases and in 12.7% of the subgroup of children with ASD and intellectual disability.
- Mutations in single genes (e.g., fragile X syndrome, Rett syndrome, tuberous sclerosis complex) require specific DNA analyses. Fragile X is the most common hereditary disorder resulting in mental retardation and may frequently occur in ASD. For families, genetic counseling to investigate this mutation is important. Boys with this mutation have symptoms; girls may exhibit a range from normal development to signs as severe as those frequently seen in boys. Rett syndrome is a genetic disorder that affects girls and is; .+

characterized by regression of mental function and loss of motor abilities (especially hand function) at an early age. Often, there is a period of autistic-like features, but these tend to decrease as girls grow older. The tuberous sclerosis complex gene aberration can give rise to various forms of developmental disorders and/or severe epilepsy. However, there are individuals with this mutation who are without symptoms.

- Many inborn metabolic disorders (usually with genetic background) cause neurological symptoms and developmental retardation, including ASD symptoms. Metabolic investigation must be considered, especially in the presence of regression, other signs of neurological dysfunction, or growth problems. Most metabolic diseases are characterized by postnatal biochemical disturbances. Disorders of cholesterol biosynthesis are also notable for their severe effects on prenatal development; an example is Smith-Lemli-Opitz syndrome, a syndrome resulting in multiple congenital anomalies.[24]

### Environmental Factors and Epigenetics

Although the basis of ASD is thought to be multifactorial, it is known to be a highly heritable disorder.[25,26] Research with new methods has described microdeletions, duplications, and other genetic variants. Some of these variations are of specific interest as a potential cause of ASD (see earlier discussion), and others may be a sign of genomic imbalances. These nonspecific variations can be found in other neuropsychiatric disorders, in cases of intellectual disability, and in psychiatric conditions. Environmental or epigenetic factors may influence the function of genes. The "second hit" hypothesis proposes that genetic factors give susceptibility but one or more environmental factors are needed for symptoms to arise. Multiplicative and/or interacting risk factors may exist.[27]

The effects of environment on phenotype are often mediated through epigenetic processes.[28] Epigenetic mechanisms can result in the silencing of particular genes and can ultimately influence the expressed phenotype.[29] Each individual's unique epigenome—the genome plus epigenetic modifications—develops as a consequence of a variety of factors. The first and likely the most important factor is the various effects exerted by the environment on the epigenome. Second, as mentioned, the epigenome is heritable: A mother can pass a methylated gene to her offspring. Third, the epigenome is subject to replication epigenetic errors, with an error rate of approximately 1 in 1000.[30] Fourth, spontaneous changes to the epigenome, apart from changes driven by environmental causes, are thought to occur and may be referred to as epigenetic drift.[31]

The role of environmental factors in the development of ASD is a crucial area of study. Examples of environmental factors that have been associated with increased risk for ASD include prenatal exposure to toxins such as thalidomide and valproic acid, shared prenatal environment in the case of twins,[32] advanced maternal or paternal age at birth, maternal prenatal medication use, and maternal migration.[33] ASD can occur after severe complications during pregnancy and in the perinatal period (e.g., congenital infections, prematurity with very low birth weight). For these children, ASD is often part of a complex developmental disorder that includes hearing and/or visual problems, intellectual disability, and cerebral palsy.

Nutritional epigenetic factors have been identified in ASD, including abnormal folic acid metabolism, which has been linked to aberrant fetal development,[34] and genetic polymorphisms of cytochrome P450, which is essential for vitamin D metabolism and thus important for neuronal growth and neurodevelopment. Defects in vitamin D metabolism and vitamin D deficiency have been implicated in ASD.[35] The period in development during which the nutritional imbalance occurs is very important in determining which disease-related gene will be affected. Different organs have critical developmental stages, and the time point at which they are compromised predisposes the individual to specific diseases. Epigenetic modifications that occur during development may not be expressed until later in life, depending on the function of the gene. Although most studies implicate prenatal periods as critical time windows, some research has shown that nutritional intake through adulthood can also affect the epigenome.[36]

## MEDICAL AND PSYCHIATRIC COMORBIDITIES

With advancements in clinical care, the appreciation that many children, adolescents, and adults with ASD have medically relevant disorders has been established. These disorders may negatively impact developmental progress and behavior and may frequently go undetected. Medical comorbidities that have been identified include hearing impairment, visual defects, seizures, sleep disorders, GI issues and disorders, food allergies, eczema, asthma, ear and respiratory infections, severe headaches, migraines, poor oral care (dental carries), metabolic disorders, hormone dysfunction, obesity, nutritional deficits, anxiety, depression, attention deficit hyperactivity disorder (ADHD), and oppositional defiant disorder.[4,22,37–45] Some of these comorbidities are common in the general population and co-occur with ASD without being part of any pathogenetic process, but some are more prevalent among children with ASD compared with their typically developing peers. Epilepsy is a common comorbid condition, affecting approximately 20% of children diagnosed with ASD, although frequency ranges vary widely, from 5% to 40%.[46,47] Maldevelopment of the cortex is a finding in many cases of epilepsy.[21]

Medical evaluation is needed to search for a possible underlying cause for ASD and to identify any comorbidities and treatable diseases. The need to investigate is especially high in cases with regression or a fluctuating course. Recognition and management of frequently occurring medical conditions often results in improved developmental gains and better quality of life for the patient and family.[48]

As a heterogeneous condition that coexists with all forms of other developmental disorders and physical disabilities or diseases, ASD may result in functional limitations that often require lifelong coordinated, interdisciplinary services and support.[49] A high rate of cognitive disabilities exists in individuals with ASD,[50,51] although the majority have intelligence in the normal range. The presence or absence of intellectual disability is considered to be the most critical factor affecting outcomes in individuals with ASD.[51] Although a small minority of individuals develop sufficient adaptive skills that they no longer meet criteria for an ASD diagnosis, children with ASD are generally considered to have lifelong developmental disabilities.[52,53]

There exists a paucity of information related to the prevalence of medical conditions among adults with ASD. In one study,[54] data from electronic medical records (but not validated by standardized clinical examinations) revealed that adults with ASD had significantly increased rates of all major psychiatric disorders, including depression, anxiety, bipolar disorder, obsessive-compulsive disorder, schizophrenia, and suicide attempts. Almost all of the medical conditions evaluated were also significantly more common among adults with ASD, including immune conditions, GI and sleep disorders, seizures, obesity, hyperlipidemia, hypertension, and diabetes.[54]

Clinicians face challenges in diagnosing medical comorbidities in patients with ASD, especially those who have impairments in communication and social interaction and deficits in sensory processing—core features of ASD. Other frequent and mainly behavioral symptoms include anxiety, aggression, agitation, irritability, impulsivity, lack of focus, disturbed sleep, self-harming, and self-stimulatory behaviors. These symptoms, sometimes called "autistic behaviors," can be a result of the neurodevelopmental disorder itself, for instance in situations with overwhelming stress, or they can be a sign of pain or other effects of underlying medical disorders. The behaviors have a substantial negative impact, not only on individuals with ASD but also on their families and society.[55] Core and co-occurring behaviors of ASD may avert a patient's ability to accurately report pain or localized discomfort and therefore can lead to missed or delayed diagnosis or opportunities for prevention or early treatment. These findings indicate an urgent need for the development of improved strategies for delivery of effective health education and health care to this growing population.[56]

### Gastrointestinal Dysfunction

A growing body of evidence suggests that a significant subset of individuals with ASD exhibit GI abnormalities,[4,57–60] and GI issues can contribute to the clinical and behavioral manifestations of ASD core-related symptoms. These symptoms include abnormal behavior, immune dysregulation, and metabolic dysfunctions that can contribute to behavioral impairment and have been significantly associated with sleep disorders and food intolerances.[61–63] Current evidence is evolving and demonstrates the importance and need to better characterize the underlying pathology of GI dysfunction and to determine whether there are any unique characteristics specific to ASD.[64] Organic GI disorders result from anatomic, metabolic, or other kinds of pathological processes that may be identified by clinical examination. The term "functional" GI disorder is used when no pathological process can be found. Organic and functional disorders may coexist in the same person. Large population-based studies with blinded methodology are needed to clearly describe the rates of GI disorders in autism.

In a large Norwegian prospective birth cohort, mothers of children with ASD were significantly more likely to report one or more GI symptom (constipation, food allergy/intolerance, or diarrhea) in either the 6- to18-month or the 18- to 36-month age period, and they were twice as likely to report at least one GI symptoms in both age periods compared with mothers of children with developmental delay or typical development.[65] Parental report of GI symptoms in ASD often requires inferences that may be limited by communication deficits.[66] Even though GI symptoms are common in young children, physicians should be mindful that children with ASD may be experiencing more GI difficulties in the first 3 years of life compared to children with typical development or developmental delay.[65] In a Danish register study based on hospital diagnoses, individuals diagnosed with infantile ASD were compared with age-matched controls. During an average observation period of 30 years, similar proportions from the ASD and comparison groups received a defined GI diagnosis (approximately 30%). In both groups, specific GI diseases occurred with low frequency.[67]

In 2010, a multidisciplinary panel of US clinicians developed a consensus report that provided clinical guidelines for the evaluation, diagnosis, and treatment of GI disorders in individuals with ASD.[68] These clinicians reviewed the extant medical literature and concluded that not enough data were available to develop evidence-based recommendations. They revealed that the most common GI symptoms and signs reported for individuals with ASD were chronic constipation, abdominal pain with or without diarrhea, and encopresis as a consequence of constipation. Other GI abnormalities that have been described in ASD include gastroesophageal reflux disease (GERD), abnormal bloating, disaccharidase deficiencies, and pathological findings such as inflammation of the GI tract and abnormalities of the enteric nervous system. Critical takeaway messages from this consensus paper were (1) that individuals with ASD deserve the same thoroughness and standard of care in the diagnostic workup and treatment of GI concerns as do other patients without ASD, and (2) that care providers should be aware that problem behavior in patients with ASD may be the primary or sole symptom of an underlying medical condition, including some GI disorders. In a follow-up publication, Buie and colleagues[69] provided examples of how general pediatric guidelines for the diagnostic workup of abdominal pain, chronic constipation, and GERD could be adapted for this patient group and recommended that supervision by an experienced care provider, such as a registered dietitian, is imperative when a diagnostic elimination diet is trialed in order to assess the clinical response appropriately. A newly developed clinical guideline from an expert panel of dietitians outlines an 11-step algorithm for the management of GI symptoms in children with ASD.[70] This algorithm and the accompanying checklist serve as a tool to individualize treatment to address GI symptoms while lessening the risk of exacerbating potential nutrient deficits. Multidisciplinary collaboration in the evaluation and treatment of GI issues is emphasized.

## Constipation

An algorithm and checklist for identification and management of constipation were published as guidance for primary practitioners.[71] They were developed by collaborative work in medical centers providing care for children with ASD. Based on the authors' combined clinical experience, a definite subset of children with ASD, especially those on the severe end of the spectrum, will fail to respond to standard therapy and should be referred to a gastroenterologist. Moreover, a change in baseline behavior is frequently the only presentation of constipation, rather than the typical hallmark characteristics such as straining, passing hard and infrequent stools, and soiling. There was a consensus opinion that the child with ASD and constipation requires a systematic evaluation for diagnosis and therapy and that after any intervention there is a need for careful follow-up.

## Gut-Brain Axis and the Microbiota

There exist hypotheses and some emerging evidence relevant to ASD in the areas of immune function, the relationship between signaling pathways of the gut and the brain, and the genome, specifically GI-microbiome interactions. Current literature supports a combination of changes in the gut microflora, intestinal permeability, inappropriate immune response, activation of specific metabolic pathways, and behavioral changes in genetically predisposed individuals.[64,72–74] Preliminary information related to gut dysbiosis may contribute to GI symptoms and may have a potential direct neurological impact in ASD.[75] Mucosal immune cells make up about 70% of the immune cells within the body, and dysfunction in these cells may have adverse consequences on GI function. Endoscopic analyses of subgroups of children with ASD and GI symptoms have revealed the presence of subtle, diffuse inflammation of the intestinal tract.[68,76] A common finding in ASD individuals and their mothers is an increased presence of autoantibodies directed toward central nervous system proteins; it is hypothesized that this may contribute to a decrease in mucosal barrier integrity.[77]

It has been hypothesized that altered intestinal permeability ("leaky gut") may play a pathogenic role in ASD.[78] Impaired intestinal barrier function in ASD may make regulating the trafficking of macromolecules between the environment and the host difficult. The intestinal epithelial barrier and its intercellular tight junctions, together with gut-associated lymphoid tissue and the neuroendocrine network, controls the trafficking of macromolecules.[79] Alterations in intestinal microflora, such as a diminished presence of certain bacteria (*Prevotella* and *Coprococcus* ssp.) that are involved in carbohydrate fermentation in the gut, were identified in children with ASD and were not altered by dietary intake patterns despite the presence or absence of GI symptoms.[80] These findings may support the idea that particular microbiome imbalances affect ASD, rather than the suggestion that imbalances occur as a result of eating behaviors or dietary differences.[75]

The protein zonulin, a component of intercellular tight junctions, is involved in regulation of gut permeability.[81] Exposure of the small intestine to either bacteria or gluten is a powerful trigger for zonulin-induced tight junction disassembly. Enteric infections have also been implicated in pathological conditions, including allergic, autoimmune, and inflammatory diseases that are associated with impairment of the intestinal barrier. In addition to bacterial exposure, gliadin, the environmental trigger of celiac disease, has been shown to alter the intestinal barrier function by releasing zonulin.[82]

## Sensitivity to Gluten

Celiac disease is an immune-mediated disorder with a prevalence of 1% to 2% in Western populations. Individuals with celiac disease typically have biopsy findings of villous atrophy and inflammation in the small intestine. They are positive for specific immunoglobulin A (IgA) antibodies (i.e., endomysium, tissue transglutaminase) but also for less specific IgG antigliadin antibodies. In Sweden, a nationwide case-control study compared ASD diagnosis in individuals with celiac disease and matched controls based on a Swedish biopsy register. There was no evidence that celiac disease was associated with ASD, but an association was found between having normal mucosa but serology results positive for celiac disease and having an ASD diagnosis. The authors discussed whether these individuals might have nonceliac gluten sensitivity.[83] In another study, Lau et al.[84] found higher levels of IgG antibodies to gliadin in children with ASD compared with controls. In a review of the relationship between autism and gluten, Buie[85] concluded that there are some gluten-sensitive patients who do not have celiac disease.

### Feeding Difficulties

The basis for any successful intervention in autism is in-depth knowledge of the neuropsychological background for behavior problems related to feeding difficulties.

#### Social-Communicative Impairment

When social interaction is impaired, ordinary motivational factors (e.g., to be one of the group during meals) might not be effective, and the use of imitation may be limited when learning new abilities (e.g., the child cannot model the behaviors of family members or peers during mealtime). Both verbal and nonverbal expressive communication is often restricted, therefore the person with ASD may have little or no ability to demonstrate what he or she wants with gestures. Impairment of receptive communication involves difficulty in understanding words as well as nonverbal communication (e.g., gestures, facial expressions). Understanding of communication in a concrete way may lead to misinterpretation.

#### Restriction of Interests and Activities

Some children have a rigid way of selecting food and are reluctant to try foods with new tastes, textures or smells. There may be rituals concerning eating, such as the way the food is arranged, the sequence in which it is served, having a specific place at the table, or a preferred noise level.

#### Sensory Differences

For some children, choosing food in a rigid, ritualistic way is an effect of hyposensitivity or hypersensitivity combined with an idiosyncratic reaction to certain stimuli. Food avoidance may be a protective mechanism in the face of an unrecognized food allergy or GI disorder; it may result from a memory of discomfort in connection with some food that, once avoided, may become impossible to reintroduce. In some instances, the child does not have the ability to understand, describe, or convey why the reaction is painful and severe. This is one example in which children with autism may exhibit behaviors consistent with the autism diagnosis that are caused by an underlying medical condition.[4]

#### Co-occurring Behavior Problems

The child who has a tendency to externalize may show disruptive behaviors at mealtime that increase stress for the whole family. Also, children with ASD may react by internalizing symptoms such as anxiety and depression. In some cases of feeding problems in ASD, identifiable organic causes can create negative behavioral responses such as fear, aggression, or escape.[86] Situation-based fears or phobias can develop that may result in swallowing difficulties. In a review, Johnson et al.[88] described links between feeding dysfunction and problematic behavior regardless of the level of functioning. They concluded that children with all forms of behavioral problems should be screened for the presence of less than optimal feeding and mealtime behaviors as well as for inadequate nutritional intake.[87]

Feeding problems often start in infancy. Barnevik Olsson et al.[88] conducted a retrospective study of young children with ASD using records from Swedish health care community referral centers. The number of consultations related to three domains were recorded: feeding problems, excessive crying, and sleeping problems. Each domain was significantly higher in the ASD group compared with age- and gender-matched controls from the same centers. All three domains were significantly positively correlated with each other. Feeding difficulties were identified as occurring in up to 25% of typically developing children during their first year of life,[89] but the rate has been reported to be as high as 80% in children with developmental disabilities[90] and 90% in preschool- and school-age children with ASD and sensory disorders.[86]

The study of childhood feeding and eating disturbances has been hampered by inconsistencies in classification and use of terminology. Parents of children with ASD often report that their children are "picky eaters," are reluctant to try new foods, are highly selective, and have a very restricted repertoire of acceptable foods[91] along with excessive intake of a few foods that can increase mealtime behavior problems and increase spousal and family stress.[92] Interestingly, picky eating is not associated with lack of appetite: These children typically have a good appetite for foods they like. This suggests that, despite increased feeding problems, children with ASD may consume an adequate volume of food to meet gross energy needs. Therefore, relying exclusively on anthropometric parameters to assess health status may mask underlying nutritional deficits.[93] Impairments of gross and fine motor skills that interfere with feeding capabilities have been associated with ASD.[94] The act of eating requires the ability to simultaneously process information from a range of sensory subtypes. Children with ASD who have problems with sensory modulation (hyporeactivity and/or hyperreactivity) that involve hearing, sight, smell, taste, and touch as well as vestibular system and proprioception[95] may exhibit a greater degree of food refusal based on food characteristics (e.g., texture or consistency, taste or smell).[96]

Marshall et al.[97] performed a systematic review and meta-analysis of interventions to improve feeding difficulties. The meta-analysis included 23 studies published between 2000 to 2013, all of which had five or fewer participants and most of which were judged to be of low-level evidence quality. The authors concluded that prospective randomized trials are needed. Health providers should avoid an exclusively behavioral approach to treating children with ASD and feeding difficulties because this management strategy could underestimate the impact of oral sensory and motor system interactions that can significantly impact feeding habits.[98]

## NUTRIENT INTAKE AND NUTRITIONAL STATUS

Individuals with ASD are nutritionally vulnerable because they exhibit selective eating patterns and have sensory sensitivities that predispose them to restricted intakes.[99] Nutritional deficiencies in children with ASD can result from co-occurring GI symptoms, organic or functional conditions, feeding problems, and psychosocial dysfunction in the family. There is a risk for growth retardation, underweight, obesity, adverse effects on psychomotor development, and increased susceptibility to infections and other diseases. In a meta-analysis of feeding problems and nutrient intake, Sharp et al.[93] identified significant specific deficits in protein and calcium intake in children with ASD compared with controls. Shmaya et al.[100] found a higher rate of nutritional deficiencies among children with ASD compared with a typically developing children; however, none of these deficiencies fell below the Dietary Reference Intakes (DRIs) with the exception of calcium. The same authors demonstrated higher weight and body mass index (BMI) Z scores in the ASD group compared with the typically developing group. The possible reasons for overweight include an unbalanced diet (e.g., preference for higher consumption of processed foods, sweets, and sweetened drinks),[101] lack of physical activity, and the frequent use of antipsychotic drugs that can cause weight gain.[102] Bandini et al noted that children with ASD compared to typically developing children engaged in fewer physical activities for less time.[103] These authors commented on the inability of standard questionnaire-based measures to capture activity in children with ASD. Growth parameters and multivitamin use in 87 children with ASD did not differ when compared to U.S. population-based age-matched cohort.[104] 32% (26/83) of the patients in that study received a multivitamin supplement.[104]

A five-center study of 288 children with ASD, of whom 12% (34/288) followed a gluten-free (GF) and casein-free (CF) diet, revealed that 56% and 78%, respectively, used dietary supplements (mostly multivitamins and fortified foods). This supplementation led to excess of several nutrients commonly consumed that could place children with ASD at risk for nutrient toxicities; however, it did not correct deficient intake of calcium or vitamin D.[105] Macronutrients such as calories and protein were not evaluated.

Attainment of peak bone mass may not occur in children with ASD.[106] Factors predisposing to an increased fracture rate include low bone mineral density (BMD), low calcium and vitamin D intake, low BMI, physical inactivity, behavioral difficulties, and use of certain drugs (e.g., proton pump inhibitors for management of GERD).[107] Vitamin D is essential for proper neurodevelopment and cognitive and behavioral function. Associations between ASD and common, functional polymorphisms in vitamin D pathways have been demonstrated, and there is preliminary evidence that vitamin D metabolism could play a role in the etiology of ASD.[108] Vitamin D deficiency has been reported in autistic children. However, data on the relationship between vitamin D deficiency and the severity of ASD are limited. Saad et al.[109] performed a case-control cross-sectional study of 122 children with ASD to assess their vitamin D status and the relationship between vitamin D deficiency and severity of autism. They found that 57% of the patients had vitamin D deficiency, and 30% had vitamin D insufficiency. The mean level of 25-hydroxyvitamin D (25-OHD) in patients with severe autism was significantly lower than in patients with mild to moderate autism. Serum 25-OHD levels were significantly negatively correlated with scores on the Childhood Autism Rating Scale (CARS). Patients with low serum 25-OHD levels participated in an open-label trial of daily vitamin $D_3$ supplementation for 3 months that resulted in significantly improved outcomes in sections of the CARS and in the aberrant behavior checklist subscales that measured behavior, stereotypy, eye contact, and attention span. Vitamin $D_3$ supplementation may have beneficial effects in ASD subjects with low serum levels.

Both calcium and vitamin D are necessary for calcium homeostasis and bone mineralization. Low bone mineralization in children, especially boys, with ASD has been reported. Bone cortical thickness (BCT), as measured on hand-wrist radiographs, was reduced in 75 boys with ASD aged 4 to 8 years.[110] In the 12% of boys who were on a CF diet, there was a significant (twofold) percent reduction in BCT, compared with boys on minimally restricted or unrestricted diets. Neumeyer et al.[106] evaluated BMD in 18 boys with ASD and 19 controls, all aged 8 to 14 years. Boys with ASD had lower BMD Z scores at the spine, hip, and femoral neck, and differences at the hip and femoral neck persisted after controlling for maturity and BMI. One-third (6/18) of the boys with ASD were on a restricted diet (GF, CF, or both [GFCF]), and almost 50% were taking supplements. Lower vitamin D intake from food, not supplements, was demonstrated in boys with ASD compared with controls, as was lower serum 25-OHD levels (<32 ng/mL). Endogenous vitamin D synthesis requires sun exposure, and it is not uncommon for children with ASD to have lower levels of physical activity and potentially less time outdoors compared with controls. Nutrient intake may be negatively impacted with the initiation of self-imposed diets (i.e., selective eating), caregiver-restricted diets (i.e., GFCF diets), or therapeutic restricted diets (i.e., antigen elimination diets for food allergies). Therapeutic restricted diets are the standard of care for managing GI diseases such as eosinophilic esophagitis (EoE), GERD, and allergies to cow milk (CMA) and multiple food proteins (MFPA). In a study by Lyall et al a significant association of food allergies was demonstrated among 560 children with ASD compared to 391 typically developing controls. Approximately 15% of children with ASD had food allergies, a 2.2-fold increase in odds compared with controls[45]). Calcium and protein are most notably deficient, and filling these nutritional gaps cannot be accomplished singularly by use of a vitamin/mineral supplement. The use of amino acid–based formula as a sole source of nutrition or as a supplement is warranted when medically indicated (e.g., CMA, GERD, MPFA, EoE).[70] Idiosyncratic nutrient deficiencies resulting from unique dietary patterns should be routinely evaluated in all children with ASD.[111]

## FEEDING AND DIETARY APPROACHES

The dietitian is an important member of the health care team who is responsible for the nutritional management of a child with ASD and assists in coordinating care with other specialists and caregivers. Each child with ASD needs routine, comprehensive longitudinal nutritional assessment that takes into account the child's individual capabilities—their strengths and challenges (e.g., oral motor skills, self-help skills, mental and chronological age) and evaluation of mealtime behaviors. An individualized nutrition care plan should be developed by a dietitian that takes into account the child's sensory and food preferences and is periodically reassessed and includes input from other team members (i.e., speech and/or feeding therapists, occupational therapist). A more controversial approach is the use of restrictive diets and dietary supplements as complementary and alternative therapies. A GFCF diet is commonly used. In a recent survey in the United Kingdom, more than 80% of parents of children with ASD reported some kind of dietary intervention for their child (GFCF diet in 29%). When asked about the effects of the GFCF diet, 20% to 29% of the parents reported significant improvements on the ASD core dimensions. The findings of this study suggested additional effects of a GFCF diet on comorbid problems of autism such as GI symptoms, concentration, and attention.[112]

A multicentered study conducted in Denmark, Norway, and England published one of the few randomized controlled trials of the GFCF diet in ASD.[113] This study demonstrated some positive behavioral improvements in a group of ASD children who received dietary treatment for 1 year. However, the large attrition rate was a notable study limitation. Many case reports of positive effects have been published, but to date there is no evidence for efficacy of GFCF diets in ASD despite frequent parental initiation of this dietary intervention. In a systematic Cochrane review, Millward et al.[114] found that because of the paucity of existing data, no meta-analysis could be conducted. These authors concluded that large-scale, randomized controlled trials were needed. Authors of later review articles[85,115,116] reached the same conclusion. A 2014 investigation indicated that several factors may be potentially pertinent regarding a positive response of symptoms to the GFCF diet.[117] Chronological age was reported to be the strongest predictor of response, and the presence of a urine compound, *trans*-indolyl-3-acryloylglycine, merited further research. It is possible that the GFCF diet is beneficial for some subset of children with ASD, but identification of this phenotype has yet to be determined. These preliminary findings should be replicated in future studies and highlight the need for a complex and sophisticated investigation of patient subgroups.

Important feasibility factors to consider related to implementing dietary intervention as an alternative to other management strategies include: a) the potential excessive diversion of available time and financial resources, b) what to do if the child strongly resists, and c) what if caregivers are unable or unwilling to embrace recommended nutrition therapy. It may be difficult to gauge how a child will react to efforts to remove or replace preferred foods, and this may result in further self-imposed dietary restriction and development of nutritional deficiencies.[70]

Early and intensive types of feeding therapies have been demonstrated positive effects in children with ASD. Various approaches are used, some based on behavioral management techniques (with prompting, shaping, and reinforcement strategies) and others on individualized pedagogical methods and adjustments of the environment to compensate for the neuropsychological difficulties characteristic of ASD. No management model has been demonstrated to be best for all children.

Regardless of what management model is implemented, facts related to the child's health and nutritional status (e.g., possible food allergies, GI issues, nutritional inadequacies) should routinely be assessed by a dietitian. A multidisciplinary approach is needed to ensure that health problems, which are often overlooked, are addressed. This ongoing surveillance and support may minimize both the child's and the family's stress and may enhance their quality of life.

### References

1. Kanner L. Autistic disturbances of affective contact. *Nervous Child.* 1943; 2:217.
2. Asperger H. Autistic psychopathy in childhood [1944]. Translated and annotated by Frith U. In: Frith U, ed. *Autism and Asperger Syndrome.* New York: Cambridge University Press; 1991.
3. World Health Organization. *The ICD-10 Classification of Mental and Behavioural Disorders: Diagnostic Criteria for Research.* Geneva: WHO; 1992.
4. Bauman ML. Medical comorbidities in autism: challenges to diagnosis and treatment. *Neurotherapeutics.* 2010; 7:320.
5. American Psychiatric Association. *Diagnostic and Statistical Manual of Mental Disorders, Fifth Edition* (DSM-5). Arlington, VA: American Psychiatric Publishing; 2013.
6. Swineford LB, Thurm A, Baird G, Wetherby AM, Swedo S. Social (pragmatic) communication disorder: a research review of this new DSM-5 diagnostic category. *J Neurodev Disord.* 2014; 6:41.
7. Yeargin-Allsopp M, Rice C, Karapurkar T, Doernberg N, Boyle C, Murphy C. Prevalence of ASD in a US metropolitan area. *JAMA.* 2003; 289:49.
8. Developmental Disabilities Monitoring Network Surveillance Year 2010 Principal Investigators; Centers for Disease Control and Prevention (CDC). Prevalence of

autism spectrum disorder among children aged 8 years—autism and developmental disabilities monitoring network, 11 sites, United States, 2010. *MMWR Surveill Summ.* 2014; 63(2):1.
9. Centers for Disease Control and Prevention. *Summary of Autism Spectrum Disorder (ASD) Prevalence Studies.* 2013. http://www.cdc.gov/ncbddd/autism/documents/asd_prevalence_table_2013.pdf. Accessed June 14, 2016.
10. Hertz-Picciotto I, Delwiche L. The rise in autism and the role of age at diagnosis. *Epidemiology.* 2009; 20:84.
11. Dawson G. Dramatic increase in autism prevalence parallels explosion of research into its biology and causes. *JAMA Psychiatry.* 2013; 70:9.
12. Idring S, Lundberg M, Sturm H, et al. Changes in prevalence of autism spectrum disorders in 2001–2011: findings from the Stockholm youth cohort. *J Autism Dev Disord.* 2015; 45:1766.
13. Baxter AJ, Brugha TS, Erskine HE, Scheurer RW, Vos T, Scott JG. The epidemiology and global burden of autism spectrum disorders. *Psychol Med.* 2015; 45:601.
14. Gliga T, Jones EJH, Bedford R, Charman T, Johnson MH. From early markers to neuro-developmental mechanisms of autism. *Dev Rev.* 2014; 34:189.
15. Sacrey LA, Zwaigenbaum L, Bryson S, et al. Can parents' concerns predict autism spectrum disorder?: a prospective study of high-risk siblings from 6 to 36 months of age. *J Am Acad Child Adolesc Psychiatry.* 2015; 54:470.
16. Lord C, Risi S, DiLavore PS, Shulman C, Thurm A, Pickles A. Autism from 2 to 9 years of age. *Arch Gen Psychiatry.* 2006; 63:694.
17. Corsello CM, Akshoomoff N, Stahmer AC. Diagnosis of autism spectrum disorders in 2-year-olds: a study of community practice. *J Child Psychol Psychiatry.* 2013; 54:178.
18. Barger BD, Campbell JM, McDonough JD. Prevalence and onset of regression within autism spectrum disorders: a meta-analytic review. *J Autism Dev Disord.* 2013; 43:817.
19. Ecker C, Spooren W, Murphy DGM. Expert review. Translational approaches to the biology of autism: false dawn or a new era? *Mol Psychiatry.* 2012; 18:435.
20. Casanova EL, Casanova MF. Genetics studies indicate that neural induction and early neuronal maturation are disturbed in autism. *Front Cell Neurosci.* 2014; 8:397.
21. Viscidi EW, Triche EW, Pescosolido MF, et al. Clinical characteristics of children with autism spectrum disorder and co-occurring epilepsy. *PLoS One.* 2013; 8(7):e67797.
22. Kohane IS, McMurry A, Weber G, et al. The co-morbidity burden of children and young adults with autism spectrum disorders. *PLoS One.* 2012; 7(4):3e33224.
23. Nicholl J, Waters W, Mulley JC, et al. Cognitive deficit and autism spectrum disorders: prospective diagnosis by array CGH. *Pathology.* 2014; 46:41.
24. Ghaziuddin M, Al-Owain M. Autism spectrum disorders and inborn errors of metabolism: an update. *Pediatr Neurol.* 2013; 49:232.
25. Hu VW, Frank BC, Heine S, Lee NH, Quackenbush J. Gene expression profiling of lymphoblastoid cell lines from monozygotic twins discordant in severity of autism reveals differential regulation of neurologically relevant genes. *BMC Genomics.* 2006; 7:118.
26. Colvert E, Tick B, McEwen F, et al. Heritability of autism spectrum disorder in a UK population-based twin sample. *JAMA Psychiatry.* 2015; 72:415.
27. Ben Itzchak E, Lahat E, Zachor DA. Advanced parental ages and low birth weight in autism spectrum disorders: rates and effect on functioning. *Res Dev Dis.* 2011; 32:2950.
28. Bell JT, Spector TD. A twin approach to unraveling epigenetics. *Trends Genet.* 2011; 27:116.
29. Feinberg AP. Epigenomics reveals a functional genome anatomy and a new approach to common disease. *Nat Biotechnol.* 2010; 28:1049.
30. Riggs AD, Xiong Z. Methylation and epigenetic fidelity. *Proc Natl Acad Sci U S A.* 2004; 101:4.
31. Petronis A, Gottesman II, Kan P, et al. Monozygotic twins exhibit numerous epigenetic differences: clues to twin discordance? *Schizophr Bull.* 2003; 29:169.
32. Hallmayer J, Cleveland S, Torres A, et al. Genetic heritability and shared environmental factors among twin pairs with autism. *Arch Gen Psychiatry.* 2011; 68:1095.
33. Sandin S, Schendel D, Magnusson P, et al. Autism risk associated with parental age and with increasing difference in age between the parents. *Mol Psychiatry.* 2016; 21:693.
34. Beaudin AE, Perry CA, Stabler SP, Allen RH, Stover PJ. Maternal Mthfd1 disruption impairs fetal growth but does not cause neural tube defects in mice. *Am J Clin Nutr.* 2012; 95:882.
35. Currenti SA. Understanding and determining the etiology of autism. *Cell Mol Neurobiol.* 2010; 30:161.
36. Mbadiwe T, Millis RM. Epigenetics and autism. *Autism Res Treat.* 2013; 2013:826156.
37. Ghaziuddin M, Weidmer-Mikhail E, Ghaziuddin N. Comorbidity of Asperger syndrome: a preliminary report. *J Intellect Disabil Res.* 1998; 42(pt 4):279.
38. Bradley E, Bolton P. Episodic psychiatric disorders in teenagers with learning disabilities with and without autism. *Br J Psychiatry.* 2006; 189:361.
39. Leyfer OT, Folstein SE, Bacalman S, et al. Comorbid psychiatric disorders in children with autism: interview development and rates of disorders. *J Autism Dev Disord.* 2006; 36:849.
40. de Bruin EI, Ferdinand RF, Meester S, de Nijs PF, Verheij F. High rates of psychiatric co-morbidity in PDD-NOS. *J Autism Dev Disord.* 2007; 37:877.
41. Simonoff E, Pickles A, Charman T, Chandler S, Loucas T, Baird G. Psychiatric disorders in children with autism spectrum disorders: prevalence, comorbidity, and associated factors in a population-derived sample. *J Am Acad Child Adolesc Psychiatry.* 2008; 47:921.
42. Joshi G, Petty C, Wozniak J, et al. The heavy burden of psychiatric comorbidity in youth with autism spectrum disorders: a large comparative study of a psychiatrically referred population. *J Autism Dev Disord.* 2010; 40:1361.
43. Levy SE, Giarelli E, Lee LC, et al. Autism spectrum disorder and co-occurring developmental, psychiatric, and medical conditions among children in multiple populations of the United States. *J Dev Behav Pediatr.* 2010; 31:267.
44. Schieve LA, Gonzalez V, Boule SL, et al. Concurrent medical conditions and health care use and needs among children with learning and behavioral developmental disabilities. National Health Interview Survey, 2006–2010. *Res Dev Disabil.* 2012; 33:467.
45. Lyall K, Van de Water J, Ashwood P, Hertz-Picciotto I. Asthma and allergies in children with autism spectrum disorders: results from the CHARGE study. *Autism Res.* 2015; 8:567.
46. Autism Genome Project Consortium. Mapping autism risk loci using genetic linkage and chromosomal rearrangements. *Nat Genet.* 2007; 39:319.
47. Bolton PF, Carcani-Rathwell I, Hutton J, Goode S, Howlin P, Rutter M. Epilepsy in autism: features and correlates. *Br J Psychiatry.* 2011; 198:289.
48. Isaksen J, Bryn V, Diseth TH, Heiberg A, Schjølberg S, Skjeldal OH. Children with autism spectrum disorders: the importance of medical investigations. *Eur J Paediatr Neurol.* 2013; 17:68.
49. Van Naarden Braun K, Christensen D, Doernberg N, et al. Trends in the prevalence of autism spectrum disorder, cerebral palsy, hearing loss, intellectual disability, and vision impairment, metropolitan Atlanta, 1991–2010. *PLoS One.* 2015; 10(4):e0124120.
50. Croen L, Grether J, Hoogstrate J, Selvin S. The changing prevalence of autism in California. *J Autism Dev Disord.* 2002; 32:207.
51. Vivanti G, Barbaro J, Hudry K, Dissanayake C, Prior M. Intellectual development in autism spectrum disorders: new insights from longitudinal studies. *Front Hum Neurosci.* 2013; 7:354.
52. Fein D, Barton M, Eigsti IM, et al. Optimal outcome in individuals with a history of autism. *J Child Psychol Psychiatry.* 2013; 54:195.
53. Anderson DK, Liang JW, Lord C. Predicting young adult outcome among more and less cognitively able individuals with autism spectrum disorders. *Child Psychol Psychiatry.* 2014; 55:485.
54. Croen LA, Zerbo O, Qian Y, et al. The health status of adults on the autism spectrum. *Autism.* 2015; 19:814.
55. Treating Autism and Autism Treatment Trust. *Medical comorbidities in autism spectrum disorders: A primer for health care professionals and policy makers.* March 2013. http://nationalautismassociation.org/pdf/MedicalComorbiditiesinASD2013.pdf. Accessed June 14, 2016.
56. Nicolaidis C, Kripke CC, Raymaker D. Primary care for adults on the autism spectrum. *Med Clin North Am.* 2014; 98:1169.
57. Ibrahim SH, Voigt RG, Katusic SK, Weaver AL, Barbaresi WJ. Incidence of gastrointestinal symptoms in children with autism: a population-based study. *Pediatrics.* 2009; 124:680.
58. Mouridsen SE, Isager T, Rich B. Diseases of the gastrointestinal tract in individuals diagnosed as children with atypical autism: a Danish register study based on hospital diagnoses. *Autism.* 2013; 17:55.
59. Chaidez V, Hansen RL, Hertz-Picciotto I. Gastrointestinal problems in children with autism, developmental delays or typical development. *J Autism Dev Disord.* 2014; 44:1117.
60. McElhanon BO, McCracken C, Karpen S, Sharp WG. Gastrointestinal symptoms in autism spectrum disorder: a meta-analysis. *Pediatrics.* 2014; 133:872.
61. Hsiao EY. Gastrointestinal issues in autism spectrum disorder. *Harv Rev Psychiatry.* 2014; 22:104.
62. Williams BL, Hornig M, Buie T, et al. Impaired carbohydrate digestion and transport and mucosal dysbiosis in the intestines of children with autism and gastrointestinal disturbances. *PLoS One.* 2011; 6(9):e24585.
63. Kang V, Wagner GC, Ming X. Gastrointestinal dysfunction in children with autism spectrum disorders. *Autism Res.* 2014; 7:501.
64. Coury DL, Ashwood P, Fasano A, et al. Gastrointestinal conditions in children with autism spectrum disorder: developing a research agenda. *Pediatrics.* 2012; 130(suppl 2):S160.
65. Bresnahan M, Hornig M, Schultz AF, et al. Association of maternal report of infant and toddler gastrointestinal symptoms with autism: evidence from a prospective birth cohort. *JAMA Psychiatry.* 2015; 72:466.
66. Gorrindo P, Williams KC, Lee EB, Walker LS, McGrew SG, Levitt P. Gastrointestinal dysfunction in autism: parental report, clinical evaluation, and associated factors. *Autism Res.* 2012; 5:101.
67. Mouridsen SE, Rich B, Isager T. A longitudinal study of gastrointestinal diseases in individuals diagnosed with infantile autism as children. *Child Care Health Dev.* 2010; 36:437.
68. Buie T, Campbell DB, Fuchs GJ III, et al. Evaluation, diagnosis, and treatment of gastrointestinal disorders in individuals with ASDs: a consensus report. *Pediatrics.* 2010; 125(suppl 1):S1.
69. Buie T, Fuchs GJ III, Furuta GT, et al. Recommendations for evaluation and treatment of common gastrointestinal problems in children with ASDs. *Pediatrics.* 2010; 125(suppl 1):S19.
70. Berry RC, Novak P, Withrow N, et al. Nutrition management of gastrointestinal symptoms in children with autism spectrum disorder: guideline from an expert panel. *J Acad Nutr Diet.* 2015; 115:1919.
71. Furuta GT, Williams K, Kooros K, et al. Management of constipation in children and adolescents with autism spectrum disorders. *Pediatrics.* 2012; 130(suppl 2):S98.
72. Samsam M, Ahangari R, Naser SA. Pathophysiology of autism spectrum disorders: revisiting gastrointestinal involvement and immune imbalance. *World J Gastroenterol.* 2014; 20:9942.
73. Mayer EA, Tillisch K, Gupta A. Gut/brain axis and the microbiota. *J Clin Invest.* 2015; 125:926.
74. Rosenfeld CS. Microbiome disturbances and autism spectrum disorders. *Drug Metab Dispos.* 2015; 43:1557.
75. Buie T. Potential etiologic factors of microbiome disruption in autism. *Clin Ther.* 2015; 37:976.
76. Gesundheit B, Rosenzweig JP, Naor D, et al. Immunological and autoimmune considerations of autism spectrum disorders. *J Autoimmun.* 2013; 44:1.

77. Onore C, Careaga M, Ashwood P. The role of immune dysfunction in the pathophysiology of autism. *Brain Behav Immun*. 2012; 26:383.
78. Liu Z, Li N, Neu J. Tight junctions, leaky intestines, and pediatric diseases. *Acta Paediatr.* 2005; 94:386.
79. Catalioto RM, Maggi CA, Giuliani S. Intestinal epithelial barrier dysfunction in disease and possible therapeutical interventions. *Curr Med Chem*. 2011; 18:398.
80. Kang DW, Park JG, Ilhan ZE, et al. Reduced incidence of *Prevotella* and other fermenters in intestinal microflora of autistic children. *PLoS One*. 2013; 8(7):e68322.
81. Fasano A. Intestinal permeability and its regulation by zonulin: diagnostic and therapeutic implications. *Clin Gastroenterol Hepatol*. 2012; 10:1096.
82. Tripathi A, Lammers KM, Goldblum S, et al. Identification of human zonulin, a physiological modulator of tight junctions, as prehaptoglobin-2. *Proc Natl Acad Sci U S A*. 2009; 106:16799.
83. Ludvigsson JF, Reichenberg A, Hultman C, Murray JA. A nationwide study of small intestinal histopathology and risk of autistic spectrum disorders. *JAMA Psychiatry.* 2013; 70:1224.
84. Lau NM, Green PHR, Taylor AK, et al. Markers of celiac disease and gluten sensitivity in children with autism. *PLoS One*. 2013; 8(6):e66155.
85. Buie T. The relationship of autism and gluten. *Clin Ther.* 2013; 35:578.
86. Nadon G, Feldman DE, Dunn W, Gisel E. Association of sensory processing and eating problems in children with autism spectrum disorders. *Autism Res Treat*. 2011; ??2011:541926.
87. Johnson CR, Turner K, Stewart PA, et al. Relationships between feeding problems, behavioral characteristics and nutritional quality in children with ASD. *J Autism Dev Disord*. 2014; 44:2175.
88. Barnevik Olsson M, Höglund Carlsson L, Westerlund J, Gillberg C, Fernell E. Autism before diagnosis: crying, feeding and sleeping problems in the first two years of life. *Acta Paediatrica*. 2013; 102:635.
89. Lindberg L, Bohlin G, Hagekull B. Early feeding problems in a normal population. *Int J Eat Disord.*1991; 10:395.
90. Bryant-Waugh R, Markham L, Kreipe RE, Walsh BT. Feeding and eating disorders in childhood. *Int J Eat Disord.* 2010; 43:98.
91. Cermak SA, Curtin C, Bandini LG. Food selectivity and sensory sensitivity in children with autism spectrum disorders. *J Am Diet Assoc*. 2010; 110:238.
92. Curtin C, Hubbard K, Anderson SE, Mick E, Must A, Bandini LG. Food selectivity, mealtime behavior problems, spousal stress, and family food choices in children with and without autism spectrum disorder. *J Autism Dev Disord.* 2015; 45:3308.
93. Sharp WG, Berry RC, McCracken C, et al. Feeding problems and nutrient intake in children with autism spectrum disorders: a meta-analysis and comprehensive review of the literature. *J Autism Dev Disord*. 2013; 43:2159.
94. Provost B, Lopez BR, Heimerl S. A comparison of motor delays in young children: autism spectrum disorder, developmental delay, and developmental concerns. *J Autism Dev Disord* 2007; 37:321.
95. Twachtman-Reilly J, Amaral SC, Zebrowski PP. Addressing feeding disorders in children on the autism spectrum in school-based settings: physiological and behavioral issues. *Lang Speech Hear Serv Sch*. 2008; 39:261.
96. Hubbard KL, Anderson SE, Curtin C, Must A, Bandini LG. A comparison of food refusal related to characteristics of food in children with autism spectrum disorder and typically developing children. *J Acad Nutr Diet*. 2014; 114: 1981.
97. Marshall J, Ware R, Ziviani J, Hill RJ, Dodrill P. Efficacy of interventions to improve feeding difficulties in children with autism spectrum disorders: a systematic review and meta-analysis. *Child Care Health Dev.* 2015; 41:278.
98. Marí-Bauset S, Llopis-González A, Zazpe-García I, Marí-Sanchis A, Morales-Suárez-Varela M. Nutritional status of children with autism spectrum disorders (ASDs): a case-control study. *J Autism Dev Disord*. 2015; 45:203.
99. Emond A, Emmett P, Steer C, Golding J. Feeding symptoms, dietary patterns, and growth in young children with autism spectrum disorders. *Pediatrics*. 2010; 126:e337.
100. Shmaya Y, Eilat-Adar S, Leitner Y, Reif S, Gabis L. Nutritional deficiencies and overweight prevalence among children with autism spectrum disorder. *Res Dev Disabil.* 2015; 38:1.
101. Evans EW, Must A, Anderson SE, et al. Dietary patterns and body mass index in children with autism and typically developing children. *Res Autism Spectr Disord.* 2012; 6:399.
102. Coury DL, Anagnostou E, Manning-Courtney P, et al. Use of psychotropic medication in children and adolescents with autism spectrum disorders. *Pediatrics*. 2012; 130(suppl 2):S69.
103. Bandini LG, Gleason J, Curtain C, et al. Comparison of physical activity between children with autism spectrum disorders and typically developing children. *Autism.* 2013; 18:376.
104. Ekvall S, Fugazzi P, Stevens F, Ekvall V. Dietary intakes, growth and other characteristics in children with autism. *J Am Diet Assoc*. 2009; 109(suppl 3):A85.
105. Stewart PA, Hyman SL, Schmidt BL, et al. Dietary supplementation in children with autism spectrum disorders: common, insufficient, and excessive. *J Acad Nutr Diet.* 2015; 115:1237.
106. Neumeyer AM, Gates A, Ferrone C, Lee H, Misra M. Bone density in peripubertal boys with autism spectrum disorders. *J Autism Dev Disord.* 2013; 43:1623.
107. Goulding A. Risk factors for fractures in normally active children and adolescents. *Med Sport Sci*. 2007; 51:102.
108. Schmidt RJ, Hansen RL, Hartiala J, et al. Selected vitamin D metabolic gene variants and risk for autism spectrum disorder in the CHARGE study. *Early Hum Dev*. 2015; 91:483.
109. Saad K, Abdel-rahman AA, Elserogy YM, et al. Vitamin D status in autism spectrum disorders and the efficacy of vitamin D supplementation in autistic children. *Nutr Neurosci*. 2015; Epub Apr 15. doi: http://dx.doi.org/10.1179/14768305 15Y.0000000019.
110. Hediger ML, England LJ, Molloy CA, Yu KF, Manning-Courtney P, Mills JL. Reduced bone cortical thickness in boys with autism or autism spectrum disorder. *J Autism Dev Disord.* 2008; 38:848.
111. Graf-Myles J, Farmer C, Thurm A, et al. Dietary adequacy of children with autism compared with controls and the impact of restricted diet. *J Dev Behav Pediatr*. 2013; 34:449.
112. Lange KW, Hauser J, Reissmann A. Gluten-free and casein-free diets in the therapy of autism. *Curr Opin Clin Nutr Metab Care*. 2015; 18:572.
113. Whiteley P, Haracopos D, Knivsberg AM, et al. The ScanBrit randomised, controlled, single-blind study of a gluten- and casein-free dietary intervention for children with autism spectrum disorders. *Nutr Neurosci*. 2010; 13:87.
114. Millward C, Ferriter M, Calver S, Connell-Jones G. Gluten- and casein-free diets for autistic spectrum disorder. *Cochrane Database Syst Rev*. 2008; (2):CD003498.
115. Whiteley P, Shattock P, Knivsberg AM, et al. Gluten- and casein-free dietary intervention for autism spectrum conditions. *Front Hum Neurosci*. 2013; 6:344.
116. Marí-Bauset S, Zazpe I, Marí-Sanchis A, Llopis-González A, Morales-Suárez-Varela M. Evidence of the gluten-free and casein-free diet in autism spectrum disorders: a systematic review. *J Child Neurol.* 2014; 29:1718.
117. Pedersen L, Parlar S, Kvist K, Whiteley P, Shattock P. Data mining the ScanBrit study of a gluten- and casein-free dietary intervention for children with autism spectrum disorders: behavioural and psychometric measures of dietary response. *Nutr Neurosci*. 2014;17:207.

# 14 The Fetal Alcohol Syndrome

AGNES M. HUBER AND SHIRLEY W. EKVALL

Ulleland et al., in Seattle, were the first in the United States to document that heavy alcohol consumption during pregnancy has a deleterious effect on the offspring.[1,2] The growth retardation, malformations, and central nervous system effects on infants exposed to alcohol in utero were identified by Jones et al.[3] as the fetal alcohol syndrome (FAS). Infants who show some symptoms of FAS but not the full constellation were defined as having fetal alcohol effects (FAE). Other terms have been proposed, such as alcohol-related birth defects (ARBD) or alcohol-related neurodevelopmental disorders (ARND). Because children with alcohol-related problems suffer from lifelong disabilities and because there is no safe level of alcohol ingestion by pregnant women, the American Academy of Pediatrics (AAP) has suggested that women who plan to become pregnant or are pregnant should abstain from alcohol during pregnancy.[4]

The incidence of FAS may be underreported. Surveys have shown variable rates of 0.9 to 1.9 per 1000 live births,[5] an incidence believed to be higher than that for Down syndrome or cerebral palsy. Newer data suggest incidence rates of 5.2 per 10,000 live births.[4] Among alcohol-abusing women, rates of FAS are on the order of 24 to 42 per 1000 for the Southwestern Apache and Ute tribes, 209 per 1000 in Ireland, and 259 per 1000 in Germany.[5] The incidence of FAE is thought to be 3 to 5 per 1000 births.[6]

Some studies have described incidence data in terms of fetal alcohol spectrum disorder (FASD), an umbrella term covering a wide range of alcohol-related birth defects of varying severity including FAS. Such studies indicate that FASD is responsible for up to 50% of disability at birth in the United Kingdom. The FASD is identified by compromised growth, health, behavior, and cognitive abilities. The analysis by Morelo in 2011 using FASD indicated underreporting in a hospital study.[7] Ospina et al. systematically reviewed the prevalence of this entity in Canada for the Institute of Health Economics.[8]

The principal features of FAS are summarized in Tables 14–1 and 14–2 based on data from Clarren and Smith.[9] Microcephaly, abnormal weight, and abnormal length are recognized at birth, as are the dysmorphic facial features.

The effects of ethanol on birth weight depend to some degree on the amount and timing of alcohol intake by the mother during pregnancy.[10] A report by Little et al.[11] on pregnancy outcome of alcoholic mothers who abstained from alcohol during pregnancy indicated that the birth weight of their infants was still decreased. Reduced birth weight is also associated with a reduced brain weight, as has been shown in an animal model of FAS.[12]

Teratogenic effects of alcohol abuse by pregnant women are thought to be most damaging during the first 8 weeks of pregnancy, when organogenesis occurs. During this period, when many women are not yet aware of their pregnancy, even a single binge-drinking episode is capable of damaging the embryo at a critical period of development. Such teratogenic effects are not reversible and can lead to lifelong compromise in growth, health, behavior, and cognitive abilities.[13]

## BIOCHEMICAL ABNORMALITIES

Alcohol readily crosses the placenta and accumulates in higher concentration in the fetus because of its high water content. Alcohol remains longer in the fetal circulation because of the low alcohol dehydrogenase level in the immature liver.[14] As is well known, alcohol has innumerable detrimental effects on metabolism and is toxic to the brain. The microcephaly of FAS infants is thought to be caused by a variety of alcohol effects during development. Olney et al.,[15] for example, showed that ethanol blocks *N*-methyl-D-aspartate (NMDA) glutamate receptors and promotes gamma-aminobutyric acid A (GABA-A) receptor activation in many parts of the brain. These processes trigger widespread neurodegeneration, causing neurons to self-destruct (apoptosis). Astroglia cells that are responsible for mitotic signaling seem particularly sensitive to the toxic effects of comparatively low levels of alcohol.[16] Such neurotoxic effects, which are nonreversible, lead to long-term dysfunction in children and adults.[17,18] The vasculature is also sensitive to alcohol. Intake by the mother of only 1½ drinks has been shown to lead to impairment of the umbilical circulation, resulting in hypoxia and hypoglycemia in the fetus.[19] The hypoglycemia in the brain is further aggravated by decreased liver storage of glycogen, resulting in hypoglycemia in the neonatal period.[20]

Alcohol can interfere with hormones, growth factors, and the immune system, and it has a variety of drug-nutrient interactions. Of special interest is the interaction between alcohol and zinc. In a study by Lillien et al.[21] of a large population of pregnant women, 48% had suboptimal zinc intakes. Low plasma zinc levels in pregnancy were reported by Flynn and co-workers.[22] Zinc deficiency has been reported to act as a co-teratogen with alcohol.[23,24] When both conditions were present at the same time, malformation and growth depression in the offspring were much more pronounced than those caused by alcohol or zinc-deficiency alone. Low zinc states in alcoholic pregnant mothers are caused not only by low dietary zinc intakes but also by decreased zinc retention due to liver damage and excess urinary loss. Children with FAS exposed to intrauterine alcohol similarly have a decreased plasma zinc level and elevated zinc excretion, probably due to liver damage caused by alcohol exposure.[25]

Many other cellular effects of alcohol have been and are still being investigated. These range from depression of adenosine triphosphate (ATP)-activated sodium transport systems, abnormal mitochondrial action, and interference with protein synthesis[26] to hormonal changes,[27] autoimmune responses,[28] potential teratogenic effects of prostaglandins,[29] and altered ganglioside-catabolizing enzymes.[30]

## FACTORS TO BE CONSIDERED IN NUTRITIONAL AND OTHER EVALUATIONS

Most of the structural and many behavioral signs of FAS can be recognized at birth.[13] However, because some features characteristic of FAS apply also to other diagnoses, the mother's drinking history during pregnancy is an important part of the clinical diagnosis. The prenatal detection of significant alcohol exposure is possible by measurement of maternal blood markers, which appears better than self-reporting methods. Stoler et al.[31] tested for blood acetaldehyde and carbohydrate-deficient transferrin, gama-glutamyl transpeptidase, and mean red blood cell volume and found that two or more positive markers were predictive of a pregnancy outcome with lower birth weight, smaller head circumference, and smaller length of the newborn infant. Some researchers have suggested that FAS can be identified with high accuracy with a standardized method of morphometric analysis.[32] A cortical gray matter asymmetry pattern in adolescents with heavy prenatal alcohol exposure revealed significant cortical abnormalities

**Table 14–1.** Principal Features of the Fetal Alcohol Syndrome

| Feature |
|---|
| Mild to moderate mental retardation |
| Microcephaly* |
| Poor coordination, hypotonia† |
| Irritability in infancy* |
| Hyperactivity in childhood† |
| Less than 2 SD for length and weight at birth* |
| Less than 2 SD for length and weight postnatally* |
| Disproportionately diminished adipose tissue† |
| Eyes—short palpebral fissures* |
| Short, upturned nose† |
| Hypoplastic philtrum* |
| Hypoplastic maxilla† |
| Mouth—thin upper vermillion, retrognathia* |
| Micrognathia or relative prognathia in adolescence* |

*in more than 80% of patients
†in more than 50% of patients
From Clarren and Smith. Used with permission.

that were consistent with cognitive dysfunction.[33] The phenotype of FAS in adolescents and older adults is often difficult to recognize.

Children affected by prenatal alcohol exposure may have cognitive problems involving memory, comprehension, and understanding. Behavioral problems including hyperactivity, aggressiveness, and destructiveness have been described, and many children with FAS are difficult to handle on a day-to-day basis.[34] Because of the variety of abnormalities in FAS and FAE, it has sometimes been difficult to diagnose the defects specifically related to alcohol, even when the amounts and timing of alcohol exposure were known from the mother's drinking history.

Four teratogenic outcomes of alcohol have been suggested: a dose-responsive effect on functional abnormalities, growth deficiency, malformations, and embryolethal effects. High alcohol exposure may produce malformations. Lower doses may produce growth abnormalities, and even lower doses produce functional abnormalities. Although FAS is related to heavy drinking throughout pregnancy, the amount and timing of binge or social drinking by pregnant women can have variable damaging effects in the offspring.[24]

## MANAGEMENT

The AAP has suggested that infants with FAS or FAE should be seen by a pediatrician who is knowledgeable and competent in the evaluation of neurodevelopmental and psychosocial problems associated with the diagnosis. This usually requires a pediatric medical specialist and referral to early intervention services. Educational services may be provided under the Individuals with Disabilities Education Act (IDEA).[4] According to Streissguth and LeDuc,[35] the developmental work should include a thorough physical examination, a family history in view of support services, a psychological/educational evaluation, and, at an appropriate age, a vocational training and developmental disability evaluation. One study found that, in order to assess the level of risk for having a child with FAS, one must conduct full behavioral, genetic, current, and lifelong nutritional history evaluations, as well as an evaluation of the body mass index.

The prenatal growth retardation of infants with FAS persists postnatally, and some infants may have failure to thrive. Infants may have a poor suck and may be difficult to feed. In severe cases in which oral food intake is insufficient, a gastrostomy tube may be needed to improve food intake and growth.

Infants with FAS are hypotonic and may exhibit irregular wake-sleep patterns. Their characteristic craniofacial features identified at birth persist throughout life. Organ and skeletal abnormalities may be identified at birth or when the child is older. Early diagnosis of FAS and FAE and definition of the child's problems are necessary to prevent secondary problems. Growth and development should be assessed throughout childhood and the teen years. Because children with FAS and FAE are highly variable in their developmental, behavioral, nutritional, and other problems, they must be assessed individually. Day et al.[37] found that at 3 years of age, children exposed to alcohol prenatally did not exhibit catch-up growth and had slower rates of growth in weight, length, and head circumference in addition to physical abnormalities. Case histories and follow-up studies of children with FAS have been published by Barnett and Shusterman,[38] Lindor et al.,[39] Streissguth et al.,[40] Gardner,[34] and Kaminski,[41] among others.

## PREVENTION AND FOLLOW-UP

The data show clearly that heavy drinking during pregnancy interferes with normal fetal growth and development. That lower intakes of alcohol and/or occasional binge drinking are harmful to the unborn is less well documented because the effects of alcohol are difficult to separate from those of nutrition, smoking, and other factors.[42] However, because alcohol intake by a pregnant mother always poses a risk for the developing embryo and fetus, the National Task Force on FAS and FAE,[43] the AAP,[4] and the Centers for Disease Control and Prevention[44] all recommend that women who are pregnant or who are planning to become pregnant should abstain from alcohol.

Prenatal exposure to alcohol is considered one of the leading preventable causes of birth defects, mental retardation, and neurodevelopmental disorders. The costs of medical, custodial, educational, and long-term follow up services to the child and the child's family and society are enormous. Because prenatal exposure to alcohol is one of the leading preventable causes of mental retardation, the AAP[4] recommends, among other points, the following:

1. When a child with FAS or FAE is diagnosed, age-appropriate evaluations, follow-up visits, and referrals such as "early intervention" and other support services should be planned by the involved health professionals and the family.
2. Efforts should be made at all levels of society (schools, colleges, adults) to educate the public about the deleterious consequences of alcohol for the unborn child.
3. Women who are pregnant or are planning to become pregnant should abstain from alcohol.

**Table 14–2.** Associated Features of the Fetal Alcohol Syndrome

| Area | Frequent* | Occasional† |
|---|---|---|
| Eyes | Ptosis, strabismus, epicanthal folds | Myopia, clinical microphthalmia, blepharophimosis |
| Ears | Posterior rotation | Poorly formed concha |
| Mouth | Prominent lateral palatine ridges | Cleft lip or cleft palate, small teeth with faulty enamel |
| Cardiac | Murmurs | Ventricular septal defect, great vessel anomalies, tetralogy of Fallot |
| Renogenital | Labial hyperplasia | Hypospadias, small rotated kidneys, hydronephrosis |
| Cutaneous | Hemangiomas | Hirsutism in infancy |
| Skeletal | Aberrant palmar | Limited joint movement, nail hypoplasia, polydactyly, radioulnar, synostosis, pectus carinatum, bifid xiphoid |
| Muscular | | Hernias of diaphragm, umbilicus or groin, distal recti |

*Reported in 26% to 50% of patients.
†Reported in 1% to 25% of patients.
From Clarren and Smith.[9] Used with permission.

4. Health professionals caring for newborns should increase their awareness of FAS and FAE including diagnosis and prevention.
5. Parents of a child with alcohol-related developmental problems should receive appropriate anticipatory guidance toward preventing similar problems in the future.

## References


1. Ulleland CN, Wenneberg RP, Igo RP, Smith NJ. The offspring of alcoholic mothers. *Pediatr Res.* 1970; 4:474.
2. Ulleland CN. The offspring of alcoholic mothers. *Ann N Y Acad Sci.* 1972; 197:167.
3. Jones KL, Smith DW, Ulleland CN, Streissguth A. Pattern of malnutrition in offspring of chronic alcoholic mothers. *Lancet.* 1973: 1:1267.
4. American Academy of Pediatrics. Committee on Substance Abuse and Committee on Children with Disabilities. Fetal alcohol syndrome and alcohol-related neurodevelopmental disorders. *Pediatrics.* 2000; 106:358.
5. Abel EL, Sokol RJ. Incidence of FAS and economic impacts of FAS-related anomalies. *Drug Alcohol Depend.* 1987; 19:51.
6. Smith DW, Jones KL, Hansen JW. Perspectives on the cause and frequency of the fetal alcohol syndrome. *Ann N Y Acad Sci.* 1976; 273:138.
7. Morelo M, Woolfall K, Dedman D, et al. Underreporting of fetal alcohol spectrum disorders and analysis of hospital episode statistics. *BMC Pediatr.* 2011; 11:14.
8. Ospina M, Dennett L. *Systematic Review on the Prevalence of Fetal Alcohol Spectrum Disorders.* Edmonton, Alberta: Council Institute of Health Economics, 2013.
9. Clarren SK, Smith DW. The fetal alcohol syndrome. *N Engl J Med.* 1978; 298:1063.
10. Mills JL, Graubard BI, Harley EE, Rhoades GG, Berendes HW. Maternal alcohol consumption and birth-weight: how much drinking during pregnancy is safe? *JAMA.* 1984; 252:1875.
11. Little RE, Streissguth AP, Barr HM, Herman CS. Decreased birth-weight in infants of alcoholic women who abstained during pregnancy. *J Pediatr.* 1980; 96:974.
12. Tran TD, Cronise K, Marino MD, Jenkins WJ, Kelly SJ. Critical periods for the effects of alcohol exposure on brain weight, body weight, activity and investigation. *Behav Brain Res.* 2000; 116:99.
13. Hannigan JH, Armant DR. Alcohol in pregnancy and neonatal outcome. *Semin Neonatal.* 2000; 5:243.
14. Pikkarainen PH, Raiha NCR. Development of alcohol dehydrogenase activity in the human liver. *Pediatr Res.* 1967; 1:165.
15. Olney JW, Wozniak DF, Jevtovic-Todorovic V, Faber NB, Bittigau P, Ikonomidou C. Drug-induced apoptotic neuro-degeneration in the developing brain. *Brain Pathol.* 2002; 12:488.
16. Costa LG, Guizzetti M. Inhibition of muscarinic receptor-induced proliferation of astroglial cells by ethanol: mechanisms and implications for the fetal alcohol syndrome. *Neurotoxicology.* 2002; 23:685.
17. Monnot M, Lovallo WR, Nixon SJ, Ross E. Neurological basis of deficits in affective prosody comprehension among alcoholics and fetal alcohol–exposed adults. *J Neuropsychiatry Clin Neurosci.* 2002; 14(3):321.
18. Day NL, Leech SL, Richardson GA, Cornelius MD, Robles N, Larkby C. Prenatal alcohol exposure predicts continued deficits in offspring size at 14 years of age. *Alcohol Clin Exp Res.* 2002; 26:1584.
19. Altura BM, Altura BT, Carella A, Chatterjee M, Halevy S, Tejani N. Alcohol produces spasms of human umbilical blood vessels: relationship to fetal alcohol syndrome. *Eur J Pharmacol.* 1982; 86:311.
20. Witek-Januseke L. Maternal ethanol ingestion: effect on maternal and neonatal glucose balance. *Am J Physiol.* 1986; 251:E178.
21. Lillien LJ, Huber AM, Rajala MM. Diet and ethanol intake during pregnancy. *J Am Diet Assoc.* 1982: 81:252.
22. Flynn A, Martier SS, Sokol RJ, Miller SI, Golden NL, Del Villano BC. Zinc status of pregnant alcoholic women: a determinant of fetal outcome. *Lancet.* 1981; 1:572.
23. Keppen LD, Pysher T, Rennert OM. Zinc deficiency acts as a co-teratogen with alcohol in fetal alcohol syndrome. *Pediatr Res.* 1985; 19:944.
24. Keppen L, Moore D, Cannon D. Zinc nutrition in fetal alcohol syndrome. *Neurotoxicology.* 1990; 11:375.
25. Assadi FK, Ziai M. Zinc status of infants with fetal alcohol syndrome. *Pediatr Res.* 1986; 20:551.
26. Abel EL. Prenatal effects of alcohol on growth: a brief overview. *Fed Proc.* 1985; 44:2318.
27. Root AW, Reiter EO, Andriola M, Duckett G. Hypothalamic-pituitary function in the fetal alcohol syndrome. *J Pediatr.* 1975; 87:585.
28. Foster JW. Possible maternal autoimmune component in the etiology of the fetal alcohol syndrome. *Dev Med Child Neurol.* 1986; 5:654.
29. Randall CL, Anton RF, Becker HC. Alcohol, pregnancy and prostaglandins. *Alcoholism.* 1987; 11:32.
30. Prasad VV. Maternal alcohol consumption and undernutrition in the rat: effects on gangliosides and their catabolizing enzymes in the CNS of newborns. *Neurochem Res.* 1989; 14:1081.
31. Stoler JM, Huntington KS, Peterson CM, et al. The prenatal detection of significant alcohol exposure with maternal blood markers. *J Pediatr.* 1998; 133:346.
32. Clarren SK, Sampson PD, Larsen J, et al. Effects of fetal alcohol exposure assessment by photographs and morphometric analysis. *Am J Med Genet.* 1987; 26:651.
33. Sowell ER, Thompson PM, Peterson BS, et al. Mapping cortical gray matter asymmetry patterns in adolescents with heavy prenatal alcohol exposure. *Neuroimage.* 2002; 17:1807.
34. Gardner J. Living with a child with fetal alcohol syndrome. *MCN Am J Matern Child Nurs.* 2000; 25:252.
35. Streissguth AP, LaDue RA. Fetal alcohol syndrome and fetal alcohol effects: teratogenic causes of mental retardation and developmental disabilities. In: Schroeder SR, ed. *Toxic Substances and Mental Retardation.* Washington, DC: American Association on Mental Deficiency; 1987.
36. May PA, Gossage JP, White-Country M, et al. Alcohol consumption and other material risk factors for fetal alcohol syndrome among three distinct samples of women before, during, and after pregnancy: the risk is relative. *Am J Med Genet.* 2004; 127C(1):10.
37. Day NL, Robles N, Richardson G, et al. The effects of prenatal alcohol use on the growth of children at three years of age. *Alcohol Clin Exp Res.* 1991; 15:67.
38. Barnett R, Shusterman S. Fetal alcohol syndrome: a review of literature and report of cases. *J Am Dent Assoc.* 1985: 111:591.
39. Lindor E, McCarthy A, McRae MG. Fetal alcohol syndrome: a review and case presentation. *J Obstet Gynecol Neonatal Nurs.* 1980; 2:222.
40. Streissguth AP, Clarren SK, Jones KL. Natural history of the fetal alcohol syndrome: a ten-year follow-up of eleven patients. *Lancet.* 1985; 2:85.
41. Kaminski M. EUROMAC: a European concerted action. Maternal alcohol consumption and its relation to the outcome of pregnancy and child development at 18 months: relation of findings to other studies. *Int J Epidemiol.* 1992; 21(suppl 1):S79.
42. Cornelius MD, Goldschmidt L, Day NL, Larkby C. Alcohol, tobacco and marijuana use among pregnant teenagers: 6-year follow-up of offspring growth effects. *Neurotoxicol Teratol.* 2002; 24:703.
43. Weber MK, Floyd RL, Riley EP, Snider DE Jr. National Task Force on Fetal Alcohol Syndrome and Fetal Alcohol Effect: defining the national agenda for fetal alcohol syndrome and other prenatal alcohol-related effects. *MMWR Morb Mortal Recomm Rep.* 2002; 51(RR-14):9.
44. Centers for Disease Control and Prevention. Surveillance for fetal alcohol syndrome using multiple sources—Atlanta, GA, 1981–1989. *MMWR Morb Mortal Wkly Rep.* 1997; 46:1118.

# 15 Down Syndrome

PATRICIA D. JACKSON, MELINDA WENDLAND, AND SHIRLEY W. EKVALL

Down syndrome (DS) is a genetic disorder that is caused when abnormal cell division results in extra chromosome 21 material. It is the most common chromosomal disorder, occurring in approximately 1 of every 700 live births.[1] The DNA sequence of human chromosome 21 was published in 2000[2] and was predicted to contain 225 genes. In 2011, 696 genes were identified on chromosome 21, and the specific functions of half of them remain unclear.[3] Despite the rapid increase in knowledge of chromosome 21, the mechanisms by which trisomy, and therefore increased gene dosage, results in the characteristic phenotype remain a research challenge.

## PHYSICAL, BIOCHEMICAL, AND OTHER ABNORMALITIES

A presumptive diagnosis of DS is usually made by a physician or other hospital staff member shortly after the child is born. Common physical findings are hypotonia; a small, brachycephalic head; facial features including upward-slanting palpebral fissures, epicanthal folds, Brushfield spots, flat nasal bridge, small ears, and small mouth; excessive skin at the nape of the neck; and a single palmar transverse crease. A karyotype performed on blood lymphocytes or skin fibroblasts is mandatory to confirm the diagnosis, even in cases in which the phenotypic appearance is obvious. Early chromosomal diagnosis, if possible within 48 hours, has been shown to be helpful for parents. For purposes of genetic counseling, it is critical to distinguish complete trisomy 21 from trisomy 21 mosaicism or an unbalanced translocation.

A number of subtle physical differences are typical of children with DS. Some, in combination, may affect the acquisition of feeding skills and may present challenges that need to be addressed in the child's intervention plan if independent feeding is to be achieved. These physical features include midfacial (maxillary) hypoplasia, a small oral cavity, a high or narrow hard palate, relative macroglossia, a small mandible, and poor oromuscular control resulting in early problems. Many babies with DS are born preterm and develop jaundice during the newborn period. The lethargy associated with jaundice can affect early feeding. The mother's feelings and positive attitude toward her newborn infant, as well as the attitude of those around her, also influences the success in establishing breast-feeding.

Delayed or abnormal dentition, malocclusion, nasal congestion, small hands, and short fingers (Fig. 15–1) can contribute to problems at later developmental stages.

Because of poor postural control and general hypotonia of the muscles, babies with DS are more commonly affected by gastroesophageal reflux, which can be painful and can result in the baby's having a negative early experience of feeding.

Additionally, certain medical conditions are more prevalent in children with DS, and these can affect their general health and ability to feed and gain weight appropriately.

The development of standardized growth charts in the United Kingdom for children with DS[4,5] has greatly enhanced clinicians' ability to properly anticipate appropriate weight gain for children in the early years and particularly as they approach adolescence.[6] In the United States, DS growth charts developed by Cronk and colleagues in 1988 were included by the American Academy of Pediatrics (AAP) in their 2001 report.[7] In 2011, however, the AAP recommended using standard weight and height growth charts in lieu of specialty charts for DS, along with monitoring the child's body mass index (BMI) and ensuring a healthy diet.[8] Some centers choose to look at both the DS growth charts and those from the Centers for Disease Control and Prevention (CDC) growth charts in comparison, for the parents' interest. Growth and weight trajectories are monitored on the World Health Organization (WHO) growth charts for 0 to 2 years of age and on the CDC charts for 2 to 20 years of age.[9]

Guidelines for regular health maintenance and preventive medical screening have been produced by the AAP and the Down Syndrome Medical Interest Group (DSMIG).[8,10] DS-specific information including growth charts is available in the United Kingdom as a supplement to standard Parent Held Record Books.[11]

These evidence-based guidelines suggest active surveillance for those health conditions known to be more common in children with DS and heightened awareness by clinicians of those health problems that may be more challenging to diagnose unless actively considered.

## ASSOCIATED MEDICAL CONDITIONS

Conditions associated with DS can be categorized as congenital, acquired, or age related.[12]

### Congenital Heart Defects

Congenital heart defects occur in 40% to 60% of newborns with DS.[13] The most common cardiac lesions are atrioventricular septal defect (50%), isolated ventricular septal defect or atrial septal defect (40%), and tetralogy of Fallot (7%).[14] Cardiac defects are responsible for significant morbidity and mortality during the first year of life, or until surgical repair can be achieved. Congenital heart disease is often associated with congestive heart failure, pulmonary hypertension, chronic valvular dysfunction, and poor growth. In adolescence, mitral stenosis or aortic regurgitation can also become apparent.[15]

### Gastrointestinal Problems

#### Gastrointestinal Tract Anomalies

Gastrointestinal tract anomalies are seen in approximately 12% of newborns with DS and commonly include tracheoesophageal fistula, esophageal atresia, duodenal atresia, imperforate anus, malrotation, and Hirschsprung disease. These conditions often require nasogastric or gastric tube feeding, parenteral nutrition, and multiple surgical procedures during the first 2 years of life.

#### Gastroesophageal Reflux

Gastroesophageal reflux, as well as causing discomfort, may contribute to cardiorespiratory problems and failure to thrive. Treatment for reflux should be the same as for all children but more prompt if suspected in a child with DS.[16]

#### Feeding Problems

Infants with DS can usually be breast-fed as well as formula-fed. Some infants require early supplementation until a successful nursing pattern is established. Some infants sleep for prolonged periods and need to be awakened for feedings to maintain adequate calorie intake.[8] In children with DS, feeding patterns should proceed according to the child's developmental readiness. Professional help from a dietitian may be

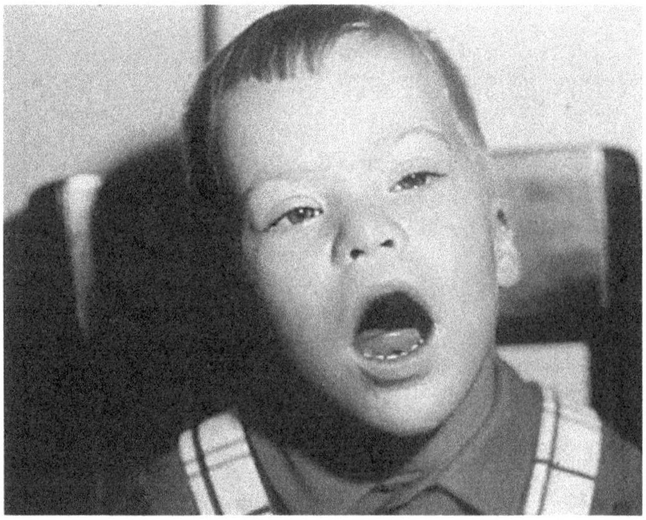

**Figure 15–1.** Boy with Down syndrome.

needed so that nutritious food is added at the proper time to facilitate oral motor development, especially when breast-feeding.

### Constipation

In children with DS, there is an increased risk of constipation related to hypotonia. If constipation is present, the child should be evaluated for restricted diet, limited fluid intake, and gastrointestinal tract malformations, including stenoses or Hirschsprung disease, for which there is an increased risk.[17] A diet with adequate fluids, fiber (particularly psyllium based), prunes or prune juice, fresh vegetables, fruits, and whole grains is required (see Chapter 36).

### Celiac Disease

Celiac disease is an immune-related disorder that is variously reported to be more common in children with DS. In any child, it results in reduction of the growth trajectory and development of gut-related symptoms.[18–21] There is debate as to whether children should be actively screened for this disorder, and a variety of practices exist in different parts of the world.

In the United States, celiac disease is thought to affect 5% of children with DS, and screening of symptomatic children is recommended[8]. Clinicians should have a high level of alertness for the condition, and children should be tested if they present with symptoms suggestive of the disorder, such as anemia, bloating or abdominal pain, diarrhea, protracted constipation, slow growth, or failure to thrive.

## Ophthalmic Problems

### Congenital Cataracts

Congenital cataracts are seen in about 2% of DS newborns; if significant in size, they require surgical removal.[22] There is also an increased incidence of ophthalmological conditions which may manifest during the first years of life, including strabismus, refractive errors, nystagmus, astigmatism, amblyopia, blepharitis, keratoconus, ptosis, and nasolacrimal duct obstruction.

## Pulmonary Problems

### Respiratory Infections

Infants (1–12 months) are susceptible to both viral and bacterial infections of the lower respiratory tract (e.g., bronchiolitis, pneumonia), which may be a significant cause of morbidity during infancy, particularly in those with uncorrected cardiac disease.[23] Recurrent upper respiratory tract infections such as otitis media, sinusitis, and rhinitis are chronic problems for many children but tend to become less common with age and growth of the craniofacial and upper respiratory structures.

### Sleep Problems

Sleep-disordered breathing, including obstructive sleep apnea is seen in 50% to 80% of children with DS.[24] Factors that predispose children with DS to obstructive sleep apnea include a small oral cavity with relative macroglossia, narrowing of the upper airway, hypotonia of the pharyngeal muscles, chronic rhinitis, enlarged tonsils or adenoids, and obesity.

## Hearing Problems

Transient or intermittent conductive hearing loss is usually the result of occult middle ear effusions, otitis media, or impacted cerumen and may affect up to 75% of children with DS in the preschool years. Sensorineural and mixed hearing loss are also seen.[25]

## Endocrine Disorders

### Congenital Hypothyroidism

Congenital hypothyroidism due to absence or aplasia of the thyroid gland occurs in about 1% of DS newborns and requires consideration of hormone replacement. The transient elevation in thyroid-stimulating hormone (TSH) sometimes observed in infants and in children up to 2 years of age may be caused by physiological dysregulation of the hypothalamic-pituitary-thyroid axis.

Disorders of thyroid function are particularly common during childhood, again related to immune dysfunction. Regular monitoring will identify any increase in TSH and any decrease in thyroxine ($T_4$), so that early replacement therapy with thyroxine can be introduced. Acquired hypothyroidism is seen in 4% to 18% of DS children.[26] Studies suggest variation internationally. Both compensated hypothyroidism (i.e., with elevated TSH and normal $T_4$) and uncompensated hypothyroidism (elevated TSH and decreased $T_4$) are seen; less commonly, hyperthyroidism leading to acute weight loss is present.

### Diabetes

As in the mainstream population, type 1 diabetes is more common in children and type 2 in adults with DS. Type 2 diabetes is associated with insulin resistance and obesity and is being seen more now at younger ages. Reports suggest that diabetes is three to four times more common in those affected with DS.[27]

Type 1 diabetes is related to autoimmune dysregulation, and has peaks at ages 2 and 12 years. Its appearance indicates the need for dietary control and insulin replacement for the child.[28]

Type 2 diabetes is influenced by the child's diet and poor weight regulation, so preventing obesity in this high-risk population should be a clear nutritional aim.

## Blood Disorders

### Leukemia

Transient myeloproliferative disorder (TMD) is sometimes seen in DS children in the first few months of life. An elevated peripheral blood leukocyte count with a predominance of "blast" forms may make this condition difficult to distinguish from true congenital leukemia.[29] Newborns with TMD are at increased risk of developing acute myeloid leukemia (AML) before 5 years of age. Ongoing studies are investigating how to predict which children may move into the high-risk group for childhood leukemia.[30]

Children with DS account for approximately 2% of all cases of acute leukemia in children. Acute myelocytic leukemia (AML) is most common in children younger than 3 years of age, whereas acute lymphocytic leukemia (ALL) is more common in older children. Within the AML group, there is an increased incidence of children with a previous history of TMD.

## Musculoskeletal Problems

### Congenital Anomalies

Children with DS are susceptible to subluxation of the hip, patella, and cervical spine. Up to 15% of children show radiographic evidence of asymptomatic C1/C2 instability, which is determined by measuring the atlantodens interval (ADI) on lateral neck radiographs. Increased atlanto-occipital instability and congenital anomalies of the craniovertebral junction and cervical spine have also been reported.

### Arthritis

Arthritis of the small joints, again an autoimmune-based disorder, is also common. Usually it is polyarticular in nature, and often the diagnosis is made late.[31]

### Epilepsy

Infantile spasms or myoclonic seizures may occur in 1% to 13% of children with DS. Seizure disorder prevalence in childhood is reported to be between 5% and 13%. Diagnosis is difficult, and false-positive diagnoses are not uncommon.

### Dental Issues

The order of appearance and distribution of teeth may vary, and dental problems are common, with teeth being more susceptible to decay related to reduced salivary flow. Attention to dental hygiene is important, as is the avoidance of sugary foods and drinks.

### Growth

The growth trajectory and final level achieved are always affected in children with DS. Early weight gain may be slow, and poor growth is often compounded by prematurity.

Growth charts in the United Kingdom have been restandardized to better characterize childhood expected growth patterns for modern, noninstitutionalized children leading active lives. (Please see Appendices 2–3 and 2–4 for UK growth charts.)

The onset and progression of puberty are the same or only slightly delayed for adolescent boys with DS. The onset of menses and the duration of menstrual cycles are about the same for girls with DS as for girls in the general population. Females of child-bearing age should be considered fertile and require educational instruction about menstruation and reproduction and access to routine gynecological care. Onset of obesity is frequently observed during the preadolescent years and may be related in part to a decreased resting metabolic rate, as well as to limited lifestyle opportunities.

## FACTORS TO BE CONSIDERED IN NUTRITIONAL EVALUATION AND INTERVENTION

### Gene Effects

The complex ways in which underlying genetic differences affect individuals with DS remain unclear, but they have an influence on growth and development of the brain and other cellular growth.

Genes in the trisomic condition are involved in brain development, in neuronal cell-cell communication, and in metabolic processes influencing the brain.[32] The ways in which these processes are controlled and interact is complex, although increasing information is emerging from studies of the Down syndrome mouse (Ts65Dn) investigating the Down syndrome critical region (DSCR) on chromosome 21 and other pathways, including DNA methylation.[33–36]

Chromosome 21 harbors at least two genes that are involved in the development of Alzheimer's disease: *APP* (which encodes amyloid precursor protein) and *BACE2* (beta-site amyloid beta A4 precursor protein-cleaving enzyme 2). APP serves as a substrate for amyloid β-peptide (Aβ), a pathogenic amino acid peptide that can precipitate in extracellular plaques in the brain. Widespread Aβ-deposition is the hallmark feature in Alzheimer's disease and results in profound neurodegeneration.[37,38]

Gene dosage effects for *APP*, copper-zinc superoxide dismutase (*SOD1*), and cystathionine β-synthase (*CBS*), have previously been researched,[39,40] SOD1 is a key enzyme in the metabolism of oxygen, catalyzing the dismutation of the superoxide free radical to oxygen and hydrogen peroxide, with the latter normally being cleared by the action of catalase and glutathione peroxidase (GPx). In the brain, however, catalase activity is low and most of the hydrogen peroxide is cleared by GPx. If excess hydrogen peroxide is present in the brain, it theoretically can react with transition metals such as iron to form the highly reactive and toxic hydroxyl radical (Fenton reaction), which may then cause or contribute to the pathogenesis of DS. This theory has not been supported in the human clinical situation. The use of antioxidants to counteract possible enzyme dysfunction has been suggested, but there is no evidence that this is effective in altering clinical outcomes.

### Developmental Expectations

Neuromotor dysfunction (generalized hypotonia with diminished primitive and deep tendon reflexes) is characteristic of most newborns with DS, and delay in the acquisition of gross motor milestones is usually apparent to physicians and parents during the first year. There is considerable individual variation in the attainment of early motor milestones. Particularly severe neuromotor dysfunction may be seen in association with infantile spasms, recurrent pulmonary infections, uncorrected congenital heart defects, or extreme ligamentous laxity. The hypotonia and ligament laxity are thought to be caused by the increase in type VI collagen genes (*COL6A1* and *COL6A2*, mapped to C21q22.3).[41] This hypotonicity also affects mastication.[42]

Delays in fine motor milestones may be apparent by the end of the first year but may go unnoticed by parents and professionals, who tend to focus on gross motor skill achievement during this time. Delays in gross and fine motor skills may persist throughout the first few years of life but rarely create a serious mobility limitation for older children. However, these children frequently demonstrate difficulty with tasks requiring precision, sequencing, and motor coordination. As expectations for language and cognitive growth increase during the second year of life, delays become apparent to parents and professionals alike. Greater deficits in expressive (speech) skills relative to comprehension or visual-spatial skills are seen, and there is considerable individual variation in the onset and complexity of spoken language. Poor speech articulation may further contribute to communication difficulties during childhood. Most children with DS test in the low-mild to moderate range on tests of cognitive function by the time they enter elementary school at 5 or 6 years of age. Development, and therefore feeding skills, can also be significantly affected by comorbid behavioral problems such as autism or attention deficit disorder.

### Growth Potential

Many chromosomal disorders are associated with disruptions in cell proliferation that lead to reductions in embryonic cell number, resulting in growth restriction and short stature. Diminished cell number and density are often observed in tissues from persons with DS. Skeletal maturation, as measured by bone age, a commonly used index of biological growth in children, is often delayed. During infancy, bone maturation may be one to two standard deviations below normal, so that by the third year, 75% of children with DS show delayed bone age compared with chronological age controls. In older children and adolescents, bone age is typically delayed by 1 to 2 years. Studies show that children with DS maintain their growth in utero during the first trimester and up to 38 weeks' gestation, when growth slows markedly.[43]

Preterm birth is common in DS. Postdelivery weight loss of greater than 10% is often seen, and recovery is slower. Throughout infancy and the preschool years, reductions (approximately 20%) in linear growth become manifest, so that by the age of 3 years, 90% of children with DS are smaller than their non-DS peers. As childhood progresses, the rate of linear growth is reduced by only 5% to 10%, but disproportionate weight gain may become problematic, particularly for females entering preadolescence. Studies have also noted the effect of lack of sleep, which often is present in children with DS because of poorly established sleep hygiene or interrupted sleep due to sleep-disordered breathing. This leads to an increased tendency to obesity resulting from an imbalance of the leptin/ghrelin control system in children.[44] Beginning in preadolescence and throughout adolescence, deceleration in the rate of growth approaches 25% to 50%, with boys being more affected. The adolescent growth spurt is less marked, and final height may be achieved earlier than in the general population.[45] Final adult height is typically two to three standard deviations lower than in the general population. Height in males typically ranges between 140 and 160 cm, whereas the typical range for adult females is between 135 and 155 cm.

At different stages of the child's life, it is important to use the correct height and weight reference charts in addition to referring to standard growth charts. (Please see Appendices 2–3 and 2–4 for details of growth charts available and which ones to use at different stages).

### Chronic Illness

Chronic illness represents an additional risk factor for growth failure in children with DS. During childhood, it is frequently associated with energy deficiency and less so with deficiency of specific nutrients. Energy deficit often results from an imbalance among energy intake, energy expenditure, and energy losses. These three factors are in balance when energy intake equals expenditure plus loss. If intake exceeds expenditure + loss, linear growth and weight gain result; if intake is less than expenditure + loss, linear growth and weight gain become suboptimal.

As an example, a child with DS and uncorrected atrioventricular septal defect (atrioventricular canal) may have poor energy balance for several reasons. Decreased intake may be caused by poor sucking, easy fatigability, dyspnea, tachypnea, and reduced gastric capacity. Increased expenditure results from higher metabolic demands due to increased cardiac workload and lack of adipose tissue. Increased losses may result from edema, gastroesophageal reflux, and malabsorption of fats and proteins. Further examples of medical conditions associated with energy imbalance are provided in Table 15–1.

## DIETARY AND OTHER TREATMENTS

### Trace Metals

There have been several investigations of the status of trace metals in DS; most have concentrated on zinc and copper, which are components of SOD1, and selenium, which is a constituent of GPx. As discussed previously, these enzymes have important antioxidant functions, but their contribution to the features seen in individuals with DS is not straightforward. Individuals with DS have presented with alterations in free zinc concentration and in some of the proteins related to zinc homeostasis. A higher number of zinc-positive spots in the cytoplasm of trisomic astrocytes is reported in the murine model, but with a decrease in total intracellular free zinc concentration. Serum selenium concentrations have also been found to be altered.[46,47] The results for plasma copper concentrations have been conflicting.

### Vitamins

There have been reports of deficiencies, malabsorption, and abnormal metabolism of a number of vitamins in DS. These studies involved small numbers of subjects and were poorly controlled. Reported malabsorption or reduced serum concentrations of vitamins may result from the increased incidence of celiac disease in DS. No significant differences in serum concentrations of vitamin D metabolites were found.[48] Decreased concentrations of vitamin E, the major fat-soluble antioxidant, have been reported in plasma and in red cells of children with DS. This could be consistent with increased utilization of antioxidants to protect against an increased oxidative stress, but it could also be explained, at least in part, by poor nutrition.

### Supplementation

As discussed earlier, there is evidence that increased oxidative stress may play a role in the pathogenesis of DS.[49,50] This means that an excess of oxygen-derived free radicals could result in increased demand for antioxidant nutrients such as vitamins C and E, β-carotene, zinc, and selenium. Despite claims in the popular press that nutritional supplements can improve some of the outcomes associated with trisomy 21, we are not aware of any convincing data to support these claims. An interest in supplementation trials was prompted by Harrell et al.,[51] who investigated the use of a megavitamin/mineral preparation in children with learning difficulties. Sixteen subjects completed the study, of whom only four had DS. The authors reported dramatic improvements in IQ, growth, physical appearance, language, educational attainment, and general health in the treated subjects. A number of small trials followed. Two reviews have critically evaluated the evidence for supplementation with antioxidant nutrients, and both concluded that most of the studies had small numbers of subjects and serious failings.[52,53] Ani et al. reviewed seven randomized controlled trials involving a total of 161 individuals with DS aged 6 months to 40 years.[53] None of these studies revealed any improvement in IQ, physical appearance, or general health with antioxidant supplementation. In a review of 53 controlled trials[54] on the effects of vitamin $B_6$, niacin, and multivitamins on mental function in different clinical groups, including individuals with DS, no evidence could be found to support vitamin supplementation; almost all of the trials showed serious failings.

Because of mounting evidence for the role of oxidative stress and folate trapping in the pathogenesis of DS, a randomized controlled trial with sufficient statistical power was designed to evaluate the effects of supplementation with antioxidant nutrients and folinic acid early in life. This study, involving 200 subjects with DS younger than 7 months of age in the United Kingdom, showed no benefit to children from vitamin supplementation.[55]

### Energy and Nutrient Needs

Energy and nutrient needs may be based on height rather than weight. The child's intake of nutrients and foods that are good for the immune system, such as protein, zinc, and vitamins C, A, E and the B vitamins, should be evaluated frequently or at least during each clinic visit.

## FOLLOW-UP

Children with DS benefit from a healthy diet and regular exercise, as do all children, to prevent excessive weight gain.[56] Whether or not there are additional health issues or ongoing disorders such as celiac disease, diabetes, or thyroid problems, the nutritional needs of the child with DS should continue to be monitored. Regular monitoring of the four areas of nutrition assessment (i.e., diet, biochemistry, feeding, and anthropometry) is needed. Behavioral support and emotional support are also recommended as required.

**Table 15–1.** Medical Conditions Associated with Energy Imbalance in Down Syndrome

| Decreased Intake | Increased Expenditures | Increased Losses |
|---|---|---|
| Prematurity | Gastrointestinal and cardiac surgery | Gastroesophageal reflux |
| Uncoordinated suck reflex | Congestive heart failure | Celiac disease |
| Oral-motor dysfunction | Pulmonary disease | Short-gut syndrome |
| Gastroesophageal reflux | Chronic infections | |
| Gastrointestinal anomaly | Chemotherapy | |
| Congenital heart disease | Hyperthyroidism | |
| Infantile spasms | | |
| Chemotherapy | | |
| Food refusal | | |

## References


1. Lejeune J, Gautier M, Turpin R. Etude des chromosomes somatique de neuf enfants mongoliens. [Study of somatic chromosomes from 9 mongoloid children.] *C R Acad Sci (Paris)*. 1959; 248:1721.
2. Hattori M, Fujiyama A, Taylor T, Watanabe H, Yada T, Park HS. The DNA sequence of human chromosome 21. *Nature*. 2000; 405:311.
3. Kahlem P. Gene-dosage effect on chromosome 21 transcriptome in trisomy 21: implication in Down syndrome cognitive disorders. *Behav Genet*. 2006; 36:416.
4. Cronk C, Crocker AC, Pueschel SM, et al. Growth charts for children with Down syndrome: 1 month to 18 years of age. *Pediatrics*. 1988; 81:102.
5. Styles ME, Cole TJ, Dennis J, Preece MA. New cross sectional stature, weight, and head circumference references for Down's syndrome in the UK and Republic of Ireland. *Arch Dis Child*. 2002; 87(2):104.
6. Down Syndrome Medical Interest Group (DSMIG); Royal College of Paediatrics and Child Health. *UK (2011) Growth Charts for Children with Down Syndrome*. Available from Harlow Healthcare, Maxwell Street, South Shields, Tyne & Wear NE33 4PU. http://www.dsmig.org.uk/information-resources/growth-charts/ Accessed June 14, 2016.
7. American Academy of Pediatrics Committee on Genetics. American Academy of Pediatrics: Health supervision for children with Down syndrome. *Pediatrics*. 2001; 107:442.
8. Bull MJ; Committee on Genetics. Clinical report: health supervision for children with Down syndrome. *Pediatrics*. 2011; 128:393. http://pediatrics.aappublications.org/content/early/2011/07/21/peds.2011-1605. Accessed June 14, 2016.
9. Centers for Disease Control and Prevention, National Center for Health Statistics. WHO growth charts and CDC growth charts. http://www.cdc.gov/growthcharts/who_charts.htm. Accessed June 14, 2016.
10. Down Syndrome Medical Interest Group. *Guidance for Essential Medical Surveillance*. http://www.dsmig.org.uk/publications/guidelines.html. Accessed June 14, 2016.
11. Down Syndrome Medical Interest Group. *PCHR Insert for Babies Born with Down Syndrome*, 3rd ed. June 2011. http://www.healthforallchildren.com/wp-content/uploads/2013/04/A5-Downs-Instrucs-chartsfull-copy.pdf.
12. Capone G. Down syndrome. In: Maria B, ed. *Current Management in Child Neurology*. Hamilton, Ontario: Decker; 1999.
13. Weijerman ME, van Furth AM, van der Mooren MD, et al. Prevalence of congenital heart defects and persistent pulmonary hypertension of the neonate with Down syndrome. *Eur J Pediatr*. 2010; 169:1195.
14. Roizen NJ, Patterson D. Down's syndrome. *Lancet*. 2003; 361:1281.
15. Baraona F, Gurvitz M, Landzberg MJ, Opotowsky AR. Hospitalizations and mortality in the United States for adults with Down syndrome and congenital heart disease. *Am J Cardiol*. 2013; 111:1046.
16. Mancchini F, Leva E, Torricelli M, Valade A. Treating acid reflux disease in patients with Down syndrome: pharmacological and physiological approaches. *Clin Exp Gastroenterol*. 2011; 4:19.
17. Amiel J, Lyonnet S. Hirschsprung disease, associated syndromes, and genetics: a review. *J Med Genet*. 2001; 38:729.
18. Bonamico M, Mariani P, Danesi HM, et al. Prevalence and clinical picture of celiac disease in Italian Down syndrome patients: a multicenter study. *J Pediatr Gastroenterol Nutr*. 2001; 33:139.
19. Pavlovic M, Radlovic N, Lekovic Z, Stojsic Z, Puleva K, Berenji K. When to screen children with Down syndrome for celiac disease? *J Trop Pediatr*. 2010; 56:443.
20. Saadah OI, Al-Aama JY, Alaifan MA, Bin Talib YY, Al-Mughales JA. Prevalence of celiac disease in children with Down syndrome screened by anti-tissue transglutaminase antibodies. *Saudi Med J*. 2012; 33:208.
21. Bhat AS, Chaturvedi MK, Saini S, et al. Prevalence of celiac disease in Indian children with Down syndrome and its clinical and laboratory predictors. *Indian J Pediatr*. 2013; 80:114.
22. Haargaard B, Fledelius HC. Down's syndrome and early cataract. *Br J Ophthalmol*. 2006; 90:1024.
23. So SA, Urbano RC, Hodapp RM. Hospitalizations of infants and young children with Down syndrome: evidence from inpatient person-records from a statewide administrative database. *J Intellect Disabil Res*. 2007; 51:1030.
24. Schott S, Amin R, Chini B, et al. Obstructive sleep apnea: should all children with Down syndrome be tested? *Arch Otolaryngol Head Neck Surg*. 2006; 132:432.
25. Park AH, Wilson MA, Stevens PT, Harward R, Hohler N. Identification of hearing loss in pediatric patients with Down syndrome. *Otolaryngol Head Neck Surg*. 2012; 146:135.
26. Popova G, Paterson WF, Brown A, Donaldson MDC. Hashimoto's thyroiditis in Down's syndrome: clinical presentation and evolution. *Horm Res*. 2008; 70:278.
27. Bergholdt R, Eising S, Nerup J, Pociot F Increased prevalence of Down's syndrome in individuals with type 1 diabetes in Denmark: a nationwide population- based study. *Diabetologia*. 2006; 49:1179.
28. American Diabetes Association. Standards of Medical Care in Diabetes—2013. *Diabetes Care*. 2013; 36(suppl 1):S11.
29. Henry E, Walker D, Wiedmeier SE, Christensen RD. Haematological abnormalities during the first week of life among neonates with Down syndrome: data from a multihospital healthcare system. *Am J Med Genet J*. 2007; 143:42.
30. James R. A study of the neonatal haematology of children with Down syndrome. PhD thesis, University of York, 2011. http://etheses.whiterose.ac.uk/4063. Accessed June 14, 2016.
31. Juj H, Emery H. The arthropathy of Down's syndrome: an underdiagnosed and underrecognized condition. *Pediatrics*. 2009; 154:234.
32. Rachidi M, Lopes C. Molecular and cellular mechanisms elucidating neurocognitive basis of functional impairments associated with intellectual disability in Down syndrome. *Am J Intellect Dev Disabil*. 2010; 115:83.
33. Olson LE, Roper RJ, Sengstaken CL, et al. Trisomy for the Down syndrome "critical region" is necessary but not sufficient for brain phenotypes of trisomic mice. *Hum Mol Genet*. 2007; 16:774.
34. Wang X, Zhao Y, Zhang X, et al. Loss of sorting nexin 27 contributes to excitatory synaptic dysfunction by modulating glutamate receptor recycling in Down's syndrome. *Nat Med*. 2013; 19:473.
35. Adorno M, Sikandar S, Mitra SS, et al. Usp16 contributes to somatic stem-cell defects in Down's syndrome. *Nature*. 2013; 501:380.
36. Kerkel K, Schupf N, Hatta K, et al. Altered DNA methylation in leukocytes with trisomy 21. *PLoS Genet*. 2010; 6(11):e1001212.
37. Rovelet-Lecrux A, Hannequin D, Raux G, et al. APP locus duplication causes autosomal dominant early-onset Alzheimer disease with cerebral amyloid angiopathy. *Nat Genet*. 2006; 38:24.
38. Webb RL, Murphy MP. β-Secretases, Alzheimer's disease, and Down syndrome. *Curr Gerontol Geriatr Res*. 2012; 2012:362839.
39. Halliwell B, Gutteridge J. Oxygen radicals and the nervous system. *Trends Neurosci*. 1985; 8:22.
40. Jovanovic S, Clements D, MacLeod K. Biomarkers of oxidative stress are significantly elevated in Down syndrome. *Free Radicals Biol Med*. 1998; 25:1044.
41. Karousou E, Stachtea X, Moretti P, et al. New insights into the pathobiology of Down syndrome: hyaluronan synthase-2 overexpression is regulated by collagen VI α2 chain. *FEBS J*. 2013; 280:2418.
42. Faulks D, Collado V, Mazlle MN, Veyrune JL, Hennequin M. Masticatory dysfunction in persons with Down's syndrome. Part 1: aetiology and incidence. *J Oral Rehabil*. 2008; 35:854.
43. Boghossian NS, Horbar JD, Murray JC, Carpenter JH. Anthropometric charts for infants with trisomies 21, 18, or 13 born between 22 weeks gestation and term: the VON charts. *Am J Med Genet A*. 2012; 158A(2):322.
44. Chen X, Beydoun MA, Wang Y. Is sleep duration associated with childhood obesity?: a systematic review and meta-analysis. *Obesity*. 2008; 16:265.
45. Kimura J, Tachibana K, Imaizumi K, Kurosawa K, Kuroki Y. Longitudinal growth and height velocity of Japanese children with Downs syndrome. *Acta Paediatrica*. 2003; 92:1039.
46. Ballestin R, Blasco-Ibanez JM, Crespo C, et al. Astrocytes of the murine model for Down syndrome Ts65Dn display reduced intracellular ionic zinc. *Neurochem Int*. 2014; 75:48.
47. Kanavan O, Aaseth J, Birketvedt, G. Thyroid hypofunction in Down's syndrome: is it related to oxidative stress? *Biol Trace Elem Res*. 2000; 78(1–3):35.
48. Stagi S, Lapi E, Romano S, et al. Determinants of vitamin D levels in children and adolescents with Down syndrome. *Int J Endocrinol*. 2015; 2015:1.
49. Lott IT. Antioxidants in Down syndrome. *Biochim Biophys Acta*. 2012; 1822:657.
50. Parisotto EB, Garlet TR, Cavalli VL, et al. Antioxidant intervention attenuates oxidative stress in children and teenagers with Down syndrome. *Res Dev Disabil*. 2014; 35:1228.
51. Harrell R, Capp R, Davis D, Peerless J, Ravitz L. Can nutritional supplements help mentally retarded children?: an exploratory study. *Proc Natl Acad Sci U S A*. 1981; 78:574.
52. Salman M. Systematic review of the effect of therapeutic dietary supplements and drugs on cognitive function in subjects with Down syndrome. *Eur J Pediatr Neurol*. 2002; 6:213.
53. Ani C, Grantham-McGregor S, Muller D. Nutritional supplementation in Down syndrome: theoretical considerations and current status. *Dev Med Child Neurol*. 2000; 42:207.
54. Kleijnen, J., Knipschild, P. Niacin and vitamin B6 in mental functioning: a review of controlled trials in humans. *Biol. Psychiatry* 1991; 29:931.
55. Ellis JM, Tan HK, Muller DP, et al. Supplementation with antioxidants and folinic acid for children with Down's syndrome: randomized controlled trial. *BMJ*. 2008; 336:594.
56. Medlen J. *The Down Syndrome Nutrition Handbook: A Guide to Promoting Healthy Lifestyles*, 2nd ed. Portland, OR: Phronesis Publishing; 2006.

# 16 Prader-Willi Syndrome

JENNIFER MILLER, HELEN McCUNE, AND DANIEL J. DRISCOLL

Prader-Willi syndrome (PWS) is a complex, multisystem syndrome that occurs with a frequency of approximately 1/10,000 to 1/30,000 and leads to significant morbidity, including central hypotonia, cognitive delay, developmental disabilities, a characteristic behavior disorder, growth deficiency, obesity compounded by a centrally driven excessive appetite (hyperphagia), growth hormone (GH) deficiency, and hypogonadism.[1] It is the most commonly recognized genetic cause of obesity.

PWS is one of the best examples of a pattern of inheritance called *genomic imprinting*. It results from loss of expression of paternally derived genes by a variety of mechanisms, including paternally inherited deletions (70–75%), maternal uniparental disomy (20–30%), and imprinting defects (2–5%).[2,3] DNA methylation analysis correctly diagnoses more than 99% of cases and is the most sensitive genetic test available.[4,5] All patients with suspected PWS should have definitive genetic testing because there is significant variability in the clinical phenotype (Table 16–1).[6]

## METABOLIC ABNORMALITIES

Individuals with PWS have a wide spectrum of metabolic abnormalities. PWS is a spectrum disorder that affects multiple body systems. The underlying pathophysiological basis of the PWS phenotype remains unclear. Current therapies for PWS show limited efficacy and are directed toward various symptoms associated with the disease process. GH deficiency is present in almost all children and in many adults with PWS. GH replacement therapy is a standard of care for children with PWS and is increasingly prescribed in infants and adults. GH replacement therapy is effective in increasing height, improving body composition, increasing bone mineral density, improving exercise endurance and quality of life, and favorably impacting development and behavior (Fig. 16–1).[7] However, it does not affect hyperphagia. Intellectual disability and neuropsychiatric issues are present to some degree in all individuals with PWS.[8,9] Additional metabolic complications frequently found in PWS include osteopenia/osteoporosis and decreased gastrointestinal motility.[10]

Individuals with PWS experience a characteristic change in food intake over time. Infants with PWS typically exhibit hypotonia, lethargy, a weak or discoordinated suck and swallow mechanism, and failure to thrive.[11] They typically do not exhibit signs of hunger and require force-feeding via gastrostomy tube, nasogastric tube, or cross-cut nipples on the bottle. Hypotonia in infants with PWS slowly resolves over time, although adults with PWS continue to exhibit some muscle hypotonia and weakness throughout their lifetime. Nutritional support is critical to optimize growth and development in infancy, but feeding skills typically improve throughout infancy. Excessive weight gain begins typically before the appetite increases, and then hyperphagia commences sometime during childhood.[11,12] All individuals with PWS will become morbidly obese as adolescents and adults if strict environmental controls are not implemented.

The underlying molecular mechanisms that contribute to excessive weight gain and hyperphagia in PWS remain incompletely understood. Appetite and satiety issues are regulated by a complex interplay among gut hormones and hypothalamic neuropeptides. Most gut-related appetite-regulating hormones are normally expressed in PWS, with the most notable exception being ghrelin, a GH secretagogue that is high in fasting states and decreases with eating. Highly elevated levels of ghrelin have been identified in individuals with PWS; although ghrelin levels decrease after intake of a meal, as is normal, they still remain comparatively high. However, it has been shown that circulating ghrelin levels are elevated in young children with PWS long before the onset of hyperphagia, especially during the early phase of poor appetite and feeding, so it seems unlikely that high ghrelin levels are directly responsible for the switch to the hyperphagic nutritional phases in PWS.[13,14] Therefore, the relationship between hyperphagia and ghrelin remains unclear, and it has been proposed that the hyperghrelinemia may be the result of hypoinsulinemia.[15] Leptin levels are appropriately elevated for the degree of obesity, indicating that leptin deficiency is not a cause of the appetite issues.

Other hormones and peptides related to appetite control in PWS have been studied. Neuropeptide Y and agouti-related protein, which cause increased feeding in animal studies, were not found to be increased in the hypothalami of individuals with PWS.[16] Animal studies have shown that the hypothalamus, particularly the parvocellular oxytocin neurons of the paraventricular nucleus (PVN), is important in the regulation of appetite.[17] In autopsy studies, the PVN of five brains of PWS individuals (aged 22–64 years) was compared with the PVN of 27 controls.[18] The PVN volume and total number of cells were lower in the brains of the individuals with PWS. The number of paravocellular oxytocin neurons was significantly decreased in the PWS brains, which suggests that these cells might be connected to decreased satiety in PWS.[18]

Some studies have suggested that the hyperphagia in PWS may be caused by abnormalities in another hypothalamic hormone, hypocretin/orexin. Orexin regulates the sleep/wake cycle, metabolism, and appetite and therefore is a viable candidate hormone to explain several of the clinical findings in PWS.[19] It is known that the sleep/wake cycle is abnormal in individuals with PWS, many of whom suffer from excessive daytime sleepiness and narcolepsy, a disorder caused by abnormally low hypocretin/orexin.[20] Within the PWS region on chromosome 15, the *SNORD116* host gene transcript has been reported to regulate expression of diurnal and circadian genes in the brain, suggesting a potential role in energy expenditure and hyperphagia in PWS.[21] However, despite considerable investigation, at this time there are no consistently identified hormone abnormalities to fully explain the hyperphagia in PWS, and the metabolic correlates of hyperphagia are still unclear.

Individuals with PWS have altered body composition with decreased muscle mass and increased fat mass compared to controls matched for body mass index (BMI). This altered body composition of children with PWS can explain the differences in energy expenditure. Basal metabolic rate (BMR) and sleeping metabolic rate (SMR) in children with PWS were found to be lower than in unaffected obese children matched for sex and bone age. However, if BMR and SMR were expressed as rate per fat-free mass, there was no difference, indicating that the lower rates resulted from the decreased fat-free mass.[22]

**Table 16–1.** Clinical Features of Prader-Willi Syndrome

| Diagnostic Criteria | % Documented* |
|---|---|
| *Major Criteria* | |
| Neonatal hypotonia | 88 |
| Feeding problems in infancy | 78 |
| Excessive weight gain | 67 |
| Facial features | 88 |
| Hypogonadism | 51 |
| Developmental delay | 99 |
| Hyperphagia | 84 |
| *Minor Criteria* | |
| Decreased fetal activity | 62 |
| Behavioral problems | 87 |
| Sleep disturbances/sleep apnea | 76 |
| Short stature | 63 |
| Hypopigmentation | 73 |
| Small hands/small feet | 88 |
| Narrow hands/straight ulnar borders | 82 |
| Eye abnormalities | 68 |
| Thick viscous saliva | 89 |
| Articulation defects | 80 |
| Skin picking | 83 |

*Based on 90 patients with molecularly confirmed diagnosis of Prader-Willi syndrome. From Holm VA, Cassidy SB, Butler MG, et al. Prader-Willi syndrome: consensus diagnostic criteria. *Pediatrics*. 1993; 91:398. Used with permission.

Adolescents with PWS had a total energy expenditure (TEE) that was only 53% of the TEE in normal obese adolescents, but the difference was only 14% when normalized for fat-free mass. This suggests that energy metabolism at the cellular level is not much diffeerent from that of children in the general population.[23]

To date, no medication has proved effective in regulating appetite in PWS. Bariatric surgery is not accompanied by a decrease in appetite such as occurs in typical individuals and is contraindicated in this population. The medications evaluated thus far in PWS have been ineffective or have been associated with unacceptable side effects.

## FACTORS TO BE CONSIDERED IN NUTRITIONAL EVALUATION

Children with PWS have different nutritional problems depending on their age. In contrast to the long-held view that there are two distinct nutritional phases in PWS (i.e., failure to thrive followed by "hyperphagia leading to obesity"), a collaborative study found that the transition between nutritional phases is much more complex, with seven different phases through which individuals with PWS typically progress[11] (Table 16–2). Phase 0 occurs in utero, with decreased fetal movements and growth restriction compared to unaffected siblings. In phase 1, the infant is hypotonic and not obese. Subphase 1a is characterized by difficulty feeding and poor appetite (age range, birth to 15 months; median age at completion, 9 months). This is followed by subphase 1b, during which the infant grows steadily along a growth curve and weight increases at a normal rate (median age at onset, 9 months; range, 5–15 months). Phase 2 is associated with weight gain; in subphase 2a, the weight increases without a significant change in appetite or caloric intake (median age at onset, 2.08 years), whereas in subphase 2b, the weight gain is associated with a concomitant increased interest in food (median age at onset, 4.5 years). Phase 3 is characterized by hyperphagia, which is typically accompanied by food-seeking and the lack of a sense of satiety (median age at onset, 8 years). Not all individuals with PWS go through all of these stages, but most do. In addition, some adults progress to phase 4, in which an individual who was previously in phase 3 no longer has an insatiable appetite and is able to feel full.

The hyperphagia that occurs in phase 3 commonly results in food-seeking behavior, with hoarding or foraging for food, eating of inedibles, and stealing of food or money to buy food. In most individuals, gastric emptying is delayed, and vomiting is rare.[24] Obesity results from these behaviors and from decreased total caloric requirement. The obesity in PWS is primarily central (abdomen, buttocks, and thighs) in both sexes, and there is less visceral fat in obese individuals with PWS than would be expected for the degree of obesity.[25,26] Obesity and its complications are the major causes of morbidity and mortality. Family, friends, and school personnel should be instructed not give the child with PWS extra food. It is helpful to include a nutrition component in the child's individualized educational plan. School meals should be monitored to ensure that the children do not obtain extra food. Because of these children's behavioral problems, they do better in a structured, consistent environment with consistent mealtimes and places.

## DIETARY MANAGEMENT

### Infants

The goal of nutrition therapy for infants is to provide adequate nutrients to promote appropriate weight gain and growth. The guidelines for feeding infants should follow the recommendations of the Academy of Pediatrics Committee on Nutrition.[27] Breast milk or infant formula should be the primary food until the infant is 6 months old. It is sometimes necessary to concentrate the formula or to add a calorie-protein supplement to breast milk to provide adequate nutrients in a smaller volume that the infant will drink. Most PWS children require oral-motor therapy to aid in the development of feeding skills. For the infant and very young child, it is important to not overly restrict fat intake; fat is still needed in the diet for adequate brain development and growth. Approximately 30% of calories should come from fat.[28]

### Children

The goal of nutritional therapy in children with PWS is to prevent excessive weight gain. Weight, height, and nutrient intake should be monitored monthly during this developmental period (Appendix 2–9). Prevention of obesity is one of the most important goals for the family of a child with PWS. Prevention of obesity is necessary to reduce the risk of breathing problems, heart disease, hypertension, fatty liver disease, and diabetes that can develop early in childhood. This goal can be accomplished with a nutrient-dense, calorie-controlled diet and consistent environmental controls that will help establish a healthy eating pattern for life. Obesity prevention requires a balance. The challenge is to help the child feel satisfied without consuming too many calories, yet to provide all of the vitamins and minerals needed to grow well.

Some parents become so fearful about potential obesity in their child that they overly restrict calories and certain food groups, which can result in growth failure. In certain situations, if weight and length have plateaued for a period of time, the degree of food restriction may need to be lessened. Parents and caregivers should monitor growth closely and should consult their physician and qualified registered dietitian for guidance on this issue.

If weight gain is greater than expected, energy intake must be restricted so that the child's weight follows the appropriate weight percentile without compromising growth. The weight-for-height ratio should be maintained between the 25th and 75th percentile, or a BMI of less than the 85th percentile on growth charts. Growth charts for PWS children have been published, but with the widespread use of GH in these children, such charts have diminished usefulness. Children with PWS need fewer calories to maintain weight gain along the appropriate growth channel. Several studies have found that children with PWS aged 4 to 14 years need 50% to 75% of the energy required by unaffected children.[29] The children

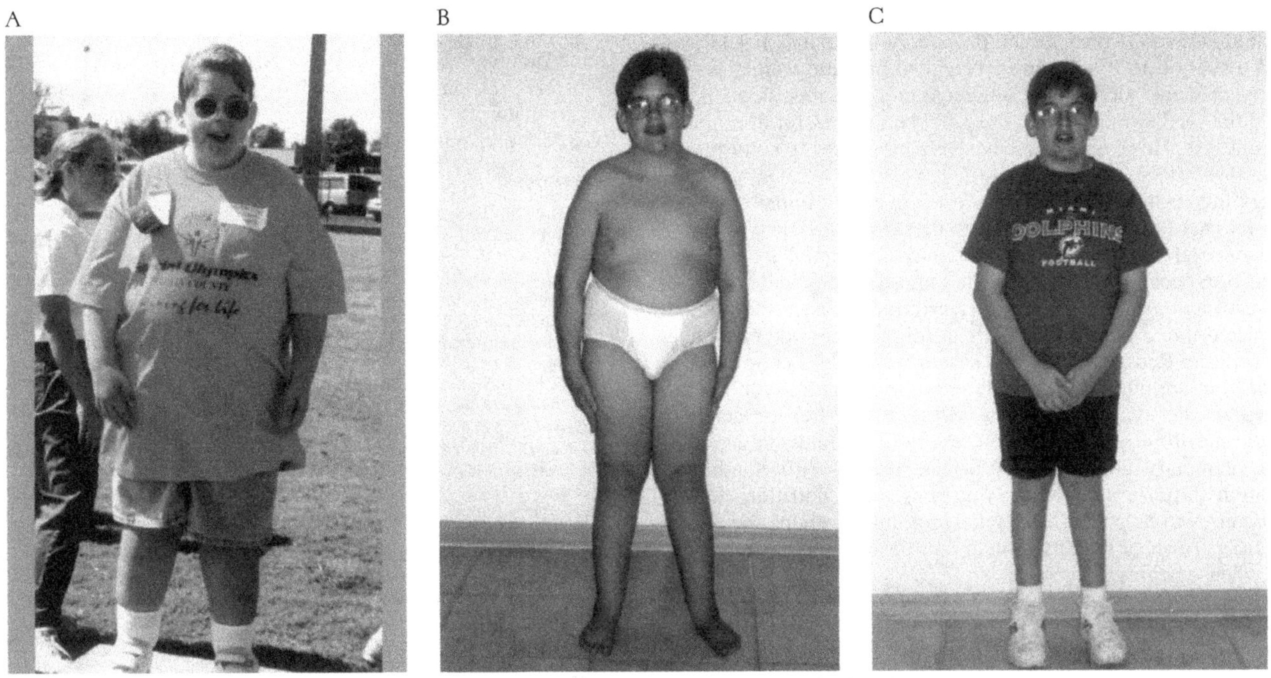

**Figure 16–1.** An adolescent male with Prader-Willi syndrome receiving growth hormone (GH) therapy at 0.033 mg/kg/day. A. Subject at 14 years of age, after 2 months of therapy. B. Subject after 9 months of therapy. C. Subject at 15 years of age, after 13 months of therapy. Notice the dramatic reduction of obesity in the waist, limbs, and face. The caloric restriction and exercise program that was in place before initiation of GH therapy was continued during the GH therapy. (Courtesy of University of Florida Health Science Center, Gainesville, Florida. Used with permission.)

needed only 8 to 11 kcal/cm of height for weight maintenance. It has been recommended that the macronutrient content of the diet be maintained at 25% protein, 45% carbohydrate, and 30% fat, with at least 20 g of fiber per day.[28] However, these ratios have to be adjusted to the individual child based on his or her weight trajectory, and many children require even fewer carbohydrates to attain adequate weight control.

Because of their limited diet, a vitamin-mineral supplement is often required to meet the needs of children with PMS. If the essential fatty acid intake is below recommendations for age, oils rich in essential fatty acids (e.g., canola, flaxseed, safflower) should be included in the child's diet. Some parents also supplement with medium-chain triglycerides because there is some evidence that they may reduce serum lipid levels, decrease body fat, and increase fatty acid oxidation.[30]

For the child who is already obese and gaining weight rapidly, an energy-restricted diet is the mainstay of treatment. If the child is already overweight, then, depending on the degree of obesity, the child be restricted to an energy intake that is adequate to maintain

**Table 16–2. (Ref 11)** Nutritional Phases in Prader-Willi Syndrome

| Phase | Description | Average Age Range (Median Age at onset) |
|---|---|---|
| Phase 0 | Decreased fetal movements in utero; lower birth rate | |
| Phase 1a | Hypotonia with difficulty feeding; may have failure to thrive | 0–9mo (birth) |
| Phase 1b | No difficulty feeding; growing appropriately on growth curve | 3–24 mo (9 mos) |
| Phase 2a | Weight increasing without an increase in appetite or excessive calories | 18 mo - 3 yr (2.08 yrs) |
| Phase 2b | Weight increasing with an increase in appetite | 3yr –12 yr (4.5 yrs) |
| Phase 3 | Hyperphagic; rarely feels full | 5 yr to adulthood (8 yrs) |
| Phase 4 | Appetite is no longer insatiable | Adulthood |

| Phase | Description | Mean Age Range |
|---|---|---|
| Phase 0 | Decreased fetal movements in utero; lower birth rate | |
| Phase 1a | Hypotonia with difficulty feeding; may have failure to thrive | 0.75 yrs |
| Phase 1b | No difficulty feeding; growing appropriately on growth curve | 2.08 yrs |
| Phase 2a | Weight increasing without an increase in appetite or excessive calories | 4.5 yrs |
| Phase 2b | Weight increasing with an increase in appetite | 8 yrs |
| Phase 3 | Hyperphagic; rarely feels full | 8.5 yrs |
| Phase 4 | Appetite is no longer insatiable | Adulthood |

Mean ages for Phases in this table – may choose which to present weight, so that he or she will "grow into" his or her present weight. If the child is severely overweight, the energy intake may need to be reduced to only 6 to 8 kcal/cm of height to promote weight loss.[31] A variety of diets, such as the ketogenic diet, the modified Atkins diet, and the Mediterranean diet, have all been successful in promoting weight loss. However, there have been no studies to confirm the safety of these diets.

Energy intake should never be so restrictive as to impair growth. It is often necessary to supplement these various diets with a vitamin-mineral supplement, calcium, and/or essential fatty acids. The nutrition education component is important to achieve normal weight gain and growth. The diet prescription for each child must be translated into a plan the family can follow. The food exchange system and the Red-Yellow-Green system for weight control have been used but are not as sustainable or well-tolerated as the lower-carbohydrate diet recommended by Miller et al.[28] Portion control, consistent mealtimes, and limited access to food are essential components of dietary control in PWS. The Prader-Willi Syndrome Association (http://www.pwsausa.org/) has many nutrition education brochures to help families. Behavioral management should be part of the nutritional therapy to help families cope with the hyperphagia when it begins.

## Other Therapies

Exercise is an important component of any weight management or weight loss program. Children with PWS have decreased levels of physical activity compared with age- and weight-matched controls.[32] Therefore, a good exercise plan is essential, and it is important to begin as early as possible. The entire family should participate because children might need extra encouragement. Not only does exercise benefit the child with PWS, but it also keeps the entire family healthier. Daily walks, bike riding, swimming, gymnastics, and martial arts such as karate and Tae Kwon Do are examples of good physical activities.

Exercise that is regularly scheduled helps burn extra calories and prevent obesity. Every effort should be made to promote physical activity because it has been shown to increase energy expenditure and muscle mass in individuals with PWS.[33] Recommendations are that individuals with PWS should perform 30 to 60 minutes of aerobic exercise per day. GH treatment in children with PWS results in improved exercise tolerance, increased linear growth, decreased percent body fat, increased lean body mass, and improved strength and agility, but it does not appear to change the children's feeling of satiety. A strict calorie-restricted diet and daily exercise are still required during treatment with GH.[28,34]

## Hydration

One of the challenges with children with PWS is their hydration status. Most young children with PWS do not like to drink water, so it is important to devise strategies to increase water intake. Adding orange, lemon, or lime juice to water can help. You can also soak apples and cinnamon overnight in water to make the water more palatable to drink. Cucumbers can be used to flavor water. Drinking juice or soda are not recommended because they provide excess calories that can cause weight gain.

## Follow-up

The nutritional therapy of children with PWS requires close monitoring of weight, height, and nutrient intake to achieve appropriate weight and growth. Children with PWS have an insatiable appetite, stubbornness, and obsessive-compulsive type behaviors that can interfere with nutritional therapy. Therefore, behavioral management should be an integral component of nutritional management. This is essential because uncontrolled obesity will lead to significant morbidity and mortality.

## ACKNOWLEDGMENTS

Grant funding was provided by NIH U54 grants HD061222 and RR019478 (DJD and JLM) and PWSA (USA). In addition, we would like to thank all of our wonderful families who have children with PWS for being our inspiration.

### References


1. Cassidy SB, Forsythe M, Heeger S, et al. Comparison of phenotype between patients with Prader-Willi syndrome due to deletion of 15q and uniparental disomy 15. *Am J Med Genet.* 1997; 68:433.
2. Driscoll DJ. Genomic imprinting in humans. In: Friedmann T, ed. *Molecular Genetic Medicine.* San Diego, CA: Academic Press; 1994.
3. Glenn CC, Driscoll DJ, Yang TP, Nicholls RD. Genomic imprinting: potential function and mechanisms revealed by the Prader-Willi and Angelman syndromes. *Mol Hum Reprod.* 1997; 3:321.
4. Driscoll DJ, Waters MF, Williams CA, et al. A DNA methylation imprint, determined by the sex of the parent, distinguishes the Angelman and Prader-Willi syndromes. *Genomics.* 1992; 13:917.
5. Glenn CC, Saitoh S, Jong MTC, et al. Gene structure, DNA methylation and imprinted expression of human *SNRPN* gene. *Am J Hum Genet.* 1996; 58:335.
6. Holm VA, Cassidy SB, Butler MG, et al. Prader-Willi syndrome: consensus diagnostic criteria. *Pediatrics.* 1993; 91:398.
7. Burman P, Ritzen EM, Lindren AC. Endocrine dysfunction in Prader-Willi syndrome: a review with special reference to GH. *Endocr Rev.* 2001; 22:787.
8. Laurier V, Lapeyrade A, Copet P, et al. Medical, psychological and social features in a large cohort of adults with Prader-Willi syndrome: experience from a dedicated centre in France. *J Intellect Disabil Res.* 2015; 59:411.
9. Woodcock KA, Oliver C, Humphreys GW. The relationship between specific cognitive impairment and behaviour in Prader-Willi syndrome. *J Intellect Disabil Res.* 2011; 55:152.
10. Butler MG, Haber L, Mernaugh R, Carlson MG, Price R, Feurer ID. Decreased bone mineral density in Prader-Willi syndrome: comparison with obese subjects. *Am J Med Genet.* 2001; 103:216.
11. Miller JL, Lynn CH, Driscoll DC, et al. Nutritional phases in Prader-Willi syndrome. *Am J Med Genet A.* 2011; 155A:1040.
12. Butler JV, Whittington JE, Holland AJ, McAllister CJ, Goldstone AP. The transition between the phenotypes of Prader-Willi syndrome during infancy and early childhood. *Dev Med Child Neurol.* 2010; 52:e88.
13. Feigerlová E, Diene G, Conte-Auriol F, et al. Hyperghrelinemia precedes obesity in Prader-Willi syndrome. *J Clin Endocrinol Metab.* 2008; 93:2800.
14. Kweh FA, Miller JL, Sulsona CR, et al. Hyperghrelinemia in Prader-Willi syndrome begins in early infancy long before the onset of hyperphagia. *Am J Med Genet A.* 2015; 167A:69.
15. Haqq AM, Farooqi IS, O'Rahilly S, et al. Serum ghrelin levels are inversely correlated with body mass index, age, and insulin concentrations in normal children and are markedly increased in Prader-Willi syndrome. *J Clin Endocrinol Metab.* 2003; 88:174.
16. Goldstone AP, Unmehopa UA, Bloom SR, Swaab DF. Hypothalamic NPY and agouti-related protein are increased in human illness but not in Prader-Willi syndrome and other obese subjects. *J Clin Endocrinol Metab.* 2002; 87:927.
17. Sabatier N, Leng G, Menzies J. Oxytocin, feeding, and satiety. *Front Endocrinol (Lausanne).* 2013; 4:35.
18. Swaab DF, Purba JS, Hofman MA. Alterations in the hypothalamic paraventricular nucleus and its oxytocin neurons (putative satiety cells) in Prader-Willi syndrome: a study of five cases. *J Clin Endocrinol Metab.* 1995; 80:573.
19. Nevsimalova S, Vankova J, Stepanova I, Seemanova E, Mignot E, Nishino S. Hypocretin deficiency in Prader-Willi syndrome. *Eur J Neurol.* 2005; 12:70.
20. Liblau RS, Vassalli A, Seifinejad A, Tafti M. Hypocretin (orexin) biology and the pathophysiology of narcolepsy with cataplexy. *Lancet Neurol.* 2015; 14:318.
21. Powell WT, Coulson RL, Crary FK, et al. A Prader-Willi locus lncRNA cloud modulates diurnal genes and energy expenditure. *Hum Mol Genet.* 2013; 22:4318.
22. van Mil EA, Westerterp KR, Gerver WJ, et al. Energy expenditure at rest and during sleep in children with Prader-Willi syndrome is explained by body composition. *Am J Clin Nutr.* 2000; 71:752.
23. Schoeller DA, Levitsky LL, Bandini LG, Dietz WW, Walczak A. Energy expenditure and body composition in Prader-Willi syndrome. *Metabolism.* 1988; 37:115.
24. Holland AJ, Treasure J, Coskeran P, Dallow J. Characteristics of the eating disorder in Prader-Willi syndrome: implications for treatment. *J Intellect Disabil Res* 1995; 39:373.
25. Brambilla P, Bosio L, Manzoni P, Pietrobelli A, Beccaria L, Chiumello G. Peculiar body composition in patients with Prader-Labhart-Willi syndrome. *Am J Clin Nutr.* 1997; 65:1369.
26. Goldstone AP, Thomas L, Brynes AE, et al. Visceral adipose tissue and metabolic complications of obesity are reduced in Prader-Willi syndrome female adults: evidence for novel influences on body fat distribution. *J Clin Endocrinol Metab.* 2001; 86:4330.
27. AAP site is: AAP facts. American Academy of Pediatrics Web site. https://www.aap.org/en-us/about-the-aap/aap-facts/Pages/AAP-Facts.aspx
28. Miller JL, Lynn CH, Shuster J, Driscoll DJ. A reduced-energy intake, well-balanced diet improves weight control in children with Prader-Willi syndrome. *J Hum Nutr Diet.* 2013; 26:2.

29. Pipes PL, Holm VA. Weight control of children with Prader-Willi syndrome. *J Am Diet Assoc.* 1973; 62:520.
30. St-Onge MP, Jones PJ. Greater rise in fat oxidation with medium-chain triglyceride consumption relative to long-chain triglyceride is associated with lower initial body weight and greater loss of subcutaneous adipose tissue. *Int J Obes Relat Metab Disord.* 2003; 27:1565.
31. Borgie KH. *Nutrition Care for Children with Prader-Willi Syndrome*. Newport Beach, CA: Prader-Willi California Foundation; 1994.
32. Eiholzer U, Nordmann Y, l'Allemand D, Schlumpf M, Schmid S, Kromeyer-Hauschild K. Improving body composition and physical activity in Prader-Willi syndrome. *J Pediatr.* 2003; 142:73.
33. Caldwell ML, Taylor RL, Bloom SR. An investigation of the use of high- and low-preference food as a reinforcer for increased activity of individuals with Prader-Willi syndrome. *J Ment Defic Res.* 1986; 30:347.
34. Carrel AL, Myers SE, Whitman BY, Allen DB. Growth hormone improves body composition, fat utilization, physical strength and agility, and growth in Prader-Willi syndrome: a controlled study. *J Pediatr.* 1999; 143:215.

# 17 Rett Syndrome

NGA HONG BRERETON, CARMEN CUFFARI, AND GENILA BIBAT

Rett syndrome (RTT), a neurodevelopmental disorder primarily involving girls, is characterized by a period of apparently normal development followed by the arrest of developmental skills. Distinctive features of RTT include deceleration in the velocity of head growth between 5 months and 4 years of age resulting in microcephaly, stereotyped hand movements, psychomotor retardation with impaired language, and loss of purposeful hand use. Most patients have electroencephalographic (EEG) abnormalities, but only half have recognizable clinical seizures. Respiratory irregularities in RTT include periodic apnea during wakefulness and intermittent hyperventilation. The incidence of RTT is approximately 1:10,000.[1] It is panethnic. Life expectancy is variable, and sudden unexplained death may occur during sleep in younger children regardless of seizure control.[2]

The necessary criteria for diagnosis of RTT are shown in Box 17–1.[3] However, a wide clinical spectrum has been recognized since the defective gene in RTT was identified. With the increase in clinical recognition and advances in the neurobiology and molecular genetics of RTT, a scoring system has been developed to facilitate comparisons among the various clinical profiles of mutation-positive children,[4] and a revised set of criteria to clarify the ambiguities in language of the current diagnostic criteria[5] has been suggested.

## GENETICS OF RETT SYNDROME

The genetic defect causing RTT has been mapped to chromosome Xq28 and identified as mutations in the methyl-CpG binding protein-2 (*MECP2*) gene.[6] The mutations cause partial or complete loss of function of the MECP2 protein, leading to a failure of repression of a variety of still unknown genes. Approximately two-thirds of clinically affected individuals have mutations in the *MECP2* gene.[7]

## PATHOBIOLOGY OF GASTROINTESTINAL SYMPTOMS IN RETT SYNDROME

Neurons appear to be more vulnerable to the gene defect as they reach maturation.[8] Generalized neuronal involvement in RTT includes the autonomic nervous system, which is believed to have a significant effect on the gastrointestinal system. This seriously interferes with aspects of gastrointestinal function and can cause oropharyngeal dysphagia, severe constipation, and gastroesophageal reflux disease (GERD).

## FACTORS TO BE CONSIDERED IN NUTRITIONAL EVALUATION

RTT presents several barriers to growth, including perturbations in feeding skills, GERD, and high basal metabolic needs.[9,10] Indeed, many females with RTT meet the criteria for moderate to severe malnutrition.[11] The decline over time in growth percentiles for weight, stature, and head size is usually uncorrected by aggressive nutritional support.[12] Decreased weight gain cannot be taken as a clinical effect of RTT because chewing, swallowing, esophagitis due to reflux, or fear of aspiration may limit intake. When these are circumvented by gastrostomy tube placement, clinically there is considerable weight gain, suggesting that the mutation in MECP2 alone does not contribute to failure to thrive Decrease in linear growth is more difficult to interpret but could be a centrally mediated effect, although there is no evidence for decreased growth hormone.[13,14] Nutrition caregivers need to recognize the eating difficulties early and initiate aggressive nutritional supportive measures, including enteral nutrition. It may be beneficial to start increasing and supplementing oral intake as early as when weight and height Z scores falls below −1.0 (personal observation). Factors that might account for these poor growth patterns include oral-motor, esophageal, digestive tract, and bowel dysfunction as well as reduced intake and alterations in energy balance.[14]

A significant number of RTT patients have poorly coordinated chewing and swallowing, resulting in dysphagia and reduced intake. In the oral-motor domain, disorders may include oropharyngeal dysfunction, sensory deficits, limited tongue mobility, and limited texture tolerance.[16] Abnormal chewing is associated with tongue thrusting and involuntary undulating tongue movements. Feeding problems are characterized by difficulty in chewing and swallowing, with associated coughing and regurgitation.[17] Esophageal problems in RTT usually are caused by GERD, but their prevalence is unknown. In a study using video-fluoroscopy,[18] oropharyngeal dysfunction was found to be present in 100% of RS patients, but only 69% had gastroesophageal dysmotility. Abnormalities of oropharyngeal function due to poor tongue mobility and reduced oropharyngeal clearance lead to laryngeal penetration of liquids and solid foods during swallowing. Absent primary or secondary waves in the esophagus, delayed emptying, atony, presence of tertiary waves, and gastroesophageal reflux characterize esophageal dysmotility, whereas diminished peristalsis characterizes gastric dysmotility. Input from a speech therapist explaining the structural elements of the food and the individual's physiological response to food in the mouth may be useful in describing the eating problems in RS. High-calorie foods, high-protein soft foods, pureed diet, and thickening of fluids can compensate for chewing and swallowing problems. Some RTT children with seizures benefit from the ketogenic diet. Others with autistic characteristics have tried a gluten-free and casein-free diet to improve bowel symptoms by inducing changes in the microbiota, which may be another mechanism to increase gut integrity.[19]

Constipation is the single most common and most distressing clinical problem. Anatomic, manometric, and histological findings are consistent with functional constipation. Barium enema shows marked distention of the colon. Rectal biopsy examinations show normal ganglion cells with negative acetylcholinesterase staining, suggesting intact innervation.[20] Although the etiology of the constipation remains unclear, it may be caused by autonomic dysfunction. If left unmanaged, constipation may decrease appetite and cause painful distention. Further, in our experience, constipation has led to thinning of the intestinal wall and a rare case of gut perforation.

In a study of actual food intake,[22] the mean energy intake of girls with RTT was 66.9% of the US recommendation according to age and 107.8% of the recommendation according to body weight. Intakes of thiamine, vitamin D, calcium, and iron were also considered low. The reduced intake has serious consequences for children's growth, nutrition, and physical health (including bone density). Radiological evidence of osteopenia was shown in 87% of patients studied, with the incidence of fractures being significantly higher than in the general population.[23]

**Box 17–1.** Current Diagnostic Criteria for Rett Syndrome

*Necessary Criteria*

1. Apparently normal prenatal and perinatal period
2. Apparently normal psychomotor development through the first 6 months
3. Normal head circumference at birth
4. Deceleration of head growth between ages 5 months and 4 years
5. Loss of acquired purposeful hand skills between the ages of 6 and 30 months, temporally associated with communication dysfunction and social withdrawal
6. Development of severely impaired expressive and receptive language and presence of apparent severe psychomotor retardation
7. Stereotypic hand movements such as handwringing or squeezing, clapping/tapping, mouthing, and "washing" or rubbing automatisms appearing after purposeful hand skills are lost
8. Diagnosis tentative until 3–5 years of age

*Supportive Criteria*

1. Breathing dysfunction: periodic apnea, intermittent hyperventilation, breath-holding spells; forced expulsion of air or saliva
2. Electroencephalographic abnormalities: slow waking background and intermittent rhythmical slowing (3–5 Hz); epileptiform discharges with or without clinical seizures
3. Seizures
4. Spasticity, often with associated with development of muscle wasting and dystonia
5. Peripheral vasomotor disturbances
6. Scoliosis
7. Growth retardation
8. Hypotrophic small feet

From Trevathan E, Naidu S. The clinical recognition and differential diagnosis of RS. *J Child Neurol.* 1988; 3:S6. Used with permission.

Alterations in energy balance may account for growth failure in girls with RTT. Metabolic rates while awake did not differ between RTT girls and normal controls; however, because of the greater time spent in involuntary motor movement, energy expenditure associated with activity is greater in the RTT girls.[21]

In a later study, Motil et al.[9] found that increased total daily energy expenditure (TEE) did not differ significantly between RS girls and controls. The repetitive movements of RTT girls were not sufficiently intense to increase the TEE. However, their lean body mass (but not body fat) was significantly less, which contributed to their lower TEE in comparison with normal controls. Platte et al.[10] reported that the resting metabolic rate (RMR) of 15 girls with RTT, aged 3 to 12 years, was approximately 160 kcal/day higher than in 13 age-matched girls with developmental delay. A study by Naidu et al.[2] found that the presence of a breathing disorder and the child's ambulatory status (i.e., whether the child walked or not) affected the basal metabolic rate, whereas the level of feeding skill and hand stereotypy did not.

## DIETARY, FEEDING, AND NUTRITIONAL MANAGEMENT

Eating problems in neurological disorders like RTT are multifaceted, with oral-motor, behavioral, nutritional, and medical components[24]. Early identification and management of the complex feeding problems in RTT individuals is essential.

Oropharyngeal dysfunction and the safety of oral feeding may be assessed by medical examination, modified barium swallowing evaluation, a sensory integration evaluation conducted by an occupational therapist, and a peripheral oral examination as part of a speech/language assessment.

Individuals with RTT who have mild chewing and swallowing problems may benefit from a variety of therapeutic techniques such as optimization of posture and seating, manipulation of texture, use of adaptive utensils, alteration of the pacing of feeding, and suggestions regarding self-feeding. In subjects with severe oropharyngeal dysfunction, oral feeding may be unsafe, leading to aspiration or penetration of material into the airway, particularly with foods that have a thin consistency. Enteral access (i.e., gastrostomy tube feeding) is indicated if there is evidence of ongoing aspiration during oral feeding causing repeated respiratory infections; inability to consume adequate calories orally due to oromotor dysfunction to meet energy requirements; increasing stressfulness of oral feeding for either the child or the caregiver; failure to supplement the diet orally; chronic food refusal; development of aversive behavior; or erratic oral intake.

GERD is best managed by consultation with a gastroenterologist. A phased therapeutic approach is usually recommended for children with motor problems.[25] In the first phase, attention is given to positioning, dietary advice, and thickening of feeds. Antacids to neutralize gastric acid may be added. The second phase includes the use of prokinetic agents to increase the tone of the lower esophageal sphincter and enhance gastric emptying. Proton pump inhibitors may also be given for persistent problems. Surgical management (fundoplication) was considered in the past for a third phase,[25] but Fortunato et al.[26] found that Nissen fundoplication had no therapeutic benefit and, surprisingly, worsened gastrointestinal symptoms. Medical management or gastrostomy tube placement would be a better alternative to Nissen fundoplication in the RTT patient population.

Functional constipation can be treated with a high-fiber diet. Fluid intake may be increased to 1.5 times normal to compensate for excessive drooling and hyperventilation. Stool softeners and lactulose have also been found to be useful. However, it is not unusual for patients with RTT to require laxative therapy with MiraLAX powder (Bayer, Whippany, NJ).

The nutritional requirements in RTT are not well defined, despite attempts to characterize the high caloric needs of these patients.[14] Routine monitoring of the nutritional status of the individual throughout the lifespan serves as a guide to nutritional intervention. Height-for-weight and weight-for-height or weight-for-age Z scores more than two standard deviations below the mean for age may indicate the need for early nutritional intervention. RTT patients usually respond to caloric intake of up to 125% of the Recommended Daily Allowance (RDA). We believe that energy requirements should be determined based on the RDA for height, age, or weight at the 25th percentile of weight-for-height or, alternatively, by using metabolic rates corrected for activity levels. World Health Organization formulas may be used for the latter; they allow for more individualized predictions based on gender, age, and body weight and also account for activity levels.[15] In the future, as more is learned about metabolism in children with RTT, a factorial approach will be based on estimation of resting energy expenditure needs, muscle tone alterations, growth needs, or nutritional repletion in malnourished children.[27]

## SUMMARY AND FOLLOW-UP

The management of feeding problems and nutrition in girls with RTT is important but poses great challenges for physicians and caregivers. Because of the wide range of nutritional concerns, interventions must be individualized. An improved understanding of the factors that contribute to growth failure in RTT will enable clinicians and researchers to develop appropriate treatment interventions.

### References


1. Hagberb B. Rett syndrome: prevalence and impact on progressive mental retardation in girls. *Acta Paediatr Scand.* 1985; 74:405.
2. Naidu S. Rett syndrome: a disorder affecting early brain growth. *Ann Neurol.* 1997; 42:3.
3. Trevathan E, Naidu S. The clinical recognition and differential diagnosis of Rett syndrome. *J Child Neurol.* 1988; 3(suppl):S6.
4. Kerr AM, Nomura Y, Armstrong D, et al. Guidelines for reporting clinical features in cases with MeCP2 mutations. *Brain Dev.* 2001; 23:208.
5. Hagberg B, Hanefeld F, Percy A, Skjeldal O. An update on clinically applicable diagnostic criteria in Rett syndrome. *Eur J Pediatr Neurol.* 2002; 6:293.
6. Cappellen D, De Oliveira C, Ricol D, et al. Rett syndrome is caused by mutations in X-linked *MeCP2* encoding methyl-CpG-binding protein 2. *Nat Genet.* 1999; 23:185.
7. Hoffbuhr K, Devaney JM, LaFleur B, et al. MeCP2 mutations in children with and without the phenotype of Rett syndrome. *Neurology.* 2001; 56:1486.
8. Jung BP, Jugloff DG, Zhang G, Logan R, Brown S, Eubanks JH. The expression of methyl CpG binding factor MeCP2 correlates with cellular differentiation in the developing rat brain and in cultured cells. *J Neurobiol.* 2003; 55:86.
9. Motil K, Schultz R, Wong W, Glaze D. Increased energy expenditure associated with repetitive involuntary movement does not contribute to growth failure in girls with Rett syndrome. *J Pediatr.* 1998; 132:228.
10. Platte P, Jaschke H, Herbert C, Korenke GC. Increased resting metabolic rate in girls with Rett syndrome compared to girls with developmental disabilities. *Neuropediatrics.* 2011; 42:179.
11. Glaze D. Commentary: the challenge of Rett syndrome. *Neuropediatrics.* 1995; 26:78.
12. Percy A, Isaacs J, Lane J. Rett syndrome: clinical experience in Alabama. *Rivista Medica.* 1998; 4:207.
13. Cooke D., Naidu;S.,Plotnick; L., Berjiwutz; G, Abnornalities of thyroid function and glucose control in subjects with Rett Syndrome. Horm Rsrch 43:273–78,
14. Huppke P.; Roth C.; Cgrusteb H,; Brockmann K.; Hanefeld F. Endocrinological sstudy on growth retardation in Rett syndrome. Acta Paeditri 2001 Nov; 90 (11):1257–61
15. Reilly S, Cass H. Growth and nutrition in Rett syndrome. *Dis Rehab.* 2001; 23:118.
16. Isaacs JS, Murdock M, Lane J, Percy AK. Eating difficulties in girls with Rett syndrome compared with other developmental disabilities. *J Am Diet Assoc.* 2003; 103:224.
17. Budden S. Rett syndrome: studies of 13 affected girls. *Am J Med Genet.* 1986; 24:99.
18. Motil KJ, Schultz RJ, Browning K, Trautwein L, Glaze DG. Oropharyngeal dysfunction and gastroesophageal dysmotility are present in girls and women with Rett syndrome. *J Pediatr Gastroenterol Nutr.* 1999; 29:31.
19. Gonzalez A, Stombaugh J, Lozupone C, Turnbaugh PJ, Gordon JI, Knight R. The mind-body-microbial continuum. *Dialogues Clin Neurosci.* 2011; 13:55.
20. Naidu S, Hyman S, Piazza K, et al. Rett syndrome: progress report on studies at the Kennedy Institute. *Brain Dev.* 1990; 12:5.
21. Motil, K., Schultz R., Brown B., Glaze D., Percy, A. Altered energy balance may account for growth failure in Rett syndrome. J Child Neurol 1994 Jul;9 (3):315–9.
22. Thommessan M, Kase B, Heiberg A. Growth and nutrition in 10 girls with Rett syndrome. *Acta Paediatr.* 1992; 81:686.
23. Naidu S, Hyman S, Piazza K, et al. A population-based approach to the investigation of osteopenia in Rett syndrome. *Dev Med Child Neurol.* 1999; 41:323.
24. Schwartzman, F. Vitolo M., Schwatzman J, Morais M. Eating practices, nutrition status and constipation in patients with Rett syndrome. Arq Gastroenterol 2008 Oct-Dec; 45 (4): 284-9.25. Lloyd D, Peirro A. The therapeutic approach to the child with feeding difficulty. III: enteral feeding. In: Sullivan P, Rosenbloom L, eds. *Feeding the Disabled Child.* Clinics in Developmental Medicine. Cambridge, UK: Cambridge University Press; 1996; 140:132.
26. Fortunato JE, Darbari A, Cuffari C, et al. Esophageal motility dysfunction in children with Rett syndrome, gastroesophageal reflux, and dysphagia. *J Appl Res.* 2007 7:84.
27. Krick J, Murphy PE, Markham JF, Shapiro BK. A proposed formula for calculating energy needs of children with cerebral palsy. *Dev Med Child Neurol.* 1992; 34:481.

# B.

# BEHAVIORAL AND EATING DISORDERS

## 18 Obesity

SHIRLEY W. EKVALL, VALLI K. EKVALL, DIANE SPEAR, AND MICHAEL FARRELL

An energy imbalance results in obesity. An individual is considered to be in energy balance when energy intake equals energy expenditure. If energy intake exceeds energy expenditure, the excess calories are stored as adipose tissue. An energy imbalance may occur when energy intake increases and energy expenditure remains the same; when energy intake remains the same and energy expenditure decreases; or when energy intake increases and energy expenditure decreases. The causes of energy imbalance are multifactorial and may include genetic, metabolic, psychological, and environmental factors.

The prevalence of overweight in children and adolescents in the United States has been increasing since the 1980s. The percentage of Americans who are obese has risen noticeably in the past few years, defying efforts by health experts and policy makers to rein in the obesity epidemic.

In 2011–2012, 35% of adults were obese, a number that had seemed to plateau since 2003 to 2004. But in 2013–2014 that number rose to 38%, based on data from the National Health and Nutrition Examination Survey (NHANES), which is released every 2 years. From 2011–2014, the prevalence of obesity in children and adolescents was 17%, a figure that had not changed significantly from 2003. In addition, adult women had higher rates of obesity (38.3%) than did men (34.3%) during that period. The results varied significantly by race: prevalence was lowest for Asian adults (11.7%), followed by white adults (34.5%), Hispanic adults (42.5%), and black adults (48.1%).

The National Center for Health Statistics (NCHS) found that children consume high quantities of fast food. The NHANES found that in 2011–2012, more than one-third of children and teens consumed fast food on a given day, and youngsters consumed on average 12.4% of their daily calories from fast-food restaurants. Children aged 12 to 19 years ate more fast food than children aged 2 to 11 years. The researchers found no differences in caloric intake from fast foods according to sex, poverty status, or weight status, but black and white children consumed more fast foods than Hispanic or Asian children.

Populations of children and adults with developmental disabilities such as myelomeningocele,[2-4] Prader-Willi syndrome,[5] and Down syndrome,[6-8] and autism[9] have been reported to have a higher prevalence of overweight than those in the general population. Some studies have involved a limited number of children. Obesity prevalences in children without and with a disability derived from NHANES, National Health Interview Survey (NHIS) and NSCH data were reported by Bandini et al.[10]

### CHILDHOOD OBESITY HISTORY

Dietz suggested that there are three critical periods during childhood development when the risk of overweight onset is elevated: the prenatal period, the period often referred to as *adiposity rebound* around 5 to 7 years of age, and adolescence.[8]

Two important determinants of the likelihood that childhood obesity will persist into adulthood are its severity and age of onset. The greater the severity of obesity, the more likely it is to persist.[11] In an animal study, the offspring of nutrient-restricted mothers during pregnancy had increased risk for obesity in later life due to the effects on adipose tissue deposition and leptin.[12] Likewise, lower birth weight was related to a higher adult subcutaneous fat mass, greater truncal distribution of that fat, and increased risk for obesity.[13] The probability that an overweight child will become an overweight adult also increases with age.[14] The likelihood that early obesity will persist into adulthood is greatest if the child is overweight during the adolescent period.[15]

There is very little information on the natural history of obesity in children with special needs. A new body of evidence is needed with stronger research designs that adhere to precise dosing characteristics for key health outcomes (e.g., pain/fatigue reduction, improved cardio-respiratory health). Multicenter trials are needed for low-prevalence populations to strengthen research designs and increase the generalizability of study findings.[16] Chumlea and Cronk suggested that overweight in children with Down syndrome becomes apparent during early childhood.[15] In a later report, they indicated that children with Down syndrome have greater body weights at statures of 105 to 110 cm than do children without mental retardation.[17] In children with Prader-Willi syndrome, obesity occurs early in development. In fact, obesity before 6 years of age is considered one of the diagnostic criteria for this condition.[5] For the child who has a physical disability, obesity may further impair mobility and the development of gross motor skills, reducing the child's ability to ambulate and increasing the likelihood that the child will remain overweight. Atencio-La Follette et al. noted that children with myelomeningocele and high lesion levels were less likely to be ambulatory.[18]

The consequences of childhood obesity are significant. As reviewed by Must and Strauss, childhood obesity is associated with elevated cardiovascular risk factor levels, type 2 diabetes, orthopedic problems, sleep apnea, and menstrual irregularities.[19] Sinha et al. reported that a significant proportion of obese children exhibit impaired glucose tolerance.[20] In addition to immediate consequences, obesity that persists into adulthood is accompanied by a substantially increased likelihood of chronic disease, including heart disease, hypertension, stroke, certain cancers, and gallbladder disease. Obesity, glucose intolerance, and hypertension in children were associated with an increased rate of premature death from endogenous causes, whereas hypercholesteremia was not a predictor of premature death from endogenous causes.[21] Obesity is a stigmatized condition in the United States, putting overweight children at risk for teasing and peer rejection. As a result, there are social and emotional consequences that can lead to depression, anxiety, and other psychological conditions. The global childhood obesity epidemic may be related to the association between social economic status and obesity.[22]

## BIOCHEMICAL, GENETIC, AND CLINICAL ABNORMALITIES

Biochemical tests rarely reveal the cause of obesity. Hypothyroidism and other endocrine disorders are not common causes of obesity in children or adolescents. However, thyroid function, fasting blood sugar, cholesterol, triglyceride, and liver function tests may be of some benefit in determining the cause of obesity in some children. Impaired glucose tolerance, a precursor of type 2 diabetes, is often detected in obese children and adolescents.[23]

There has been increasing interest in the role of the human microbiome in the pathogenesis of obesity and its complications such as the metabolic syndrome, nonalcoholic liver disease and nonalcoholic steatohepatitis. The human microbiome is composed of trillions of bacteria that live in and on the human body, mostly in the intestinal tract. Studies suggest that gut microbiota are involved in the control of weight, energy homeostasis, and inflammation. Therefore, they may play a previously underappreciated role in obesity for both children[24] and adults.

The human microbiome has two prominent bacterial phyla: Firmicutes and Bacteroidetes. Numerous studies have shown a difference in the composition and the ratio of these two groups in lean versus obese individuals. Diet composition also affects the microbiome. The microbiome is established early in life. The major initial inoculum is maternal flora. Maternal flora can be affected by diet and antibiotic administration. Probiotics change the maternal microbiome and thus affect the infant microbiome. The route of delivery, vaginal versus caesarean delivery, and type of feeding (breast milk or formula) affect the microbiome of the infant. Repeated antibiotic exposure also affects the microbiome. Once a microbiome is established, it tends to stay the same.

The composition of the microbiome affects the ability to ferment nondigestible carbohydrates in the colon. This fermentation produces short-chain fatty acids such as acetate, propionate, and butyrate, which are the preferred fuels of the colonocyte. Fermentation results in increased "scavenging" of ingested carbohydrates and thus affects energy intake. Alterations in the microbiome also affect gastrointestinal hormones, particularly glucagon-like peptide 1 (GLP-1) and peptide YY. These hormones inhibit gastric motility via the ileal brake, thus decreasing energy intake.

## GENETICS

Evidence suggests that there is a genetic component to obesity. Studies examining fatness similarities among twins and other biological siblings have shown that similarities are strongest for monozygotic twins, less so for dizygotic twins, and still less for other siblings.[25] Heritability of fatness has been examined by assessing monozygotic and dizygotic twins living in similar or different environments and in adoptees separated from their biological parents.[26,27] The twin study and the adoptive study both found that heredity was a major determinant of body mass index (BMI). These observations support a strong genetic component to fatness. However, because families share the same environment, it is difficult to determine how much of the similarity in fatness results from genetic factors and how much from environmental factors. A study of children whose parents were obese suggests that children with one or more obese parents have a significantly greater risk of becoming obese than children with two lean parents.[15] In this study, for both overweight and non-overweight children younger than 10 years of age, the risk of obesity in adult life with an obese parent was more than twice that of children with lean parents.

## FACTORS TO BE CONSIDERED IN NUTRITIONAL EVALUATION

### Energy Expenditure

Studies have been done to determine whether the energy expenditure of obese persons is less than that of nonobese persons. In this section, the literature on the resting metabolic rate (RMR) and the thermic effect of food is briefly reviewed. The other two components of energy expenditure in children are the energy spent on physical activity, which is voluntary, and the energy cost of growth. Studies examining the relationship of physical activity to obesity are discussed later in the chapter (see "Environmental Factors").

### Resting Metabolic Rate

The RMR is the amount of energy required to maintain life processes; it comprises 60% to 75% of the total energy expenditure (TEE). The RMR can be measured by indirect calorimetry or predicted on the basis of body size, body weight, and body height. Studies in both children[28,29] and adults[30] have shown that RMR is higher in obese compared with nonobese persons when expressed in absolute terms (kcal/day) (see Appendix 1–4). This can be attributed to the greater body size of the obese person. When RMR is adjusted for body composition, it has not been found to be lower in obese children[28,30] or adults.[31,32] However, in children and adults with Prader-Willi syndrome,[33] myelodysplasia,[34,35] or Down syndrome,[36] RMR was found to be lower than in typically developing children. Fat-free mass (FFM) was decreased in all these groups of children and adolescents and accounted for the decrease in RMR. However, in the children with Down syndrome, the lower RMR could not be explained by a decrease in FFM.

### Thermic Effect of Food

The thermic effect of food (TEF) is the increase in energy expenditure observed after a meal. Studies on the TEF are equivocal; some suggest that energy expenditure may be decreased in obese persons,[37–39] whereas others show no differences between obese and nonobese people.[40–43] Although the TEF represents only a small percentage of the daily energy expenditure (6–10%), small differences over a long period could potentially lead to a significant energy imbalance. Overall, the studies to date of energy expenditure do not support the hypothesis that RMR or TEF is reduced in the already obese state in typically developing children and adults. However, children with disabilities who have decreased resting energy expenditure may have an increased risk of obesity. Longitudinal studies are presently underway to determine whether low energy expenditure is a risk factor for obesity.

## Environmental Factors

Although genetic factors may increase the susceptibility of an individual to obesity, obesity is ultimately caused by a positive energy balance, which occurs when energy intake exceeds energy expenditure for a prolonged period. Thus, the interaction between genetics—that is, an increased susceptibility to obesity—coupled with an environment that promotes increased energy intake and/or decreased energy expenditure can lead to obesity. Environmental factors that may contribute to obesity are those that influence either energy intake or energy expenditure.

### Energy Intake

Many studies have been conducted to compare the energy intake of obese and nonobese children and adults. However, because of the significant underreporting of energy intake in both obese and nonobese persons,[31,44] these studies have not been useful in determining whether obese people eat more than nonobese people.

Dietary factors that may increase energy intake include increased accessibility to food, the lower cost of fast foods, and increased availability of food outside the home. Moreover, portion sizes in restaurants are often large, and fast-food restaurants typically provide high-fat, high-calorie meals. In the United States, many high-energy food items are more readily accessible and less costly than fresh fruits and vegetables. Vending machines are frequently located in recreational facilities and schools and tend to sell high-energy, low-nutrient-dense foods or carbonated soft drinks and juices in 12- to 20-oz (560 mL) portions, each providing 1.5 to 2.5 servings. In a longitudinal study of children 11 to 17 years of age, Ludwig et al. reported an association between consumption of sugar-sweetened beverages and overweight.[45] Use of sugar substitutes such as stevia or monk fruit extracts appears to be acceptable, plain water is even better. The way food is packaged and sold often makes it more economical to buy the larger size of an item, although the larger portion may be excessive. Young and Nestle reported increases in portion size for many foods since the 1970s.[46] Marketing strategies and advertising on television and billboards also encourage the consumption of high-energy, low-nutrient-dense foods. All of these environmental factors can promote a positive energy balance.

### Physical Activity and Total Daily Energy Expenditure

The energy spent on physical activity is a major determinant of daily energy expenditure. Decreases in physical activity lead to decreases in energy expenditure. If the energy spent on physical activity is decreased without a concomitant decrease in energy intake, a positive energy imbalance will result. Although the energy cost of physical activity cannot be measured directly, it can be calculated from measures of TEE and RMR. The TEE/RMR ratio is the amount of energy spent above resting and is often referred to as the *physical activity level*, although it also includes the energy associated with the TEF. Studies of the energy spent on physical activity by obese and nonobese children have not found obese children to use less energy than nonobese children.[29,47] This may be a result of the increased energy cost of moving a greater body weight (see Appendix 1–4 for equations).

Studies of daily energy expenditure have been conducted in populations of children and adolescents with disabilities. In a study by Bandini et al.,[34] TEE and the TEE/RMR ratio (Fig. 18–1) were significantly lower in nonambulatory adolescents with myelodysplasia than in typically developing adolescents but were not lower in children who could ambulate. Similar studies in nonambulatory children with

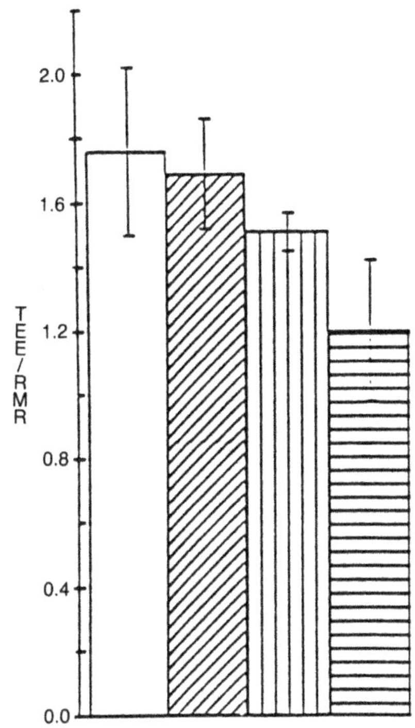


**Figure 18–1.** Comparison of energy expenditure above resting levels in normal obese adolescents and adolescents with myelodysplasia. TEE/RMR = ratio of total energy expenditure to resting metabolic rate. (From Bandini LG, Schoeller DA, Fukagawa NK, Wykes LJ, Dietz WH. Body composition and energy expenditure in adolescents with cerebral palsy or myelodysplasia. *Pediatr Res.* 1991; 29:70; and Schoeller DA, Levitsky LL, Bandini LG, Dietz WH, Walczak A. Energy expenditure and body composition in Prader-Willi syndrome. *Metabolism.* 1988; 37:115.)

cerebral palsy have also reported a lower daily energy expenditure compared with controls.[34,48,49] In persons with Prader-Willi syndrome, the TEE was found to be lower than that in obese or nonobese individuals; the differences were attributed to decreases in both FFM and physical activity.[33]

### Inactivity

The more time children spend engaged in sedentary behavior, the less time they spend being physically active. In Australia, additional green space in neighborhoods provided improved weight status in a study of more than 4000 children aged 6 to 13 years. Waist circumference and waist-to-height ratio were used as the methodology.[50] Children who spend significant amounts of time in sedentary behaviors will use less energy. Gortmaker et al. showed a significant relationship between obesity and hours of television watching.[51] Playing video games and using a computer are also common sedentary behaviors of children. Safety issues may limit physical activity in some children; many live in areas where it is unsafe to walk to school or play outside, contributing to a decrease in physical activity and an increase in sedentary behavior. For children with disabilities, structured activities are limited. Children with disabilities often do not have the opportunity to play on a sports team or engage in community programs. Physical disabilities may further limit involvement in after-school activities.

## Clinical Assessment

Identification of obesity in the child and adolescent depends on the criteria used. Because laboratory measures of body composition, such as underwater weighing, dual energy X-ray absorptiometry (DEXA), potassium 40 ($^{40}$K) counting, and measures of total body water are too expensive and laborious to be used in clinical settings, anthropometric measures have been used to assess obesity in children and adolescents. Measures of weight-for-height, BMI, and triceps skinfold (TSF) are the most commonly used anthropometric indices to monitor growth and to identify children who are overweight. BMI is calculated by dividing weight in kilograms by height in meters squared (wt/ht$^2$). Charts prepared by the NCHS have been used to identify children who are overweight—that is, above the 95th percentile of weight-for-height.[52] The Centers for Disease Control and Prevention has published revised growth charts (http://www.cdc.gov/growthcharts) that include new reference charts for BMI based on age and gender and are recommended for the identification of overweight children. They provide percentile curves for BMI and include the 3rd and 97th percentiles for age and gender.

Because BMI is not a measure of body fatness, persons who have large amounts of muscle may be overweight without having excess fat. If the diagnosis of obesity is questionable, a measure of skinfold thickness should be made. Sex- and age-specific standards for skinfold thickness are available. A method of calculating body fat percentage from the sum of biceps, triceps, subscapular, and suprailiac skinfold thickness is presented in Table 18–1. In adults, a measure of waist circumference is useful to determine the risk of associated morbidity with increased body weight[53]; waist circumference standards for children are not available but are being developed by Ekvall et al.[54]

Diagnosis of overweight in the child with a developmental disorder is complicated by the fact that growth often differs significantly from that of typically developing children. Because of alterations in body composition in children with disabilities, BMI may not be a valid measure of overweight. Validation studies on the use of BMI to assess body fatness in children with disabilities are lacking. Therefore, caution must be used when interpreting BMI percentiles for children with disabilities. Although there is a lack of validation studies on BMI, several studies have evaluated the use of skinfold thickness as a measure of body fatness in children with disabilities. Luke et al. found no difference in body composition determined by skinfold measures and by isotopic dilution techniques in children with Down syndrome.[55] However, Lee showed that fatness increases over paralyzed limbs,[56] suggesting that TSF may not be an accurate assessment of body fatness in children with paraplegia because there may be an alteration in fat distribution. In small studies of subjects with Prader-Willi syndrome,[33] cerebral palsy,[34] or myelodysplasia,[34] skinfold thickness underestimated body fatness measured primarily by isotopic dilution techniques. Grogan and Ekvall examined body composition in children with myelomeningocele or myelodysplasia and observed a significant correlation of abdominal skinfold thickness and TSF, with the child's percentage of FFM determined by $^{40}$K counting. Body fat correlated significantly with waist circumference but not with BMI in this population.[35]

These data suggest that although equations for determining body fatness for typically developing children may be acceptable, they may be less accurate in children with disabilities, especially those with atrophy of the lower extremities (because height is squared in the BMI calculation). These findings emphasize the need for specific anthropometric references to accurately assess fatness in children with disabilities. Because of the morbidity associated with adult obesity and the increased risk of impaired glucose tolerance and other consequences discussed earlier, identification and treatment for overweight children and adolescents is essential. Treatment goals for children at risk of overweight (84th–95th percentile) and those actually overweight (>95th percentile) are presented in Table 18–2.[55]

**Table 18–1.** Skinfold Thickness* at Different Body Fat Percentages in Children Aged 0–18 Years

| | Percent Body Fat, Male (mm) | | | | | Percent Body Fat, Female (mm) | | | | |
|---|---|---|---|---|---|---|---|---|---|---|
| Age (yr) | 15 | 20 | 25 | 30 | 35 | 15 | 20 | 25 | 30 | 35 |
| 0† | 17 | 22 | 30 | 40 | 52 | 17 | 22 | 30 | 40 | 52 |
| 1‡ | 18 | 24 | 32 | 43 | 58 | 18 | 24 | 32 | 43 | 58 |
| 2 | 18 | 25 | 34 | 45 | 60 | 18 | 25 | 34 | 45 | 60 |
| 4 | 20 | 27 | 37 | 51 | 68 | 18 | 25 | 34 | 46 | 62 |
| 6 | 22 | 30 | 41 | 57 | 78 | 19 | 25 | 35 | 47 | 63 |
| 8 | 23 | 33 | 46 | 64 | 88 | 19 | 26 | 35 | 47 | 65 |
| 10 | 25 | 36 | 51 | 72 | 101 | 19 | 27 | 37 | 51 | 69 |
| 12 | 27 | 40 | 57 | 81 | 115 | 21 | 30 | 42 | 58 | 80 |
| 14 | 27 | 44 | 63 | 92 | 132 | 23 | 33 | 47 | 66 | 92 |
| 16 | 32 | 48 | 71 | 104 | 152 | 25 | 37 | 53 | 75 | 106 |
| 18 | 34 | 52 | 79 | 117 | 175 | 27 | 40 | 58 | 85 | 122 |

*Sum of bicipital, tricipital, suprailiac, and subscapular thicknesses.
†Mean age was used (6 mo).
‡Mean age was used (18 mo).
Modified from Yanovski JA. Pediatric obesity. *Rev Endoc Metab Disord.* 2001; 2:371. Used with permission.

**Table 18–2.** Recommended Weight Goals

| BMI Percentile | Complications* | Goal |
|---|---|---|
| 85th–94th | No | Weight maintenance |
| 95th | No | Weight maintenance |
| | Yes | Weight loss |
| 85th–94th | No | Weight maintenance |
| | Yes | Weight loss |
| 95th | No | Weight loss |

*Indicates mild complications such as mild hypertension, insulin resistance, and dyslipidemias. More acute complications, such as orthopedic problems, sleep apnea, obesity, hypoventilation syndrome, or pseudotumor cerebri, should be referred to a pediatric obesity center. BMI = body mass index.
Adapted from Barlow SE, Dietz WH. Obesity evaluation and treatment: expert committee recommendations. The Maternal and Child Health Bureau, Health Resources and Services Administration, and the Department of Health and Human Services. *Pediatrics.* 1998; 102:E29, Figure 2. Copyright © 1998 American Academy of Pediatrics.

Criteria for selecting patients for a weight control program vary among facilities. The guidelines used by the Nutrition Department at the Cincinnati Children's Hospital Medical Center's Division of Developmental Disabilities (CCDDD) for identifying children at high risk for overweight are as follows:

- Children with one or both parents and/or siblings who are obese
- Children with a family history of heart disease
- Children who show a tendency toward a discrepancy of weight-for-height (>10% overweight for height or weight >50th percentile), especially those from birth to 4 years of age and those entering adolescence (9 to 13 years of age).
- Children with >25% immobility determined from the physical activity score (see Chapter 4) and >25th percentile in weight for age
- Children with Down syndrome, Prader-Willi syndrome, cretinism, myelomeningocele, spastic cerebral palsy, Rubinstein-Taybi syndrome, Klinefelter syndrome, or other endocrine disorders

## NUTRITIONAL COUNSELING AND FAMILY EMOTIONAL SUPPORT

Diet remains the cornerstone of effective weight reduction. Although caloric restriction is necessary to promote a negative energy balance, it should be initiated with caution in the overweight child. Growing children require energy to support adequate growth. Therefore, the key is to provide the right number of calories that will allow for weight loss and/or weight maintenance while at the same time supporting growth. Recommended amounts of nutrients are vital for proper physical maturation, and the diet must contain adequate amounts of carbohydrate, fat, protein, vitamins, and minerals to promote good health.[57]

Several investigators have expressed energy needs of children with disabilities in terms of kilocalories per centimeter of height (kcal/cm). For children with Down syndrome, caloric intakes were estimated to be 16.1 kcal/cm for boys and 14. 3 kcal/cm for girls (Table 18–3).[58] Bandini et al.[34] reported 9.0 to 12.5 kcal/cm for those with spastic quadriparesis and 10.6 to 16.1 kcal/cm for two adolescents with athetosis. Culley and Middleton did not measure energy expenditure directly in children with cerebral palsy but categorized energy needs based on caloric intake in 5- to 11-year-old children according to the degree of motor dysfunction.[59] Children with cerebral palsy who are ambulatory but have mild to moderate motor dysfunction needed 13.9 kcal/cm of height, whereas those who were nonambulatory needed 11.1 kcal/cm. Bandini et al.[60] reported a significant correlation of RMR with body height in adolescents and young adults with severe CNS impairment. These numbers should be interpreted cautiously because

**Table 18–3.** Estimated Caloric Requirements for Children with Specific Developmental Disabilities (based on height)*

| Developmental Disability | Guide for Caloric Intake |
|---|---|
| *Down Syndrome*[17,55,58,59]<br>Results from the presence of an extra chromosome 21, which causes developmental problems such as congenital heart disease, mental retardation, small stature, and decreased tone | Boys, 16.1 kcal/cm (40.9 kcal/in.)<br>Girls, 14.3 kcal/cm (36.3 kcal/in.) |
| *Prader-Willi Syndrome*[5,33]<br>A disorder characterized by uncontrollable eating habits, inability to distinguish hunger from appetite, severe obesity, poorly developed genitalia, and moderate to severe mental retardation | For maintenance, 10–11 kcal/cm (26.7 kcal/in.)<br>For weight loss, 8.5 kcal/cm (21.6 kcal/in.) |
| *Spina Bifida (Myelomeningocele)*[16,34,35]<br>Results from a midline defect of the skin, spinal column, and spinal cord; characterized by hydrocephalus, mental retardation, and lack of muscular control | For maintenance, 9–11 kcal/cm (25.0 kcal/in.) or estimate LBM or AT<br>For weight loss, 7 kcal/cm (17.78 kcal/in.) or about 50% of the level for a child without myelomeningocele if weight is >50th percentile, activity is minimal, and age is >3 yr; after age 6 yr, determine by AT or LBM. Keep weight at <25th percentile for age. |
| *Cerebral Palsy*[34,59]<br>A disorder of muscle control or coordination resulting from injury to the brain during its early stages of development; there may be associated problems with intellectual, visual, or other functions. | 13.9 kcal/cm (35.3 kcal/in.) for age 5–11 years with mild to moderate activity level<br>11.1 kcal/cm (28.2 kcal/in.) for age 5–11 years with severe restrictions |

*References to guides for caloric intake can be found in the chapters on individual disorders.
AT = adipose tissue; LBM = lean body mass.
Modified from Rokusek C, Heindrichs E, eds. *Nutrition and Feeding for the Developmentally Disabled: A How-To Manual.* Vermillion, SD: South Dakota University Affiliated Facility Center for the Developmentally Disabled; 1985. Used with permission.

they are based on very small groups of children. In the Grogan and Ekvall study, the lean body mass (LBM) of 14 children with myelomeningocele averaged 50% of LBM in children without that condition. Caloric needs, which are largely based on FFM or active tissue, would be only 9 to 11 kcal/cm height, and about 7 kcal/cm height would be required for weight loss after age 3.[35]

Use of the familiar four food groups model (www.choosemyplate.gov/kids) with reduced amounts of fat, sugar, and sodium is suggested (see Appendix 7). Use of skim milk or low-fat dairy products for children older than 2 years of age and consumption of fresh fruits and vegetables and foods high in fiber (e.g., legumes) are fundamental principles for promoting good health. Likewise, limiting the consumption of processed foods and foods high in sodium that are available within the home, at work, at school, or in restaurants is recommended. Among other things, increased sodium intake can cause thirst and increased snacking, contributing to weight gain. Fast food can be a strong contributor to weight gain.

A child with a disability creates special challenges for the family, both practically and emotionally. The child's development and his or her success in participating effectively in day-to-day life are directly related to the ability of the family to adapt to the child's special needs, which include nutrition and weight control. The family must be an integral part of any intervention plan. A child with special needs may have language or cognitive delays, behavior problems, poorly developed play skills, social deficits, weak self-help skills, and other difficulties, all which may have a significant impact on the family and may have implications for nutrition counseling.

Nutrition counseling, like other forms of counseling, must adhere to the basic principles of good practice:

1. Establish positive, nonjudgmental rapport with the child and family
2. Assume a role of consultant rather than expert; this acknowledges the strengths of the child and family and their ability to be partners in the child's own care
3. Conduct a comprehensive assessment to determine the best course of action
4. Design interventions that are individualized and respect the family's values
5. Provide information and advice that are appropriate and not too technical or too basic
6. Set realistic and achievable goals
7. Offer ongoing support and encouragement throughout the process

The dietitian plays a crucial role in providing support and encouragement to the child and family as they attempt to change long-held behavior patterns. Initiating and sustaining behavioral changes are most likely accomplished when the child and family feel respected and accepted.

Conducting a comprehensive history is the first step in understanding the evolution of a child's eating patterns. Many children with special needs have early feeding problems, which may have an impact on current habits. An assessment of whether feeding problems have been a result of physiological, functional, or social-interactive factors is important. Physiological problems include chewing and swallowing difficulties, low tone, and oral-motor difficulties. Functional difficulties include gastroesophageal reflux, a history of ear or upper respiratory tract infections, and avoidance of certain food textures. Social-interactive factors include oppositional behavior at mealtimes and parental anxiety about feeding. These factors must be understood so that interventions can be appropriately tailored to meet the child's and family's needs. For example, a child who had an early feeding problem in which maintaining sufficient caloric intake was problematic may now have a healthy and, at times, too large appetite. This child's parents may have a very difficult time restricting foods for the child when earlier years were spent anxiously trying to encourage the child to eat. Likewise, parent-child interactions in which food issues have resulted in power struggles require special attention if the nutrition plan is to be carried out successfully. Cultural and family values must also be taken into consideration because food is often used as a means of nurturing the child. For children who are difficult to nurture and soothe because of their special needs, families may turn to food as a way to calm, praise, or reward the child. The dietitian must be aware and respectful of these issues and devise strategies that promote healthful eating while not dismissing the ways in which the family is trying to support the child.

The most effective way in which a child can be helped to engage in healthy eating patterns and physical exercise is to encourage all family members to adopt these habits. This creates an environment where messages and practices become consistent and decreases the likelihood that special eating rules apply only to the child who is overweight. It reduces the probability that the overweight child will be singled out or identified as the "problem." Moreover, because many overweight children have overweight parents, the benefits of adopting healthy eating and physical exercise habits are experienced by all family members. It is important that the dietitian assess the family's readiness to change and the extent to which they are prepared to change menus, snacks, and physical activity routines. Research has shown that there are stages of change that can be identified in individuals or families,[61] and that motivational interviewing techniques can be employed to increase readiness to adopt new behaviors.[62] If the dietitian determines that the family is not ready to change, then it is advisable not to try to institute a comprehensive weight management plan. Such a plan will likely fail and may contribute to the child's and family's sense of personal failure and hopelessness. A health-centered rather than weight-centered perspective, with parents as the central agents, may be more effective.[63]

For families who are motivated to change their eating and physical activity behaviors, the dietitian's goal is to help the family understand the relationship between energy intake and energy expenditure in easy-to-understand terms and to assist them to make changes in eating and activity habits. The first step is to help families understand their current eating and physical activity behaviors and to appreciate the ways in which these contribute to the child's (and other family members') overweight or obesity. Identifying particular problematic practices (e.g., high-fat/high-calorie snacks, excessive television viewing) can help the family recognize those habits that need to be changed or modified. The dietitian plays a strong educational role in teaching the family about healthful eating practices and the benefits of physical exercise. The dietitian can also assist the family to make changes in the structure of their eating habits, such as when meals are eaten, what kinds and amounts of food are consumed, "temptation foods" that remain in the household, and ways in which food may be used to praise or reward the child. Helping the family to substitute more nutritionally balanced foods for high-calorie, high-fat foods, identifying new ways to engage the entire family in physical activity, and devising new ways to praise and reward children other than the use of food are a few examples of concrete changes that can be made.[60] Weight management and physical activity should begin in young children as preventive measures.[64,65]

Helping parents to change daily routines within the household can promote weight loss and control for all members. Examples of areas to focus on include

- Encouraging physical activity, with an emphasis on fun and enjoyment
- Establishing specific times for meals and snacks on a daily basis
- Making healthful snacks (e.g., fruits, vegetables) readily available in the home and eliminating unhealthful snacks that serve as temptations
- Avoiding the use of food as a reward
- Allowing children developmentally appropriate control of food and food choices
- Praising desirable behavior (both related to and not related to eating)
- Limiting the amount of time spent watching television or playing computer games
- Modeling healthy eating and physical activity behaviors
- Supporting and assisting the child to manage any teasing or hurtful social situations that occur because of overweight

## Behavior Modification

As described earlier, a family-based treatment program that combines nutrition education, exercise, behavior modification, and family support has been shown to be effective. Epstein et al. showed that in families with an obese parent, treatments targeted at both the parent and the child have resulted in more successful weight loss and weight maintenance than programs in which only the child is targeted.[65] If a child is older than 9 years of age and is capable of understanding, he or she should be interviewed separately from the parent, if possible. Moreover, long-term weight control is more successfully achieved by exercise attained through lifestyle changes than by structured exercise programs.[66] Examples of lifestyle changes include walking to school instead of driving, doing housework, taking the stairs instead of an elevator, parking farther away from one's destination and walking, and other such changes that increase energy expenditure as part of daily activities. Other studies conducted by Epstein et al. suggested that both decreasing sedentary behavior and increasing physical activity are effective tools to promote weight loss in overweight children.[67] In a review of behavioral treatments for obesity, Robinson emphasized the need for self-monitoring of diet and activity during the treatment program and suggested that parents often need help with parenting skills to follow through with behavioral modification programs.[68] For children with developmental disorders, achieving increased physical activity may be difficult. The assistance of a physical therapist may be useful in designing activities that are appropriate for specific individual needs. For example, the level of the lesion

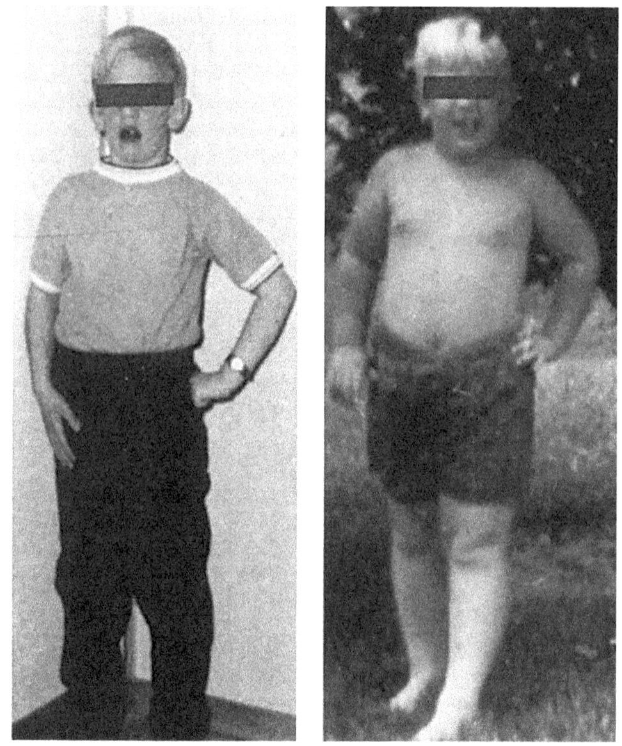

**Figure 18–2.** Picture of a child after weight loss *(left)* and before weight loss *(right)*. The child was rewarded for behavioral changes and resulting weight loss with a watch. (From Cincinnati Children's Hospital Medical Center, Division of Developmental Disabilities, Department of Nutrition. Used with permission.)

may have some effect on ambulation in children with myelomeningocele. A "Wheelies Club" for those in wheelchairs with this condition appears helpful. (See Chapter 4 for physical activity/caloric expenditure and Appendix 4 for the physical activity record.) The behavior modification reward for weight loss, such as a watch, may be given by the family (Fig. 18–2).

Success is most likely when weight loss goals are set as small steps within a long-term process. Each step involves the alteration of an undesirable behavior and should be reinforced through rewards that promote adoption and retention of a new, desired behavior. For children, the most common types of reinforcement are verbal praise delivered immediately after the desired behavior is performed and simple tangible rewards such as a small toy or an outing with a parent. Individuals, including children, often benefit from receiving feedback about their progress when trying to adopt a new behavior or achieve a new goal. Devising a chart that tracks healthful eating and increased physical activity can be reinforcing in itself, or a chart can be used in combination with other small, motivating rewards. For older children and adolescents, participation in group programs that provide peer support can also have positive outcomes. A low score on the Healthy Eating Index–2010, based on the *Dietary Guidelines for Americans* from the US Department of Agriculture, was associated with overweight and obesity, and this index may be used as a tool.[69]

## Follow-up

For a weight reduction program to be successful, it is necessary to provide continued supportive therapy after the program has been completed. The components of follow-up counseling are similar to those used in the actual treatment. Follow-up individualized nutrition counseling, exercise encouragement, and behavioral and emotional support are all important for promoting adherence. Many successful weight reductions are short term; to improve the overall long-term effectiveness of a weight loss program, a follow-up program is required.

## GUIDELINES FOR THE DIETETIC PROFESSIONAL

The following guidelines were adapted from those of the Academy of Nutrition and Dietetics.[70] In general, dietitians can improve the overall health and well-being of children by

- Promoting the *Dietary Guidelines for Americans* for healthy children after the age of 2 years
- Endorsing the use of the four food groups model (www.choosemyplate.gov/kids) as a guide for meeting the dietary recommendations
- Using the Mediterranean diet or the Dietary Approaches to Stop Hypertension (DASH) diet (see Appendix 1)
- Encouraging use of the Kid's Activity Model (see "Resources for the Dietitian") to promote physical activity among children
- Conducting effective nutrition education training programs for physicians, child nutrition personnel, and other health care providers
- Fostering communication and partnerships across all health-related disciplines
- Developing and implementing strategies for the education of parents and caregivers on how to foster a more healthful lifestyle in the home environment
- Advocating for the need to increase federal and state funding of nutrition education programs
- Putting physical activity back in the schools as a requirement[71]

Programs for prevention of obesity need to focus on reaching a better balance between caloric intake and energy expenditure for the whole family. This is especially important because the fatness level of children with two obese parents is reportedly three times that of children with two lean parents.[72] The pedometer, developed in Japan, can be an important tool to educate parents and children on the steps needed in physical activity and weight loss.

The Academy guidelines[70] recommend that children 2 years of age and older and adolescents select a healthy assortment of foods including vegetables, fruits, grains (especially whole grains), fat-free or low-fat milk products, and protein foods such as fish, lean meat, poultry, and beans. Some specific ways to reach these goals are increasing exercise and active play; decreasing the fast food and sodium in the diet; eating at the table during meals and while snacking; increasing the use of fruits and vegetables at meals and as snacks; and considering bringing lunch from home rather than buying it at school. The Guidelines also recommend that children get at least 1 hour of physical activity daily and that nonactive forms of play, such as watching television or playing video games, be limited. This is especially true for children with special health-care needs.[73]

Research[74,75] focusing on weight management practices used by pediatricians found that the greatest barriers to improving management of obesity were lack of client compliance, time, and interest. Physicians did use the new pediatric growth charts and used weight-for-height (for younger children), weight-for-age, and visual determination to assess overweight and obesity. However, BMI was not routinely used, despite its known usefulness as an assessment measure for children in the general population and, less so, for those with disabilities. Most pediatricians did discuss weight with the parent and/or the child, discussed the diet and physical activity history for overweight or obese children, and provided some form of diet and exercise counseling. These pediatricians looked to dietitians as a credible source of information, services, and expertise to manage obesity.

Ideally, dietitians should be present in pediatric offices for a good long-range investment in health. They can employ strategies for the development of better and more culturally appropriate educational materials and can conduct seminars on wellness and pediatric obesity for both physicians and parents. However, this can be achieved only if the profession advocates strongly for increased reimbursement for dietetic services.

## FUTURE RESEARCH

Further research is needed to better understand the regulation of body weight. Research on the energy needs of special populations is needed to provide optimal nutrition and prevention of obesity. Prevention and intervention programs for high-risk populations are needed to improve health and well-being. Policy changes and new thinking, tracking obesity into adulthood, are required.[76–79] Nutrition food label regulations are being updated by the US Food and Drug Administration with the requirement for listing percent daily values for added sugars.

## RESOURCES FOR THE DIETITIAN

Websites that may be helpful for the dietitian include the following:

- The Kid's Activity Pyramid: www.learningzonexpress.com/poskidacpyr.htm
- National Center on Health, Physical Activity and Disability: www.nchpad.org
- Obesity Education Initiative of the National Heart, Lung, and Blood Institute Information Center: www.nhlbi.nih.gov/about/oei/index.htm or (301)592-8573
- President's Council on Physical Fitness, Sports and Nutrition: www.fitness.gov or (202)690-9000
- Weight Control Information Network (WIN) of the National Institute of Diabetes and Digestive and Kidney Diseases (NIH): www.niddk.nih.gov or 1-877-946-4627

### References


1. Ogden CL, Carroll MD, Kit BK, Flegal KM. Prevalence of obesity and in body mass index among US children and adolescents, 1999–2010. *JAMA*. 2012; 307:483.
2. Shepherd K, Roberts DW, Golding S, Thomas BJ, Shepherd RW. Body composition in myelomeningocele. *Am J Clin Nutr*. 1991; 53:1.
3. Hayes-Allen MC, Tring FC. Obesity: another hazard for spina bifida children. *Br J Prev Social Med*. 1973; 27:192.
4. Ekvall S, Ekvall V, Beck C, et al. Childhood obesity: myelomeningocele chart. In: Ekvall S, Ekvall V, eds. *Pediatric and Nutrition in Chronic Disorder and Development Disorders*. New York: Oxford University Press, 2005:403, 404.
5. Holm VA, Cassidy SB, Butler MG, et al. Prader-Willi syndrome: consensus diagnostic criteria. *Pediatrics*. 1993; 91:398.
6. Rubio SS, Rimmer JH, Chicoine B, Braddock D, McGuire DE. Prevalence of overweight and obesity in persons with Down syndrome. *Mental Retard*. 1998; 36:175.
7. Bell AJ, Bhate MS. Prevalence of overweight and obesity in Down's syndrome and other mentally handicapped adults living in the community. *J Intellect Disabil Res*. 1992; 36:359.
8. Dietz WH. Critical periods in childhood for the development of obesity. *Am J Clin Nutr*. 1994; 59:955.
9. Bandini LG, Gleason J, Curtain C, et al. Comparison of physical activity between children with autism spectrum disorders and typically developing children. *Autism*. 2013; 18:376.
10. Bandini L, Curtain C, Hamad C, Tybor D, Must A. Prevalence of overweight in children with developmental disorders in the continuous national Health and Nutrition Examination Survey (NHANES) 1999–2002. *J Pediatr*. 2005; 146:738.
11. Guo SS. Predicted overweight and obesity in adulthood from body mass index values in childhood and adolescence. *Am J Clin Nutr*. 2002; 76:653.
12. Bispham J, Gopalakrishnan GS, Dandrea J, ET AL. Maternal endocrine adaptation throughout pregnancy to nutritional manipulation: consequences for maternal plasma leptin and cortisol and the programming of fetal adipose tissue development. *Endocrinology*. 2003; 144:3575.
13. Te Velde SJ, Twisk JW, van Mechelen W, Kemper Han C. Birth weight, adult body composition, and subcutaneous fat distribution. *Obes Res*. 2003; 11:202.
14. Whitaker RC, Wright JA, Pepe MS, Seidel KD, Dietz WH. Predicting obesity in young adulthood from childhood and parental obesity. *N Engl J Med*. 1997; 337:869.
15. Chumlea WC, Cronk CE. Overweight among children with trisomy 21. *J Ment Defic Res*. 1981; 25:275.
16. Rimmer JH., Chen MD., McCubbin JA., Drum C., Peterson J. Exercise intervention research on persons with disabilities: what we know and where we need to go. *Am J Med Rehabil*. 2010; 89:249.
17. Cronk CE, Chumlea WC, Roche AF. Assessment of overweight children with trisomy 21. *Am J Ment Defic*. 1985; 89:433.
18. Atencio-La Follette P, Ekvall S, Oppenheimer S, Grace E. Effect of level of lesion and quality of ambulation on growth chart measurements in children with myelomeningocele. *J Am Diet Assoc*. 1992; 92:858.
19. Must A, Strauss RS. Risks and consequences of childhood and adolescent obesity. *Int J Obes*. 1999; 23(Suppl):S2.
20. Sinha R, Fisch G, Teague B, et al. Prevalence of impaired glucose tolerance among children and adolescents with marked obesity. *N Engl J Med*. 2002; 346:802.
21. Franks PW, Hanson RL, Knowler LC, Sievers MI, Bennett PH, Looker HC. Childhood obesity, other cardiovascular risk factors, and premature death. *N Engl J Med*. 2010; 362:485.
22. Wang Y, Lim H. The global childhood obesity epidemic and the association between socio-economic status and childhood obesity. *Int Rev Psychiatry*. 2012; 24:176.
23. Yanovski JA. Pediatric obesity. *Rev Endocr Metab Disord*. 2001; 2:371.
24. Sanchez M, Panahi S, Termblay A. Childhood obesity: a role for gut microbiota? *Int J Environ Res Public Health*. 2015; 12:162.
25. Bouchard C, Savard R, Despres JP, Tremblay A, Leblanc C. Body composition in adopted and biological siblings. *Hum Biol*. 1985; 57:61.
26. Stunkard AJ, Thorkild TIA, Hanis C, et al. An adoption study of human obesity. *N Engl J Med*. 1986; 314:193.

27. Stunkard AJ, Harris JR, Pedersen NL, McClearn GE. The body-mass index of twins who have been reared apart. *N Engl J Med.* 1990; 322:1483.
28. Maffeis C, Schultz Y, Micciolo R, Zocacante L, Pinelli L. Resting metabolic rate in six- to ten-year-old obese and nonobese children. *J Pediatr.* 1993; 122:556.
29. Bandini LG, Schoeller DA, Dietz WH. Energy expenditure in obese and nonobese adolescents. *Pediatr Res.* 1990; 27:198.
30. Delany JP, Bray GA, Harsha DW, Volaufova J. Energy expenditure in preadolescent African American and white boys and girls: the Baton Rouge Children's Study. *Am J Clin Nutr.* 2002; 75:705.
31. Prentice AM, Black AE, Coward WA, et al. High levels of energy expenditure in obese women. *Br Med J.* 1986; 292:983.
32. Ravussin E, Burnand B, Schutz Y, Jequier E. Twenty-four-hour energy expenditure and resting metabolic rate in obese, moderately obese and control subjects. *Am J Clin Nutr.* 1982; 35:566.
33. Schoeller DA, Levitsky LL, Bandini LG, Dietz WH, Walczak A. Energy expenditure and body composition in Prader-Willi syndrome. *Metabolism.* 1988; 37:115.
34. Bandini LG, Schoeller DA, Fukagawa NK, Wykes LJ, Dietz WH. Body composition and energy expenditure in adolescents with cerebral palsy or myelodysplasia. *Pediatr Res.* 1991; 29:70.
35. Grogan CB, Ekvall SM. Body composition of children with myelomeningocele, determined by K40, urinary creatinine and anthropometric measures. *J Am Coll Nutr.* 1999; 18:316.
36. Luke A, Roizen NJ, Sutton M, Schoeller DA. Energy expenditure in children with Down syndrome: correcting metabolic rate for movement. *J Pediatr.* 1994; 125:829.
37. Bessard T, Schutz Y, Jequier E. Energy expenditure and postprandial thermogenesis in obese women before and after weight loss. *Am J Clin Nutr.* 1983; 38:680.
38. Segal KR, Gutin R, Nyman AM, Pi-Sunyer FX. Thermic effect of food at rest, during exercise, and after exercise in lean and obese men of similar body weight. *J Clin Invest.* 1985; 76:1107.
39. Shetty PS, Jung RT, James WPT, Bawand MA, Callingham BA. Postprandial thermogenesis in obesity. *Clin Sci.* 1981; 60:519.
40. Molnar D, Varga P, Rubecz I, Hamar A, Mestyan J. Food-induced thermogenesis in obese children. *Eur J Pediatr.* 1985; 144:27.
41. Bandini LG, Schoeller DA, Cyr H, Yong VR, Oh S, Dietz WH. Energy expenditure during carbohydrate overfeeding in obese and nonobese adolescents. *Am J Physiol.* 1989; 256:E357.
42. Felig P, Cunningham J, Levitt M, Hendler R, Nadel E. Energy expenditure in obesity in fasting and postprandial state. *Am J Physiol.* 1983; 244:E45.
43. Blaza S, Garrrow JS. Thermogenic response to temperature, exercise and food stimuli in lean and obese women, studied by 24 hour direct calorimetry. *Br J Nutr.* 1983; 49:171.
44. Bandini LG, Schoeller DA, Cyr H, Dietz WH. Comparison of energy intake and energy expenditure in obese and nonobese adolescents. *Am J Clin Nutr.* 1990; 52:421.
45. Ludwig DS, Peterson KE, Gortmaker SL. Relation between consumption of sugar-sweetened drinks and childhood obesity: a prospective, observational analysis. *Lancet.* 2001; 357:505.
46. Young LR, Nestle M. The contribution of expanding portion sizes to the U.S. obesity epidemic. *Am J Public Health.* 2002; 92:246.
47. Maffeis C, Zaffanello M, Pinelli L, Schutz Y. Total energy expenditure and patterns of activity in 8–10-year-old obese and nonobese children. *J Pediatr Gastroenterol Nutr.* 1996; 23:256.
48. Stallings VA, Zemel BS, Davies JC, Cronk CE, Charney EB. Energy expenditure of children and adolescents with severe disabilities: a cerebral palsy model. *Am J Clin Nutr.* 1996; 64:627.
49. van den Berg-Emons HJG, Saris WHM, de Barbanson DC, Westerterp KR, Huson A, van Baak MA. Daily physical activity of school children with spastic diplegia and of healthy control subjects. *J Pediatr.* 1995; 127:578.
50. Sanders T, Feng X, Fahey PP, Lonsdale C, Astell-Burt T. Green space and child weight status: does outcome measurement matter? Evidence from an Australian longitudinal study. *J Obes.* 2015; 2015:194838.
51. Gortmaker SL, Must A, Sobol AM, Peterson K, Colditz GA, Dietz WH. Television viewing as a cause of increasing obesity among children in the United States, 1986–1990. *Arch Pediatr Adolesc Med.* 1996; 150:356.
52. Hamill PV, Drizd TA, Johnson CL, Reed RB, Roche AF. NCHS growth curves for children, birth–18 years, United States. *Vital Health Stat.* 1977; 11:165.
53. National Heart, Lung, and Blood Institute. *Clinical Guidelines on the Identification, Evaluation, and Treatment of Overweight and Obesity in Adults: The Evidence Report.* Publication No. 98-4083. Bethesda, MD: National Institutes of Health; September 1998.
54. Ekvall S, Ekvall V, Frondorf J, et al. The development of a standardized waist circumference growth chart for children as a tool in predicting weight change (abstract). *J Intellect Disabil Res.* 2000; 44(3–4):189.
55. Luke A, Sutton M, Schoeller DA, Roizen NJ. Nutrient intake and obesity in prepubescent children with Down syndrome. *J Am Diet Assoc.* 1996; 96:1262.
56. Lee MMC. Thickening of the subcutaneous tissues in paralyzed limits in chronic hemiplegia. *Hem Biol.* 1959; 31:187.
57. Barlow SE, Dietz WH. Obesity evaluation and treatment: expert committee recommendations. The Maternal and Child Health Bureau, Health Resources and Services Administration, and the Department of Health and Human Services. *Pediatrics.* 1998; 102:E29.
58. Culley WJ, Goyal K, Jolly DH, Mertz ET. Caloric intake of children with Down's syndrome (mongolism). *J Pediatr.* 1965; 66:772.
59. Culley WJ, Middleton TO. Caloric requirements of mentally retarded children with and without motor dysfunction. *J Pediatr.* 1969; 75:380.
60. Bandini LG, Puelzl-Quinn H, Morelli JA, Fukagawa NK. Estimation of energy requirements in persons with severe central nervous system impairment. *J Pediatr.* 1995; 126:828.
61. Prochaska JO, Crawley B. *Changing for Good*, reprint ed. New York: Avon Publishers; 1995.
62. Miller WR, Rollnick S, Conforti K. *Motivational Interviewing: Preparing People for Change*, 2nd ed. New York: Guilford Press; 2002.
63. Golan A, Crows M. Parents are key players in the prevention and treatment of weight-related problems. *Nutr Rev.* 2004; 62:39.
64. Ekvall S, Ekvall V. Diets in infants and children and obesity development. In: Moya M, Sawatzki G, Motulsky A, Moran J, eds. *Infant Nutrition in the Prevention of Chronic Pathology.* 3rd International Satellite Symposium, European Society of Pediatric Research. Madrid: Edicoines Ergon, S.A.; 1996.
65. Epstein LH, Valoski A, Wing RR, McCurley J. Ten-year follow-up of behavioral, family-based treatment for obese children. *JAMA.* 1990; 264:2519.
66. Epstein LH, Wing RR, Koeske R, Ossip DJ, Beck S. A comparison of lifestyle change and programmed aerobic exercise on weight and fitness changes in obese children. *Behav Ther.* 1982; 13:651.
67. Epstein LH, Valoski AM, Vara LS, et al. Effects of decreasing sedentary behavior and increasing activity on weight change in obese children. *Health Psychol.* 1995; 14:109.
68. Robinson TN. Behavioural treatment of childhood and adolescent obesity. *Int J Obes.* 1999; 23(Suppl 2):S52.
69. Hiza H, Guenther P, Rihane C. *Diet Quality of Children Age 2–17 Years as Measured by the Healthy Eating Index–2010.* Nutrition Insight 52. Washington, DC: USDA Center for Nutrition Policy and Promotion; July 2013.
70. Ogata BN, Hayes D. Position of the Academy of Nutrition and Dietetics: nutrition guidance for healthy children ages 2 to 11 years. *J Acad Nutr Diet.* 2014; 114:1257.
71. Farias ES., Paula F, Carvalho WR, Goncalves EM, Baldin AD, Guerra-Junior G. Influence of programmed physical activity on body composition among adolescent students. *J Pediatr (Rio J).* 2009; 85:28.
72. Garn SM, Clark DC. Trends in fatness and the origins of obesity. *Pediatrics.* 1976; 57:443.
73. Position of the Academy of Nutrition and Dietetics: Nutrition services for individuals with intellectual and developmental disabilities and special health care needs. *J Acad Nutr Diet.* 2015; 115;593.
74. Salcedo AF, Martinez-Vizcaino V, Sanchez LM, et al. Impact of an afterschool physical activity program on obesity in children. *J Pediatr.* 2010; 157:36.
75. Allen M, Touger-Decker R, Maillet-O'Sullivan J, Holland B. A survey of obesity management practices of pediatricians in New Jersey. *Top Clin Nutr.* 2003; 18:3.
76. Gortmaker SL, Swinburn BA, Levy D, et al. Changing the future of obesity: science, policy, and action. *Lancet.* 2011; 384:838
77. Roberto CA, Swinburn B, Hawkes C, et al. Patchy progress on obesity prevention: emerging examples, entrenched barriers, and new thinking. *Lancet.* 2015; 385:2400.
78. Singh AS, Mulder C, Twisk JW, van Mechelen W, Chinapaw MJ. Tracking of childhood overweight into adulthood: a systematic review of the literature. *Obes Rev.* 2008; 9:474.
79. Hampl S, Stough C, Cordts K, Best C, Blackburn K, Gillette M. Effectiveness of a hospital-based multidisciplinary pediatric weight management program: two year outcomes of PHIT Kids. *Childhood Obesity.* 2016; 12:20.

# 19 Attention Deficit Hyperactivity Disorder

ERIC K. BONSALL, VALLI K. EKVALL, AND SHIRLEY W. EKVALL

Attention deficit hyperactivity disorder (ADHD) is a complex and common neurodevelopmental disorder that occurs in approximately 5% of children and 2.5% of adults. Left untreated, this disorder can negatively impact social and academic performance in children and interpersonal relationships and workplace performance in adults. There is a gender bias toward males, with a ratio of approximately 2:1 in children and 106:1 in adults.[1] ADHD occurs more commonly among first-degree biological relatives of those with ADHD.[2] Approximately 20% to 30% of children with ADHD have one parent with the disorder. ADHD is frequently comorbid with mood and anxiety disorders, learning disorders, and oppositional defiant disorder.[3,4] The symptoms commonly persist into adulthood.[1] The diagnostic criteria for ADHD, from the fifth edition of the American Psychiatric Association's *Diagnostic and Statistical Manual of Mental Disorders* (DSM-5), are listed in Box 19-1.

## DIAGNOSIS AND CLINICAL PRESENTATION

The hallmark features of the disorder are inappropriate degrees of impulsiveness, hyperactivity, and inattention. Mood dysregulation, irritability, and secondary emotional problems such as low self-esteem are frequently seen. ADHD is cross-situational, and manifestations of the disorder appear in the school, at home, and in social situations. Symptoms must appear in at least two different settings for a diagnosis to be made. At school, the child may give the impression that he or she is not listening or make comments out of turn. At home, the child may fail to follow through with requests or interrupt other family members. With peers, excessive talking or failure to follow the rules of the game are common. Evidence of the disorder may be minimal or absent when the child is receiving frequent rewards for appropriate behavior, is under close supervision, is in a novel environment, is engaged in especially interesting activities, or is in a one-to-one situation. Therefore, it is important that the clinician gather data from a variety of sources (e.g., parents, teachers) and ask about the child's behavior in a variety of situations within each setting (e.g., doing homework, during meals).[1] Signs of the disorder also may be reduced if the child is receiving appropriate psychotropic medication and consistent behavior management techniques are being implemented.

A comprehensive clinical evaluation by a specialist (psychologist, child psychiatrist, developmental pediatrician, or pediatric neurologist) is needed to diagnose ADHD. The evaluation should be based on multiple sources (i.e., parent, teacher, and child) using multiple instruments. The following clinical findings should be present to diagnose ADHD: (1) the parent, teacher, and child report a history and current symptoms of ADHD; (2) clinical observations of the child indicate inattention, impulsivity, and overactivity; (3) a review of school records from kindergarten to the present with the elementary teacher includes comments such as "can't stay seated," "difficulty listening," "talks out of turn," and "rushes through assignments"; (4) elevated parent and teacher rating scale scores on ADHD subscales; and (5) low scores relative to IQ on performance tests designed to evaluate attention, such as the Gordon Diagnostic System (a computerized continuous performance test) and the Wechsler Intelligence Scale for Children-IV (WISC-IV) Working Memory or the WISC-III Freedom from Distractibility factors. Research demonstrates that these performance tests have a 91% accuracy rate in identifying children with and without ADHD.[5,6]

Behavior rating scales offer a practical, quick, and inexpensive means of screening for ADHD and for augmenting a clinical evaluation. Many behavior rating scales have significant validity, reliability, and normative and factor analytic data. However, the scales are subjective and therefore susceptible to rater bias. Also, ADHD cannot be diagnosed or ruled out based on scale scores alone. Two types of rating scales are available. One focuses only on ADHD symptomatology, and the other evaluates multiple areas of psychopathology including ADHD. The latter type assists in making a differential diagnosis and provides a comprehensive overview of the child's psychological functioning in several areas.

One of the most widely tested and empirically sound instruments for evaluating psychopathology is the *Child Behavior Checklist* (CBCL; by T. M. Achenbach, 1981, from the University of Vermont, Burlington). The CBCL assesses multiple mood and behavior disorders and provides scores in such categories as hyperactive, depressed, anxious, and aggressive. The American Academy of Pediatrics has endorsed the adapted Vanderbilt Rating Scale developed by M. Wolraich for the Parent Informant (see Appendix 9). Another rating scale is the *Conners Teacher Rating Scale* (by C. K. Conners, from Western Psychological Services, Los Angeles), a 39-item measure that assesses multiple areas of psychopathology in children aged 4 through 12 years, with empirical data on more than 15,000 children. Still another is the *Pediatric Behavior Scale* (PBS; by S.D. Lindgren, from Linden Press, Solon, Iowa), an instrument for 6- to 16-year-olds especially designed for use in a medical setting (see Appendix 9). The PBS comprises 165 items rated by an adult on a four-point scale and requires about 15 minutes to complete. It yields scores in six categories: conduct problems, ADHD, depression and anxiety, deviant behavior, health concerns, and cognitive and academic difficulties.

A specific ADHD scale is the *Attention Deficits Disorders Evaluation Scale* (ADDES; by C. B. McCarney, from Hawthorn Educational Services, Columbia, Missouri; 1-800-542-1673). The ADDES has two versions: a 47-item parent scale and a 60-item teacher scale. The scales each take about 12 to 15 minutes to complete. The ADDES has excellent empirical support. Scores on three subscales (inattentive, impulsive, and hyperactive) are plotted on a profile graph and converted into standard scores. The ADDES School Version has an accompanying manual providing intervention strategies for teachers. Computerized versions are available for scoring and to generate a printout of individualized strategies.

### Differential Diagnosis

It is imperative to consider a differential diagnosis for children with ADHD because other disorders may manifest with similar features. Some children have multiple diagnoses. ADHD is more common in children with multiple handicaps than in nondisabled children, with prevalence rates as high as 25% to 50%.[7] Iron deficiency anemia in young children has been linked to decreased cognitive and psychomotor performance and should be ruled out when evaluating for ADHD.[8] Also, school-age children who are malnourished or who skip breakfast may perform less well on academic tests and should be evaluated if they show symptoms of ADHD.[9] Other disorders to be considered are oppositional defiant disorder, autism spectrum disorder, intermittent explosive disorder, specific learning disabilities, and disruptive mood dysregulation disorder.

**Box 19–1.** Diagnostic Criteria for Attention Deficit Hyperactivity Disorder

A. A persistent pattern of inattention and/or hyperactivity-impulsivity that interferes with functioning or development, as characterized by (1) and/or (2):
1. **Inattention:** Six (or more) of the following symptoms have persisted for at least six months to a degree that it is inconsistent with developmental level and that negatively impacts directly on social and academic/occupational activities:
**Note:** The symptoms are not solely a manifestation of oppositional behavior, defiance, hostility, or failure to understand tasks or instructions. For older adolescents and adults (age 17 and older), at least five symptoms are required.
a. Often fails to give close attention to details or makes careless mistakes in schoolwork, at work, or during other activities (e.g., overlooks or misses details, work is inaccurate).
b. Often has difficulty sustaining attention in tasks or play activities (e.g., has difficulty remaining focused during lectures, conversations, or lengthy reading).
c. Often does not seem to listen when spoken to directly (e.g., mind seems elsewhere, even in the absence of any obvious distraction).
d. Often does not follow through on instructions and fails to finish schoolwork, chores, or duties in the workplace (e.g., starts tasks but quickly loses focus and is easily sidetracked).
e. Often has difficulty organizing tasks and activities (e.g. difficulty managing sequential tasks; difficulty keeping materials and belongings in order; messy, disorganized work; has poor time management; fails to meet deadlines).
f. Often avoids, dislikes, or is reluctant to engage in tasks that require sustained mental effort (e.g., schoolwork or homework; for older adolescents and adults, preparing reports, completing forms, reviewing lengthy papers).
g. Often loses things necessary for tasks or activities (e.g., school materials, pencils, books, tools, wallets, keys, paperwork, eyeglasses, mobile telephones).
h. Is often easily distracted by extraneous stimuli (for older adolescents and adults, may include unrelated thoughts).
i. Is often forgetful in daily activities (e.g., doing chores, running errands; for older adolescents and adults, returning calls, paying bills, keeping appointments).
2. **Hyperactivity and impulsivity:** Six (or more) of the following symptoms have persisted for at least six months to a degree that is inconsistent with developmental level and that negatively impacts directly on social and academic/occupational activities:
**Note:** The symptoms are not solely a manifestation of oppositional behavior, defiance, hostility, or a failure to understand tasks or instructions. For older adolescents and adults (age 17 and older), at least five symptoms are required.
a. Often fidgets with or taps hands or feet or squirms in seat.
b. Often leaves seat in situations when remaining seated is expected (e.g., leaves his or her place in the classroom, in the office or other workplace, or in other situations that require remaining in place).
c. Often runs about or climbs in situations where it is inappropriate. (**Note**: In adolescents and adults may be limited to feeling restless.)
d. Often unable to play or engage in leisure activities quietly.
e. Is often "on the go," acting as if "driven by a motor" (e.g., is unable to be or uncomfortable being still for extended time, as in restaurants, meetings; may be experienced by others as being restless or difficult to keep up with).
f. Often talks excessively.
g. Often blurts out an answer before a question has been completed (e.g., completes people's sentences; cannot wait for turn in conversation).
h. Often has difficulty waiting his or her turn (e.g., while waiting in line).
i. Often interrupts or intrudes on others (e.g., butts into conversations, games, or activities; may start using other people's things without asking or receiving permission; for adolescents and adults, may intrude into or take over what others are doing).

B. Several inattentive or hyperactive-impulsive symptoms were present prior to age 12 years.
C. Several inattentive or hyperactive-impulsive symptoms are present in two or more settings (e.g., at home, school, or work; with friends or relatives; in other activities.)
D. There is clear evidence that the symptoms interfere with, or reduce the quality of, social, academic, or occupational functioning.
E. The symptoms do not occur exclusively during the course of schizophrenia or another psychotic disorder and are not better explained by another mental disorder (e.g., mood disorder, anxiety disorder, dissociative disorder, personality disorder, substance intoxication or withdrawal.)

*Specify* whether:

**314.01 (F90.2) Combined presentation:** If both Criterion A1 (inattention) and Criterion A2 (hyperactivity-impulsivity) are met for the past 6 months.
**314.00 (F90.0) Predominantly inattentive presentation:** If Criterion A1 (inattention) is met but Criterion A2 (hyperactivity-impulsivity) is not met for the past 6 months.
**314.01 (F90.1) Predominantly hyperactive/impulsive presentation:** If Criterion A2 (hyperactivity-impulsivity is met and Criterion A1 (inattention) is not met for the past 6 months.

*Specify* if:

**In partial remission:** When full criteria were previously met, fewer than the full criteria have been met for the past 6 months, and the symptoms still result in impairment in social, academic, or occupational functioning.

*Specify* current severity:

**Mild**: Few, if any, symptoms in excess of those required to make the diagnosis are present, and symptoms result in no more than minor impairment in social or occupational functioning.
**Moderate:** Symptoms or functional impairment between "mild" and "severe" are present.
**Severe:** Many symptoms in excess of those required to make the diagnosis, or several symptoms that are particularly severe, are present or the symptoms result in marked impairment in social or occupational functioning.

American Psychiatric Association. *Diagnostic and Statistical Manual of Mental Disorders, Fifth Edition* (*DSM-5*). Washington, DC: American Psychiatric Association; 2013.

## Neurological and Biochemical Factors

Predisposing factors, such as abnormalities of the central nervous system (CNS), may be present with ADHD. These conditions include cerebral palsy, epilepsy, neurological disorders caused by neurotoxins, and other difficulties that may affect the transmission of neurotransmitters such as serotonin and catecholamines.[2] Because the attention system is widespread throughout the brain, it is sensitive to a variety of potential insults, including malnutrition. A 5-year prospective study involving more than 23,020 mothers and their childres demonstrated a clear increased risk for externalizing behavioral problems in children exposed to unhealthy diets in utero.[10] In addition, prenatal exposure to maternal obesity has been linked to hyperactivity.[11] The effects of prolonged protein and calorie restrictions on the developing CNS are of particular concern. The amino acid transmitter is the predominant substance needed in transmission in the CNS, whereas monoamines and peptides function as neuromodulators.[12] Each of these classes of neurochemical messages has been implicated in the regulation of food intake[13,14] (see Chapter 12).

Malnutrition at an early age is associated with cognitive and behavioral deficits such as impairments in language and motor skills, interpersonal relationships, and adaptive and motivational behavior. However, it is often difficult to separate nutrition from other environmental and socioeconomic problems. Two substances, docosahexanoic acid (DHA) and radioiodine, may be associated with ADHD. DHA is the active component found in fish and has been lacking in formula diets for infants over the past 50 years. Its deficiency may be associated with ADHD.[15] Supplementation of formulas may be helpful in overcoming this deficiency. The therapeutic delivery of radioiodine to a mother during pregnancy can result in fetal hypothyroidism and may be associated with ADHD and memory impairment in the infant.[16] Lactating mothers who have been given standard diagnostic doses of radioiodine should stop breast-feeding their infants after its administration.[16]

Increased lead levels may be associated with hyperactivity, impulsiveness, learning problems, and other behavioral dysfunctions. Lead levels were shown to be elevated in children admitted to a residential psychiatric treatment facility.[17] The initial evaluation of ADHD should include a screening for potentially elevated blood lead levels.[18–20]

## FACTORS TO BE CONSIDERED IN NUTRITIONAL AND OTHER EVALUATIONS

### Medication

An interdisciplinary team consisting of a psychologist, physician, nutritionist, and educator can provide the most comprehensive clinical evaluation for ADHD. It is essential that standardized measures and set diagnostic criteria be used in this process. Pharmacological therapy, particularly stimulant medication, is a major component of treatment. The most widely used medications are stimulants that include methylphenidate components (Ritalin, Concerta, Metadate, Focalin, Daytrana Methylin) and dextroamphetamine/amphetamine medications (Adderall, Vyvanse, Dexedrine). Stimulants have been used safely to treat ADHD since 1937.

In 14 studies of school-age children with ADHD reviewed by Barkley et al., the average response rate to stimulant medication was 77%.[21,22] A similar response rate has been reported for multiply handicapped and intellectually disabled preschool children with ADHD.[23] The use of stimulant medications in elementary, middle, and junior high schools almost doubled during the 1990s.[24]

Stimulants are short-acting medications. They take effect in about 20 minutes and last for 3 to 8 hours. The longer-acting stimulants, such as Adderall and Concerta, may eliminate the need for a noon dosage in school. The primary action of stimulant drugs may be to restrict or lessen the variability of behavioral patterns or responses to environmental stimuli, thereby tending to restore the homeostasis of the monoamine-related neurotransmission process.[25,26] These medications usually are well tolerated, although there are a few adverse reactions, which typically subside within 1 to 2 weeks; irritability, decreased appetite, and insomnia are the most common side effects. If they do not subside, a change in the dosage or type of medication is indicated.

Stimulant medications may also act as growth suppressants (perhaps affecting growth hormone) in children receiving long-term treatment. Weight loss usually occurs first, with a later decrease in height (especially after 2 to 4 years of treatment).[27–31] Roche et al.[29] noted a temporary retardation in the rate of weight increase, suggesting a temporary slowing in growth and stature; yet, this slowing did not affect adult stature or weight. This temporary effect was present in the first few years of treatment during pre puberty and appeared to be related to drug dosage and the absence of drug holidays (e.g., cessation of medication during the summer vacation). The total dosage for summer holidays affected weight deficits more than growth deficits. If stimulants lead to significant appetite suppression, it is important to advise families to have the child eat a breakfast containing most food groups before taking the morning medication. Children who experience a decrease in appetite with stimulants may also benefit from a high-calorie nutritional snack before bed. The effect of the stimulant usually wears off by bedtime. For children who are clear responders to stimulants but who have ongoing problems with weight loss or failure to make expected weight gain, collaboration with a registered dietitian is warranted.

Children who do not respond to stimulant therapy or who experience significant side effects may benefit from nonstimulant medications. Atomoxetine (Strattera) is a highly selective norepinephrine reuptake inhibitor that enhances norepinephrine and dopamine in the frontal cortex. In clinical trials, Strattera significantly reduced symptoms of ADHD. Its advantage over stimulants is that Strattera is effective for 24 hours. Other nonstimulant medications include clonidine (Catapres, Kapvay) and guanfacine (Tenex, Intuniv).

Because ADHD is not a benign disorder usually outgrown, it is important to combine drug therapy with counseling, educational accommodations, behavior management strategies, and close communication among parents, school personnel, and professionals—a multimodal approach. It is important for the family to be involved as part of the process. In families of children with ADHD, relationships may be characterized by resentment and antagonism, especially because the variability in the child's symptomatic status often leads others to believe that all of his or her troublesome behavior is willful. Family discord and negative parent-child interactions may be present. Such negative interactions may diminish with successful treatment.[1]

In summary, the treatment of ADHD involves (1) using medication to eliminate the symptoms as much as possible, (2) helping the child and others to manage effectively and compensate for the remaining symptoms, and (3) modifying the environment and making accommodations to enhance the child's potential for success at home and in school. The last component is very important. Children with ADHD are entitled to accommodations in school under federal law (i.e., Individuals with Disabilities Education Act, 1999). Accommodations may include, for example, preferential seating (up front near the teacher and between students who are attentive), a backpack check at the end of each school day to make sure that the child has not forgotten papers and materials, and two sets of books—one for home and one for school.

### Megavitamins and Supplements

Megavitamins have been shown to produce no significant decrease in ADHD and may produce toxic effects in the child.[32,33] Haslam et al.[34] studied 41 subjects with ADHD using a double-blind, repeated crossover design. Initially, 12 (29%) of the children using megavitamins—3 g niacin amide, 3 g ascorbic acid, 1.2 g calcium pantothenate, and 0.6 g pyridoxine[32]—showed significant behavioral improvement during stage 1. However, only 7% of these same subjects (all boys) elected to participate in stage 2 of the study. The subjects actually showed more disruptive classroom behavior when treated with vitamins versus placebo during stage 2. The results showed that megavitamins were ineffective in the management of ADHD and should not be used because of the potential for gastrointestinal complaints and hepatotoxicity. Vitamin supplementation is indicated only for children with a verified deficiency.

Omega 3 fatty acids are found in flaxseed and fish (especially tuna and salmon) and can be given as supplements. Studies have found low levels of these long-chain fatty acids in individuals with ADHD.[35,36] Moreover, there are studies that demonstrate the benefits of supplementation of omega fatty aids in ADHD treatment.[37] However, others have failed to replicate this finding. Further research is needed in this area.

### Food Allergies

Allergies to food may be considered a potential cause of hyperactivity. Some children show allergic reactions, such as gastrointestinal upset or skin eruptions, to certain foods; however, food allergies are seldom the sole cause of hyperactivity. Feingold and others proposed that certain food additives, synthetic food colors and flavorings, and naturally occurring salicylates could cause hyperactivity.[38] Controlled, double-blind experimental investigations have not shown Feingold's low-salicylate diet to dramatically improve behavior. However, 3% of children with ADHD, particularly those of preschool age, responded positively to the Feingold diet,[33] so it may be useful in a small subgroup of children. In general, parental ratings revealed more positive behavior changes with the experimental diet than did the school ratings when children were tested with food colors and diet.[40,42] Importantly, 35% to 39% of children with ADHD responded to a placebo. This high rate of placebo response needs to be taken into account when evaluating dietary and other interventions.[39–41]

Feingold's low-salicylate diet is a defined diet with several modifications. The diet involves avoiding foods containing natural salicylates, such as almonds, apples, apricots, blackberries, cherries, gooseberries, grapes or raisins, nectarines, oranges, plums or prunes, raspberries, strawberries, cucumbers or pickles, and tomatoes. Also avoided are foods containing artificial flavors and colors, such as ice cream, oleomargarine, cake mixes, bakery goods (except plain bread), Jell-O, candies, gum, cloves, oil of wintergreen, toothpaste and toothpowder, mint flavors, lozenges, mouthwash, jams or jellies, luncheon meats (e.g., salami, bologna), and frankfurters. Beverages to avoid are cider (and cider vinegars), wine (and wine vinegars), Kool-Aid and similar beverages, soda pop (all soft drinks), all teas, and diet drinks and supplements. Salicylates are also found in all medicines containing aspirin (e.g., Bufferin, Anacin, Excedrin, Alka-Seltzer, Empirin, Darvon Compound) and perfumes. All labels of prepared foods and drugs should be checked for artificial flavorings and colorings.[39] The low-salicylate diet is not harmful but does limit the food sources of vitamin C (which should be supplemented). Other modifications in the diet may involve the exclusion of items such as milk, corn, wheat, and sucrose, which may then added back to the diet individually. Diets and other treatment approaches that have not been empirically proven should not be substituted for techniques that are scientifically proven, such as stimulant medication and behavior modification. More conclusive research is needed on nutrition and hyperactivity.

A significant proportion of patients with celiac disease present with comorbid ADHD symptoms and show a dimunition in those symptoms on a gluten-free diet.[43] Foods high in gluten include foods containing barley, wheat, and rye. A gluten-free diet should have no harmful effects and is relatively easy to implement (see Chapter 54).

### Sugar

A popular misconception among parents is that sugar causes hyperactivity. However, a placebo-controlled study of young children who were thought to be sugar sensitive by their parents demonstrated that sugar did not affect behavior.[44] Reviews of published double-blind, placebo-controlled sugar challenge studies by other authors[45,46] also demonstrated that ingestion of sugar does not result in hyperactivity. Although sugar has not been definitively linked to ADHD,[47] reduction in the consumption of sweets, increased intake of complex carbohydrates, and 50% reduction of sugar in recipes may be beneficial to overall health. A recent study noted an increased risk for obesity and physical inactivity in adolescents with ADHD.[48] Sugar intake and physical activity levels need to be monitored in this group of patients.

## DIETARY AND OTHER MANAGEMENT

Many factors, such as medications, weight gain, and dietary habits, should be taken into consideration when conducting a complete nutritional assessment. A 24-hour food recall with a food frequency cross-check should be completed first, followed by a 3-day diet diary to ensure that the nutritional assessment is as complete as possible (see Chapter 4). Information should be obtained about behavior at mealtimes, food habits, food allergies, and food likes and dislikes. The best dietary treatment may be to discuss with the family the lack of proven usefulness of a defined diet or unconventional diet therapy while being willing to evaluate the effects of the diet if the family insists on its use. For example, one should advise the family not to give too much attention to a special diet at the cost of neglecting scientifically proven treatments.

If the family insists on a defined diet, the child should be evaluated monthly, if possible, with a complete nutritional assessment including dietary, biochemical, anthropometric, and physical signs (see Appendix 7–1, "Nutrition Quality Assurance Criteria, Development Disorders"). If medication is administered, a complete nutritional assessment should be done periodically, with special attention given to growth parameters. Reducing or eliminating medication during weekends or summer holidays should be considered if the child is in the prepubertal period.

### Diet, Nutrients, and Neurotransmitters

Improved study designs using random, double-blind trials to evaluate empirically the effectiveness of proposed treatments should be conducted, as has been done in assessing the impact of stimulant medication on ADHD symptoms. The adverse effects of dietary interchange should be evaluated because they affect the family psychologically and biologically.[49] Research is needed on the synthesis of brain neurotransmitters that respond to dietary fluctuations and fat in relation to neuronal function. Studies linking diet, brain transmission, and brain dysfunction should be pursued[45] (see Chapter 12). The effects of vitamin $B_{12}$ and folate on transmethylation reactions and the effects of ascorbic acid on hydroxylation reactions continue to be of interest, as are the behavioral effects of trytophan, tyrosine, thiamine (vitamin $B_1$), pyridoxine (vitamin $B_6$), carbohydrate, protein, and caffeine[50] (see Chapter 12).

The trace minerals iron, copper, and zinc may influence neurotransmitter metabolism. For example, iron is a cofactor for tyrosine hydroxlase and serum zinc; copper-deficient rats have shown decreased brain tyrosine hydroxolase activity.[50] Benner[47] noted that children who responded to the Feingold diet had an elevated serum copper concentration. The reason for this is unclear. Zinc status also has an impact on catecholamine and hypothalamic pituitary activity. Zinc deficiency in gestation has been found to impair learning, reduce the attention span, and produce poor memory in mouse, rat, and rhesus monkey offspring. Calcium is known to be involved in nerve conditions.[50] DHA has been shown to improve visual acuity and mental development in small-for-gestational-age human infants.[15] This provides some evidence that micronutrients beyond iron and iodine may be needed for brain development and growth; however, better-controlled studies involving human subjects are needed. Data have been limited and often inconclusive in this area.

## SUMMARY

ADHD is a common neurobehavioral disorder that, if left untreated, can have deleterious effects in multiple areas across the lifespan. Treatment must be multimodal, involving a team of qualified professionals. Medication management and cognitive behavioral techniques are the standard of care.[51] However, nutritional strategies are an important complement to these treatments. The nutritionist should be involved with the initial assessment, management of medication side effects, and ongoing treatment of individuals with ADHD across the lifespan.

### References

1. American Psychiatric Association. *Diagnostic and Statistical Manual of Mental Disorders, Fifth Edition (DSM-5)*. Washington, DC: American Psychiatric Association; 2013.
2. Braaten EB, Beiderman J, Monuteaux MC, et al. Revisiting the association between attention-deficit/hyperactivity disorder and anxiety disorders: a familial risk analysis. *Biol Psychiatry.* 2003; 53:93.
3. Bond W. Recognition and treatment of attention deficit disorder. *Clin Pharmacol.* 1987; 6:617.
4. Mayes SD, Calhoun SL, Crowell EW. Learning disabilities and ADHD: overlapping spectrum disorders. *J Learn Dis.* 2000; 33:417.
5. Mayes SD, Calhoun SL, Crowell EW. WISC-III Freedom from Distractibility as a measure of attention in children with and without attention deficit hyperactivity disorder. *J Atten Disord.* 1998; 2:217.
6. Mayes SD, Calhoun SL, Crowell EW. Clinical validity and interpretation of the Gordon Diagnostic System in ADHD assessments. *Child Neuropsychol.* 2001; 7:32.
7. Fisher W, Burd L, Kuna DP, Berg D. Attention deficit disorders and the hyperactivities in multiply disabled children. *Rehabil Lit.* 1985; 46:250.
8. Pollitt E, Saco-Pollitt C, Leibel RL, Viteri FE. Iron deficiency and behavioral development in infants and preschool children. *Am J Clin Nutr.* 1986; 43:555.
9. Meyers AF, Sampson AE, Weitzman M, Rogers BL, Kayne H. School breakfast program and school performance. *Am J Dis Child.* 1989; 143:1234.
10. Jacka FN, Ystrom E, Brantsaeter AL, et al. Maternal and early postnatal nutrition and mental health of offspring by age 5 years: a prospective cohort study. *J Am Acad Child Adolesc Psychiatry.* 2013; 52:1038.

11. Fernondes C, Grayton H, Poston L. Prenatal exposure to obesity leads to hyperactivity in offspring. *Mol Psychiatry.* 2012; 17:1159.
12. Iverson L. Amino acids and peptides: fast and slow chemical signals in the nervous system? *Proc R Soc Lond B.* 1984; 221:245.
13. Morely J. The neuroendocrine control of appetite: the role of the endogenous opiates, cholecystokinin, TRH, gamma-aminobutyric acid and the diazepam receptor. *Life Sci.* 1980; 27:355.
14. Morely J, Levine A. Pharmacology of eating behavior. *Annu Rev Pharmacol Toxicol.* 1985; 25:127.
15. Spencer T, Biederman J, Wilens T. Growth deficits in children with attention deficit hyperactivity disorder. *Pediatrics.* 1998; 102(2 pt 3):501.
16. Gorman CA. Radioiodine and pregnancy. *Thyroid.* 1999; 9:721.
17. Bonsall EK, Heinley M, Bixler EO. Blood lead levels in children admitted for residential treatment (abstract). Presented at the American Academy of Child and Adolescent Psychiatry Annual Meeting, Washington, DC, 1996.
18. Graff C, Murphy L, Ekvall S, Magnon M. In-home toxic chemical exposures. *Pediatr Nurs.* 2006; 36:597.
19. Tyler C, White-Scott S, Ekvall S, Abulafe L Environmental health and developmental disabilities: a life span approach. *Fam Commun Health.* 2008; 30:287.
20. Brockel BJ, Cory-Sletcha DA. The effects of postweaning low-level Pb exposure on sustained attention: a study of target densities, stimulus presentation rate, and stimulus predictability. *Neurotoxicology.* 1999; 20:921.
21. Barkley RA, Fischer M, Smallish L, Fletcher K. Does the treatment of attention-deficit/hyperactivity disorder with stimulants contribute to drug use/abuse?: a 13-year prospective study. *Pediatrics.* 2003; 111:97.
22. Barkley RA. Issues in the diagnosis of attention-deficit/hyperactivity disorder in children. *Brain Dev.* 2003; 25:77.
23. Mayes SD, Sanderson DL, Bixler EO, Humphery EJ, Mattison RE. Methylphenidate and ADHD: influence of age, IQ and neurodevelopmental status. *Dev Med Child Neurol.* 1994; 36:1099.
24. Zito JM, Safer DJ, DosReis S, et al. Psychotropic practice patterns for youth: a 10-year perspective. *Arch Pediatr Adolesc Med.* 2003; 157:17.
25. Thomson JB, Varley CK. Prediction of stimulant response in children with attention-deficit/hyperactivity disorder. *J Child Adolesc Psychopharmacol.* 1998; 8:125.
26. Vitiello B, Severe JB, Greenhill LL, et al. Methylphenidate dosage for children with ADHD over time under controlled conditions: lessons from the MTA. *J Am Acad Child Adolesc Psychiatry.* 2001; 40:188.
27. Holtkamp K, Peters-Wallraf B, Wuller S, Pfaaffle R, Herpertz-Dahlmann B. Methylphenidate-related growth impairment. *J Child Adolesc Psychopharmacol.* 2002; 12:55.
28. Schertz M, Adesman AR, Alfieri NE, Bienkowski RS. Predictors of weight loss in children with attention deficit hyperactivity disorder treated with stimulant medication. *Pediatrics.* 1996; 98(4 pt 1):763.
29. Roche AF, Lipman RS, Overall JE, Hung W. The effects of stimulant drugs on the growth of hyperactive children. *Pediatrics.* 1979; 63:847.
30. Poulton A, Cowell CT. Slowing of growth in height and weight on stimulants: a characteristic pattern. *J Paediatr Child Health.* 2003; 39:180.
31. Spencer TJ, Biederman J, Harding M, O'Donnell D, Faraone SV, Wilens TE. Growth deficits in ADHD children revisited: evidence for disorder-associated growth delays? *J Am Acad Child Adolesc Psychiatry.* 1996; 35:1460.
32. Feingold B. Food additives and hyperactivity. *Hosp Pract.* 1973; 8:11.
33. Harley JP, Matthews CG, Eichman P. Synthetic food colors and hyperactivity in children: a double blind challenge experiment. *Pediatrics.* 1978; 62:975.
34. Haslam RH, Dalby JT, Rademaker AW. Effects of megavitamin therapy on children with attention deficit disorders. *Pediatrics.* 1984; 74: 103.
35. Mitchell EA, Aman MG, Turbotte SH, Manku M. Clinical characteristics and serum essential fatty acid levels in hyperactive children. *Clin Pediatr (Phila).* 1987; 26:406.
36. Colter A, Cutler C, Mecking K. Fatty acid status and behavioral symptoms of attention deficit hyperactivity disorder in adolescents: a case control study. *Nutr J.* 2008; 7:8.
37. Richardson AJ, Montgomery P. The Oxford-Durham study: a randomized, controlled level of dietary supplementation with fatty acids in children with developmental coordination disorder. *Pediatrics.* 2005; 115:1860.
38. Swanson JM, Kinsbourne M. Food dyes impair performance of hyperactive children on a laboratory learning test. *Science.* 1980; 207:1485.
39. Wolraich ML, Lindgren SD, Stumbo PJ, et al. Effects of diets high in sucrose or aspartame on behavior and cognitive performance of children. *N Engl J Med.* 1994; 330:301.
40. Hoover DE, Milich R. Effects of sugar ingestion expectancies on mother-child interactions. *J Abnorm Child Psychol.* 1994; 22:501.
41. Krummel DA, Seligson FH, Guthrie HA. Hyperactivity: is candy causal? *Crit Rev Food Sci Nutr.* 1996; 36:31.
42. Lucas B. Nutrition for school-age children. In: Trahms CT, Pipes PL, eds. *Nutrition in Infancy and Childhood*, 6th ed. Columbus, OH: WCB/McGraw-Hill; 1997.
43. Niederhofer H, Pittschieder K. A preliminary investigation of ADHD symptoms in person with celiac disease. *J Atten Disord.* 2006; 10:200.
44. Lipton M, Mayo J. Diet and hyperkinesis: an update. *J Am Diet Assoc.* 1983; 83:132.
45. Lipton MA, Golden RN. Nutritional therapies in the psychiatric therapies. In: Karasu TB, ed. *The Somatic Therapies*. Washington, DC: The Psychiatric Association; 1984.
46. Greenwood CEL, Anderson GH. An overview of the mechanism by which diet affects brain function. *Food Tech.* 1986; 50:132.
47. Benner A. Trace mineral levels in hyperactive children responding to the Feingold diet. *J Pediatr.* 1979; 94:944.
48. Khalife N, Kantomaa M, Glover V, et al. Childhood attention deficit hyperactivity disorder symptoms are risk factors for obesity and physical inactivity in adolescence. *J Am Acad Child Adolesc Psychiatry.* 2014; 53:425.
49. Lipton M, Mayo J. Diet and hyperkinesis: an update. *J Am Diet Assoc.* 1983; 83:132.
50. Greenwood CEL, Anderson GH. An overview of the mechanism by which diet affects brain function. *Food Tech.* 1986; 50:132.
51. MTA Cooperative Group. A 14-month randomized clinical trial of treatment strategies for attention-deficit/hyperactivity disorder. *Arch Gen Psychiatry.* 1999; 56:1073.

# 20 Failure to Thrive

SALISA LEWIS, BARBARA NIEDBALA, DIANE SPEAR, AND SHIRLEY W. EKVALL

Inadequate growth of infants and young children has traditionally been called *failure to thrive* (FTT). Historically, diagnostic criteria for FTT distinguish infants and children with chronic inadequate growth (weight for age <5th percentile) from those in whom there is a recognizable retardation of growth velocity (usually a shift of two or more major growth percentiles).[1,2] The American Academy of Pediatrics Committee on Nutrition has defined FTT as "A significantly prolonged cessation of appropriate weight gain compared with recognized norms for age and gender after having achieved a stable pattern."[3,4] In more recent literature, undernutrition and/or pediatric malnutrition has been deinfed as "an imbalance between nutrient requirement and intake, resulting in cumulative deficits of energy, protein or micronutrients that may negatively affect growth, development and other relevant outcomes. The child's inability to consume sufficient nutrients to sustain adequate growth is the fundamental cause of FTT. This inadequate intake may stem from a variety of diseases (historically called organic FTT), environmental causes (historically called nonorganic FTT), or both. It is now recognized that almost all cases of failure to thrive stem from multiple factors, both disease-specific and psychosocial.[5] Growth failure affects 10% to 30% of children in indigent populations.[3,6,7] In the United States, FTT accounts for 1% to 5% of hospital admissions of children younger than 2 years of age, and up to 80% of children with FTT present before 18 months of age.[1,8] Inadequate growth has been closely linked with behavioral, developmental, and intellectual problems that persist even after growth velocity resumes.[3,9–11]

## ETIOLOGY

Disease states or physical impairments that lead to decreased calorie intake, excessive caloric losses, increased nutrient requirements, or impaired utilization of nutrients may cause temporary delay in growth until the condition is recognized and treated. Common medical conditions associated with FTT include gastrointestinal disorders, central nervous system problems, cardiac abnormalities, pulmonary disease, endocrinopathies, inborn errors of metabolism, chronic kidney disease, chronic liver disease, cancer, inflammatory bowel disease, short bowel syndrome, Duchenne muscular dystrophy, human immunodeficiency virus (HIV) infection, and lead poisoning.[12] Growth failure in these conditions is outside the scope of this chapter. It is estimated that major organic disease accounts for no more than 5% of FTT cases.[8,13]

Poverty is the major risk factor for FTT. FTT can be caused by breast-feeding difficulties, improper formula preparation, poor parental diet offering, poor feeding techniques, oral-motor dysfunction, food aversion, subtle neurological and/or behavioral problems with child or parent, and dysfunctional parent-child interactions and behaviors.[3] Often, a failing infant is hospitalized, a voracious appetite and daily growth are observed, and the cause is found to be simply lack of adequate intake. However, inadequate intake may result from conditions such as lactation failure, low birth weight or prematurity, oral-motor dysfunction, extreme poverty, neglect, or abuse. In two population studies, only 5% to 10% of FTT cases were registered for abuse or neglect.[14,15]

The child obviously depends on the family to supply an adequate diet and a nurturing environment, yet infants and children also determine their intake of what is offered. Differences in eating behaviors and feeding patterns between children with FTT and controls have been documented, including poor feeding skills and undemanding behavior,[14] delayed weaning, and less liking for food in general,[16] and eating a narrower range of food.[2] Some children lack normal responses to internal hunger or satiation cues.[17] In a small group of children with nonorganic FTT ($n$ = 47), Reilly and colleagues[18] found that 36% of the children had measurable oral-motor dysfunction. Poor suck, difficulty chewing and swallowing, and poor motor abilities contribute to growth failure by interfering with nutrient intake. Oral sensorimotor impairments, ranging from mild to severe, may be present from birth.[19]

*Inadequate* or *inappropriate* diets provided by the parents or caregivers, such as improper infant formula choice or dilution,[20] increased use of fruit juice,[21] or prolonged use of elimination diets may be causes of malnutrition. In young infants, the reality of inadequate breast milk intake should be investigated. True breast-feeding failures due to insufficient lactation (from retained placenta, mammary gland hypoplasia, or severe maternal illness) or due to the infant's inability to stimulate lactogenesis are not uncommon.[22]

## PREMATURE BIRTH

Premature birth is also a risk factor for FTT: 19.7% of 914 premature infants enrolled in a prospective study developed FTT by 30 months.[23] More than 80% of these cases did not involve chronic medical disorders. Instead, several biological and environmental differences were found between those who developed FTT and those who did not. Dysfunction in the mother-child relationship has been well studied and is continually being researched.[24,25] Black and Krishnakumar[26] found that maternal perceptions and behaviors were not in synchrony with children's growth, suggesting that growth depends on the maternal relationship. This again supports a multifactorial etiology, including both disease-specific and psychosocial factors. The psychosocial factors can be multiplied by the stress of poverty and maternal or caregiver undernutrition, which is especially prevalent in underserved areas and populations. In the current medical era of reimbursement, knowing and documenting pediatric undernutrition in growth failure is a critical component of nutrition assessment and monitoring.[4]

## UNDERNUTRITION

FTT can be synonymous with, or an acute sign of, pediatric undernutrition. Pediatric undernutrition is defined as "an imbalance between nutrient requirement and intake, resulting in cumulative deficits of energy, protein or micronutrients that may negatively affect growth, development and other relevant outcomes."[4] Again, poverty is the leading cause of pediatric undernutrition. Pediatric undernutrition can be divided into acute, chronic, and severe cases. Severe acute undernutrition, experienced by children ages 6 to 60 months, is defined as a very low weight for height (−3 standard deviations [SD] on Z scores) compared with the median growth standards recognized by the World Health Organization (WHO); as visible wasting (a mid-upper arm circumference [MUAC] ≤115 mm); or by the presence of nutritional edema. Wasting is differentiated from severe acute undernutrition by a weight-for-age Z score of –2 SD. Stunting, or chronic undernutrition, is defined by WHO as a height-for-age or length-for-age Z score of

−2 SD on the National Center for Health Statistics/WHO reference. Stunting is most closely associated with socioeconomic problems such as food insecurity, neglect, and poor care. Use of the Academy of Nutrition and Dietetics/American Society for Parenteral and Enteral Nutrition diagnostic indicators to identify and document pediatric undernutrition in FTT children will provide a standardized definition for care, and qualitative information on the cost-effectiveness of nutrition care.[4]

## BIOCHEMICAL ABNORMALITIES

Although growth failure evidenced by anthropometric values is the main diagnostic criterion for pediatric undernutrition, some practitioners order serum chemistry studies to support a diagnosis of FTT, growth failure, and or undernutrition. Biochemical abnormalities consistent with malnutrition are found with FTT. Levels of serum proteins may be either depressed or maintained, depending on the duration and consistency of protein and calorie deprivation. The child may show iron deficiency anemia or have laboratory evidence of decreased vitamin D intake (i.e., increased serum alkaline phosphatase). Lead levels may be increased because lead is more readily absorbed when body calcium, zinc, iron, and protein stores are low.[27,28]

## FACTORS TO BE CONSIDERED IN NUTRITIONAL EVALUATION

### Medical History

The maternal medical history should include a pregnancy history with weight gain, prenatal care, complications, labor, and delivery information. The neonatal history should include gestational age and birth weight, intrauterine growth rate, Apgar scores, any neonatal illness, jaundice or feeding difficulties, and the results of newborn screening. An infant's or toddler's current medical history should include the immunization record, allergies, current medications, and any history of weight loss, vomiting, diarrhea, food refusal, dysphagia, coughing, gagging, snoring, recurrent respiratory illness, malabsorption, or developmental delays.[29] Maternal health during and after pregnancy can have a significant impact on the mother-infant pair.

### Diet History

In addition to detailed maternal and child medical histories, a detailed diet history should elicit information about the infant's or child's daily meal routine and behavior: what is prepared, the setting in which it is offered, the response, and the actual intake. Included should be questions about sucking, chewing, swallowing, and refusal of certain food textures, thicknesses, or major groups of food. Determining a family's access to food is vital, including forms of public assistance and availability of groceries, transportation, and finances. The type of housing and whether refrigeration, cooking, baking, and sanitation areas are available are important factors. A cultural food history to discover any unusual food practices, beliefs, or restrictions can be helpful. Identifying who shops for food, who cooks, and who cares for the child can also be important. A detailed food record, including measured amounts of food, breast milk (prefeeding and postfeeding weights), or formula is a good way to determine actual caloric intake. The nutritionist should primarily identify potential areas for tailored intervention rather than merely diagnosing dietary deficiencies.[2]

FTT in a breast-feeding infant must be evaluated quickly and carefully. The infant should be observed by a professional specifically trained in lactation counseling and assessment for ability to latch on at the breast, efficient suck, length of time nursing, number of nursing periods per 24 hours, and hydration status.[5] Information about supplemental formula, juice, water, and solid foods needs to be obtained, as well as pacifier use. The mother's interest in breast-feeding, her ability to lactate, and her overall health and nutrient intake should also be assessed. If possible, a feeding should be observed, and a prefeeding and postfeeding weight check should be conducted to assess milk intake from the breast.

Infant weight parameters provide highly reliable criteria for assessing the effectiveness of breast-feeding in the neonate. Weight loss of up to 10%[5] (or ≥7% from birth weight), failure to surpass birth weight by 2 weeks of age, and failure to begin weight gain of approximately 28 g/day by 5 days of age are "red flags" to look for when assessing breast-fed neonates.[22] Neifert stated that whenever doubt exists about the infant's ability to extract milk efficiently, the mother should be instructed to use a fully automatic electric breast pump to express the residual milk that remains after feedings so as to prevent diminished milk production.[22]

For a formula-fed infant, the formula type, exact preparation methods, and amounts and types of supplemental water, juice, and other foods should be determined. If the infant is receiving Women, Infants and Children Supplemental Food Program (WIC) benefits, the type of formula, amount, and date of last visit can be verified with the issuing office. Because WIC is a supplemental food program, the infant's or child's needs are not totally met by the program; information about the formula and foods bought by the family is also necessary. The parent should be interviewed carefully about what is prepared and offered versus what is actually taken in by the infant. Often, an observed intake in the clinic or hospital is an indication of this.

When the infant is old enough to begin taking solid foods, the diet history must become more detailed. The caregivers may complete a 3-day diet history at home. When the most reliable history of food offered and consumed is obtained, the diet is evaluated for energy, protein, carbohydrate, fat, vitamins and minerals, and fiber content. Of special concern is the day-to-day consistency of the intake. A 24-hour recall or even a 3-day history may reflect adequate intake, but the provision of nutrients may be inconsistent over a greater period. If the child is not gaining weight, regardless of the theoretical amount consumed, the current diet is not meeting his or her needs for growth.

### Feeding Assessment

The feeding assessment, both behavioral and oral-motor, is described in detail in Chapter 24. Whenever possible, the child should be observed at mealtime with the usual caregiver. Observation of the child and caregiver at mealtime by a multidisciplinary team including a dietitian/nutritionist, speech therapist, and social worker can help identify psychosocial issues or more subtle feeding problems. In children with FTT, oral-motor dysfunction may be subtle, and the child may present as merely fussy, irritable, or difficult or, conversely, as undemanding and with a low appetite—both of which can affect the reaction of those caring for the child.

### Growth Assessment

The child's current weight, length or height, head circumference, MUAC, and triceps skinfold should be measured.[4] Serial measurements should be obtained from previous medical records if possible, to provide a more complete picture of growth velocity over time. Measurements for children born 4 or more weeks premature should be age-adjusted until the child is 2 years old. No single anthropometric parameter can predict the degree of risk for a child,[30] and clinical judgment must be used. Measurements should be plotted on the appropriate curve: WHO 0–3 years growth curves for children 0–2 years of age; CDC 2–20 years growth curves for children older than 2 years. Z scores for pediatric undernutrition should be obtained and tracked. Z scores are more precise than percentile charts because a Z score is always the same standard deviation below the mean. The Z scores are especially important in children who fall below the percentile charts. Plotting weight-for-height on the growth chart gives an objective measure of the thinness of the child, as does measuring the triceps skinfold and the MUAC.[4,31] These measurements are the first to reflect positive changes when nutritional intervention begins. Information on the growth patterns of the father, mother, and siblings is also helpful. For any child with FTT, growth velocity may be an important calculation because it can be compared with reference data for age.[1,13] Growth failure with weight-for-length less than 70% of the expected value in an infant or young toddler should be considered a medical emergency.[32]

## GROWTH

### Normal Growth in Term Infants

The average birth weight for a term infant is 3.3 kg. Weight drops as much as 10% in the first few days of life, secondary to loss of excess fluid. By 10 to 14 days of life, birth weight should be regained. Breast-fed infants who are fed smaller volumes of colostrum for the first few days regain their birth weight a little later than bottle-fed infants.

On average, infants gain 1 kg/mo during the first 3 months of life, 0.5 kg/mo from age 3 to 6 months, 0.33 kg/mo from age 6 to 9 months, and 0.25 kg/mo from age 9 to 12 months. Term infants double their birth weight by age 4 to 6 months and triple it by age 12 months. An alternative schema to use is that term infants gain almost 30 g (1 oz) per day for the first 3 months and then almost 15 g (0.5 oz) per day for the next 6 months. From age 9 months until the child is a toddler, the average weight gain is roughly 0.25 kg/mo (or 0.5 lb/mo). After that point, the weight gain is about 2 kg/yr through early school age.

Caloric intake to ensure adequate intake in a normal infant is 100 to 110 kcal/kg/day for the first 6 months and 100 kcal/kg/day for the second half of the first year. Beyond 10 kg, 50 kcal/kg/day is required until 20 kg is reached; beyond 20 kg, 20 kcal/kg/day is necessary.

Term infants grow 25 cm in length during the first year and 12.5 cm during the second year; growth then slows to approximately 5 or 6 cm between age of 4 years and the onset of puberty, at which time growth can increase to as much as 12 cm/yr.

The average head circumference is 35 cm at birth and rapidly increases to 47 cm by 1 year of age. The rate of growth then slows, reaching an average of 55 cm by age 6 years.[10]

### Biochemical Assessment

In making a differential diagnosis of FTT, the physician may order a multitude of laboratory tests, such as stool studies for malabsorption, blood urea nitrogen and creatinine in renal dysfunction, or glucose in diabetes. Biochemical tests helpful in determining the nutritional status of the child include the complete blood count, serum electrolytes, lead levels, serum transferrin, total protein and albumin, zinc, and alkaline phosphatase. The physician's diagnosis will direct the need for more specific nutrient deficiency tests.[1]

### Clinical Assessment

Physical examination can be an important part of the nutrition assessment. Many micronutrient deficiencies have physical symptoms that may be the first sign of a nutrient deficit.[31] Obvious signs of malnutrition are noted. Muscle wasting, very thin arms and legs, and decreased subcutaneous fat (especially in the child's face, arms, and, in toddlers, buttocks) are seen in chronic malnutrition. Look for signs of temporal wasting.[31] Examine the hair for thickness, color, and texture and the eyes for brightness; look for moist, pink membranes. The lips and tongue should also appear moist and pink. Skin and nails should be inspected for signs of nutritional deficiency. Any signs of abuse or neglect must be noted.

## DIETARY MANAGEMENT

A multidisciplinary approach that includes medical, nursing, nutritional, and social services, as well as referrals to physical and occupational therapy, child development, gastroenterology, or other medical specialties, is most often used. Each member of the multidisciplinary team provides initial assessments, and then a unified treatment plan is devised. Hospitalization may be necessary in some cases to confirm the diagnosis, perform specific laboratory tests, monitor weight, provide optimal nutritional intake, and observe caregiver-child interactions.[34]

FTT clinics are most often used to bring pertinent health professionals together to consult and to monitor children. Evaluation teams in early intervention clinics often use the Peach Survey Form to determine the depth of nutrition counseling required (see Appendix 5). The family may need help in obtaining resources such as WIC, food stamps, public welfare, visiting nurses, support groups, educational programs for parents, child care, or transportation. Nutrition management includes (1) assessment of nutrition status and rate of growth; (2) provision of adequate calories, protein, and other nutrients for optimum growth; (3) nutritional instruction to the parents and other caregivers about exact amounts, types, and preparation of food; and (4) long-term monitoring of nutrition status and growth[35] (Table 20–1).

*Catch-up growth* is the phenomenon of increased growth velocity in a child whose growth has faltered.[36] It begins with a period of growth acceleration followed by a slowing of growth until the normal percentile for the child is reached. In cases of poverty or overt neglect, catch-up growth may be seen when the child is given ad lib amounts of age-appropriate foods. In most cases, however, the nutritionist must plan for a target amount of nutrients. When calories and protein are provided in amounts that are equal to normal age-specific requirements[37] (see Table 20–1), the growth of the child will continue along the low percentile rank to which he or she has fallen. A method to determine appropriate amounts is illustrated in Box 20–1. Individual needs of each child must also be considered in relation to the medical condition, gastrointestinal tolerance, and renal solute load. Any nutritional treatment plan must be integrated into the overall care of the FTT patient and be developed in consultation with the primary physician.[36] If foods are fortified by using a more concentrated infant formula or by adding more carbohydrate, fat, or protein sources, instructions to the caregivers should be both verbal and written. Demonstrations of proper formula mixing may be done in the hospital or clinic. Feeding problems and misconceptions will need to be corrected by ongoing nutritional instruction.

### Prognosis and Follow-up

In acute stages, severe malnutrition causes children to become more apathetic, to be less active, and to explore their environments less.[38] Developmental levels are extremely low in multiple areas during this acute stage. There is some suggestion that extremely malnourished children younger than 6 months of age have a poorer prognosis than those who experience severe malnutrition at an older age. Because most children treated for severe malnutrition return to the same under-nourishing and unstimulating environment from which they came, it is difficult to ascribe the consistently found deficits in cognitive skills, motor skills, and behavior to acute malnutrition or chronic food deprivation versus understimulation alone. The highest risk occurs when these conditions take place in combination.

The mechanism by which severe malnutrition affects brain function acutely and chronically is still under investigation. Kwashiorkor and marasmus seem to have similar negative effects on mental development.[39]

**Table 20–1.** Brief Sketch of Dietary Reference Intakes, 2001

| Age (yr) or Condition | Calories (kcal/day) | Protein (g/kg/day) | Calcium (mg/day) | Iron (mg/day) | Zinc (μg/day) | Vitamin D (IU/day) |
|---|---|---|---|---|---|---|
| 0–0.5 | | 1.0–1.52 (EAP-AI for 0–6 mo) | 210 | 0.27 | 2 | 400 |
| 0.5–1.0 | | 1.0–1.2 (EAP-AI for 7–12 mo) | 270 | 11 | 3 | 400 |
| 1–3 | | 13 (0.87–0.95) | 700 | 7 | 3 | 400 |
| 4–8 | | 19 | 1000 | 10 | 5 | 400 |

Adapted from Otten J, Helwig JP, Meyers LD. *Dietary Reference Intakes: The Essential Guide to Nutrient Requirements*. Washington, DC: National Academy Press; 2006.

**Box 20–1.** Estimating Catch-up Growth Requirements*

Catch-up Growth Requirement (kcal/kg/day) =
Calories Required for Weight Age (kcal/kg/day)
× Ideal Weight for Age (kg) ÷ Actual Weight (kg)

1. Plot the child's height and weight on the NCHS growth charts.
2. Determine at what age the present weight would represent at the 50th percentile (weight age).
3. Determine recommended calories for weight age.
4. Determine the ideal weight (50th percentile) for the child's present age.
5. Multiply the value obtained in step 3 by the value obtained in step 4.
6. Divide the value obtained in step 5 by the child's actual weight.

Estimated protein requirements during catch-up growth can be calculated similarly:

*Guidelines are used to estimate catch-up growth requirements; precise individual needs vary and are mediated by the medical status and diagnosis.

NCHS = National Center for Health Statistics.

From Rathburn JM, Peterson KE. Nutrition in failure to thrive. In: Grand RJ, Sutphen JL, Dietz WH, eds. *Pediatric Nutrition*. Boston: Butterworths; 1987. Used with permission.

Most studies have looked at global IQ measures. Specific effects on reasoning and perceptual-spatial function have been found consistently,[40–42] but effects on other cognitive skills remain to be determined. Motor skills seem to be affected, with clumsiness, motor delay, and sensory integration problems noted in different studies.[41,43,44] Behavior problems seem to be characterized by poor attention, greater distractibility, and less emotional control.[45–47]

The mammalian brain has been proven to have a great capacity for rehabilitation after proper nutrition is restored. However, it is likely that some effects of early malnutrition are mediated through an alteration in neurotransmitter metabolism. There are strong suggestions from animal research that the neurotransmission system is permanently altered. The response to endogenous and exogenous neurotransmitter chemicals may be permanently decreased. The hippocampus, a midline brain structure that is important in modulating activity between the two hemispheres, is irreversibly damaged. The cerebellum, important in balance and motor function, can be severely affected. Delays in psychomotor development have been consistently observed in children with FTT.[30,40–42] More of the changes in the cerebellum appear to be reversible with nutritional rehabilitation than was previously suspected.[48,49] Other recent approaches for assisting with FTT relate to hypertension and celiac disease in the young child.[50,51]

FTT is a multifactorial set of symptoms of pediatric malnutrition (undernutrition). The primary cause of FTT and pediatric malnutrition is poverty. The severity of the undernutrition, as outlined previously, warrants intervention. A multidisciplinary team approach that evaluates maternal and infant medical history, psychosocial history, growth and feeding history, and observation of the child-caregiver feeding interaction is essential for optimal outcome. The dietitian/nutritionist should carefully assess history, physical findings, and psychosocial factors when creating a feeding rehabilitation plan.

## Adult Failure to Thrive

All cases of FTT stem from multiple factors, both disease-specific and psychosocial,[5] in the pediatric population and also in adults. Pediatric patients with FTT have not achieved their expected functional level, whereas adults with FTT are unable to maintain their functional status; the symptom complex is similar at both ends of the age spectrum.[52] The National Institute of Aging describes FTT as a syndrome manifested by weight loss greater than 5% of baseline, decreased appetite, poor nutrition, and inactivity, often accompanied by dehydration, depressive symptoms, impaired immune function, and low cholesterol levels.[53] Such conditions describe a syndrome of global decline that occurs in older adults as a worsening of physical frailty that is frequently compounded by cognitive impairment and/or functional disability.[53,54] These conditions can easily lead to inadequate food intake, malnutrition, unintended weight loss, weakness, functional decline, and other complicating factors such as falls, impaired immune response, and poor wound healing. In adults with preexisting disability, including intellectual and developmental disability (IDD), aging may result in increased risk factors and earlier onset of symptoms than is typically seen in people without IDD. Identifying cognitive decline in individuals with IDD can be especially challenging because cognitive difficulties can be related to lifelong deficits or to changes resulting from dementia.[55]

FTT, both disease-specific and psychosocial, can appear at any point within the lifespan of an adult with IDD. Obtaining a baseline of performance is critical for assessing functional ability and cognitive and behavioral changes. Studies suggest conducting a detailed assessment between the ages of 25 and 40 years to establish a baseline level of performance for individuals with Down syndrome[56–58] and at age 50 years for those with other intellectual disability.[56,59] Periodic reassessments, after baseline are recommended so that substantial changes can be identified.[60]

## References


1. Careaga MC, Kerner JA. A gastroenterologist's approach to failure to thrive. *Pediatr Ann.* 2000; 29:558.
2. Wright CM. Identification and management of failure to thrive: community perspective. *Arch Dis Child.* 2000; 82:5.
3. Block RW, Krebs NF, Committee on Child Abuse and Neglect, Committee on Nutrition. Failure to thrive as a manifestation of child neglect. *Pediatrics.* 2005; 116:1234.
4. Becker PJ, Carney LN, Corkins MR, et al. Consensus statement of the Academy of Nutrition and Dietetics/American Society for Parenteral and Enteral Nutrition: indicators recommended for the identification and documentation of pediatric malnutrition (undernutrition). *J Acad Nutr Diet.* 2014; 114:1988.
5. Rabinowitz S, Rogers G, Unnikrishnan N. Nutritional considerations in failure to thrive. Article 985007. Last update April 24, 2014. http://emedicine.medscape.com. Accessed June 21, 2016.
6. Gahagan S. Failure to thrive: a consequence of undernutrition. *Pediatr Rev.* 2006; 27:e1.
7. Zenel JA. Failure to thrive: a general pediatrician's perspective. *Pediatr Rev.* 1997; 18:371.
8. Cole SZ, Lanham JS. Failure to thrive: an update. *Am Fam Physician.* 2011; 83:829.
9. Hufton IW, Dates K. Non-organic failure to thrive: a long-term follow-up. *Pediatrics.* 1977; 59:73.
10. Singer L. Long-term hospitalization of failure-to-thrive infants: developmental outcome at three years. *Child Abuse Neglect.* 1986; 10:479.
11. Sidebotham P. Failure to thrive. *Arch Dis Child.* 2000; 82:428.
12. Kyle GK, Shekerdemian LS, Coss-Bu JA. Growth failure and nutrition considerations in chronic childhood wasting diseases. *Nutr Clin Pract.* 2015; 30:227.
13. Wright C, Callum J, Birks E, Jarvis S. Community-based management of failure to thrive: a randomized control trial. *BMJ.* 1998; 317:571.
14. Skuse D, Gill D, Reilly S, Wolke D, Lynch M. Failure to thrive and the risk of child abuse: a prospective population study. *J Med Screen.* 1995; 2:145.
15. Wright C, Birks E. Risk factors for failure to thrive: a population-based survey. *Child Care Health Dev.* 2000; 26:5.
16. Wright C, Loughridge J, Moore G. Failure to thrive in a population context: two contrasting studies of feeding and nutritional status. *Proc Nutr Soc.* 2000; 59:37.
17. Kasese-Hara M, Wright C, Drewett R. Energy compensation in young children who fail to thrive. *J Child Psychol Psychiatry.* 2002; 43:449.
18. Reilly SM, Skuse DH, Wolke D, Stevenson J. Oral-motor dysfunction in children who fail to thrive: organic or non-organic? *Dev Med Child Neurol.* 1999; 41:115.
19. Ramsay M, Gisel EG, Boutry M. Non-organic failure to thrive: growth failure secondary to feeding skill disorder. *Dev Med Child Neurol.* 1993; 35:285.
20. Massa G, Vanoppen A, Gillis P, Aerssens P, Alliet P, Raesm M. Protein malnutrition due to replacement of milk by rice drink. *Eur J Pediatr.* 2001; 160:382.
21. Smith MM, Lifshitz F. Excess fruit juices consumption as a contributing factor in nonorganic failure to thrive. *Pediatrics.* 1994; 93:438.
22. Neifert MR. Prevention of breastfeeding tragedies. *Pediatr Clin North Am.* 2001; 48:273.
23. Kelleher KJ, Casey PH, Bradley RH, et al. Risk factors and outcomes for failure to thrive in low birth weight preterm infants. *Pediatrics.* 1993; 91:941.
24. Skuse DH. Non-organic failure to thrive: a reappraisal. *Arch Dis Child.* 1985; 60:173.
25. Vietze PM, Falsey S, O'Connor S, Sandler H, Sherrod K, Altemeier WA, eds. *High-Risk Infants and Children: Adult and Peer Interactions.* New York: Academic Press; 1980.
26. Black MM, Krishnakumar A. Predicting longitudinal growth curves of height and weight using ecological factors for children with and without early growth deficiency. *J Nutr.* 1999; 129:539.
27. Mahaffey KR. Nutritional factors in lead poisoning. *Nutr Rev.* 1981; 39:353.
28. Bithoney WG. Elevated lead levels in children with nonorganic failure to thrive. *Pediatrics.* 1986; 78:891.
29. Sirotnak AP, Chiesa A. Failure to thrive clinical presentation. Article 915575. Last update November 4, 2015. http://emedicine.medscape.com. Accessed June 21, 2016.
30. Raynor P, Rudolf MCJ. Anthropometric indices of failure to thrive. *Arch Dis Child.* 2000; 82:364.

31. Green Corkins KG. Nutrition-focused physical examination in pediatric patients. *Nutr Clin Pract.* 2015; 30:203.
32. Oates RK, Kempe RS. Growth failure in infants. In: Helfer MA, Kempe RS, Krugman RD, eds. *The Battered Child*, 5th ed. Chicago: University of Chicago Press; 1997: 374.
34. Showers J, Mandelkorn R, Coury DL, McCleery J. Non-organic failure to thrive: identification and intervention. *J Pediatr Nurs.* 1986; 1:240.
35. Peterson KE, Washington J, Rathbun JM. Team management of failure to thrive. *J Am Diet Assoc.* 1984; 84:810.
36. Rathbun JM, Peterson KE. Nutrition in failure to thrive. In: Grand RJ, Sutphen JL, Dietz WH, eds. *Pediatric Nutrition*. Boston: Butterworths; 1987.
37. National Research Council. *Recommended Dietary Allowances*, 10th ed. Washington, DC: National Academy Press; 1989.
38. Grantham-McGregor S. A review of studies of the effect of severe malnutrition on mental development. *J Nutr.* 1995; 125(8 Suppl):2233S.
39. Galler JR, Ramsey FC, Forde V, Salt P, Archer E. Long-term effects of early kwashiorkor compared with marasmus: II. Intellectual performance. *J Pediatr Gastroenterol Nutr.* 1987; 6:847.
40. Champakam S, Srikantia S, Gapalan C. Kwashiorkor and mental development. *Am J Clin Nutr.* 1968; 21:844.
41. Hoorweg J, Stanfield J. The effects of protein energy malnutrition in early childhood on intellectual and motor abilities in later childhood and adolescence. *Dev Med Child Neurol.* 1976; 8:130.
42. Nwuga V. Effect of severe kwashiorkor on intellectual development among Nigerian children. *Am J Clin Nutr.* 1977; 30:1423.
43. Cravioto J. Not by bread alone: effect of early malnutrition and stimuli deprivation on mental development. In: Ghai O, ed. *Perspectives in Pediatrics*. New Delhi: Interprint; 1977.
44. Galler JR, Ramsey FC, Salt P, Archer E. Long-term effects of early kwashiorkor compared with marasmus: III. Fine motor skills. *J Pediatr Gastroenterol Nutr.* 1987; 6:855.
45. Galler JR, Ramsey F, Solimano G, Lowell WE. The influence of early malnutrition on subsequent behavioral development: II. Classroom behavior. *J Am Acad Child Psychiatry.* 1983; 22:16.
46. Richardson SA, Birch HG, Grabie E, Yoder K. The behavior of children in school who were severely malnourished in the first two years of life. *J Health Social Behav.* 1972; 13:276.
47. Richardson S, Birch H, Ragbeer C. The behavior of children at home who were severely malnourished in the first two years of life. *J Biosocial Sci.* 1975; 7:255.
48. Drewett R, Corbett S, Wright C. Cognitive and educational attainments at school age of children who failed to thrive in infancy: a population-based study. *J Child Psychol Psychiatry.* 1999; 40:551.
49. Boddy J, Skuse D, Andrews B. The developmental sequelae of non-organic failure to thrive. *J Child Psychol Psychiatry.* 2000; 41:1003.
50. Phillips AR, Eliason JL, Stanley JC, Coleman DM. Infantile renovascular hypertension with failure to thrive, *Ann Vasc Surg.* 2016; 227:e5.
51. Khalab M, Baker RD, Ly EK, et al. Presenting pattern of celiac disease. *J Pediatr Gastroenterol Nutr.* 2016:121:66.
52. Sarkisian CA, Lachs MS. Failure to thrive in older adults. *Ann Intern Med.* 1996; 124:1072.
53. Institute of Medicine Committee on a National Research Agenda on Aging, Division of Health Promotion and Disease Prevention. *Extending Life, Enhancing Life: A National Research Agenda on Aging*. Washington, DC: National Academies Press; 1991.
54. Hamerman D. Toward an understanding of frailty. *Ann Intern Med.* 1999; 130:945.
55. Devenny DA, Krinsky-McHale SJ, Sersen G, Silverman WP. Sequence of cognitive decline in dementia in adults with Down's syndrome. *J Intellect Disabil Res.* 2000; 44:654.
56. Jokinen MP, Janicki SM, Keller P, McCallion LT; National Task Group on Intellectual Disabilities and Dementia Practices. *Guidelines for Structuring Community Care and Supports for People with Intellectual Disabilities Affected by Dementia*. 2013. Washington, DC: American Academy of Developmental Medicine and Dentistry. http://aadmd.org/sites/default/files/NTG_Guidelines-posting-version.pdf. Accessed June 21, 2016.
57. Kirk LJ, Hick R, Laraway A. Assessing dementia in people with learning disabilities: the relationship between two screening measures. *J Intellect Disabil.* 2006; 10:357.
58. O'Caoimh R, Clune Y, Molloy W. Screening for Alzheimer's disease in Down syndrome. *J Alzheimer Dis Parkinsonism.* 2013; 3(3):S7:1.
59. Krinsky-McHale SJ, Silverman W. Dementia and mild cognitive impairment in adults with intellectual disability: issues of diagnosis. *Dev Disabil Res Rev.* 2013; 18:31.
60. Otten J, Helwig JP, Meyers LD. *Dietary Reference Intakes: The Essential Guide to Nutrient Requirements*. Washington, DC: National Academy Press; 2006.

# 21 Rumination

VALLI K. EKVALL AND SHIRLEY W. EKVALL

The American Psychiatric Association has specified the diagnostic criteria for rumination in infancy in the *Diagnostic and Statistical Manual of Mental Disorders, Fifth Edition* (DSM-5).[1] These criteria are outlined in Box 21–1.

**Box 21–1.** Diagnostic Criteria for Rumination Disorder

A. Repeated regurgitation of food over a period of at least 1 month. Regurgitated food may be rechewed, reswallowed, or spit out.
B. The repeated regurgitation is not attributable to an associated gastrointestinal or other medical condition (e.g., gastroesophageal reflux, pyloric stenosis).
C. The eating disturbance does not occur exclusively during the course of anorexia nervosa, bulimia nervosa, binge-eating disorder, or avoidant/restrictive food intake disorder.
D. If the symptoms occur in the context of another mental disorder, such as intellectual disability (intellectual developmental disorder) or another neurodevelopmental disorder, they are sufficiently severe to warrant additional clinical attention.

*Specify* if:

**In remission:** After full criteria for rumination disorder were previously met, the criteria have not been met for a sustained period of time.

American Psychiatric Association. *Diagnostic and Statistical Manual of Mental Disorders, Fifth Edition (DSM-5)*. Washington, DC: American Psychiatric Association; 2013.

Although 84% of ruminators described in the literature have problems with weight, 16% are not underweight or losing weight.[2] Most ruminators, particularly those with developmental delays, are clearly not normal before the onset of rumination. The rationale for the diagnostic requirement of rumination being present "for at least 1 month" is unclear and may interfere with prompt diagnosis and treatment of this potentially life-threatening disorder. A definition of rumination consistent with the existing literature is "the voluntary and pleasurable repeated regurgitation of stomach contents without an organic cause."

Rumination disorder is seen in infants but has been described more frequently in mentally retarded children and adults. Of the 123 cases of rumination reported in the literature, 38% involved infant ruminators, and 62% of ruminators were mentally retarded individuals of any age. Rumination can be found in up to 10% of institutionalized individuals with severe or profound mental retardation.[3]

Rumination—the regurgitation or backward flow of stomach contents—must be distinguished from vomiting, which is the forcible expulsion of stomach contents. Involuntary vomiting is a common symptom in young children and may be associated with infections such as salmonella, tonsillopharyngitis, and septicemia. Psychogenic vomiting can be a symptom of a variety of psychological problems, including anorexia, bulimia nervosa, and anxiety disorder. However, it differs from rumination in that it is not a pleasurable or self-stimulating act. The diagnosis can be made on the basis of symptoms alone.[4]

Rumination in infants differs from ordinary regurgitation or other organic problems that are involuntary and do not require effort on the part of the infant to induce regurgitation. Deliberate regurgitation is often achieved by thrusting the fingers into the mouth, by a series of vigorous thrusting movements of the tongue backward and forward, or by tightening of the abdominal muscles. Rumination may be a willed effort. It usually begins within 30 minutes after completion of a meal and continues for up to 1 hour or longer, gradually decreasing. The decline with time may be related to the process of gastric emptying (i.e., a gradual decrease in the amount of food to ruminate) and to the increasingly unpleasant or acidic taste of the stomach contents.

Age at onset for rumination in infants is usually between 3 weeks and 12 months (mean, 5.7 months); for rumination in mentally retarded individuals, it is 3 months to 21 years (mean, 5.7 years).[2] The disorder is about 3.5 times more common in males than in females. Infants also frequently exhibit other self-stimulating behaviors, such as head rolling, head banging, body rocking, and excessive finger and thumb sucking. Satiation treatment has been effective in reducing or eliminating ruminative vomiting in persons with developmental disorders. White bread was made available for 1 hour after each daily meal and assured satiety, therefore preventing rumination.[5] Infants with rumination are often described as quiet, sad, and singularly wide-eyed, and some are irritable and hungry between episodes. These infants seem to be lost in inner contemplation and are very detached from the environment but are quick to respond to external stimulation. However, infant ruminators do not comprise a homogeneous group in terms of social, emotional, and behavioral functioning, and much variation is described in the literature.[2]

## ETIOLOGY

Etiological theories of rumination that have had some currency at various times include heredity, dilation of the lower end of the esophagus or the stomach, overaction of the sphincter muscles in the upper portions of the alimentary canal, cardiospasm, pylorospasm, gastric hyperacidity, achlorhydria, movements of the tongue, insufficient mastication, a pathological conditioned reflex, aerophagy, finger sucking, neuropathic constitution, motility neurosis, gastric neurosis, lack of occupation, and boredom. These theories received only limited acceptance, mainly because they did not generate effective treatment strategies or because they described involuntary or organic problems, not true rumination, which is voluntary and nonorganic.

Current theories—the psychodynamic or psychogenic theory in infants and a learning or self-stimulation theory in adults and in children who are mentally retarded—implicate different rewarding consequences for seeking stimulation.[6]

The psychodynamic explanation has two central assumptions. The first links ruminating behavior to infant characteristics such as anxiety, depression, or neurotic tendencies. The second emphasizes maternal characteristics and the mother-child interaction. Psychodynamic theory holds that, as a result of the mother's personality problems or psychosocial stress that influence her ability to interact with the baby, she cannot form an appropriate bond and interaction pattern with the infant. The infant seeks internal gratification because of a lack of external stimulation. An infant who is unable to evoke appropriate responses from his or her mother is thought to resort to rumination as a tension-releasing or stimulation-producing activity. Several studies have also shown that those who engage in ruminative responses have higher levels of depression. Rumination is predictive of depressive and anxiety disorders.[7]

The main emphasis of the behavioral approach, based on the learning or self-stimulation theory, is on the consequences of the behavior.

Rumination is thought to be maintained as a result of positive reinforcement. In contrast to psychodynamic theories, which focus on the origin of the behavior, the behavioral theories emphasize its maintenance. Chronic rumination is thought to be a self-stimulatory behavior, independent of social reinforcement or nurturing parents, in individuals who are mentally retarded.

Rumination occurs most frequently when the infant is alone. By the time the diagnosis is made, the child may be severely malnourished and may have undergone extensive medical evaluations to rule out organic causes.

Although rumination does not appear to be linked to any organic abnormality, it is often confused with a variety of other disorders. A lack of awareness often leads to delay in diagnosis.[8] Because rumination is uncommon, many erroneous diagnoses may be made before the physician, by a process of elimination, labels the problem as rumination. Some diagnoses commonly considered before the symptom complex was recognized as rumination included adrenal insufficiency, pyloric stenosis, food allergy, duodenal ulcer, esophageal achalasia, and severe feeding problems of unknown origin. Rumination was initially considered to be a symptom of gastroesophageal reflux caused by a physical disorder, such as achalasia or hiatal hernia. It was believed that activities associated with ruminating behavior (e.g., tongue thrusting) are initiated as the result of an attempt to empty the esophagus of refluxed gastric contents or as a response to abnormal esophageal dilation. However, when a child with rumination is admitted to an inpatient facility with another diagnosis (e.g., failure to thrive), close observation by clinicians, in conjunction with a detailed social history, usually enables the diagnosis of rumination to be made. Another method of diagnosis is the use of duodenal manometry.[9]

## COMPLICATIONS

The chronic vomiting associated with rumination can lead to a rapid breakdown in bodily functions with serious repercussions such as dehydration and malnutrition, resulting in lowered resistance to disease. It may result in weight loss, failure to thrive, electrolyte imbalance, dehydration, malnutrition, anemia, depressed immunocompetence, aspiration, aspiration pneumonia, gastric disorders, and even death. Rumination is a syndrome characterized by repetitive regurgitation of small amounts of food from the stomach. The food is then partially or completely rechewed, reswallowed, or expelled. This syndrome is relatively common in infants and mentally retarded persons, but it also occurs in adults with normal intelligence. Rumination syndrome is frequently misdiagnosised in adults as vomiting due to gastroparesis or gastroesophageal reflux. This syndrome must be considered in the differential diagnosis of a patient with regurgitation, vomiting (especially postprandially), and weight loss. Reassurance, explanations, and behavioral therapy are the mainstays of treatment in adults with normal intelligence who have the rumination syndrome. Appropriately controlled trials are needed to establish the best therapy.

The mortality rate attributed to individuals with chronic rumination ranges from 12% to 20%, although it has been declining.[10] Progression of this condition may also detract from a child's physical appearance, lead others to avoid the child, impede developmental progress, and cause tooth decay. The dental manifestations are the result of exposure to acids and are commonly seen in patients with eating disorders.[1] The importance of screening for rumination among these patients has been stressed, as well as screening for eating disorders among individuals who ruminate.[11]

## BIOCHEMICAL AND BEHAVIORAL ABNORMALITIES

The behavioral approach to the etiology and maintenance of rumination states that rumination is a conditioned behavior and can be eliminated by altering the antecedents or consequences of the behavior. Behavioral techniques have often been used to treat rumination, and the results have been quick, effective, and enduring when a rigorous behavioral program has been used. However, these techniques usually require one-to-one attention during the period of implementation, and they may be constrained by legal and regulatory restrictions.

Behavioral treatments that have been used successfully to eliminate rumination include aversive conditioning (e.g., administering a taste-aversive substance or an electric shock immediately after rumination), overcorrection, and the presentation or withdrawal of reinforcement contingent on rumination behavior. Several studies have shown that those who engage in ruminative responses have higher levels of depression. Rumination is predictive of depressive and anxiety disorders. The data collected by Rast et al.[10] revealed that rumination decreased significantly in frequency when ruminators were allowed to eat to satiation (three to eight times the normal meal volume) and increased again when smaller standard portions were eaten. A satiation diet must be maintained indefinitely to control rumination, unlike behavior modification strategies that can be faded, often without recurrence of rumination. Studies of persons with Prader-Willi syndrome have shown that rumination becomes more frequent with increased caloric restriction.[12]

Although not as effective as high-calorie satiation programs, satiation achieved through the consumption of low-calorie foods also has been found to decrease rumination. It has been suggested that oropharyngeal and esophageal stimulation from chewing and swallowing may contribute to the etiology and maintenance of ruminating behavior. One study examined the role of chewing in rumination and found that moderate decreases in rumination occurred after the consumption of normal meals that were preceded by supplementary gum chewing.[13]

The frequency of rumination in a 12-year-old boy with profound mental retardation was investigated over a 4-week period. Less frequent rumination was significantly associated with individual attention (versus independent play or group activity), special education programming (versus programming during nonschool hours), time spent with caregivers who liked the child (versus those who liked him less), earlier time of the day (versus later in the day), and increasing time after meals.[14]

The relationship between the assumed etiology and the method of treatment is complex. Those who see rumination as a learned conditioning problem are likely to recommend only behavioral treatment, particularly if the patient is mentally retarded. Those who believe rumination to be a disturbance in the mother-child relationship may opt to arrange for a stimulating environment, a nurturing mother substitute, and therapy for the mother, particularly when the ruminator is an infant. An interdisciplinary team approach often is required in cases of severe rumination.[15]

## FACTORS TO BE CONSIDERED IN NUTRITIONAL EVALUATION

### Nutritional Assessment

Particular attention should be given to calorie and protein intake. In nutritional assessments to measure malnutrition, anthropometric data such as height, weight, waist circumference, and triceps skinfold (including muscle mass) measurements should be obtained during the initial evaluation, and periodically throughout the treatment program, to provide a baseline against which to monitor future developmental gains. Biochemical tests should include routine blood and urine analysis and serum nutrient analysis to identify any suspected nutrient deficiencies. Mothers of infants who ruminate are typically described as immature, dependent, and depressed and may not provide adequate simulation, which the infant requires for proper development. The parent-child interaction should be assessed during the evaluation.

### Treatment

Because of confusion about the various theories of causation in rumination, several methods of treatment have been identified. Placing the child in a prone position at a 30- to 45-degree angle with the head up on an antireflux board may be somewhat effective after meals. However, this approach is more appropriate for treatment of involuntary gastroesophageal reflux than for rumination. Similarly, medications that improve lower esophageal sphincter tone and accelerate gastric emptying (metoclopramide and bethanechol) may reduce rumination. However, if these medications are discontinued, rumination is likely to resume. The medications do not prohibit rumination but make it more difficult for the ruminator to regurgitate purposefully. Rumination still occurs while the individual is taking these medications, but its frequency may be reduced.

A surgical treatment—a Nissen fundoplication used for the treatment of involuntary gastroesophageal reflux—also has been used in an attempt to control rumination. However, this procedure has a significant rate of postoperative morbidity and mortality. Additionally, one of us has treated a patient who continued to ruminate after fundoplication. The procedure makes it difficult but not impossible to ruminate. Considering these limitations and the existence of safer and more effective procedures (e.g., behavioral techniques), medication and surgery are not advised.

Psychodynamic or psychogenic treatment methods may involve one of two approaches. The first is aimed at changing the parent-child interaction. Substitute or surrogate mothers, who provide a stimulating and nurturing environment, have been used with success. At the same time, the mother may be treated with psychotherapy and trained in parenting skills. Because rumination is relatively rare but potentially fatal for infants, environmental changes and enhanced mothering skills can be critical to correction of the rumination and promotion of appropriate weight gain in the child.

A review of the behavioral literature reveals several effective interventions based on the principles of reinforcement and punishment. These include delivery of an aversive stimulus contingent on rumination (most commonly a taste-aversive substance, such as lemon juice or Tabasco sauce, or an electric shock), overcorrection (requiring the ruminator to practice oral hygiene for an extended period after each episode of rumination, which is experienced as aversive), time out from positive reinforcement, and differential reinforcement of other or incompatible behaviors. Other treatment approaches have involved contingent or noncontingent increased social attention and stimulation, satiation, providing peanut butter after consumption of food (which works in the same way as satiation by increasing caloric intake), changing the consistency of food, and decreasing the rate of feeding.[16,17] Satiation treatment has also been effective in reducing or eliminating ruminative vomiting in persons with developmental disabilities. These techniques have been successful in some but not all cases. What is effective with one ruminator may not work with another.

In choosing interventions, one should consider ethical issues, the client's rights, and social validation data. The factors that promote or hinder generalization of treatment effects and maintenance of effects after treatment are poorly understood and merit systematic research. Treatment needs to be individualized according to the ruminator's symptoms, rumination frequency, complications (which may justify aggressive treatment), and family or caregiver dynamics.

## DIETARY MANAGEMENT

A very promising new area of investigation is the nutritional and mechanical management of rumination. Previously, nutritional management consisted of decreasing the amount of food presented at each meal, giving clear liquids, and withholding fluids during mealtime. However, these procedures proved ineffective in improving nutritional status and instead produced weight loss and dehydration to the point of hospitalization. A different approach, supported Khan et al.[9] and Mousa et al.,[18] postulated that rumination is best treated by a multidisciplinary team. A combined effort of the team, which included both psychologists and dietitians, was reported to provide the highest degree of success.

Providing large quantities of food has resulted in a decrease in rumination, an increase in weight, and an improvement in nutritional status. Although consumption to the point of satiation reduces rumination, it can cause weight gain above the estimated ideal body weight. Weight should be monitored accordingly. After satiation is discontinued, rumination often recurs. Environmental changes and enhanced mothering skills can be critical, particularly for infants.[19–21]

Children who ruminate are typically found to consume their food ravenously. This condition is managed by providing the proper eating environment in which to decrease the rate of consumption and maintain a high-calorie, high-protein intake. Management techniques to be considered during treatment include the following:

- Avoid stimulation or excitement at mealtimes.
- Provide relaxed, quiet mealtimes to promote slow eating and adequate mastication of food.
- Avoid excessive fluid intakes during and soon after meals.
- Avoid consumption of raw or coarse foods.
- Decrease stimulation of the gastric mucosa by providing bland foods only (not acidic, spicy, or greasy foods).[22]
- Avoid highly concentrated fat, which may cause diarrhea and dehydration.
- Avoid overloading the stomach or prolonged stomach emptiness.
- Provide thicker liquids, which are more difficult to regurgitate.

A high-protein, high-calorie diet is usually needed; sometimes it may be as high as 33% above the Dietary Reference Intake levels (DRI).

### Follow-up

During treatment and follow-up, anthropometric measurements such as weight, height, waist circumference, and triceps skinfold (with muscle mass) should continue to be monitored and documented. Food intake and loss must be recorded daily, with particular attention given to calorie and protein intake. If rumination recurs, both the frequency and the amount of loss should be determined, and treatment should be resumed immediately.

### References


1. American Psychiatric Association. *Diagnostic and Statistical Manual of Mental Disorders, Fifth Edition*. Washington, DC: American Psychiatric Association; 2013.
2. Mayes SD. Eating disorders of infancy and early childhood. In: Hooper SR, Hynd GW, Mattisons RE, eds. *Child Psychopathology: Diagnostic Criteria and Clinical Assessment*. Hillsdale, NJ: Erlbaum; 1992.
3. Fredericks DW, Carr JE, William's WL. Overview of the treatment of rumination disorder for adults in a residential setting. *J Behav Ther Exp Psychiatry*. 1998; 29:31.
4. Talley NJ. Rumination syndrome. *Gastroenterol Hepatol*. 2011:7:117.
5. Thibadeau S, Blew P, Reedy P, Luiselli JK. Access to white bread as an intervention for chronic ruminative vomiting. *J Behav Ther Exp Psychiatry*. 1999; 30:137.
6. Mayes SD, Humphrey JJ, Hanford HA, Mitchell JF. Rumination disorder: differential diagnosis. *J Am Acad Child Adolesc Psychiatry*. 1988; 27:300.
7. Nolen-Hoeksema S. The role of rumination in depressive disorders and mixed anxiety/depressive symptoms. *J Abnorm Psychol*. 2000; 109:504.
8. Malcolm A, Thumshirn MB, Camilleri M, Williams DD. Rumination syndrome. *Mayo Clin Proc*. 1997; 72:646.
9. Kahn S, Hyman P, Cocjin J, Di Lorenzo C. Rumination syndrome in adolescents. *J Pediatr*. 2000; 136:528.
10. Rast J, Johnston JM, Drum C, Conrin J. The relation of food quantity to rumination behavior. *J Appl Behav Anal*. 1981; 14:121.
11. Eckern M, Stevens W, Mitchell J. The relationship between rumination and eating disorders. *J Eat Disord* 1999; 26:414.
12. Alexander RC, Greenswag LR, Nowak AJ. Rumination and vomiting in Prader-Willi syndrome. *Am J Med Genet*. 1987; 28:889.
13. Rast J, Ellinger-Allen JA, Johnston JM. Dietary management of rumination: four case studies. *Am J Clin Nutr*. 1985; 42:95.
14. Humphrey F, Mayes SD, Bixier EO. Variables associated with frequency of rumination in a boy with profound mental retardation. *J Autism Dev Disord*. 1989; 19:435.
15. Green AD, Alioto A, Mousa H, Di Lorenzo C. Severe pediatric rumination syndrome: successful interdisciplinary inpatient management. *J Pediatr Gastroenterol Nutr*. 2011; 52:414.
16. Greene KS, Johnston JM, Rossi M, Rawal A, Winston M, Barron S. Effects of eating peanut butter on ruminating. *Am J Ment Retard*. 1991; 95:631.
17. Johnson J, Greene K. Relation between ruminating and quantity of food consumed. *Ment Retard*. 1992; 30:07.
18. Mousa H, Montgomery M, Alioto A. Adolescent rumination syndrome. *Curr Gastroenterol Rep*. 2014; 16:398.
19. Franco K, Campbell N, Tamburrino M, Evans C. Rumination: the eating disorder of infancy. *Child Psychiatry Hum Dev*. 1993; 24:91.
20. Thame MM, Burton KA, Forrester TE. The human ruminant. *West Indian Med J*. 2000; 49:172.
21. Chial H, Camilleri M, Williams D, Litzinger K, Perrault J. Rumination syndrome in children and adolescents: diagnosis, treatment, and prognosis. *Pediatrics*. 2003; 111:158.
22. Academy of Nutrition and Dietetics. *Pediatric Nutrition Care Manual: Gastroesophageal Reflux*. http://www.nutritioncaremanual.org. Accessed June 20, 2016.

# 22 Anorexia Nervosa, Bulimia Nervosa, and Eating Disorders

VALLI K. EKVALL, SHIRLEY W. EKVALL, MICHAEL FARRELL, AND ASAD DALIA

Eating disorders (EDs) are psychiatric disorders with diagnostic criteria based on psychological, behavioral, and physiological characteristics.[1] They involve abnormal behavior related to weight control, accompanied by an intense preoccupation with food, a great fear of gaining weight, and an obsession with becoming thinner.[2] The three classic categories of EDs are anorexia nervosa (AN), bulimia nervosa (BN), and eating disorders not otherwise specified (EDNOS). The catch-all EDNOS category has now been divided into Binge Eating Disorder (BED), Other Specified Feeding or Eating Disorder (OSFED), and Unspecified Feeding and Eating Disorder (UFED).[3] EDs are not limited by socioeconomic class and are found in a wide demographic range.[2,4,5]

The term *anorexia nervosa* was coined in 1874 by Sir William Gull to describe a nervous disease characterized by a loss of appetite and severe wasting.[6] The most notable features of AN are marked weight loss and the maintenance of low body weight.[7] The fourth edition of the *Diagnostic and Statistical Manual of the American Psychiatric Association, Fifth Edition* (DSM-5)[3] establishes the criteria for AN as given in Box 22–1. In the early literature, AN was often seen as a form of rebellion against sexuality. Through maintenance of a low body weight, a young girl was able to delay sexual maturation. This view is still held today, although there is a higher prevalence of married women with AN today. AN has been divided by some authors into primary and secondary or atypical forms. Patients with primary AN fear becoming obese, perhaps because of a disturbed body image, and make a variety of attempts to lose weight. Secondary or atypical AN often results from psychiatric disorders, such as conversion reaction, depression (unipolar or bipolar), or schizophrenia, or from other medical diseases involving a true loss of appetite.[6] The person with AN may be brought to the health professional when the body weight is 15% below normal. By that time, the person may have bradycardia, edema, hypotension, neonatal-like or lanugo hair, and amenorrhea but may deny having symptoms.[3] The person with AN may prepare elaborate meals but limit food intake to a few low-calorie foods.

BN occurs generally between the ages of 12 and 28 and affects approximately 2% to 5% of the population.[8] BN is defined in DSM-5 by the diagnostic criteria given in Box 22–2. The individual at risk for BN may have a biological vulnerability to depression that is exacerbated by chaotic and conflicting family and social role expectations. Society's emphasis on thinness often helps the person identify weight loss as the solution. Dieting leads to binging, and then the cyclic disorder begins again.[9] Intake restriction can be the physiological or psychological trigger for subsequent binge eating.[10,11] A *binge* is not defined by the amount of food intake alone, but also by its accompanying behaviors, such as an intense feeling of being out of control during the binge episode. Any subjective or objective sensation of stomach fullness may cause the person to purge. After purging, the person may feel some initial relief, but it is often followed by guilt and shame. Resuming normal eating patterns commonly leads to gastrointestinal complaints such as bloating, constipation, and flatulence. Although the focus is on the food, the binge/purge behavior is often a means of regulating and managing emotion and medicating emotional pain.[11]

Certain factors suggest a favorable prognosis for BN, including early age at onset, hysterical personality structure, short duration of symptoms, and diminution of body perception disturbances after weight increase.[12] The following factors suggest an unfavorable prognosis: vomiting, abuse of purgatives, compulsive personality traits, numerous physical complaints, and psychological test results that are suggestive of psychosis.[12]

Currently, a person cannot be diagnosed as having both AN and BN at the same time. Half of all patients with EDs do not fit the criteria for either AN or BN, and a significant portion of them are now classified as having BED. Those who have a feeding or eating disorder that causes significant impairment or distress but does not meet the criteria for a diagnostic eating disorder are categorized as having OSFED (Box 22–3) or UFED.[3]

Although some investigators believe that EDs have a single cause, they are more likely to be the result of a multifactorial chain of events. The interacting causes have roots in three spheres: biological, psychological, and social.[13] Certain early experiences and family influences may create intrapsychic conflicts that produce a psychological predisposition toward an ED. A stressful life and striving for perfection, particularly in a family of achievers, can initiate some of the problems in this disorder. The biological factors that initiate AN may be mediated by pubertal endocrine changes. Psychological conflicts lead to personality and behavioral changes that promote and support dieting. Data indicate that about 60% of the families of children with AN are rigid, overprotective, and enmeshed; 20% display extreme chaos and disorganization; and 20% appear normal.[13]

By some reports, up to 70% of young women feel fat, and 33% are dieting at any given time; dieting may even exist in school-age children. Of children surveyed in grades 3 through 6, 45% wanted to be thinner, and 37% had tried to lose weight; 7% scored in the AN range on the questionnaire.[14] If nutrient intake is decreased sufficiently, amenorrhea and other metabolic disturbances may occur. The occurrence of amenorrhea is associated with a combination of hypothalamic dysfunction, weight loss, decreased body fat, stress, and excessive exercise.[15] The fear syndromes can be distinguished from AN by the lack of body image distortion and the prompt response to nutrition counseling. A study by Tovée et al.[16] examined the perception of body mass by women with AN, women with BN, and control subjects. They were asked to estimate the body mass index (BMI) of women in photographs and their own BMI. The women with EDs consistently underestimated the BMI of women in photographs. They also overestimated their own BMI, and as the BMI of the observer declined, its overestimation increased.[16]

There is less of an increase in AN as girls approach 14 years of age, so those who gain 20 to 30 lb as a result of earlier maturation may tend to be more vulnerable to AN or BN.[17] The process often begins with relatively innocent dieting. Initial success in losing weight may fuel the desire to lose even more. The person may become more secretive, compulsive, and particular about his or her dietary habits. Physical and mental signs of AN begin to develop but often are ignored or denied. The person withdraws increasingly from social interaction and becomes immersed in achievement-oriented activities as family and friends become worried. Eventually, the individual becomes hostile toward his or her family. School performance may decline, despite excessive studying, as the person becomes easily distractible, preoccupied, and, ultimately, depressed and apathetic. Nonsuppressible hunger (i.e., BN) may also ensue as a reaction to chronic semistarvation; 50% of people with AN also develop BN. This urge ultimately may lead to rapid weight gain and obesity before stabilization at normal weight occurs. The person with BN who continues to desire to be thin will resort to vomiting or purging through abuse of laxatives and diuretics. This practice leads to

**Box 22–1.** Criteria for Anorexia Nervosa

A. Restriction of energy intake relative to requirements, leading to a significantly low body weight in the context of age, sex, developmental trajectory, and physical health. *Significantly low weight* is defined as a weight that is less than minimally normal or, for children and adolescents, less than that minimally expected.
B. Intense fear of gaining weight or of becoming fat, or persistent behavior that interferes with weight gain, even though at a significantly low weight.
C. Disturbance in the way in which one's body weight or shape is experienced, undue influence of body weight or shape on self-evaluation, or persistent lack of recognition of the seriousness of the current low body weight.

**Coding note:** The ICD-9-CM code for anorexia nervosa, 307.1, was assigned regardless of the subtype. The current ICD-10-CM code depends on the subtype.

*Specify* whether:

**(F50.01) Restricting type:** During the last 3 months, the individual has not engaged in recurrent episodes of binge eating or purging behavior (i.e., self-induced vomiting or the misuse of laxatives. diuretics, or enemas). This subtype describes presentations in which weight loss is accomplished primarily through dieting, fasting, and/or excessive exercise.

**(F50.02) Binge-eating/purging type:** During the last 3 months, the individual has engaged in recurrent episodes of binge eating or purging behavior (i.e., self-induced vomiting or the misuse of laxatives, diuretics, or enemas).

*Specify* if:

**In partial remission:** After full criteria for anorexia nervosa were previously met, Criterion A (low body weight) has not been met for a sustained period, but either Criterion B (intense fear of gaining weight or becoming fat or behavior that interferes with weight gain) or Criterion C (disturbances in self-perception of weight and shape) is still met.

**In full remission:** After full criteria for anorexia nervosa were previously met, none of the criteria have been met for a sustained period of time.

*Specify* current severity:

The minimum level of severity is based, for adults, on current body mass index (BMI) or, for children and adolescents, on BMI percentile. The ranges below are derived from World Health Organization categories for thinness in adults; for children and adolescents, corresponding BMI percentiles should be used. The level of severity may be increased to reflect clinical symptoms, the degree of functional disability, and the need for supervision.

**Mild:** BMI >17 kg/m$^2$
**Moderate:** BMI 16–16.99 kg/m$^2$
**Severe:** BMI 15–15.99 kg/m$^2$
**Extreme:** BMI <15 kg/m$^2$

From American Psychiatric Association. *Diagnostic and Statistical Manual of Mental Disorders, Fifth Edition* (DSM-5). Washington, DC: American Psychiatric Association; 2013. Used with permission.

chronic AN and BN with serious consequences. Bulimarexia, a specific category involving binging followed only by purging, is a disorder that may persist considerably longer than AN[18] (Table 22–1).

AN occurs most often among young (<25 years), affluent white women of at least normal intelligence but is not limited to that group. Students in disciplines that require an increased focus on body image (e.g., dancing, drama) or exercise (e.g., physical education) have a greater risk of developing AN.[19] One study found anorexic-like behaviors to be significantly higher among college students taking an elective nutrition course than among dietetic majors.[20] The commonly cited female-to-male ratio in both AN and BN is 10:1. Males with EDs are often in professions or activities that require a lean body (e.g., dancing, modeling, athletics); dieting or purging may be performed in order to weigh in at a lower weight class for wrestling.[21] Adolescent males below the 25th percentile for BMI, upper arm circumference, and subscapular and triceps skinfold thickness should be considered to be in an unhealthy, malnourished state.[21]

The course of AN may be episodic or unremitting, but most commonly it consists of a single episode. With BN, the course is usually chronic or intermittent over many years. The mortality rate for AN is between 5% and 20%, one of the highest among psychiatric disorders.[6,19] Risk factors for the development of EDs include having a family member with AN or BN and a family history of affective disorder or substance abuse. Weight loss can occur in individuals with depression, but there is no disturbance in body image or intense fear of obesity, as is seen in AN.[8] In BN, parents of the person affected are often obese, or the child may be obese in adolescence.

**Box 22–2.** Criteria for Bulimia Nervosa

A. Recurrent episodes of binge eating. An episode of binge eating is characterized by both of the following:
   1. Eating, in a discrete period of time (e.g., within any 2-hour period), an amount of food that is definitely larger than what most individuals would eat in a similar period of time under similar circumstances.
   2. A sense of lack of control over eating during the episode (e.g., a feeling that one cannot stop eating or control what or how much one is eating).
B. Recurrent inappropriate compensatory behaviors in order to prevent weight gain, such as self-induced vomiting; misuse of laxatives, diuretics, or other medications; fasting; or excessive exercise.
C. The binge eating and inappropriate compensatory behaviors both occur, on average, at least once a week for 3 months.
D. Self-evaluation is unduly influenced by body shape and weight.
E. The disturbance does not occur exclusively during episodes of anorexia nervosa.

*Specify* if:

**In partial remission:** After full criteria for bulimia nervosa were previously met, some, but not all, of the criteria have been met for a sustained period of time.

**In full remission:** After full criteria for bulimia nervosa were previously met, none of the criteria have been met for a sustained period of time.

*Specify* current severity:

The minimum level of severity is based on the frequency of inappropriate compensatory behaviors (see below). The level of severity may be increased to reflect other symptoms and the degree of functional disability.

**Mild:** An average of 1–3 episodes of inappropriate compensatory behaviors per week.
**Moderate:** An average of 4–7 episodes of inappropriate compensatory behaviors per week.
**Severe:** An average of 8–13 episodes of inappropriate compensatory behaviors per week.
**Extreme:** An average of 14 or more episodes of inappropriate compensatory behaviors per week.

From American Psychiatric Association. *Diagnostic and Statistical Manual of Mental Disorders, Fifth Edition* (DSM-5). Washington, DC: American Psychiatric Association; 2013. Used with permission.

**Box 22–3.** Criteria for Other Specified Feeding or Eating Disorders

This category applies to presentations in which symptoms characteristic of a feeding or eating disorder that cause clinically significant distress or impairment in social, occupational, or other important areas of functioning predominate but do not meet the full criteria for any of the disorders in the feeding and eating disorders diagnostic class. The Other Specified Feeding or Eating Disorder (OSFED) category is used in situations in which the clinician chooses to communicate the specific reason that the presentation does not meet the criteria for any specific feeding or eating disorder. This is done by recording "Other specified feeding or eating disorder" followed by the specific reason (e.g., "Bulimia nervosa of low frequency"). Examples of presentations that can be specified using the OSFED designation include the following:

1. **Atypical anorexia nervosa:** All of the criteria for anorexia nervosa are met, except that despite significant weight loss, the individual's weight is within or above the normal range.
2. **Bulimia nervosa (of low frequency and/or limited duration):** All of the criteria for bulimia nervosa are met. except that the binge eating and inappropriate compensatory behaviors occur, on average, less than once a week and/or for less than 3 months.
3. **Binge-eating disorder (of low frequency and/or limited duration):** All of the criteria for binge-eating disorder are met, except that the binge eating occurs, on average. less than once a week and/or for less than 3 months.
4. **Purging disorder:** Recurrent purging behavior to influence weight or shape (e.g., self-induced vomiting; misuse of laxatives, diuretics, or other medications) in the absence of binge eating.
5. **Night eating syndrome:** Recurrent episodes of night eating, as manifested by eating after awakening from sleep or by excessive food consumption after the evening meal. There is awareness and recall of the eating. The night eating is not better explained by external influences such as changes in the individual's sleep-wake cycle or by local social norms. The night eating causes significant distress and/or impairment in functioning. The disordered pattern of eating is not better explained by binge eating disorder or another mental disorder, including substance use, and is not attributable to another medical disorder or to an effect of medication.

From American Psychiatric Association. *Diagnostic and Statistical Manual of Mental Disorders, Fifth Edition* (DSM-5). Washington, DC: American Psychiatric Association; 2013. Used with permission.

**Table 22–1.** Biochemical and Physical Manifestations of Anorexia Nervosa and Bulimia

| Manifestation | Anorexia Nervosa | Bulimia |
|---|---|---|
| Endocrine/metabolic | Amenorrhea | Menstrual irregularities |
| | Osteoporosis | |
| | Decreased norepinephrine secretion | |
| | Low somatomedin C | |
| | Functional hypothyroidism, high $RT_3$, normal $T_4$ and TSH | |
| | Elevated cortisol | |
| | Decreased/erratic vasopressin secretion | |
| | Prepubertal gonadotropin levels (LH, FSH) | |
| Cardiovascular | Bradycardia | |
| | Hypotension | |
| | Arrhythmias | |
| Renal | Renal calculi | Hypokalemia—diuretic-induced |
| | Edema | Ipecac poisoning |
| Gastrointestinal | Early satiety | Acute gastric dilation, rupture |
| | Constipation | Dental enamel erosion |
| | | Esophagitis |
| | | Mallory-Weiss tears (esophageal rupture) |
| | | Parotid enlargement |
| Biochemical | Hypokalemia | Hypokalemia—laxative-induced |
| | Metabolic alkalosis | |
| | Hypophosphatemia | |
| | Elevated bilirubin (Gilbert's disease) | |
| | Azotemia | |
| | Hypercarotenemia | |
| Hematological | Bone marrow hypoplasia | |
| | Leukopenia | |
| | Thrombocytopenia | |
| Immunological | Hypocomplementemia anergy | |
| Pulmonary | | Aspiration pneumonia |

FSH = follicle-stimulating hormone; LH = luteinizing hormone; $RT_3$ = resin triiodothyronine; $T_4$ = thyroxine; TSH = thyroid-stimulating hormone.
Courtesy of Michael Farrell, MD, Department of Gastroenterology, Cincinnati Children's Hospital Medical Center, Cincinnati, Ohio.
Used with permission

## BIOCHEMICAL AND CLINICAL ABNORMALITIES

The signs and symptoms and laboratory findings in AN and BN are understood most easily in the context of the stage of the illness and the dietary pattern. After onset, adipose tissue becomes depleted, but laboratory tests show no abnormalities. AN and BN are often associated with potentially serious medical complications.[6,22] Physicians need to become more familiar with EDs, especially because many of these people appear to be healthy on initial examination, and frequently they deny having any illness and minimize their symptoms.[6] A significant number of people with BN have normal body weight or weight above the normal range; only suspicion will lead to the diagnosis of the disorder. People with AN may wear baggy clothes to hide their thinness. Persons with AN and BN may have brittle hair and nails, lanugo-like body hair, asteatodic skin, and carotendermia as a result of malnutrition. They may have dental erosion, gingivitis, hand calluses due to self-induced vomiting; and other concomitant psychiatric illnesses such as hand dermatitis due to compulsive hand washing.[23–25] Other obsessive-compulsive behaviors also may be present.

### Complications

Long-term complications of AN and BN include cardiovascular arrhythmia leading to heart failure, renal complications caused by dehydration, and demineralization of bone (osteoporosis), especially if the individual is not physically active. Self-induced starvation can also lead to delayed gastric emptying, decreased gut motility, and severe constipation. There is evidence of structural brain abnormalities early in the disease process, and it is uncertain whether these are reversible.[26–28] There may be difficulty in urination, causing elevated serum amylase levels.[29] The skeletal system may be involved as a result of ipecac abuse or hypokalemia in BN.[30] Water and electrolyte imbalances are major complications. Restoration of muscle electrolytes, particularly potassium and sodium, produces a greater positive effect on muscle function in AN than does repletion of body nitrogen.[31] Cytokine production may be abnormal.[32] Prolonged undernutrition usually decreases serum cholesterol, although patients with AN may have hyperlipidemia. People with AN can have elevated serum carotene and vitamin A levels, although overt vitamin deficiencies are rare. Adolescent AN patients with more than 12 months' duration of the disorder, more than 6 months of amenorrhea, a BMI less than 12, a calcium intake less than 600 mg/day, and physical activity for less than 3 hours/week are at a high risk of reduced bone mineral density.[33] Ghrelin levels correlate negatively with the BMI and normalize after a 25% increase in BMI. Densitometry is recommended to determine the degree of osteopenia.[34] Treatment for osteoporosis associated with AN includes weight gain, restoration of gonadal function, and calcium supplementation. Estrogen alone has proved inadequate for increasing bone density.[34] In patients with AN, constipation, bradycardia, hypothermia, and orthostatic changes may be present, and exercise tolerance and cardiac function may be decreased.[35]

## FACTORS TO BE CONSIDERED IN NUTRITIONAL EVALUATION

A detailed history, including onset of the disorder, early childhood nutrition, and a current history, is essential. The person with AN may be using a low-calorie or other restrictive diet, have a distorted self-image, exercise obsessively, occasionally abuse alcohol or other drugs, use body weight to determine self-worth, talk and think about food constantly, and be afraid of being unable to stop eating. Possible warning signs of AN or BN in adolescents are shown in Table 22–2. Patients with BN often show strong feelings of guilt and anger when taking in large amounts of fat calories.[36]

### Behavior

A study by Vaz et al.[37] found that patients with EDs often have an aversion to food with a high protein content (e.g., meat, fish, milk, eggs). In another study, all subjects restricted their caloric intake, but 38% maintained a diet of satisfactory quality. Of the 62% whose diets were unsatisfactory in quality, most had irregular meal patterns, and a large proportion of this group indulged in binge eating, fasting, or vomiting.[6]

### Laboratory Values

Serum albumin, prealbumin, and retinol-binding protein levels may be normal or reduced if severe depression is present due to either primary or secondary malnutrition.[38] Polito et al.[39] concluded that basal metabolic rates as well as plasma leptin concentrations were lower in women with AN. Body potassium may be elevated, and growth hormone and urinary zinc excretion may be increased. A complete blood cell count, electrolytes, blood urea nitrogen/creatinine or transferrin tests, and osmolality tests of both serum and urine may be performed (Fig. 22–1).[40] Laboratory studies are most helpful in documenting the degree of physiological adaptation to undernourishment and the complications of AN and BN and in differentiating the symptoms of these conditions from those of other illnesses resembling EDs. Consideration of the stage of the disorder is important in evaluating the laboratory findings. People with BN have abnormalities in the hypothalamic-pituitary-thyroidal axis, as seen by the response of triiodothyronine ($T_3$) to thyrotropin-releasing hormone.[41] This response differs from hypothroidism in that a 25% body weight loss, increased growth hormone level, and normal results for gonadotropin, protein-bound iodine, and $T_3$ are seen. Magnetic resonance imaging findings provide further evidence of pituitary abnormalities in patients with EDs, but the deficiencies may result from endocrine-related nutritional dysregulation.[42] The higher C-peptide excretion per kilogram body weight in children with AN compared with normal-weight children indicates that insulin secretion is increased in relation to body weight.[43] Serum electrolyte values tend to be in the normal range except when vomiting or laxative abuse is a feature. In the latter case, the reported values may be high because of dehydration, which may be serious and can cause death. Because of changes due to dehydration, the hematological picture is variable. Vomiting may result in decreased extracellular blood values, metabolic alkalosis, and a shift of blood potassium into the cells. Laxative abuse produces hypovolemia, hypokalemia, metabolic acidosis, and up to 60 mEq/L loss of potassium ion in the stool.[40] The presence of hypophosphatemia indicates the need for hospitalization.

**Table 22–2.** Warning Signs of Anorexia Nervosa or Bulimia

| Category of Warning Signals | Anorexia Nervosa | Bulimia Nervosa |
|---|---|---|
| Eating and related behaviors | Caloric intake <100 kcal/day | Binge eating at least twice a week |
| | Calorie counting | Eating used as coping strategy |
| | Denial of hunger cues | Fasting or restrictive dieting |
| | Extreme physical activity | Feels lack of control over eating |
| | Fasting or restrictive dieting | Frequent cravings for sweets, starches |
| | Feels controlled by food | Frequent thoughts about food |
| | Food avoidances or hoarding | Guilt after eating, secret eating |
| | Food seen as good or bad | Purging behavior |
| | Frequent meal skipping | Regular alcohol use |
| | Frequent thoughts about food | Wide variation in caloric intake |
| Body image and body | Body-image disturbance | Current or previous obesity satisfaction |
| | Fear of weight gain | Fear of weight gain |
| | Previously overweight | Overly concerned with weight or shape |
| | Thinness as valued goal | Thinness as valued goal |
| | Weight goal ≤85% expected weight | Unrealistic weight goal |
| | Amenorrhea (≥3 mo with no menses) | Bloating, nausea, abdominal pain |
| | Bloating, nausea | Frequent menses (<21 days or >45 days) |
| | Cold intolerance | |
| Personal functioning | Delayed psychosexual development | Depressed affect |
| | Depressed affect | Negative self-identity |
| | Individuation difficulties | Perfectionist |
| | Poor coping with life events | Recent withdrawal from friends |
| | Perfectionist | Substance use, early sexual activity |
| | Recent withdrawal from friends | |
| Environmental influences | Enmeshed or overinvolved family | Chaotic or uninvolved family |
| | Family history of obesity, eating disorder, or weight focus | Family history of obesity, eating disorder, or weight focus |
| | Few close friends | High achievement expectations |
| | Participation in body-focused activity | Participation in body-focused activity |

From Adams LB, Shafer MB. Early manifestations of eating disorders in adolescents: defining those at risk. *J Nutr Educ.* 1988; 20:307. Used with permission.

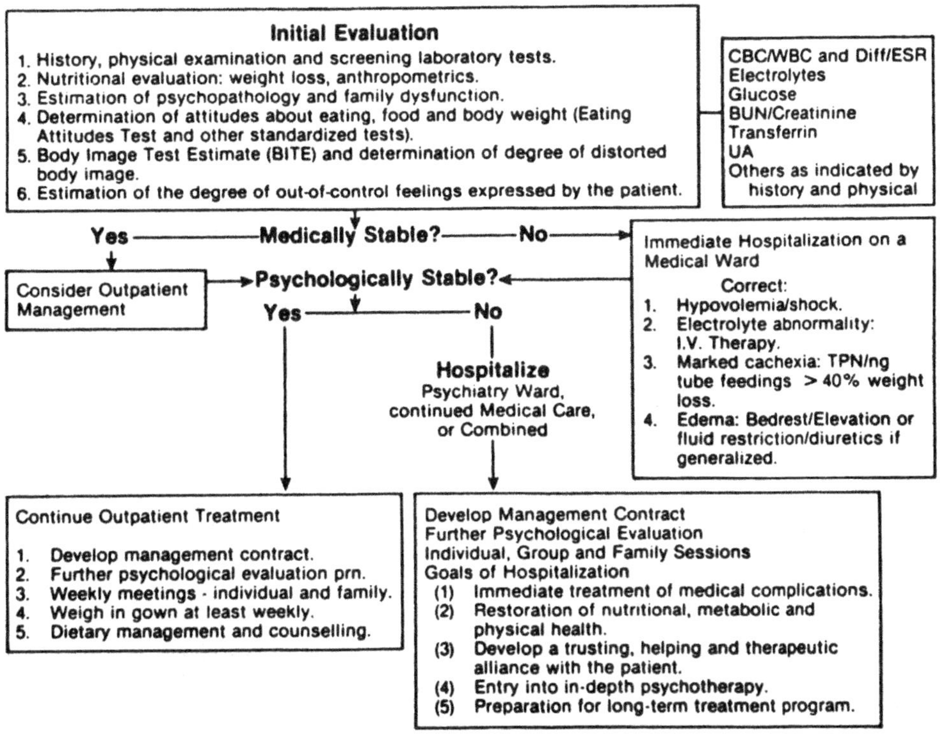


**Figure 22–1.** Initial triage and management of the eating disorder patient. BUN = blood urea nitrogen; CBC/WBC = complete blood cell count with white blood cell count; Diff/ESR = differential cell count with erythrocyte sedimentation rate; ng = nasogastric; TPN = total parenteral nutrition; UA = urine analysis.

Serum protein or albumin values tend to remain normal until advanced stages of starvation are reached. Zinc, copper, and iron-binding protein deficiencies reflect starvation.[44] The ratio of total body potassium to total body water is not decreased, nor is the ratio of total exchangeable sodium to total potassium elevated in persons with AN, as they are in clinical malnutrition.[45] Body composition measures should not be evaluated as malnutrition in the nutritional management of people with AN.[45] The level of cortisol in the brain is decreased in AN. Increased levels of cortisol fuel the body and shrink the fronto-temporal lobe.[46] This may cause the rejection or gorging of food and produce a preoccupation with food.[47] The candidate genes for AN are located in the chromosome 1p33–36 linkage region.[48]

### Anthropometric Measures

Height, weight, muscle mass, triceps fatfold, and physical activity should be measured and records kept regularly. Weight loss appears to be a major marker (rather than other anthropometric measures), especially if depression is present.[38] According to research by Trocki and Sheperd, a change in BMI is not an accurate indicator of change in body composition in adolescent girls experiencing AN, so its use in a clinical setting for this purpose is questionable.[49] Prolonged undernutrition in early adolescence may affect the adolescent growth spurt and depress growth in stature.

### Physical Signs

It is important to evaluate the skin, hair, nails, lips and tongue, and skeletal appearance of individuals with suspected EDs (see Table 22–1).

## DIETARY MANAGEMENT

Both AN and BN require a multifaceted treatment approach encompassing medical management and behavioral, individual, cognitive, and family therapy. Becker et al.[12] stated that an interdisciplinary team can be most beneficial to those with an ED.[50] The dietitian is a key member of this team because nutrition intervention is a main concern in these disorders (Box 22–4). In EDs, the immediate aim should be to restore the person's nutritional state to normal. Dietitians can identify disordered eating patterns through use of assessment instruments such as the Eating Disorder Inventory (EDI) and the Eating Attitude Test (EAT). Skilled clinicians use DSM-5 diagnostic criteria to categorize candidates properly for the multifaceted treatment approach.

### Nutrition

The dietitian's responsibility is to determine the immediate and long-term goals in nutrition rehabilitation during hospital and follow-up care. The dietitian also may serve as a general practitioner in working with the psychotherapist in the areas of body image, fitness, relaxation, assertiveness, problem solving, and anger management. The outpatient dietitian prescribes, evaluates, and monitors the dietary regimen. The hospital dietitian works with patients who have severe medical, psychological, and nutritional risks. Dietitians working with persons who have EDs must understand healthy patterns of eating, the consequences of EDs, proper screening tools, drug-nutrient interactions, and the needs of this vulnerable population. Counseling tools, standards of care and quality assurance standards, research in nutrition rehabilitation, and compliance education using statistical tools are also needed.[51] In particular, the dietitian must have good counseling and listening skills. Mere weight loss can cause irritability, depression, preoccupation with food, and sleep disturbance. A good relationship with the therapist is essential before nutrition intervention can take place.[51]

It is best to encourage weight gain through normal self-feeding rather than with artificial products. However, liquid supplements have been useful as an intermediate step if the patient is unwilling to eat ordinary food.[51] In cases of severe AN (weight loss 40–60%), total parenteral nutrition (TPN) with close monitoring of electrolytes has been found to be a successful method of treatment until the patient is able to regain normal oral uptake in 3 to 8 weeks[52] (see Box 22–4). TPN may be accepted more readily than nasogastric tube feedings and can produce rapid correction in electrolyte balance and protein and mineral levels, although enteral nutrition with nasogastric tube feedings is often the first line of treatment. However, TPN is expensive and requires close monitoring because of the possible risks of sepsis and air embolus due to deliberate tampering with the TPN line, especially if the patient is depressed.[53,54] It should not be considered a

**Box 22–4.** Nutritional Management of Eating Disorders

I. Nutritional assessment
  A. Anthropometry
    1. Height/weight; ideal weight range
    2. Skinfold measurements; percent body fat
  B. Laboratory tests
    1. Hematocrit, hemoglobin
    2. Transferrin, albumin
  C. Physical signs of possible nutritional deficiencies
    1. Hair, skin, lips, tongue, gums, and nails
  D. Dietary history
    1. Restrictive eating pattern, binging/fasting cycle
    2. Binging/fasting cycle
    3. Binging/purging
II. Nutritional support
  A. Establishing nutrient needs
    1. Calories, protein, vitamins
  B. Choosing feeding modality
    1. Parenteral, enteral, or oral
  C. Guidelines for nutritional therapy
    1. Gradual increase in caloric intake; controlled carbohydrate load; small, frequent stools
  D. Goals for nutritional support
    1. Restoration or preservation of nutrition status
    2. Weight maintenance/controlled gain or loss
    3. Independently maintained nutritional intake
  E. Treatment plan
    1. Inpatient: behavior program
    2. Outpatient
      a. Weekly or biweekly weight checks
      b. Intake and vomiting/laxatives
    3. Outcome goals
      a. Cessation of vomiting/laxatives
      b. Weight maintenance; controlled loss or gain
      c. Ability to maintain adequate and balanced intake
      d. Incorporation of exercise as tolerated

Protocol of the Arizona Health Science Center, University Hospital Nutrition Service. From Comerci GD. Setting standards of care for diagnosis and treatment of adolescents with eating disorders. *J Adolesc Health.* 1995; 16:416. Used with permission.

routine treatment for AN but rather a last resort for those who do not respond to reasonable corrective measures such as enteral nutrition.[40] TPN must be combined with psychosocial treatment. Estimated basal caloric requirements should be adjusted based on the measured basal metabolic rate.[6] Abnormal cardiac function often occurs in asymptomatic patients with AN undergoing refeeding therapy.[54] Improved cardiac function may lag weight gain.[55]

Key nutrition therapies require expertise in nutritional requirements for the life stage of the affected individual, nutritional rehabilitation treatments, and modalities to restore normal eating patterns.[1] Multiple components of nutrition assessment performed by dietitians can contribute to treatment plans. The diet plan should emphasize behavior strategies that require self-care and self-monitoring[6] and should achieve weight maintenance and incorporate variety and regularity into eating. The person may be instructed to keep a diet record and to record the number of laxatives, diuretics, and binge vomiting episodes. Giving high-potassium foods to correct electrolyte imbalance and high-calcium foods for bone density and gradually adding foods that were recently omitted from the diet should be considered. Constipation may result from slowed gut motility caused by energy conservation and a small intake (this should subside with increased food intake). The person may engage in laxative abuse to relieve constipation. An effective way to decrease laxative abuse may be to contract with the patient to decrease the use of laxatives by a specified amount while increasing fiber and fluid intake. The focus should be on the food preferences and nutritional needs of the entire family, not just the person with AN. Mealtimes should be pleasurable and filled with conversation so that the person with AN will associate food with pleasantness. The person with AN also should be involved in meal planning. The caretaker should sit with the child once a week and use recipe cards, cookbooks, and supermarket advertisements to devise menus for meals and snacks for the following week.

Outpatient therapy may be tried if the person has lost less than 25% of body weight. Gowers et al.[55] found that an inpatient stay at a hospital did not improve self-esteem or social confidence in those with AN. The goal of dietary treatment is to reestablish a normal weight pattern with an individualized approach. The common problems of bloating and early satiety may require extensive counseling and medication. The patient must also be convinced that weight gain will not be excessive or too rapid. Therapy should also include a psychological component, focusing on the inner conflicts of the patient, family dynamics, and supportive counseling of the parents. Successful drug-dependency treatment programs using a 12-step recovery method have been used by Overeaters Anonymous (OA).[56] The focus of OA is on group therapy, peer support, honesty (spiritual awakening), and abstinence from specific trigger foods and other compulsive eating behaviors that reduce binging, starving, and graze-type eating.[56] Because those with combined AN and BN are more prone to chemical dependency, the effects of alcohol and drugs on nutritional status must be evaluated and treated.[1,57]

Nutrition education is also needed to help the person understand the relationship of food to growth and weight so that he or she can make appropriate food choices. Nutritional rehabilitation along with some form of re-educative psychotherapy remains the mainstay of management of AN. In BN, both fluoxetine and cognitive behavior therapy have been found to be effective.[58]

## Hospital Treatment

It is generally believed that psychological disturbances underlie the severe dieting and food restrictions that form the basis of AN. Self-starvation affects physiological processes as well as psychological functions, thereby creating a self-perpetuating cycle that maintains the disorder.[59] Ending the secrecy of the ED may be the first step in treatment. Because of the interactions between psychological and physiological areas, an interdisciplinary approach is necessary in the treatment of both AN and BN in the hospital. The required members of the interdisciplinary team include a physician specializing in behavioral health, a nutritionist/dietitian, a registered nurse, a clinical social worker, and a consulting psychologist or psychiatrist.[40]

Weight loss of 30% to 40% of the predisorder body weight, decreased growth over a 3-month period, hypophosphatemia, or significant abnormalities of electrolytes indicate the need for hospitalization.[40] Severe depression or attempted suicide, severe binging and purging, psychosis, family crisis, and lack of response to outpatient therapy are other reasons for hospitalization.[7] Initially, the dietitian or nutritionist should obtain a detailed diet, weight, and behavior history. The protocol of care should specify the parameters of nutrition rehabilitation, itemizing caloric requirements, activity level, weight goals, and supervision of meals. Restricting exercise during the initial refeeding of AN clients may be necessary.

The hospital plan should include the family to help them understand the ED and what is involved in the patient's treatment. Family involvement also greatly eases the transition from the hospital to the home (see Fig. 22–1). Use of nasogastric tube feeding or peripheral intravenous feeding should be limited to those who need both calories and medical treatment or those who have severe electrolyte imbalance, hypophosphatemia, and fluid retention.[1] A weight gain of 3 lb/wk for 8 to 12 weeks on a regular diet is ideal. Gradual weight gain is important; rapid weight gain may put undue stress on the heart. A maintenance diet must be determined a few weeks before discharge. Amenorrhea often is the last symptom seen before recovery.

## Medications

Under certain circumstances, some medications appear to be helpful; however, they should not be administered as the sole treatment for ED. Fluoxetine is part of a common adjunctive treatment regimen in AN or BN when obsessive-compulsive traits are present. Reboxetine, a selective norephinephrine reuptake inhibitor, was found to decrease the frequency of binge eating and vomiting episodes among bulimic patients.[60] Weight or food nutrient changes may occur with some antidepressant, antianxiety, and antipsychotic agents (see Chapter 27). Further research is needed in this area of treatment.

## Behavior Modification

Behavior therapy forms the basis for most treatment regimens. In behavior modification, symptoms, rather than the possible underlying disturbances, are treated by reinforcing patient behaviors that increase weight. Patients are given reasonable, specific goals for which to aim and are rewarded with positive reinforcement. Behavior modification treatment programs demonstrate short-term benefits, but their long-term outcome is unknown. The person with AN must learn coping and interpersonal skills through the help of family, friends, and self-help groups and avoid relapsing by choosing one or two confidants. Healthy exercise three times per week for 20 to 30 minutes must replace the obsessive exercise regimen. The person with BN must learn new eating habits to replace the alternating pattern of overfeeding and underfeeding and may also need medication to accomplish this change.[61] The nutritionist must be aware of the magnitude of the change required during treatment and be knowledgeable about the relevant behavioral tools,[62] such as the Multidimensional Inventory, the Depression Inventory, the Eating Attitudes Test, and the Twelve-Step Approach for Eating Disorders.

Cognitive behavioral therapy (CBT), a leading therapy for individuals with BN, places a primary emphasis on reduction of binge eating and a secondary emphasis on weight loss. CBT helps an individual to identify and restructure maladaptive cognitions, such as faulty beliefs and thought patterns about the relationship between eating patterns and physical symptoms and perceptions of body weight changes.[1] Dialectical behavior therapy has become increasingly popular as an ED treatment; emotional dysregulation is considered an influencing factor for the ED, and symptomatic behaviors are considered to be maladaptive coping skills.[1] New coping skills are practiced, aimed at replacing ED behaviors with more constructive ones while enhancing self-respect.

According to the Academy of Nutrition and Dietetics (AND), those who wish to work with this population need advanced training to gain the required expertise.[1] The AND Practice Groups, including the Behavioral Health Nutrition (BHN) group; the Sports, Cardiovascular and Sports Nutrition (SCAN) group; and the Pediatric Nutrition Practice Group (PNPG), as well as other EDs organizations (e.g., International Association of Eating Disorders Professionals, Academy of Eating Disorder Professionals, National Eating Disorders Association), provide many important resources for the registered dietitian, including newsletters, workshops, and conferences. Russell reviewed other management techniques for AN.[63]

## Follow-up

The treatment plan should be reevaluated and updated periodically[64] (see Box 22–4). Strober et al.[65] conducted a long-term follow-up study of severely anorexic patients who had been hospitalized. Almost 76% met the criteria for full recovery, but recovery took place over 57 to 79 months. Coverage for clients with AN in managed care is a challenge,[66] although partial hospitalization is of benefit for some clients.[66,67] New targets for treatment should include neurotransmitters and imaging studies[68] (see Chapter 12).

For outpatient therapy, encouraging moderation of intake, a variety of foods, regulation in mealtimes, and reintroduction of feared foods will give the patient confidence in weight control and food selection. The dietitian/nutritionist can provide nutrition and behavior interventions to correct the cognitive distortions concerning food.[69] Providing ongoing nutrition education regarding nutrient needs for growth, rather than restriction for weight control, can help the patient make proper food choices and should encourage recovery.

Because the development of ED behaviors may begin with unsafe diets and unproven diet products, the patient should be made aware of the dangers of fad diets and diet products. The major organs affected in the long term—the brain and skeletal system—both respond to improved nutrition, with maintenance of body weight the best predictor of recovery.[70] Likewise, extreme dieting behavior in female elementary, junior high, and high school students, as well as in the general public, should be examined and treated as early as possible. The person with AN must learn to recognize stressful events or people that trigger AN and must have an emergency plan for such occurrences. If a weight loss of more than 5 lb occurs during the follow-up period, the physician should be notified. It is the position of the AND that nutrition intervention, including nutrition counseling by a registered dietitian nutritionist (RDN), is an essential component of team treatment of patients with AN, BN, and other EDs during assessment and treatment across the continuum of care.[1]

## ACKNOWLEDGMENT

We wish to acknowledge Shelly Bellman for her helpful assistance in typing this chapter.

### References

1. American Dietetic Association. Position of the American Dietetic Association: nutrition intervention in the treatment of eating disorders *J Am Diet Assoc.* 2011; 111:1236.
2. Kreipe RE, Churchill BH, Strauss J. Longer-term outcome of adolescent with anorexia nervosa. *Am J Dis Child.* 1989; 43:1233.
3. American Psychiatric Association. *Diagnostic and Statistical Manual of Mental Disorders, Fifth Edition* (DSM-5). Washington, DC: American Psychiatric Association; 2013.
4. Fisher M, Golden NH, Datzman KD, et al. Eating disorders in adolescents: a background paper. *J Adolesc Health Care.* 1995; 16:420.
5. Rogers L, Resnick MD, Mitchell JE, Blum RW. The relationship between socioeconomic status and eating-disordered behaviors in a community sample of adolescent girls. *Int J Eating Disord.* 1997; 22:15.
6. Korndorfer SR, Lucas AR, Suman VJ, Crowson CS, Krahn LE, Melton LJ 3rd. Long-term survival of patients with anorexia nervosa: a population-based study in Rochester, Minn. *Mayo Clin Proc.* 2003; 78:278.
7. Abraham SF, Beumont PJV. How patients describe bulimia or binge eating. *Psychol Med.* 1982; 12:625.
8. Hudson JI, Pope HG. *The Psychobiology of Bulimia.* Washington, DC: American Press; 1987.
9. American Psychiatric Association Work Group on Eating Disorders. Practice guideline for the treatment of patients with eating disorders (revision). *Am J Psychiatry.* 2000; 157(Suppl 1):1.
10. Heatherington MM, Altemus M, Nelson ML. Eating behavior in bulimia nervosa: multiple meal analyses. *Am J Clin Nutr.* 1994; 60:864.
11. Wegner KE, Smyth JM, Crosby RD, Wittrock D, Wonderlich SA, Mitchell JE. An evaluation of the relationship between mood and binge eating in the natural environment using ecological momentary assessment. *Int J Eat Disord.* 2002; 32:352.
12. Becker AE, Grinspoon SK, Klibanski A, Herzog DB. Eating disorders. *N Engl J Med.* 1999; 340:1092.
13. Anderson AE. Anorexia nervosa and bulimia: a spectrum of eating disorders. *J Adolesc Health Care.* 1983; 4:15.
14. Maloney MJ, McGuire J, Daniels SR, Specker B. Dieting behavior and eating attitudes in children. *Pediatrics.* 1989; 84:842.
15. Fisher M. Medical complications of anorexia and bulimia nervosa. *Adolesc Med Stat Art Rev.* 1992; 3:481.
16. Tovée MJ, Emery JL, Cohen-Tovée EM. The estimation of body mass index and physical attractiveness is dependent on the observer's own body mass index. *Proc Biol Sci R Soc.* 2000; 267:1987.
17. Crisp AH. Premorbid factors in adult disorders of weight, with particular reference to primary anorexia nervosa (weight phobia): a literature review. *J Psychosom Res.* 1970; 14:1.
18. Harris RT. Bulimia anorexia, and related serious eating disorders with medical complications. *Ann Intern Med.* 1983; 99:800.
19. Joseph A, Wood IK, Goldberg SC. Determining populations at risk for developing anorexia nervosa based on selection of college major. *Psychiatr Res.* 1982; 7:53.
20. Johnston CS, Christopher FS. Anorexic-like behavior in dietetic majors and other student populations. *J Nutr Ed.* 1991; 23:148.
21. Abrams SA, Silber TJ, Esteban NV. Mineral balance and bone turnover in adolescents with anorexia nervosa. *J Pediatr.* 1993; 123:326.
22. Golden N, Sacker IM. An overview of the etiology, diagnosis, and management of anorexia nervosa. *Clin Pediatr.* 1984; 23:209.
23. Williams JF, Freidman IM, Steiner H. Hand lesions characteristic of bulimia. *Am J Dis Child.* 1986; 140:28.
24. Joseph AB, Herr B. Finger calluses in bulimia. *Am J Psychiatry.* 1985; 5:655.
25. Schwartz B, Clendenning W. A cutaneous sign of bulimia. *J Am Acad Dermatol.* 1985; 12:725.
26. Katzman DK, Zipursky RB. Adolescents with anorexia nervosa: the impact of the disorder on bones and brains. *Ann N Y Acad Sci.* 1997; 817:127.
27. Artmann H, Grau H, Adelmann M. Reversible and non-reversible enlargement of cerebrospinal fluid spaces in anorexia nervosa. *Neuroradiology.* 1985; 27:304.
28. Nusabum M, Shenker I, Marc J. Cerebral atrophy in anorexia nervosa. *Psychiatr Med.* 1980; 96:869.
29. Bachrach LK, Guido D, Katzman D, Litt IF, Marcus R. Decreased bone density in adolescent girls with anorexia nervosa. *Pediatrics* 1990; 86:440.

30. Mitchell JE, Fletcher L, Hanson K, et al. The relative efficacy of fluoxetine and manual-based self-help in the treatment of outpatients with bulimia nervosa. *J Clin Psychopharmacol.* 2001; 21:298.
31. Russell DM, Prendergast PJ, Darby PL, Garfinkel PE, Whitewell J, Jeejeebhoy KN. A comparison between muscle function and body composition in anorexia nervosa: the effect of refeeding. *Am J Clin Nutr* 1983; 38:229.
32. Raymond NC, Dysken M, Bettin K, et al. Cytokine production in patients with anorexia nervosa, bulimia nervosa, and obesity. *Int J Eat Disord.* 2000; 28:293.
33. Soriano-Guillen L, Barrios V, Campos-Barro A, Argente J. Ghrelin levels in obesity and anorexia nervosa: effect of weight reduction or recuperation. *J Pediatr.* 2004; 144:36.
34. Grinspoon S, Herzog D, Klibanski A. Mechanisms and treatment options for bone loss in anorexia nervosa. *Psychopharmacol Bull.* 1997; 33:399.
35. Romano C, Chimali C, Panasi S, Greco R. Reduced hemodynamic load and cardiac hypertrophy. *Am J Clin Nutr* 2003; 77:308.
36. Sunday S, Einhorn A, Holmi K. Relationship of perceived macronutrient and caloric content to affective cognitions about food in eating-disordered, restrained, and unrestrained subjects. *Am J Clin Nutr.* 1992; 55:362.
37. Vaz FJ, Alcaina T, Guisado JA. Food aversions in eating disorders. *Int J Food Sci Nutr.* 1998; 49:181.
38. Maes M, Vandewoude M, Scharpe S, et al. Anthropometric and biochemical assessment of the nutritional state in depression: evidence for lower visceral protein plasma levels in depression. *J Affect Disord.* 1991; 23:25.
39. Polito A, Fabbri A, Ferro-Luzzi A, et al. Basal metabolic rate in anorexia nervosa: relation to body composition and leptin concentrations. *Am J Clin Nutr.* 2000; 71:1495.
40. Comerci GD. Setting standards of care for diagnosis and treatment of adolescents with eating disorders. *J Adolesc Health.* 1995; 16:416.
41. Kiyohara K, Tamai H, Bobayashi N, Nakagawa T. Hypothalamic-pituitary-thyroidal axis alterations in bulimic patients. *Am J Clin Nutr.* 1988; 47:805.
42. Doraiswamy P, Krishnan R, Boyko OB, et al Pituitary abnormalities in eating disorders: further evidence from MRI studies. *Prog Neuropsychopharmacol Biol Psychiatry.* 1991; 15:351.
43. Wallensteen M, Ginburg BE, Dahlquist G. Urinary C-peptide excretion in obese and anorexic children. *Acta Paediatr Scand.* 1991; 80:521.
44. Casper RC, Kischner B, Sanstead HH, Jacob RA, Davis JM. An evaluation of trace metals, vitamins, and taste function in anorexia nervosa. *Am J Clin Nutr.* 1980; 33:1801.
45. Dempsey DT, Crosby LO, Lusk E, Oberlander JL, Pertschuk MJ, Mullen JL. Total body water and total potassium in anorexia nervosa. *Am J Clin Nutr.* 1984; 40:260.
46. Uhe A, Szmuckler G, Collier G, Hansky J, O'Dea K, Young G. Potential regulators of feeding behaviors in anorexia nervosa. *Am J Clin Nutr.* 1992; 55:28.
47. Kaye WH, Lilenfeld LR, Berrettini WH, et al. A search for susceptibility loci for anorexia nervosa: methods and sample description. *Biol Psychiatry.* 2000; 47:794.
48. Bergen AW, van den Bree MB, Yeager M, et al. Candidate genes for anorexia nervosa in the 1p33-36 linkage region: serotonin 1D and delta opioid receptor loci exhibit significant association to anorexia nervosa. *Mol Psychiatry.* 2003; 8:397.
49. Trocki O, Sheperd R. Change in body mass index does not predict change in body composition in adolescent girls with anorexia nervosa. *J Am Diet Assoc.* 2000; 100:457.
50. Lock J, Le Grange D. Family-based treatment of eating disorders. *Int J Eat Disord.* 2005; 37:564.
51. Krey SH, Palmer K, Porcelli KA. Eating disorders: the clinical dietitian's role. *J Am Diet Assoc.* 1989; 89:41.
52. Croner S, Larson J, Schildt B, Symreng T. Severe anorexia nervosa treated with total parenteral nutrition: clinical course and influence on clinical chemical analyses. *Acta Paediatr Scand.* 1985; 74:230.
53. Hill KK, Hill DB, Humphries LL, Maloney MJ, McClain CJ. A role for *Helicobacter pylori* in the gastrointestinal complaints of eating disorder patients? *Int J Eat Disord.* 1999; 25:109.
54. Gold PN, Goodwin FK, Chrousos GP. Clinical and biochemical manifestations of depression: relation to neurobiology of stress. *N Engl J Med.* 1988; 319:348.
55. Gowers S, Weetman A, Hossain F, Elvins R. Impact of hospitalization on the outcome of adolescent anorexia nervosa. *Br J Psychol.* 2000; 176:138.
56. Devlin CL. Twelve step intervention in compulsive eating. *J Am Diet Assoc.* 1991; 91:A81.
57. Delvenne V, Goldman S, Biver F, et al. Brain hypometabolism of glucose in low-weight depressed patients and in anorexic patients: a consequence of starvation? *J Affect Disord.* 1997; 44:69.
58. Chakraborty K, Basu D. Management of anorexia and bulimia nervosa: an evidence-based review. *Indian J Psychiatry.* 2010; 52: 174.
59. Wakeling A. Neurobiological aspects of feeding disorders. *J Psychiatr Res.* 1985; 19:A81.
60. El-Giamal N, de Zwaan M, Bailer U, et al. Reboxetine in the treatment of bulimia nervosa: a report of seven cases. *Int Clin Psychopharmacol.* 2000; 15:351.
61. Greene GW, Acterberg C, Crumbaugh J, Soper J. Dietary intake and dieting practices of bulimic and non-bulimic female college students. *J Am Diet Assoc.* 1990; 90:576.
62. Gray GE, Gray LK. Nutritional aspects of psychiatric disorders. *J Am Diet Assoc.* 1989; 89:1492.
63. Russell J. Management of anorexia nervosa. *BMJ.* 2004; 328:479.
64. Garfinkel PE, Kennedy SH, Kaplan AS. Views on classification and diagnosis of eating disorders. *Can J Psychiatry.* 1995; 40:445.
65. Strober M, Freeman R, Morrell W. The long-term course of severe anorexia nervosa in adolescents: survival analysis of recovery, relapse and outcome predictors over 10–15 years in a prospective study. *Int J Eat Disord.* 1997; 22:339.
66. Hill KK, Maloney MJ. Treating anorexia nervosa patients in the era of managed care. *J Am Acad Child Adolesc Psychiatry.* 1997; 36:1632.
67. American Psychiatric Association. Practice guidelines for the treatment of patients with eating disorders (revision). American Psychiatric Association Work Group on Eating Disorders. *Am J Psychiatry.* 2000; 157(Suppl);1.
68. Barbarich NC, Kaye WH, Jimerson D. Neurotransmitter and imaging studies in anorexia nervosa: new targets for treatment. *Curr Drug Target CNS Neurol Disord.* 2003; 2:61.
69. Roch CL. Nutritional and medical assessment and management of eating disorders. *Am J Clin Nutr.* 1999; 2:332.
70. Starr T, Kreipe R. Anorexia nervosa and bulimia nervosa: brains, bones and breeding. *Curr Psychiatry Rep.* 2014; 16:441.

# 23 Lead Toxicity and Pica

AGNES M. HUBER AND SHIRLEY W. EKVALL

Lead (Pb), a heavy metal, has increased in the environment as a result of industrialization, causing an increased lead burden in children and adults. Pica, the ingestion of nonfood items such as paint chips by children during the mouthing stage, can lead to frank lead toxicity. The relationship between lead toxicity and pica is complicated because it involves several nutrients. Lead toxicity and pica can each occur independently.

## LEAD EXPOSURE

Subclinical lead exposure and frank lead toxicity in children is a worldwide problem. The first national data on blood lead levels in US children were obtained by second National Health and Nutrition Examination Survey (NHANES II) between 1976 and 1980.[1] The data showed that 4% of children between 6 months and 5 years old had blood lead levels greater than 39 µg/dL. The high-risk children in this group were black inner-city children, 12% of whom had increased blood lead levels, and children of low-income families. However, increased blood levels were also found in some children in rural and high-income families. The major source of lead in the environment was thought to be lead-containing fuels and flaking lead paint in old houses. However, lead was also obtained from drinking water and foods. All of these sources were able to increase the lead burden in children and adults.

With the decreased use of leaded gasoline beginning in the early 1980s, the average blood lead level in US children fell. However, there were still many children, mostly black, with blood lead levels greater than 40 µg/dL. A further decline in blood lead concentration in children occurred after the elimination of lead solder from canned foods and the ban on leaded paint in housing. However, despite the dramatic decline in children's blood levels, lead toxicity has remained epidemic among impoverished children who live in older rental housing predominantly in the northeastern and midwestern regions of the United States.[2] Because evidence is accumulating that even blood levels lower than 10 µg/dL are associated with cognitive defects and learning problems, and because there is no safe level of exposure, it has become paramount to control and prevent childhood exposure to lead. In 2012, the Centers for Disease Control and Prevention (CDC) reported that 5 µg/dL of lead was found in the blood of 2.5% of children aged 1 to 5 years.[3]

## PATHOPHYSIOLOGICAL EFFECT OF LEAD

Lead has a variety of effects and interferes with many metabolic processes (Tables 23–1 and 23–2). Whereas the anemia caused by lead toxicity and the effects on the kidney appears to be reversible, the neurological consequences to lead exposure are not.

Lead is a divalent cation that can displace iron and/or zinc, elements that are necessary for heme synthesis. In studies on low-level lead effects on hematological parameters,[4] reduced mean corpuscular volume (MCV) and mean corpuscular hemoglobin (MCH) levels were found, and the suggestion was made that these parameters might be a sensitive measure of low-level lead exposure. However, such data are ambiguous because they do not distinguish between iron deficiency anemia and anemia caused by lead toxicity only. Bergdahl et al.[5] and others[6] have suggested a highly significant association of blood lead levels with protoporphyrin and with blood hemoglobin. The detrimental effect of lead on the kidney is well known. Chronic low-level lead exposure in children had effects on glomerular, proximal and distal tubular, and interstitial markers similar to those occurring in adults but at lower concentrations of lead exposure. Excretion losses of prostaglandins, thromboxane $B_2$, and epidermal growth factor were more pronounced than in adults.[7]

The developing brain of a child is at greater risk than the adult brain for the detrimental effects of lead. Cross-sectional and longitudinal studies measuring functional deficits have found that lead effects during early development extend into adulthood. With a doubling of blood lead concentration from 10 to 20 µg/dL in early life, an average loss of 1 to 3 IQ points was estimated, indicating that early exposure to lead has long-term consequences.[8] A study of an asymptomatic group of children aged 3 to 7 years who were enrolled in a Head Start program showed a linear negative relationship between the IQ and blood lead levels. This suggested that lead at any level has a detrimental effect.[9]The mechanisms of the neurotoxicity of lead on the developing brain, like those of other toxicants such as mercury, polychlorinated biphenyls, alcohol, and nicotine, are largely unknown.[10] Suggestions have related to interference of lead with the dopaminergic system,[11] reduced plasticity of neurons,[12] or disruption of calcium homeostasis in the immature brain.[8] Studies of lead on oxidative stress have shown that lead in the brain has a distinctive distribution with a preferential accumulation in thalamus, hippocampus, and parietal cortex, indicating that lead has a complex regional distribution and correlation with lipid oxidation.[13]

## NUTRITIONAL FACTORS

Optimal nutrition is vital to the prevention and treatment of lead toxicity. Children who are deficient in iron absorb a greater proportion of a lead dose than children who are not. A similar increased intestinal absorption of lead occurs when dietary calcium is low.[16] Deficiencies of body calcium, zinc, iron, and protein are all associated with decreased resistance to lead exposure. The high prevalence of lead toxicity among inner-city and poor children is attributed to exposure to flaking lead paint in dilapidated housing. A contributing factor, usually overlooked, is that many of these children are lactose intolerant, with low calcium intakes and generally suboptimal nutrition. Even with comparatively low blood lead levels of 10 to 15 µg/dL, a significant reduction in serum 1,25-dihydroxyvitamin D has been observed, further worsening the child's calcium status.[17,18]

Because of their high metabolic rate, young children absorb more lead from the air they breathe, compared with adults. Because of their increased growth rate, the gastrointestinal absorption of mineral nutrients, including lead, is also more efficient. The high growth rate with concomitant food intake plus exposure to hand dust obtained from mouthing behavior may be the primary source of lead during the first year of life and may explain problems with lead toxicity in this young age group. For all these reasons, preschool children are at the highest risk for lead intoxication. The other high-risk group for increased lead absorption is pregnant women. Lead crosses the placenta and is detrimental to the developing fetus.[19] Children and pregnant women should be exposed to the least amount of lead possible, and their nutrient status should be optimal for protection.

**Table 23–1.** Influence of Nutritional Status on Lead Toxicity

| Nutritional Factor | Effect |
|---|---|
| Fasting | Increases GI lead absorption |
| High-fat diets | Increases body lead burden |
| Lecithin | Increases GI lead absorption |
| Calcium | Liberal dietary intake protects |
| Iron deficiency | Increases susceptibility to lead toxicity |
| Zinc | Liberal dietary intake protects |

GI, gastrointestinal.

The long-term effects on growth of children with chronic low-level lead exposure, as measured by lead deposition in dentin, have shown a significant association between lead burden with body mass index. This suggests that lead exposure in childhood can result in adulthood obesity.[20]

## SCREENING, TREATMENT, PREVENTION, AND FOLLOW-UP

An understanding of the detrimental effects of subclinical lead levels in children has resulted in lowering of the blood lead cutoff level over the years, from 60 to 40, then 25, and finally 10 µg/dL. However, in 2012, 2.5% of children between 1 and 5 years of age still showed 5 µg/dL of lead in their blood.[3] Reductions were also found for protoporphyrin (erythrocyte protoporphyrin from 50 µg/dL to lower concentrations).

The full effects of chronic exposure to low levels of lead are not known. There is some evidence linking learning problems, dental caries, and delinquency to early lead exposure.[2] Community assessments by geostatistical methods have shown that learning disabilities in school children are associated with chronic low levels of lead exposure.[21] There is even a suggestion that chronic low-level lead exposure in early life may be an etiological factor in Alzheimer's disease.[22] All of these results indicate that there is no safe cutoff level for lead exposure, and public health measures should focus on primary prevention.

All children should be screened[23] for blood lead concentration, especially those with pica, anemia, growth failure, or developmental or behavioral problems. Information should be obtained on other risk factors, such as living in old, poorly maintained housing or low socioeconomic status of the family. Controlling the environment, strengthening the family's support system, enhancing nutrition, and offering remedial education are essential to a successful therapeutic outcome. An impoverished environment may accentuate, and an enriched environment may ameliorate, neurobehavioral and neurotoxic developmental effects due to lead exposure.[24] In one study, Bithoney found significant higher lead level in abused children as compared with controls.[25]

Children who are diagnosed with lead toxicity need to be detoxified. Vigorous chelation therapy can reduce the morbidity and mortality. Chelation agents bind lead, and the resultant chelate is excreted in urine. However, there are side effects, and special attention must be given to mineral nutrients. An effort must be made to remove the lead from the child's environment. As shown in Figure 23–1, chelation treatment alone had no lasting effect. Only after removal of the child from the high lead environment did blood lead values stay in the lower ranges.[26] States have enacted laws about remediation of older residences that contain lead paint to protect children and pregnant women from exposure to flaking lead paint. To prevent exposure to lead dust during this procedure, children and women of child-bearing age should leave the premises until lead remediation is complete.[27] Urban soils may also contain a considerable amount of lead.[28] Grass covers on playgrounds help to decrease formation of lead-containing dust.

Lead is part of our modern environment, and we are exposed to it through the air we breathe and the dust we inhale. We can get lead in our drinking water if the water is brought to us in lead pipes, as it is in many old houses. Lead can be a contaminant in food, and can be obtained through nonfood items ingested when a child or adult practices pica. Because there are detrimental effects on health, especially in children during neurodevelopment, we need to be vigilant to keep our environment as free of lead as possible and to prevent children and pregnant women from being exposed to lead. In 2000, Markowitz[29] called lead poisoning "a disease for the next millennium" and claimed that there were almost a million preschool children with elevated blood lead levels in the United States. Only by eliminating lead exposure, providing a good diet with sufficient essential mineral elements, screening children for lead, and using chelation therapy for children with high lead burdens, with subsequent follow-up to maximize the intervention, can we make an impact in lowering the lead burden in children and adults.

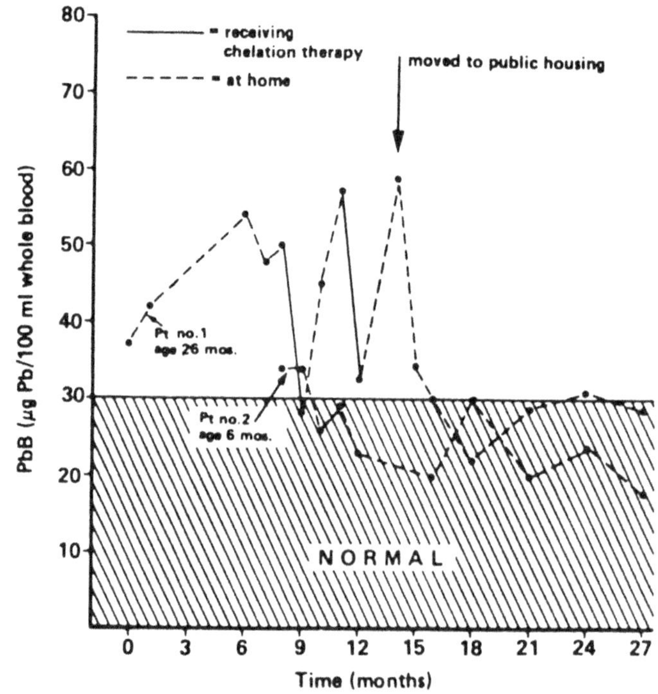


**Figure 23–1.** Serial changes in blood lead levels (PbB) in siblings as related to changes in housing. Patient no.1, the older sibling, received chelation therapy, twice in the hospital *(solid lines)*. After each treatment course, this child returned to the same, older housing. Patient no.2, the younger sibling, was first tested at 6 months of age, when the older sibling was hospitalized, and was sent immediately to stay with an aunt in a public, lead-free housing unit. When the PbB of patient no. 1 spiked for a third time, the family, including both siblings, moved to public housing. Patient no. 1's PbB promptly declined without additional chelation therapy. The shaded portion of the figure indicates the "normal" PbB range. (From Chisholm JJ Jr. Pediatric exposure to lead, arsenic, cadmium, and methyl mercury. In: Chandra RK, ed. *Trace Elements in Nutrition of Children*. New York: Vevey/Raven; 1985. Used with permission.)

**Table 23–2** Effects of Lead on Health

| |
|---|
| *Hematopoiesis* |
| Anemia due to increased heme synthesis |
| Elevated amino levulinic acid and protoporphyrin in urine and erythrocytes |
| *Immune System* |
| Decreased host resistance to bacteria and viral infections |
| Other effects possible |
| *Kidney* |
| Aminoaciduria |
| Glucosuria |
| Reduced synthesis of calcitriol (1,25-dihydroxycholecalciferol) |
| *Nervous System* |
| Peripheral nervous system damage (in adults) |
| Central nervous system damage (in children) |
| Low-level exposure |
| Impaired psychological, behavioral, and intellectual function |

## PICA INCIDENCE

Various definitions of pica are in use, such as indiscriminate craving, clay eating, or stomach illness. Pica that is practiced during pregnancy has been referred to as "hunger of pregnant women." One author described pica a repetitive search for and ingestion of nonfood substances. Others apply the term to a pathological craving for items normally considered food and for substances normally not regarded as food, such as clay or coal. The types of pica described include geophagia, the ingestion of clay and dirt; pagophagia, the consumption of refrigerator frost; and coprophagia, the ingestion of fecal matter. Other pica substances include string, putty, plaster, ashes, crayons, laundry starch, cigarette butts, oak leaves, paper, cloth, and even insects. For young children who are living in environments with a high lead content, such as old lead-painted houses, pica may lead to frank lead intoxication during the mouthing stage of development.

Pica is most prevalent among children between the ages of 1 and 3 years. Among psychotic and mentally retarded children, the incidence exceeds 50%. In a group of 991 adults with mental retardation, the incidence of pica was found to be 26% greater than that of any other eating dysfunction, including anorexia, rumination, and hyperphagia.[30] Pica may also occur in pregnant women. The craving for particular food items during pregnancy is widely recognized. In addition to craving for fruit and other sweet, sour, or bitter foods, pregnant women crave nonfood substances. Some pregnant women from the southern United States eat clay and starch. This type of pica has been reported in other populations of black, white, and Mexican pregnant women. The incidence during pregnancy ranges from 0% to 68%, depending on the population studied.[31]

## ETIOLOGY OF PICA

Pica has been explained as a craving due to a deficiency of calcium, vitamin D, phosphorus, or vitamin C. However, the incidence of pica did not decline among children given vitamin and mineral supplements.

Most attempts to link pica with nutritional states have concentrated on iron. Pagophagia in pregnant women consuming large quantities of ice (average, 700 g/day) has been associated with iron deficiency. The low hemoglobin and low serum iron levels in these women responded to iron therapy, after which the pagophagia disappeared.[32] Other theories explaining pica are psychological, specifically persistence of the infantile hand-to-mouth behavior pattern, a need to chew something solid, or a craving sensation related to texture, color, odor, or taste. Pica also may be cultural or familial; for example, clay eating was encouraged among male youths of Greece. Pica may also be practiced in an effort at self-medication. Pharmacological effects have been sought from consuming extraordinary amounts of ground coffee, cigarette butts, oak leaves, and other substances.

## FACTORS TO BE CONSIDERED IN EVALUATION OF PICA AND LEAD

The health risks in pica are many. They range from ingestion of toxic substances such as lead, to interference with normal digestion and absorption of nutrients, to ingestion of life-threatening substances such as glass. Surgery for foreign bodies, gastrointestinal obstruction, and vomiting after eating foreign substances has been frequently reported. Of special concern in children and adults are pinworms and other parasitic infections and the risk of lead toxicity, especially in children and pregnant women. In children and adults with developmental disabilities, and in children with suspected abuse, lead levels must be very closely monitored.[33–36]

Nutritional assessments of children and adults with pica have revealed dietary inadequacies. Iron deficiency anemia is frequently associated with geophagia and pagophagia. People with pica often consume less meat and milk, fewer vitamin C–rich foods, and a less varied diet. Geophagia has been associated with ingestion of fewer calories, less thiamine and niacin, and lower iron intake. When pica is complicated by lead toxicity, the nutritional status of children is compromised further by the detrimental effects of lead on hemoglobin and vitamin D metabolism. If lead toxicity is severe, urinary losses of many nutrients will occur as a result of kidney damage.

The theory that some individuals may practice pica as self-medication has led to the belief that pica is a treatment for mineral deficiencies. The suggestion has been made that iron and other essential trace elements may be obtained from clay and earths. However, this has not been born out. Clays and earths consumed are cation exchangers that bind minerals, making them unavailable for intestinal absorption. The studies by Danford et al.[32] in adults practicing geophagia showed that, although calcium, iron, and zinc intakes were adequate according to the US Dietary Reference Intakes (DRIs), hemoglobin, serum iron, and serum zinc levels were low, indicating a decreased efficiency of absorption.

## DIETARY MANAGEMENT

The treatment of pica involves many health disciplines. The dietitian and physician are involved because pica is frequently associated with nutrient deficiency, specifically deficient mineral absorption, and risks for gastrointestinal obstruction, parasitic infections, and, in some cases, lead toxicity. Pica represents a behavioral challenge to the psychiatrist and psychologist. An anthropologist may be interested in the study of pica as related to cultural patterns ingrained in the food habits of a region and possibly to an ancestral food shortage. A public health nurse may be involved in screening and identification of increased lead burdens in children and pregnant women with pica. The dietician must assess the diet, anthropometrics, and blood values, especially those relating to iron and zinc status. Not all types of pica are affected by diet, especially if they relate to a possible addictive behavior (e.g., consumption of cigarette ends). However, improvement of the diet, intake of sufficient fluid, and supplementation with minerals and vitamins may lessen the pica behavior.

### References


1. Mahaffey RK, Annest JL, Roberts J, Murphy RS. National estimates of blood lead levels: United States, 1976–80: association with selected demographic and socioeconomic factors. *N Engl J Med*. 1982; 307:573.
2. Lanphear BP, Dietrich KN, Berger O. Prevention of lead toxicity in U S children. Ambul Pediatr. 2003; 3:27.
3. Centers for Disease Control and Prevention. Childhood Lead Poisoning Prevention Program: What Do Parents Need to Know to Protect Their Children? 2012. https://www.cdc.gov/nceh/lead/acclpp/blood_lead_levels.htm. Accessed June 20, 2016.
4. Jacob B, Ritz B, Heinrich J, Hoelscher B, Wichmann HE. The effect of low-level blood lead on hematologic parameters in children. *Environ Res*. 2000; 82:150.
5. Bergdahl IA, Vahter M, Counter SA, et al. Lead in plasma and whole blood from lead exposed children. *Environ. Res*. 1999; 80:25.
6. Hammad TA, Sexton M, Langenberg P. Relationship between blood lead and dietary iron intake in preschool children. *Ann Epidemiol*. 1996; 6:30.
7. Fels, LM, Wunsch M, Baranowski J, et al. Adverse effects of chronic low level lead exposure on kidney function: a risk group study in children. *Nephrol Dial Transplant*. 1998; 13:2248.
8. Winneke G, Lillienthal H, Kramer U. The neurobehavioral toxicology and teratology of lead. *Arch Toxicol Suppl*. 1996; 18:57.
9. Dietrich KM, Kraft KM, Shukla R, Bornschein RL, Succop PA. The neurobehavioral effects of early lead exposure. In: Schroeder SR, ed. *Toxic Substances and Mental Retardation*. AAMD Monographs. Washington, DC: American Association on Mental Deficiency; 1987.
10. Schettler T. Toxic threats to neurologic development of children. *Environ Health Perspect*. 2001; 109:813.
11. Leite EM, Leroyer A, Nisse C, et al. Urinary homovanillic acid and serum prolactin levels in children with low environmental exposure to lead. *Biomarkers*. 2002; 7:49.
12. Gilbert ME, Mack CM, Laskey SM. Chronic developmental lead exposure and hippocampal long-term potentiation: biphasic dose-response relationship. *Neurotoxicology*. 1999; 20:71.
13. Villeda-Hernandez J, Barroso-Moguel R, Mendez-Armenta M, Nava-Ruiz C, Huerta-Romero R, Rios C. Enhanced brain regional lipid peroxidation in developing rats exposed to low-level lead acetate. *Brain Res Bull*. 2001; 55:247.
14. Mushak P, Crocenti AF. Lead and nutrition I: biologic interactions of lead with nutrients. *Nutr Today*. 1996; 31:12.
15. Mahaffey KR. Nutrition and lead: strategies for public health. *Environ Health Perspect*. 1995; 103:191.
16. Long GJ, Rosen JF. Lead perturbs epidermal growth factor (EGF) modulation of intracellular calcium metabolism and collagen synthesis in clonal rat osteoblastic (ROS 17/2.8) cells. *Toxicol Appl Pharmacol*. 1992; 114:63.
17. Mahaffey KR, Rosen JF, Chesney RW, Peeler JT, Smith CM, DeLuca HF. Association between age, blood lead concentrations, and serum 1,2-dihydroxycholechalciferol levels in children. *Am J Clin Nutr*. 1982; 35:1327.

18. Schanne FA, Gupta RK, Rosen JF. Lead inhibits 1,25-dihydrovitamin D-3 regulation of calcium metabolism in osteoblastic osteosarcoma cells (ROS 17/2.8) *Biochim Biophys Acta.* 1992; 1180:187.
19. Hackley B, Katz-Jacobson A. Lead poisoning in pregnancy: a case study with implications for midwives. *J Midwifery Womens Health.* 2003; 48:30.
20. Kim R, Hu H, Rotnitzky A, Bellinger D, Needleman H. A longitudinal study of chronic lead exposure and physical growth in Boston children. *Environ Health Perspect.* 1995; 103:952.
21. Margai F, Henry N. A community-based assessment of learning disabilities using environmental contextual risk factors. *Soc Sci Med.* 2003; 56:1073.
22. Prince M. Is chronic low-level lead exposure in early life an etiologic factor in Alzheimer's disease? *Epidemiology.* 1998; 9:618.
23. Centers for Disease Control and Prevention. *Screening Young Children for Lead Poisoning: Guidance for State and local Public Health Officials.* Atlanta: CDC; 1997.
24. Schneider JS, Lee MH, Anderson DW, Zuck L, Lidsky TI. Enriched environment during development is protective against lead-induced neurotoxicity. *Brain Res.* 2001; 896:48.
25. Bithoney W, Vandeven A, Ryan A. Elevated lead levels reported in abused children. *J Pediatr.* 1993; 122:719.
26. Chisholm JJ Jr. Pediatric exposure to lead, arsenic, cadmium, and methyl mercury. In: Chandra RK, ed. *Trace Elements in Nutrition of Children.* New York: Vevey/Raven; 1985.
27. Centers for Disease Control and Prevention. Children with elevated blood lead levels attributed to home renovation and remodeling [editorial]. *JAMA.* 1997; 277:1030.
28. Mielke HW, Gonzales CR, Smith MK, Mielke PW. The urban environment and children's health: soils as an integrator of lead, zinc, and cadmium in New Orleans, Louisiana, USA. *Environ Health Perspect.* 1999; 81:117.
29. Markowitz M. Lead poisoning: a disease for the next millennium. *Curr Probl Pediatr.* 2000; 30:62.
30. Danford DE, Huber AM. Eating dysfunction in an institutionalized mentally retarded population. *Appetite.* 1981; 2:281.
31. Smullian JC, Motiwala S, Sigman RK. Pica in a rural obstetric population. *South Med J.* 1995; 88:1236.
32. Danford DE, Smith JC, Huber AM. Pica and mineral status. *Am J Clin Nutr.* 1982; 35:958.
33. Graff C, Murphy L, Ekvall, S, Magnon M. In-home toxic chemical exposure and children with developmental disabilities. *Pediatr Nurs.* 2006; 32:597.
34. Tyler C, White-Scott S, Ekvall S, Abulafa L. Environmental health and developmental disabilities: a lifespan approach. *Fam Commun Health J.* 2008; 34:4.
35. Harper E, Ekvall S, Ekvall V, Wei P. The nutritional status of children with suspected abuse. In: Atroski F, ed. *Pharmacology and Nutritional Intervention in the Treatment of Disease.* Croatia: InTech; 2014.
36. Bithoney W, Vandeven A, Ryan A. Elevated lead levels in reportedly abused children. *J Pediatr.* 1993; 122:719.

# C.

# FEEDING DISORDERS

## 24 Feeding and Eating Problems of the Child or Adult with Intellectual and Developmental Disabilities and Special Health Care Needs

DIANE SPEAR, HARRIET CLOUD, SHIRLEY W. EKVALL, PAULA CUSHING, LINDA HICKS, AND JULIA WAHOFF

The nutritional health of an infant, child, or adult is determined by adequate intake of food or other nutritional products by feeding and/or eating. The amount of food intake depends on the infant's ability to suckle, suck, progress to the cup and solid food, and eventually self-feed the recommended mix of protein, fat, carbohydrates, vitamins, minerals, and water. Infants and children with special health care needs are frequently at risk for feeding problems that impact their growth, energy needs, and immunity to disease.[1] In children and adults with intellectual and developmental disabilities (IDD), there is a high incidence of dysphagia and eating issues acquired in infancy and/or developed with the progression of physical and neurological problems and aging.[2,3] Other consequences of feeding and eating problems may include anemia, vitamin and mineral deficiencies, dental caries, increased risk for dehydration, aspiration and choking, developmental delays, and psychosocial problems. Feeding and eating problems have been defined as the inability or refusal to eat certain foods because of neuromotor dysfunction, obstructive lesions, and/or psychosocial factors. Problems are classified as oral-motor, positioning, or behavioral.[1]

Feeding and eating problems are frequently found in infants, children, and adults with cerebral palsy, cleft lip and palate, Down syndrome, seizures, spina bifida, prematurity, Prader-Willi syndrome, hypotonia, and other chronic medical disorders.[1,2] Feeding and eating problems should be assessed with an understanding of the normal development of feeding and the physical makeup of the mouth and pharynx.

### NORMAL DEVELOPMENT OF FEEDING

Feeding is a multidimensional process that follows the infant's development and also influences it. It is part of the infant's interaction with the environment that promotes learning and development. The feeding process involves the development of oral-motor, gross motor, fine motor, and behavioral skills.[4]

Oral-motor skills include suckling, sucking, swallowing, chewing, biting, gagging, tongue elevation, and lateralization. The oral cavity consists of the upper jaw or maxilla, the lower jaw or mandible, upper and lower lips, cheeks, tongue, teeth, floor of the mouth, hard and soft palates, uvula, and anterior and posterior facial arches (Fig. 24–1). These structures are necessary for sucking and suckling, biting, and chewing. The structures involved in swallowing are the pharyngeal structures and the larynx. Pharyngeal structures include the superior, medial, and inferior pharyngeal constrictors, which function as a valve at the top of the esophagus.[5] The juncture of the pharynx and the

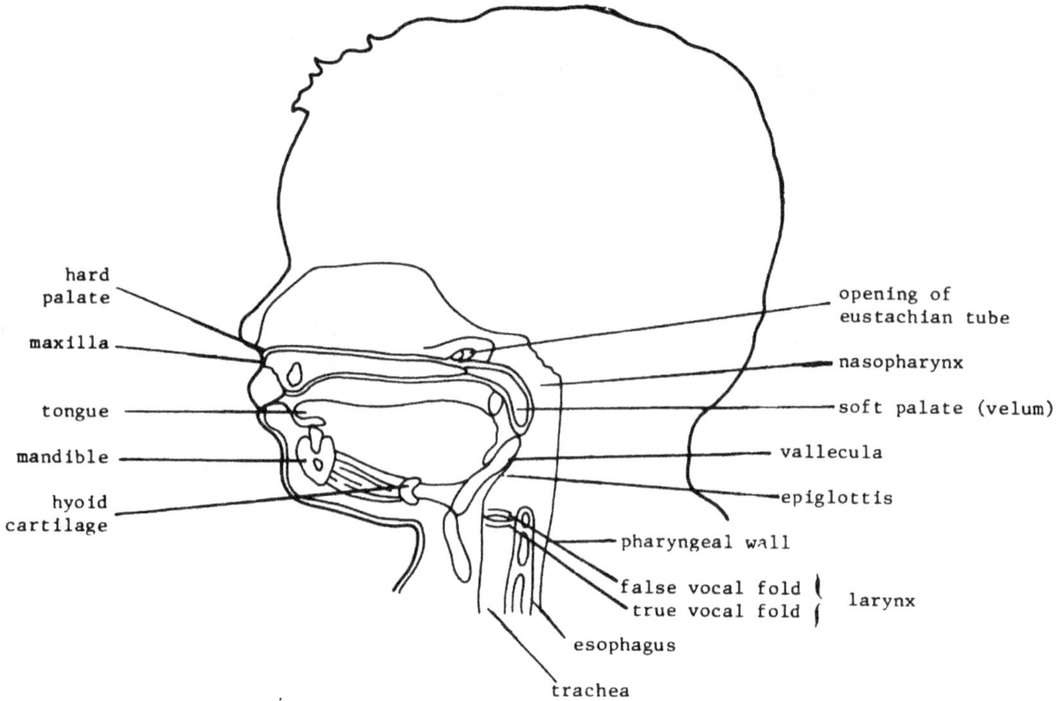


**Figure 24–1.** The mouth and pharynx of the newborn (sagittal section). (From Morris SE, Klein MD. *Pre-feeding Skills: A Comprehensive Resource for Mealtime Development,* 2nd ed. Tucson, AZ: Therapy Skills Builders; 2000. Used with permission.)

esophagus is known as the *P-E juncture* of the cricopharyngeal sphincter. The larynx functions to keep food from entering the airway. The esophagus is a thin, muscular tube that distends as food boluses are propelled through it by peristaltic movements.[5,6] It is approximately 23 to 25 cm long and is closed by a sphincter at each end. The esophagus passes through the diaphragm and terminates in the stomach at the lower esophageal sphincter, sometimes referred to as the *cardiac sphincter* or the *gastroesophageal sphincter*.

The normal infant is born ready to suck. The normal development of feeding is presented in Table 24–1. Swallowing is a complex motor sequence involving the coordination of a large number of muscles in the mouth, pharynx, larynx, and esophagus. Swallowing by the fetus plays a significant role in the regulation of amniotic fluid volume during a normal pregnancy.[6] The swallowing process is divided into three phases: oral, pharyngeal, and esophageal. During the *oral phase*, the food or liquid is organized into a bolus and moved from the front to the back of the mouth. The bolus is held and released to the pharynx as the swallow is triggered. Three cranial nerves provide efferent control of the oral phase of swallowing. These nerves affect the motor control of the lips, cheeks, and mouth, as well as tongue and jaw movements.[6] The *pharyngeal phase* of swallowing involves the closure of the nasal, laryngeal, and oral openings to prevent fluid leakage and to channel the direction of the bolus; the opening of the cricopharyngeal sphincter; and the creation of a sufficient pharyngeal pressure gradient to

**Table 24–1.** Feeding Development in Normal Infants

| Age | Oral-Motor Skills | Self-Feeding |
|---|---|---|
| 0–4 wk | Rooting reflex<br>Suckling pattern<br>Suck-swallow reflex<br>Jaw and tongue move up and down | |
| 8 wk | Tongue moves forward and back<br>Suckling still primary action | |
| 12 wk | Corners of lips become active in sucking<br>Tongue is extended out of the mouth in anticipation of feeding | |
| 16 wk | Sucking stage begins<br>Tongue thrust still present | Sees bottle and becomes excited |
| 20 wk | Munching stage begins<br>Smacks lips together<br>Strained foods introduced | Pat or puts hands on bottle |
| 24 wk | Lips begin to close around spoon<br>Progression of solid food continues | |
| 28 wk | Lips begin to move while chewing<br>Vertical chewing stage begins<br>Jaw and tongue move up and down | Plays with spoon<br>May help spoon find mouth |
| 32–36 wk | Lip closure achieved<br>Cup drinking begins | Feeds self crackers, cookies, etc.<br>Holds bottle |
| 40–52 wk | Tongue lateralization leads to rotary chewing<br>Licks food from lower lip | Can hold own bottle well<br>Can hold cup but may spill contents |

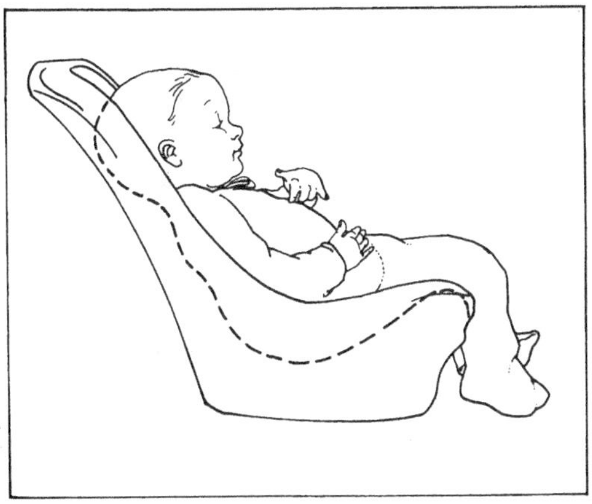

Figure 24–2. Proper feeding position for an infant. (From Cloud H. *Team Approach to Pediatric Feeding Problems.* Chicago: American Dietetic Association; 1987. Used with permission.)

transport the bolus from the oral cavity to the opening of the esophagus. Twenty-six muscles and six cranial nerves must be coordinated for the pharyngeal swallow to occur safely and efficiently.[6] The *esophageal phase* of swallowing is the final segment in the transfer of nutrients from the mouth to the stomach. Peristaltic contractions move the fluid or bolus along the esophagus toward the stomach.[5,6] The growth and development of all oral skills is believed to continue until about the age of 3 years. At that point, the normal child should have all the basic components of oral skills that will be needed throughout life.[7] This may not be true, however, in the child with developmental disabilities and special needs.

## GROSS MOTOR DEVELOPMENT

At birth, all infants are motorically dependent, receiving all stability from physiological flexion and external support.[5,6] They are held for feeding in a position with the head and upper body elevated to less than 45 degrees. By 3 months of age, infants gain head control, allowing them to lift and turn the head while lying on the stomach. By 6 months, infants begin to sit without support, grasp for objects, and discover the world through their mouths, exploring tastes, shapes, weights, and textures. At that point, they may be fed in a highchair or infant feeding seat. As a stable feeding position develops at 6 to 8 months, infants are able to hold a small cup.[7] Feeding position is an important consideration for all children. The child must have adequate support for the head, trunk, and legs. The ideal position of a child for is with hip flexion of 90 degrees or more, the thighs in neutral alignment or slight

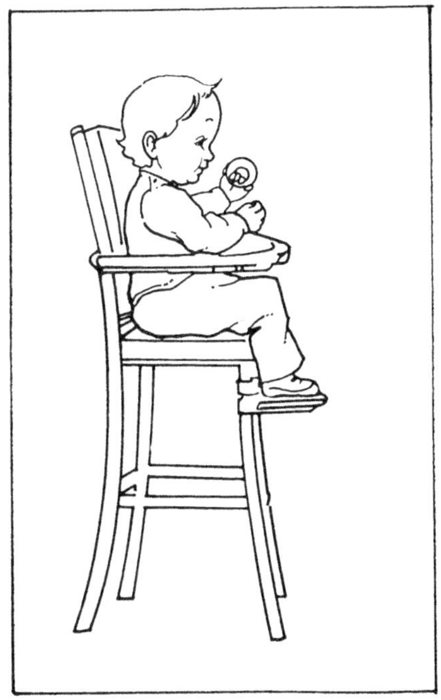

Figure 24–3. Good feeding position for a child aged 6 to 24 months, showing hip flexion and trunk and head in the midline. Good foot support with a stool should continue throughout childhood. (From Cloud H. *Team Approach to Pediatric Feeding Problems.* Chicago: American Dietetic Association; 1987. Used with permission.)

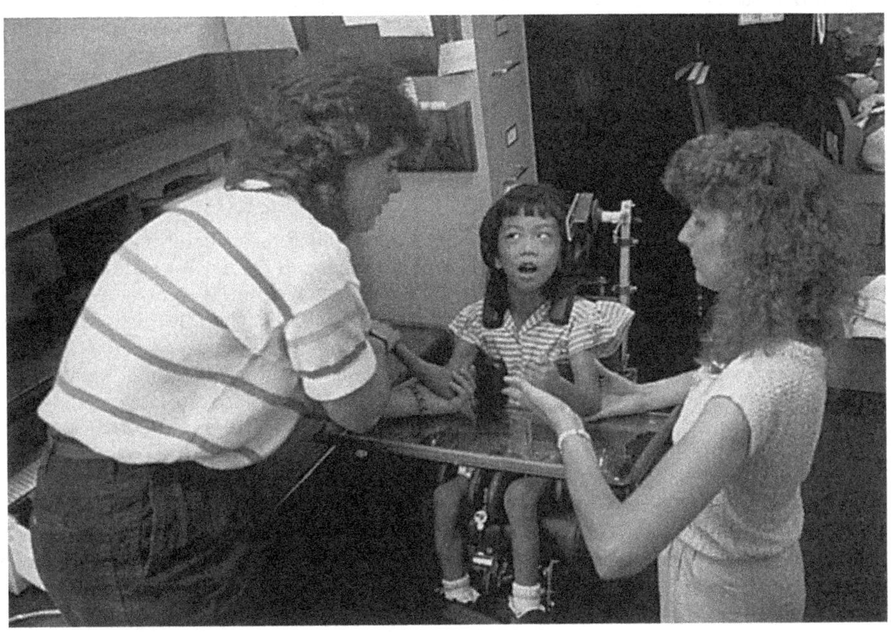

Figure 24–4. A positioning chair provides good trunk support, proper hip placement, and head control, all of which are necessary for working with children who have oral-motor problems. Used with permission.

abduction, ankles in dorsiflexion matching the degree of hip flexion, the trunk in the midline, elbows flexed and resting in a tray, and head in the midline with the chin slightly ventroflexed[5] (Figs. 24–2 and 24–3). When an infant or child has an oral-motor problem, positioning the child in the appropriate position for feeding is mandatory for comfort and safety[5,6] (Fig. 24–4). For safe swallowing, it is important to maintain the appropriate position, especially head and body alignment, throughout the feeding or eating process.

## BEHAVIORAL ASPECTS OF FEEDING AND EATING

Feeding is an important element of parent-child relations, beginning in infancy and continuing through adolescence[7] and into adulthood. In a normal feeding situation, the child or infant is in control of food or fluid intake and should communicate to the mother or feeder by furnishing cues related to satiety.[6–8] As infants mature, they respond to the feeder's reaction to the cues they provide. This response may be positive or negative, causing either a decrease or an increase in a certain feeding behavior, depending on the feeder's reaction to the infant or child. Positive behaviors that accompany feeding include accepting a wide variety of foods and textures, remaining seated, keeping hands off other people, self-feeding at the appropriate level, eating at a moderate pace, eating and drinking quietly, using utensils appropriately, and chewing and swallowing with the mouth closed.[8] Negative behaviors include crying, refusing to accept an item of food, gagging and vomiting in response to food offered, and inability or unwillingness to sit still during mealtime.[6] Studies of normal parent-infant interactions have highlighted mealtime as a major venue for parenting and bonding, playing, and learning social games.[7]

Environmental factors also influence the feeding behaviors of infants and children.[9] These factors can include feeding the child in a highly distractible location, such as in front of a television or near a radio; providing little or no structure in the timing of meals; and not permitting the child the autonomy of intake that his or her developmental level demands. Appetite can also influence feeding behavior. As the child matures after the first year of life, the growth rate is reduced, and the appetite may reflect this. Often, the serving size for various foods is too great, overwhelming the child with a small appetite.

## FEEDING AND EATING PROBLEMS

Infants, children, and adults with IDD such as Down syndrome, cerebral palsy, Prader-Willi syndrome, autism, and Rett syndrome are at risk for a number of feeding and eating problems.[1,2] Feeding and eating problems include oral-motor problems, problems with sensory processes, and problems with the feeding or eating process.

### Oral-Motor and Swallowing Problems

Oral-motor problems were described by Lane and Cloud as exaggeration of normal neuromotor mechanisms that disrupt the rhythm and organization of oral-motor function and interfere with the feeding process (Table 24–2).[9] These problems include tonic bite reflex, tongue thrust, jaw thrust, tongue retraction, lip retraction, and sensory defensiveness. Whenever oral-motor problems occur, food intake is limited and the possibility of severe nutritional problems exists. Slow growth and inadequate weight gain are common among children with oral-motor feeding problems and are often attributed to fatigue on the part of both the child and the feeder. Oral-motor dysfunction often causes a disturbance in the normal progression of feeding development and food textures which may carry over into adulthood, especially for the child with IDD. Oral-motor problems frequently are found in people with cerebral palsy and seriously interfere with adequate intake of calories, protein, fat, carbohydrates, vitamins, and minerals.[10,11]

The incidence of dysphagia is high in the population with IDD, increasing the risk of choking and aspiration, which can lead to poor nutrition status, dehydration, and death.[12,13] Ensuring adequate and safe intake is essential. No two people are alike in their eating and swallowing ability. Each should have an individualized eating plan based on their oral motor and functional ability to consume food and liquids safely and adequately.[2,12]

**Table 24–2.** Common Feeding Problems

| Problem | Description |
|---|---|
| Tonic bite reflex | Strong jaw closure when teeth and gums are stimulated |
| Tongue thrust | Forceful and often repetitive protrusion of an often bunched or thick tongue in response to oral stimulation |
| Jaw thrust | Forceful opening of the jaw to the maximal extent during eating or drinking, in attempts to speak, or in general excitement |
| Tongue retraction | Pulling back the tongue within the oral cavity on the presentation of food, spoon, or cup |
| Lip retraction | Pulling back the lips in a very tight smile-like pattern at the approach of the spoon or cup toward the face |
| Sensory defensiveness | A strong adverse reaction to sensory input (e.g., touch, sound, light) |

Modified from Lane S, Cloud HH. Feeding problems and intervention: an interdisciplinary approach. *Top Clin Nutr*. 1988; 3:23.

### Problems with Sensory Processes

Sensory processes can be perturbed in the neurologically impaired infant and child with seizure disorders, spina bifida, cerebral palsy, or autism, and this often carries over into adulthood. The two broad categories are hypersensitivity and hyposensitivity.[6] The infant, child, or adult with hypersensitivity has strong reactions to a variety of stimuli, resulting in increases in postural tone and abnormal reflex patterns. Behaviors that may be observed are gagging, grimacing, arching, turning away, crying, and/or vomiting. For example, turning the head away or pushing objects away may occur when oral exploration is encouraged and when the lips are touched with the nipple of a bottle, a spoon, or a toothbrush. Hypersensitive and aversive responses can be part of a global tactile processing problem, or they can be localized to the face and mouth or, more specifically, to a certain part of the mouth, most frequently the tongue.[6] Some causes of hypersensitivity are immaturity, chronic illness, unpleasant oral-tactile experiences, delayed introduction of oral feeding, and neurological impairment. Premature infants and sick infants who have been intubated repeatedly or for long periods may learn a pattern of defensive behavior in response to stimulation in and around the oral area.[14]

Hyporeactions frequently are encountered in people who are hypotonic or who have poor swallowing cues. Reductions in taste acuity, smell, and touch-pressure sensitivity in the mouth may occur. These sensory impairments contribute to severe motor feeding disorders and indifference to eating. An additional problem with either hyperreaction or hyporeaction is sensory overload. When placed in an environment filled with many distractions (or even a normal environment), the neurologically damaged person may react with hyperactivity and display no attention to feeding.[15] Control of the feeding environment to decrease sensory input is a key factor in nutrition intervention. Some ideas to improve the sensory process can be included in the sensory diet (Box 24–1).

### Problems with the Feeding Process

The feeding process involves suckling, sucking, swallowing, biting, chewing, and self-feeding. Problems in the suckling and sucking processes involve a suckle that may be arrhythmic, weak, poorly sustained, inefficient, or rapid, resulting in inadequate intake of formula or breast milk. The infant may be unable to develop a firm

**Box 24–1.** Sensory Diet

A balanced sensory diet consists of a planned, scheduled, and executed activity program. The sensory diet is geared to the individual's nervous system needs. The advantage of a good sensory diet is that it helps the child become more focused, adaptable, and skillful and less agitated, and it makes the child more willing to sense his or her world. It also may help with feeding problems.

A good sensory diet should include combinations of alerting, calming, and organizing activities. The order depends on the child's needs. The diet should be individualized and should consist of tactile, vestibular, and proprioceptive sensory activities.

A. **Alerting or awaking activities:** These activities help the undersensitive child to become more active by energizing the child with stimulation.
   1. Loud, crunchy foods
   2. Bouncing on a knee, beach ball, therapy ball, large ball, or inflatable toy.
   3. Jumping up and down on an a ~~Moose Mountain~~ inflatable toy, cushion, or mattress (placed flat on the floor for safety)
   4. Taking a shower for the water-on-skin stimulation, using plain water first and then adding bubbles or colored soap
   5. Playing with navy beans, lima beans, sand, pebbles, or water
   6. Finger painting with plain paint, then adding sand, cereal, rice, or other textures
   7. Finger painting with shaving cream (supervised only)

B. **Relaxing activities:** These activities are great for the oversensitized individual and help to decrease hyperresponsiveness or overresponsiveness to stimulation by calming aggression, redirecting focus, and relaxing the child after each session.
   1. Cuddling, deep pressure hugging, back rubbing, lap rocking, or swaying
   2. Listening to relaxing music or music videos
   3. Pushing on walls with the back, buttocks, hands, head, or shoulders
   4. Rocking on teeter totters or glider rockers; rocking back and forth in slow motion
   5. Swinging in any form, back and forth in slow motion
   6. Sucking on a pacifier, sugar-free hard candy, frozen fruit bar, frozen Pedialyte pop, or flavored ice bar
   7. Taking a bath
   8. Watching a relaxing movie

C. **Organizing activities:** These activities help to adjust the child's responses for better regulation by temporarily altering the sensory system for proper functioning.
   1. Eating chewy foods—bagels, bakery foods, bread or pizza crust, dried fruits, cheese, fruit bars or roll-ups, granola bars, gum, licorice, shrimp, or clams
   2. Assuming an upside-down position—standing on the head, hanging from the legs on uneven bars, wheelbarrow walking, walking on the hands
   3. Hanging from a chin-up bar by the hands or climbing heights on a rope
   4. Pushing or pulling heavy items—furniture, vacuum cleaner, wheelbarrow, or stroller with toys or books in it
   5. **Progression of activities:** Routines are important, so start simple and work up. Use activities in which the child has an interest and change activities every 2 to 4 hours. Try counting to 5 before making a transition from one activity to another. Watch for signs that the child is starting to relax (e.g., facial expressions). Crying, whimpering, and laughing can mean that it is time to cool off or calm down. If the child tries to jump from a high place, he or she probably needs a jumping experience. If the child is running back and forth, a moving activity will work best. If the child is fidgety, redirect to another activity such as painting.

D. **Tactile integration activities:**
   1. Box play—Use boxes of various sizes and shapes to build, paint, fill and unfill; sit in them, rearrange them, and put stickers on them.
   2. Back rubs—Rub the child's back in a downward motion, always using firm, deep pressure (a light touch sensation may stay with the child for minutes to hours after the back rub has been completed and may cause pain); the arm and legs can also be rubbed using this method.
   3. Cut a hole in a shoe box and fill it with a few small items (e.g., small doll, ring with keys, toy airplane, toy car). Have the child place a hand inside the box and guess what is in it. This helps the child improve the ability to discriminate between items without using the eyes.
   4. Finger painting with plain paints first, then added textures
   5. Other sensory finger items (e.g., peanut butter, chocolate syrup, pancake syrup, pudding, Jell-O, jelly) can be used to make items or shapes in the mixtures for an added learning experience.
   6. Guess the item—Using a finger or the end of a pencil, draw a letter, shape, number, or picture on the child's back or hand.
   7. Cooking play—When cooking, let the child play with the cookie dough, bread dough, meatloaf mixture, cake mix, or muffin dough for added textures.
   8. Have the child use washcloths, body sponges, body scrubbers, or nail brushes to scrub his or her body.
   9. Wrap the child tightly in a sheet, blanket, or bedspread to create a deep pressure that is pleasurable for the child's sensory system.
   10. Touch an electric toothbrush externally and internally to the cheeks and tongue to desensitize the child who demonstrates hypersensitivity or tactile defensiveness.

E. **Taste activities**
   1. Blowing bubbles—This helps to prevent pain from eating by strengthening mouth and tongue muscles.
   2. Drinking from a straw to strengthen muscles
   3. Sensory silverware—wide-handled spoons and forks that have knobs or spirals
   4. Sensory cups with straws
   5. **Eating ideas**: Make sure that the child's elbows are at table height and the feet are flat on the floor or supported. Offer a variety of foods, textures, and different ways to eat them. Use crunchy, soft, chewy, or lumpy foods at each meal, allowing finger feeding and use of utensils. Check to be sure that the child does not have food allergies or intolerances.

F. **Vestibular activities**
   1. Ball bouncing using handles
   2. Somersaults or spinning with a Sit 'n Spin toys, merry-go-round, tire swing, or swivel chair
   3. Swinging with a slow motion, which can be very relaxing
   4. Sliding sitting up and lying down, front and back
   5. Walking on unstable or moving surfaces
   6. Riding Big Wheel or other tricycles, bikes, or scooters

G. **Proprioceptive activities**
   1. Have the child carry heavy or large items, push furniture back and forth, or carry light- to medium-weight loads on his or her back like a camel.
   2. Press both hands down on the child's head carefully.
   3. Paper ripping—Let the child tear strips, squares, or circles from paper.
   4. Toss a ball back and forth.
   5. Play leapfrog.
   6. Roughhousing—push, pull, tug, roll, and tumble

H. **Fine motor skills:** Develop by flour sifting, playing with Lego building blocks, or putting together a jigsaw puzzle.

I. **Motor planning:** Use tunnels, stepping stones, stairs, or ladders.

J. **Bilateral coordination:** ball rolling and clapping

K. **Visual skills:** finding the flashlight dot on the wall; making shapes, mazes, dot-to-dot puzzles, or a geoboard

L. Consider where, when, how often, and how many activities the child needs and which activities are best for the child.

Adapted from *Autism Awakening 4 Therapy*. Autism Awakening, 1900 K Street, SW, Cedar Rapids, IA, 52404.

seal around the nipple, with milk lost from the mouth.[5] As the infant matures even into adulthood, oral-motor problems such as delays in control of lips, tongue, cheeks, and jaw may contribute to inability to remove food from a spoon with the upper lip or difficulty using the tongue to propel the food to the back of the mouth for swallowing. Other problems include choking, abnormal swallowing patterns caused by absent or delayed swallowing reflexes, gagging on increased textures, and inability to chew in a developmentally appropriate manner.[5]

## ASSESSMENT OF FEEDING AND EATING PROBLEMS

Assessment of feeding and eating problems is most effectively done with a team approach.[1] In many clinics that address feeding, the team consists of a nutritionist, an occupational therapist, a speech pathologist, a nurse, and, in some instances, a special educator and a dentist. Ideally, the team will have an interdisciplinary approach and function in both assessment and management. One example of an interdisciplinary assessment form was developed by the Boling Center at the University of Tennessee in Memphis (Box 24–2).[16] Most feeding teams observe the child during feeding carried out by the parent or caregiver.

In a community home or residential setting for adults with IDD, dietitian nutritionists have varying roles in the management of eating problems depending on the setting and accessible resources. Good communication and collaboration among disciplines is important in helping a person to eat safely and effectively.[17] The evaluation and management of eating problems begins with mealtime observation in a person's usual environment and includes observation of food preparation and eating assistance provided by caregivers. Dietitian nutritionists are often instrumental in identifying eating and swallowing problems, the need for an eating or mealtime evaluation with a team of professionals, and appropriate diet orders.[18,19] Whatever the setting, pursuing more training in the area of dysphagia management can assist the dietitian nutritionist in becoming more proficient in eating assessment and intervention.[20]

## ASSESSMENT OF ORAL-MOTOR PROBLEMS

Assessment of the oral-motor process is usually completed by the occupational therapist or speech pathologist and is influenced by the expertise available to the agency, school, or developmental center (Table 24–3). Some assessments require specific tests, such as videofluoroscopy using the barium swallow to evaluate swallowing problems. The transit time, oral-motor skills, and amount of aspiration are identified by this process.[6] The barium swallow is an excellent tool to assess esophageal function, structural abnormalities, and gastroesophageal reflux. The modified barium swallow is specifically designed to evaluate the pharyngeal swallow. It can depict the initiation of swallowing; duration of the pharyngeal swallow; adequacy, presence, and amount of aspiration; and protective reactions in response to aspiration. Positioning in a normal feeding position is necessary for this test. The modified barium swallow does not identify gastroesophageal reflux or esophageal structural problems well.[6]

## ASSESSMENT OF POSITIONING PROBLEMS

Assessment of positioning problems should include observation of head control, trunk control, foot stability, placement of the hips and pelvis, shoulder girdle, knee flexion, and sitting base.[5] Appropriate positioning varies, depending on the problem identified, and could include reclining on the stomach, lying on the side, sitting, or standing. Numerous therapeutic positioning devices are available that provide adequate trunk support, place the hips and pelvis in a stable position, prevent shoulder retraction, and promote head control. Proper positioning also improves visual control, which will increase food intake because the individual may be better able to see the food being offered, enhancing the ability to self-feed.[6] Positioning provides the physical supports needed for optimal use of the arms and hands to self-feed and to chew and swallow to the best of the person's ability. Proper positioning of a person with postural challenges is specific to the individual and is best determined with the assistance of a physical therapist or occupational therapist.

## BEHAVIORAL AND ENVIRONMENTAL PROBLEMS

Observing a person's behavior provides information on how well the individual deals with the environment. Behavioral responses can range from social engagement to self-regulatory, stress, or avoidance behaviors. Some of the indicators of early behavioral problems include a sleepy baby, poor cues related to when to feed, difficulty with feeding transitions, agitation, frequent crying, difficulty initiating sucking, and poor rhythm.[6] As the child matures, the need for control of feeding progresses, requiring an assessment of developmental readiness for transition.[15] Assessment factors should include the daily routine, structured meal and snack times, nap time, bedtime, and emphasis placed on food intake by the parent or other caregiver. Some toddlers are discouraged from self-feeding because of the messiness of that activity even though their need for autonomy is evident. Behavioral cues related to transitioning from a bottle to a cup can be missed, making weaning more difficult, especially with a full set of teeth. The sensory diet uses certain assessments and treatments for behavioral problems in autism, attention-deficit hyperactivity disorder, and other conditions (see Box 24–1 and Chapter 19).

As the toddler begins walking and climbing, mealtime structure may become a battle between the parent and child over sitting still in the highchair or at the toddler table and completing the meal. Exposure to distractions such as television, radio, or other people will seriously interfere with intake. Medications can distort taste and dull the appetite.

Assisting an adult with eating encompasses the same behavioral aspects that may interfere with eating safely and effectively in childhood. Such issues include a lack of focus during mealtime, refusal to eat, spitting out food, and eating too much or too fast, resulting in gagging or choking. Behavioral therapy interventions may be necessary and may include finding a quiet place to eat without distractions, adjusting mealtimes, and reducing portion sizes and/or the number of foods served at one time. When assessing behavioral problems, it is important to consider the etiology of the behavioral response and to differentiate among responses that are neurologically based, those that are caused by physical pain or discomfort, and issues concerning the ability to communicate.[17]

## FACTORS TO BE CONSIDERED IN NUTRITIONAL ASSESSMENT AND INTERVENTION

Numerous studies have identified inadequate nutritional intake in infants, children, and adults with IDD and special health care needs due to feeding problems.[2,10] Assessment of the nutritional status of the infant or child is an important part of the feeding evaluation. Nutrition assessment for the child or adult with a feeding or eating problem is similar to that of any child with special health care needs.[1,2] In general, it includes obtaining anthropometric information, dietary information, biochemical values when available, cultural indicators, family values related to food, and clinical indicators such as elimination, medications, frequency of illnesses, and special foods the family may be purchasing (see Appendix 5).

Determination of the nutrient and fluid needs of the child or adult with a feeding problem is part of the nutrition assessment and the plan for intervention.[6] Determination of energy need is essential in counseling the parent or caregiver who may be reluctant to follow intervention

**Box 24–2.** Developmental Feeding Tool

Parent/Guardian__________
Address__________
City______ State______ Zip______
County______ Telephone______
Referrer__________

Date__________
Staff member__________
Child's name__________
Birth date______ Age____ Sex____ Race____
Head circumference (cm)____ (%ile NCHS)____ Hand dominance____
Height (cm)____(%ile NCHS)____ Weight (kg)____ (%ile NCHS)____
Weight for height (%ile NCHS)____ Hematocrit____ Urine screen____

*Physical*

Yes No

Size

1. Weight (Avg. %ile NCHS)
2. Underweight
3. Overweight
4. Stature (Avg. %ile NCHS)
5. Short (<5th %ile for ht. NCHS)
6. Tall (>95th %ile for ht. NCHS)
7. Abnormal body proportions*
8. Head circumference (Avg. %ile NCHS)
9. Microcephalic
10. Macrocephalic

Laboratory

11. Hematocrit (Normal)
12. Urine screen (Normal)*

Health Status

13. Bowel problems*
14. Diabetes
15. Vomiting
16. Dental caries
17. Anemia
18. Food allergies/intolerance*
19. Medications*
20. Vitamin/mineral supplements*
21. Ingests nonfood items
22. Therapeutic diet*
23. General appearance (Normal)*
24. Head (Normal)*
25. Eyes (Normal)*
26. Ears (Normal)*
27. Nose (Normal)*
28. Teeth/gums (Normal)*
29. Palate (Normal)*
30. Skin (Normal)*
31. Muscles (Normal)*
32. Arms/hands (Normal)*
33. Legs/feet (Normal)*

*Neuromotor/Muscular*

Yes No

Tonicity

34. Body tone (Normal)*

Head and Trunk Control

35. Head control (Normal)*
36. Lifts head in prone
37. Head lags when pulled to sitting
38. Head drops forward
39. Head drops backward
40. Trunk control (Normal)*

Upper Extremity Control

41. Range of motion (Normal)*
42. Approach to object (Normal)*
43. Grasp of object (Normal)*
44. Release of object (Normal)*
45. Brings hands to mouth
46. Dominance established

Reflexes

47. Grossly normal
48. Asymmetrical tonic neck reflex*
49. Symmetrical tonic neck reflex*
50. Moro reflex*
51. Grasp reflex*

Body Alignment

52. Scoliosis
53. Kyphosis
54. Lordosis
55. Hip subluxation or dislocation suspected

Position in Feeding

56. Mother's lap
57. Infant seat
58. High chair
59. Table and chair
60. Wheelchair
61. Other adaptive chair*

*Oral/Motor*

Yes No

Facial Expression

62. Symmetrical structure/function*
63. Muscle tone lips/cheeks (Normal)
64. Hypertonic muscle tone of lips
65. Hypotonic muscle tone of lips

Oral Reflexes

66. Gag (Normal)*
67. Bite (Normal)*
68. Rooting (Normal)*
69. Suck/swallow (Normal)*

Respiration

70. Mouth
71. Nose
72. Thoracic
73. Abdominal
74. Regular rhythm*

Oral Sensitivity

75. Inside mouth (Normal)*
76. Outside mouth (Normal)*
77. Hypersensitivity*
78. Hyposensitivity*
79. Intolerance to brushing teeth

*Feeding Patterns*

Bottle-feeding

80. Suckling tongue movements
81. Sucking tongue movements
82. Firm lip seal*
83. Coordinated suck-swallow-breathing
84. Difficulty swallowing*

Cup-Drinking

85. Adequate lip closure*
86. Loses less than ½ total amount*

Yes No

Size

87. Wide up-and-down jaw movements
88. Stabilizes jaw by biting edge of cup
89. Stabilizes jaw through muscle control
90. Drinks through a straw Feeding patterns—Spoon-feeding

Yes No

Tonicity

91. Suckles as food approaches
92. Cleans food off lower lip
93. Cleans food off spoon with upper lip
94. Munching pattern

Lateralizes tongue:

95. When food placed between molars

Yes No

Facial Expression

96. When food placed center of tongue
97. To move food from side to side
98. Vertical jaw movements
99. Rotary jaw movements

Feeding patterns—Chewing

100. Lip closure during chewing*

(continued)

**Box 24–2.** Continued

*Physical*

Isolated Voluntary Tongue Movements

101. Protrudes/retracts tongue
102. Elevates tongue outside mouth
103. Elevates tongue inside mouth
104. Depresses tongue outside mouth
105. Depresses tongue inside mouth
106. Lateralizes tongue outside mouth
107. Lateralizes tongue inside mouth

Special Oral Problems

108. Drools*
109. Thrusts tongue when utensil placed in mouth*
110. Thrusts tongue during chewing/swallowing*
111. Other oral-motor problem*

*Nutrition History*

Past Status

112. Feeding problems birth—1 year*
113. Breast-fed
114. Bottle-fed
115. Weaned

Current Status

116. Eats blended food
117. Eats limited texture
118. Eats chopped table foods
119. Eats table foods
120. Feeds unassisted
121. Feeds with partial guidance
122. Feeds with complete guidance
123. Drinks from a cup unassisted
124. Drinks from a cup assisted
125. Finger-feeds
126. Uses a spoon
127. Uses a fork
128. Uses a knife

*Neuromotor/Muscular*

129. Average rate of eating
130. Fast rate of eating
131. Slow rate of eating

*Diet Review*

132. Appetite normal
133. Eats 3 meals/day
134. Snacks daily Dietary Intake, Current
135. Milk/dairy products, 3–4/ day
136. Vegetables, 2–3/day
137. Fruit, 2–3/day
138. Meat/meat substitute, 2–3/day
139. Bread/cereal, 3–4/day
140. Sweets/snacks, 1–2/day
141. Liquids, 2 cups/day

*Social/Behavioral*

Child-Caregiver Relationship

142. Child responds to caregiver
143. Caregiver affectionate to child

Social Skills

144. Eye contact
145. Smiles
146. Gestures (e.g., waves bye-bye)
147. Clings to caregiver
148. Interacts with examiner
149. Responds to simple directions
150. Seeks approval
151. Toilet trained
152. Knows own sex Behavior Problems
153. Self-abusive
154. Hyperactive
155. Aggressive
156. Withdrawn
157. Other* play
158. Plays infant games (e.g., pat-a-cake)
159. Solitary play
160. Parallel play
161. Cooperative play
162. Additional comments*

*Oral/Motor*

Number Comments

*List or specify in comments section.

From Smith, MH, Connolly P, McFadden S, et al. Developmental feeding tool. In: Smith MH, ed. *Feeding Management for Child with a Handicap: A Guide for Professionals*. Memphis, TN: Boling Child Development Center, University of Tennessee Center for the Health Sciences; 1982. Used with permission.

**Table 24–3.** Cincinnati Children's Hospital Medical Center Strategies for Identification and Intervention of Oral-Motor Problems

| Reflex | Diagnosis | Stimulation Mechanics |
|---|---|---|
| Gag | 1. Walk tongue blade to back tongue until tongue bumps/elicit gag. | 1. When spoon feeding, apply gentle pressure on tongue with spoon.<br>2. Place spoon lateral to tongue. |
| Suck | 1. Place pacifier or finger in mouth. Lips should close around it with strong suction applied. | 1. Offer pacifier dipped in cold fruit juice/formula.<br>2. Experiment with various nipple types.<br>3. Use gloved finger to stimulate by pushing gently downward on tongue to encourage initiation of sucking.<br>4. Encourage use of straw; use cold liquids. |
| Swallow | 1. Offer drink of water (observe for initiation of swallowing; observe for signs of gagging, coughing, wet vocalizations<br>2. Modified barium swallow. If there is concern regarding swallowing, check positioning, develop tongue control. | 1. Ensure good positions and alignment.<br>2. Keep head stable and in a downward position/chin tuck.<br>3. Position cup centrally; use other hand under chin to apply gentle upward pressure to minimize fluid loss.<br>4. Offer cold/sour items (e.g., lemon ice). |
| Tongue thrust | 1. Use pretzel stick or small tongue blade dipped in fruit; can also use pretzel stick if bite reflex is not overdeveloped. Place in mouth and observe.<br>2. Tongue section will push out solid food placed on anterior third of tongue. | 1. Vibrate (carefully) under tongue on either side of frenulum with pretzel stick.<br>2. Place foods in corners of mouth between teeth<br>3. (a) When spoon feeding, use spoon with shallow bowl (small amounts of food); (b) when spoon is placed in mouth, produce a slight downward pressure on tongue with spoon.<br>4. Use jaw control activities at noneating times. |
| Tongue lateralization | 1. *Place peanut butter/cream cheese at corners of mouth/in cheeks and ask patient to lick mouth. | 1. Press against lateral sides of tongue with tongue blade or use popsicle stick several times ½ to 1 hour before feeding time.<br>2. Play games—make faces, lick peanut butter, or lick ice cream cone.<br>3. Exercise tongue—place gauze on tongue and use fingers to gently move tongue.<br>4. Place food over lateral molars to encourage tongue lateralization. |
| Tongue elevation | 1. *Place peanut butter at center of upper lip and ask patient to lick mouth. | 1. Using a small, soft brush, tongue blade, or pacifier, touch roof of mouth.<br>2. Play games—make faces, lick peanut butter, or lick ice cream cone. |
| Bite | 1. Overreactive: strong clamping on the feeding spoon.<br>2. Underreactive: drooling. | 1. Stimulate the gums to stimulate bite reflex (use index finger or ear swab).<br>2. Offer cracker, bread, or vegetables in pieces that do not fit into the mouth unless bitten off. |
| Loose (slack) jaw | 1. Place small pieces of cracker between molars.<br>2. Observe chewing action for rotary movement. | 1. Using fingers, vibrate over zygotic arch, near frontal ear lobe.<br>2. Use hands to guide jaw up and inward while child chews.<br>3. Have child imitate adult while feeling adult's jaw.<br>4. Use jaw control technique when child is a passive player. |
| Stable jaw—poor action | 1. Place small pieces of cracker between molars.<br>2. Observe chewing action for rotary movements. | 1. Using fingers, vibrate masseters.<br>2. Introduce firm foods gradually; start with well-cooked to soft-raw foods (easily dissolved crunchy foods).<br>3. Have child imitate adult while feeling adult's jaw. |
| Chewing | 1. Observe chewing for rotary motion—not loose vertical motion. | 1. Massage gums with index finger before feeding.<br>2. Have child imitate adult while feeling adult's jaw.<br>3. Play games before mirror: yawn, blow kisses.<br>4. Foods: progress slowly from well-cooked to raw (easily dissolved, crunchy foods) |
| Finger feeding | 1. Serve thin slices of fresh, peeled fruits and vegetables.<br>2. Serve cubes of cheese.<br>3. Serve crackers/various shapes. | 1. Play with stacking toys.<br>2. Play pegboards, push-pull toys, and pointing games (nose, eyes, ears, etc.).<br>3. Pour water or sand from cup to cup.<br>4. Hand-over-hand techniques. |
| Cup drinking | 1. Offer drink of water and observe: (a) cup should rest on lower lip, not teeth; (b) upper lip should close over cup rim. | 1. Begin with weighted cup with handles and progress to plastic cup without handles.<br>2. Stand behind child and use hand to close lower jaw. |
| Spoon feeding | 1. Offer applesauce/mashed potatoes/yogurt in bowl and observe: does spoon turn over or reach the mouth in the upright position? | 1. Offer foods that stay on the spoon: cooked cereal, mashed potatoes, puddings/custards, squash (cooked and mashed), or sweet potatoes.<br>2. Work from behind child when assisting him/her in grasping and using spoon, hand-over-hand technique.<br>3. Do not let spoon touch teeth. |
| Drooling | 1. Accompanies poor swallowing reflex and/or jaw control. | 1. Use jaw control actions at feeding and nonfeeding times—provide gentle input to lower jaw anteriorly.<br>2. Stimulate swallowing reflex. |

*May not use this technique in some children with cerebral palsy.

suggestions addressed to oral-motor problems. The reluctance may stem from concern about a change that may result in decreased food intake and subsequent weight loss. In the adult, reluctance to follow intervention suggestions may be associated with individual choice or preference and caregiver perception. The Dietary Reference Intakes (DRIs) promulgated by the National Academy of Science[21] are not always applicable because of differences in physical development, growth rate, and activity level. See Table 18–3 in Chapter 18 for a list of recommended energy needs for children with Down syndrome, cerebral palsy, Prader-Willi syndrome, and spina bifida or myelomeningocele. This information can be used in planning feeding interventions for children with these syndromes.

Assessment of eating and mealtime activities should result in individualized interventions related to texture and consistency of food and liquids, eating position, oral motor and swallowing skills, environmental and behavioral factors, and the level of assistance needed to keep the person safe during eating.[2] Terminology and methods of modifying the texture and consistency of foods and liquids may vary across health care settings and among health care professionals.[22,23] Dietitians and nutritionists need to stay abreast of current standards and issues in implementation of dysphagia diets such as the National Dysphagia Diet (Box 24–3). Thickened liquids can be prescribed for people who are at risk for aspiration.[23] Thickening agents are also used to stabilize the liquid in certain foods, such as soups and pureed fruit. People receiving thickened liquids need increased monitoring for adequate fluid intake. People who are nonverbal may be at risk of dehydration due to inability to ask for liquids. Education and training of the patient, the family, and/or care providers on all aspects of feeding and eating assistance is essential to ensure adequate and safe intake of food and fluids.[22]

Another important nutritional consideration is medication and its impact on appetite, elimination, and nutrient utilization. Many children and adults with IDD take medications that may cause increased or depressed appetite, nausea, mouth dryness, dental problems, gastrointestinal irritation, constipation or diarrhea, and weight change. Anticonvulsant medications may interfere with the absorption of vitamins and minerals.[24] Timing of meals or certain foods in relation to medication needs to be considered, as does method of administration when the person has swallowing problems.

## Tube Feeding

Children with severe feeding problems that interfere with growth and are the result of malabsorption, failure to thrive, or hypermetabolism may require enteral support, either orally or in the form of tube feeding.[25] Increasing numbers of children who have gastroesophageal reflux may require fundoplication surgery accompanied by a gastrostomy to provide adequate nutrition[26–30] (see Chapter 35). Formula selection for tube feeding depends on caloric density, nutrient composition and source, digestibility, osmolality, viscosity, accessibility, taste, and cost.

All of these factors are influenced by the age and clinical needs of the child or adolescent (see Appendix 9) and are equally applicable

**Box 24–3.** The National Dysphagia Diet: Key Food Highlights

The National Dysphagia Diet (NDD) was created to set standard terminology for a progressive diet to be used nationally in the treatment of dysphagia. The NDD requires specification of both the diet consistency and liquid viscosity. The NDD diet levels require customization to the patients' individual preferecnes and ablilities.

*Dysphagia Pureed (NDD 1)*

This diet consists of smooth pureed, homogeneous, and cohesive foods, requiring little to no chewing. Foods should be "pudding-like."

- Avoid gelatin, fruited yogurt, unblenderized cottage cheese, peanut butter, and any food with lumps, including hot cereal and soup.
- Avoid scrambled, fried, or hard-boiled eggs; soufflés are allowed.
- Mashed potatoes should be served with gravy, butter, margarine, or sour cream.
- Pre-gelled, slurried breads are allowed.
- ***Dysphagia Mixed:*** This Inova Mount Vernon Hospital diet is a customized pureed diet with one mechanically altered item. That item will not be meat or large entrees such as spaghetti with meat sauce. The diet is used within the hospital setting only.

*Dysphagia Mechanically Altered (NDD 2)*

This level consists of foods that are moist, soft-textured, and easily formed into a bolus, requiring some chewing; moist, tender ground or finely diced meats; soft tender-cooked vegetables; soft ripe or canned fruits; and slightly moistened dry cereal with little texture. No bread, dry cake, rice, cheese cubes, corn, or peas is allowed.

- Meats should be ground or minced no larger than ¼ inch pieces and moistened with gravy or sauce.
- Canned fruit is allowed (except pineapple, which is stringy); cooked fruits and fresh banana are allowed. Avoid skins, dried fruits, coconut, and seeds.
- Scrambled, poached, and soft-cooked eggs are allowed.
- Cooked vegetables should be less than ½ inch in size and fork mashable.
- ***Mechanical Soft:*** This diet allows the same foods as the mechanically altered diet but also allows bread, cakes, and rice.

*Dysphagia Advanced (NDD 3)*

This level consists of foods that have almost regular textures, are generally soft, and easy to chew with the exception of very hard, sticky, or crunchy foods. It allows bread, rice, moist cakes, shredded lettuce, and tender, moist whole meats cut into bite-size pieces. It avoids hard fruits and vegetables, corn skins, nuts, and seeds.

*Liquid Consistency*

Spoon-thick
Honey-like
Nectar-like
Thin—Includes all beverages, such as water, ice, milk, milkshakes, juices, coffee, teas, sodas, carbonated beverages, and liquid supplements, as well as frozen desserts and gelatin.

Adapted from McCallum SL. The National Dysphagia Diet: implemented at a regional rehabilitation center and hospital system. *J Am Diet Assoc.* 2003; 103:381. Used with permission.

to adults with severe eating and swallowing problems. The transition from tube feeding to oral feeding can be achieved more easily if oral-motor and positioning treatments are initiated when the tube feeding is begun.[5] Such treatments are important to counteract the problems that necessitated the initiation of the tube feeding. Treatment for the oral-motor problem may include working on lip closure, tongue lateralization, sucking, and other aspects (see Tables 24–2 and 24–3 for treatment therapies). All oral-motor treatments should be carried out before the transition from tube to mouth feeding is made. Some programs approach this event aggressively, whereas others concentrate on a gradual transition to reintroduce oral feeding as a pleasant experience.

Two major nutrients need to be monitored during the weaning process: calories and fluids. The registered dietitian or nutritionist calculates energy and protein needs and sets up an exchange list for food and tube-feeding formulas. As the amount of food ingested by mouth increases, the amount of formula per tube may be decreased, especially if 100% of the fluid and 80% of the nutrient requirements are maintained. Successful transition from tube to oral feeding requires variable amounts of time to achieve. Parents and caregivers may become discouraged and may need a great deal of support from professionals working with them.[31] If problems in swallowing persist, a dysphagia diet with different levels of food texture and liquid consistency may be needed (see Box 24–3).

## Self-feeding

Self-feeding is defined as the willingness and ability to use a cup, fingers, or spoon to pick up a cracker or bite of cereal and bring it to the mouth.[32] The ability to self-feed may be limited because of muscle control problems. An array of adaptive eating utensils, cups, and plates exists to help overcome these limitations. Many types of spouted cups are available to help initiate the weaning process and encourage holding of the cup (a two-handled cup or one with no handles usually is preferred). A "nosy cup" or cutout cup may be helpful for someone who tilts his or her head back during the drinking process, which opens the airway and increases the risk for aspiration during swallowing. Spoons in many shapes and sizes are available to assist in moving from finger feeding to use of the spoon and in adapting to various motor issues. Nylon- and plastic-covered spoons are available for protecting the teeth and lips, as well as spoons that can be strapped onto the hand. Spoons and utensils for someone who has difficulty grasping may need built-up handles and Velcro slings to be positioned over the hand. Bowls and plates are also available in a variety of sizes and shapes to assist in self-feeding. Sides should be high to enable scooping, and the plate or bowl may require anchoring to the highchair, tray, or table with a nonslip substance such as a Dycem non-skid mat, clay, or suction cups. People with physical challenges may require some level of assistance to eat, but they should be encouraged to self-feed as much as possible to make eating a pleasant experience.

## Follow-up

After the initial assessment, the infant or child with special health care needs must be seen on a regular basis, either weekly or monthly, for treatment and monitoring of the feeding program. Anthropometric measures should be obtained on a regular basis, along with evaluation of the child's and family's reaction to the program. Close monitoring of growth and trends in the child's special health care needs can indicate the overall adequacy of energy intake and prevent weight loss.[17] The success of the feeding intervention is determined by the coordination of services between the home and the program (at school or in the developmental center) and inclusion of the parent or care provider as an active member of the feeding team. Coordination with agencies such as the WIC program or insurance programs in the provision of tube-feeding products and transportation to feeding appointments may be required. Developing good working relationships with individuals, families, and their personal support teams is crucial for obtaining positive outcomes.

Education and training are essential in all steps of implementing the feeding or eating plan, not just for the person but also for the family, care providers, educators, and other health care professionals.[17] Depending on the applicable state Medicaid and Medicaid waiver programs, community resources, and residential settings, follow-up services for adults may be available for needed implementation, training and monitoring of eating/mealtime interventions and related nutritional health outcomes. Dietitian nutritionists practicing in the field of IDD need to be knowledgeable about funding sources and coverage of nutrition services by individual state and private payment programs.

Tables 24–1 through 24–3 and Boxes 24–1 are taken from Ekvall SW, Ekvall VK. *Pediatric Nutrition in Chronic Diseases and Developmental Disorders: Prevention, Assessment, and Treatment,* 2nd Edition. Oxford: Oxford University Press; 2005.

### References


1. Cloud HH. Nutrition services for children with developmental disabilities and special health care needs. *Top Clin Nutr*. 2001; 16:28.
2. Cushing P, Spear D, Geerts S, et al. *The Adult with Intellectual and Developmental Disabilities: A Resource Tool for Nutritional Professionals.* Chicago: Academy of Nutrition and Dietetics; 2008.
3. Rosenzweig LY. Serving the aging developmentally disabled population. *Top Clin Nutr*. 2008; 23:98.
4. Humphrey R. Feeding problems and the mother-infant relationship. In: Wolf L, ed. *Problems with Eating: Intervention for Children and Adults with Developmental Disabilities*. Rockville, MD: American Occupational Therapy Association; 1987.
5. Morris SE, Klein MD. *Pre-feeding Skills: A Comprehensive Resource for Mealtime Development*, 2nd ed. Tucson, AZ: Therapy Skill Builders; 2000.
6. Wolf L, Glass R. Functional anatomy and physiology of the suck/swallow/breathe triad, In: Wolf LS, Glass RP, eds. *Feeding and Swallowing Disorders in Infancy, Assessment and Management*. Tucson, AZ: Therapy Skill Builders; 1992.
7. Carruth BR, Skinner JD. Feeding behaviors and other motor development in healthy children (2–24 months). *J Am Coll Nutr*. 2002; 21:88.
8. Cloud HH. Developmental disabilities. In: Samour PQ, King K, eds. *Pediatric Nutrition*, 4th ed. Sudbury, MA: Jones & Bartlett Learning; 2012.
9. Lane S, Cloud HH. Feeding problems and intervention: an interdisciplinary approach. *Top Clin Nutr*. 1988; 3:23.
10. Fung EB, Samson-Fang L, Stallings VA, et al. Feeding dysfunction is associated with poor growth and health status in children with cerebral palsy. *J Am Diet Assoc*. 2002; 102:361.
11. Waterman ET, Koltai PJ, Downey JC, Cacace AT. Swallowing disorders in a population of children with cerebral palsy. *Int J Pediatr Otorhinolaryngol*. 1992; 24:63.
12. Ball SL, Patner SG, Redley M. The extent and nature of need for mealtime support among adults with intellectual disabilities. *J In. Dis Res Rev*. 2012; 56:382.
13. Chadwick DD, Jolliffe J. A descriptive investigation of dysphagia in adults with intellectual disabilities. *Int Dis Res Rev*. 2009; 53:118.
14. Anderson DM. Nutrition for premature infants. In: Samour PQ, Helm KK, Lang C, eds. *Pediatric Nutrition*, 4th ed. Sudbury, MA: Jones & Bartlett Learning; 2012.
15. Blissett J, Harris G. A behavioral intervention in a child with a feeding problem. *J Hum Nutr Diet*. 2000; 15:255.
16. Smith, MH, Connolly P, McFadden S, et al. Developmental feeding tool. In: Smith MH, ed. *Feeding Management of the Child with a Handicap*. Memphis, TN: Boling Child Development Center, University of Tennessee Center for Health Sciences; 1982.
17. Ptomey LT, Wittenbrook W. Position of the Academy of Nutrition and Dietetics: nutrition services for individuals with intellectual and developmental disabilities and special health care needs. *J Acad Nutr Diet*. 2015; 115;593.
18. Cushing P, Spear D, Novak P, et. al. Academy of Nutrition and Dietetics: standards of practice and standards of professional performance for registered dietitians (competent, proficient, and expert) in intellectual and developmental disabilities. *J Acad Nutr Diet*. 2012; 112;1454.
19. Steward L. Development of nutrition and swallowing check list, a screening tool for nutrition and swallowing risk in people with intellectual disability. *J Int Dev Dis*. 2003; 28:171.
20. Brody RA, Touger-Decker R, VonHagen S, Maillet JD. Role of registered dietitians in dysphagia screening. *J Am Diet Assoc*. 2000; 100:1029.
21. National Research Council Food and Nutrition Board. *Recommended Dietary Allowances*, 10th ed. Washington, DC: National Academy of Sciences Press; 1989.
22. New York State Office for People with Developmental Disabilities. *Choking Prevention Training Resources*. http://www.opwdd.ny.gov/opwdd_careers_training/training_opportunities/choking_prevention_training_resources. Accessed June 20, 2016
23. National Dysphagia Diet Task Force, American Dietetic Association. *National Dysphagia Diet: Standardization for Optimal Care*. Chicago: American Dietetic Association; 2002.
24. Pronsky ZM, ed. *Food and Medication Interactions*, 17th ed. Birchrunville, PA: Food-Medication Interactions; 2012.
25. Wadie GM, Lobe TE. Gastroesophageal reflux disease in neurologically impaired children: the role of the gastrostomy tube. *Semin Laparosc Surg*. 2002; 9:180.
26. Stevenson RD. Measurement of growth in children with developmental disabilities. *Dev Med Child Neurol*. 1996; 38:855.
27. Stallings VA, Zemel BS, Davies JC, Cronk CE, Charney EB. Energy expenditure of children and adolescents with severe disabilities: a cerebral palsy model. *Am J Clin Nutr*. 1996; 64:627.
28. Isaacs JS, Georgeson KE, Cloud HH, Woodall N. Weight gain and triceps skinfold fat mass after gastrostomy placement in children with developmental disabilities. *J Am Diet Assoc*. 1994; 94:849.

29. Cowin DS, Isaacs JS, Georgeson KE, Bartolucci AA, Cloud HH, Craig CB. Weight and length changes in children after gastrostomy placement. *J Am Diet Assoc.* 1996; 96:874.
30. Lewis G, Ekvall S, Ekvall V. Neurologic handicapping conditions. In: *Nutrition Support Practice Manual.* Silver Spring, MD: American Society for Parenteral and Enteral Nutrition; 1998.
31. Dunitz-Scheer M, Levine A, Roth Y, et al. Prevention and treatment of tube dependency in infancy and early childhood. *Infant Child Adolesc Nutr.* 2009; 1:73.
32. Boehme R. Significant aspects of self-feeding. In: *Problems with Eating: Intervention for Children and Adults with Developmental Disorders.* Rockville, MD: American Occupational Therapy Association; 1987.

# 25 Cleft Lip and Cleft Palate

HOWARD M. SAAL

Cleft lip occurring either with or without cleft palate (CL/P) and cleft palate by itself (CP) are among the most common birth defects. These orofacial clefts result from incomplete merging and fusion of embryonic processes during formation of the face.[1,2] The annual incidence of CL/P in the United States between 2004 and 2006 was 1 in 940 live births; for CP in the same time period, the incidence was 1 in 1574 live births.[3] Microforms of orofacial clefts are also known to occur, the best example being submucous CP. In this condition, there is incomplete fusion of the muscular layers of the velum (soft palate) with fusion of the overlying mucosa. In children and adults with submucous CP, the clinical features are highly variable, ranging from an isolated clinical finding of bifid uvula to severe difficulties of speech (hypernasality) and of feeding, often with attendant chronic otitis media.[4] Orofacial clefts are classified by anatomic involvement. They include unilateral cleft lip, bilateral cleft lip, midline cleft lip, cleft lip with cleft palate (usually indicating involvement of both the primary and secondary palates), and cleft palate secondary to Pierre Robin sequence[1,5] (Figs. 25–1, 25–2, and 25–3).

Hundreds of disorders have been associated with orofacial clefts, including both genetic and teratogenic conditions. The authoritative catalog, Online Mendelian Inheritance in Man, lists 747 single gene disorders that are associated with CL/P or CP.[6] Among the most common causes of cleft palate is the Pierre Robin sequence. This specifically refers to disruption of normal elevation and fusion of the palatal shelves secondary to micrognathia and a posteriorly placed tongue[1] (Fig. 25–2). Like all orofacial clefts, Pierre Robin sequence can be caused by multiple underlying disorders.[7]

Lip and palate development occurs between 5 and 10 weeks' gestation. Lip development typically begins at 5 weeks' gestation with rapid proliferation of the maxillary prominences, which leads to nasal, cheek, and upper lip formation, including formation of the maxillary incisors. This development extends to the incisive foramen,[1] completing the primary palate. The secondary palate extends back from the incisive foramen and includes the hard and soft palates. Fusion of the palate is completed by 10 weeks' gestation.[1]

## INCIDENCE

In the United States between the years 2004 and 2005, approximately 4437 infants with CL/P were born annually.[3] The incidence of CL/P varies depending on ethnicity, gender, and socioeconomic factors. Native Americans have the highest reported prevalence at birth, with 3.6 CL/P cases per 1000 births. Asians have the second highest prevalence, with 2.1 cases per 1000 Japanese births and 1.7 cases per 1000 Chinese live births.[8] Gender also plays a role in the etiology of CL/P because males predominate by a 2:1 ratio.[5] In contrast, CP occurs equally across all racial and ethnic groups.

In nonsyndromic CL/P, unilateral clefts are more common than bilateral ones (Figs. 25–1 and 25–2). Among cases of unilateral CL/P, there is a predominance of left-sided clefts. The ratio of left-sided to right-sided to bilateral CL/P is 6:3:1. Boys are more likely than girls to be born with CL/P, with a 3:2 ratio.[3]

## GENETIC AND ENVIRONMENTAL FACTORS

CP and CL/P are etiologically distinct conditions. In both, it is essential to distinguish between syndromic and nonsyndromic (isolated) cases. Approximately 50% of children with CP (including those with Pierre Robin sequence) and 30% of those with CL/P have an underlying syndrome or multiple anomalies.[5,9] Nonsyndromic CL/P and CP are probably best described as orofacial clefts that occur in the absence of any other underlying genetic disorders or major malformations.[10] Isolated CL/P and CP are inherited as multifactorial conditions, meaning that the condition is caused by both genetic predisposition and nongenetic maternal and fetal environmental factors.[11] These factors may include alterations in nutrition, in utero exposures (including viral illnesses), use of tobacco or alcohol products, and others yet to be defined.[12–14] Fetal factors may include fetal crowding or changes in umbilical blood flow. There have been many studies of the role of maternal folic acid supplementation in both causation and prevention of orofacial clefts.[15–19] Other associated risk factors include maternal smoking, especially in the presence of specific genotypes, alcohol use, anticonvulsant use, and some maternal illnesses.[12,15,20,21]

The role of genetic factors in CL/P and CP is further underscored by the racial differences noted within specific populations. The recurrence risk for a family that has had one child with orofacial cleft or for an individual with an orofacial cleft is between 3% and 5% with each pregnancy. These recurrence risks are greater for families with increased numbers of affected individuals; for example, a family with two affected children has a 5% to 10% recurrence risk.

Several genes have been implicated as possibly predisposing to isolated CL/P and CP, including transforming growth factor-α (*TGFA*), transforming growth factor-β3 (*TGFB3*), *MSX1*, and *TFAP2A*, which encodes the transcription factor AP-2α.[14] Mutations in *IRF6*, the gene that encodes interferon regulatory factor-6, have been shown to cause Van der Woude syndrome, the most common inherited syndrome associated with orofacial clefts, and popliteal pterygium syndrome, which has also been identified as a cause of nonsyndromic CL/P.[22]

All studies performed to date have documented that several genes predispose to isolated multifactorial CL/P and CP, and no single gene predominates. If mutations of a single gene caused most cases of isolated CL/P or CP, the expected recurrence risks would be 25% in autosomal recessive inheritance and 50% in autosomal dominant inheritance. However, with a recurrence risk in the range of 3% to 5%, it is clear that other genes must play a causative role. There are approximately 19,000 human protein-coding genes,[23] many of which are involved in craniofacial development. This underscores the need to look at craniofacial development, especially with respect to the lip and palate, as a complex developmental process requiring the spatial and temporal interactions of multiple genetic and nongenetic factors.

## MATERNAL NUTRITION

Just as a great deal of work has been done in identifying the genes that predispose to orofacial clefts, much effort has been made to identify nongenetic factors that are also important in the etiology of oral facial

A

B

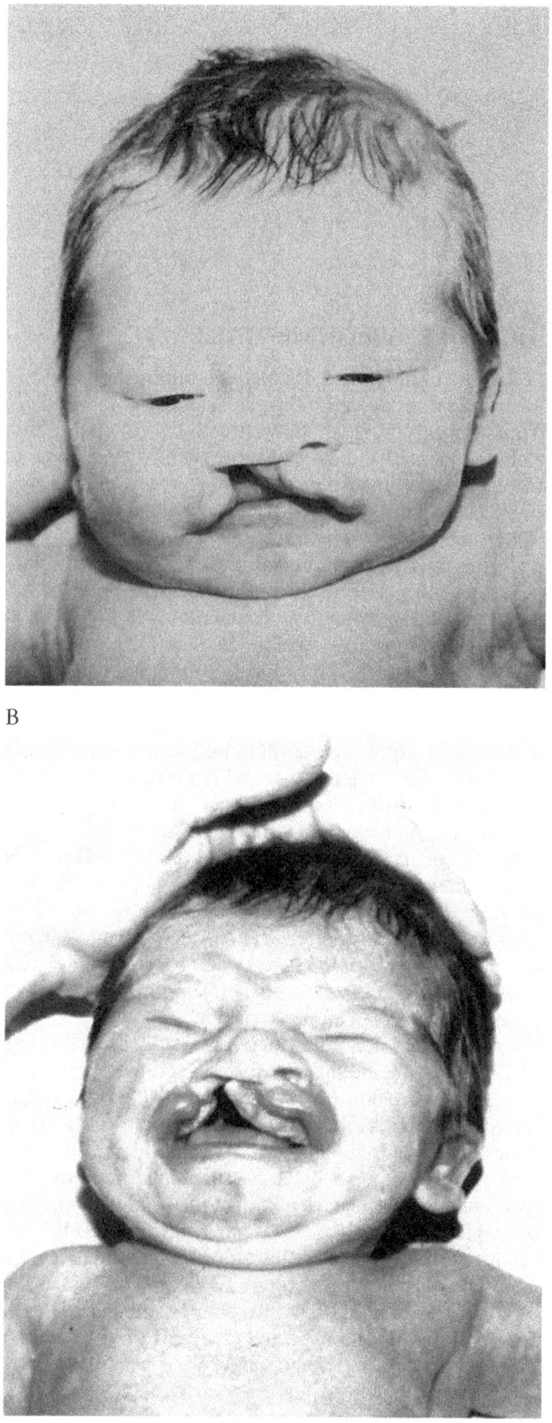

**Figures 25-1.** A and B, A male infant with isolated unilateral complete cleft lip and cleft palate. Notice the nasal deformity and the deformity of the alveolus secondary to normal muscular forces. (Courtesy of Howard Saal, MD, Division of Human Genetics, Cincinnati Children's Hospital Medical Center, Cincinnati, OH.)

clefts and appear to modify the effects the genetic factors. Probably the best-studied nutrient is folic acid. It has been clearly documented that women who take folic acid before conception and during early gestation dramatically decrease their risk of having a child with a neural tube defect.[16–19,24] The exact mechanism by which folic acid decreases this risk is not known. One possible mechanism is that elevated levels of folic acid may be needed in women who have a known variant of the gene for the enzyme methylene tetrahydrofolate reductase

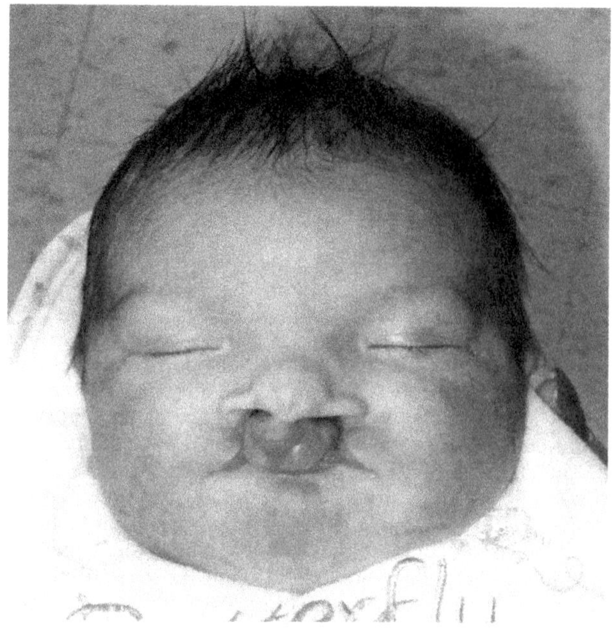

**Figure 25–2.** A female infant with bilateral cleft lip and cleft palate. The cleft lip causes a flattened nasal bridge. She also has hypertelorism (increased interorbital distance). (Courtesy of Howard Saal, MD, Division of Human Genetics, Cincinnati Children's Hospital Medical Center, Cincinnati, OH.)

(*MTHFR*). This thermolabile variant of *MTHFR* is caused by a base substitution at nucleotide 677, from cytosine to thymine.[25,26] In one study from Ireland, 98 children with CL/P and 848 control infants were tested for this thermolabile variant. The children with CL/P were significantly more likely to be homozygous for the C677T variant of *MTHFR* compared with the control population (odds ratio, 2.06; $P = .02$), and similar findings were reported for the CP-only group (odds ratio, 3.23; $P = .02$).[27] One meta-analysis showed a decreased risk for having a child with orofacial clefts among women who took multivitamins early in pregnancy.[28] However, in the most recent review and meta-analysis, although the use of periconceptional folic acid and other supplements played a role in prevention of neural tube defects,

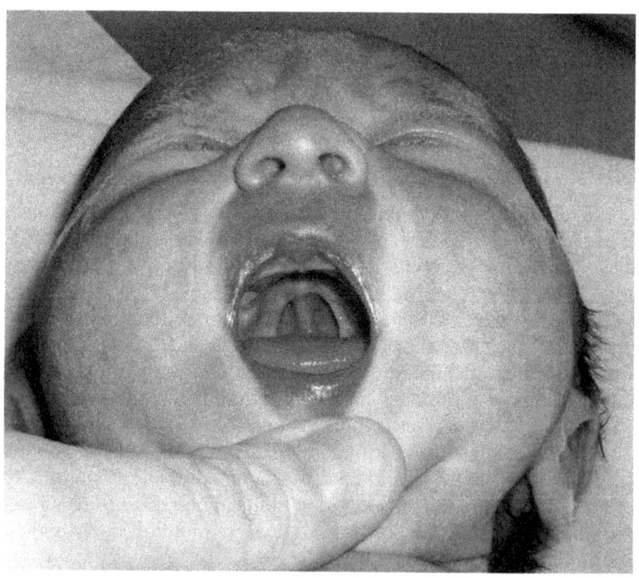

**Figure 25–3.** A male infant with a cleft palate. This child has Pierre Robin sequence, and the cleft is U-shaped. (Courtesy of Howard Saal, MD, Division of Human Genetics, Cincinnati Children's Hospital Medical Center, Cincinnati, OH.)

there was no evidence for prevention of other birth defects, including CL/P or CP.[29]

Animal studies have demonstrated possible protective effects of vitamin $B_6$ (pyridoxine) against teratogen-induced oral clefts. There are several potential pathways by which pyridoxine may protect against oral clefts. Pyridoxine supplementation reduced the occurrence of corticosteroid-induced oral clefts in mice. When the diet of certain strains of mice was depleted of vitamin $B_6$, there was an increased incidence of isolated oral clefts in 20% of offspring; this rose to more than 60% when deoxypyridoxine (a vitamin $B_6$ antagonist) or cortisone was administered to the pyridoxine-deficient mothers. It should be noted that corticosteroid-induced oral clefting in mice is strain dependent, suggesting that the protective effects of vitamin $B_6$ may depend on a genotype.

## TERATOGENIC CAUSES

Multiple teratogens that are known to cause orofacial clefts; however, these substances typically cause other congenital anomalies as well. Several studies have shown an association between maternal cigarette smoking and orofacial clefts. A meta-analysis found that the overall odds ratio for CL/P was 1.29 and that for CP was 1.32, indicating a weak association between maternal smoking and orofacial clefts.[13] Children with fetal alcohol syndrome also have a much higher risk for orofacial clefts. A study of the Iowa State Birth Defects Registry showed that there was a slightly statistically significant increase in risk of having offspring with CL/P among women who had more than 10 alcoholic drinks per month (odds ratio, 4.0; 95% confidence interval, 1.1 to 15.1). No significant odds ratios were recorded for lower-consumption groups (4–10 drinks per month), and there was no significantly increased risk of CP.[31]

Anticonvulsants have also been associated with CL/P and CP, one example being phenytoin. Children exposed prenatally to phenytoin who have oral clefts appear to have a higher incidence of other birth defects as well. Valproic acid is another potent teratogen. Several studies have shown that, in addition to causing neural tube defects, valproic acid is associated with increased risk for CP, metopic suture synostosis, and developmental disabilities.[20,32] Lamotrigine is a newer-generation anticonvulsant that has been associated with CP.[33]

Some maternal illnesses, including diabetes, are associated with an increased risk for having a child with an orofacial cleft. Diabetic embryopathy can be associated with a wide range of birth defects, including cardiovascular malformations, brain anomalies, vertebral anomalies, and renal anomalies in addition to orofacial clefts. In a Canadian epidemiologic study, the incidence of malformations seen in in women with prepregnancy diabetes was 93.4 per 1000 live births, compared with 41.5 per 1000 live births in women who did not have prepregnancy diabetes.[34] The odds ratio for having a child with an orofacial cleft was 2.48 for women with type 1 diabetes mellitus and 2.77 for women with type 2 diabetes mellitus.[34]

## FACTORS TO BE CONSIDERED IN NUTRITIONAL EVALUATION AND MANAGEMENT

The immediate action to take when a child is born with an orofacial cleft is to reassure the parents that the child can be fed an adequate diet. Unfortunately, breast-feeding is almost never successful in children with orofacial clefts (the exception being some cases of cleft lip). Many women decide to express breast milk, and this should be encouraged. Because children with CL/P or CP tend to swallow excess air, they should be burped frequently to diminish the risk of reflux, emesis, and colic.

In a study of parents who had a child with an orofacial cleft, the main concerns identified were feeding success, the possibility of airway obstruction, and normal development. The issues most frequently addressed in this study were (1) use of proper medical terminology for cleft lip and cleft palate; (2) discussion of feeding issues and interventions; (3) demonstration of special CP bottles and nipples; (4) explanation of the normal aspects of the physical examination; (5) addressing the cause of the orofacial cleft and alleviating guilt; (6) reassurance that the child was not in pain or discomfort; (7) review of the signs and symptoms of illness, such as choking and airway obstruction; and (8) arranging for appropriate follow-up appointments with specialists who can address important issues at the appropriate times of development.[35]

The initial feeding problem in children with orofacial clefts is insufficient suction. For nutritive sucking, negative pressure must be held in the mouth while the nipple is pressed; a defect in the palate makes this impossible for children with orofacial clefts. In most centers, attention is focused on the use of specialized bottles and nipples for feeding. Regular nipples can also be used, but often the opening of the nipple must be enlarged for adequate flow of breast milk or formula. Under most circumstances, children with CL/P or CP are unlikely to breast-feed successfully. A trial of breast-feeding may be offered for a short time (24 hours), but adequate fluid intake and potential dehydration must be very closely monitored. If breast-feeding is unsuccessful, breast pumping and nonnutritive sucking should be encouraged. The primary goal of feeding any child should be to ensure adequate nutrition and fluid intake.

There are many approaches to feeding an infant with an orofacial cleft, and these should be individualized to the needs of the infant. Gavage feeding is almost never necessary in a child with an isolated CL/P or CP. It is more commonly needed in children with Pierre Robin sequence who have some respiratory difficulty or obstruction during feeding. Children with underlying genetic disorders, especially those with neurological difficulties and abnormal oral facial tone, may have more significant feeding difficulties and may require gavage feeding. Children with isolated multifactorial CL/P or CP can follow normal schedules for initiating solids; they should not be treated any differently from children who do not have orofacial clefts. In some centers, surgeons prefer that children stop bottle feeding after cleft lip or cleft palate surgery for a predetermined period. Drinking from a cup may be encouraged before palate closure. In most centers, lip repair is performed at approximately 3 months of age and palate repair at 9 months.

### Growth

Because there are numerous concerns with regard to feeding and nutrition in children with orofacial clefts, growth may be an issue for these children. Older studies showed lower mean weight gain per week in infants with CL/P compared with matched controls.[36] One study found that girls born with orofacial clefts were shorter than controls and boys with orofacial clefts were taller than controls after 3 years.[37] However, these studies did not control for syndromic CL/P and CP. A more recent study looking at growth of infants with isolated CL/P and CP found that weight and growth percentiles decreased during the first year of life but not to a clinically significant extent, and this was followed by statistically significant recovery. No child demonstrated failure to thrive.[38]

Children with orofacial clefts should be monitored closely by their primary care physician and by the cleft palate team with regard to growth and development. Children who demonstrate any signs of failure to thrive should be evaluated for adequate nutritional intake as well as the possibility that there may be other health-related conditions including underlying syndromes. Growth disturbance in most children with orofacial clefts can be avoided with adequate feeding instruction for the family, use of appropriate bottles, and close follow-up.

### Treatment

Treatment for CL/P and CP is primarily directed toward nutrition, growth, and family support. Children should be managed at centers that offer a multidisciplinary approach to the treatment of orofacial clefts and other craniofacial disorders. In the United States and Canada, information on such centers is available from the Cleft Palate Foundation via their Cleftline (www.cleftline.org). Management of the infant with orofacial clefts involves primarily experienced pediatricians, clinical geneticists, plastic surgeons, pediatric dentists, otolaryngologists, nutritionists, and audiologists. As the child gets older, there is a need for evaluation and treatment by speech pathologists and psychologists. Standards for comprehensive management of children with CL/P, CP, and other craniofacial conditions have been delineated by the American Cleft Palate-Craniofacial Association.[39]

The initial focus of management for a newborn infant with an orofacial cleft is appropriate management of feeding. This is usually best accomplished with the use of special bottles that allow the person feeding the child to squeeze formula into the child's mouth to overcome the lack of negative pressure needed for normal sucking. Children with isolated CL/P or CP should reach their birth weight by age 2 weeks. It is often important to involve a dietitian in the management of an infant with an orofacial cleft in order to assess appropriate caloric intake and, in some cases, assist with caloric supplementation.

The other factor in early management for a child with orofacial cleft is to work closely with the family and provide appropriate support. Having a child with an obviously visible birth defect can be devastating to a family. Although most of these children have an excellent prognosis, helping families overcome their guilt and their grieving is an essential component of early management.

## Follow-up and Summary

Feeding a child with an orofacial cleft requires an individualized approach. Use of special bottles is encouraged, but this must be accompanied by appropriate instruction and support for the parents and close follow-up of infant growth and development. Every child with an orofacial cleft should be monitored by a craniofacial team or cleft palate team. The child's parents and the pediatrician or family physician are important members of this team. Growth parameters should be assessed every 3 months during the first year of life and every 6 months thereafter.

Women who are contemplating pregnancy should be encouraged to take a multivitamin with folic acid before conception and during pregnancy because of the known positive benefits in preventing neural tube defects and possibly orofacial clefts.

### References


1. Sperber GH, Sperber SM, Guttmann GD. *Craniofacial Embryogenetics and Development*. Shelton, CT: People's Medical Publishing House; 2010.
2. Centers for Disease Control and Prevention. *Facts about Cleft Lip and Cleft Palate*. http://www.cdc.gov/ncbddd/birthdefects/cleftlip.html. Accessed June 20, 2016.
3. Parker SE, Mai CT, Canfield MA, et al. Updated national birth prevalence estimates for selected birth defects in the United States, 2004–2006. *Birth Defects Res A Clin Mol Teratol*. 2010; 88:1008.
4. Nasser M, Fedorowicz Z, Newton JT, Nouri M. Interventions for the management of submucous cleft palate. *Cochrane Database Syst Rev*. 2008; (1):CD006703.
5. Tolarova MM, Cervenka J. Classification and birth prevalence of orofacial clefts. *Am J Med Genet*. 1998; 75:126.
6. McKusick-Nathans Institute of Genetic Medicine, Johns Hopkins University School of Medicine. *Online Mendelian Inheritance in Man (OMIM)*. http://www.ncbi.nlm.nih.gov/omim/?term=cleft+lip+and%2For+cleft+palat Accessed June 20, 2016.
7. Bookman LB, Melton KR, Pan BS, et al. Neonates with tongue-based airway obstruction: a systematic review. *Otolaryngol Head Neck Surg*. 2012; 146:8.
8. Croen LA, Shaw GM, Wasserman CR, Tolarova MM. Racial and ethnic variations in the prevalence of orofacial clefts in California, 1983–1992. *Am J Med Genet*. 1998; 79:42.
9. Jugessur A, Farlie PG, Kilpatrick N. The genetics of isolated orofacial clefts: from genotypes to subphenotypes. *Oral Dis*. 2009; 15:437.
10. Leslie EJ, Marazita ML. Genetics of cleft lip and cleft palate. *Am J Med Genet C Semin Med Genet*. 2013; 163C:246.
11. Stanier P, Moore GE. Genetics of cleft lip and palate: syndrome genes contribute to the incidence of non-syndromic clefts. *Hum Mol Genet*. 2004; 13:R73.
12. Shaw GM, Wasserman CR, Lammer EJ, et al. Orofacial clefts, parental cigarette smoking, and transforming growth factor-alpha gene variants. *Am J Hum Genet*. 1996; 58:551.
13. Schutte BC, Murray JC. The many faces and factors of orofacial clefts. *Hum Mol Genet*. 1999; 8:1853.
14. Rahimov F, Jugessur A, Murray JC. Genetics of nonsyndromic orofacial clefts. *Cleft Palate Craniofac J*. 2010; 49:73.
15. Shaw GM, Lammer EJ. Maternal periconceptional alcohol consumption and risk for orofacial clefts. *J Pediatr*. 1999; 134:298.
16. Butterworth CEJr, Bendich A. Folic acid and the prevention of birth defects. *Annu Rev Nutr*. 1996; 16:73.
17. Mills JL, Kirke PN, Molloy AM, et al. Methylenete-trahydrofolate reductase thermolabile variant and oral clefts. *Am J Med Genet*. 1999; 86:71.
18. Shaw GM, Todoroff K, Finnell RH, Rozen R, Lammer EJ. Maternal vitamin use, infant C677T mutation in MTHFR, and isolated cleft palate risk. *Am J Med Genet*. 1999; 85:84.
19. Werler MM, Hayes C, Shapiro S, Mitchell AA. Multivitamin supplementation and risk of birth defects. *Am J Epidemiol*. 1999; 150:675.
20. Wlodarczyk BJ, Palacios AM, George TM, Finnell RH. Antiepileptic drugs and pregnancy outcomes. *Am J Med Genet A*. 2012; 158A:2071.
21. Saal HM. The genetics evaluation and common craniofacial syndromes. In: Kummer AW, ed. *Cleft Palate and Craniofacial Anomalies: Effects on Speech and Resonance*, 2nd ed. Clifton Park, NY: Thomson Delmar Learning; 2008.
22. Schutte BC, Saal HM, Goudy S, et al. *IRF6-Related Disorders*. http://www.ncbi.nlm.nih.gov/books/NBK1407/. Accessed June 20, 2016.
23. Ezkurdia D, Juan JM, Rodriguez A, et al. Multiple evidence strands suggest that there may be as few as 19,000 human protein-coding genes. *Hum Mol Genet*. 2014; 23:5866.
24. Birnbacher R, Messerschmidt AM, Pollak AP. Diagnosis and prevention of neural tube defects. *Curr Opin Urol*. 2002; 12:461.
25. Shaw GM, Rozen R, Finnell RH, Todoroff K, Lammer EJ. Infant C677T mutation in *MTHFR*, maternal periconceptional vitamin use, and cleft lip. *Am J Med Genet*. 1998; 80:196.
26. Shaw GM, Todoroff K, Finnell RH, Rozen R, Lammer EJ. Maternal vitamin use, infant C677T mutation in *MTHFR*, and isolated cleft palate risk. *Am J Med Genet*. 1999; 85:84.
27. Mills JL, Kirke PN, Molloy AM, et al. Methylenete-trahydrofolate reductase thermolabile variant and oral clefts. *Am J Med Genet*. 1999; 86:71.
28. Johnson CY, Little J. Folate intake, markers of folate status and oral clefts: is the evidence converging? *Int J Epidemiol*. 2008; 37:1041.
29. De-Regil LM, Peña-Rosas JP, Fernández-Gaxiola AC, Rayco-Solon P. Effects and safety of periconceptional oral folate supplementation for preventing birth defects. *Cochrane Database Syst Rev*. 2015; (12):CD007950.
30. Jacobsson C, Granstrom G. Effects of vitamin B6 on beta-amino-propionitrile-induced palatal cleft formation in the rat. *Cleft Palate Craniofac J*. 1997; 34:95.
31. Munger RG, Romitti PA, Daack-Hirsch S, Burns TL, Murray JC, Hanson J. Maternal alcohol use and risk of orofacial cleft birth defects. *Teratology*. 1996; 54:27.
32. Meador KJ, Baker GA, Browning N, et al. Foetal antiepileptic drug exposure and verbal versus non-verbal abilities at three years of age. *Brain*. 2011; 134(Pt 2):396.
33. Holmes LB, Baldwin EJ, Smith CR, et al. Increased frequency of isolated cleft palate in infants exposed to lamotrigine during pregnancy. *Neurology*. 2008; 70(Pt 2):2152.
34. Liu S, Rouleau J, León JA, et al. Impact of pre-pregnancy diabetes mellitus on congenital anomalies, Canada, 2002–2012. *Health Promot Chronic Dis Prev Can*. 2015; 35:79.
35. Young JL, O'Riordan M. What information do parents of newborns with cleft lip, palate, or both want to know? *Cleft Palate Craniofac J*. 2001; 38:55.
36. Jones WB. Weight gain and feeding in the neonate with cleft: a three center study. *Cleft Palate J*. 1988; 25:379.
37. Felix-Schollaart B, Hoeksma JB, Prahl-Anderson B. Growth comparison between children with cleft lip and/or palate and controls. *Cleft Palate Craniofac J*. 1992; 29:475.
38. Zarate YA, Martin LJ, Hopkin RJ, Bender PL, Zhang X, Saal HM. Evaluation of growth in patients with isolated cleft lip and/or cleft palate. *Pediatrics*. 2010; 125:e543.
39. American Cleft Palate-Craniofacial Association. *Parameters for Evaluation and Treatment of Patients with Cleft Lip/Palate or Other Craniofacial Anomalies*. 2009. http://www.acpa-cpf.org/uploads/site/Parameters_Rev_2009.pdf.

# D.

# DRUGS

## 26 Use of Botanicals in Children and Adults

GAIL B. MAHADY, SHEILA M. WICKS, AND RUDOLF BAUER

Complementary and alternative medicine (CAM) use in the United States continues to grow, with about 75% of adults using some form of CAM therapy.[1,2] CAM includes exercise therapies (e.g., yoga); music therapies; mind-body interactions; manipulations (e.g., massage); hydrotherapy, and herbal medicines and dietary supplements.

CAM use in pediatric populations also continues to increase. Between 1% and 89% of children use some type of CAM therapy, including botanical dietary supplements (BDS), to treat a wide range of medical conditions.[1–3] Use of CAM therapies is prevalent among 20% to 40% of healthy children, 46% to 84% of children with cancer, 33% to 89% of children with asthma, 19% of children with diabetes, 44% of children with epilepsy, 49.6% of children with irritable bowel disease, and 54% of children with sickle cell disease.[1–3] More than 50% of children with rheumatoid arthritis, 50% to 75% of children with autism spectrum disorders, and about 33% of children with neurological disorders are reportedly using a wide range of CAM therapies, including BDS, which are also known as herbal medicinal products.[1] Results from CAM surveys have suggested that the use of CAM by parents and caretakers is the single best predictor of CAM use in children.[2]

In the United States, dietary and herbal supplements are one of the most commonly used forms of CAM, with annual sales in the range of $11.5 to $32.4 billion, of which BDS sales make up about $5.5 billion.[1–4] Surveys indicate that between 50% and 68% of the US population uses dietary supplements, and about 30% using BDS to treat or prevent a wide array of common ailments and diseases, including the common cold, depression, and other non–life-threatening medical conditions.[4,5] Approximately 72% of US adult women claim to use dietary supplements.[4] Because women make up the largest percentage of BDS users, it is not unexpected that many of these women also administer herbal medicines or BDS to their children. National and international surveys indicate that BDS administration to children is increasing, and it is estimated that between 22% and 89% of children are exposed to dietary supplements and herbal preparations for management of a wide range of acute and chronic ailments including asthma, anxiety, attention deficit hyperactivity disorders (ADHD), insomnia, and respiratory infections.[3,6]

Ethnic differences also play a role in the use of herbal and dietary supplements. One study reported much higher use of dietary supplements among Hispanic children compared with Caucasian children and further suggested that the number of supplements used in Hispanic children was also higher.[6]

Unfortunately, many of these treatments are never discussed with the child's attending pediatrician. Using the 2007 National Health Interview Survey data for individuals younger than 18 years of age ($N$ = 9417), Birdee and coworkers[3] compared CAM and BDS use in pediatric populations and examined independent associations of CAM use with sociodemographic factors, prescription medication use, delays in health care caused by access difficulties, and common medical conditions or symptoms. Children receiving CAM or BDS were more likely to be adolescents rather than infants or toddlers, to live in Western states, to have a parent with a college education, and to use prescription medication.[3] These pediatric patients were also more likely to have anxiety or stress, dermatologic conditions, musculoskeletal conditions, and sinusitis. Use of CAM by a parent was strongly associated with the child's use, and as in other studies, many of these treatments were never discussed with the pediatrician.[3] This trend presents both interesting opportunities and dilemmas for health care professionals and parents because many of these treatments have not been clinically tested for safety and efficacy in children. It further suggests that health care professionals must ask their patients about use of these therapies and, if possible, obtain a complete medical history that includes the use of dietary supplements and herbal medicines.

## FACTORS TO BE CONSIDERED IN EVALUATING HERBAL MEDICINES

In European countries such as Germany, numerous clinical investigations have focused on herbal medicine use in pediatric patients, whereas in the United States there is still very little clinical research being performed in this population. The reasons for this disparity lie in legal and regulatory issues. The German Drug Law for the approval and marketing of an herbal medicinal product (HMP) states that, in addition to sufficient justification of the efficacy, proof of safety (i.e., no negative effects beyond the measure acceptable according to current knowledge of medical science) is needed.[7] European companies are required to have data to demonstrate the safety and efficacy of herbal products before marketing them. In the United States, the Dietary Supplements Health and Education Act of 1994 classified botanicals (herbal preparations) as dietary supplements; as a consequence, most of the BDS on the US market have never been tested for safety or efficacy. Nevertheless, the media distribute information about efficacy without supporting documentation. Published research on dietary supplements is available, but much of the data is preclinical and not even translated into the English language. This is particularly concerning when it comes to the pediatric use of botanical products because there are still no US guidelines for the safe use of botanicals in pediatric populations.

BDS dosages are a concern because there are no guidelines that take age-dependent variations into account. One study indicated that adverse reactions to drug therapy were a significant cause of death and injury among infants and children younger than 2 years of age.[8] Feasible models for regulatory reform can be found in Europe, particularly Germany, where herbs and phytomedicines are accepted and integrated into medicine and pharmacy. According to European Union definitions, HMPs are "medicinal products containing as active ingredients exclusively plant material and/or vegetable drug preparations." Vegetable drugs are "plant material used for a medicinal purpose. An herbal drug or a preparation thereof is regarded as one active ingredient in its entirety whether or not the constituents with therapeutic activity are known."[9]

## MANAGEMENT

In Germany, recommended dosages for infants and children up to 16 years of age have been developed by the Kooperation Phytopharmaka (i.e., Cooperation on Phytopharmaceuticals), a private company that assesses the efficacy, safety, and quality of HMPs, taking into consideration body weight, body surface, and age. Recommended dosages for adults are developed by Commission E, a scientific advisory board that is the German equivalent of the US Food and Drug Administration. The recommendations are for single-entity herbal products.

Average values for body weight, height, and body surface are calculated for girls and boys in four age groups (0 to 1, 1–4, 4–10, and 10–16 years). The results are used to calculate dosages for each age group based on the recommendations for adults. These age-stratified calculations, as a theoretical statement, are supported by product-specific and representative surveys on the dosages applied in practice by doctors prescribing these medications to children and contribute to justifying the therapeutically optimum dosage for the various age groups before the German Health Authorities (Bundesinstitut für Arzneimittel und Medizinprodukte—BfArM). In 1998 and again in 2002, the Kooperation Phytopharmaka published *Kinderdosierungen von Phytopharmaka*, a handbook of pediatric dosage for single-entity herbal preparations.[10] This book currently is available only in the German language. A review of the use of HMPs in pediatrics was published by Schilcher in 1999 but this also is not available in English.

### Treatment and Safety

This chapter provides an overview of some of the more commonly used botanicals for which clinical studies on efficacy and safety for pediatric use are available. Botanicals include *Andrographis paniculata*, butterbur, cranberry, *Echinacea*, evening primrose oil, fennel, garlic, German chamomile, ivy leaf, thyme, and valerian (Table 26-1). These herbs have been extensively used in children, and they have a relatively high safety profile when used correctly.

A standardized 60% ethanol extract from the aerial parts of *Andrographis paniculata* containing 4% andrographolides, as well as other products, has shown efficacy in clinical studies and can be recommended for treatment and prevention of the common cold.[11–13] The daily dose depends on the product used.

Butterbur (*Petasites hybridus*) has been shown in randomized controlled clinical trials to be effective for the treatment of pediatric migraine.[14,15] The daily dose in these studies was 50 to 150 mg daily for 4 months of a specialized, semipurified extract from Europe. This is the only extract that has been shown to be effective in clinical studies.

Juice and extracts from cranberries (*Vaccinium macrocarpon*) are often used for prevention and symptomatic treatment of urinary tract infections (UTIs).[16–19] However, the data from controlled clinical trials are conflicting. Some studies performed in pediatric populations have suggested that cranberry ingestion does not reduce bacteriuria or symptomatic urinary tract infections,[18] whereas others showed a significant reduction in the risk of recurrent UTIs.[16,17,19] Cranberry products may not be useful for treatment of UTIs but may be of benefit as prophylaxis in children with recurrent UTIs. Some case studies have suggested an interaction of cranberry juice with warfarin.

Oral preparations of *Echinacea* (*E. purpurea*, *E. angustifolia*, and *E. pallida*) are frequently used to prevent and treat upper respiratory tract infections (URTIs) and UTIs. Data from clinical trials are conflicting; some suggest a reduction in the symptoms of URTIs in children, but, depending on the quality of the preparation and the mode of application, negative results also have been reported.[20–25] Echinacea administration was associated with a borderline increased risk of having at least one more episode of acute otitis media during 6-month follow-up, compared with placebo.[25] German Commission E monographs have indicated that *Echinacea* products should be avoided in patients with autoimmune disease because of their purported immune-stimulating effects.[9] They reported contraindications to the use of *Echinacea* that included progressive systemic diseases such as tuberculosis, leukosis, collagenosis, multiple sclerosis, acquired immunodeficiency syndrome (AIDS) or human immunodeficiency virus (HIV) infection, and other autoimmune diseases. Serious toxicities due to echinacea have not been reported. Echinacea preparations should not be administered to children who have allergies to members of the Asteraceae family (e.g., daisy, chamomile, ragweed).

Evening primrose (*Oenothera biennis*) seed oil (EPO) is rich in γ-linoleic acid and therefore is used for the treatment of atopic eczema, cyclic and noncyclic mastalgia, premenstrual syndrome, psoriasis, rheumatoid arthritis, chronic fatigue syndrome, and diabetic neuropathy.[26–31] Based on the results of clinical trials, EPO may have some benefit for the treatment of atopic dermatitis in children, but a relatively high dose (0.5 g/kg/day) is needed for a clinical response.[26,27,31] In clinical studies, EPO supplementation produced minimal or little improvement in hyperactive children.[28,29] However, it might have a preventive effect on diabetic vascular complications due to altered essential fatty acids and triglyceride metabolism.[30]

Fennel oil preparations (*Foeniculum vulgare* var. *vulgare*) are considered useful for mild spastic disorders of the gastrointestinal tract, feelings of fullness, and flatulence, as well as for catarrhs of the upper respiratory tract.[32] Clinical pediatric studies with fennel or its preparations are not yet available. The suggested dosages of crushed or ground seeds for teas, tea-like products, and other galenical preparations for internal use per day by age group are as follows: 0 to 1 year, 1 to 2 g;

**Table 26–1.** Clinical Studies with Commonly Used Botanicals in Children and Adults

| Herb | Therapeutic Use | Clinical Studies | | | | | | Ref. No. |
|---|---|---|---|---|---|---|---|---|
| | | Study Design | Target Parameter | Formulation | Cases | Dose/Duration | Outcome | |
| *Andrographis paniculata* Burm f. Nees, Acanthaceae | Treatment and prevention of common cold, influenza, other infectious diseases | RCT, double-blind study | Prophylaxis of common colds | Standardized extract of the aerial parts, 4% andrographolides | 107 school children | 200 mg/day for 3 mo | No difference after first or second month, but significant decrease in common colds after third month | 11 |
| *A paniculata* and *Eleuthrococcus* combination | Treatment of common cold | RCT, three parallel group study comparing an *Andrographis* combination with *Echinacea* | Adjunct treatment of common cold | Standardized *A. paniculata* extract, with Immunal, a preparation containing *Echinacea purpurea* | 130 children ages 4–11 yr | Standardized extract of *A. paniculata* and extract of *Eleuthrococcus senticosus*, 2 tablets tid | *Andrographis* significantly more effective than Immunal when started at an early stage of uncomplicated common cold | 12 |
| *A. paniculata* and *E. senticosus* | Acute respiratory viral infection | RCT | Efficacy in acute respiratory illness | Combination product containing *A. paniculata* and *E. senticosus* | 53 children | Same as above | Reduced symptoms of early acute uncomplicated respiratory disease | 13 |
| Butterbur: roots of *Petasites hybridus* | Migraine headache | Prospective, randomized, partly double-blind, placebo-controlled, parallel-group trial | Pediatric migraine | Butterbur root extract compared with music therapy | 58 primary school children (ages 8–12 yr) | 8 wk baseline, 12 wk treatment, 8 wk and 6 mo follow-up visits | Butterbur root extract and music therapy both superior to placebo in reducing migraine | 14 |
| Butterbur: roots of *P. hybridus* | Migraine headache | Two placebo-controlled, parallel-group, randomized trials | Migraine prevention in children and adolescents with severe migraines | Root extract | 289 children and adolescents | 50–150 mg/day for 4 mo | 77% of patients reported reduction in frequency of migraine attacks by ≥50%; attack frequency was reduced by 63% | 15 |
| Cranberry: fruits of *Vaccinium macrocarpon*, Ericaceae | Prevention and symptomatic treatment of UTI | Uncontrolled | Reduction of white and red blood cell counts and *Escherichia coli* cultures in the urine | Cranberry juice | 17 catheterized children with spina bifida | 1–3 glasses for 2 wk | Reduction of white and red blood cell counts in almost all urine samples; no reduction in *E. coli* cultures | 16 |
| Cranberry fruit juice | UTI | Randomized, placebo-controlled comparison study | Prevention of UTI recurrences | Cranberry juice contained 7.5 g cranberry concentrate and 1.7 g lingonberry concentrate in 50 mL water without added sugars | 84 girls (ages 3–14 yr) with recurrent UTIs | 50 mL/day cranberry versus *Lactobacillus* or placebo for 6 mo | Treatment with cranberry led to significant reduction in risk of repeated UTIs vs *Lactobacillus* or control | 17 |
| Cranberry fruit juice | UTI | RCT, double-blind, placebo-controlled | Prevention of UTI recurrences | Cranberry juice, containing 41 g cranberry concentrate, including flavoring, in 1 L of juice | 263 children (129 in cranberry group) | 5 mL/kg, up to 300 mL/day, of either cranberry juice or placebo in 1 or 2 daily doses for 6 mo | No significant reduction in number of children experiencing recurrence of UTI, but effective in reducing actual number of recurrences and related antimicrobial use | 18 |
| Cranberry fruit | Prevention of UTIs | RCT, double-blind comparison study with trimethoprim | Prophylaxis of recurrent UTI | 3% cranberry extract in glucose syrup | 85 infants (<1 yr) and 107 children >1 yr of age | 0.2 mL/kg cranberry syrup at bedtime | Safe and effective prophylaxis for recurrent UTI in infants and children; at this dose, efficacy was similar to trimethoprim in subjects >1 yr old | 19 |
| *Echinacea*: aerial parts and roots of *E. purpurea* (L.) Moench, *E. angustifolia* D.C., *E. pallida* (Nutt.), Asteraceae | Internal: prevention and treatment of URTIs and UTIs | Controlled studies | Treatment of pertussis | Pressed juice of the aerial, flowering parts of *E. purpurea* | 63 received *Echinacea* only; 77, *Echinacea* and antibiotics; 30, antibiotics only | Injection of 2 mL/day in children or 1 mL/day in infants for 3 days | Particularly successful in early stage of disease | 20 |
| | External: poorly healing wounds and chronic ulcers | Case reports | Angina lacunaris, otitis media, pertussis, spastic bronchitis | Pressed juice of the aerial, flowering parts of *E. purpurea* | | | Reduction in symptoms | 21 |
| | | Observational study | Effectiveness on recurring URTIs | Pressed juice of the aerial, flowering parts of *E. purpurea* | 1322 adults and children | | Reduction in symptoms after 10 days | 22 |
| | | Placebo-controlled | Early treatment of URTIs to prevent recurrent otitis media | 50% Alcoholic extract of *E. purpurea* root and seed, herb strength 1:1 | | 15–30 drops tid for 3 days, then half the dose for 7 days | Not effective | 23 |

*(continued)*

**Table 26–1.** Continued

| Herb | Therapeutic Use | Clinical Studies | | | | | | Ref. No. |
|---|---|---|---|---|---|---|---|---|
| | | Study Design | Target Parameter | Formulation | Cases | Dose/Duration | Outcome | |
| *E. purpurea* | Acute URTI | RCT, double-blind, placebo-controlled | Treatment of acute URTI to reduce risk of subsequent URTI | | 524 children (ages 2–11 yr) | Various doses depending on age, monitored over 4 mo | *Echinacea* was associated with a 28% decreased risk of subsequent URTI | 24 |
| *E. purpurea* | Otitis media | RCT, two-by-two factorial trial | Efficacy of *E. purpurea* and/or OMT to prevent acute otitis media in otitis-prone children | Alcohol extract of *Echinacea* roots and seeds | 90 children (12–60 mo) | 10 days | Not effective. *Echinacea* was associated with a borderline increased risk of having at least one episode of acute otitis media during 6-mo follow-up compared with placebo | 25 |
| Evening primrose oil (EPO): oil of the seeds of *Oenothera biennis*, Onagraceae | Atopic eczema, ADHD, diabetes, mastalgia, premenstrual syndrome, psoriasis, rheumatoid arthritis, chronic fatigue syndrome, diabetic neuropathy | Double-blind, placebo-controlled, parallel-group trial | Atopic dermatitis | EPO or placebo containing sunflower oil (similar spectrum of essential fatty acids) | 58 children | 2–3 g/day for 16 wk | Symptomatic improvements in both groups, but no significant difference for EPO vs placebo.<br>Significant flaw: placebo also contained essential fatty acids | 26 |
| | | Double blind, placebo-controlled clinical trial | Atopic dermatitis | EPO or placebo | 51 children | Placebo, EPO (0.5 g/kg/day), or a combination of 50% placebo and 50% EPO (0.5 g/kg/day) for 16 wk | Significant improvement in clinical symptoms with 100% EPO; increased n-6 fatty acids in erythrocyte cell membranes | 27 |
| | | Double-blind, placebo-controlled, crossover design | ADHD | Seed oil capsules, each containing 360 mg linoleic acid (LA) and 45 mg γ-linoleic acid (GLA) | 31 children | 3 caps bid for 4 wk | Higher blood concentration of DGLA, minimal or no improvement in behavioral problems | 28 |
| | | Latin-square, double-cross-over design with random assignment of sequence | ADHD | Capsules, each containing 500 mg EPO (40 mg GLA and 350 mg LA) | 18 boys | 1 cap D-amphetamine and 4 caps EPO or placebo in the morning, 4 caps EPO or placebo in the afternoon for 1 mo | EPO effect only a trend, perhaps due to small sample size and possible neutralization of EPO effect caused by the amphetamine | 29 |
| | | Double-blind, placebo-controlled | Effect on serum essential fatty acid and plasma $PGE_2$ and $PGF_{2\alpha}$ levels in children with insulin-dependent diabetes mellitus | Capsules, each containing 45 mg GLA and 360 mg LA | 11 children | 2 caps daily for 4 mo, then 4 caps daily for 4 mo | 2 caps daily showed no effect; 4 caps daily significantly increased DGLA and significantly decreased $PGE_2$ levels | 30 |
| Evening primrose oil (EPO) | Atopic dermatitis (AD) | RCT, dose and duration study | Serum fatty acid level and EASI scores of all AD patients at weeks 0, 2, 4, and 8 | Evoprim, 40 mg EPO per capsule | 40 children | 160 mg/day for 8 wk or 320 mg/day for 8 wk | EASI scores improved in both groups but greater with higher dose; no adverse effects reported | 31 |
| Fennel: fruits of *Foeniculum vulgare* Miller var. *vulgare*, Apiaceae | Mild spasmodic GI complaints, bloating, flatulence, catarrh of the upper respiratory tract | No clinical studies available | | | | | German Commission E: promotion of GI motility and an antispasmodic | 32 |
| Garlic: bulb of *Allium sativum*, Alliaceae | Hyperlipidemia, coronary heart disease; prevention of atherosclerosis | Randomized, double-blind, placebo-controlled | Efficacy in children with familial hyperlipidemia and a minimum fasting total cholesterol level >4.8 mmol/L | Commercially available garlic extract | 30 children | 300 mg tid for 8 wk | No significant effect on cardiovascular risk factors such as total, LDL, or HDL cholesterol or triglycerides; small effect on apolipoprotein A-1 | 33 |
| Garlic bulb | Acute respiratory illness | Safety study and RCT, double-blind, placebo-controlled, allicor versus benzimidazole | Prevention of acute viral respiratory infections in children | Allicor (long-acting garlic tablets) | 42 children (ages 10–12 yr), with 41 garlic treated, and 73 treated with benzimidazole | 300 mg/day | Morbidity reduced 2- to 4-fold vs controls in the treated group. In the second study, allicor reduced morbidity 1.7-fold vs placebo and 2.4-fold vs benzimidazole | 34 |
| German chamomile: flower heads of *Matricaria recutita* L., Asteraceae | Internal: spasms or inflammatory GI diseases<br>External: skin and membrane inflammations, irritations and inflammations of the respiratory tract | Prospective, double-blind, randomized, multicenter, parallel-group study | Acute, noncomplicated diarrhea | Apple pectin-chamomile extract or placebo in addition to usual rehydration and alimentation diet | 79 (ages 6 mo to 5.5 yr) | Dose not stated | Significant reduction ($P < .05$) in duration of diarrhea by ≥5.2 hr in the herb group; continuous recovery in the chamomile group | 35 |

| | | | | | | | | |
|---|---|---|---|---|---|---|---|---|
| German chamomile flavonoid | Autism spectrum disorders (ASD) | Open-label pilot study | ASD symptoms: age-equivalent scores on VABS, ABC, ATEC, and CGI Improvement scale | Dietary supplement capsule containing flavonoids (>95% pure), luteolin (100 mg/cap, from chamomile), quercetin (70 mg/cap), and the quercetin glycoside rutin (30 mg/cap) | 50 children (ages 4–10 yr) | 1 cap per 10 kg weight daily with food for 26 wk | Significant improvement in adaptive functioning on VABS age-equivalent scores and reduction (26.6–34.8%) in ABC subscale scores; transient (1–8 wk) increased irritability in 27 of the 50 participants | 36 |
| *Ginkgo biloba* L., Ginkgoaceae | Primary headaches (migraine and tension-type) | Open-label study | Prevention of migraine | Complex of ginkgolide B, coenzyme Q10, riboflavin, and magnesium | 119 school children | Dosed for 3 mo | Mean frequency per month of migraine significantly decreased | 37 |
| *G. biloba* leaves | Dementia and memory impairment | Double-blind, randomized, parallel comparison study | Treatment of children with DSM-IV-TR diagnosis of ADHD | *G. biloba* extract (Ginkgo T.D., Tolidaru, Iran) and methylphenidate | 50 children (39 boys and 11 girls) with ADHD diagnosis | Ginkgo T.D. 80 mg/day for weight <30 kg, 120 mg/day for >30 kg (group 1) or methylphenidate | Ginkgo T.D. less effective than methylphenidate on the Teacher and Parent ADHD Rating Scale-IV | 38 |
| *G. biloba* leaves | Nootropic and cholinergic drug | Open-label study | Treatment of children with DSM-IV-TR diagnosis of dyslexia | *Ginkgo* leaf extract: EGb 761 | 15 children (ages 5–13 yr) | 80 mg/day for 35 days | Statistically significant time and effect with decrease in several indexes of dyslexia severity | 39 |
| *G. biloba* leaves | Reduction of cholesterol | Randomized, comparison controlled clinical trial | Treatment of hypercholestrolemia in children with primary nephritic syndrome | *Ginkgo* leaf extract | 35 children | Prednisone plus *G. biloba* leaf extract (18 cases) or prednisone plus dipyridamole (17 cases) for 8 wk | Lowered blood lipid levels and urinic protein plus improved clinical symptoms and renal function in children with nephritic syndrome | 40 |
| *G. biloba* leaves | ADHD | Open-label | Quality of life, ADHD symptoms | *G. biloba* leaf extract: EGb 761 | 20 children | 240 mg/day for 3–5 wk | Improved quality of life, ADHD core symptoms, and CPT score | 41 |
| Ivy leaf: leaves of *Hedera helix* L., Araliaceae | Acute and chronic respiratory tract infections, spastic cough | Randomized, double-blind, placebo-controlled, crossover study | Effect on airway resistance, intrathoracic gas volume, and other spirometric parameters in children with bronchial asthma | Water-ethanol solution (30% ethanol; herb-to-extract ratio, 5–7:1) | 24 children (ages 4–12 yr) | 35-mg extract (equivalent to 210 mg crude drug) daily for 3 days, washout period of 3–5 days | Statistically significant and clinically relevant improvement, especially in airway resistance and intrathoracic gas volume in ivy-treated group | 42 |
| | | Randomized, crossover | Comparison of orally vs rectally administered formulation | Water-ethanol solution, extract as a suppository formulation | 26 children (ages 5–11 yr) | | Oral and rectal forms equivalent if given in a dose ratio of 1:5 | 43 |
| | | Double-blind crossover | Dose comparison of an alcohol-free juice preparation vs the water-ethanol solution | Alcohol-free juice preparation, water-ethanol solution | 25 (ages 10–16 yr) | | Water-ethanol solution ~2.5 times more effective than alcohol preparation | 44 |
| | | Multicenter, prospective postmarketing surveillance | Chronic bronchitis | Tablets containing 65 mg dried ivy leaf extract (herb-to-extract ratio, 5–7.5:1) | 1350 patients (ages ≥4 yr) | 1 (1/2) or 2 tablets per day depending on age (corresponding to 97.5 or 130 mg dried extract) for 4 wk | Improvement or cure of cough (92%), expectoration (94%), dyspnea (83%), respiratory pain (86%); each symptom group with >38% cured patients | 45 |
| Ivy leaf | Bronchitis | Postmarketing surveillance | Assessment of safety and efficacy in the treatment of bronchitis | Syrup containing dried ivy leaf extract | 9657 patients (5181 children) | 1–2 tsp/day for 7 days | 95% of patients showed reduced symptoms; safety was very good | 46 |
| Ivy leaf and thyme (*Thymus vulgaris* L.) | Bronchitis | Postmarketing surveillance study | Acute bronchitis and productive cough | Syrup containing dried ivy leaf and thyme extract | 1234 children (ages 2–17 yr) | Age-appropriate dosages for 10 days, prescribed by doctor on a case-by-case basis | Reduction in coughing and BSS in treated children; two mild adverse events | 47 |

*(continued)*

**Table 26–1.** Continued

| Herb | Therapeutic Use | Clinical Studies | | | | | | Ref. No. |
|---|---|---|---|---|---|---|---|---|
| | | Study Design | Target Parameter | Formulation | Cases | Dose/Duration | Outcome | |
| Ivy leaf | Acute bronchitis | Double-blind, randomized comparison study | Acute bronchitis | Ivy leaf extract | 590 patients (~40% children); 66% were >10 yr old, 23% were 4–10 yr, and 11% were 2–4 yr old | Age >10 yr, 24 drops; 4–10 yr, 16 drops; 2–4 yr, 12 drops | Reduction in BSS in treated children | 48 |
| Ivy leaf | Bronchitis and cough | Two open-label trials | Cough and bronchitis | Ivy leaf extracts | 268 (ages 0–12 yr) | Varying doses for up to 14 days | Global effect rated "good" or "very good" in 96.5% of cases; good tolerability | 49 |
| Ivy leaf | Add-on therapy for bronchial asthma | Double blind, placebo-controlled, randomized crossover study | Symptoms of asthma | Ivy leaf dry extract plus inhaled corticosteroids or placebo | 30 children (ages 6–11 yr) with partial or uncontrolled mild persistent allergic asthma | Varying doses; 4 wk run-in and 4 wk treatment | Significant improvement of symptoms after treatment with ivy vs placebo | 50 |
| Thyme: *T. vulgaris* L., *T. zygis* L., Lamiaceae | Bronchitis, whooping cough, upper respiratory inflammation | Controlled, multicenter, postmarketing surveillance | Acute bronchitis | Combination of 60 mg cowslip root extract and 160 mg thyme | 7783 patients (2000 <12 yr, remainder >12 yr) | Combination or reference drug (N-acetylcysteine or ambroxol) for 10 days | Herbal combination marginally better than reference medicine; significantly better in tolerance | 51 |
| Valerian: roots of *Valeriana officinalis* L. and other *Valeriana* species, Valerianaceae | Insomnia, anxiety | Randomized, double-blind, placebo-controlled, crossover trial | Intransigent sleep difficulties in children with an intellectual deficit | *Valeriana edulis* product | 5 children | 20 mg/kg body weight daily for 2 wk | Significant reductions in sleep latencies and nocturnal time awake, lengthened total sleep time, and improved sleep quality in valerian group | 52 |
| Roots of *V. officinalis* and leaves of *Melissa officinalis* L. | Anxiety, insomnia | Open, multicenter | Restlessness and nervous dyskoimesis | Each tablet contained 160 mg valerian root dry extract and 80 mg lemon balm leaf dry extract | 918 children | 3.5–4 tablets per day | Core symptoms of dyssomnia and restlessness reduced from "moderate/severe" to "mild" or "absent" in most patients | 53 |
| Roots of *V. officinalis* and leaves of *M. officinalis* L. | Anxiety, insomnia, hyperactivity | Observational | Hyperactivity, sleep, impulsiveness, focus, and social behavior | 640 mg valerian root extract WS 1014 and 320 mg lemon balm extract WS 1303 (Sandrin) | 169 primary school children with hyperactivity and concentration difficulties but not meeting ADHD criteria | 640 mg valerian and 320 mg lemon balm per day | Increased focus, reduced hyperactivity and impulsiveness; significant improvements in sleep quality and social behavior | 54 |

ABC = Aberrant Behavior Checklist; ADHD = attention-deficit hyperactivity disorder; ATEC = Autism Treatment Evaluation Checklist; bid = two times daily; BSS = Bronchitis Severity Score; CGI = Clinical Global Impression; CPT = Continuous Performance Test; DGLA = dihomo-γ-linolenic acid; DSM-IV-TR = *Diagnostic and Statistical Manual of Mental Disorders*, 4th edition, text rev.; EASI = Eczema Area Severity Index; GI = gastrointestinal; HDL = high-density lipoprotein; LDL = low-density lipoprotein; OMT = osteopathic manipulative treatment; $PGE_2$ = prostaglandin $E_2$; $PGF_{2\alpha}$ = prostaglandin $F_{2\alpha}$; RCT = randomized placebo-controlled trial; tid = three times daily; URTI = upper respiratory tract infection; UTI = urinary tract infection; VABS = Vineland Adaptive Behavior Scales.

1 to 4 years, 1.5 to 3 g; 4 to 10 years, 3 to 5 g; 10 to 16 years, 5 to 7 g. The dosages by age for fennel syrup or honey are 1 to 4 years, 3 to 6 g; 4 to 10 years, 6 to 10 g; 10 to 16 years, 10 to 20 g.[10] Fennel oil is contraindicated for infants and toddlers. The daily dosages for internal use by age group are 4 to 10 years, 0.05 to 0.2 mL; 10 to 16 years, 0.1 to 0.6 mL. Unless otherwise advised by a physician or pharmacist, fennel oil should not be consumed for an extended period. Diabetics must consider the sugar content in fennel syrup and fennel honey.[10]

Garlic (*Allium sativum*) is used in adults and children for prevention and treatment of hyperlipidemia and coronary heart disease as well as various respiratory illnesses.[33,34] In a clinical study with pediatric patients who had familial hyperlipidemia and a minimum fasting total cholesterol level greater than 4.8 mmol/L (>185 mg/dL), a commercially available garlic extract (300 mg three times daily) had no significant relative attributable effect on fasting total cholesterol, low-density lipoprotein cholesterol, high-density lipoprotein cholesterol, triglycerides, apolipoprotein B100, lipoprotein(a), fibrinogen, homocysteine, or blood pressure but also no adverse effects.[33] Garlic extract therapy had no significant effect on cardiovascular risk factors in pediatric patients with familial hyperlipidemia.[33]

German chamomile (*Matricaria recutita*) is used to aid digestion; ease gas, bloating, and intestinal cramps; and calm stress-related stomach complaints, but it may also be useful for long-term management of chronic digestive conditions such as irritable bowel syndrome, gastritis, and ulcers.[35] In German pediatric medicine, chamomile preparations are the first choice in caring for the sensitive skin of infants and young children, especially for inflammatory skin conditions such as diaper rash and milk crust.[10] Following the Kooperation Phytopharmaka for oral application, the dosages of the herb are given by age group: 0 to 1 year, 0.5 to 1 g; 1 to 4 years, 1 to 2 g; 4 to 10 years, 2 to 3 g; 10 to 16 years, 3 g. For the preparation of chamomile tea, about 150 mL of boiling water is poured over the herb; it is covered and steeped 5 to 10 minutes, after which it is passed through a tea strainer. For gastrointestinal complaints, unless otherwise prescribed, a cup of the freshly prepared tea is drunk three or four times daily between meals. For poultices and rinses, 3% to 10% infusions are used; as a bath additive, 10, 30, or 50 g is used in 10 L of water. Semisolid formulations are also used, with preparations corresponding to 3% to 10% herbal content.[10] German chamomile has also been shown to have some positive effects on children with autism spectrum disorders.[36] In one study, children treated with German chamomile showed significant improvements in adaptive functioning, as measured by Vineland Adaptive Behavior Scales (VABS) age-equivalent score, and in overall behavior, as indicated by the reduction (26.6–34.8%) in Aberrant Behavior Checklist (ABC) subscale scores; however, there was a transient (1–8 weeks) increased irritability in 27 of the 50 participants.[36]

The leaves of *Ginkgo biloba* have been recommended for memory impairment, primary headaches (migraines and stress headaches), dyslexia, hypercholesterolemia, and ADHD.[37–41] Treatment of children aged 5 to 13 years who were diagnosed with dyslexia using the DSM-IV-TR criteria with 80 mg of *G. biloba* extract for 35 days significantly decreased several indices of dyslexic severity.[39] In another trial, *G. biloba* reduced stress headaches, and improved quality of life in children with ADHD in clinical trials.[38,39,41] *G. biloba* extract, in combination with prednisone, was also shown to lower blood lipid levels and urinic protein in children with nephritic syndrome and to improve their renal function.[40]

Ivy leaf (*Hedera helix*) is recommended for diseases of the respiratory tract such as acute and chronic infections, asthma, bronchitis, and spastic cough.[42–50] In clinical trials, ivy leaf syrup and other preparations reduced symptoms such as cough and significantly and clinically improved airway resistance and intrathoracic gas volume.[42–50] The suggested daily dosages for oral administration are 0 to 1 year, 0.02 to 0.05 g herb; 1 to 4 years, 0.05 to 0.15 g; 4 to 10 years, 0.1 to 0.2 g; 10 to 16 years, 0.2 to 0.3 g. Because of the very low single doses, the Kooperation Phytopharmaka[10] strongly advises users not to prepare infusions for oral administration. It is better to use standardized products. Eructation and nausea are rare adverse effects.

Preparations containing thyme (*Thymus vulgaris* or *Thymus zygis*) have been used for treatment of bronchitis, whooping cough, and upper respiratory tract inflammation.[51] Topically, thyme is used as a gargle or mouthwash, or for inunctions or baths. Pure thyme oil is extremely toxic; the signs of toxicity range from nausea to respiratory arrest. The Kooperation Phytopharmaka[10] suggests the following dosages for internal use of the dried herb or an equivalent amount of fresh herb for infusions to be drunk several times each day: 0 to 1 years, 0.5 to 1 g/150 mL of water; 1 year or older, 1 to 2 g/150 mL of water. The dose information for the internal use of the fluid extract are given by age group: 1 to 4 years, 0.3 to 1.0 g; 4 to 10 years, 0.5 to 1.3 g; 10 to 16 years, 1.0 to 2.0 g. Because of its alcohol content, the fluid extract is contraindicated for infants before 1 year of age.

Extracts of valerian root (*Valeriana officinalis*), alone or in combination with other plant extracts, are often prescribed in Europe and other parts of the world as a substitute for the benzodiazepines in the treatment of insomnia and anxiety.[9] Several clinical trials have evaluated the safety and efficacy of commercial valerian products containing standardized extracts.[52–54] However, only one clinical trial has assessed the effects of a valerian product (*Valeriana edulis*) alone in a pediatric population (dose, 20 mg/kg body weight).[52] A combination of extracts from the roots of *Valeriana officinalis* and leaves of *Melissa officinalis* L. (lemon balm) have been used for management of anxiety, insomnia, and hyperactivity in children.[53,54] Open and observational studies have suggested that this combination, at a daily dosage of 640 mg valerian and 320 mg lemon balm, may increase focus, reduces hyperactivity and impulsiveness and significantly improves sleep quality and social behavior.[53,54] The preliminary findings suggest that valerian may be safe and effective for long-term treatment of intransigent sleep difficulties in children with intellectual deficits, and it therefore warrants further investigation.

As well as the herbs commonly used in pediatrics, there are herbs on the market that are particularly contraindicated for infants and children younger than 12 years of age, according to the German Commission E.[10] These include aloe (*Aloe barbadensis* and *Aloe carpensis*), buckthorn bark (*Frangulae cortex*) and buckthorn berry (*Rhamni cathartici fructus*), *Cascara sagrada* bark (*Rhamni purshianae cortex*), rhubarb root (*Rhei radix*), senna leaf (*Sennae folium*), and senna pod (*Sennae fructus*). Because of their content of 1,8-dihydroxyanthracene derivatives, these drugs have a strong laxative effect. For infants and small children, preparations of the following leaves and oils should not be applied to the facial area, especially the nose: cajeput oil (*Cajeputi aetheroleum*; contains cineol, which has a hyperemic effect), camphor (*Camphora*), eucalyptus leaf and oil (*Eucalypti folium/aetheroleum*), mint oil (*Menthae arvensis aetheroleum*), peppermint oil (*Menthae piperitae aetheroleum*), and niauli oil (*Niauli aetheroleum*). Fennel oil (*Foeniculi aetheroleum*, a volatile oil containing anethole and fenchone) should not be administered to infants or toddlers.

Horseradish (*Armoraciae rusticanae radix*) and watercress (*Nasturtii herba*), both of which contain mustard glycosides and mustard oil, should not be administered to children younger than 4 years of age.

Because of its high estragole content, basil oil (*Basilici aetheroleum*) preparations should not be used with infants and small children or for extended periods of time. Medicinal and/or clinical reports and other material on empirical medicinal use of basil oil are not available.

Nasturtium (*Tropaeolum majus*), which contains mustard oil, should not be used for infants and small children. White mustard seed (*Sinapis albae semen*), which contains mustard oil glycosides and mustard oil, should not be used in children younger than 6 years of age.

The Chinese herb ma huang (*Ephedra sinica*) cannot be recommended for children as a supplement because of its possible adverse cardiovascular effects.[55]

## References

1. Barnes PM, Bloom B, Nahin RL. Complementary and alternative medicine use among adults and children, United States, 2007. *Natl Health Stat Rep.* 2008; 12:1.
2. Post-White J, Fitzgerald M, Hageness S, Sencer SF. Complementary and alternative medicine use in children with cancer and general and specialty pediatrics. *J Pediatr Oncol Nurs.* 2009; 26:7.

3. Birdee GS, Phillips RS, Davis RB, Gardiner P. Factors associated with pediatric use of complementary and alternative medicine. *Pediatrics*. 2010; 125:249.
4. Council for Responsible Nutrition (CRN). 2013 CRN Consumer Survey on Dietary Supplements: A Snapshot of the Nutritional Supplement User. 2014. http://robinsonpharma.com/Health-Industry-Insights/2013-CRN-Consumer-Survey-on-Dietary-Supplements-A-Snapshot-of-the-Nutritional-Supplement-User. Accessed June 21, 2016.
5. Nicastro HL, Bailey RL, Dodd KW. Using 2 assessment methods may better describe dietary supplement intakes in the United States. *J Nutr*. 2015; 145:1630.
6. Guenther E, Mendoza J, Crouch BI, Moyer-Mileur LJ, Junkins EP Jr. Differences in herbal and dietary supplement use in the Hispanic and non-Hispanic pediatric populations. *Pediatr Emerg Care*. 2005; 21:507.
7. Keller K. Phytotherapy at a European level. Presented at the third international European Scientific Cooperative on Phytotherapy (ESCOP) symposium. In: *Phytomedicine*. Stuttgart: Gustav Fischer Verlag;1994: 40.
8. Moore TJ, Weiss SR, Kaplan S, Blaisdell CJ. Reported adverse drug events in infants and children under 2 years of age. *Pediatrics*. 2002; 110:53.
9. Blumenthal M, Busse WR, Goldberg A, Gruenwald J. *The Complete German Commission E Monographs*. Austin, TX: American Botanical Council; 1998.
10. Kooperation Phytopharmaka. *Kinderdosierungen von Phytopharmaka*: Part 2. Bonn, Germany: Kooperation Phytopharmaka; 2002.
11. Cáceres DD, Hancke JL, Burgos RA, Sandberg F, Wikman G. Prevention of common colds with *Andrographis paniculata* dried extract: a pilot double-blind study. *Phytomedicine*. 1997; 4:101.
12. Spasov AA, Ostrovskij OV, Chernikov MV, Wikman G. Comparative controlled study of *Andrographis paniculata* fixed combination, Kan Jang and an *Echinacea* preparation as adjuvant in the treatment of uncomplicated respiratory disease in children. *Phytother Res*. 2004; 18:47.
13. Shakhova EG, Spasov AA, Ostrovskiĭ OV, Konovalova IV, Chernikov MV, Mel'nikova GI. Effectiveness of using the drug Kan-Yang in children with acute respiratory viral infection (clinico-functional data) [in Russian]. *Vestn Otorinolaringol*. 2003; 3:48.
14. Oelkers-Ax R, Leins A, Hillecke T, et al. Butterbur root extract and music therapy in the prevention of childhood migraine: an explorative study. *Eur J Pain*. 2008; 12:301.
15. Pothmann R, Danesch U. Migraine prevention in children and adolescents: results of an open study with a special butterbur root extract. *Headache*. 2005; 45:196.
16. Rogers J. Pass the cranberry juice. *Nursing Times*. 1991; 87:36.
17. Ferrara P, Romaniello L, Vitelli O, Gatto A, Serva M, Cataldi L. Cranberry juice for the prevention of recurrent urinary tract infections: a randomized controlled trial in children. *Scand J Urol Nephrol*. 2009; 43:369.
18. Salo J, Uhari M, Helminen M, et al. Cranberry juice for the prevention of recurrences of urinary tract infections in children: a randomized placebo-controlled trial. *Clin Infect Dis*. 2012; 54:340.
19. Fernández-Puentes V, Uberos J, Rodríguez-Belmonte R, Nogueras-Ocaña M, Blanca-Jover E, Narbona-López E. Efficacy and safety profile of cranberry in infants and children with recurrent urinary tract infection [in Spanish]. *An Pediatr (Barc)*. 2015; 82:397.
20. Baetgen D. Erfolge in der Keuchhusten-Behandlung mit Echinacin®. *Therapiewoche*. 1984; 36, 34:5115.
21. Sprockhoff O. Erfahrungen aus einer kinderärztlichen Praxis mit Myo-Echinacin. *Landarzt*. 1964; 27:1173.
22. Götte, K., Roschke, I. Unterstützende Behandlung von akuten Atemwegsinfekten bei Kindern mit rezidivierenden Infekten im Bereich der oberen Atemwege. *Prakt Pädiatr*. 2001; 95.
23. Mark JD, Grant KL, Barton LL. The use of dietary supplements in pediatrics: a study of *Echinacea*. *Clin Pediatr*. 2001;40:265.
24. Weber W, Taylor JA, Stoep AV, Weiss NS, Standish LJ, Calabrese C. *Echinacea purpurea* for prevention of upper respiratory tract infections in children. *J Altern Complement Med*. 2005; 11:1021.
25. Wahl RA, Aldous MB, Worden KA, Grant KL. *Echinacea purpurea* and osteopathic manipulative treatment in children with recurrent otitis media: a randomized controlled trial. *BMC Complement Altern Med*. 2008; 8:56.
26. Biagi PL, Bordoni A, Masi M, et al. A long-term study on the use of evening primrose oil (Efamol) in atopic children. *Drugs Exp Clin Res*. 1988; 14:285.
27. Hederos CA, Berg A. Epogam evening primrose oil treatment in atopic dermatitis and asthma. *Arch Dis Child*. 1996; 75:494.
28. Aman MG, Mitchell EA., Turbott SH. The effects of essential fatty acid supplementation by Efamol in hyperactive children. *J Abnorm Child Psychol*. 1987; 15:75.
29. Arnold LE, Kleykamp D, Votolato NA, et al. Gamma-linolenic acid for attention-deficit hyperactivity disorder: placebo-controlled comparison to D-amphetamine. *Biol Psychiatry*. 1989; 25:222.
30. Arisaka M, Arisaka O, Yamashiro Y. Fatty acid and prostaglandin metabolism in children with diabetes mellitus: II. The effect of evening primrose oil supplementation on serum fatty acid and plasma prostaglandin levels. *Prostaglandins Leukot Essent Fatty Acids*. 1991; 43:197.
31. Chung BY, Kim JH, Cho SI, et al. Dose-dependent effects of evening primrose oil in children and adolescents with atopic dermatitis. *Ann Dermatol*. 2013; 25:285.
32. ESCOP, European Scientific Cooperative on Phytotherapy, 1996.
33. McCrindle BW, Helden E, Conner WT. Garlic extract therapy in children with hypercholesterolemia. *Arch Pediatr Adolesc Med*. 1998; 152:1089.
34. Andrianova IV, Sobenin IA, Sereda EV, Borodina LI, Studenikin MI. Effect of long-acting garlic tablets "allicor" on the incidence of acute respiratory viral infections in children [in Russian]. *Ter Arkh*. 2003;75:53.
35. De la Motte D, Bose-O'Reilly SS, Heinisch M, Harrison F. Double-blind comparison of an apple pectin-chamomile extract preparation with placebo in children with diarrhea [in German]. *Arzneimittelforschung*. 1997; 47:1247.
36. Taliou A, Zintzaras E, Lykouras L, Francis K. An open-label pilot study of a formulation containing the anti-inflammatory flavonoid luteolin and its effects on behavior in children with autism spectrum disorders. *Clin Ther*. 2013; 35:592.
37. Esposito M, Carotenuto M. Ginkgolide B complex efficacy for brief prophylaxis of migraine in school-aged children: an open-label study. *Neurol Sci*. 2011; 32:79.
38. Salehi B, Imani R, Mohammadi MR, et al. *Ginkgo biloba* for attention-deficit/hyperactivity disorder in children and adolescents: a double blind, randomized controlled trial. *Prog Neuropsychopharmacol Biol Psychiatry*. 2010; 34:76.
39. Donfrancesco R, Ferrante L. *Ginkgo biloba* in dyslexia: a pilot study. *Phytomedicine*. 2007; 14:367.
40. Zhong ZM, Yu L, Weng ZY, et al. Therapeutic effect of *Ginkgo biloba* leaf extract on hypercholestrolemia in children with nephrotic syndrome [in Chinese]. *Nan Fang Yi Ke Da Xue Xue Bao*. 2007; 27:682.
41. Uebel-von Sandersleben H, Rothenberger A, Albrecht B, Rothenberger LG, Klement S, Bock N. *Ginkgo biloba* extract EGb 761® in children with ADHD. *Z Kinder Jugendpsychiatr Psychother*. 2014; 42:337.
42. Mansfeld HJ, Höhre H, Repges R, Dethlefsen U. Sekretolyse und Bronchospasmolyse. *TW Padiatr*. 1997; 10:155.
43. Mansfeld H, Höhre H, Repges R, Dethlefsen U. Therapie des Asthma bronchiale mit Efeublätter-Trockenextrakt. *Münch Med Wochenschr*. 1998; 140:26.
44. Gulyas A, Repges R, Dethlefsen U. Konsequente Therapie chronisch-obstruktiver Atemwegserkrankungen bei Kindern. *Atemwegs Lungenkrankh*. 1997; 23:291.
45. Hecker M. Runkel F, Voelp A. Treatment of chronic bronchitis with ivy leaf special extract—multicenter post-marketing surveillance study in 1,350 patients [in German]. *Forsch Komplementarmed Klass Naturheilkd*. 2002; 9:77.
46. Fazio S, Pouso J, Dolinsky D, et al. Tolerance, safety, and efficacy of *Hedera helix* extract in inflammatory bronchial diseases under clinical practice conditions: a prospective, open, multicentre postmarketing study in 9657 patients. *Phytomedicine*. 2009; 16:17.
47. Marzian O. Treatment of acute bronchitis in children and adolescents. Non-interventional postmarketing surveillance study confirms the benefit and safety of a syrup made of extracts from thyme and ivy leaves [in German]. *MMW Fortschr Med*. 2007; 149(Suppl):69.
48. Cwientzek U, Ottillinger B, Arenberger P. Acute bronchitis therapy with ivy leaves extracts in a two-arm study: a double-blind, randomised study vs. an other ivy leaves extract. *Phytomedicine*. 2011; 18:1105.
49. Schmidt M, Thomsen M, Schmidt U. Suitability of ivy extract for the treatment of paediatric cough. *Phytother Res*. 2012; 26:1942.
50. Zeil S, Schwanebeck U, Vogelberg C. Tolerance and effect of an add-on treatment with a cough medicine containing ivy leaves dry extract on lung function in children with bronchial asthma. *Phytomedicine*. 2014; 21:1216.
51. Wichtl M, Bisset NG, eds. *Herbal Drugs and Phytopharmaceuticals*. Stuttgart: Medpharm Scientific Publishers; 1994.
52. Francis AJ, Dempster RJ. Effect of valerian, *Valeriana edulis*, on sleep difficulties in children with intellectual deficits: randomized trial. *Phytomedicine*. 2002; 4:273.
53. Müller SF, Klement S. A combination of valerian and lemon balm is effective in the treatment of restlessness and dyssomnia in children. *Phytomedicine*. 2006; 13:383.
54. Gromball J, Beschorner F, Wantzen C, Paulsen U, Burkart M. Hyperactivity, concentration difficulties and impulsiveness improve during seven weeks' treatment with valerian root and lemon balm extracts in primary school children. *Phytomedicine*. 2014; 21:1098.
55. Lanski SL, Greenwald M, Perkins A, Simon HK. Herbal therapy use in a pediatric emergency department population: expect the unexpected. *Pediatrics*. 2003; 111:981.

# 27 Drug Therapy and Nutrition

MARSHAL SHLAFER AND REBECCA J. SHLAFER

Drug therapy and nutrition for developmentally disabled and mentally retarded individuals living in intermediate care facilities are regulated by federal guidelines, which are based on symptoms rather than diagnoses.[1] Some drugs, including vitamins in pharmacologic doses (i.e., doses greater than those typically used to correct deficiency states) can cause undesirable food-drug or nutrient-drug interactions.[2] This needs to be differentiated from the generally low doses used for supplemental replacement of vitamins and minerals, as described in several sections of this chapter. Supplements used in this context sometimes can compensate for adverse drug effects; amounts used are based on individual needs determined during nutrition assessment (see Chapter 4).

Drugs used in the treatment of chronic diseases are too diverse and too numerous to discuss in this chapter or to cite as references. The more important ones, including drugs used for management of developmental disabilities and substances that are commonly misused, are summarized in Table 27–1. In most cases, the table lists only drugs that are considered prototypes of a class. If there are important differences among other members of a class, individual drugs that are noteworthy are listed separately.

This chapter focuses on several commonly prescribed drugs or drug groups and their nutritional consequences and interactions. This includes drugs used mainly in children and adolescents with developmental disorders and those given for a variety of common medical conditions in adults.

## NUTRITION, BIOCHEMICAL ABNORMALITIES, AND PHARMACOKINETICS

*Pharmacokinetics* encompasses four major processes that affect the entry of exogenous substances into the systemic circulation, their ability to reach sites of action, and their elimination from the body. These processes, which are related both directly and indirectly, are absorption, distribution, metabolism, and excretion. The integrity of each process is an important determinant of the effects of drugs as well as nutrients. The textbook by Brunton et al.[3] provides a comprehensive table showing complete pharmacokinetic properties of a host of drugs and useful information from which one may assess how those properties are affected by altered renal and hepatic status.

### Absorption

The most common route for administration of drugs and nutrients is oral. Like most drugs, many nutrients are absorbed by passive diffusion through cell membranes. Some, however, are absorbed by other processes. For example, iron is absorbed mainly by active (adenosine triphosphate [ATP]-dependent) transport, and glucose is absorbed by ATP-independent, carrier-mediated, facilitated diffusion.

Three key characteristics of drug and nutrient molecules affect their absorption: lipid solubility, ionization (local pH and the pKa of the molecule), and molecular size. Absorption is also influenced by gut motility and by other factors affecting the local environment in various parts of the gastrointestinal tract. For example, absorption of fat-soluble vitamins (i.e., vitamins A, D, E, K) depends heavily on the presence of adequate amounts of bile salts. Absorption of vitamin $B_{12}$, a large water-soluble molecule, depends on the presence of intrinsic factor and normally low gastric acidity.

Gut motility, and the effect of motility changes on absorption, is less a factor with respect to nutrients. With nutrients, the most important (and most common) issues arise with ingestion of polyvalent cations—particularly calcium (in supplements) and aluminum salts (a common source being antacids). Calcium and aluminum reduce gut motility (i.e., increase gut transit time), which may allow more complete absorption of oral drugs. Conversely, magnesium salts (again, mainly in antacids) increase motility and give less time for certain drugs to be absorbed. The same results can occur with constipation or diarrhea, respectively, especially if prolonged, and regardless of the etiology.

Normally, the stomach is an acidic environment, and the duodenum is alkaline; significant alterations of pH from the norm as a result of drugs, disease, or certain nutrient deficiencies, can affect the absorption of drugs and nutrients.

Age may also affect absorption of oral drugs through pH- and motility-related effects. Normal gastric pH is not achieved until about 3 years of age, and pH rises again in older adults due to lessened activity of acid-secreting parietal cell pumps; these "proton pumps" may also be inhibited by esomeprazole (Nexium) and many other drugs that are widely used and widely misused. As gastric pH rises, a greater proportion of drugs that are weak acids is in the ionized and poorly diffusible form; absorption is reduced, diminishing the effects of these drugs. Conversely, gastric absorption of weak bases is increased, with the potential for excessive effects or frank toxicity.

Generalized and clinically significant malnutrition can have a profound impact on pharmacokinetics. Changes in the gut, mucosal cells, and specific membrane transporters can affect absorption of a variety of drugs and nutrients. Although the changes described here apply to many drugs, some specific consequences may occur. For example, vitamin $B_{12}$ deficiency may be caused by diminished vitamin absorption due to achlorhydria or, more often, by profound inhibition of gastric acid secretion due to use of proton pump inhibitors. Celiac disease can result in lower plasma zinc levels in persons with Down syndrome.[4]

Three variables are most affected by changes in drug or nutrient absorption. One is the rate of absorption—the amount absorbed per unit time. The second is the extent of absorption, which encompasses the total amount of drug absorbed from a particular dose over some stated time span. Either or both of these variables can be altered to a clinically significant degree, together or independently of one another. Collectively, these two variables affect what is perhaps the most important variable: bioavailability. This discussion focuses on oral bioavailability because the oral route is the most common mode of administration.

A working definition of *bioavailability* is the fraction (or percentage) of a dose that reaches the systemic circulation in a form that is capable of causing pharmacologic effects, good or bad. The variable known as the area under the curve (AUC) provides the best indication of bioavailability overall. The plasma concentration of a drug is measured at intervals starting just before and then periodically after drug administration; the data are plotted on a graph, and the integral (AUC) is calculated.

### Distribution

Just as important as processes that affect the entry of drug molecules into the bloodstream are those that affect their ability to leave the blood for ultimate distribution to, and effects on, parenchymal cells.

**Table 27–1.** Potential Adverse Nutritional and Other Significant Side Effects of Selected Drugs

| Drug Category or Class | Generic Name (Brand Name) | Adverse Reactions | Comments |
|---|---|---|---|
| ***Drugs Used for Arthritis or Other Inflammatory States*** | | | |
| Analgesics (nonnarcotic; includes most "traditional" NSAIDs, excludes disease-modifying antirheumatic drugs such as methotrexate, TNF modifiers) | Aspirin | 1. GIdistress (variable incidence, severity)<br>2. Gastric mucosal damage may cause bleeding, iron deficiency anemia<br>3. Potential ↑ urinary vitamin C excretion<br>4. Urinary acidification by high doses of vitamin C causes ↓ renal salicylate excretion, ↑ risk of toxicity | 1. May alter taste<br>2. Administration with food or antacids may reduce GI distress; may also reduce absorption and therapeutic effects<br>3. Buffered aspirin products may increase serum sodium levels<br>4. Severe GI intolerance may depress appetite and subsequent nutrient intake<br>5. Gastric damage with oral administration may cause blood loss, anemia |
| | Colchicine | See 1 and 2 for aspirin above<br>1. ↓ Vitamin $B_{12}$ absorption<br>2. Gastric mucosal damage may ↑ fecal blood loss, iron deficiency | |
| Corticosteroids (all administered orally or parenterally) | Prednisone | 1. Hyperglycemia<br>2. Hypernatremia<br>3. Hypokalemia<br>4. Hypertriglyceridemia, hypercholesterolemia<br>5. ↓ Protein synthesis, ↑ protein catabolism<br>6. Potential deficiencies of vitamins C, D, $B_2$ (pyridoxine), and folate | 1. With systemic steroids, hyperglycemia is a significant concern for patients with prediabetes or frank diabetes owing to glucocorticoid activity<br>2. ↑ Renal sodium reabsorption accompanied by water retention due to mineralocorticoid actovotu may be sufficient to cause or worsen edema, heart failure, hypertension<br>3. ↑ Renal potassium loss (mineralocorticoid effect) and subsequent reduced blood potassium ($K^+$) concentrations may be significant<br>4. ↑ Protein catabolism contributes to muscle wasting with long-term therapy<br>5. Hypophosphatemia, combined with hypocalcemia, may contribute to bone fragility with long-term high-dose use; if phosphorus supplements are indicated, use sodium-free preparations to avoid exacerbating hypernatremia |
| Uriocosuric drugs | Probenecid (Benemid), sulfinpyrazone (Anturane) | 1. Potential ↑ in renal excretion of calcium, magnesium, sodium | |
| ***Drugs Used for Neoplastic Diseases*** | | | |
| Alkylating agents | Cyclophosphamide (Cytoxan) | 1. Metallic taste, nausea, and vomiting | 1. Ideally, avoid in malnutrition<br>2. High fluid output needed to prevent sterile hemorrhagic cystitis |
| Antimetabolites | Methotrexate (Folex) | 1. ↓ Dihydrofolate reductase<br>2. Nausea, anorexia, stomatitis | 1. Administer reduced folate (leucovorin) when needed<br>2. Monitor fluid intake and output |
| Antitumor antibiotics | Doxorubicin (Adriamycin) | 1. Nausea, vomiting, and mucositis | 1. Use suitable antiemetic (e.g., ondansetron) for nausea, vomiting |
| Hormonal and antihormonal agents | Diethystilbestrol (Stilphostrol) | 1. Nausea and occasional vomiting, constipation | 1. Monitor sodium intake, blood pressure, and cardiac status<br>2. Use stool softeners, mild laxatives; ↑ dietary fiber and fluid |
| ***Drugs Used for Cardiovascular Conditions*** | | | |
| Aldosterone receptor antagonists | Spironolactone (Aldactone), eplerenone (Inspra) | 1. Hyperkalemia, hyponatremia | 1. Of particular concern if used with potassium (K)-sparing diuretics or oral K supplements (avoid) because aldosterone receptor blockade induces renal K wasting |
| Angiotensin modifiers (ACE inhibitors; angiotensin receptor blockers) | Captopril (Capoten), others; losartan (Cozaar), others | 1. Hyperkalemia, hyponatremia | 1. See aldosterone receptor antagonists |
| Anticoagulants, oral | Warfarin (Coumadin) | 1. Prolongs prothrombin time (and INR) effects ↓ by vitamin K, resulting in ↑ risk of thromboembolism and its consequences | 1. Avoid intake of large amounts of vitamin K in foods such as green leafy vegetables; maintain consistent daily vitamin K intake to avoid fluctuations in INR; does not apply to newer warfarin alternatives (e.g., dabigatran [Pradaxa])<br>2. Anemia, iron deficiency during pregnancy |
| ***Cholesterol-Lowering Drugs*** | | | |
| Bile acid sequestrants | Colesevelam (Welchol) (Questran), Colestipol Cholestyramine (Colestid) | 1. ↓ Absorption of fat-soluble vitamins (A, D, E, K) | 1. Colesevelam is far less likely to interfere with oral absorption of vitamins, other drugs and is preferred to cholestyramine and other older agents<br>2. Colesevelam has intrinsic beneficial effects (particularly in conjunction with other antidiabetic drugs) for type 2 diabetes mellitus (lowers plasma glucose) |

| | | | |
|---|---|---|---|
| Statins | Atorvastatin (Lipitor), others | 1. Risk of myositis—potentially severe and complicated by myopathy, rhabdomyolysis, and renal failure<br>2. ↑ Risk of type 2 diabetes | 1. Monitor for muscle tenderness, aches, pains; may be early indicators of drug-induced skeletal muscle inflammation or frank damage<br>2. Risks of skeletal muscle damage and rhabdomyolysis increased when statins are administered with any other classes of lipid-lowering agents, so combined therapy should be avoided if possible<br>3. Coenzyme Q supplementation appears to have no benefit in reducing myositis, myopathy, rhabdomyolysis |
| ***Antihypertensive Drugs*** | | | |
| Vasodilators | Hydralazine (Apresoline), diazoxide (Hyperstat) | 1. Probable ↓ serum vitamin $B_6$ levels; peripheral neuritis, neuropathy<br>2. Hyperglycemia | 1. May be symptomatic (neuropathy, paresthesias) with long-term therapy, whether used for hypertension or heart failure; prophylactic pyridoxine supplementation is advised; IV pyridoxine may be indicated for severe, acute neuropathies<br>2. Consequences of hyperglycemia caused by diazoxide may be transiently important for diabetic patients even when used short-term by parenteral routes for hypertension and/or heart failure |
| Catecholamine depletors | Guanfacine (Tenex) | 1. Gastric hyperacidity, dyspepsia, diarrhea, urinary frequency due to unmasking of opposing parasympathetic nervous system on gut and urinary tract | 1. GI distress often sufficient to cause prolonged anorexia leading to inadequate nutrient intake over the long run |
| ***Diuretics*** | | | |
| Thiazides (benzothiazides) and thiazide-like agents (e.g., metolazone, chlorhalidone, indapamide) | Hydrochlorothiazide (and many others) | 1. Hyponatremia<br>2. Hypokalemia<br>3. Hypercholesterolemia, hypertriglyceridemia<br>4. Hyperglycemia, ↓ glucose tolerance<br>5. Hypercalcemia | 1. Thiazides and thiazide-like diuretics rank high on lists of drugs "most likely to cause hyponatremia," and may occur with usual therapeutic doses.<br>2. Diuretic-induced hypokalemia, whether thiazide or loop diuretic (e.g., furosemide), contributes to digoxin toxicity. Use potassium ($K^+$)-rich foods, prescription oral $K^+$ supplements, or K-sparing diuretics (e.g., amiloride, triamterene, spironolactone, eplerenone) for prophylaxis or treatment of asymptomatic hypokalemia; avoid concomitant use of oral K supplements and K-sparing diuretics, ACE inhibitors, or angiotensin receptor blockers (hyperkalemia risk)<br>3. Thiazides and thiazide-like diuretics cause cellular (skeletal muscle, adipocyte) resistance to insulin, already a problem for many patients with type 2 diabetes mellitus. Administration to diabetic patients often requires modifications to diet, exercise, and/or antidiabetic drug therapy<br>4. Reduced renal calcium excretion accounts for hypercalcemia; monitor accordingly, especially in patients taking digoxin |
| Loop ("high ceiling") diuretics | Furosemide (Lasix), bumetanide, torsemide, ethacrynic acid | 1. Hypokalemia<br>2. Hyperglycemia<br>3. Hypocalcemia<br>4. Hypomagnesemia<br>5. Dehydration, hypochloremic, hypokalemic (metabolic) alkalosis | 1. Volume depletion is more likely to occur and to be severe than with any other diuretic classes, is dose dependent, and may be symptomatic (e.g., hypotension)<br>2. Risk of hyponatremia far less than with thiazides<br>3. Effects of loop diuretics on renal calcium handling are the opposite of those of the thiazides |
| Carbonic anhydrase inhibitors | Acetazolamide (Diamox) | 1. Hypokalemia<br>2. Hyperglycemia<br>3. Metabolic acidosis | 1. See thiazides; may occur after diuretic effect subsides; treatment is continued (as for treatment of glaucoma, seizures)<br>2. See thiazides<br>3. Urine is alkalinized, causing blood base deficit with systemic carbonic anhydrase inhibitors |

(*continued*)

**Table 27–1.** Continued

| Drug Category or Class | Generic Name (Brand Name) | Adverse Reactions | Comments |
|---|---|---|---|
| Potassium-sparing diuretics | Triamterene (Dyrenium), amiloride (Midamor) | 1. Hyponatremia<br>2. Hyperkalemia | 1. Risk of hyponatremia and its consequences (e.g., excessive fluid depletion) mainly when used adjunctively with potassium (K)-wasting diuretics, as is often done<br>2. Avoid use of K-sparing diuretics (especially in absence of a K-wasting agent) in combination with ACE inhibitor (captopril, others) or angiotensin receptor blocker (e.g., losartan) to avoid risk of severe hyperkalemia<br>3. Do not administer oral K supplements to patients who are receiving a K-sparing diuretic (to reduce risk of hyperkalemia) |
| ***Drugs with Predominant CNS Effects or Uses*** | | | |
| Alcohol (ethanol) | | 1. Gastric irritation; high dose can cause ulcers, inhibit drug metabolism; low dose stimulates hepatic metabolizing enzymes<br>2. Organ damage and malnutrition when large amounts are ingested in place of a well-balanced diet<br>3. Malabsorption of vitamins A, C, $B_1$, $B_{12}$, and folic acid; ↑ excretion of folic acid, calcium, magnesium, zinc<br>4. Fetal alcohol syndrome<br>5. Hepatic necrosis, largely with long-term high-dose intake<br>6. Wernicke encephalopathy with either long-term or acute high-dose intake (risks increased by, acutely managed with, thiamine) | 1. Rapidly absorbed; milk products slow absorption<br>2. Enters fetal circulation and maternal milk<br>3. Give diet of high nutritional quality<br>4. Low dose stimulates hepatic metabolizing enzymes |
| Nicotine | | 1. ↓ Appetite, ↑ physical activity; can lead to weight loss, generalized nutritional deficiencies<br>2. ↓ Intake of sweets, ↑ intake of fatty foods<br>3. ↑ LDL and VLDL, favors atherogenesis<br>4. ↑ Hepatic metabolism, lowers blood levels of many other drugs (e.g., theophylline, propranolol, many AEDs) | 1. Alters taste sensation<br>2. Clear link with carcinogenesis<br>3. Cardiovascular, metabolic effects |
| Marijuana (THC) | | 1. ↑ Appetite, food intake, weight gain | |
| CNS stimulants or anorexigenics | Methylphenidate (Ritalin), amphetamines and mixtures (Adderall), cocaine, phenytoin (Dilantin) | 1. Nervousness, insomnia, headache, dizziness<br>2. Anemia, alopecia<br>3. ↓ Appetite, abdominal pain, nausea, weight loss | 1. Avoid use with nonselective MAO inhibitors<br>2. Inhibit metabolism of AEDs, tricyclic antidepressants |
| Anticonvulsants, antiepileptic drugs (AEDs) | | 1. Nausea, vomiting, constipation<br>2. Megaloblastic anemia<br>3. Gingival hyperplasia<br>4. Hyperglycemia<br>5. Insomnia, dizziness, headache, fatigue | 1. Administer drug with or immediately after meal<br>2. Poor water solubility<br>3. Excessive folate supplementation may counteract desired anticonvulsant effects |
| | Valproic acid (Depakene, Depakote) | 1. Transient nausea, vomiting, and indigestion at initiation of therapy<br>2. Diarrhea, abdominal cramps, and constipation<br>3. Hair loss | 1. Allegedly most teratogenic of all common AEDs<br>2. Capsules should be swallowed, not chewed |
| | Carbamazepine (Tegretol) | 1. Drowsiness, dizziness, unsteadiness, nausea, diplopia<br>2. Blood dyscrasias | 1. Excreted in breast milk<br>2. Use with extra care during pregnancy |
| Barbiturates | Phenobarbital | 1. Nausea. vomiting, constipation<br>2. ↑ Breakdown of vitamin D<br>3. Vitamin D and calcium deficiency may lead to osteomalacia or rickets<br>4. ↑ Incidence of fractures<br>5. Alters hepatic synthesis of vitamin K; hemorrhage of newborn when taken during third trimester<br>6. Fetal malformation when high doses are taken during early pregnancy | 1. Not very lipid soluble; enters CNS and tissues slowly<br>2. Unmetabolized drug excreted via kidneys and breast milk<br>3. Long half-life; can inhibit seizures without causing marked sedation (dose dependent)<br>4. Give drug with meals<br>5. Give high fiber and fluid diet<br>6. Give vitamin K supplements to baby and mother just before and just after birth to reduce bleeding risks<br>7. Excreted in breast milk |

| | | | |
|---|---|---|---|
| Benzodiazepines | Diazepam (Valium), many others | 1. Commonly reported: drowsiness, fatigue, and ataxia<br>2. Infrequent: constipation, nausea, changes in salivation, skin rash, tremor, insomnia | |
| Antidepressants, SSRIs, tricyclics, others | Fluoxetine (Prozac) | 1. Insomnia, dry mouth, constipation, paralytic ileus, skin rash, nausea, vomiting, anorexia, epigastric distress, diarrhea or constipation, peculiar taste, stomatitis, abdominal cramps, fatigue, headache, alopecia<br>2. ↑ or↓ Weight<br>3. In enuretic children receiving amitriptyline: nervousness, sleep disorders, tiredness, and mild GI disturbance that usually disappears during continued drug therapy or when dosage is ↓ | 1. Peripheral autonomic side effects much more common with amitriptyline and other tricyclic antidepressants, which are now seldom used for depression (SSRIs or atypical antidepressants preferred); more commonly used as adjunct to pain management with an opioid; also used for reducing enuresis in children; not recommended for children younger than 6 years of age<br>2. Safe use in pregnancy not established<br>3. Excreted in breast milk<br>1. Effects on appetite and subsequent changes in body weight vary among agents in this class<br>2. Generally lack autonomic side effects associated with most tricyclic/ tetracyclic antidepressants (hypotension, tachycardia, reductions in bowel and bladder function) |
| Antidepressants, MAO inhibitors | Pargyline (Eutonyl) | 1. Dizziness, constipation, dry mouth, hypotension (especially postural), drowsiness, weakness and fatigue, edema, GI disturbances, tremors, twitching | 1. MAO inhibitor class may result in serious or fatal hypertensive crisis if patient ingests tyramine-rich foods or beverages or decongestants containing pseudoephedrine |
| Antimanic drug | Lithium (Cibalith, others) | 1. Early effects related to blood drug levels include nausea, dry mouth, diarrhea, thirst, diabetes insipidus– like state<br>2. Effects unrelated to blood levels include weight gain, metallic taste, altered taste of some foods, edema of hands and ankles<br>3. Constipation | 1. Absorbed quickly and well<br>2. Metabolism closely associated with serum sodium balance: sodium deficiency of any cause ↑ risk of lithium side effects and toxicity, so consistency in daily dietary intake (and loss) of sodium is essential)<br>3. Give with meals to reduce nausea<br>4. Monitor electrolyte loss<br>5. Monitor exercise for fluid loss<br>6. Give high fiber and fluid diet |
| Antiparkinson drugs, dopaminergic agents | Levodopa (Dopar, Larodopa) alone or in combination with carbidopa (Sinemet) | 1. Nausea, vomiting, dry mouth, dysphagia<br>2. Anorexia<br>3. Headaches, dizziness, insomnia, fatigue | 1. Give drug with meals; however, high-protein diet will compromise effectiveness<br>2. Monitor weight; allow adequate time to eat<br>3. Encourage high fiber and fluid diet; laxatives and stool softener may be indicated |
| Opioids | Morphine, others | 1. Constipation, nausea, vomiting<br>2. Hypotension, mainly orthostatic | |
| Antipsychotics (neuroleptics), traditional agents (phenothiazines, butyrophenones) | Chlorpromazine (Thorazine) | 1. Drowsiness<br>2. Dry mouth, blurred vision, constipation, nausea, vomiting, nasal stuffiness, pallor<br>3. Dermatitis (photosensitivity) | 1. Reproductive studies in animals failed to show teratogenic effect |
| | Haloperidol (Haldol) | 1. Tardive dyskinesia<br>2. Lethargy<br>3. Decreases thirst sensation | 1. Possible fetal damage during pregnancy |
| ***Drugs Used for Endocrine-Metabolic Disorders*** | | | |
| Antidiabetic drugs | Insulins (all) | 1. Hypoglycemia resulting from hyperinsulinism; hunger, weakness<br>2. ↓ Serum potassium | 1. Give calorie-modified diet planned according to individual nutritional needs |
| | Sulfonylureas (glimepiride, others) | 1. Risk of hypoglycemia<br>2. Nausea, vomiting, diarrhea, heartburn, or abdominal pain<br>3. Occasional GI bleeding | 1. ↑ By excessive exercise, skipping of meals, poor nutrition; carry source of simple sugar for emergencies<br>2. Age and excessive alcohol intake ↑ risk of hypoglycemia; give drug with meals |
| | Biguanides: metformin (Glucophage) | 1. Anorexia (appetite suppression may contribute to weight loss) | 1. Risk of lactic acidosis, the incidence of which is rare but is fatal about 50% of the time when it develops in response to metformin |
| | Sodium/glucose cotransporter 2 (SGT2) inhibitors (“gliflozins”): canigliflozin (Invokana) | 1. Hypoglycemia (excessive effect); hyponatremia, hypotension from excess renal fluid loss (glucose- mediated osmotic diuresis) | 1. In addition to routine checks of plasma glucose, monitor blood pressure and body weight for indications of excessive diuresis |

*(continued)*

**Table 27–1.** Continued

| Drug Category or Class | Generic Name (Brand Name) | Adverse Reactions | Comments |
|---|---|---|---|
| Thyroid, antithyroid drugs | Levothyroxine (Synthroid); propylthiouracil, ("PTU"; Propacil) | 1. ↑ Bowel activity if doses are excessive or increased too rapidly<br>2. Fever<br>3. Nausea | 1. Monitor frequency and consistency of stool |
| | Iodine, iodides (Lugol solution) | 1. Staining of teeth<br>2. Diarrhea; pain in throat, mouth, and gums; vomiting | 1. Sip medication through straw; also helps mask bad taste<br>2. May indicate iodism; assess immediately, avoid iodine-containing foods and drugs<br>3. Bloody diarrhea or vomitus may indicate acute iodine poisoning |
| Drugs that alter serum calcium levels | Calcitonin, salmon | 1. Nausea with or without vomiting | |
| | Bisphosphonates (e.g., etidronate) | 1. Hypocalcemia, hypophosphatemia | 1. Use for osteoporosis depends on increased uptake of serum calcium and phosphorous from blood into bone |
| Androgens and anabolic drugs | Testosterone (Andro 100), others | 1. Hypercalcemia, renal calcium stones<br>2. Constipation, vomiting | 1. Hepatotoxicity a major concern with long-term misuse/abuse |
| | Conjugated estrogens (Premarin) | 1. Anorexia or increased appetite, weight gain<br>2. Nausea, bloating, vomiting<br>3. Diarrhea, abdominal cramping<br>4. Edema | |
| | Medroprogesterone acetate (Provera) | 1. Changes in appetite, nausea, edema, weight gain | |
| Oral contraceptives, estrogen-progestin combinations | Many | 1. Low serum vitamin C; possible low vitamins $B_1$, $B_{12}$, $B_6$, $B_2$, folate, magnesium, zinc<br>2. High hematocrit, hemoglobin, serum iron, calcium, vitamins A and E<br>3. ↑ Absorption of vitamin A and calcium<br>4. May cause hyperglycemia | |
| ***Drug Used for GI Disorders*** | | | |
| Antacids | All | 1. May interfere with absorption of any orally administered vitamins<br>2. ↑ Gastric pH; may reduce iron absorption<br>3. May ↑ serum sodium levels unless low-sodium or sodium-free products are used | 1. Discourage frequent or excessive use unless use can be monitored or supervised<br>2. Sodium-free products preferred for chronic, intensive therapy, especially when hypernatremia is an added risk<br>3. Magnesium-aluminum combination products generally preferred for long-term use (e.g., for ulcers) to minimize altered gut motility |
| | Aluminum salts (e.g., aluminum hydroxide gel) | 1. Potential hypercalcemia, hypophosphatemia with chronic high-dose use<br>2. Constipation possible unless used in combination with magnesium salt | 1. Used in combination with magnesium salt to reduce risk of constipation |
| | Calcium carbonate | 1. Risk of hypercalcemia with frequent or high-dose use<br>2. Constipation probable unless used in combination with magnesium salt; fecal impaction possible | 1. Calcium salts usually used in combination with magnesium salt to reduce risk of constipation when the therapeutic goal is an antacid effect |
| | Magnesium hydroxide, oxide (e.g., milk of magnesia) | 1. Risk of hypermagnesemia frank magnesemia persons with renal dysfunction magnesium<br>2. Diarrhea (dose-related) probable unless used in combination with constipating antacid (aluminum or calcium salt), with potential generalized fluid and electrolyte loss | 1. Discourage use of products containing only magnesium, especially high-dose use and/or by persons with poor renal function and the elderly<br>2. Assess for excessive fluid and electrolyte loss and neurological evidence of hypermagnesemia |
| | Sodium bicarbonate | 1. Risk of hypernatremia and associated hypertension, circulating fluid overload, edema<br>2. Metabolic alkalosis | |
| Antihistamines ($H_2$ blockers; "H2RAs") | Ranitidine (Zantac), nizatidine (Axid), famotidine (Pepcid), cimetidine (Tagamet) | 1. ↓ Gastric acid secretion, increased gastric pH, may interfere with absorption of iron, vitamin $B_{12}$ | 1. ↓ Hepatic metabolism of many other drugs (cimetidine only) |

| | | | |
|---|---|---|---|
| Laxatives, cathartics | All | 1. Excessive and potentially significant fluid, electrolyte loss (especially of potassium) with laxative/cathartic abuse<br>2. ↓ Absorption of orally administered drugs and vitamins<br>3. ↓ Spontaneous bowel rhythm, especially if abused as part of laxative-antidiarrheal drug cycle | 1. Discourage routine use as antacid unless under physician's supervision<br>2. If interacting drugs or nutrients must be administered (orally), separate administration by at least 2 hr if possible |
| | Bisacodyl, enteric- coated tablets (Dulcolax) | 1. Gastric mucosal irritation if taken with antacids, alkaline foods | 1. Avoid interaction |
| | Bulk-forming agents (e.g., calcium polypsyllium), stool softeners (e.g., docusate) | 1. Potential constipation or gut obstruction; dysphagia | 1. Administer with ample amounts of water or juice as recommended on label |
| | Magnesium salts (citrate, hydroxide, sulfate) | See antacids | |
| Proton pump inhibitors | Esomeprazole (Nexium) | 1. Profound ↓ gastric acid secretion, increased gastric pH, may interfere with absorption of iron, vitamin $B_{12}$<br>2. Diarrhea | 1. Generally mild, self-limiting; frequent and long-lasting loose stools >6/day may indicate serious *Clostridium difficile* superinfection, fluid/electrolyte loss |
| | Mineral oil | 1. ↓ Absorption of fat-soluble vitamins (A, D, E, K)<br>2. Aspiration may cause severe lipid pneumonitis<br>3. Nausea, vomiting, diarrhea | 1. Discourage use |
| ***Drugs Used for Infectious Diseases*** | | | |
| Antibiotics | Penicillins | 1. Nausea, epigastric distress<br>2. Vomiting, diarrhea<br>3. Glossitis or black hairy tongue | 1. Not absorbed well after oral administration; decreased acidity increases absorption |
| | Erythromycins | 1. GI distress (may be severe) | |
| | Tetracyclines | 1. Staining of teeth in newborn if administered during pregnancy or in children before deciduous teeth develop | 1. Avoid administering with any polyvalent cation salts (Al, Ca, Fe, Mg), which bind drug in gut and reduce absorption. Applies to foods/beverages rich in any of the above (especially calcium-rich dairy); antacids, which commonly contain Al + Mg (some contain only Ca); individual or combination mineral or vitamin/mineral supplements |
| | Fluoroquinolones (e.g., ciprofloxacin) | 1. Tendonitis, tendon rupture, mainly Achilles (from drug-induced impairment of collagen metabolism) | 1. See tetracyclines<br>2. Avoid administering to children unless no reasonable antibiotic alternatives are available (risk of tendon issues) |
| | Isoniazid ("INH") | 1. Peripheral neuropathy resulting from ↓ of pyridoxine's effect on nervous tissue<br>2. Hypoglycemia<br>3. Nausea and vomiting from gastric irritation<br>4. ↓ Absorption of folic acid; vitamins $B_{12}$, E; niacin depletion<br>5. ↑ Excretion of vitamin $B_{12}$ and folic acid | 1. Give pyridoxine ($B_6$) supplements |

↑ = increased, increases, stimulated, stimulates; ↓ = decreased, decreases, inhibited, inhibits; ACE = angiotensin-converting enzyme; AED = antiepileptic drug; CNS = central nervous system; GI = gastrointestinal; $H_2$ = histamine 2 receptor; IV = intravenous; LDL = low-density lipoprotein; MAO = monoamine oxidase; NSAIDs = nonsteroidal anti-inflammatory drugs; SSRI = selective serotonin reuptake inhibitor; THC = tetrahydrocannabinol; TNF = tumor necrosis factor; VLDL = very-low-density lipoprotein. From Mohs ME, Watson RR, Leonard-Green R. Nutritional effects of marijuana, cocaine, and nicotine. *J Am Diet Assoc.* 1990; 90:1261[51]; Roe DA. *Nutrient and Drug Interactions.* New York: Van Nostrand Reinhold/AVI; 1988; Bray J. Drug treatment of obesity. *Am J Clin Nutr.* 1992; 55:538S; Wellman P. Overview of adrenergic anorectic agents. *Am J Clin Nutr.* 1992; 55:193S; Pronsky ZM, Crowe JP. *Food-Medication Interactions*, 18th ed. New York: Food Medication Interactions Publishing; 2015.

Not all nutrient or drug molecules circulating in the bloodstream are free at any given time to interact with the cells of the body; instead, a portion of the total molecules are bound to plasma proteins. Only free (unbound) molecules can produce effects, and only they are capable of being metabolized or otherwise eliminated. The percentage of drug molecules bound to plasma protein, which is determined by a drug-dependent equilibrium, depends on the drug's chemical structure, other physicochemical properties (e.g., the pKa), and the plasma albumin content. Some liver and kidney diseases cause hypoalbuminemia, requiring drug dosage adjustments (usually reductions) based on total and free serum drug levels for highly plasma protein–bound drugs. Brunton et al.[3] provides specific information about many drugs.

### Elimination 1: Metabolism

The two major processes that are largely responsible for eliminating drugs or nutrients in the body are metabolism and excretion. The liver is the major site of metabolism, and the hepatocyte's microsomal cytochrome P450 enzyme system is the major means for biotransformation. Overall, metabolism transforms a drug to one or more metabolites that are less active pharmacologically or biologically and therefore potentially less toxic to the body; it also generally converts drugs or nutrients to metabolites that are more soluble in water and therefore can be eliminated more readily by the kidneys. Various nutrients are required for normal metabolic functions of the liver or are themselves substrates for metabolic reactions.

Several factors can alter the activity of the P450 system and dramatically influence drug responses. Enzyme activities peak at puberty and remain high until about 60 years of age. With some drugs such as theophylline, however, the metabolic rate is highest at about 8 to 13 years of age. In old age, enzyme activity gradually declines. Age-related decreases in renal function may accompany declines in hepatic function. Marked and prolonged nutrient deficiencies can seriously impair liver function, including those functions necessary to eliminate therapeutic agents. Any disease or chemical (including many drugs) that damages hepatocytes, reduces hepatic blood flow, or directly inhibits the P450 system has the potential to reduce drug or nutrient metabolism. Deficiencies or excesses of hormones, particularly insulin and thyroxine, can have marked effects on hepatic drug metabolism overall.

### Elimination 2: Excretion

The kidneys are the main organ for eliminating drugs and drug metabolites. Their effectiveness in this regard depends on renal blood flow (influenced by cardiac output) and the integrity of transporters (i.e., molecular pumps) located in various parts of the nephron. Conditions that decrease cardiac output or blood pressure to levels sufficient to reduce renal blood flow can decrease the glomerular filtration rate and hinder drug elimination. Just as local pH and the pKa of a drug affect absorption, urine pH influences tubular secretion and, more importantly, tubular reabsorption. Medical disorders and the drugs used to treat them can affect urine pH, producing dramatic effects on the biological fate of drugs. For example, alkalization of the urine by sodium bicarbonate increases the elimination of salicylate (i.e., aspirin) by favoring the formation of ionized and poorly diffusible molecules that cannot undergo tubular reabsorption. The effects on amphetamine and amphetamine-like drugs such as methylphenidate, which are weak bases, are the opposite: alkalization of the urine reduces excretion. The interaction of amphetamine with urinary acidification is particularly problematic because of the widespread use of these drugs in the treatment of attention-deficit hyperactivity disorder (ADHD). If dosages are not titrated properly or not timed properly with respect to meals, anorexia and nutritional deficits may occur (the desired result when amphetamines are given for anorexigenic effects in grossly obese persons).

## ADVERSE NUTRITIONAL EFFECTS OF PSYCHOACTIVE DRUGS

### Anticonvulsants (Antiepileptic Drugs)

Because of their many adverse effects on metabolism, antiepileptic drugs (AEDs) have been a subject of research for many years.[5–11] Numerous adverse effects on nutrition or metabolism have been reported, including abnormalities in mineral and bone metabolism (resulting in rickets or osteomalacia), folate deficiency with or without macrocytosis, congenital malformations, and connective tissue disorders. Phenytoin, a strong inducer of the P450 system with a host of clinically significant drug interactions, causes gingival hyperplasia ("Dilantin hyperplasia"). Neural tube defects can occur among infants of mothers taking any of several common AEDs, the biggest offender being valproic acid, a strong P450 inhibitor. Abnormal fat and protein metabolism and low blood levels of vitamins E and K, pyridoxine, vitamin $B_{12}$, biotin, and thyroid hormones have also been reported. Bone metabolism is affected, as shown by decreased levels of serum phosphate, calcitonin, calcium, and various vitamin D moieties, which depend on the drug dose and duration of treatment. The pathophysiology of rickets and osteomalacia has been attributed to induction (stimulation) of the hepatic P450 enzyme system that results in vitamin D deficiency or increased skeletal turnover of minerals.[11] Most reports point to the need for ensuring an adequate vitamin D serum level by supplementation or sunlight exposure.

According to Dawson-Hughes,[12] dietary protein has both positive and negative effects on calcium metabolism. Protein stimulates the production of insulin-like growth factor 1 (IGF-1), which promotes osteoblast-mediated bone formation; protein also increases urinary calcium loss but reduces bone calcium loss.[13] A study of the vitamin D, calcium, and bone status in 338 developmentally delayed children receiving AEDs showed ambulatory status to be an important risk factor for low serum calcitriol and osteopenia; physical activity and prophylactic vitamin D supplementation were recommended for those at risk.[13]

Studies of folate deficiency after AED use are continuing, and several hypotheses have been proposed. One is that intestinal folic acid absorption is inhibited by AEDs. Others postulate that folate acts as a cofactor for phenytoin metabolism.[14] Causes of folate deficiency include decreased folate absorption, decreased metabolic activation of folate, and decreased induction of drug-metabolizing enzymes for which certain AEDs can act as substrates, inducers (e.g., phenytoin, ethosuximide), or inhibitors (e.g., valproic acid). Although various mechanisms can result in folate deficiency and impaired hematopoiesis, induction of drug enzymes may increase not only the requirement for the enzymes but also the rate of drug metabolism, resulting in an increase in the drug dosage given and an increased risk of other drug side effects and adverse responses. Folate deficiency and the resultant increased homocysteine level have been linked to neurodegenerative disorders by Mattson and Shea and others,[14–17] and to cognitive diseases by Miller.[18] Alterations in folic acid metabolism are of most consequence to pregnant women because folate deficiency has been reported to cause congenital malformations and stillbirths.[19] According to Suarez et al.,[20] insufficient levels of serum vitamin $B_{12}$ also may be an important etiologic factor leading to neural tube defects. For pregnant women taking phenytoin, another nutritional risk is the possibility of hemorrhagic disease or other coagulopathies in the newborn, which have been attributed to decreased levels of vitamin K–dependent clotting factors. This is a major reason why pregnant women taking phenytoin should be given supplemental vitamin K shortly before delivery, and the baby should be given the drug prophylactically immediately after birth.

Gingival hyperplasia during phenytoin therapy is another, widely known adverse effect of AEDs; it is reported in approximately 60% of pediatric patients taking phenytoin. The mechanism probably involves altered collagen metabolism rather than altered drug metabolism per se. In severe cases, phenytoin-induced gingival hyperplasia can indirectly alter the dietary intake of many nutrients because it becomes difficult or impossible to chew properly. There is no known cure or treatment, but frequent oral health care, preferably by a dentist with considerable experience in proper prevention and treatment of gingival disease, can minimize the problems.

Largely because of hepatotoxicity, hyperammonemia is a common side effect of valproic acid therapy for epilepsy.[21] Treatment with a medium-length, straight-chain fatty acid diet was reported to abolish valproate-induced hyperammonemia. Hypocarnitinemia, related to an alteration in fatty acid metabolism in persons receiving valproate, has also been reported.[22,23] Carnitine deficiency from altered fatty acid metabolism, insufficient endogenous carnitine synthesis, or both, may be a mechanism for valproic acid hepatotoxicity.[24] Castro-Gago et al.[25] studied serum amino acids in 22 epileptic children treated with valproic acid. Hypocarnitinemia was found in all 22, and hyperammonemia in 16 (73%). Levels of glutamic acid, arginine, glycine, serine, and alanine were higher in valproic acid–treated patients than in controls, whereas levels of aspartic acid and ornithine were lower. Urea cycle dysfunction was suggested as a contributing factor in these findings, and the authors recommended avoidance of a high-protein diet. Abnormal fat metabolism resulting from AED therapy includes increased serum triglycerides and/or cholesterol in persons on long-term multidrug therapy. Blood folic acid levels remain unchanged. Lower thyroxine and higher retinol-binding capacity were found among children with delayed cognitive development who received phenytoin (diphenylhydantoin), phenobarbital, or AED combinations, but vitamin A was higher among those receiving phenytoin. Vitamin A and retinol-binding protein were lower in children with infections, and vitamin A was lower in those with serum zinc levels lower than 70 μg/dL.

## Neuroleptics

Neuroleptics, mainly the phenothiazines (chlorpromazine and many others), are antipsychotic drugs that are widely used, largely because of their relatively low cost; they are linked to abnormalities in nutrient metabolism. Whereas the typical use of neuroleptics is for patients with schizophrenia or dementia of various etiologies, they are gaining a more accepted role in the treatment of patients with autism spectrum disorder (ASD) who have prominent behavioral issues. Drug-related nutritional issues and problems seem to apply mostly to phenothiazines and not the newer, "nontraditional" antipsychotics such as risperidone and olanzapine. The nontraditional antipsychotics are noteworthy mainly because they carry a very low risk of extrapyramidal side effects and tardive dyskinesia and a low risk of peripheral autonomic (particularly antimuscarinic) side effects. However, these advantages may sometimes be outweighed by the disadvantages of cost and a higher risk of neutropenia.

Pyridoxine may alleviate certain toxicities resulting from phenothiazines, and ascorbic acid may play an important role in modulating the behavioral effects of haloperidol (a butyrophenone) and virtually all phenothiazines. Tardive dyskinesia[26] and the accompanying xerostomia caused by thickening of saliva due to peripheral antimuscarinic effects can reduce the desire or ability to eat, with the expected pannutritional deficiencies ensuing. Reduced saliva volume and increased viscosity caused by traditional antipsychotics can lead to dental caries and tooth loss if adequate dental care is not provided. Weight loss is not uncommon in patients during long-term neuroleptic use, but the causes are far-ranging and can encompass the expected drug effects as well as anorexia from physiological, pharmacologic, and psychological (i.e., depression) issues. Problems with inadequate food lubrication, chewing, and swallowing resulting from reduced salivary secretions can be exacerbated by dysfunction of oropharyngeal skeletal muscles and the attendant difficulties and dangers. Zarate and Quiroz recommended increased study of combination treatments to determine the most efficacious and safe combinations.[27] Fernandez and Friedman noted that the severity of tardive dyskinesia and the absolute need for antipsychotic therapy often dictate the treatment approach for tardive dyskinesia.[28] However, most therapies aimed at tardive dyskinesias are prophylactic and provide only symptomatic relief, meaning that they do not halt or reverse the underlying brain biochemical abnormalities. Once tardive dyskinesias develop, regardless of the cause, they cannot be reversed by any known medications.

Chlorpromazine promotes weight gain, which is attributed to an increased appetite (in some patients) and water retention from both direct and indirect renal effects. A factor contributing to or accompanying weight gain is glucose intolerance due to inhibited insulin release. Persons who are prediabetic or diabetic are at greater risk.

## Central Nervous System Stimulants

Methylphenidate and related drugs such as amphetamine mixtures (e.g., Adderall) are classified as stimulants; however, they have a dose-dependent sedating effect on children (and many older patients) with ADHD. Although there seems to be no evidence that methylphenidate or amphetamines specifically interfere with the metabolism of any particular nutrient, the nutritional effects of these drugs have not been investigated fully beyond the widespread awareness that they are anorexigenic and therefore may cause nutritional issues as a result of decreased food or nutrient intake. There is also the potential for significant suppression of growth in height and weight, usually preceded by reduced appetite. Rebound weight gain is often observed during summer months when medication is discontinued. The same effects, and their underlying mechanisms, apply to amphetamines used in lieu of methylphenidate.

Central nervous system stimulants are sometimes prescribed to patients with ASD, mainly to counteract the generalized sedation and certain other side effects often associated with neuroleptics. However, doing so often results in problems with drug interactions, such as when one drug counteracts the desired effects of another. The same issue applies when stimulants are used to reduce sedation and other key side effects of antidepressants.

## Antidepressants and Mood-Elevating Drugs

Appetite and body weight can be affected by antidepressants, depending on the drug class, just as they can be affected by depression itself. The subclass of antidepressants known as nonselective monoamine oxidase (MAO) inhibitors (e.g., pargyline) is responsible for a unique and potentially lethal interaction with foods and beverages that are rich in tyramine, drugs that are classified as mixed-acting sympathomimetics (e.g., pseudoephedrine) or indirect-acting sympathomimetics (e.g., amphetamines), and meperidine. Today, because of these dangers and the typically excellent efficacy and side effect profiles of the newer selective serotonin reuptake inhibitors (SSRIs) such as citalopram, escitalopram, fluoxetine, fluvoxamine, and paroxetine, nonselective MAO inhibitors are seldom used. The newer, brain-selective MAO inhibitors (e.g., selegiline) that are used for conditions such as Parkinson disease are far less likely to participate in the food and drug interactions described, but caution is still advised.

The SSRIs have become first-line drugs for depression, but far less is known about them with respect to drug-nutrient interactions. SSRIs are used in the treatment of postpartum depression. Spillmann et al. reported marked declines in platelet 5-hydroxytryptamine (5-HT) levels in treated mothers, whereas infants showed little or no change after exposure through breast-feeding.[29] They also found that tryptophan depletion increased depressive symptoms in medicated, formerly depressed patients. Epperson et al. reported that mothers taking SSRIs can breast-feed their infants without appreciably affecting peripheral or central 5-HT transport in the infants.[30] Nordeng et al.[31] investigated the level of excretion in breast milk and listed the then-available SSRIs in order from highest to lowest: citalopram, fluoxetine, paroxetine, fluvoxamine, and sertraline.

Tricyclic antidepressants (e.g., imipramine) were the mainstay of depression therapy until use of SSRIs became widespread. However, drugs such as imipramine still play an important role in managing nocturnal enuresis in some children. The benefit with this use arises from rather strong antimuscarinic (atropine-like) effects, not from relief of depression. The main adverse potential nutritional effects are largely identical to those of any antimuscarinic drug. Xerostomia leads to difficulties in chewing, swallowing, and initiating oral digestion of foods and consequent issues of food or nutrient intake. Reduction of gut motility leads to constipation, and bladder motility also is reduced.

Lithium is a naturally occurring element that has long been used for prevention of manic episodes in patients with bipolar illness, although antidepressants have now assumed a greater role. Because lithium therapy is still sometimes used, it is important to note the importance of periodic monitoring of serum sodium levels during lithium therapy. The cations $Na^+$ and $Li^+$ are chemically similar and compete with one another in various cell regulatory events. When there is a positive sodium balance (i.e., excessive sodium intake or reduced renal sodium loss), lithium blood levels and effects are reduced. A negative sodium balance prolongs the half-life of lithium, increasing the risk of excessive or toxic blood levels and effects. Drugs that elevate serum sodium levels (e.g., systemic corticosteroids, many antihypertensive drugs) may reduce lithium effects. Dietary sodium restriction or administration of sodium-wasting drugs (that is, *all* diuretics) can raise serum lithium levels and increase the risk of potentially serious lithium toxicity. Because of the relatively high risks of side effects and adverse responses with lithium, SSRIs and other classes of drugs have taken on a major role as lithium alternatives in the mood-stabilizing therapy of bipolar disorder.

## ADRENAL CORTICOSTEROIDS (GLUCOCORTICOIDS)

Glucocorticoids are a crucial element for successful treatment of the number one cause of chronic disease, physician and emergency visits, and hospitalizations among children with or without developmental disorders: asthma. Glucocorticoids have a host of applications and are used in a wide range of dosages. Replacement doses are given for hypocortisolism (e.g., Addison disease). Pharmacological dosages are used for suppression of inflammation, including various arthritic conditions and asthma. Prednisone is one of the most widely prescribed oral agents, and despite its classification as a glucocorticoid, it has clinically significant mineralocorticoid (aldosterone-like) actions. Metabolic effects due to glucocorticoid activity are diverse. Most importantly and most commonly, they include hyperglycemia, alterations of fat metabolism, and increased protein (muscle) catabolism, with protein synthesis diverted to carbohydrate synthesis (i.e., gluconeogenesis) at the expense of muscle wasting. Stimulated appetite, a common outcome of systemic corticosteroid therapy, may be inadequate to prevent weight loss and various dietary nutrient deficiencies.

Orally inhaled corticosteroids (e.g., beclomethasone) are used in the management of well-controlled asthma far more than oral agents, which are largely reserved for frequent and poorly controlled asthma or asthma flare-ups. Depending on the actual drug and dose, metabolic effects may occur with prednisone use. However, as a class, the oral agents are poorly absorbed, and effects on metabolism are usually slight if they occur at all.

## VITAMINS USED IN PHARMACOLOGICAL DOSES (MEGAVITAMINS)

During the early 20th century, the importance of niacin (nicotinic acid) in the diet was recognized when it was found to prevent or cure pellagra. The ostensible similarities of the mental symptoms of pellagra to those of schizophrenia led to the use of niacin megadoses for treating the latter condition. The term *megavitamin* or *orthomolecular therapy* encompasses the use of vitamins such as thiamine, pyridoxine, vitamin $B_{12}$, biotin, vitamin E, ascorbic acid, and folic acid, singly or in combination, to treat nonspecific mental retardation, psychosis, ASD, hyperactivity, dyslexia, Down syndrome, and other learning and developmental disorders. Although remarkable benefits of megavitamin therapy have occasionally been reported, objective data have not provided sufficient documentation to allow endorsement of this type of therapy by the American Psychiatric Association or other applicable and respected professional groups.

Use of vitamins in pharmacologic doses (i.e., greater than recommended supplemental or replacement doses) raises questions of safety and side effects. The toxic effects of excessive amounts of the fat-soluble vitamins A, D, E, and K, which tend to sequester in adipose tissue, have long been established, whereas water-soluble vitamins are generally considered harmless because excess amounts tend to be excreted. However, the latter generalization is not always correct, especially when up to 1000 times the normal requirement are used therapeutically. Until evidence of a long-term reduction in cardiovascular events was shown to be lacking with niacin, pharmacologic doses were often used as a first-line approach (along with diet and exercise) to raise high-density lipoprotein (HDL) cholesterol; however, such doses commonly cause erythema, pruritus, and generalized cutaneous flushing. There were also worrisome reports of liver damage, hyperglycemia, and increased hemoglobin $A_{1C}$ and uric acid levels. Another water-soluble vitamin, pyridoxine ($B_6$), was shown to cause neuropathy after daily consumption of 2 to 6 g, despite the fact that it has been used widely and rather successful to reduce neuritis and neuropathy from such drugs as the antihypertensive/heart failure medicine hydralazine.

Birth defects associated with vitamin A occurred with maternal intake of 25,000 IU/day. Pfeiffer et al.[32] reviewed and summarized outcomes on the efficacy of vitamin $B_6$ and magnesium in the treatment of autism and found that a majority of the studies reported a favorable response; many studies were thought to have methodologic shortcomings.

## COMPLEMENTARY AND ALTERNATIVE MEDICINES

A quickly growing area of discussion and concern is the use of complementary and alternative medicines (CAMs). CAMs have been self-prescribed (and sometimes prescribed by a care provider) for a host of conditions, but in many situations proof of efficacy is lacking or, at best, unclear or equivocal. Teenagers, adolescents, and young adults have probably accounted for a major portion of the growth in CAM use, and in many cases these medicines are chosen because of fear of adverse effects from traditional drugs or a real or perceived lack of efficacy of the prescription medications.

Use of herbal (botanical) and dietary supplement (HDSs) accounts for almost one-half of all CAM use in the United States.[33] In recent years, HDS use has grown in excess of 50%, and in approximately 95% of cases, HDSs were self-prescribed, mainly to maintain or improve health.[34–37] To complicate matters somewhat, it has been estimated that fewer than 40% of patients using CAMs, or particularly HDSs, disclosed such use to their health care providers.[33,38,39] A prevailing reason may be the perception that herbal and other "natural" medicines are safe, free of adverse or unwanted side effects, and free of interactions with other drugs. Chapter 26 provides for more information about specific botanicals.

Efficacy and safety are often more apparent than real with CAMs or HDSs. For example, St. John's wort has gained popularity among many people as a mood elevator. However, it is a powerful inducer of several members of the cytochrome P450 enzyme system (e.g., CYP1A2, CYP2C9, CYP2C19, CYP3A4) that are responsible for metabolizing a host of diverse drugs with low therapeutic indices or unfavorable side effects and drug-interaction profiles. (The therapeutic index is the ratio of average lethal dose or blood concentration to average effective dose or concentration.) St John's wort interacts with many other drugs. It also strongly induces P-glycoprotein, a major cell membrane efflux pump for many drugs, leading to greater elimination or inhibited uptake of many drugs that exert their therapeutic effects only after gaining access to the intracellular compartment.

At least 1000 medicines, including herbals, have been linked to the development of drug-induced hepatic damage or frank hepatotoxicity. Aside from general illness arising from liver damage (with potentially fatal outcome or requirement for liver transplantation), hepatotoxicity or simple hepatic dysfunction can cause impaired metabolic inactivation or detoxification of many drugs; impaired activity of drugs that must be metabolically activated first (these are called prodrugs, an example of which is the widely used antiplatelet drug, clopidogrel); and impaired synthesis of albumin, which plays a crucial role in carrying drug molecules through the circulation and maintaining a normal equilibrium between bound and free (active) drug molecules. Two good references for information on these issues are Stirrimann et al.[40] and Bunchorntavakul and Reddy.[41] The US Food and Drug Association has an excellent website with a searchable database identifying drugs and supplements associated with hepatotoxicity,[42] as will as other sites with information on HDSs.[43,44]

## FACTORS TO BE CONSIDERED IN NUTRITIONAL ASSESSMENT

Individuals on drug therapy who are at risk for nutrient deficiencies require nutrition screening and/or assessment, including a dietary study, anthropometric measurements, physical examination, suitable biochemical analyses, and observation of feeding and eating skills and behaviors. The dietary assessment focuses on nutrients (e.g., thiamine[45]) that carry a risk of deficiency because of nutrient intake quantity or of drug therapy. For example, the emphasis of the dietary study for a person taking AEDs would be on intake of foods rich in calcium, vitamins D and K, and folic acid. Nonfood sources of activated vitamin D (e.g., exposure to sunlight) and amount of activity (which increases utilization of vitamin D) should also be considered. Commonly used anthropometric measurements for children are height, weight, and triceps skinfold. These are useful in assessing growth and development. Monitoring of height and weight is recommended for children who are taking methylphenidate or an amphetamine mixture for attention deficit disorder or ADHD, whereas monitoring of weight is recommended for persons taking lithium or neuroleptics. The physical examination includes screening for signs and symptoms of nutrient deficiencies, such as megaloblastic anemia accompanying folic acid deficiency or skeletal abnormalities observed in rickets. Laboratory analysis of blood or urine for nutrient or enzyme levels could detect subclinical nutrient deficiencies. Low serum levels of inorganic phosphorus and elevated alkaline phosphatase may be indicative of rickets or osteomalacia.

## DIETARY SUPPLEMENTATION AND MANAGEMENT

Drug therapy is a first-line mode of intervention for a host of illnesses, and it is important to understand the physiological mechanisms that cause or contribute to adverse drug effects in providing nutritional care. In most cases, dietary modification or nutrient supplementation and regulation of the dosage and timing of drug administration can partially compensate for the relevant adverse effects.

Improving the overall quality of the diet is often preferred to supplementation with specific nutrients. However, supplementation with vitamin D and folic acid has been recommended for persons taking AEDs. Reversal of an abnormal serum profile with vitamin $D_2$ treatment has been demonstrated. Although bone mass values were unchanged in vitamin $D_3$–treated patients taking phenobarbital or phenytoin,[46] slow, gradual improvement in bone mass has been achieved.[47,48] Long-term, low-dose supplementation 400 IU of vitamin $D_3$ daily) is recommended for epileptic pregnant women on AED therapy.[49] Studies in sunny regions of the world have found that adequate ultraviolet light exposure, diet, and activity can prevent the development of AED-induced osteomalacia.[50] Because toxic effects of megadoses of vitamin D have been reported, a cautious combination of these approaches is recommended.

Prophylactic vitamin K therapy has become the norm for pregnant women taking phenytoin or other barbiturates. Although folic acid supplementation has resulted in improved mental status in some persons with epilepsy, routine supplementation is not recommended, and there is some suggestion that supplementing the diet with even small amounts of oral folate may reduce serum concentrations of some anticonvulsants. This can contribute to an associated loss of seizure control unless the drug dosage is increased and/or the dosing intervals are shortened. The best option is to avoid folate supplementation to prevent related changes in drug dosages. Periodic measurements of serum drug concentrations is essential whenever adjustments in dosages of AEDs seem warranted.

Among pregnant epileptic women, supplementation decreased the incidence of folate deficiency and negative outcomes, particularly fetal neural tube defects (see Chapter 10). Folate supplementation has also been suggested during lithium therapy. Fasting blood glucose levels must be monitored in patients taking chlorpromazine or systemic corticosteroids (e.g., prednisone). There is also growing evidence that 3-hydroxy-3-methylglutaryl–coenzyme A (HMG-CoA) reductase inhibitors (i.e., statins such as atorvastatin), the first-line drugs for most dyslipidemias, pose a risk of prediabetes or diabetes.

Appropriate exercise and dietary modifications assist in limiting weight gain. In healthy volunteers, high-carbohydrate foods were found to enhance and protein-rich foods to reduce phenytoin absorption; fatty foods had no measurable influence.

Some anorexigenic effects of drugs can be offset by modifying the dose and by administering the drug with meals. Weekly monitoring of weight and energy intake is recommended so that drug therapy may be adjusted as needed. Additional suggestions for management of the adverse effects of specific drugs are presented in Table 27–1.

In the specific context of children with developmental disorders, a host of dietary modifications have been tried, not so much to prevent or correct unwanted side effects of prescription drugs but as actual treatments for the developmental disorder. Common dietary modifications have included drastically reducing (or abolishing) intake of casein and/or gluten. Most studies have failed to show any consistent or statistically significant beneficial effects of such approaches in the development or symptoms of ASD, nor any ability to augment the effects of drugs traditionally used to treat it. One major drawback to chelation therapy of any kind, aside from questionable rationales and efficacy, is that common chelators are nonselective. They bind not only target heavy metals but also important polyvalent cations such as calcium, magnesium, and zinc and therefore can cause a host of neurological, neuromuscular, and cardiovascular toxicities.

### References


1. MedLine Plus. *Developmental Disabilities.* U.S. National Library of Medicine. Last update, May 2016. http://www.nlm.nih.gov/medlineplus/developmentaldisabilities.html Accessed June 23, 2016.
2. McCabe BJ, Wolfe JJ, Frankel EH. *Handbook of Food-Drug Interactions.* Boca Raton, FL: CRC Press; 2003.
3. Brunton LL, Chabner BA, Knollmann BC, eds. *Goodman and Gilman's the Pharmacological Basis of Therapeutics*, 12th ed. New York: McGraw-Hill; 2011.
4. LiCastro F, Ariani RA, Faldella G, et al. Immune-endocrine status and coeliac disease in children with Down's syndrome: relationships with zinc and cognitive efficiency. *Brain Res Bull.* 2001; 55:313.
5. Pavlakis SG, Chusid RL, Roye DP, Nordli DR. Valproate therapy: predisposition to bone fracture? *Pediatr Neurol.* 1998; 19:143.
6. Pedrera JD, Canal ML, Carvajal J, et al. Influence of vitamin D administration on bone ultrasound measurements in patients on anticonvulsant therapy. *Eur J Clin Invest.* 2000; 30:895.
7. Pluskiewicz W, Nowakowska J. Bone status after long-term anticonvulsant therapy in epileptic patients: evaluation using quantitative ultrasound of calcaneus and phalanges. *Ultrasound Med Biol.* 1997; 23:553.
8. Filardi S, Guerreiro CA, Magna LA, Marques Neto JF. Bone mineral density, vitamin D and anticonvulsant therapy. *Arq Neuropsiquiatr.* 2000; 58:616.
9. Bischof F, Basu D, Pettifor JM. Pathological long-bone fractures in residents with cerebral palsy in a long-term care facility in South Africa. *Dev Med Child Neurol.* 2002; 44:119.
10. De Marco P, Calevo MG, Moroni A, et al. Reduced folate carrier polymorphism (80A → G) and neural tube defects. *Eur J Hum Genet.* 2003; 11:245.
11. Alderman CP, Hill CL. Abnormal bone mineral metabolism after long-term anticonvulsant treatment. *Ann Pharmacother.* 1994; 28:47.
12. Dawson-Hughes B. Interaction of dietary calcium and protein in bone health in humans. *J Nutr.* 2003; 133:852S.
13. Baer MT, Kozlowski BW, Blyler EM, Trahms CM, Taylor ML, Hogan MP. Vitamin D, calcium, and bone status in children with developmental delay in relation to anticonvulsant use and ambulatory status. *Am J Clin Nutr* 1997; 65:1042.
14. Mattson MP, Shea TB. Folate and homocysteine metabolism in neural plasticity and neurodegenerative disorders. *Trends Neurosci.* 2003; 26:137.
15. Wilson RD, Davies G, Desilets V, Reid GJ, et al. The use of folic acid for the prevention of neural tube defects and other congenital anomalies. *J Obstet Gynaecol Can.* 2003; 25:959.
16. Yerby MS. Management issues for women with epilepsy: neural tube defects and folic acid supplementation. *Neurology.* 2003; 61(Suppl 2):S23.
17. Yerby MS. Clinical care of pregnant women with epilepsy: neural tube defects and folic acid supplementation. *Rev Neurol.* 2002; 15:34:236.
18. Miller AL. The methionine-homocysteine cycle and its effects on cognitive diseases. *Altern Med Rev.* 2003; 8:7.
19. Stumpf DA. Symptoms of B(12) deficiency can occur in women of childbearing age supplemented with folate. *Neurology.* 2003; 60:353.
20. Suarez L, Hendricks K, Felkner M, Gunter E. Maternal serum $B_{12}$ levels and risk for neural tube defects in a Texas-Mexico border population. *Ann Epidemiol.* 2003; 13:81.
21. Matsui K, Iwamoto H, Ohtsuki N, Kobayashi T, Miyake S, Yamada M. The problems of valproate therapy in severely handicapped children: valproate induced hyperammonemia and hypocarnitinemia. *No To Hattatsu.* 1991; 23:32.
22. Miyamoto T, Miyamoto M, Hirata K, Katayama S. A case report of valproate encephalopathy [in Japanese]. *Rinsho Shinkeigaku.* 1999; 39:1075.
23. Chung S, Choi J, Hyun T, Rha Y, Bae C. Alterations in the carnitine metabolism in epileptic children treated with valproic acid. *J Korean Med Sci.* 1997; 12:553.
24. De Vivo DC, Bohan TP, Coulter DL, et al. L-Carnitine supplementation in childhood epilepsy: current perspectives. *Epilepsia.* 1998; 39:1216.

25. Castro-Gago M, Rodrigo-Saez E, Novo-Rodriguez I, Camina MF. Hyperaminoacidemia in epileptic children treated with valproic acid. *Childs Nerv Syst.* 1990; 6:434.
26. Kulkarni SK, Naidu PS. Tardive dyskinesia: an update. *Drugs Today.* 2001; 37:97.
27. Zarate CA, Quiroz JA. Combination treatment in bipolar disorder: a review of controlled trials. *Bipolar Disord.* 2003; 5:217.
28. Fernandez HH, Friedman JH. Classification and treatment of tardive syndromes. *Neurology.* 2003; 9:16.
29. Spillmann MK, Van der Does AJ, Rankin MA, et al. Tryptophan depletion in SSRI-recovered depressed outpatients. *Psychopharmacology (Berl).* 2001; 155:123.
30. Epperson N, Czarkowski KA, Ward-O'Brien D, Weiss E, Gueorguieva R, Jatlow P. Maternal sertraline treatment and serotonin transport in breast-feeding mother-infant pairs. *Am J Psychiatry.* 2001; 158:1631.
31. Nordeng H, Bergsholm YK, Bohler E, Spigset O. The transfer of selective serotonin reuptake inhibitors to human milk. *Tidsskr Nor Laegeforen.* 2001; 20;121:199; comment 1156.
32. Pfeiffer SI, Norton J, Nelson L, Shott S. Efficacy of vitamin $B_6$ and magnesium in the treatment of autism: a methodology review and summary of outcomes. *J Autism Dev Disord.* 1995; 25:481.
33. Tindle HA, Davis RB, Phillips RS, Eisenberg DM. Trends in use of complementary and alternative medicine by US adults: 1997–2002. *Altern Ther Health Med.* 2005; 11:42.
34. Barnes PM, Bloom B, Nahin RL. Complementary and alternative medicine use among adults and children: United States, 2007. *Natl Health Stat Rep.* 2008; 10:1.
35. Unützer J, Klap R, Sturm R, et al. Mental disorders and the use of alternative medicine: results from a national survey. *Am J Psychiatry.* 2000; 157:1851.
36. Snyder J, Brown P. Complementary and alternative medicine in children: an analysis of the recent literature. *Curr Opin Pediatr.* 2012; 24:539.
37. Bailey RL, Gahche JJ, Miller PE, et al. Why US adults used dietary supplements. *JAMA Intern Med.* 2013; 173:355.
38. Institute of Medicine Committee on the Use of Complementary and Alternative Medicine by the American Public. *Complementary and Alternative Medicine in the United States.* Washington, DC: National Academies Press; 2005.
39. Eisenberg DM, Kessler RC, VanRompay MI, et al. Perceptions about complementary therapies relative to conventional therapies among adults who use both: results from a national survey. *Ann Intern Med.* 2001; 135:344.
40. Stirrimann G, Kessebohm K, Lauterburg B. Liver injury caused by drugs: an update. *Swiss Med Wkly.* 2010; 140:13080.
41. Bunchorntavakul C, Reddy KR. Herbal and dietary supplement toxicity. *Aliment Pharmacol Ther.* 2013; 37:3.
42. LiverTox database. *Clinical and Research Information on Drug-induced Liver Injury.* http://www.livertox.nih.gov Accessed June 21, 2016.
43. US Food and Drug Administration. *Information for Consumers on Use of Dietary Supplements.* http://www.fda.gov/food/dietarysupplements/usingdietarysupplements/ Accessed June 21, 2016.
44. U.S. Food and Drug Administration. *Dietary Supplements.*http://www.fda.gov/Food/DietarySupplements/default.htm Accessed June 21, 2016.
45. Ke ZJ, DeGiorgio LA, Volpe BT, Gibson GE. Reversal of thiamine deficiency: induced neurodegeneration. *J Neuropathol Exp Neurol* 2003; 62:195.
46. Shibley IA, Pennington SN. Metabolic and mitotic changes associated with the fetal alcohol syndrome. *Alcohol.* 1997; 32:423.
47. Carrel AL, Myers SE, Whitman BY, Allen DB. Benefits of long-term therapy in Prader-Willi syndrome: a 4-year study. *J Clin Endocrinol.* 2002; 87:1581.
48. Cohen S, Glazewski R, Khan S, Khan A. Weight gain with risperidone among patients with mental retardation: effect of calorie restriction. *J Clin Psychiatry.* 2001; 62:114.
49. Glick NR, Fischer MH, Adkins WN. The influence of nutrition on IGF-1 in tube-fed profoundly retarded adults. *J Am Coll Nutr.* 2001; 20:81.
50. Hals J, Ek J, Svalastog AG, Nilsen H. Studies on nutrition in severely neurologically disabled children in an institution. *Acta Paediatr.* 1996; 85:1469; comment in *Acta Paediatr.* 1997; 86:670.

# E.

# MISCELLANEOUS CHRONIC DISEASES

## 28 | Allergy and Immunological Disorders

CHRISTINA C. LEWIS, CAROL J. HENDERSON, AND AMAL H. ASSA'AD

There is a powerful interplay between the human immune system and nutrition. The integrity of the immune system depends in part on a healthy nutrition status, and congenital or acquired defects in immunity may lead to disturbances in nutrition, such as cachexia or malnutrition. Abnormalities of the immune response, such as those that lead to an allergic reaction to foods, may impair the nutrition status of the individual. This chapter provides an overview of the immune system, immunodeficiencies, and the interactions between nutrition and immunity. The development of food allergy in children is described, as an example of an immune disorder that directly impacts nutrition.

### OVERVIEW OF THE IMMUNE SYSTEM

The human immune system is sophisticated and powerful, but depends on adequate nutrition to function optimally. Even minor alterations in nutrition can result in defective immunity, and deficiencies of trace elements can predispose to life threatening infections.[1,2] The human immune system has several layers of protection against invading microorganisms and other pathogens. The various cells and mediators of the immune system are components of and confer either innate or adaptive immunity (Table 28-1).

#### Innate Immunity

Innate immunity consists of primary, nonspecific immune protection that is conferred by physical barriers (e.g., epithelial surfaces) and by certain cells (e.g., macrophages) and proteins (e.g., cytokines). The function of innate immunity is to combat pathogens immediately (within hours), before an infection becomes robust. However, because of its ability to react rapidly, the innate immune system has a limited repertoire of action.

The physical barriers of the body provide the first line of defense. Intact skin forms a highly effective and almost impermeable barrier to microorganisms and pathogens. Secretions of the sweat and sebaceous glands can inhibit the growth of bacteria. Secretions of the eyes (tears), the respiratory tract (mucus), and the gastrointestinal tract (saliva and stomach acid) work in concert with mechanical processes to clear microorganisms from the epithelium. These physical barriers, along with the person's individual repertoire of commensal bacteria, greatly reduce the likelihood of infection.

The primary cells involved in innate immune responses are neutrophils, macrophages, and natural killer (NK) cells. The principal proteins of innate immunity are those of the complement system, which are manufactured by the liver. Complement proteins elicit innate immunity by marking cells and microorganisms for phagocytosis and lysis. In the event that a microorganism is able to bypass these basic defenses of innate immunity, the host has additional, more sophisticated mechanisms that can be employed to stop the spread of infection.

#### Adaptive Immunity

Adaptive immunity is the most sophisticated arm of the immune system; it has humoral and cellular components, which collectively give rise to the memory and specificity that are its hallmarks. Adaptive immunity has the ability to remember and respond more vigorously with repeated exposures to the same microbe, and it is able to recognize

**Table 28–1.** The Components of the Human Immune System

| Innate Immunity | Adaptive Immunity |
|---|---|
| **Characteristics** | |
| *Natural, native (no memory)*<br>• First line of defense<br>• Nonspecific responses against microbial pathogens<br>• Immediate, maximal responses<br>• Does not confer long-lasting immunity (i.e., no immunological memory) | *Acquired, specific (has memory)*<br>• Mechanisms stimulated by microbes to adapt<br>• Pathogen- and antigen-specific responses<br>• Exposure leads to immunological memory<br>• More powerful mechanisms develop later |
| **Activity** | |
| Defenses in place *before* infection occurs | Recognition of specific microbes *after* initial exposure |
| **Components** | |
| 1. Epithelial barriers<br>2. Phagocytic cells<br>• Neutrophils<br>• Macrophages<br>3. Inflammation<br>• Complement<br>4. Antiviral defense<br>• Dendritic cells<br>• Natural killer (NK) cells | 1. Lymphocytes<br>• B cells<br>• T cells<br>2. *Humoral or antibody-mediated immunity*<br>• Immunoglobulins (IgG, IgA, IgM, IgE) produced by differentiated B cells (plasma cells)<br>3. *Cellular or cell-mediated immunity (CMI)*<br>• T cells |

or distinguish between two very closely related macromolecules that are present on pathogens. The *humoral* and *cellular components* of adaptive immunity produce antibodies and activate lymphocytes, respectively, when foreign and altered proteins have been identified. Immune cells produce circulating antibodies and communicate with one another via secreted and circulating cytokines and chemokines. In its normal function, the cellular and humoral components of adaptive immunity are intact and simultaneously contribute to an immunologic reaction.

B lymphocytes are the effector cells of the humoral response. They produce antibodies whose main function is to neutralize extracellular microorganisms. These antibodies are proteins with very high specificity for their target. The antibodies produced are immunoglobulins (Ig): IgG, IgA, IgM, and IgE. IgA occurs in serum and secretory forms; the latter of which is the humoral immune system's main defense in the gut. In addition to the immunoglobulins produced by the humoral arm of adaptive immunity, cell-mediated immunity (CMI) is also conferred by activation of T lymphocytes, which are directed specifically toward intracellular pathogens such as viruses and certain bacteria.

The cellular components that inhabit mucosal surfaces, although traditionally identified as the mediators of innate immunity, are now also recognized for their ability to engage in adaptive immunity. They can capture, process, and present foreign antigens, or produce inflammatory cytokines that act as chemoattractants, inviting circulating immune cells to the site of inflammation. The adaptive immune system interacts intricately with the innate immune system to combat infection. Cells from the innate immune system interact with T and B lymphocytes in lymph nodes to coordinate a highly effective defense against invading microbes (Fig. 28-1).

## PRIMARY AND SECONDARY IMMUNODEFICIENCIES

Human immunodeficiency disorders predispose individuals to a range of immunologic dysfunctions and complications, including infections, autoimmunity, and cancer. These disorders are classified by etiology (Table 28–2). *Primary* immunodeficiency diseases are a group of relatively rare (1/500 to 1/500,000) inherited disorders that are described in terms of the main immune component that is deficient, absent, or defective. One or more abnormalities in the immune system can result in the inability to fight infections and/or increased susceptibility to various malignancies.

*Severe combined immunodeficiency (SCID)* represents a group of conditions that are primary immune deficiencies in which intrinsic defects in T- and B-lymphocyte intracellular signaling systems occur, leading to disrupted immunity, (especially CMI) and susceptibility to serious infections.[3–5] For instance, X-linked agammaglobulinemia (XLA) is caused by a defect in the enzyme tyrosine kinase. This defect leads to an arrest in maturation of the B cells and to a lack of antibody production, thereby affecting humoral immunity.[6] In addition, some primary immunodeficiencies may arise from a defective complement cascade. Complement proteins normally lyse and kill invading microorganisms by themselves or in conjunction with antibodies, and

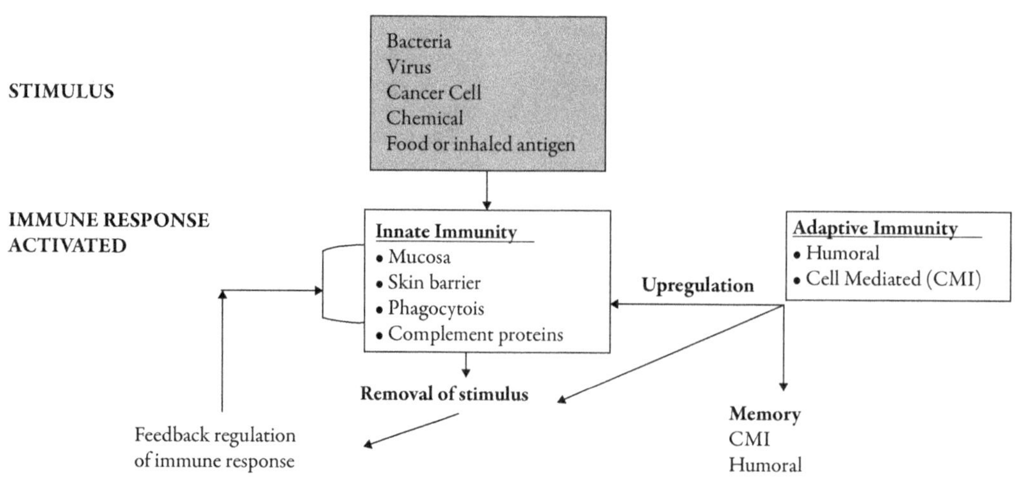


**Figure 28–1.** Overview of adaptive and innate immune response.

**Table 28–2.** Human Immunodeficiences

| Primary Immunodeficiency | Secondary Immunodeficiency |
|---|---|
| **Characteristics** | |
| *Hereditary, genetically determined*: part of normal immune system is deficient, absent, or defective, causing increased susceptibility to infection<br>• Many autosomal recessive or X-linked<br>• >200 rare, chronic disorders described<br>• Typically manifest during infancy and childhood as recurrent or unusual infections<br>• Classified by immune component affected:<br>1. Humoral immune deficiency<br>2. Cellular immune deficiency<br>3. Combined humoral/ cellular immunity<br>4. Phagocytic cells<br>5. Complement proteins | *Acquired, environmentally determined*: immune system becomes defective as a result of exposure to some environmental immunosuppressive agent or force:<br>• Prolonged serious illness<br>• Systemic disorders<br>• Immunosuppression<br>• Elderly<br>• Hospitalized patients<br>• Cancer<br>• Chronic infections |
| **Specific Examples** | |
| • Chronic granulomatous disease (CGD)<br>• DiGeorge syndrome (DGS)<br>• X-linked agammaglobulinemia (XLA)<br>• Severe combined immune deficiency (SCID)<br>• Common variable immunodeficiency (CVID) | • Acquired immunodeficiency syndrome (AIDS) caused by human immunodeficiency virus (HIV)<br>• Autoimmune diseases (e.g., rheumatoid arthritis, Crohn's disease)<br>• Organ transplantation<br>• Aging<br>• Splenectomy due to trauma<br>• Diabetes mellitus<br>• Severe malnutrition<br>• Leukemia, lymphoma, multiple myeloma<br>• Chemotherapy<br>• Steroid therapy<br>• Severe burns |

therefore a defective or missing complement protein may predispose an individual to infection. Complement deficiency is an example of a defect in the innate immune system that also affects the humoral arm of adaptive immunity.[7] Chronic granulomatous disease is caused by a defect in the killing of bacteria phagocytosed by neutrophils, which are part of innate immunity.[8]

*Secondary* or *acquired* forms of immunodeficiency are considerably more common than primary or genetic forms. Secondary immunodeficiency states are found in newborns and in patients receiving immunosuppressive therapy. They may develop in patients with prolonged serious illnesses such as infectious diseases (e.g., human immunodeficiency virus [HIV] infection), malignancies (e.g., leukemia), and a variety of systemic diseases (e.g., diabetes mellitus), or even after surgery or trauma. The relationship among nutrition, immunocompetence, and health is very complex. While patients with a secondary immunodeficiency have an intact immune system, their immunologic defense mechanisms may become transiently or permanently impaired during or after a primary disease or insult.

## INTERACTION OF THE IMMUNE SYSTEM AND NUTRITION

### Mucosal Immunity

The gastrointestinal (GI) tract represents the largest immunologic surface in the body. The small intestine has the largest surface area in the GI tract because of its structural features such as the villi and microvilli, which are designed to facilitate nutrient absorption from ingested foods and to neutralize foreign antigens. The GI lumen contains innumerable microorganisms and dietary proteins. From an immune perspective, the challenge is to guard the extensive surface area of the GI tract against breaches by microorganisms, especially those that are pathogenic. In the small intestine, the greatest source of antigenic load is from ingested food. However, while the antigen load decreases as ingested food is digested and absorbed, the microbial load increases. The intestinal immune system is tightly regulated. It must remain nonreactive or tolerant to antigens from food or commensal flora, while also retaining the ability to mount a protective immune response to guard against pathogenic entry into the circulation and the inflammatory consequences of immune activation by bacterial molecules. Enzymes from salivary, gastric, pancreatic, and intestinal secretions, combined with mastication and peristalsis, reduce ingested substances to small sugars, peptides, and fats. A single layer of columnar epithelial cells lines the GI lumen, protecting against microbes from the external environment and preventing foreign antigens from entering the circulatory pathways. In addition, nonspecific (mucin coat) and specific (secretory IgA) mechanisms block potentially harmful antigenic substances from penetrating the intestinal barrier.

Dietary antigens that do not undergo proteolysis in the lumen can be taken up by the intestine in various ways. Intact molecules that remain after digestion are deposited in the extracellular space by exocytosis.[9] Approximately 2% of intact proteins reach the intestinal lymph and portal circulation under physiological conditions.[10] Antigen transport across the intestinal barrier has been shown to be altered by immunization or allergic sensitization, thereby either enhancing or inhibiting uptake. Many of the immunological and mechanical barriers involved in this process are immature at birth, leaving the infant at risk. Large amounts of immunologically intact food proteins penetrate the gut barrier in children and adults and enter into the circulation, but clinical tolerance prevents pathological reactions. A failure to develop tolerance or a breakdown in tolerance results in excessive production of food-specific IgE antibodies. Mast cells line the GI tract, spanning from the lips to the rectum. Food antigens are most rapidly absorbed from the small intestine, colon, and rectum and more slowly from the esophagus and stomach. When food allergens penetrate mucosal barriers and reach specific IgE antibodies bound to mast cells, mediators such as histamine, leukotrienes, and prostaglandins are released, inducing an immediate hypersensitivity reaction manifested by vasodilatation, smooth muscle contraction, and other alterations in normal physiology (Fig. 28–2).

### Influence of Diet on Mucosal Immunity

The two factors with the strongest impact on the mucosal immune system are diet and the microbiota. The microbiota is significantly altered by changes in the diet,[11] revealing an indirect mechanism of dietary regulation of the mucosal immune system. Dietary components can also have direct effects on the mucosal immune system. Retinoic acid, a vitamin A metabolite, is best known for promoting the generation of regulatory T cells, although its impact is not always regulatory. In the presence of the inflammatory cytokine interleukin 15 (IL-15), retinoic acid can amplify inflammatory responses, and it can contribute to intestinal damage in the murine model of celiac disease.[12] Vitamin D promotes migration of lymphocytes to the GI tissue, significantly

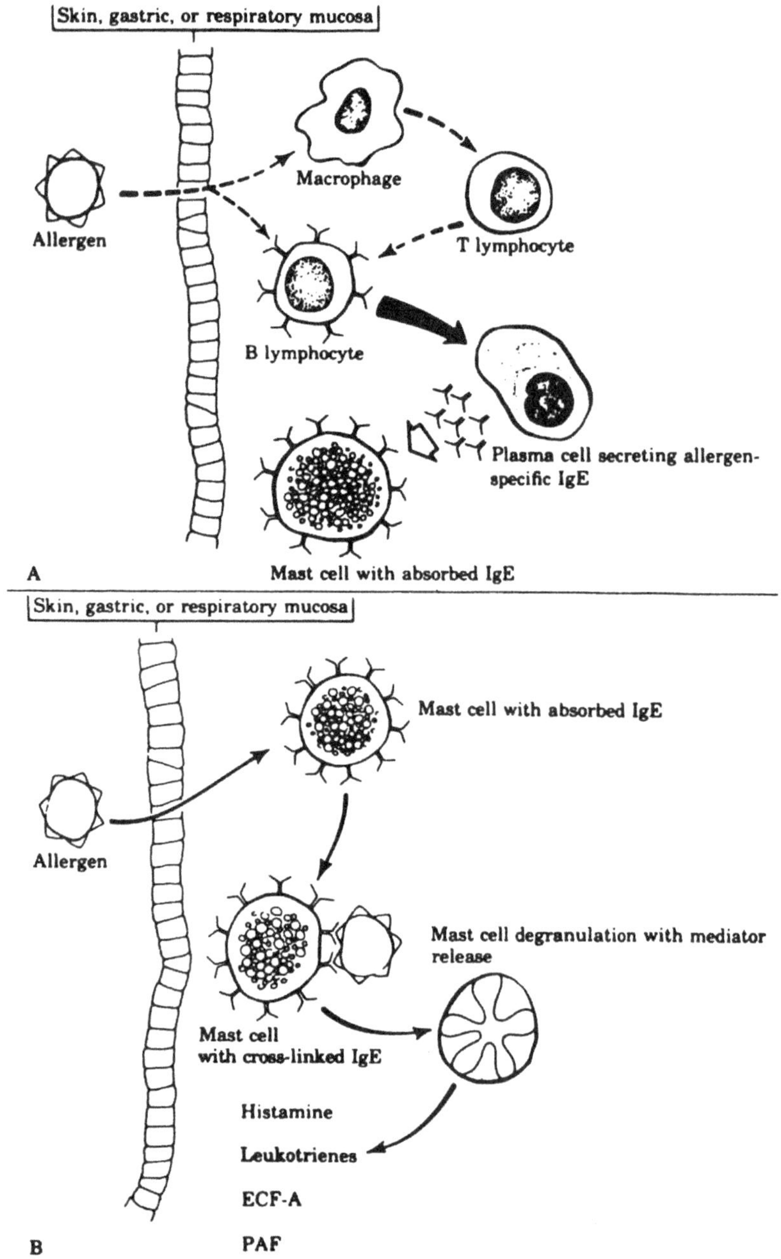


**Figure 28–2.** **A.** Allergen sensitization. On first exposure, the allergen is absorbed. A macrophage takes up the allergen, processes it, and presents it to the T lymphocyte. A B lymphocyte exposed to the allergen is influenced by the T lymphocyte to mature into an allergen-specific immunoglobulin E (IgE)-secreting plasma cell. These IgE antibodies are absorbed onto the surface of a mast cell (sensitization). **B.** Allergen stimulation of mediator release. On subsequent exposure, the allergen is absorbed and cross-links with specific IgE antibody on sensitized mast cell. The mast cell degranulates, and mediators are released. ECF-A = eosinophil chemotactic factor of anaphylaxis; PAF = platelet activating factor. (From Lawlor GJ, Fischer TJ, eds. *Manual of Allergy and Immunology,* 2nd ed. Boston: Little, Brown, and Company; 1988. Used with permission.)

reducing a unique population of regulatory intraepithelial lymphocytes whose function is to protect the epithelium against pathogen- and immune-induced pathology. In contrast to these regulatory dietary elements, a high-fat diet has proinflammatory effects because it alters cytokines that regulate the epithelial barrier function.[13,14]

It has long been recognized that malnourished individuals are more susceptible to infection than those who are adequately nourished. Various proteins, carbohydrates, fats, vitamins, and minerals act as building blocks and substrates by which the immune system gains its strength. Any deficiency in the supply lines of these nutrients creates a weakness that microbes may exploit to gain a foothold in their invasion of the host. Similarly, individuals with a primary or secondary immune defect fare worse when they are malnourished. The fate of the immune system is so closely tied to nutrition status that it has been suggested that immune system studies be used as a barometer of nutrition status.[14]

## Immunologic Changes in the Chronically Malnourished

Anorexia nervosa and bulimia nervosa are psychiatric illnesses in which the patients have abnormal eating patterns that result in chronic protein-calorie malnutrition. Studies have indicated that anorexia and bulimia patients have fewer lymphocytes than normal control subjects.[15,16] Anorexia patients had impaired CMI as evidenced by abnormal delayed-type hypersensitivity skin tests.[15] Despite these findings, it has been recognized that increased vulnerability to infection is less common in people with anorexia nervosa than in other malnourished patients. Protein-energy malnutrition (PEM) is said to be the most common cause of immunodeficiency world wide. It includes kwashiorkor, marasmus, and nutritional dwarfism of childhood.[17] PEM is used as an example of the extensive effects of malnutrition on the immune system.

### Cellular Immunity

Patients with PEM have atrophy of lymphoid tissue including lymph nodes, tonsils, and thymus. In the thymus, there is loss of corticomedullary differentiation and fewer lymphoid cells. CMI appears to be more affected than humoral immunity. Delayed-type hypersensitivity cutaneous responses, both to recall and to new antigens, are markedly depressed, and some PEM patients have complete anergy to many antigens.[17] Malnourished children have a significant decrease in numbers of both $CD4^+$ and $CD8^+$ T cells; the decrease is more pronounced for $CD4^+$ T cells, leading to a lower $CD4^+$-to-$CD8^+$ ratio.[1]

### Humoral Immunity

Experiments in patients with PEM show a reduction in the number of antibody-producing cells and in the amount of immunoglobulin secreted. Co-culture experiments suggest that this is in part due to a result of poor T-cell function in PEM patients.[17] Patients with kwashiorkor have impaired ability to produce antibodies of all types; this is reversed after a few days of protein therapy.[18] Secretory IgA levels are lower in PEM patients who have been immunized with viral vaccines, compared with healthy controls.[19]

### Phagocytosis

In order for phagocytosis to occur efficiently, foreign matter must be coated (opsonized) with particles recognized by the phagocyte. One such group of opsonins are the proteins of complement. Patients with PEM make less complement, and it has lower activity and decreased phagocytosis.[17] Specifically, reductions of C3, C5, factor B, and total complement activity appear to be the cause for poor phagocytosis. Kielmann and Curcio showed that poorly nourished children in India had an inability to produce C3 in response to infection.[20]

### Cytokines

Patients with PEM have decreased production of the cytokines IL-1, IL-2, and interferon-γ. These cytokines are involved in upregulation of the immune system in response to infection. Some foods stimulate cytokine production. Solis-Pereyra et al.[13] reported that yogurt bacteria induced plasma interferon-α and interferon-β production in mice. In the same study, they observed that, although there was no direct evidence of increased cytokine production in humans consuming yogurt bacteria, they did exhibit an increase in activity of an enzyme induced by interferon, called 2′-5′-synthetase. In addition, blood mononuclear cells from healthy subjects incubated in the presence of yogurt bacteria had detectable levels of interferon-γ in plasma.[13]

## IMMUNOLOGIC CHANGES IN SPECIFIC MALNUTRITION SYNDROMES

### Cystic Fibrosis

Cystic fibrosis is a somewhat common chronic illness that affects approximately 1 in 2500 Caucasian children in the United States. Among other issues, patients develop a pancreatic exocrine insufficiency resulting in protein and fat malabsorption, which causes distention and frequent bulky, greasy, foul-smelling stools. Without correction, the malabsorption may result in failure to gain weight and ultimately in linear growth deficits. Malabsorption may negatively affect the immune system by causing a lack of vital trace elements, minerals, and vitamins.

### Vitamin, Mineral, and Trace Element Deficiency

Animal and human studies have evaluated the effects of vitamin and trace mineral deficiencies on immunity. Table 28–3 summarizes the impact of these deficiencies.

Breast-feeding has long been recommended for the prevention of allergic diseases, but existing epidemiologic evidence is highly controversial.[21] Likewise, the optimum age for introduction of solid foods has been greatly debated, and there exists no conclusive evidence that permits general recommendations. A diversity of solid foods introduced during the first year of life has been linked to less atopic dermatitis and asthma later in life.[22]

## FOOD ALLERGY

### Overview

As mentioned previously, the main function of the immune system is to detect and eliminate foreign proteins from the body. The largest protein load that the immune system encounters is that of food intake. In this situation, the immune system has to take a stance opposite its main mission, which is to detect and eliminate pathogens. In handling food proteins, the immune system has to detect the foreign protein and subsequently learn to become tolerant; otherwise, food allergies will develop. Food allergies are typically characterized by type I hypersensitivity immune reactions.[23,24] Type I hypersensitivity reactions entail the robust production of IgE antibodies by activated B lymphocytes and subsequent activation of mast cells and basophils, which causes release of vasoactive amines such as histamine. This series of events is mediated by the T lymphocytes. Although absorption from the gut of intact food proteins, which are considered foreign proteins, continues throughout life, an estimated 98% of adults and 92% of children develop oral tolerance to all food proteins ingested.[25] The process of recognizing food proteins and developing tolerance to them is accompanied by the production of serum food protein–specific IgG, which does not mediate allergic reactions.

Food allergy is defined as "an adverse health effect arising from a specific immune response that occurs reproducibly on exposure to a given food."[26] These immune responses may be IgE-mediated, non–IgE-mediated, or some combination of both mechanisms. Sensitization indicates that an individual has demonstrated IgE or other antibodies or antigen-reactive cells in the absence of clinical symptoms. An immune-mediated food allergy requires both the presence of sensitization and clinical responsiveness when the food is ingested. The prevalence of clinically proven allergic reactions to food is on the rise, now affecting up to 5% of adults and 6% to 8% of children in the United States.[27–30]

**Table 28–3.** Effects of Trace Element Deficiencies on the Immune System

| Trace Element | Function | Deficiency |
|---|---|---|
| Zinc | Development and maintenance of immune system | • Failure of wound healing<br>• Negative effect on CMI, lymphoid atrophy, and lower thymic hormone levels with potential for increased susceptibility to pathogens |
| Iron | Part of hemoglobin and myoglobin | • Lymphoid atrophy, fewer lymphocytes, and decreased proliferation to stimuli<br>• Decrease in secretory IgA<br>• Monocyte function, inflammatory response, and delayed skin hypersensitivity reaction are decreased |
| Copper | Cofactor for multiple enzymes | • Negative impact on CMI, phagocytosis, and antibody production in rodent studies |
| Magnesium | DNA synthesis and functions in many metabolic pathways | • Negative impact on CMI, phagocytosis, and antibody production in rodent studies |
| Vitamin A | Vision, cell growth and development | • Decreased thymic size, natural killer cell activity, and lymphocyte response to mitogens in animal studies |
| B vitamins | Cofactors in many metabolic pathways | • Pyridoxine deficiency and folic acid deficiency cause anemia associated with reduced CMI |
| Vitamin C | Antioxidant | • Negative impact on neutrophil function, delayed cutaneous hypersensitivity, abnormal complement levels, and reduced phagocytic function in humans and animals |
| Vitamin D | Calcium homeostatsis and immunity | • Decreases in delayed-type hypersensitivity |
| Vitamin E | Protects cell membranes from oxidants | • Decreased phagocyte function and lymphocyte proliferation |

CNI = cell-mediated immunity; IgA = immunoglobulin A.
Data from references 2, 19, 84–86.

Food allergy management frequently requires avoidance of food antigens and therefore can negatively impact nutrient intake. Longitudinal comprehensive nutrition assessment provided by a dietitian who can devise appropriate intervention strategies is warranted for all children with food allergies. Nutrition assessment may also be indicated for adults with food allergy.[31] Commonly, an elimination diet is necessary to prevent potentially life-threatening anaphylaxis. Allergen elimination can also improve chronic symptoms (e.g., atopic dermatitis) when a food is proven to trigger the symptoms. The goal of allergen elimination is to prevent acute and chronic food-allergic reactions in the safest and least restrictive environment while supplying a balanced diet that promotes health in children and adults.

## Symptoms Related to Food Allergy

### Dermatological Symptoms

Food allergy–induced skin symptoms fall into two categories: atopic dermatitis (eczema) and urticaria (hives). Urticaria typically begins promptly after the ingestion of a known food allergen; usually, it is diagnosed early and the offending food is identified. Atopic dermatitis has an interesting relationship to food allergy. Patients with atopic dermatitis are at high risk for acute reactions to the common food allergens. They are also typically sensitized to multiple food allergens, although many of these do not cause clinical symptoms. However, patients often report that some foods, when consumed frequently, exacerbate itching and precipitate atopic dermatitis flare-ups.

### Respiratory Symptoms

Respiratory symptoms of a food-allergic reaction include upper respiratory tract symptoms—sneezing, rhinorrhea, congestion, and tearing. Lower respiratory tract signs and symptoms include stridor, hoarse voice, cough, dyspnea, and wheezing. Although these symptoms are severe and could be life-threatening, they are less common than other food allergy symptoms.

### Gastrointestinal Symptoms

GI symptoms including nausea, abdominal pain and cramps, vomiting, and diarrhea are often immediate and may occur while the food is being consumed. Resolution of symptoms is often rapid, and return of appetite frequently occurs after a GI food reaction. Diarrhea may occur immediately or be delayed for several hours.

### Pollen-Food Syndrome

Pollen-food syndrome, also called oral allergy syndrome, is a form of urticaria confined to the lips and oropharynx that most commonly occurs in individuals with pollen allergy. Symptoms include itching of the throat with or without facial angioedema and/or tingling or the lips, tongue, palate, and throat. Mild oral edema may occur immediately after ingestion of certain foods, most commonly raw fruits and vegetables. This result is caused by specific IgE antibodies directed to the aeroallergens that cross-react with certain proteins in foods.

## Non–IgE-Mediated Reactions to Food

Not all GI food-allergic disorders are associated with food-specific IgE antibodies. Non–IgE-mediated reactions, which are poorly defined clinically and scientifically, are thought to be T-cell mediated. They are typically delayed in onset, occurring 4 to 28 hours after ingestion of the offending food. Nonimmune or nonallergic adverse reactions are referred to as *food intolerance, and may* include pharmacological reactions and lactose intolerance.

Cell-mediated (non–IgE-mediated) food hypersensitivity disorders that affect the GI tract include allergic proctocolitis, food protein–induced proctocolitis (FPIES), enterocolitis, and enteropathies. These disorders have overlapping symptoms and represent well-characterized immunologic responses to dietary proteins that are clinically distinguishable. Diagnosis requires a history, physical examination, exclusion of alternative diagnoses, dietary elimination and oral food challenge, biopsy, and selected laboratory evaluations.

### Allergic Proctocolitis

Allergic proctocolitis, also known as dietary protein proctocolitis, is characterized by the presence of mucoid, frothy, and bloody stools in an otherwise healthy infant.[32] It occurs in exclusively breast-fed infants and is caused by food proteins derived from the maternal diet that are transferred through lactation. Diagnosis is based on clinical features and recovery after dietary therapy.[33] The mean age at diagnosis is about 60 days (range, 1 day to 6 months), and resolution usually occurs within 1 year, although symptoms may continue longer in some patients. In most cases, a maternal diet free of cow's milk leads to prompt resolution of rectal bleeding; in some patients, a multiple food allergy occurs, with sensitization to soy, egg, rice, and wheat.[34]

The definitive diagnosis requires withdrawal of the presumed allergen and monitoring for resolution of symptom. Rectal bleeding usually resolves within 72 to 96 hours of maternal avoidance of cow's milk protein. However, in about 7% of cases, an extensively hydrolyzed formula must be used, and 5% of affected infants require an amino acid–based formula.[35] Infants who develop this condition while ingesting protein hydrolysate formula experience resolution of bleeding after substitution of an amino acid-based formula. Because there is usually no risk of a severe reaction, trigger foods that have been eliminated may be gradually reintroduced. However, if there is a suspicion of mild enterocolitis (e.g., vomiting in addition to hematochezia) or history of IgE-mediated reactions, dietary advancement may require caution, with allergy testing (e.g., skin or serum testing for specific IgE to the causal food) and medically supervised oral food challenges.

### Food Protein–Induced Enterocolitis Syndrome

Onset of FPIES symptoms occurs early in life and is uncommon after 1 year of age. FPIES typically occurs after the introduction of cow's milk- or soy-based formulas. Children with detectable milk-specific IgE antibodies have a more protracted course than do those without IgE antibodies. Some individuals convert to immediate IgE-mediated milk allergy. Additional common food triggers (e.g., rice, oats, barley) and symptoms often occur after an infant starts eating solid foods. Other foods that have been documented as triggers for FPIES include meats, fish, fruits, vegetables, and eggs. Unlike some food-allergy reactions that can trigger an allergic response throughout the body, the symptoms of FPIES are typically confined to the GI system. Inflammation involves both the small and the large intestine. Vomiting and diarrhea may not occur until several hours after the offending food is consumed, so a link between the symptom and the food may not be apparent. Acute symptoms may mimic those of sepsis and can include severe protracted projectile vomiting and watery or bloody diarrhea, dehydration, lethargy, leukocytosis, hypotension, thrombocytosis, and methemoglobinemia. Chronic symptoms include weight loss, failure to thrive, anemia, hypoalbuminemia, and fecal leukocytes. FPIES typically resolves within 1 to 5 years.

### Enteropathy

Enteropathy occurs in infancy and has symptoms related to protein malabsorption, most commonly diarrhea. It is most commonly caused by cow's milk proteins and usually resolves by age 1 to 3 years. Gluten-sensitive enteropathy is discussed in another chapter.

## IgE-Mediated Reactions to Food

IgE-mediated immediate hypersensitivity reactions to foods are most common in young children. Fifty percent of these reactions develop during the first year of life and are largely driven by food-specific antigens. The IgE-mediated reactions are usually divided into immediate-onset reactions and immediate plus late phase reactions (in which the immediate-onset symptoms are followed by prolonged or ongoing symptoms). IgE-mediated anaphylactic reactions to foods occur immediately after ingestion. These reactions are acute, life-threatening events and can cause GI, pulmonary, and cardiovascular symptoms.

## ALLERGIC AND EOSINOPHILIC GASTROINTESTINAL DISEASE

Eosinophilic gastrointestinal disorders (EGIDs) involve an accumulation of eosinophils, a type of white blood cell that often increases when an allergic reaction occurs. Most of these disorders are rare (an exception being eosinophilic esophagitis). They are characterized by eosinophil-dominant inflammation in various segments of the GI tract and are almost always associated with immune sensitization to multiple foods.[16] Many affected patients have a history of an atopic disease.

EGID diagnoses are confirmed histologically and are defined by the number of eosinophils (EOS) per high-power field (hpf) in the relevant tissue:

- Eosinophilic esophagitis (EoE): ≥15 EOS/hpf[36,37]
- Eosinophilic gastritis: ≥30 EOS/hpf in at least 5 hpfs of the gastric mucosa[38]
- Eosinophilic duodenitis/jejunitis: ≥26 EOS/hpf[39]
- Eosinophilic ileitis: ≥28 EOS/hpf
- Eosinophilic colitis: ≥50 EOS/hpf in the colonic mucosa[39]

### Eosinophilic Esophagitis

EoE is an emerging GI disorder characterized by marked esophageal eosinophilia that is etiologically linked to immune hypersensitivity to foods (i.e., dietary antigens)[36]; it is a chronic disorder that persists from childhood into adulthood.[40,41] The high rate of response to food-elimination diets, especially amino acid–based elemental diets,[42–45] and the frequent recurrence of disease after food reintroduction imply that EoE is mediated by allergic sensitization to foods.[46–48] Esophageal biopsies are mandatory for the diagnosis of EoE, though clinical manifestations and responsiveness to proton pump inhibitors must be taken into consideration. The diagnosis of EOE requires clinicopathological correlation.

EoE is the most common type of EGID, occurring in approximately 1 of every 4000 children.[49] EoE is more commonly diagnosed in boys (male-to-female ratio, 3:1), in children of Caucasian ethnicity, and in children who have a personal or family history of atopy. The male predominance is also observed in adults.[50] The reported median age at diagnosis ranges from 5.4 to 9.6 years. The presenting symptoms of EoE vary by age. Young children are more likely to have vomiting and feeding disorders as compared to older children, who often present with abdominal pain, dysphagia, or food bolus impaction.[49] The predominant symptom of EoE in young adults is dysphagia. Many children with EoE have an IgE-mediated food allergy and atopy; however, the underlying pathogenic mechanism of EoE is not entirely IgE mediated, and routine allergy tests (i.e., skin or atopy patch) are usually not helpful in identifying foods that provoke symptoms.[51] The pathogenesis of EoE is unknown, but it is multifactorial, involving genetic, immunologic, and environmental factors. There is evidence that EoE is more prevalent in patients with food allergy, rhinitis, asthma, or atopic dermatitis.[52,53] All of these pathologies are characterized by an altered immune response to common antigens that creates an aberrant T helper type 2 (Th2) lymphocyte response and, hence, uncontrolled activation of eosinophils, mast cells, and basophils.[54–58]

The dietary approach (i.e., elimination diets) and topical corticosteroids are considered first-line therapies[59]; they aim to resolve symptoms and prevent long-term complications such as formation of strictures. Both therapies are effective in the management of EoE in teens and young adults.[45,60–64] Elimination diets are more often favored over topical corticosteroid therapy because they can identify the root cause of the EoE,[60,62,65] and after histologic remission (≤14 EOS/hpf) is attained,[36] a wide and varied diet can often be resumed.[62] Elimination diets can help achieve sustained drug-free disease remission without exposure to the potential risks of topical corticosteroids[60] (e.g., candidiasis, bone demineralization). Discontinuation of topical corticoids typically results in recurrence of eosinophilic inflammation and associated symptoms. The empiric six-food elimination diet (SFED), described later, has been demonstrated to be more cost-effective than topical steroids in management of EoE after the first year.[63]

Three commonly prescribed diet therapies are used to manage EoE: the elemental diet, the SFED, and the allergy test–directed elimination diet. A fourth diet has been described in adults—the four-food elimination diet,[66] which empirically eliminates milk, egg, wheat, and legumes. An elemental diet is defined as one that eliminates all foods and provides complete nutrition by the exclusive use of an amino acid–based formula. The SFED empirically eliminates the six most common allergenic foods—milk, soy, wheat, egg, peanuts or tree nuts, and fish or shellfish—regardless of allergy test results. A skin test–directed elimination diet is defined as one that eliminates only those foods that elicited positive results on allergy testing. The only study to date comparing the efficacy of these diets demonstrated that the odds of histologic remission were 5.6-fold higher with elemental diets versus SFEDs and 12.5-fold higher with elemental diets versus directed diets; the results for SFEDs versus directed diets were not significantly different. Among a total of 98 patients, histologic remission was achieved in 96% of 49 patients on the elemental diet, 81% of 26 patients on the SFED, and 65% of 23 patients on the allergy test–directed diet. Remission was achieved in 54% of adult patients with EoE who were treated with the four-food elimination diet.[66]

The decision to proceed with dietary therapy should be based on patient preference and available resources. A collaborative and multidisciplinary approach including gastroenterologists, allergists, nurses, and dietitians is essential for the success of this approach. Any restricted diet can pose significant nutritional risks including both micronutrient and macronutrient deficiencies. Patients are at high nutritional risk based on the number and types of food proteins that are being removed from the diet. Nutrient deficits on the SFED can significantly negatively impact serum levels of zinc, B vitamins, calcium, vitamin D, magnesium, selenium, as well as dietary fiber and proteins, if alternative sources of these vitamins are not incorporated.[61] Nutrient needs change throughout the life cycle.

The dietitian's role is essential in determining ongoing nutritional adequacy, providing patient and family education (e.g., reading food labels), assessing barriers and creating solutions for dietary adherence, and promoting adequate linear growth and weight gain.[67] To ensure adequate nutritional intake while on any type of elimination diet, supplementation with an amino acid–based formula is recommended. Approximately one-third of patients on an elimination diet required daily amino acid–based formula supplementation to achieve adequate nutritional intake.[33] Details on how to reintroduce foods after achieving remission and current recommendations for nutritional management of EoE are available for children[67] and adults.[61]

## PATHOGENESIS OF FOOD ALLERGY

In persons with food allergy, the absorption of highly sensitizing food proteins (such as cow's milk, peanut, or shrimp protein) is associated with the production of IgE antibodies. The food protein–specific IgE antibodies remain attached to IgE receptors on mast cells until a second exposure to the food protein (allergen) occurs (see Fig. 28–2). The food allergen links to the IgE antibodies attached to their receptors, causing the receptors to signal the mast cells to degranulate and release their preformed mediators, mainly histamine. Histamine released locally causes wheal-and-flare reactions in the skin, known as hives. Histamine released into the circulation causes smooth muscle contraction of the GI tract, resulting in vomiting or diarrhea, contraction of the bronchial smooth muscles resulting in wheezing, and relaxation of the vascular bed resulting in hypotension and shock. This constellation of symptoms in its severest form is known as *anaphylaxis*.

Allergic responses occur when the immune system becomes skewed toward a tendency to become sensitized, or atopic. *Atopy* includes patients who have allergic rhinitis in response to environmental allergens, allergic asthma, or eczema. Food allergy occurs in a high percentage of children who have eczema, and children with eczema commonly have allergies to multiple foods.[68] Food allergy occurs in response to food proteins that are inherently sensitizing and to which there is a large exposure in early childhood. The most common food allergens in childhood are cow's milk proteins,[69–72] hen's egg proteins,[73] and, in the United States and European countries, peanuts.[74,75] Less frequently, children suffer from allergy to soy or wheat proteins. Common allergenic proteins in adults are peanut, fish, shellfish, and tree nuts.

Contrary to popular belief, food allergy is not caused by simple sugars or carbohydrates (e.g., lactose), and rarely do small-molecular-weight compounds such as food additives, preservatives, and dyes cause true food allergy symptoms.[43,76] The nonallergenic adverse reactions to these types of foods are collectively referred to as *food intolerance*.

The diagnosis of food allergy is based on three elements: a medical history compatible with an acute immediate allergic reaction after ingestion of a food, evidence of the presence of IgE to the food in question by skin testing or measurement of circulating IgE, and a food challenge.

## FACTORS TO BE CONSIDERED IN NUTRITION EVALUATION AND DIAGNOSIS

A rational diagnostic approach is needed for the patient with suspected food hypersensitivity. This approach includes an accurate history, a detailed physical examination, and appropriate application of proven *in vitro* and *in vivo* testing.

The history should pay close attention to the nature, severity, and duration of symptoms. Other important historical factors are age at onset, suspected precipitating foods, and the temporal relationship between ingestion of the suspected food and onset of symptoms. Important points in the history include (1) the suspected food, (2) the amount of food that causes a reaction, (3) the form of the food that causes a reaction, (4) the timing of the reaction, (5) the reproducibility of the reaction, (6) the most recent occurrence of an adverse food reaction, (7) an accurate description of the symptoms and the severity of the reaction, (8) the current diet, and (9) any other medical or psychiatric condition that would preclude performing a food challenge.

Organ systems commonly involved in food allergy reactions are the skin, the GI tract, the respiratory tract, and the cardiovascular system. Observable symptoms may include vomiting, diarrhea, hypotension, hives, flushed appearance, itching of skin or mucous membranes, rhinorrhea, coughing, wheezing, and throat clearing. A thorough physical examination focusing on the previously discussed organ systems is important. Pediatric patients with eczema are much more likely to have food allergy than those without eczema.

Patients with multiple food allergies who have had extensive dietary restriction may demonstrate evidence of malnutrition. In the evaluation of malnutrition, the examiner should pay close attention to muscle mass and the amount of subcutaneous tissue. Patients with malabsorption often demonstrate a protuberant abdomen, thin extremities, and wasting of the buttocks. Sparse hair growth and the appearance of lanugo on the back indicate continued caloric deprivation. Peripheral edema suggests hypoproteinemia. Hepatomegaly occurs with fatty infiltration of the liver during malnutrition.

## TESTING FOR FOOD HYPERSENSITIVITY

After a careful history and physical examination, laboratory tests can help document food hypersensitivity. These tests include methods designed to detect IgE antibodies to the foods in question and to exclude other causes for the symptoms. For example, a patient with diarrhea requires a stool culture to exclude common pathogens, a complete blood count looking for anemia, and analysis of stool for occult blood loss. In patients with poor weight gain, frequent sinopulmonary infections, abnormal greasy stools, and a sweat chloride concentration should be obtained to exclude cystic fibrosis. In patients with suspected lactose intolerance, measurement of stool reducing substances or a lactose tolerance test is indicated. In complex cases, invasive procedures such as esophagoscopy or intestinal biopsies may be required.

### In Vitro Tests

The serum specific IgE test is designed to detect the presence of serum IgE directed toward a specific antigen. The test is currently performed using one of several automated platforms approved by the US Food and Drug Administration (FDA), including the ImmunoCAP System (Thermo Fischer Scientific, Waltham, MA), the Immulite System (Siemens Healthcare, Iselin, NJ), and a small portable device manufactured by Optigen (Hitachi Chemical Diagnostics, Mountain View, CA). The measurements provide a serum specific IgE in kU/L units (1 kU/L = 2.4 ng/mL). Depending on the system, the measurements can be quantitative or semiquantitative, and results from different systems are not comparable. The test can be used to detect serum specific IgE in patients who are unable to undergo skin testing for various reasons such as recent antihistamine therapy or an eczema outbreak, and in physician's offices where skin testing expertise is not available. The tests are usually more expensive than skin testing, and they differ from skin tests in sensitivity and specificity. A negative serum specific IgE test result (<0.1 kU/L) has a high negative predictive value when compared with oral food challenges, but positive test results vary in their positive predictive value and do not always correlate with skin test results or clinical allergy diagnosis.[77]

The ability to produce either natural or recombinant components of a food allergen has allowed increased specificity of results and detection of cross-sensitization between inhalant allergens from plants and food allergens. Such tests are called component-resolved diagnostics. An example is the peanut component test by Thermo Fischer Scientific, in which the result of peanut sensitization is obtained by testing its components allergens, ara h 1, 2, 3, 8, and 9. Positive results to ara h 1, 2, and 3 are likely consistent with clinical reactivity, whereas positive results to ara h 8 and 9 may indicate cross-sensitization to plant proteins including pathogen-related proteins (PR-10) and lipid transfer proteins (LTP).[78]

### Skin Tests

Skin tests demonstrate that the allergen-specific IgE is bound to mast cells in the skin and that bridging the IgE receptor with allergen leads to mast cell degranulation. Skin testing with commercially available food extracts is done by the prick method. Intradermal skin testing should be avoided because of the greater danger of systemic reactions and of nonspecific irritant reactions.[79,80] If the patient has IgE antibody to a food, a local hive reaction will be produced at the site of the skin test, usually within 15 minutes.

### Application of Skin Tests and In Vitro Tests

A negative prick skin test or failure to detect antigen-specific IgE in the circulation indicates greater than 95% negative predictive accuracy for a clinically significant reaction on challenge. A negative skin test or negative in vitro test result in response to a food can be used as a guide to help determine which food is less likely to cause an IgE-mediated reaction on food challenge when multiple foods are suspected. However, these tests do not exclude a non–IgE-mediated reaction or a nonimmunologic reaction. On the other hand, the positive predictive value of these tests in detecting a clinical reaction is rather low, less than 50%.[46]

In summary, evidence of IgE sensitization by prick skin tests or by *in vitro* tests, which is sometimes obtained when screening panels of skin tests or serum specific IgE tests are used, should not be the sole basis for diagnosis of adverse food reactions. Likewise, it should not be a substitute for diagnostic challenge procedures in the presence of a suggestive clinical history.

### Food Challenges

#### Blind Challenge

At present, the gold standard test to confirm food allergy is the double-blind placebo-controlled food challenge. The clinicians and the patient are unaware of whether a placebo or the suspected food is being fed to the patient during this procedure. This method has the advantage of objectivity; it eliminates any bias that knowledge of the food would have on the patient or observer. As a research tool, it has become the gold standard to which other methods of evaluating adverse reactions to foods are compared. In clinical practice, it is the clinician's most

**Table 28–4.** Examples of Food Items and Ingredients To Be Avoided in a Cow's Milk Elimination Diet

| Artificial Butter Flavor | Cottage Cheese | Whey Protein | Milk Protein | Goat's Milk |
|---|---|---|---|---|
| Butter | Curds | Lactalbumin | Milk solids | Nougat |
| Butter fat | Custard | Lactalbumin phosphate | Malted milk | Pudding |
| Butter oil | Ghee | Lactoglobulin | Condensed milk | Rennet casein |
| Buttermilk | Half & Half | Lactose† | Evaporated milk | Sour cream |
| Casein | Casein hydrolysate | Lactulose | Dry milk | Whey in all forms |
| Caseinates (all) | Milk protein hydrolysate | Milk-based infant formula | Whole milk | Yogurt |
| Cheese | Protein hydrolysate* | Milk derivative | Nonfat milk | |
| Cream | Whey hydrolysate | Milk powder | 2%, 1%, or skimmed milk | |

Note: Deli meats may contain or be contaminated with milk protein.
*Although protein hydrolysate does not directly indicate milk hydrolysate, the vagueness of the term does not allow for identification of the protein source, which could be an allergenic protein.
†Lactose, which is the carbohydrate in cow's milk, is not an allergen. However, the presence of lactose in a product may indicate that it is made with cow's milk or is possibly contaminated with cow's milk.

reliable procedure for diagnosing an adverse food reaction and serves as the basis for prescribing a food-specific elimination diet. It is also the procedure by which the clinician can confidently dismiss the role of foods as causative agents for the patient's symptoms.[81] However, because this challenge is costly and time-consuming, many clinicians perform open food challenges or single-blinded challenges. A single-blind challenge removes the element of patient bias but not potential observer bias.

### Open Challenge

An open challenge is performed in a physician's office under monitored conditions, which usually lessens patient anxiety and the accompanying subjective complaints. It is also an easy way to document objective symptoms such as urticaria. A positive open challenge with adequate documentation of objective symptoms is diagnostic of an adverse food reaction, and a negative challenge excludes the diagnosis. A challenge that results in only subjective symptoms should be confirmed by a blinded challenge. Open challenges are particularly useful in infants and small children because the procedure time is markedly shortened. A positive food challenge by itself does not prove that an immunological mechanism is responsible for the adverse food reaction; adverse reactions to foods can result from other conditions, such as lactase deficiency in lactose-intolerant patients. The food challenge results, the history, and the results of IgE testing complement each other in the diagnosis of food allergy.[82]

## MANAGEMENT

### Elimination of Specific Food Allergens

Currently there is no cure for food allergy. Avoidance of the foods that have been proven to cause adverse reaction is the mainstay of management. There is no place for rotational diets in the management of food allergy. The food allergen should be eliminated from the diet in all hidden and obvious forms. This usually requires meticulous label reading and knowledge of the various names under which a food may be listed. For example, milk proteins may be listed on a label as casein, whey, or lactoglobulin, and egg proteins may be listed as ovalbumin. Food allergy patients may be sensitive to minute amounts of the protein in processed foods, so patients may be advised to eliminate from their diet foods that are processed with their food allergen. For example, patients with peanut allergy are usually advised to avoid tree nuts because they are typically processed on the same manufacturing line as peanuts, and cross-contamination is common.

A comprehensive list of food allergen diets is beyond the scope of this text, but Table 28–4 gives an example of the food labels to be avoided in a cow's milk elimination diet. Further information may be obtained from Food Allergy Research and Education (FARE) http://www.foodallergy.org/. A useful classification of foods from plant and animal sources is presented in Appendix 6. The help of a well-trained nutritionist is extremely valuable for patients and their families, to assist them in learning about label reading and how to avoid nutritional deficiencies in cases of multiple food allergies in children.

### Treatment of Acute Reactions

If IgE-mediated food allergy is proven, the patient should be issued an injectable form of epinephrine and trained on how and when to use the medication. In case of an acute reaction, immediate medical attention is necessary for monitoring of vital signs and treatment with injectable epinephrine, antihistaminics, fluid resuscitation, and bronchodilators if needed. Oral steroids are usually given to prevent a late phase reaction.

### Recent Advances in Management

Research in food allergy centers on desensitization and the induction of tolerance. The common food allergens are being studied, mainly cow's milk, eggs, and peanuts. Approaches being tested in human subjects to induce desensitization include oral, sublingual, and epicutaneous immunotherapy.[78,83] Oral immunotherapy is also in clinical trials using pretreatment with an anti-IgE antibody, omalizumab, which is currently approved by the FDA for treatment of allergic asthma. These approaches are based on the theory that repeated exposure to small amounts of a specific food allergen through the oral mucosa, the gut, or the skin can cause the immune system to switch from immune activation to immune tolerance. Use of omalizumab has been associated with decreased side effects of oral immunotherapy when a subject is fed various amounts of a food to which he or she is allergic.[27]

#### References


1. Chandra RK. Nutrition and the immune system from birth to old age. *Eur J Clin Nutr.* 2002; 56(Suppl 3):S73.
2. Beisel WR, Edelman R, Nauss K, Suskind RM. Single-nutrient effects on immunologic functions. Report of a workshop sponsored by the Department of Food and Nutrition and its nutrition advisory group of the American Medical Association. *JAMA.* 1981; 245:1.
3. Chinn IK, Shearer WT. Severe combined immunodeficiency disorders. *Immunol Allergy Clin North Am.* 2015; 35:4.
4. Rivers L, Gaspar HB. Severe combined immunodeficiency: recent developments and guidance on clinical management. *Arch Dis Child.* 2015; 100:7.
5. Buckley RH. Primary cellular immunodeficiencies. *J Allergy Clin Immunol.* 2002; 109:5.
6. Tsukada S, Rawlings DJ, Witte ON. Role of Bruton's tyrosine kinase in immunodeficiency. *Curr Opin Immunol.* 1994; 6:4.
7. O'Neil KM. Complement deficiency. *Clin Rev Allergy Immunol.* 2000; 19:2.
8. Kamani NR, Infante AJ. Chronic granulomatous disease and other disorders of neutrophil function. *Clin Rev Allergy Immunol.* 2000; 19:2.
9. Mazo VK, Shaternikov VA, Gmoshinskii IV. Proteolysis of dietary protein antigens in in vivo and in vitro systems [in Russian]. *Usp Fiziol Nauk.* 1986; 17:2.
10. Cunningham-Rundles C. Dietary antigens and immunologic disease in humans. *Rheum Dis Clin North Am.* 1991; 17:2.
11. Lopetuso LR, Petito V, Scaldaferri F, Gasbarrini A. Gut microbiota modulation and mucosal immunity: focus on rifaximin. *Mini Rev Med Chem.* 2015; 16:3.
12. Nanda S. Celiac disease: retinoic acid and IL-15 jointly implicated in reversal of oral tolerance. *Nat Rev Gastroenterol Hepatol.* 2011; 8:4.
13. Solis-Pereyra B, Aattouri N, Lemonnier D. Role of food in the stimulation of cytokine production. *Am J Clin Nutr.* 1997; 66:2.
14. Chandra RK. 1990 McCollum Award lecture. Nutrition and immunity: lessons from the past and new insights into the future. *Am J Clin Nutr.* 1991; 53:5.
15. Marcos A, Varela P, Toro O, et al. Interactions between nutrition and immunity in anorexia nervosa: a 1-y follow-up study. *Am J Clin Nutr.* 1997; 66:2.
16. Marcos A, Varela P, Toro O, Nova E, Lopez-Vidriero I, Morande G. Evaluation of nutritional status by immunologic assessment in bulimia nervosa: influence of body mass index and vomiting episodes. *Am J Clin Nutr.* 1997; 66:2.

17. Batool R, Butt MS, Sultan MT, Saeed F, Naz R. Protein-energy malnutrition: a risk factor for various ailments. *Crit Rev Food Sci Nutr.* 2015; 55:2.
18. Scrimshaw NS, San Giovanni JP. Synergism of nutrition, infection, and immunity: an overview. *Am J Clin Nutr.* 1997; 66:2.
19. Chandra RK. Nutrition and the immune system: an introduction. *Am J Clin Nutr.* 1997; 66:2.
20. Kielmann AA, Curcio LM. Complement (C3), nutrition, and infection. *Bull World Health Organ.* 1979; 57:1.
21. Dogaru CM, Nyffenegger D, Pescatore AM, Spycher BD, Kuehni CE. Breastfeeding and childhood asthma: systematic review and meta-analysis. *Am J Epidemiol.* 2014; 179:10.
22. Roduit C, Frei R, Depner M, et al. Increased food diversity in the first year of life is inversely associated with allergic diseases. *J Allergy Clin Immunol.* 2014; 133:4.
23. Patel BY, Volcheck GW. Food allergy: common causes, diagnosis, and treatment. *Mayo Clin Proc.* 2015; 90:10.
24. Oettgen HC, Burton OT. IgE receptor signaling in food allergy pathogenesis. *Curr Opin Immunol.* 2015; 36:109.
25. Commins SP. Mechanisms of oral tolerance. *Pediatr Clin North Am.* 2015; 62:6.
26. Boyce JA, Assa'ad A, Burks AW, et al. Guidelines for the diagnosis and management of food allergy in the United States: report of the NIAID-sponsored expert panel. *J Allergy Clin Immunol.* 2010; 126(Suppl):S1.
27. Sicherer SH, Sampson HA. Food allergy: epidemiology, pathogenesis, diagnosis, and treatment. *J Allergy Clin Immunol.* 2014; 133:2.
28. Gupta RS, Springston EE, Warrier MR, et al. The prevalence, severity, and distribution of childhood food allergy in the United States. *Pediatrics.* 2011; 128:1.
29. Branum AM, Lukacs SL. Food allergy among children in the United States. *Pediatrics.* 2009; 124:6.
30. Rona RJ, Keil T, Summers C, et al. The prevalence of food allergy: a meta-analysis. *J Allergy Clin Immunol.* 2007; 120:3.
31. Nowak-Wegrzyn A, Groetch M. Nutritional aspects and diets in food allergy. *Chem Immunol Allergy.* 2015; 101:209.
32. Kaya A, Toyran M, Civelek E, Misirlioglu E, Kirsaclioglu C, Kocabas CN. Characteristics and prognosis of allergic proctocolitis in infants. *J Pediatr Gastroenterol Nutr.* 2015; 61:1.
33. Atanaskovic-Markovic M. Refractory proctocolitis in exclusively breast-fed infants. *Endocr Metab Immune Disord Drug Targets.* 2014; 14:1.
34. Lucarelli S, Di Nardo G, Lastrucci G, et al. Allergic proctocolitis refractory to maternal hypoallergenic diet in exclusively breast-fed infants: a clinical observation. *BMC Gastroenterol.* 2011; 11:82.
35. Lake AM. Food-induced eosinophilic proctocolitis. *J Pediatr Gastroenterol Nutr.* 2000; 30(Suppl):S58.
36. Liacouras CA, Furuta GT, Hirano I, et al. Eosinophilic esophagitis: updated consensus recommendations for children and adults. *J Allergy Clin Immunol.* 2011; 128:1.
37. Dellon ES, Gonsalves N, Hirano I, et al. ACG clinical guideline: evidenced based approach to the diagnosis and management of esophageal eosinophilia and eosinophilic esophagitis (EoE). *Am J Gastroenterol.* 2013; 108:5.
38. Lwin T, Melton SD, Genta RM. Eosinophilic gastritis: histopathological characterization and quantification of the normal gastric eosinophil content. *Mod Pathol.* 2011; 24:4.
39. DeBrosse CW, Case JW, Putnam PE, Collins MH, Rothenberg ME. Quantity and distribution of eosinophils in the gastrointestinal tract of children. *Pediatr Dev Pathol.* 2006; 9:3.
40. DeBrosse CW, Franciosi JP, King EC, et al. Long-term outcomes in pediatric-onset esophageal eosinophilia. *J Allergy Clin Immunol.* 2011; 128:1.
41. Assa'ad AH, Putnam PE, Collins MH, et al. Pediatric patients with eosinophilic esophagitis: an 8-year follow-up. *J Allergy Clin Immunol.* 2007; 119:3.
42. Kelly KJ, Lazenby AJ, Rowe PC, Yardley JH, Perman JA, Sampson HA. Eosinophilic esophagitis attributed to gastroesophageal reflux: improvement with an amino acid-based formula. *Gastroenterology.* 1995; 109:5.
43. Markowitz JE, Spergel JM, Ruchelli E, Liacouras CA. Elemental diet is an effective treatment for eosinophilic esophagitis in children and adolescents. *Am J Gastroenterol.* 2003; 98:4.
44. Liacouras CA, Spergel JM., Ruchelli E, et al. Eosinophilic esophagitis: a 10-year experience in 381 children. *Clin Gastroenterol Hepatol.* 2005; 3:12.
45. Kagalwalla AF, Sentongo TA, Ritz S, et al. Effect of six-food elimination diet on clinical and histologic outcomes in eosinophilic esophagitis. *Clin Gastroenterol Hepatol.* 2006; 4:9.
46. Spergel JM, Beausoleil JL, Mascarenhas M, Liacouras CA. The use of skin prick tests and patch tests to identify causative foods in eosinophilic esophagitis. *J Allergy Clin Immunol.* 2002; 109:2.
47. Wang FY, Gupta SK, Fitzgerald JF. Is there a seasonal variation in the incidence or intensity of allergic eosinophilic esophagitis in newly diagnosed children? *J Clin Gastroenterol.* 2007; 41:5.
48. Nielsen RG, Husby S. Eosinophilic oesophagitis: epidemiology, clinical aspects, and association to allergy. *J Pediatr Gastroenterol Nutr.* 2007; 45:3.
49. Noel RJ, Putnam PE, Rothenberg ME. Eosinophilic esophagitis. *N Engl J Med.* 2004; 351:9.
50. Sealock RJ, Rendon G, El-Serag HB. Systematic review: the epidemiology of eosinophilic oesophagitis in adults. *Aliment Pharmacol Ther.* 2010; 32:6.
51. Henderson CJ, Abonia JP, King EC, et al. Comparative dietary therapy effectiveness in remission of pediatric eosinophilic esophagitis. *J Allergy Clin Immunol.* 2012; 129:6.
52. Philpott H, Nandurkar S, Royce SG, Thien F, Gibson PR. Risk factors for eosinophilic esophagitis. *Clin Exp Allergy.* 2014; 44:8.
53. Virchow JC. Eosinophilic esophagitis: asthma of the esophagus? *Dig Dis.* 2014; 32:54.
54. Simon D, Straumann A, Simon HU. Eosinophilic esophagitis and allergy. *Dig Dis.* 2014; 32:30.
55. Straumann A, Bauer M, Fischer B, Blaser K, Simon HU. Idiopathic eosinophilic esophagitis is associated with a T(H)2-type allergic inflammatory response. *J Allergy Clin Immunol.* 2001; 108:6.
56. Lucendo AJ. Cellular and molecular immunological mechanisms in eosinophilic esophagitis: an updated overview of their clinical implications. *Expert Rev Gastroenterol Hepatol.* 2014; 8:6.
57. Rieder F, Nonevski I, Ma J, et al. T-helper 2 cytokines, transforming growth factor beta1, and eosinophil products induce fibrogenesis and alter muscle motility in patients with eosinophilic esophagitis. *Gastroenterology.* 2014; 146:5.
58. Abdulnour-Nakhoul SM, Al-Tawil Y, Gyftopoulos AA, et al. Alterations in junctional proteins, inflammatory mediators and extracellular matrix molecules in eosinophilic esophagitis. *Clin Immunol.* 2013; 148:2.
59. D'Alessandro A, Esposito D, Pesce M, Cuomo R, De Palma GD, Sarnelli G. Eosinophilic esophagitis: from pathophysiology to treatment. *World J Gastrointest Pathophysiol.* 2015; 6:4.
60. Doerfler B, Bryce P, Hirano I, Gonsalves N. Practical approach to implementing dietary therapy in adults with eosinophilic esophagitis: the Chicago experience. *Dis Esophagus.* 2015; 28:1.
61. Gonsalves N, Yang GY, Doerfler B, Ritz S, Ditto AM, Hirano I. Elimination diet effectively treats eosinophilic esophagitis in adults; food reintroduction identifies causative factors. *Gastroenterology.* 2012; 142:7.
62. Wolf WA, Jerath MR, Sperry SL, Shaheen NJ, Dellon ES. Dietary elimination therapy is an effective option for adults with eosinophilic esophagitis. *Clin Gastroenterol Hepatol.* 2014; 12:8.
63. Lucendo AJ. Meta-analysis-based guidance for dietary management in eosinophilic esophagitis. *Curr Gastroenterol Rep.* 2015; 17:10.
64. Arias A, Gonzalez-Cervera J, Tenias JM, Lucendo AJ. Efficacy of dietary interventions for inducing histologic remission in patients with eosinophilic esophagitis: a systematic review and meta-analysis. *Gastroenterology.* 2014; 146:7.
65. Wechsler JB, Schwartz S, Amsden K, Kagalwalla AF. Elimination diets in the management of eosinophilic esophagitis. *J Asthma Allergy.* 2014; 7:85.
66. Molina-Infante J, Arias A, Barrio J, et al. Four-food group elimination diet for adult eosinophilic esophagitis: a prospective multicenter study. *J Allergy Clin Immunol.* 2014; 134:5.
67. Feuling MB, Noel RJ. Medical and nutrition management of eosinophilic esophagitis in children. *Nutr Clin Pract.* 2010; 25:2.
68. Eigenmann PA, Sicherer SH, Borkowski TA, Cohen BA, Sampson HA. Prevalence of IgE-mediated food allergy among children with atopic dermatitis. *Pediatrics.* 1998; 101:3.
69. Bock SA. Prospective appraisal of complaints of adverse reactions to foods in children during the first 3 years of life. *Pediatrics.* 1987; 79:5.
70. Host A, Halken S. A prospective study of cow milk allergy in Danish infants during the first 3 years of life: clinical course in relation to clinical and immunological type of hypersensitivity reaction. *Allergy.* 1990; 45:8.
71. Schrander JJ, van den Bogart JP, Forget PP, et al. Cow's milk protein intolerance in infants under 1 year of age: a prospective epidemiological study. *Eur J Pediatr.* 1993; 152:8.
72. Hide DW, Guyer BM. Cows milk intolerance in Isle of Wight infants. *Br J Clin Pract.* 1983; 37:9.
73. Nickel R, Kulig M, Forster J, et al. Sensitization to hen's egg at the age of twelve months is predictive for allergic sensitization to common indoor and outdoor allergens at the age of three years. *J Allergy Clin Immunol.* 1997; 99:5.
74. Sicherer SH, Munoz-Furlong A, Burks AW, Sampson HA. Prevalence of peanut and tree nut allergy in the US determined by a random digit dial telephone survey. *J Allergy Clin Immunol.* 1999; 103:4.
75. Tariq SM, Stevens M, Matthews S, Ridout S, Twiselton R, Hide DW. Cohort study of peanut and tree nut sensitisation by age of 4 years. *BMJ.* 1996; 313:7056.
76. Young E, Patel S, Stoneham M, Rona R, Wilkinson JD. The prevalence of reaction to food additives in a survey population. *J R Coll Physicians Lond.* 1987; 21:4.
77. Amin MR, Khoury JC, Assa'ad AH. Food-specific serum immunoglobulin E measurements in children presenting with food allergy. *Ann Allergy Asthma Immunol.* 2014; 112:2.
78. Nanda MK, Assa'ad AH, Khoury J, Lierl MB. What is the role of component IgE: analysis by ImmunoCAP and microarray compared to food-specific IgE in peanut and egg allergy? *J Allergy Clin Immunol.* 2015; 135(2 Suppl):AB31.
79. Bock SA, Lee WY, Remigio L, Holst A, May CD. Appraisal of skin tests with food extracts for diagnosis of food hypersensitivity. *Clin Allergy.* 1978; 8:6.
80. Lockey RF. Adverse reactions associated with skin testing and immunotherapy. *Allergy Proc.* 1995; 16:6.
81. Nowak-Wegrzyn A, Assa'ad AH, Bahna SL, et al. Work group report: oral food challenge testing. *J Allergy Clin Immunol.* 2009; 123(Suppl):S365.
82. Fiocchi A, Schunemann HJ, Brozek J, et al. Diagnosis and rationale for action against cow's milk allergy (DRACMA): a summary report. *J Allergy Clin Immunol.* 2010; 126:6.
83. Sampson HA, Agbotounou W, Thébault C, et al. Epicutaneous immunotherapy (EPIT) is effective and safe to treat peanut allergy: a multi-national double-blind placebo-controlled randomized phase IIb trial. *J Allergy Clin Immunol.* 2015; 135(2 Suppl):AB390.
84. Zhao Z, Ross AC. Retinoic acid repletion restores the number of leukocytes and their subsets and stimulates natural cytotoxicity in vitamin A-deficient rats. *J Nutr.* 1995; 125:8.
85. Carman JA, Hayes CE. Abnormal regulation of IFN-gamma secretion in vitamin A deficiency. *J Immunol.* 1991; 147:4.
86. Wiedermann U, Hanson LA, Kahu H, Dahlgren UI. Aberrant T-cell function in vitro and impaired T-cell dependent antibody response in vivo in vitamin A-deficient rats. *Immunology.* 1993; 80:4.

# 29 HIV Infection in Children

KEITH-THOMAS AYOOB

Acquired immune deficiency syndrome (AIDS) is caused by the human immunodeficiency virus type 1 (HIV-1) and is usually transmitted through the exchange of blood or blood products or by sexual contact. In children, HIV is typically acquired perinatally from high-risk HIV-infected mothers (85%) or through receipt of contaminated blood products. High-risk mothers are identified as injecting drug users, sexual partners of infected persons, or recipients of HIV-contaminated blood or blood products. Breast milk is also known to transmit HIV. Antiretroviral drug therapy (ART) has been used to dramatically reduce the rate of mother-to-child transmission.[1] The first cases of pediatric HIV were in the United States were diagnosed in 1982.[2,3] The number of HIV and AIDS cases increased dramatically during the 1980s and early 1990s. As of December 2010, the latest date for which statistics are available from the Centers for Disease Control and Prevention (CDC), there were 10,798 persons living with perinatally acquired HIV infection in the United States and six dependent territories; 5134 of them had been classified as having stage 3 (AIDS) at some point.[4]

Between 2008 and 2011, approximately 70% of new diagnoses of HIV infection in children younger than 13 years of age occurred in African Americans, followed by Hispanic/Latino children at approximately 15%. Five states—New York, New Jersey, Florida, California, and Texas—accounted for most children younger than 13 years of age who were living with perinatally acquired HIV infection.[4]

## DIAGNOSIS OF HIV/AIDS IN CHILDREN AND ADULTS

Human immunodeficiency is diagnosed by blood analysis for the HIV virus. The virus and its antibodies can be detected in blood. The test can be done at birth, allowing pharmacological intervention immediately, if necessary.

In 2008, the CDC modified its classification system for HIV and AIDS for children younger than 18 months old and for those between the ages of 18 months and 13 years. For adolescents older than 13 years and adults, HIV and AIDS were reclassified into a single case definition for HIV infection with three stages (plus a fourth category, stage unknown).[5] The CDC classification is detailed in Box 29–1; Table 29–1 compares the CDC classification with that of the World Health Organization (WHO). Box 29–2 lists the 2008 AIDS-defining criteria.

## MANIFESTATIONS OF CHRONIC HUMAN IMMUNODEFICIENCY VIRUS

HIV formerly was characterized by a plethora of opportunistic infections (see Box 29–2). Better treatment and prevention protocols and the use of ART beginning in the mid-1990s have resulted in a dramatic decrease in morbidity, mortality, and the incidence of opportunistic infections and maternal-child transmission of HIV.[6] Because of these advances, HIV infection in children has evolved from a terminal disease into a chronic one, albeit one that can affect multiple organ systems.

Despite advances in medication, not everyone can tolerate or respond to ART, and opportunistic infections are of heightened concern in such persons. When opportunistic infections do manifest, control rather than cure is often the most realistic goal. Growth failure and failure to thrive are common features of HIV and may be the primary presenting signs in children who were not diagnosed during infancy.

One study found an early decline in the linear growth rate, but weight for height was preserved until HIV disease was advanced.[7] A delayed onset of pubertal development has also been found among children with perinatally acquired HIV infection.[8] A large European study comparing infected and uninfected children born to HIV-infected mothers and followed for 10 years found that infected children grew more slowly than uninfected children and that the differences increased with age, with severely symptomatic children experiencing poorer growth at all ages.[9] Another study found that children born to HIV-infected mothers were small for age, but uninfected children caught up; infected children experienced a more pronounced decrease in height for age than in weight for age.[10] A high HIV viral load is associated with poor growth.[11] Some studies have shown positive results on growth with pharmacological therapies such as ART and other antiretroviral therapies,[12,13] although a larger study found that protease inhibitors were associated with only minor improvements in height and weight.[14] In another study, catch-up growth was observed after the introduction of ART but was limited to children in whom stunting had occurred before the introduction of ART and who were younger than 3 years of age.[15]

Increasingly common in surviving HIV-infected children is significant, progressive neurological disease or *HIV-1 progressive encephalopathy*, which manifests as developmental delays, including feeding problems, motor dysfunction, loss of developmental milestones, and psychiatric and behavioral manifestations.[16–18] Aggressive intervention with ART is now common, and it may halt or even reverse the encephalopathy in some cases. The viral load appears to be an indicator of encephalopathy risk.[19] Gastrointestinal problems are common with HIV infection, especially in developing countries and where access to medication is limited. Diarrhea is common, but malabsorption can occur even in the absence of chronic diarrhea.[20,21]

## COMORBID CONDITIONS IN PEDIATRIC HIV INFECTION

As beneficial as ART has been to both adults and children with HIV, it is not without some drawbacks, including a significant risk of comorbidities. Long-term ART has been shown to be an independent predictor of chronic renal impairment in HIV-infected adults.[22,23] In children on long-term ART, decreased renal function and hypophosphatemia can occur over time.[24] However, one study that followed vertically infected children and young adults for 132 months after commencement of ART found that hypophosphatemia is not always be clinically significant.[23]

Lipid abnormalities in chronic pediatric HIV infection are well documented in adults but have been less studied in children. Significant dyslipidemia in children has been associated with the use of protease inhibitors and has included hypercholesterolemia and hypertriglyceridemia.[25–29] The multicenter Perinatal AIDS Collaborative Transmission Study (PACTS) and its follow-up (PACTS-HOPE) found that children receiving ART, specifically protease inhibitor regimens, had an increased risk of hypercholesterolemia and hypertriglyceridemia. Research shows that changing ART regimens may not improve hypercholesterolemia.[30]

Adults with HIV infection who are receiving ART also have an increased risk of cardiovascular events such as myocardial infarction, stroke, bypass surgery,[31] and atherosclerosis.[32] Increased risk of

**Box 29–1.** 2008 Surveillance Case Definitions for HIV Infection and AIDS in Children and Adults

### *Children <18 Months of Age*

A child aged <18 months is categorized for surveillance purposes as definitively or presumptively HIV infected if born to an HIV-infected mother and if the laboratory criterion or at least one of the other criteria is met.

#### LABORATORY CRITERION FOR DEFINITIVE HIV INFECTION

A child aged <18 months is categorized for surveillance purposes as definitively HIV infected if born to an HIV-infected mother and the following laboratory criterion is met:

- Positive results on two separate specimens (not including cord blood) from one or more of the following HIV virologic (nonantibody) tests:
  - HIV nucleic acid (DNA or RNA) detection**
  - HIV p24 antigen test, including neutralization assay, for a child aged ≥1 month
  - HIV isolation (viral culture)

#### LABORATORY CRITERION FOR PRESUMPTIVE HIV INFECTION

A child aged <18 months is categorized for surveillance purposes as presumptively HIV infected if (1) born to an HIV-infected mother, (2) the criterion for definitively HIV infected is not met, and (3) the following laboratory criterion is met:

- Positive results on one specimen (not including cord blood) from the three HIV virologic tests listed for definitive HIV infection and no subsequent negative results from HIV virologic or HIV antibody tests

#### OTHER CRITERIA (FOR CASES THAT DO NOT MEET LABORATORY CRITERIA FOR DEFINITIVE OR PRESUMPTIVE HIV INFECTION)

- HIV infection diagnosed by a physician or qualified medical-care provider based on the laboratory criteria and documented in a medical record. Oral reports of prior laboratory test results are not acceptable.

  *or*
- When test results regarding HIV infection status are not available, documentation of a condition that meets the criteria in the 1987 pediatric surveillance case definition for AIDS (*1*) (see Box 29-2: "AIDS-defining Conditions")

### *Children Aged 18 Months to <13 Years*

Children aged 18 months to <13 years are categorized as HIV infected for surveillance purposes if at least one of laboratory criteria or the other criterion is met. Laboratory-confirmed evidence of HIV infection is now required for all reported cases of HIV infection among children aged 18 months to <13 years.

#### LABORATORY CRITERIA

- Positive result from a screening test for HIV antibody (e.g., reactive enzyme immunoassay [EIA]), confirmed by a positive result from a supplemental test for HIV antibody (e.g., Western blot, indirect immunofluorescence assay);

*or*

- Positive result or a detectable quantity by any of the following HIV virologic (nonantibody) tests***:
  - HIV nucleic acid (DNA or RNA) detection (e.g., polymerase chain reaction [PCR])
  - HIV p24 antigen test, including neutralization assay
  - HIV isolation (viral culture)

#### OTHER CRITERION (FOR CASES THAT DO NOT MEET LABORATORY CRITERIA)

- HIV infection diagnosed by a physician or qualified medical-care provider based on the laboratory criteria and documented in a medical record. Oral reports of prior laboratory test results are not acceptable.

### *Adolescents ≥13 Years and Adults*

The CDC case definition of HIV is now classified into three stages of increasing severity—Stage 1, Stage 2, and Stage 3 (AIDS)—and a fourth category, Stage Unknown. Table 29–1 compares the stages of HIV infection as defined by the CDC and the World Health Organization (WHO).

Laboratory-confirmed evidence is now required for an HIV diagnosis; the laboratory criteria are the same as for the age group 18 months to <13 years. Laboratory evidence is definied in the following table:

TABLE. Comparison of World Health Organization (WHO) and CDC stages of human Immunodeficiency virus (HIV) Infection,* by CD4+ T-lymphocyte Count and percentage of otal lymphocytes

| who stage[†] | WHO T-lymphocyto count and percentage[§] | CDC stage[¹] | CDC T-lymphocyte count and perecentage |
|---|---|---|---|
| Stage 1 (HIV infection) | CD4+ T-lymphocyte count ≥500 colls/μL | Stage1 (HIV infection) | CD4+ T-lymphocyto cojunt of ≥500 Cells/μL or CD4+ T-lymphocyte percentage of ≥29 |
| Stage 2 (HIV infection) | CD4+ T-lymphocyte count 350–499 colls/μL | Stage2 (HIV infection) | CD4+ T-lymphocyto count of 200–499 cells//μL or cd CD4+ T-lymphocyto cojunt of 14–28 |
| Stage 3 (advanced HIV disease (AHD]) | CD4+ T-lymphocyte count 200–349 colls/μL | Stage2 (HIV infection) | CD4+ T-lymphocyto count of 200–499 cells//μL or cd CD4+ T-lymphocyto percentage of 14–28 |
| Stage 3 (acquired Immunodeficiency syndrome (AIDS]) | CD4+ T-lymphocyto count of<200 cells//μL or CD4+ T-lymphocyto cojunt of <15 | Stage 3(AIDS) | CD4+ T-lymphocyto count of<200 cells/μL or CD4+ T-lymphocyto percentage of <14 |

* For reporting purpose only.

(*continued*)

**Box 29–1.** Continued

† Amoung adults and children aged ≥5 years.

§ Percentage applicable for stage 4 only.

¶ Among adults and adolegcents (aged≥13 years). CDC also indudes a fourth stage. Stage unknown: laboratory confirmation of HIV infection but no information on CD4+ T-lymphocyte count or percentage and no information on AIDS-defining conditions.

(Retrieved August 6, 2015 from: http://www.cdc.gov/mmwr/preview/mmwrhtml/rr5710a2.htm)

Merely having an AIDS-defining condition alone is no longer sufficient for classification as HIV-infected. AIDS-defining conditions are listed in Box 29–2.

From Centers for Disease Control and Prevention (CDC). Revised surveillance case definitions for HIV infection. *MMWR Morb Mortal Wkly Rep.* 2008; 57(RR10):1. Available at http://www.cdc.gov/mmwr/preview/mmwrhtml/rr5710a1.htm. Accessed June 21, 2016.

**HIV nucleic acid (DNA or RNA) detection tests are the virologic methods of choice for the diagnosis or exclusion of infection in children aged <18 months. Although HIV culture can be used, culture is less standardized and less sensitive than nucleic acid detection tests. The use of p24 antigen testing to exclude infection in children aged <18 months is not recommended because of poor sensitivity, especially in the presence of HIV antibody. Commercial tests for RNA and DNA detection have become widely available. Quantitative RNA tests have been approved by the Food and Drug Administration (FDA) for monitoring HIV infection, and qualitative RNA tests have been approved to aid diagnosis. The quantitative and qualitative RNA tests meet FDA standards for high analytic and clinical sensitivity and specificity (*14–16*). All available tests detect the subtypes of group M and strains of group O. HIV-2 can be diagnosed with HIV-2 DNA PCR. HIV RNA tests sometimes do not detect HIV-2 because the viral loads in some HIV-2–infected persons are below detectable levels. Because of the possibility of mutation or recombination involving the sequences detected by a particular test, occasionally, virus might not be detected in a specimen from an HIV-2 infected individual. If HIV-2 infection seems likely but results are negative, testing with a different assay might be advisable.

*** For HIV screening among children aged 18 months to <13 years infected through exposure other than perinatal exposure, HIV virologic (non-antibody) tests should not be used in lieu of approved HIV antibody screening tests. A negative result (i.e., undetectable or nonreactive) by an HIV virologic test (e.g., viral RNA nucleic acid test) does not rule out the diagnosis of HIV infection.

atherosclerotic cardiovascular disease has been seen in children and adolescents who on long-term ART.[33] A review of studies in adults with HIV infection showed that dietary intervention and supplementation with omega-3 fatty acids was more beneficial in lowering triglycerides than in lowering low-density lipoprotein (LDL) cholesterol or raising high-density lipoprotein (HDL) cholesterol.[34]

Lipodystrophy syndrome has been defined as redistribution of body fat by means of peripheral lipoatrophy or centripetal lipohypertrophy or both processes; both types of redistribution may occur with or without laboratory abnormalities (e.g., dyslipidemia).[35]One or more of four physical characteristics, alone or in combination, can be observed in affected individuals[36]:

- Lipoatrophy: loss of fat in the extremities
- Lipohypertrophy: fat accumulation in the abdomen and trunk regions
- "Buffalo humps: large dorsocervical fat accumulation on the back of the neck
- Breast hypertrophy: seen mostly in women

The presence of lipodystrophy has been found to occur in 27% to 33% of children receiving ART.[37,38] Lipodystrophy syndrome characteristics were associated with dosing regimens, with children receiving adult regimens significantly more likely to develop these characteristics. Longer duration of treatment has been found to be a primary risk factor for lipodystrophy.[38]

Insulin resistance has been associated with lipodystrophy in children.[39–43] Several studies have found elevated fasting insulin levels in the absence of obesity, with and without abnormal fasting glucose levels.[43–45] Hepatic abnormalities have been identified in HIV-infected children, specifically abnormal liver structure and hepatic steatosis.[46] Antiretroviral medications can be harsh on the systems of children and have been associated with impaired liver function due to mitochondrial toxicity.[47] Osteoporosis has also surfaced as a risk factor in HIV-infected children. Arpadi et al. found children with HIV to have significantly reduced bone density compared with uninfected children.[48]

## FACTORS TO BE CONSIDERED IN NUTRITIONAL EVALUATION

Although malnutrition is no longer inevitable in every situation, and although opportunistic infections are less of a risk in developed countries where medications are available, nutrition status takes on a new but equally important significance. Suboptimal intakes of nutrients have become more of a concern because of the negative impact of ART on the appetite. Most ART medications are associated with some level of decreased appetite and nausea, which are common complaints of persons taking them. For children who must take these medications, perhaps for their entire lives and starting often in infancy, food and

**Table 29–1.** Comparison of World Health Organization (WHO) and Centers for Disease Control and Prevention (CDC) Stages of Human Immunodeficiency Virus (HIV) Infection*

| WHO stage† | WHO T-lymphocyte count and percentage§ | CDC stage¶ | CDC T-lymphocyte count and percentage |
|---|---|---|---|
| Stage 1 (HIV infection) | $CD4^+$ T-lymphocyte count of ≥ 500 cells/μL | Stage 1 (HIV infection) | $CD4^+$ T-lymphocyte count of ≥500 cells/μL *or* $CD4^+$ T-lymphocyte percentage of ≥29 |
| Stage 2 (HIV infection) | $CD4^+$ T-lymphocyte count of 350–499 cells/μL | Stage 2 (HIV infection) | $CD4^+$ T-lymphocyte count of 200–499 cells/μL *or* $CD4^+$ T-lymphocyte percentage of 14–28 |
| Stage 3 (advanced HIV disease [AHD]) | $CD4^+$ T-lymphocyte count of 200–349 cells/μL | Stage 2 (HIV infection) | $CD4^+$ T-lymphocyte count of 200–499 cells/μL *or* $CD4^+$ T-lymphocyte percentage of 14–28 |
| Stage 4 (acquired immunodeficiency syndrome [AIDS]) | $CD4^+$ T-lymphocyte count of <200 cells/μL *or* $CD4^+$ T-lymphocyte percentage of <15 | Stage 3 (AIDS) | $CD4^+$ T-lymphocyte count of <200 cells/μL *or* $CD4^+$ T-lymphocyte percentage of <14 |

*For reporting purpose only.

†Among adult and children aged ≥5 years.

§Percentage application for stage 4 only.

¶Among adult and adolescent (aged ≥13 years). CDC also includes a fourth stage, stage unknown: laboratory confirmation of HIV infection but no information on $CD4^+$ T-lymphocyte count or percentage *and* no information on AIDS-defining condition.

From Centers for Disease Control and Prevention (CDC). Revised surveillance case definitions for HIV infection, Appendix B. *MMWR Morb Mortal Wkly Rep.* 2008; 57(RR10):1. Available at http://www.cdc.gov/mmwr/preview/mmwrhtml/rr5710a3.htm. Accessed June 21, 2016.

**Box 29–2.** Aids-Defining Conditions

- Bacterial infections, multiple or recurrent*
- Candidiasis of bronchi, trachea, or lungs
- Candidiasis of esophagus†
- Cervical cancer, invasive§
- Coccidioidomycosis, disseminated or extrapulmonary
- Cryptococcosis, extrapulmonary
- Cryptosporidiosis, chronic intestinal (>1 month's duration)
- Cytomegalovirus disease (other than liver, spleen, or nodes), onset at age >1 month
- Cytomegalovirus retinitis (with loss of vision)†
- Encephalopathy, HIV related
- Herpes simplex: chronic ulcers (>1 month's duration) or bronchitis, pneumonitis, or esophagitis (onset at age >1 month)
- Histoplasmosis, disseminated or extrapulmonary
- Isosporiasis, chronic intestinal (>1 month's duration)
- Kaposi sarcoma†
- Lymphoid interstitial pneumonia or pulmonary lymphoid hyperplasia complex*†
- Lymphoma, Burkitt (or equivalent term)
- Lymphoma, immunoblastic (or equivalent term)
- Lymphoma, primary, of brain
- *Mycobacterium avium* complex or *Mycobacterium kansasii*, disseminated or extrapulmonary†
- *Mycobacterium tuberculosis* of any site, pulmonary,†§ disseminated,† or extrapulmonary†
- *Mycobacterium*, other species or unidentified species, disseminated† or extrapulmonary†
- *Pneumocystis jirovecii* pneumonia†
- Pneumonia, recurrent†§
- Progressive multifocal leukoencephalopathy
- *Salmonella* septicemia, recurrent
- Toxoplasmosis of brain, onset at age >1 month†
- Wasting syndrome attributed to HIV

*Only among children aged <13 years. (CDC. 1994 Revised classification system for human immunodeficiency virus infection in children less than 13 years of age. MMWR 1994;43[No. RR-12].)
†Condition that might be diagnosed presumptively.
§Only among adults and adolescents aged ≥13 years. (CDC. 1993 Revised classification system for HIV infection and expanded surveillance case definition for AIDS among adolescents and adults. MMWR 1992;41[No. RR-17].)

From Centers for Disease Control and Prevention (CDC). Revised surveillance case definitions for HIV infection, Appendix A. *MMWR Morb Mortal Wkly Rep.* 2008; 57(RR10):1. Available at http://www.cdc.gov/mmwr/preview/mmwrhtml/rr5710a2.htm. Accessed June 21, 2016.

eating may never have the same appeal as for normally developing children not taking the medications.

Nutrient deficiencies can result from increased need, decreased intake, malabsorption, or some combination of these mechanisms. In children with HIV infection, the causes of these conditions may be multifactorial and even additive. Recovery from normal childhood infections and diseases may take longer, and low-grade intermittent or persistent fever may occur, increasing the demand for nutrients and using up needed energy and nutrient stores. Children who are ill seldom have optimal appetites, and this leads to inadequate intake. An additional complicating factor is the volume of fluid required for the number of medications children are often taking, which can displace nutrient-dense foods and hamper energy intake. Malabsorption, which may or may not be symptomatic, compounds the nutritional needs of the HIV-infected child. The nutritional status of children with HIV infection needs to be monitored regularly, starting with a basic nutrition assessment as soon as an HIV diagnosis is made.[49]

## NUTRITION ASSESSMENT

Appropriate guidelines for assessing and monitoring children with HIV infection have been established.[50] The 2010 HIV/AIDS evidence-based nutrition practice guideline developed by the American Dietetic Association (now the Academy of Nutrition and Dietetics),[51] is summarized in Box 29–3.

The daily recommended intakes (DRIs) can be used as a guide, but realistically, energy and protein needs have to be adjusted based on activity level, clinical symptoms, and individual variance.

Nutrition assessment of children with HIV infection is facilitated by an experienced registered dietitian who specializes in the nutritional care of children with special health care needs.[49,52] In addition to a detailed dietary history and the usual questions dealing with food preferences, use of supplements, and food allergies and intolerances, information regarding methods of feeding, developmental milestones, and usual appetite and bowel habits should be obtained.

Laboratory values relevant for assessment of the nutrition status of the child with HIV infection include albumin, prealbumin, transferring, $CD4^+$ and $CD8^+$ T lymphocyte count, viral load, hemoglobin, hematocrit, cholesterol, and triglycerides.[50] Anthropometric, dietary, and medical data are reliable indicators of nutritional risk for children with HIV, and a useful instrument combining these factors has been developed.[49,53] General assessment techniques are discussed in greater detail in Chapter 4 and nutrition support in Chapter 35. Body composition can also be assessed to determine its components, but this approach has some drawbacks in children. Skinfold measurements can detect localized fat deposits, but they cannot detect acute changes in body composition, and measurements can vary between examiners. Bioelectrical impedance analysis (BIA) is simple, but the equipment is expensive and not readily available in many clinics where HIV-infected children are examined. BIA has not been validated for the detection of lipodystrophy in children.

The guidelines state that medical nutrition therapy should be provided by a registered dietitian/nutritionist once or twice annually for asymptomatic persons and in two to six or more visits annually for symptomatic persons, based on symptoms or complications.

Psychosocial problems affect the maintenance of nutrition status. Most children with HIV infection come from homes where one or both parents are infected; parents may be deceased, uninvolved with the child, or in various stages of the disease themselves. Children with HIV infection may be exposed to more subjective stresses and years of negative life events and mental health issues.[54] They are often in foster or kinship care and are often from lower socioeconomic backgrounds in inner-city areas where family and environmental stressors compete for the attention of the caregiver, making care at home erratic. Because care at home may be influenced by cultural background and social mores, nutrition evaluation of the HIV-infected child should include a search for any nonphysical barriers to optimal management.

## DIETARY MANAGEMENT

The goal of dietary management is to optimize the dietary contribution to the child's growth and development and to prevent or delay nutrient deficiencies. An initial baseline nutrition assessment, performed as soon as possible after an HIV diagnosis is made, should address the child's growth and developmental levels, including feeding skill milestones.[49,50,55] A healthful eating plan for the child with HIV must consider a variety of factors, including family income, caregiver competence, developmental feeding skills, family culture, access to food supplies, and cooking facilities.

If failure to thrive has been determined, the following formulas[56] are used to determine the minimum and maximum energy needs and optimal calorie intake:

Minimum:

$$\text{Weight (kg) at 50th percentile for actual height} \times \frac{\text{DRI for calories per kg based age}}{\text{Actual weight (kg)}} = \text{kcal/kg}$$

Maximum:

$$\text{Weight (kg) for age at 50th percentile} \times \frac{\text{DRI for calories per kg based age}}{\text{Actual weight (kg)}} = \text{kcal/kg}$$

**Box 29–3.** HIV/AIDS Evidence-Based Nutrition Practice Guideline

***HIV/AIDS: Assessment of Food- and Nutrition-Related History??stet??***

The Registered Dietitian (RD) should assess the food- and nutrition-related history of people with HIV infection, including but not limited to

- Food and nutrient intake, focusing on energy, protein, fat, fiber, sodium, calcium, and vitamin D
- Medications herbal supplements taken and their potential negative interactions
- Knowledge, beliefs, and attitudes
- Behavior
- Factors affecting access to food and food- and nutrition-related supplies
- Physical activity and function
- Nutrition-related patient- and client-centered measures

***HIV/AIDS: Anthropometric Assessment***

The RD should include the following anthropometric measurements in the initial assessment:

- Weight, height and body mass index; for children, growth pattern indices
- In addition, body compartment estimates should be included, such as circumference measurements (midarm muscle, waist, hip, and waist-to-hip ratio) or measurements of body cell mass and body fat (by dual-energy x-ray absorptiometry [DXA], bioelectrical impedance analysis [BIA], bioimpedance spectroscopy or skinfold thickness measurements).

Baseline anthropometric measurements provide information for the nutrition assessment. Most studies in men, women, children, and adolescents have reported that fat-free mass and fat mass are altered in people with HIV infection.

***HIV/AIDS: Determining Energy Needs***

The RD should use clinical judgment and consider several factors when determining the energy needs of adults and children with HIV infection to maintain a healthy body weight. Factors related to energy needs in people with HIV infection include age, gender, stage of disease, nutritional status, opportunistic infections and comorbidities, inflammation, and effects of medications. Although research reports increased resting energy expenditure (as much as 5–17%) in people with HIV infection, total energy expenditure may be similar to that of healthy control subjects.

***HIV/AIDS: Macronutrient Composition***

- The RD should prescribe an individualized diet with a macronutrient composition based on the Dietary Reference Intakes (DRI): 20–35% of calories from fat, 45–65% from carbohydrate, and 10–35% from protein, with 14 g fiber per 1000 kcal
- In people with HIV infection, protein needs are highly individualized. Low-fiber/high-fat diets are associated with fat deposition, insulin resistance, and obesity. Studies indicate that diets low in saturated fat and total fat result in reduced triglyceride levels, increased high-density lipoprotein (HDL)-cholesterol levels, and a lower risk of lipohypertrophy.

***HIV/AIDS: Macronutrient Composition for Hyperlipidemia***

- For people with HIV infection who have hyperlipidemia, the RD should encourage consumption of a cardioprotective dietary pattern tailored to the individual's needs to provide a fat intake of 25–35% of calories, >7% of calories from saturated fat, <1% of calories from *trans*-fatty acids, and <200 mg of cholesterol per day.
- Studies on several lifestyle modification interventions for the treatment of hyperlipidemia in people with HIV infection report improvements in serum lipid profile. Research indicates that diets that are low in saturated fat and total fat and include omega-3 fatty acids result in reduced triglyceride levels, increased HDL-cholesterol levels, and a lower risk of lipohypertrophy.

***HIV/AIDS: Vitamin and Mineral Supplementation***

If people with HIV infection cannot meet their Recommended Dietary Allowance (RDA) levels for micronutrients through diet, the RD should recommend vitamin and mineral supplements, especially for calcium and vitamin D. Micronutrient deficiencies are common in HIV-infected individuals, and studies report increased morbidity and mortality in those not taking vitamin supplementation.

Adapted from American Dietetic Association. HIV/AIDS evidence-based nutrition practice guideline. Chicago: American Dietetic Association, December 2010.

For example, a 9-month-old girl with a weight of 5 kg and a length of 63 cm would require 702 to 928 kcal, or 140 to 185 kcal per kilogram of body weight. More calories are needed for catch-up growth (see Chapter 20). The resting energy expenditure may be increased in HIV, but decreased caloric intake may be a more influential cause of short-term weight loss, especially if malabsorption is present.[21] A simpler method of calculation for children and adolescents who are asymptomatic or have mild signs or symptoms is to increase calories to 150% to 200% of the DRI if growth velocity is slow for age.[57] Close follow-up is necessary because feeding the child with HIV-related growth failure may result in a gain of weight but not height.[58]

Protein requirements in the HIV-infected child with growth failure can be estimated by substituting the DRI for protein into the same formulas. Another method is to increase the DRI for protein by 50% to 100% to provide for the increased needs and nitrogen losses the body may incur due to HIV infection as long as renal function is satisfactory.[59] Regarding micronutrient intake, the DRI is intended to meet the needs of most normal healthy people but may not meet the needs of the child whose body is chronically fighting an HIV infection. For such children, a thorough multivitamin and mineral supplement may be recommended. The supplement should be in an easily consumed form and should provide no more than 100% of the DRI.[50]

A multidisciplinary approach is required for comprehensive care of the HIV-infected child, especially if the child's intake is inadequate due to developmental delays or feeding skill difficulties. A feeding evaluation by a multidisciplinary dysphagia team focused on proper positioning and textural and oral desensitization issues showed improved intake in most of the children studied.[60] When appropriate, caregivers should be taught appropriate techniques for feeding the developmentally delayed child to help ensure adequate intake and to facilitate a more positive caregiver-child interaction during feeding. When children cannot support their needs with regular foods alone, enteral formulas or other medical foods may be considered.

Nasogastric or gastrostomy feedings are options when children cannot obtain adequate nutrition with oral feedings alone. Nasogastric tubes are better used only on a short-term basis. The weight gained by placing gastrostomy tube feeding in these children may be mostly fat weight rather than muscle mass.[61] When adherence to ART is poor, a gastrostomy tube can be used successfully to deliver medication and improve viral load and CD4+ T-cell percentages[62] (see Chapter 35).

The interaction of medications with foods is a constant challenge to the nutrition professional working with HIV-infected children. These children are likely to be taking numerous medications, any of which may have adverse effects on appetite.[63] Drug-nutrient interactions, including effects of meal timing, must be considered when making dietary recommendations because many medications must be taken with (or without) food for optimal effectiveness. Food and water safety must also be considered when making recommendations because the child with a compromised immune system is more vulnerable to opportunistic bacteria such as *Cryptosporidium* and other water-borne organisms.[49] Weakened immune systems may also be more vulnerable to food-borne contamination and may take longer to recover from food poisoning episodes. Proper food handling and water safety practices deserve emphasis when counseling the caregivers of children with HIV.

The use of supplements in children and adults with HIV infection has received increased focus in developing and developed countries. A 2013 review of studies primarily in African countries concluded that multiple micronutrients may be clinically beneficial for poorly nourished children but also noted the lack of an evidence base and suggested that more trials studying single-nutrient supplementation were indicated.[64] A review on bone health in vertically infected children and adolescents reported evidence of disrupted vitamin D metabolism with ART and found that supplementation may be needed to achieve functional vitamin D sufficiency. Supplemental calcium was also suggested if the dietary history indicates insufficient intake.[65]

## FOLLOW-UP

The *vulnerable child syndrome* becomes a greater possibility as children live longer with a chronic illness such as HIV infection, and it can play a role in establishing poor eating habits and nutrition risks. Often, parents and caregivers feel guilty about, or sorry for, the child and may be reluctant to set limits for the child that can establish lifelong positive eating habits. A lack of appropriate dietary guidance and limit-setting can set the stage for eating behavior problems and power struggles focused on food issues. Poor eating habits that are established in childhood and allowed to continue may be more difficult to change when HIV-related symptoms develop years later. The importance of good nutrition and a healthy age-appropriate and developmentally appropriate eating style at all stages of this disease needs to be emphasized to caregivers.[66]

Attention must be given to the issue of confidentiality and disclosure. As children with HIV grow, they become increasingly aware of their environment but caregivers may not want them to know their diagnosis. In counseling caregivers when the child is present, it is important to avoid using the terms *HIV* or *AIDS* when the content of the conversation applies to the child. Even other family members may not be aware of the child's HIV diagnosis. Any documents sent from the child's records to clinics, schools, or other places should not mention HIV or AIDS unless the parent or legal guardian has given permission for disclosure.

### References


1. Brocklehurst P, Volmink J. Antiretrovirals for reducing the risk of mother-to-child transmission of HIV infection. *Cochrane Database Syst Rev.* 2002; (2):CD003510.
2. Oleske J, Minnefor A, Cooper R Jr, et al. Immune deficiency syndrome in children. *JAMA.* 1983; 249:2345.
3. Rubenstein A. Acquired immune deficiency syndrome in infants. *Am J Dis Child.* 1983; 137:825.
4. Centers for Disease Control and Prevention. *Pediatric HIV Surveillance.* http://www.cdc.gov/hiv/pdf/statistics_surveillance_Pediatric.pdf. Accessed June 21, 2016.
5. Schneider E, Whitmore S, Glynn MK, Dominguez K, Mitsch A, McKenna MT. Revised surveillance case definitions for HIV infection among adults, adolescents, and children aged <18 months and for HIV infection and AIDS among children aged 18 months to <13 years—United States, 2008. *MMWR Morb Mortal Wkly Rep.* 2008; 57(RR10):1. Available at http://www.cdc.gov/mmwr/preview/mmwrhtml/rr5710a1.htm. Accessed June 21, 2016.
6. Gortmaker SL, Hughes M, Cervia J, et al. The impact of protease inhibitor combination therapy on mortality among children and youth infected with HIV-1. *N Engl J Med.* 2002;345:1522.
7. Mintz M. Clinical features and treatment interventions for human immunodeficiency virus–associated neurologic disease in children. *Semin Neurol.* 1999; 19: 165.
8. Buchacz K, Rogol AD, Lindsey JC, et al. Delayed onset of pubertal development in children and adolescents with perinatally acquired HIV infection. *J Acquir Immune Defic Syndr.* 2003; 33:56.
9. Chase C, Ware J, Hittleman J, et al. Early cognitive and motor development among infants born to women infected with human immunodeficiency virus. Women and Infants Transmission Study Group. *Pediatrics.* 2000; 106:E25.
10. Mitchell W. Neurological and developmental effects of HIV and AIDS in children and adolescents. *Ment Retard Dev Disabil Res Rev.* 2001; 7:211.
11. Peters VB, Rosh JR, Mugrditchian L, et al. Growth failure as the first expression of malnutrition in children with human immunodeficiency virus infection. *Mt Sinai J Med.* 1998; 65:1.
12. Newell ML, Borja MC, Peckham C. Height, weight, and growth in children born to mothers with HIV-1 infection in Europe. The European Collaborative Study. *Pediatrics.* 2003; 111:e52.
13. Saavedra JM, Henderson RA, Perman JA, Hutton N, Livingston RA, Yolken RH. Longitudinal assessment of growth in children born to mothers with human immunodeficiency virus infection. *Arch Pediatr Adolesc Med.* 1995; 149:497.
14. Nachman SA, Lindsey JC, Pelton S, et al. Growth in human immunodeficiency virus–infected children receiving ritonavir-containing antiretroviral therapy. *Arch Pediatr Adolesc Med.* 2002; 156:497.
15. Verweel G, van Rossum AMC, Hartwig NG, Wolfs TFW, Sherpbier HJ, DeGroot R. Treatment with highly active retroviral therapy in human immunodeficiency virus type 1–infected children is associated with a sustained effect on growth. *Pediatrics.* 2002; 109:e25.
16. Dreimane D, Nielsen K, Deveikis A, Bryson YJ, Geffner ME. Effect of protease inhibitors combined with standard anti-retroviral therapy on linear growth and weight gain in human immunodeficiency virus type 1–infected children. *Pediatr Infect Dis J.* 2001; 20:315.
17. Buchacz K, Cervia JS, Lindsey JC, et al. Impact of protease inhibitor–containing combination antiretroviral therapies on height and weight growth in HIV-infected children. *Pediatrics.* 2001; 108:E72.
18. Steiner F, Kind C, Aebi C, et al. Growth in human immunodeficiency virus type 1–infected children treated with protease inhibitors. *Eur J Pediatr.* 2001; 160:611.
19. Perez Mato S, Van Dyke RB. Pulmonary infections in children with HIV infection. *Semin Respir Infect.* 2002; 17:33.
20. Knox TA, Spiegelman D, Skinner SC, Gorbach S. Diarrhea and abnormalities of gastrointestinal function in a cohort of men and women with HIV infection. *Am J Gastroenterol.* 2000; 95:3482.
21. Carbonnel F, Beaugerie L, Abou Rached A, et al. Macronutrient intake and malabsorption in HIV infection: a comparison with other malabsorptive states. *Gut* 1997; 41:805.
22. Ryom L, Mocroft A, Kirk O, et al. Association between antiretroviral exposure and renal impairment among HIV-positive persons with normal baseline renal function: the D:A:D study. *J Infect Dis.* 2013, 207:1359.
23. Giacomet V, Nannini P, Vigano A, et al. Long-term renal effects of tenofovir-disoproxil-fumarate in vertically HIV-infected children, adolescents, and young adults: a 132-month follow-up study. *Clin Drug Invest.* 2015, 35:419.
24. Pontrelli G, Cotugno N, Amodio D, et al. Renal function in HIV-infected children and adolescents treated with tenofovir disoproxil fumarate and protease inhibitors. *BMC Infect Dis.* 2012, 12:18.
25. Lainka E, Oezbeck S, Falck M, Ndagijimana J, Niehaus T. Marked dyslipidemia in human immunodeficiency virus–infected children in protease inhibitor–containing antiretroviral therapy. *Pediatrics.* 2002; 110:e56.
26. Melvin AJ, Lennon S, Mohan KM, Purnell JQ. Metabolic abnormalities in HIV-type 1–infected children treated and not treated with protease inhibitors. *AIDS Res Hum Retroviruses.* 2001; 17:1117.
27. Arpadi SM, Cuff PA, Horlick M, Wang J, Kotler DP. Lipodystrophy in HIV-infected children is associated with high viral load and low CD4+-lymphocyte percentage at baseline and use of protease inhibitors and stavudine. *J Acquir Immune Defic Syndr.* 2001; 27:30.
28. Farley J, Gona P, Crain M, et al. Prevalence of elevated cholesterol and associated risk factors among perinatally HIV-infected children (4-19 years old) in Pediatric AIDS Clinical Trials Group 219C. *J Acquir Immune Defic Syndr.* 2005; 38:480.
29. Tassiopoulos K, Williams PL, Seage GR III, et al. Association of hypercholesterolemia incidence with antiretroviral treatment, including protease inhibitors, among perinatally HIV-infected children. *J Acquir Immune Defic Syndr.* 2008; 47:607.
30. Jacobson DL, Williams P, Tassiopoulos K, et al. Clinical management and follow-up of hypercholesterolemia a perinatally HIV-infected children enrolled in the PACTG 219C study. *J Acquir Immune Defic Syndr.* 2011; 57:413.
31. Desai M, Joyce V, Bendavid E, et al. Risk of cardiovascular events associated with current exposure to HIV antiretroviral therapies in a US veteran population. *Clin Infect Dis.* 2015; 61:445.
32. Aragones G, Pardo-Reche P, Fernandez-Sender L, et al. The deleterious influence of tenofovir-based therapies on the progression of atherosclerosis in HIV-infected patients. *Mediators Inflamm.* 2012; 2012:372305.
33. Patel K, Wang J, Jacobson DL, et al. Aggregate risk of cardiovascular disease among adolescents perinatally infected with the human immunodeficiency virus. *Circulation.* 2014; 129:1204.
34. Stradling, C., Chen, Y.F., Russell, T., Connock, M., Thomas, G.N., Taheri, S. The effects of dietary intervention on HIV dyslipidemia: a systematic review and meta-analysis. PLoS One. 2012;7(6):e38121. doi: 10.1371/journal.pone.0038121. Epub 2012 Jun 11.

35. Papi L, Menezes AC, Rocha H, et al. The presence of lipodystrophy and risk factors for dyslipidemia in HIV-infected children in Brazil. *Braz J Infect Dis.* 2014; 18:394.
36. *What defines HIV lipodystrophy?: a Roundtable Organized by the Forum for Collaborative HIV Research.* San Diego, CA: September 23, 2002. George Washington University Medical Center, Center for Health Services Research and Policy.
37. Piloya T, Bakeera-Kitaka S, Kekitiinwa A, Kamya MR. Lipodystrophy among HIV-infected children and adolescents on highly active antiretroviral therapy in Uganda: a cross sectional study. *J Int AIDS Soc.* 2012, 15:17427.
38. Bhutia E, Hamal A, Pal Yadav T, Ramesh KL. Lipodystrophy syndrome among HIV infected children on antiretroviral therapy in northern India. *Afr Health Sci.* 2014; 14:408.
39. Amaya RA, Kozinetz CA, McMeans A, Schwarzwald H, Kline MW. Lipodystrophy syndrome in human immunodeficiency virus–infected children. *Pediatr Infect Dis J.* 2002; 21:405.
40. Miller TL. Nutritional aspects of HIV-infected children receiving highly active antiretroviral therapy. *AIDS.* 2003; 17(Suppl 1):S130.
41. Miller TL. Nutrition in paediatric human immunodeficiency virus infection. *Proc Nutr Soc.* 2002; 59:155.
42. Jaquet D, Levine M, Ortega-Rodriguez E, et al. Clinical and metabolic presentation of the lipodystrophic syndrome in HIV-infected children. *AIDS.* 2002; 14:2123.
43. Blazquez D, Ramos-Amador JT, Sainz T, et al. Lipid and glucose alterations in perinatally-acquired HIV-infected adolescents and young adults. *BMC Infect Dis.* 2015; 15:119.
44. Dapena M, Jimenez B, Noguera-Julian A, et al. Metabolic disorders in vertically-HIV infected children: future adults at risk for cardiovascular disease. *J Pediatr Endocrinol Metab.* 2012; 25:529.
45. Aldrovandi GM, Lindsey JC, Jacobson DL, et al. Morphologic and metabolic abnormalities in vertically-HIV-infected children and youth. *AIDS.* 2009; 23:661.
46. Albisetti M, Braegger CP, Stallmach T, Willi UV, Nadal D. Hepatic stenosis: a frequent non-specific finding in HIV-infected children. *Eur J Pediatr.* 1999; 158:971.
47. Avi Lemberg D, Palasanthiran P, Goode M, Ziegler JB. Tolerabilities of antiretrovirals in paediatric HIV infection. *Drug Saf.* 2002; 25:973.
48. Arpadi SM, Horlick M, Thornton J, Cuff PA, Wang J, Kotler DP. Bone mineral content is lower in prepubertal HIV-infected children. *J Acquir Immune Defic Syndr.* 2002; 29:450.
49. Position of the American Dietetic Association and the Dieticians of Canada. Nutrition intervention in the care of persons with human immunodeficiency virus infection. *J Am Diet Assoc.* 2000; 100:708.
50. Heller L, Rothpletz-Puglia P, Morris V, Papthakis P. HIV/AIDS children/adolescents' medical nutrition therapy protocol. In: Gilbreath J, Inman-Felton AE, Johnson EQ, Robinson G, Smith K, eds. *Medical Nutrition Therapy Across the Continuum of Care.* Chicago: American Dietetic Association and Morrison Health Care; 1998.
51. American Dietetic Association. HIV/AIDS evidence-based nutrition practice guideline. Chicago: American Dietetic Association, December 2010. https://www.guidelinecentral.com/summaries/hivaids-evidence-based-nutrition-practice-guideline/#h2_scope. Accessed June 21, 2016.
52. Shevitz AH, Knox TA. Nutrition in the era of highly active antiretroviral therapy. *Clin Infect Dis.* 2001; 32:1769.
53. Heller L, Fox S, Hell KJ, Church JA. Development of an instrument to assess nutritional risk factors for children with human immunodeficiency virus. *J Am Diet Assoc.* 2000; 100:323.
54. Brown LK, Lourie KJ, Pao M. Children and adolescents living with HIV and AIDS: a review. *J Child Psychol Psychiatry* 2000; 41:81.
55. Story M, Holt K, Sofka D, eds. *Bright Futures in Practice: Nutrition*, 2nd ed. Arlington, VA: National Center for Education in Maternal and Child Health; 2002.
56. Bentler M, Stanish M. Nutrition support of the pediatric patient with AIDS. *J Am Diet Assoc.* 1987; 87:488.
57. Rothpletz-Puglia P. Nutrition management of the child with HIV infection. *Nutr Focus Child Special Health Care Needs.* 1999; 14:1.
58. Henderson RA, Saavedra JM, Perman JA, Hutton N, Livingston RA, Yolken RH. Effect of enteral tube feeding on growth of children with symptomatic human immunodeficiency virus infection. *J Pediatr Gastroenterol Nutr.* 1994; 18:429.
59. Scott G. Clinical manifestations of HIV infection in children. *Pediatr Ann.* 1988; 17:365.
60. Pressman H, Morrison S. Dysphagia in the pediatric AIDS population. *Dysphagia.* 1988; 2:166.
61. Miller TL, Awnetwant EL, Evans S, Morris VM, Vazquez IM, McIntosh K. Gastrostomy tube supplementation for HIV-infected children. *Pediatrics.* 1995; 96:696.
62. Shingadia D, Viani RM, Yogev R, et al. Gastrostomy tube insertion for improvement of adherence to highly active antiretroviral therapy in pediatric patients with human immunodeficiency virus. *Pediatrics.* 2000; 105:E80.
63. Pronsky Z, Elbe D, Ayoob KT, Crowe JP, Epstein S, Roberts WH. *Food Medication Interactions.* Birchrunville, PA: Food Medication Interactions, 2015.
64. Irlam JH, Siegfried N, Visser ME., Rollins, N.C. Micronutrient supplementation for children with HIV infection. *Cochrane Database Syst Rev.* 2013; (10):CD010666.
65. Puthanakit T, Siberry GK. Bone health in children and adolescents with perinatal HIV infection. *J Int AIDS Soc.* 2013; 16:18575.
66. Ayoob K. Nutrition issues in children with HIV/AIDS. *Diet Dev Psychol Disord.* 1996; 14:1.

# 30 Malnutrition in Juvenile Idiopathic Arthritis

INEZ MARTINCEVIC, RAYFEL SCHNEIDER, AND DANIEL LOVELL

## DIAGNOSIS AND PREVALENCE OF JIA

Juvenile idiopathic arthritis (JIA) is the most common form of chronic arthritis in childhood and an important cause of disability in children and adolescents. The term JIA includes a heterogeneous group of diseases that have in common chronic inflammation of the synovial membranes and articular structures. Joint inflammation causes swelling, pain, and stiffness of the affected joints, which can limit the range of movement of individual joints and cause disability. Some children with JIA have systemic manifestations such as fever, rash, fatigue, poor appetite, and weight loss. The diagnosis of JIA is based entirely on the clinical examination and is made when a child younger than 16 years of age is found to have arthritis in one or more joints for at least 6 weeks and all other causes of arthritis have been excluded.[1] The prevalence rates in various countries range from 4 to 400 cases per 100,000 people at risk.[2]

## CLASSIFICATION OF JIA

The International League of Associations for Rheumatology (ILAR) classification criteria, revised in 2001, are universally accepted and include six major subtypes of JIA.[1] The classification is based on the distinctive features of each subtype in the first 6 months of the disease (Table 30–1). The major clinical distinguishing features of the subtypes are the number of affected joints ($\leq$4 in oligoarthritis; $\geq$5 in polyarthritis), the presence or absence of systemic symptoms (e.g., fever, rash), enthesitis (inflammation at the sites of attachment of ligaments, tendons, fascia, or joint capsule to bone), and features of psoriasis. The most common extraarticular manifestation of JIA is uveitis, a form of inflammatory eye disease that is seen most frequently in the oligoarthritis, polyarthritis, and psoriatic subtypes. Overall, JIA affects girls twice as commonly as boys, but the sex ratio differs among the subtypes. Although arthritis occurs in 10% to 15% of children with inflammatory bowel disease, this type of arthritis is not included in the ILAR classification of JIA.[3]

## TREATMENT OF JIA

The optimal treatment of children and adolescents with JIA involves a multidisciplinary team whose efforts are tailored to the individual needs of patients and families to induce remission of the disease and to help patients achieve their full physical growth and psychosocial development. With the availability of modern treatments, achievement of disease remission is a realistic goal for many patients.

Recommendations for the pharmacological treatment of JIA endorsed by the American College of Rheumatology were published in 2011 and 2013.[4,5] Nonsteroidal antiinflammatory drugs (NSAIDs) may be effective in reducing joint pain and stiffness, but most patients with JIA do not respond adequately to NSAIDs alone. Intraarticular corticosteroids have been shown to be safe and effective in children and may be the only pharmacological treatment needed for oligoarthritis. Pediatric rheumatologists try to avoid systemic corticosteroids, but these are sometimes needed, particularly for systemic JIA and for severe refractory arthritis in other subtypes of JIA.

Of the traditional disease-modifying antirheumatic drugs (DMARDs), methotrexate has remained the first choice for polyarticular-course arthritis and for arthritis refractory to NSAIDs or intraarticular corticosteroids, given its proven efficacy, safety, and affordability.[6] Other traditional DMARDs include leflunomide, which has similar efficacy to methotrexate,[7] and sulfasalazine,[8] which may be most effective in enthesitis-related arthritis. Access to biological agents has dramatically improved outcomes for patients with JIA whose disease is unresponsive to traditional DMARDs. Tumor necrosis factor (TNF) inhibitors (i.e., etanercept, adalimumab, and infliximab)[9–11] have the longest track record of efficacy in polyarticular-course JIA, but a host of newer, effective biological agents has now been studied in JIA, including a T-cell costimulatory modulator (abatacept),[12] an interleukin 6 (IL-6) inhibitor, tocilizumab,[13] and the interleukin 1 (IL-1) inhibitors, anakinra[14] and canakinumab.[15] Moreover, biological agents have become the first choice of DMARDs for certain subtypes of JIA, particularly TNF inhibitors for some patients with enthesitis-related arthritis[4] and IL-1 and IL-6 inhibitors for systemic JIA.[5]

Although there is evidence that vitamin D has immunomodulatory and antiinflammatory properties in its hormone form (1,25-dihydroxyvitamin D),[16,17] data correlating 25-hydroxyvitamin D levels with JIA onset or disease activity are limited.[18]

## FACTORS TO BE CONSIDERED IN NUTRITIONAL EVALUATION

The term *malnutrition* embodies a spectrum of manifestations ranging from severe undernutrition to overnutrition, including overweight and obesity. Patients with JIA are at risk for all types of malnutrition (Table 30–2).

The prevalence of poor nutritional status in JIA ranges between 4% and 50%.[19–28] This wide range can be explained by the various definitions of compromised nutritional status. Undernutrition in JIA has been described based on several parameters such as standard anthropometric measures (weight, height, weight-for-height index, and body mass index [BMI]),[19–32] dimensions of body composition (midarm circumference, triceps skinfold thickness, and midarm muscle circumference),[19,23,25,29] and four-site skinfolds (biceps, triceps, subscapular, and suprailiac) to calculate total fat mass and fat free mass,[24] as well as bioelectrical impedence,[26] abnormal levels of visceral proteins (including albumin, prealbumin, and retinol-binding protein),[19–25,27] and subpar nutrient consumption.[20,24,28,30]

However, there are limitations with traditional methods of assessing protein-energy malnutrition in autoimmune diseases like JIA (Table 30–3). The shortcomings of weight, height, and related BMI are that they do not provide information about body composition. Cachexia and sarcopenia have been associated with increased morbidity and mortality rates, poor quality of life, and limited physical functioning of patients with rheumatoid arthritis (RA)[33] and other chronic conditions[34,35] that may parallel JIA. Low levels of albumin, prealbumin, and retinol-binding protein may be related to inadequate protein intake. However, abnormal visceral protein levels also correlate with active inflammation and do not necessarily indicate a deficiency in protein consumption.[36] Ferritin is an intracellular protein that reflects iron stores and can be low in cases of undernutrition. As an acute phase protein, it is elevated during periods of inflammation and therefore may not accurately reflect iron stores in patients with active JIA.[36] Collecting reliable and accurate dietary data for children and adolescents is challenging. Studies report that children are unable

**Table 30–1.** International League of Associations for Rheumatology (ILAR) Classification Subtypes of Juvenile Idiopathic Arthritis (JIA)

| ILAR Subtype | Percentage (%) of all JIA Cases | Age and Sex Predominance | Joints Involved | Other Features |
|---|---|---|---|---|
| Systemic | 10 | Any age<br>F = M | Oligoarticular or polyarticular | Fever<br>Rash<br>Lymphadenopathy<br>Hepatosplenomegaly<br>Serositis (especially pericarditis)<br>Fatigue<br>Anorexia<br>Weight loss |
| Oligoarthritis:<br>Persistent<br>Extended | 40–50 | Early childhood; peak at 1–3 yr<br>F > M | Persistent: ≤4 joints, large joints<br>Extended: ≥5 joints after initial 6 mo of oligoarthritis | Uveitis (asymptomatic)<br>ANA positive in 60–80% |
| Polyarthritis, RF negative | 15–25 | Bimodal; peaks at 1–3 and 9–14 yr<br>F > M | ≥5 joints | Uveitis (asymptomatic)<br>ANA positive in 50% |
| Polyarthritis, RF positive | 5 | Late childhood or adolescence<br>F > M | ≥5 joints<br>Symmetric arthritis of small and large joints, often erosive | Rheumatoid nodules<br>ANA positive in 50% |
| Enthesitis-related arthritis | 5–10 | Late childhood or adolescence<br>F < M | Lower limb joints<br>Sacroiliac joints and inflammatory back pain | Enthesitis<br>HLA-B27 positive in >60%<br>Family history of HLA-B27–related disease<br>Uveitis (symptomatic) |
| Psoriatic arthritis | 5–10 | Early childhood; peak at 9–11 yr<br>F > M | Oligoarticular or polyarticular<br>Dactylitis | Psoriasis<br>Nails pits<br>Onycholysis<br>Family history of psoriasis |
| Undifferentiated | 5–10 | | | Does not fulfill criteria for any subtype, or fulfills criteria for more than one category |

ANA = antinuclear antibodies; F = female; HLA = human leukocyte antigen; M = male; RF = rheumatoid factor.

to estimate portion sizes or frequency of food consumed, and parents are often proxy reporters, which affects intake results. Recall data and food records are also flawed in that underreporting and overreporting of intake are common.[37]

Overweight and obesity are on the opposite side of the malnutrition spectrum. The reported prevalence of overweight and obesity in JIA is between 5% and 30%.[38–40] This range reflects the use of different definitions for these conditions, which are based on percentile cut-offs on growth charts for weight and BMI[29] (see Table 30–3).

There is no validated tool to determine and classify the nutritional status of patients with JIA. Nevertheless, because of the prevalence of nutritional abnormalities reported in this population, it is imperative that patients with JIA be screened and evaluated for malnutrition so as to optimize health, growth, and development.

## UNDERNUTRITION

Compromised nutritional status in JIA has been associated with disease subtype and duration.[26,28,29,31,32,41–43] Moreover, malnutrition in JIA, as in other autoimmune conditions, is related to disease activity and severity.[29] Studies suggest that proinflammatory cytokines may alter nutritional status through their impact on body composition, appetite regulation, joint involvement, energy expenditure, and bone growth and remodeling.[41–49] Elimination diets may also lead to undernutrition. Although some studies suggest that fasting, particularly when followed by a vegetarian diet, may reduce inflammation in RA,[50] there are no data to support elimination diets in children with JIA. Similarly, reports associating arthritis with food allergy in children are rare[51] and do not provide support for widespread recommendation of elimination diets.

**Table 30–2.** Factors That Contribute to Malnutrition in Juvenile Idiopathic Arthritis

| Undernutrition | Overnutrition |
|---|---|
| Disease subtype | Medication (primarily corticosteroids) |
| Disease duration | Functional disability |
| Active disease | Lack of physical activity |
| Poor nutrient intake: anorexia (cytokine mediated) | Excess nutrient intake |
| Joint damage | Accessibility/food insecurity |
| Accessibility/food insecurity | |

### Body Composition

Depleted muscle stores and reduced lean body mass have been reported in JIA.[24,26,29] Based on studies in RA and animal models, it is likely that these indicators of malnutrition are related to active disease. Among patients with RA, lean body mass has been inversely associated with the number of swollen joints, and evidence suggests that proinflammatory cytokines such as tumor necrosis factor alpha (TNF-α) and interleukins facilitate muscle wasting.[44,45] It has been postulated that cytokines activate pathways in skeletal muscle cells that cause increased proteolysis, myocyte apoptosis, and decreased amino acid transport and regeneration within the tissue, triggering muscle breakdown.[46,47] Studies of the pathogenesis of cytokine-mediated muscle wasting are ongoing, and it would be interesting to investigate whether therapies targeting cytokine pathways improve altered body composition and nutritional status in JIA.

### Appetite

Undernutrition is also influenced by suboptimal macronutrient and micronutrient intake, which have been described in JIA.[20,21,30] It is thought that cytokines mediate anorexia in inflammatory conditions, thereby reducing intake. Production of TNF-α and IL-1β was shown to be higher in patients with RA compared with healthy controls, and IL-1β levels have been inversely associated with energy intake.[45] Studies in rats have shown that IL-1 interacts with hypothalamic appetite pathways and may be involved in inducing anorexia.[48,49] Therapies in RA that block TNF-α lessen inflammation and affect gut hormones that are thought to be involved in appetite control.[52] The role of cytokines in arthritis and appetite regulation is unclear. However, studying changes in eating patterns during periods of inflammation and remission may provide more insight into the relationship between poor nutritional status and disease activity in JIA.

**Table 30–3.** Parameters Used to Assess Malnutrition

| Parameter | Risk of Malnutrition: Undernutrition | Risk of Malnutrition: Overnutrition |
|---|---|---|
| *Anthropometric* | | |
| Height | <3rd %tile or >–2 Z score | N/A |
| Weight | <3rd %tile or >–2 Z score | N/A |
| BMI (kg/m$^2$) | <3rd %tile | Overweight >85th %tile; Obese >97th %tile |
| Adjusted weight-for-height index* | <0.80 | N/A |
| Triceps skinfold thickness | <5th %tile | N/A |
| Arm circumference | <5th %tile | N/A |
| Midarm muscle circumference | <5th %tile | N/A |
| *Biochemical* | | |
| Serum albumin | <35 g/L | N/A |
| Serum prealbumin | <10.9 mg/dL | N/A |
| Serum retinol-binding protein | <2.6 mg/dL | N/A |
| Ferritin | <10 μg/L | N/A |
| *Dietary Intake* | | |
| Estimated macronutrient needs for gender and age | Inadequate intake, less than estimated calories/day | Intake that is greater than estimated calories/day |
| Micronutrient intake | May be reduced compared to DRI | May be greater than or compromised† compared to DRI |

Adapted from Promoting Optimal Monitoring of Child Growth in Canada. Using the New WHO Growth Charts; Collaborative Public Policy Statement: Dietitians of Canada; 2010. From Frisancho AR. New norms of upper limb fat and muscle areas for assessment of nutritional status. American Journal of Clinical Nutrition; 34: 25-40; 1981

*Actual weight divided by ideal body weight.

†Micronutrient intake may be inadequate in overweight or obesity. This is most often related to a poor diet that is low in fruits and vegetables and other nutrient-dense foods.

N/A = not applicable; BMI = body mass index; DRI = Dietary Reference Intakes.

### Joint Involvement

Poor eating may also be related to the specific joints involved. Between 18% and 40% of patients with JIA develop arthritis of the temporomandibular joint (TMJ), which contributes to painful mastication and restricts opening of the mouth.[53,54] Both symptoms are associated with decreased caloric intake and changes in the texture of foods consumed.[22] Similarly, inflammation of small joints of the hands may impact hand dexterity, which may affect self-feeding and food preparation. These limitations may hinder optimal nutrient intake in active JIA and should be considered when nutritional status is assessed.

### Energy Expenditure

Malnutrition in JIA may also be affected by metabolic processes. Knops et al.[55] demonstrated that correction for changes in body composition increased the resting energy expenditure of patients with systemic JIA by up to 21%. Hypermetabolism is also seen in patients with oligoarticular or polyarticular JIA, although to a lesser extent. In RA, TNF-α and IL-1β production correlates significantly with increased resting energy expenditure.[45] It is thought that cytokines stimulate the release of catecholamines from the adrenal gland, leading to an increase in resting metabolic rate.[56] In active disease, hypermetabolism may exacerbate malnutrition in JIA. However, no studies have suggested that resting energy expenditure is elevated in JIA in remission. Considering the changes in energy requirements and the lack of disease-specific equations that accurately predict energy expenditure in JIA, indirect calorimetry should be used, if available, to determine energy requirements, especially if the disease is not well controlled, and to reduce the risk of malnutrition.

### Growth

Growth impairment occurs in 10% to 40% of patients with JIA,[20,23,41,42,57] with the most prominent reduction in height velocity in systemic JIA. The variability in prevalence of growth failure can be attributed to use of different definitions of short stature.[58] There are also challenges associated with accurately measuring height in patients with JIA and joint contractures, which should be taken into account. Clinicians can use other tools to assess growth in the setting of active joint disease, such as midarm span, ulna length, or knee height. Limitations of these approaches include instrument accessibility and reliable extrapolated data for children and adolescents.[59,60]

Compromised growth velocity can be influenced by diet, systemic glucocorticoid (GC) therapy, and active disease.[29] Although nutrients are essential for bone health, studies in JIA have not found any statistically significant relationship between inadequate intake and short stature.[24,28] The pathophysiology of GC-induced bone loss and growth retardation is complex. GC may suppress osteoblastogenesis, promote apoptosis of osteoblasts, and even increase bone resorption via osteoclast activity.[61] Although observational studies have demonstrated a correlation between the duration and dose of GC use and impaired growth,[29,60] some studies have not shown a significant association between cumulative doses of corticosteroids and short stature.[29,41,43] Nevertheless, GC dose and duration of use remain important factors in assessing growth of patients with JIA.

Active disease and related circulating cytokines have been implicated in the etiology of short stature in JIA. Bone growth is regulated by the growth hormone (GH)–insulin-like growth factor 1 (IGF-1) axis.[62] IGF-1 is produced by the liver in response to GH stimulation and is the main effector of GH action at the growth plate of bones.[62] Low IGF-1 levels have been reported in 9% to 35% of patients with JIA.[29,60] Reduced IGF-1 levels have been associated with disease activity and elevated erythrocyte sedimentation rate (ESR), and they negatively correlate with increased IL-6 production.[29,62] These findings are consistent with results found in other autoimmune diseases, such as inflammatory bowel disease, and support the notion that disease activity and severity interact with normal growth pathways, leading to short stature in JIA.[29,60,62]

Evidence strongly suggests that early and good control of disease is of the utmost importance in preventing and correcting poor nutritional status in children with JIA. During periods of inflammation, aggressive nutrition interventions may be warranted. Calorie-rich diets and supplements may reduce significant catabolism, meet higher energy demands, and potentially minimize growth failure in patients with active JIA.

## OVERWEIGHT AND OBESITY

Unlike undernutrition, overweight and obesity have not been found to be associated with JIA subtype or disease activity[39,40] but have been associated with GC use, functional disability, and reduced physical activity.[29,38,40] There is also a strong correlation between increased markers of inflammation and obesity in childhood,[37] but it may be difficult to determine whether elevated inflammatory markers in obese children with JIA are the result of obesity or of active inflammation associated with JIA. GCs are thought to cause overweight and obesity by increasing appetite, which increases caloric intake, and alters body composition, including excess adiposity and development of Cushing syndrome.[63] The mechanisms by which GCs cause overweight and obesity in JIA have not been well elucidated. Table 30–4 lists dietary recommendations for patients with JIA who are prescribed GCs; they are also useful for patients who require counseling for weight loss

Although the literature pertaining to overweight and obesity is vast, and much of the information related to management can be applied to JIA, more studies are needed to understand these conditions and the related altered body composition in JIA. Clinicians identifying JIA patients at risk of becoming overweight should encourage appropriate eating behaviors early to prevent continued weight gain, changes to fat and muscle mass, and development of metabolic syndrome.[64] Strategies to foster safe but effective exercise in JIA, despite functional limitations, are vital for conditioning, developing muscle strength, and preventing overweight and obesity. Studies of psychosocial factors that contribute to overweight and obesity in JIA are also warranted.

## EFFECT OF JIA TREATMENTS ON GROWTH AND NUTRITION

Treatments used for JIA can have both detrimental and beneficial effects on growth and nutrition in children with JIA. Corticosteroids have known negative effects on bone mineralization and linear growth. They also commonly result in excessive weight gain, muscle mass loss, and increased fat mass, as described earlier. NSAIDs such as naproxen, meloxicam, and celecoxib commonly cause nausea, abdominal pain, and decreased appetite. Methotrexate commonly causes nausea, abdominal pain, and mouth ulcers around the time of the weekly dosing. However, by controlling the inflammatory process, methotrexate, anti-TNF therapies (e.g., etanercept, infliximab, adalimumab), anti–IL-6 therapy (tocilizumab), and anti–IL-1 therapies (e.g. anakinra, canakinumab) have been shown to increase linear growth in children with JIA.[2]

## SEQUELAE OF JIA

### Osteoporosis

Low bone mineral content has been described in 15% to 55% of children with JIA.[65] The cause is usually multifactorial, including poor dietary intake of calcium, decreased physical activity limiting bone density, decreased muscle mass exerting rotational forces on the bone, and inflammatory cytokines that induce increased bone turnover. In addition, chronic corticosteroid use can negatively influence bone mineralization. The key to minimizing or avoiding poor bone mineralization is effective control of the arthritis without the use of corticosteroids so that physical function is normal or near normal, the inflammatory cascade is normalized, and appetite is improved. If low bone density is observed, treatment with bisphosphonates has been shown to be beneficial.[66]

### Anemia

Little has been published on the incidence or prevalence of anemia in JIA. However, anemia associated with arthritis is well known and is most often diagnosed as iron deficiency anemia, which may be related to inadequate dietary intake of iron, or anemia of chronic disease, which results from disease activity. Because ferritin is an acute phase reactant, levels may be elevated when there is true iron deficiency. Elevated levels of soluble transferrin receptor or the transferrin receptor-ferritin index may be helpful in identifying iron deficiency in this setting.[67] In the setting of methotrexate use, folate deficiency anemia may develop if folic acid supplementation is not prescribed. In the absence of effective treatment, proinflammatory cytokines, including TNF-α, interferon-γ, IL-1, and IL-6, are thought to influence anemia of chronic disease. Anemia of chronic disease is usually mild-to-moderate, normochromic, normocytic (and less often microcytic) and is usually not associated with elevated reticulocytes.[68] Differentiating the causes of anemia in JIA can be challenging but is important because it has implications for treatment.

## COMPLEMENTARY AND ALTERNATIVE MEDICINE

Complementary and alternative medicine (CAM) has been reported to be used in 34% to 92% of patients with JIA.[69–71] CAM has various definitions and in general includes practices and/or products that are not considered part of conventional medicine.[69–71] CAM can include naturopathy, homeopathy, acupuncture, chiropractic, osteopathy, hypnosis, reiki, music therapy, meditation, dietary supplements (including calcium and vitamin D), massage, traditional or folk remedies, and copper bracelets.[69–71] Although CAM may have beneficial and therapeutic effects, concerns exist about potential interactions with medicines, toxicity, and organ damage, as well as lack of evidence pertaining to dosage and use in specific patient groups, and overall underreporting.[71]

Rouster-Stevens et al.[71] found that parents of children with JIA viewed conventional medications as being helpful but also used a

**Table 30–4.** Dietary Recommendations for Patients with Juvenile Idiopathic Arthritis (JIA) Who Are Prescribed Glucocorticosteroids or Who Require Nutrition Counseling for Weight Loss

| Recommendation | Nutrient Guideline | Rationale |
|---|---|---|
| Lower sodium | 1.5–2.0 g/day<br><200 mg sodium per serving | Prevent hypertension and edema |
| Monitor total fat | <30% of total calories | Prevent weight gain and hyperlipidemia |
| Monitor saturated fat* | Approximately10% of total fat | Prevent weight gain and hyperlipidemia |
| Reduce simple starches | Choose complex and fiber-rich carbohydrates for approximately 75% of total carbohydrate intake | Prevent weight gain |
| Protein rich | 1.0–1.5 g/kg of body weight or adjusted body weight | Support growth<br>Prevent significant catabolism, especially at the time of diagnosis or in active disease |
| Monitor caloric intake | Caloric goals are gender- and age-based<br>Caloric intake still sufficient to support linear growth | Prevent weight gain or support weight loss |
| Calcium | Meet age-based requirements<br>Recommended adequate intake (AI) for calcium:<br>1–3 yr: 700 mg/day<br>4–8 yr: 1000 mg/day<br>9–18 yr: 1300 mg/day | Prevent osteoporosis<br>Use supplements as needed |
| Vitamin D | Supplement with at least 600 IU/day as recommended by Dietary Reference Intakes† | Support optimal vitamin D status<br>Future research is needed regarding potential effects in JIA and disease outcomes |

Adapted from Pediatric Nutriton Practice Group. *Pediatric Manual of Clinical Dietetics.* Chicago: American Dietetic Association (1998).
*Review of saturated fats as part of healthy diet under review by Dietary Guidelines Advisory Committee (2015).
†Some experts recommend higher doses of vitamin D supplementation daily.

variety of CAMs, which they perceived as being useful and would recommend to other families of children with JIA. They also found that dietary restrictions used to improve pain or manage JIA were common, identifying an area for future research regarding the impacts of elimination diets on comorbidities and malnutrition in JIA.[71] Although there is no evidence that any form of CAM can mitigate, treat, or cure JIA, it is important to engage parents, guardians, and extended family in discussions about the use of CAM because it can affect management and nutritional status in JIA.

Malnutrition is prevalent in JIA, and its pathogenesis is multifactorial. Robust evidence indicates that disease activity plays a major role in the development of abnormal nutritional status, thus appropriate disease control is important to support a well nourished state. As well patients with JIA should routinely be screened for risks and evidence of malnutrition so that adequate and timely nutrition interventions can be implemented and optimize overall health.

## References


1. Petty RE, Southwood TR, Manners P, et al. International League of Associations for Rheumatology classification of juvenile idiopathic arthritis: second revision, Edmonton 2001. *J Rheumatol.* 2004; 31:390.
2. Thierry S, Fautrel B, Lemelle I, Guillemin F. Prevalence and incidence of juvenile idiopathic arthritis: a systematic review. *Joint Bone Spine.* 2014; 81:112.
3. Passo MH, Fitzgerald JF, Brandt KD. Arthritis associated with inflammatory bowel disease in children: relationship of joint disease to activity and severity of bowel lesion. *Dig Dis Sci.* 1986; 31:492.
4. Beukelman T, Patkar NM, Saag KG, et al. 2011 American College of Rheumatology recommendations for the treatment of juvenile idiopathic arthritis: initiation and safety monitoring of therapeutic agents for the treatment of arthritis and systemic features. *Arthritis Care Res.* 2011; 63:465.
5. Ringold S, Weiss PF, Beukelman T, et al. 2013 Update of the 2011 American College of Rheumatology recommendations for the treatment of juvenile idiopathic arthritis: recommendations for the medical therapy of children with systemic juvenile idiopathic arthritis and tuberculosis screening among children receiving biologic medications. *Arthritis Rheum.* 2013; 65:2499.
6. Giannini EH, Brewer EJ, Kuzmina N, et al. Methotrexate in resistant juvenile rheumatoid arthritis: results of the U.S.A.-U.S.S.R. double-blind, placebo-controlled trial. The Pediatric Rheumatology Collaborative Study Group and The Cooperative Children's Study Group. *N Engl J Med.* 1992; 326:1043.
7. Silverman E, Mouy R, Spiegel L, et al. Leflunomide or methotrexate for juvenile rheumatoid arthritis. *N Engl J Med.* 2005; 352:1655.
8. van Rossum MA, Fiselier TJ, Franssen MJ, et al. Sulfasalazine in the treatment of juvenile chronic arthritis: a randomized, double-blind, placebo-controlled, multicenter study. Dutch Juvenile Chronic Arthritis Study Group. *Arthritis Rheum.* 1998; 41:808.
9. Lovell DJ, Giannini EH, Reiff A, et al. Etanercept in children with polyarticular juvenile rheumatoid arthritis. Pediatric Rheumatology Collaborative Study Group. *N Engl J Med.* 2000; 342:763.
10. Lovell DJ, Ruperto N, Goodman S, et al. Adalimumab with or without methotrexate in juvenile rheumatoid arthritis. *N Engl J Med.* 2008; 359:810.
11. Ruperto N, Lovell DJ, Cuttica R, et al. A randomized, placebo-controlled trial of infliximab plus methotrexate for the treatment of polyarticular-course juvenile rheumatoid arthritis. *Arthritis Rheum.* 2007; 56:3096.
12. Ruperto N, Lovell DJ, Quartier P, et al. Abatacept in children with juvenile idiopathic arthritis: a randomised, double-blind, placebo-controlled withdrawal trial. *Lancet.* 2008; 372:383.
13. De Benedetti F, Brunner HI, Ruperto N, et al. Randomized trial of tocilizumab in systemic juvenile idiopathic arthritis. *N Engl J Med.* 2012; 367:2385.
14. Quartier P, Allantaz F, Cimaz R, et al. A multicentre, randomised, double-blind, placebo-controlled trial with the interleukin-1 receptor antagonist anakinra in patients with systemic-onset juvenile idiopathic arthritis (ANAJIS trial). *Ann. Rheum. Dis.* 2011; 70:747.
15. Ruperto N, Brunner HI, Quartier P, et al. Two randomized trials of canakinumab in systemic juvenile idiopathic arthritis. *N Engl J Med.* 2012; 367:2396.
16. Adorini L, Penna G. Control of autoimmune diseases by the vitamin D endocrine system. *Nature Clin Pract Rheum.* 2008; 4:404.
17. Cutolo M, Otsa K, Uprus M, Paolino S, Seriolo B. Vitamin D in rheumatoid arthritis. *Autoimmunity Rev.* 2007; 7:59.
18. Nisar MK, Masood F, Cookson P, Sansome A, Ostor AJ. What do we know about juvenile idiopathic arthritis and vitamin D?: a systematic literature review and meta-analysis of current evidence. *Clin Rheum.* 2013; 32:729.
19. Henderson CJ, Lovell DJ. Assessment of protein-energy malnutrition in children and adolescents with juvenile rheumatoid arthritis. *Arthritis Care Res.* 1989; 2:108.
20. Miller ML, Chacko JA, Young EA. Dietary deficiencies in children with juvenile rheumatoid arthritis. *Arthritis Care Res.* 1989; 2:22.
21. Bacon MC, White PH, Raiten DJ, et al. Nutritional status and growth in juvenile rheumatoid arthritis. *Semin Arthritis Rheum.* 1990; 20:97.
22. Haugen MA, Hoyeraal HM, Larsen S, Gilboe IM, Trygg K. Nutrient intake and nutritional status in children with juvenile chronic arthritis. *Scand J Rheum.* 1992; 21:165.
23. Henderson CJ, Lovell DJ, Gregg DJ. A nutritional screening test for use in children and adolescents with juvenile rheumatoid arthritis. *J Rheum.* 1992; 19:1276.
24. Strano CG, Polito C, Alessio M, et al. Nutritional status in active juvenile chronic arthritis not treated with steroids. *Acta Paediatr.* 1995; 84:1010.
25. Unsal E, Buyukgebiz B, Cevik N. Assessment of protein-energy malnutrition in children with chronic arthritis. *Turk J Pediatr.* 2001; 43:191.
26. Lofthouse CM, Azad F, Baildam EM, Akobeng AK. Measuring the nutritional status of children with juvenile idiopathic arthritis using the bioelectrical impedance method. *Rheumatology.* 2002; 41:1172.
27. Garcia-Consuegra Molina J, Merino Munoz R, Lama More R, Coya Vina J, Gracia Bouthelier R. Growth in children with juvenile idiopathic arthritis. *An Pediatr (Barc).* 2003; 58:529.
28. Cleary AG, Lancaster GA, Annan F, Sills JA, Davidson JE. Nutritional impairment in juvenile idiopathic arthritis. *Rheumatology.* 2004; 43:1569.
29. Souza L, Machado SH, Bredemeier M, Brenol JC, Xavier RM. Effect of inflammatory activity and glucocorticoid [corrected] use on nutritional variables in patients with juvenile idiopathic arthritis. *J Rheum.* 2006; 33:601.
30. Caetano MC, Ortiz TT, Terreri MT, et al. Inadequate dietary intake of children and adolescents with juvenile idiopathic arthritis and systemic lupus erythematosus. *J. Pediatr.* 2009; 85:509.
31. Shin ST, Yu HH, Wang LC, et al. Nutritional status and clinical characteristics in children with juvenile rheumatoid arthritis. *J Microbiol Immunol Infect.* 2010; 43:93.
32. Mondal R, Sarkar S, Das NK, et al. Growth of children with juvenile idiopathic arthritis. *Indian Pediatr.* 2014; 51:199.
33. Engvall IL, Elkan AC, Tengstrand B, Cederholm T, Brismar K, Hafstrom I. Cachexia in rheumatoid arthritis is associated with inflammatory activity, physical disability, and low bioavailable insulin-like growth factor. *Scand J Rheum.* 2008; 37:321.
34. Kovesdy CP, Kalantar-Zadeh K. Accuracy and limitations of the diagnosis of malnutrition in dialysis patients. *Semin Dialysis.* 2012; 25:423.
35. Montano-Loza AJ. Clinical relevance of sarcopenia in patients with cirrhosis. *World J Gastroenterol.* 2014; 20:8061.
36. Fleck A. Clinical and nutritional aspects of changes in acute-phase proteins during inflammation. *Proc Nutr Soc.* 1989; 48:347.
37. Burrows TL, Martin RJ, Collins CE. A systematic review of the validity of dietary assessment methods in children when compared with the method of doubly labeled water. *J Am Diet Assoc.* 2010; 110:1501.
38. Schenck S, Niewerth M, Sengler C, et al. Prevalence of overweight in children and adolescents with juvenile idiopathic arthritis. *Scand J Rheum.* 2015; 44:288.
39. Pelajo CF, Lopez-Benitez JM, Miller LC. Obesity and disease activity in juvenile idiopathic arthritis. *Pediatr Rheum.* 2012; 10:3.
40. Gronlund MM, Kaartoaho M, Putto-Laurila A, Laitinen K. Juvenile idiopathic arthritis patients with low inflammatory activity have increased adiposity. *Scand J Rheum.* 2014; 43:488.
41. Liem JJ, Rosenberg AM. Growth patterns in juvenile rheumatoid arthritis. *Clin Exp Rheum.* 2003; 21:663.
42. Zak M, Muller J, Karup Pedersen F. Final height, armspan, subischial leg length and body proportions in juvenile chronic arthritis: a long-term follow-up study. *Hormone Res.* 1999; 52:80.
43. Saha MT, Verronen P, Laippala P, Lenko HL. Growth of prepubertal children with juvenile chronic arthritis. *Acta Paediatr.* 1999; 88:724.
44. Roubenoff R, Roubenoff RA, Ward LM, Holland SM, Hellmann DB. Rheumatoid cachexia: depletion of lean body mass in rheumatoid arthritis—possible association with tumor necrosis factor. *J Rheum.* 1992; 19:1505.
45. Roubenoff R, Roubenoff RA, Cannon JG, et al. Rheumatoid cachexia: cytokine-driven hypermetabolism accompanying reduced body cell mass in chronic inflammation. *J Clin Invest.* 1994; 93:2379.
46. Argiles JM, Busquets S, Stemmler B, Lopez-Soriano FJ. Cachexia and sarcopenia: mechanisms and potential targets for intervention. *Curr Opin Pharmacol.* 2015; 22:100.
47. Reid MB, Li YP. Tumor necrosis factor-alpha and muscle wasting: a cellular perspective. *Respir Res.* 2001; 2:269.
48. Hellerstein MK, Meydani SN, Meydani M, Wu K, Dinarello CA. Interleukin-1-induced anorexia in the rat: influence of prostaglandins. *J Clin Invest.* 1989; 84:228.
49. El-Haj T, Poole S, Farthing MJ, Ballinger AB. Anorexia in a rat model of colitis: interaction of interleukin-1 and hypothalamic serotonin. *Brain Res.* 2002; 927:1.
50. Muller H, de Toledo FW, Resch KL. Fasting followed by vegetarian diet in patients with rheumatoid arthritis: a systematic review. *Scand J Rheum.* 2001; 30:1.
51. Schrander JJ, Marcelis C, de Vries MP, van Santen-Hoeufft HM. Does food intolerance play a role in juvenile chronic arthritis? *Br J Rheum.* 1997; 36:905.
52. Chen CY, Tsai CY. From endocrine to rheumatism: do gut hormones play roles in rheumatoid arthritis? *Rheumatology.* 2014; 53:205.
53. Henderson CJ, Lovell DJ. Nutritional aspects of juvenile rheumatoid arthritis. *Rheum Dis Clin North Am.* 1991; 17:403.
54. Cannizzaro E, Schroeder S, Muller LM, Kellenberger CJ, Saurenmann RK. Temporomandibular joint involvement in children with juvenile idiopathic arthritis. *J Rheum.* 2011; 38:510.
55. Knops N, Wulffraat N, Lodder S, Houwen R, de Meer K. Resting energy expenditure and nutritional status in children with juvenile rheumatoid arthritis. *J Rheum.* 1999; 26:2039.
56. Morley JE, Thomas DR, Wilson MM. Cachexia: pathophysiology and clinical relevance. *Am J Clin Nutr.* 2006; 83:735.
57. Simon D, Fernando C, Czernichow P, Prieur AM. Linear growth and final height in patients with systemic juvenile idiopathic arthritis treated with longterm glucocorticoids. *J Rheum.* 2002; 29:1296.
58. Gibson RS. Anthropometric assessment of body size. In: Gibson RS, ed. *Principles of Nutritional Assessment.* New York: Oxford University Press; 2005:250.
59. Gauld LM, Kappers J, Carlin JB, Robertson CF. Height prediction from ulna length. *Dev Med Child Neurol.* 2004; 46:475.
60. Aitman TJ, Palmer RG, Loftus J, et al. Serum IGF-1 levels and growth failure in juvenile chronic arthritis. *Clin Exp Rheum.* 1989; 7:557.
61. Mushtaq T, Ahmed SF. The impact of corticosteroids on growth and bone health. *Arch Dis Child.* 2002; 87:93.

62. Walters TD, Griffiths AM. Mechanisms of growth impairment in pediatric Crohn's disease. *Nat Rev Gastroenterol Hepatol.* 2009; 6:513.
63. Berthon BS, MacDonald-Wicks LK, Wood LG. A systematic review of the effect of oral glucocorticoids on energy intake, appetite, and body weight in humans. *Nutr Res.* 2014; 34:179.
64. Zanette Cde A, Machado SH, Brenol JC, Xavier RM. Metabolic syndrome and juvenile idiopathic arthritis. *Rev Brasil Reumatol.* 2010; 50:190.
65. Soybilgic A, Tesher M, Wagner-Weiner L, Onel KB. A survey of steroid-related osteoporosis diagnosis, prevention and treatment practices of pediatric rheumatologists in North America. *Pediatr Rheum.* 2014; 12:24.
66. Bianchi ML, Cimaz R, Bardare M, et al. Efficacy and safety of alendronate for the treatment of osteoporosis in diffuse connective tissue diseases in children: a prospective multicenter study. *Arthritis Rheum.* 2000; 43:1960.
67. Infusino I, Braga F, Dolci A, Panteghini M. Soluble transferrin receptor (sTfR) and sTfR/log ferritin index for the diagnosis of iron-deficiency anemia: a meta-analysis. *Am J Clin Pathol.* 2012; 138:642.
68. Masson C. Rheumatoid anemia. *Joint Bone Spine.* 2011; 78:131.
69. Hagen LE, Schneider R, Stephens D, Modrusan D, Feldman BM. Use of complementary and alternative medicine by pediatric rheumatology patients. *Arthritis Rheum.* 2003; 49:3.
70. Nousiainen P, Merras-Salmio L, Aalto K, Kolho KL. Complementary and alternative medicine use in adolescents with inflammatory bowel disease and juvenile idiopathic arthritis. *BMC Complement Altern Med.* 2014; 14:124.
71. Rouster-Stevens K, Nageswaran S, Arcury TA, Kemper KJ. How do parents of children with juvenile idiopathic arthritis (JIA) perceive their therapies? *BMC Complement Altern Med.* 2008; 8:25.

# 31 Cancer in Children and Young Adults

ELIZABETH WELIN AND INGRID ORA

Childhood cancer is a leading cause of death in children older than 6 weeks of age, second only to accidental deaths. The overall incidence of cancer is 13 cases per 100,000 white children and 10 cases per 100,000 black children younger than 15 years.[1] In 2014, an estimated 15,780 children between 0 and 19 years of age were diagnosed with cancer, and 1960 of these children eventually died of their disease.[2]

Pediatric cancers are different from those found in adults in terms of type, biology, treatment, and prognosis. The most common pediatric cancers are acute leukemias and brain tumors. Other types of pediatric cancers include Hodgkin's and non-Hodgkin's lymphomas, neuroblastoma (i.e., tumor arising from the sympathetic nervous system), Wilms' tumor (i.e., kidney cancer), rhabdomyosarcoma (i.e., cancer arising from soft muscle tissue), retinoblastoma (i.e., eye tumor), bone tumors (i.e., osteosarcoma and Ewing's sarcoma), hepatoblastoma (i.e., liver cancer), germ cell tumors, and less common tumors.

## TREATMENT AND PROGNOSIS OF CHILDHOOD CANCERS: AN OVERVIEW

The prognosis and outcome for children with cancer have improved dramatically over recent decades. In 1975, about 50% of children diagnosed with cancer before the age of 20 years survived at least 5 years, but between 2010 and 2014, almost 80% survived at least 5 years.[2] In the past 30 years, the death rate for childhood cancer has decreased by 50% (from 50 to approximately 25 deaths per 1 million people), with a 25% decrease in the childhood cancer mortality rate.[3]

The dramatic increases in survival rates for children with cancer reflect the introduction of multimodal treatment with chemotherapy, radiation therapy, and surgery and improvements in supportive care. They are the direct result of hypothesis-driven clinical trials by large cooperative oncology groups. The Children's Oncology Group (COG), the American Society of Pediatric Hematology/Oncology (ASPHO), and the International Society of Paediatric Oncology (SIOP) are three of the largest pediatric cooperative groups in the United States and internationally. Other treatment groups in the United States include the Intergroup Rhabdomyosarcoma Study (IRS) and the National Wilms Tumor Study (NWTS).

In addition to refinements of the treatment protocols, an important factor in improved survival has been more aggressive supportive care management. More than 95% of pediatric patients diagnosed with cancer are treated at major pediatric oncology centers that have all the pediatric subspecialty services necessary to care for patients undergoing aggressive cancer therapy. Nutritional support has been one of the pivotal supportive care areas.

## INCIDENCE AND SIGNIFICANCE OF CACHEXIA

The incidence of cachexia has been reported to be as high as 50% among newly diagnosed pediatric cancer patients.[3] The percentage of children with cachexia at the time of diagnosis ranges from 5.6% to 50%, depending on the type of cancer, the time from onset of symptoms to diagnosis, and the socioeconomic status of the family.[4–7]

Malnutrition has an adverse effect on pediatric and adult patients undergoing cancer therapy. It may manifest as an inability to tolerate aggressive chemotherapy or radiation therapy, frequent delays in therapy due to myelosuppression, increased rates of infections, or decreased overall survival rates. Malnutrition and weight loss are associated with decreased median survival and decreased performance status.[8,9] Specifically, data have shown that patients with acute lymphoblastic leukemia (ALL) are at risk for relapse and decreased overall survival if they are underweight at diagnosis or have a decrease in body mass index (BMI) during the early phases of treatment.[10,11] The goals for nutritional support are to reverse nutritional deficits, prevent further deficits, allow for normal growth and development, minimize morbidity, and maximize quality of life.

For many years, oncologists were hesitant to provide aggressive nutritional support to oncology patients for fear that tumor growth would be enhanced.[12] Before the availability of central venous access, parenteral nutrition was not a practical option. Many studies have now shown that nutritionally replete patients tolerate therapy well and that nutrition intervention leads to an improved quality of life and fewer interruptions in therapy.[13] The nutrition status at the time of diagnosis may predict the child's ability to tolerate aggressive treatment. This underscores the importance of nutrition staging at the time of diagnosis as well as during treatment.[4,12,14,15] The systems most readily affected by protein-energy malnutrition (PEM) are the hematopoietic, gastrointestinal, and immunological systems, which are also the organ systems most affected by traditional chemotherapy and radiation therapy. Ongoing nutritional assessment and evaluation in patients at high nutritional risk provide data for altering nutrition strategies or modifying nutrition regimens.

## BIOCHEMICAL ABNORMALITIES AND NUTRITIONAL SCREENING

Several biochemical abnormalities may be associated with the patient's diagnosis or with the treatment of cancer. These include low levels of serum proteins (albumin, transferrin, prealbumin, and retinol-binding protein) associated with malnutrition; electrolyte and phosphate abnormalities (usually associated with tumor lysis syndrome); and antibiotic therapy or kidney function abnormalities. Liver function values may be elevated due to the primary tumor or the treatment. Serum albumin and prealbumin levels can be indicative of visceral protein status, but several variables can affect their accuracy, including hydration status, liver function, and renal function.[16] Prealbumin is likely a better indicator of nutrition status because its half-life is 2 to 3 days, whereas the half-life of albumin is 21 days.[16]

## DETERMINATION OF NUTRITION STATUS AND RELATED NUTRITIONAL RISK

The determination of nutrition status and of the nutritional risk related to cancer treatment provides the basis for planning and modifying nutritional support. The initial nutrition screening should focus on the identification of children with clear evidence of PEM. Criteria for PEM are a weight loss of at least 5%, or weight-for-height below the 5th percentile when height is equal to or greater than the 10th percentile for age, or a serum albumin concentration lower than 3.2 g/dL.[17,18] Serum albumin is used as a biochemical indicator of protein nutrition, and a concentration lower than 3.2 g/dL (the lowest percentile for healthy children)[19] is an indicator of PEM. However, serum albumin is affected by many variables and may not be the most sensitive marker of nutrition status in pediatric oncology patients.

Recently published criteria outlining how to identify pediatric malnutrition (undernutrition) can also be used to determine the nutrition status of pediatric oncology patients.[20] Using these criteria, the variables to be monitored are weight-for-height Z scores, BMI Z scores, length-for-height Z scores, mid-upper arm circumference, weight gain velocity, weight loss, deceleration in weight-for-length or weight-for-height Z scores, and inadequate nutrient intake. Tables 31–1 and 31–2 describe how these criteria are used to classify patients as mildly, moderately, or severely malnourished.[20] Different criteria are used when only one data point is available to the practitioner and when two or more data points are available.

## NUTRITION SCREENING

Initial screening for PEM includes determination of body weight, a brief dietary history, selected anthropometric measurements, at least one biochemical measure of protein status (usually albumin or prealbumin), and information related to recent changes in weight, appetite, energy, or activity levels and complications associated with treatment (e.g., mucositis, nausea). Past growth records, which can be obtained from the primary care physician, can be quite helpful. Skinfold measurements obtained by trained examiners can provide additional information on depletion of fat reserves.[21,22]

## DETERMINATION OF NUTRITIONAL RISK RELATED TO CANCER TREATMENT

PEM commonly occurs in certain high-risk children with neoplastic diseases.[5] The incidence is greater in children with certain tumor types and in patients with advanced stages of disease (stages III and IV).[6] It varies from 6% in children with newly diagnosed leukemia[6] to as high as 50% in children with newly diagnosed stage IV neuroblastoma.[4] Children being treated with more aggressive or intensive therapies are more likely to develop PEM or to have further worsening of PEM.[17,23–25] Other factors that may contribute to the development or worsening of PEM are surgery, fever, infection, and pain—which may decrease the child's appetite and oral intake despite increased calorie and protein needs. Patients can develop significant PEM several months after the start of therapy compared with their status at diagnosis.[26] Between 25% and 40% of children undergoing abdominal or pelvic irradiation or chemotherapy can be expected to become malnourished.[27]

PEM may be associated with other nutrient inadequacies during cancer treatment. For example, a group of seven young children with advanced Wilms' tumors who averaged an intake of 62 kcal/kg/day—64% of the Recommended Daily Allowance [RDA—during initial intense treatment also had low intakes of calcium, phosphate, iron, vitamin A, thiamine, and niacin.[28] At least five of these children had nutrient intakes of less than 66% of the RDA, and three had intakes of calcium and iron less than 33% of the RDA. Various chemotherapeutic agents can cause renal losses of elements such as calcium, magnesium, and potassium.

## CRITERIA FOR NUTRITION INTERVENTION

Children can be classified based on their diagnosis, stage of disease, and intensity of treatment as having a low or high nutritional risk. Children with a low nutritional risk may be effectively supported with intensive nutrition counseling and oral supplements, whereas high-risk patients should be considered for either enteral or parenteral nutritional supplementation. A small group of children initially assessed as having a low risk of nutritional deficits develop significant weight loss during their treatment. These children should be considered for more aggressive nutritional support. Criteria for nutrition intervention are outlined in 31–1 and 31-2.

## DIETARY AND NUTRITION MANAGEMENT

### Goals for Nutritional Repletion

The goal for nutritional repletion is adequate reversal of PEM and continued nutritional support during the highest nutritional risk periods of cytotoxic chemotherapy and abdominal irradiation. Reasonable nutrition goals include achieving a weight that is 1 kg above the 50th percentile of weight for height.[29] Allow for fluid readjustment after cessation of parenteral nutrition fluids, triceps skinfold measurements greater than the 5th percentile,[30] or subscapular skinfolds greater than the 10th percentile.[31,32] Ensure that the patient has some energy reserves and normalized serum protein concentrations.

A dietary history includes complications associated with cancer treatment, such as nausea, vomiting, mucositis of the gastrointestinal tract, taste alterations, food aversions, diarrhea, constipation, altered periods of eating and sleeping, and impaired mobility (Box 31–1). Children may have little desire to eat during chemotherapy infusions even if nausea is not a problem. If nausea is significant, there are a variety of antiemetic agents that can be used to ameliorate this side effect of therapy. During periods when white blood cell counts are low due to chemotherapy, patients may develop painful mouth sores and/or irritations or mucositis of the esophagus or stomach. They may be unable to eat because of the pain or unable to absorb nutrients during episodes of mucositis. Diarrhea may result from irritation of the intestinal mucosa caused by chemotherapy or radiation therapy. Alternatively, constipation may be a problem because of low dietary fiber intake, lack of activity, use of narcotic analgesics, or administration of some chemotherapeutic agents. Other complications that can result from intensive cancer therapy and reduce the child's ability to take in adequate nutrition include enterocolitis (mostly due to *Clostridium difficile*), jaw pain, and typhlitis. Typhlitis is an infection of the bowel wall in a patient who is profoundly neutropenic. Treatment includes antibiotic therapy and bowel rest (nothing by mouth).

### Methods for Nutritional Support

#### Oral Feeding and Supplements

With less aggressive cancer therapy, oral feeding can be done successfully in many patients. Individual nutrition counseling emphasizes use of the patient's favorite nutrient-dense foods during periods when nutrient intakes are likely to be the best and food aversions are least likely. In addition to an understanding of the treatments, an in-depth nutrition history is helpful to learn the specific eating habits of the child and the family's lifestyle. Nutrition counseling provides information regarding the kinds and amounts of foods that are appropriate for child's age and specific suggestions to improve energy and protein intake. It should also include guidance regarding the time of eating in relation to treatments and information about fluctuations in appetite secondary to treatments. Appetite recovery occurs 3 to 5 days after chemotherapy.[18] Food preferences during

**Table 31–1.** Indicators When Only a Single Data Point Is Available as a Criterion for Identification and Diagnosis of Undernutrition

| Primary Indicators | Mild Malnutrition | Moderate Malnutrition | Severe Malnutrition |
|---|---|---|---|
| Weight-for-height Z score | −1 to −1.9 Z score | −2 to −2.9 Z score | ≥−3 Z score |
| BMI for age Z score | −1 to −1.9 Z score | −2 to −2.9 Z score | ≥−3 Z score |
| Length/height Z score | No data | No data | −3 Z score |
| Mid-upper arm circumference | ≥−1 to −1.9 Z score | ≥−2 to −2.9 Z score | ≥−3 Z score |

From Becker PJ, Nieman-Carney L, Corkins MR, et al. Consensus statement of the Academy of Nutrition and Dietetics/American Society for Parenteral and Enteral Nutrition: indicators recommended for the identification and documentation of pediatric malnutrition (undernutrition). *J Acad Nutr Diet.* 2014; 114:1988.

**Table 31–2.** Primary Indicators When Two or More Data Points are Available for Use as Criteria for Identification and Diagnosis of Malnutrition Related to Undernutrition

| Primary Indicators | Mild Malnutrition | Moderate Malnutrition | Severe Malnutrition |
|---|---|---|---|
| Weight gain velocity (age <2 yr) | <75% of the norm for expected weight gain | <50% of the norm for expected weight gain | <25% of the norm for expected weight gain |
| Weight loss (age 2–20 yr) | 5% of usual body weight | 7.5% of usual body weight | 10% of usual body weight |
| Deceleration in weight-for-length/height Z score | Decline of 1 Z score | Decline of 2 Z scores | Decline of 3 Z scores |
| Inadequate nutrient intake | 51–75% of estimated energy/protein need | 25–50% estimated energy/protein need | ≤25% of estimated energy/protein need |

From Becker PJ, Nieman-Carney L, Corkins MR, et al. Consensus statement of the Academy of Nutrition and Dietetics/American Society for Parenteral and Enteral Nutrition: indicators recommended for the identification and documentation of pediatric malnutrition (undernutrition). *J Acad Nutr Diet.* 2014; 114:1988.

treatments often change because of changes in taste associated with treatment.[33] Children tend to like salty or spicy foods and strongly flavored foods while they are undergoing therapy.

## Enteral Feeding

For patients whose therapy prevents them from taking in adequate calories and protein due to decreased appetite and/or nausea and vomiting but whose gastrointestinal tract is functional, enteral feeding via a nasogastric (NG) tube, nasojejunal (NJ) tube, gastrostomy tube (GT), or gastrojejunal (GJ) tube is an option. More and more data are supporting the great value of NG feeding.[34] Often, one of the family's and patient's major concerns about NG or NJ feeds is the discomfort related to passing the tube and the gagging and feeling of irritation at the back of the throat. Some very sensitive children have associated vomiting. There is also a small risk of bleeding if the treatment-related platelet count is low or the patient has a coagulopathy. An increased risk of sinus infections has been observed in those patients whose treatments cause prolonged periods of neutropenia.

GT feedings have been used successfully and safely in children with cancer.[35] Complications included insertion site reactions, inflammation, and infection, especially during times of neutropenia[35]; exuberant granulation tissue; mechanical problems such as leaking, obstruction, breakage, and accidental dislodgment; insertion site bleeding; and feeding intolerance. GT feedings are associated with minor complications but permit effective and cost-effective nutritional support for pediatric cancer patients.[28] Postpyloric feedings using NJ or GJ tubes can be beneficial to patients who have obstructions of the stomach or other parts of the gastrointestinal tract due to tumor burden, which may result in poorly tolerated oral or gastric feeding via GT or NG tubes. It can also be beneficial in patients with significant nausea to bypass the stomach and provide feeds via NJ or GJ tubes; this maintains use of the gastrointestinal tract to provide nutrition but avoids large volumes of feeds to be vomited from the stomach.

**Box 31–1.** Types of Pediatric Cancer Associated with High and Low Nutritional Risks

***High Nutritional Risk***

Acute myeloid leukemia
Stage III and IV neuroblastoma
Some non-Hodgkin's lymphomas
Stage III and IV rhabdomyosarcoma
Stage III and IV Wilms' tumor
Some brain tumors
Relapsed cancers of various types
Other widespread tumors of various types

***Low Nutritional Risk***

Stage I and II neuroblastoma
Stage I and II Wilms' tumor
Acute lymphoblastic leukemia in maintenance therapy
Other localized, nonmetastatic tumors

Enteral feeds can be provided in the home setting, and this is often required because patients' nutritional needs tend to be very high for the duration of therapy. Providing enteral feeds at home can often decrease the number of days spent in the hospital and improve quality of life. Enteral feeding tubes can also be used for medication administration.

## Parenteral Nutrition

Parenteral nutrition via a central venous catheter can be used as an adjunct to enteral feeds. It should be used intermittently, when the patient is experiencing too much nausea to tolerate enteral feeds or when enteral feeds are not an option, such as during episodes of enterocolitis, severe mucositis, or typhlitis. Patients' full nutritional and fluid needs can be provided with the use of total parenteral nutrition and intralipids.

Parenteral nutritional support using peripheral veins is of limited value because peripheral veins cannot tolerate hyperosmolar solutions. Numerous studies have demonstrated the limitations of peripheral nutritional support compared with central nutritional support. Most pediatric patients receiving chemotherapy have a central venous catheter placed for chemotherapy administration and for supportive care. Home hyperalimentation is feasible for patients who need ongoing nutritional support. Side effects of central nutritional support include complications related to the central venous catheter, such as infections and thrombosis, and abnormalities in liver function studies.

## Overweight and Obesity

The prevalence of overweight and obesity among certain populations of pediatric oncology patients has increased in recent years. Especially among patients with ALL, overweight and obesity after successful completion of therapy continues to be a growing problem. A recent study in patients with ALL found that Hispanic patients had a high propensity for being overweight or obese after completion of therapy.[36] Such data can help identify patients with a high likelihood for becoming overweight or obese and allow practitioners time for early dietary interventions. Providing education on maintaining a diet that is high in protein and low in simple sugars and encouraging appropriate physical activity can help to prevent obesity.

## Adolescents and Young Adults

It has been found that cancer develops more often in young people aged 15 to 25 years than in those younger than 15 years of age.[37] The cancers most commonly diagnosed in children aged 15 to 19 years are Hodgkin's disease, germ cell tumors, central nervous system tumors, non-Hodgkin's lymphoma, thyroid cancer, malignant melanoma, and ALL.[37] Psychological and social factors can contribute to delayed diagnosis in adolescents and young adults because they often are too embarrassed to bring their problem to anyone's attention.[37] These patients also can have nutritional deficiencies that are difficult to address and manage given their frequent refusal of enteral and parenteral nutritional support due to social stigma, psychological stress, or other factors. The nutritional needs and goals of these patients are not different from those of their younger counterparts, and their outcomes can likewise be affected by poor nutrition status during therapy, so aggressive nutrition interventions should be implemented.

## SUMMARY

The benefits of nutritional support in a child with cancer are an improved ability to withstand the sometimes aggressive treatment regimens, better maintenance of normal or near-normal growth, improved organ function, better ability to resist or fight infections, and improved overall quality of life while going through treatment.

### References


1. Pizzo PA, Poplack DG. *Principles and Practice of Pediatric Oncology*, 4th ed. Philadelphia: Lippincott, Williams & Wilkins; 2002.
2. National Cancer Institute. *Cancer in Children and Adolescents*. www.cancer.gov/types/childhood-cancers/child-adolescent-cancers-fact-sheet. Accessed June 21, 2016.
3. Van Eys J. Nutrition and cancer: physiological interrelationships. *Annu Rev Nutr*. 1985; 4:435.
4. Rickard K, Detamore CM, Coates TD, et al. Effect of nutrition staging on treatment delays and outcome in stage IV neuroblastoma. *Cancer*. 1983; 52:587.
5. Smith D, Stevens MI, Booth I. Malnutrition at diagnosis of malignancy in childhood: common but mostly missed. *Eur J Pediatr*. 1991; 150:318.
6. Richard K, Baehner RL, Coates TD, Weetman RM, Provisor AJ, Grosfeld JL. Supportive nutritional intervention. *Cancer Res*. 1982; 42(Suppl):766.
7. Ramirez I, Van Eys J, Carr D, Arter P, Coody D, Taylor G. Malnutrition in children with malignancies. *Proc Am Assoc Cancer Res*. 1980; 21:378.
8. Dewys WD, Begg C, Lavin P, et al. Prognostic effect of weight loss prior to chemotherapy in cancer patients. *Am J Med*. 1980; 69:491.
9. Donaldson S, Wesley MN, DeWys WD, Suskind RM, Jaffe N, Van Eys J. A study of the nutritional status of pediatric cancer patients. *Am J Dis Child*. 1981; 135:1107.
10. den Hoed MAH, Pluijm SMF, de Groot-Kruseman HA, et al. The negative impact of being underweight and weight loss on survival of children with acute lymphoblastic leukemia. *Haematologica*. 2015; 100:62.
11. Yazbeck N, Samia L, Saab R, Abboud MR, Solh H, Muwakkit S. Effect of malnutrition at diagnosis on clinical outcomes of children with acute lymphoblastic leukemia. *J Pediatr Hematol Oncol*. 2016; 38:107.
12. Andrassy R, Chwals W. Nutritional support of the pediatric oncology patient. *Nutrition*. 1998; 14:124.
13. Van Eys J. Benefits of nutritional intervention on nutritional status, quality of life and survival. *Int J Cancer Suppl*. 1998; 11:66.
14. Murry D, Riva L, Poplack D. Impact of nutrition on pharmacokinetics of antineoplastic agents. *Int J Cancer Suppl*. 1998; 11:48.
15. Ladas EJ, Sacks N, Brophy P, Rogers PC. Standards of nutritional care in pediatric oncology: results from a nationwide survey on the standards of practice in pediatric oncology. A Children's Oncology Group study. *Pediatr Blood Cancer*. 2006; 46:339.
16. Ladas EJ, Sacks N, Meacham L, et al. A multidisciplinary review of nutrition considerations in the pediatric oncology population: a perspective from Children's Oncology Group. *Nutr Clin Pract*. 2005; 20:377.
17. Rickard K, Lohgmani ES, Grosfeld JL, et al. Short- and long-term effectiveness of enteral and parenteral nutrition in reversing or preventing protein energy malnutrition in advanced neuroblastoma: a prospective randomized study. *Cancer*. 1985; 56:2881.
18. Rickard K, Grosfeld JL, Coates TD, Weetman RM, Baehneret RL. Advances in nutrition care of children with neoplastic diseases: a review of treatment, research and application. *J Am Diet Assoc*. 1986; 86:1666.
19. Trevorrow V. Serum proteins. In: McCammon RW, ed. *Human Growth and Development*. Springfield, IL: Charles C. Thomas; 1970.
20. Becker PJ, Nieman-Carney L, Corkins MR, et al. Consensus statement of the Academy of Nutrition and Dietetics/American Society for Parenteral and Enteral Nutrition: indicators recommended for the identification and documentation of pediatric malnutrition (undernutrition). *J Acad Nutr Diet*. 2014; 114:1988.
21. Heymsfield S, McManus C, Smith J, Stevens V, Nixon D. Anthropometric measurement of muscle mass: revised equations for calculation of bone free arm muscle area. *Am J Clin Nutr*. 1982; 36:680.
22. Elhasid R, Laor A, Lischinsky S, Postovsky S, Arush M. Nutritional status of children with solid tumors. *Cancer*. 1999; 86:119.
23. Rickard K, Grosfeld JL, Kirksey A, Ballantine TVN, Baehner RL. Reversal of protein-energy malnutrition in children with advanced neoplastic disease. *Ann Surg*. 1979; 190:771.
24. Richard K, Kirksey A, Baehnewet RL, et al. Effectiveness of enteral and parenteral nutrition in the nutritional management of children with Wilms' tumors. *Am J Clin Nutr*. 1980; 33:2622.
25. Rickard K, Godshall BJ, Loghmani ES, et al. Integration of nutrition support into oncologic treatment protocols for high and low nutritional risk children with Wilms' tumor: a prospective randomized study. *Cancer*. 1989; 64:491.
26. Yaris N, Wesley MN, Ghavimiet F. Nutritional status of children with cancer and its effects on survival. *Turk J Pediatr*. 2002; 44:35.
27. Donaldson S, Wesley M, Ghavimi F, Shils M, Suskind R, DeWys W. A prospective review, clinicopathologic correlation and dietary management. *Med Pediatr Oncol*. 1982; 10:129.
28. Mathew P, Bowman L, Williams R, et al. Complications and effectiveness of gastrostomy feedings in pediatric cancer patients. *J Pediatr Hematol Oncol*. 1996; 18:81.
29. Hamill P, Drizd TA, Johnson CL, Reed R, Roche A, Moore W. Physical growth: National Center for Health Statistics percentiles. *Am J Clin Nutr*. 1979; 32:607.
30. Frisancho A. New norms of upper limb fat and muscle area for assessment for nutrition status. *Am J Clin Nutr*. 1981; 34:2540.
31. Owen GM. Measurement, recording and assessment of skinfold thickness in childhood and adolescence: report of a small meeting. *Am J Clin Nutr*. 1982; 35:629.
32. Karlberg P, Karlverb P, Taranger J, Engstrom I, Lichtenstein H, Svennberg-Redemunity I. The somatic development of children in a Swedish urban community. *Acta Paediatr Scand*. 1976; 258:1.
33. DeWys W. Changes in taste sensation and feeding behaviour in cancer patients: a review. *J Hum Nutr*. 1978; 32:447.
34. Nitenberg G. Nutritional support of the cancer patient: issues and dilemmas. *Crit Rev Oncol Hematol*. 2000; 34:137.
35. Aquino V, Smyrl CB, Hagg R, McHard KM, Prestridge L, Sandler ES. Enteral nutritional support by gastrostomy tube in children with cancer. *J Pediatr*. 1995; 127:58.
36. Brown AL, Lupo PJ, Danysh HE, Okcu MF, Scheurer ME, Kamdar KY. Prevalence and predictors of overweight and obesity among a multiethnic population of pediatric acute lymphoblastic leukemia survivors: a cross-sectional assessment. *J Pediatr Hematol Oncol*. 2016; 3:S27
37. Bleyer WA. Cancer in older adolescents and young adults: epidemiology, diagnosis, treatment, survival, and importance of clinical trials. *Med Pediatr Oncol*. 2002; 38:1.

# 32 Congenital Heart Disease and Lipid Disorders

ALAN B. LEWIS, STEPHANIE SANBORN, AND VIOLET HSIEH

## CONGENITAL HEART DISEASE

Congenital heart disease (CHD) has an incidence of 8 to 10 cases per 1000 live births and represents 12% of all congenital malformations.[1–3] Approximately 40,000 infants are born annually in the United States with congenital heart abnormalities. Just over one-fourth of these defects are severe enough to result in cardiac catheterization, surgery, or death within the first year of life.[4] With the improvements in surgical techniques and survival over the past several decades, it is estimated that 2 to 3 million American children and adults with CHD are alive today. Between 1989 and 1999, deaths rates from CHD declined by 31.5%.[2]

Congenital heart anomalies may be divided into two broad categories: acyanotic and cyanotic. Within the former group, defects may be further classified into left-to-right shunt lesions, such as atrial septal defects (ASD) and ventricular septal defects (VSD), or obstructive lesions, such as aortic or pulmonary valve stenosis or coarctation of the aorta. Cyanotic heart malformations include complete transposition of the great arteries (TGA) and tetralogy of Fallot. Table 32–1 lists the more common malformations in each of these categories.

### Acyanotic Congenital Heart Defects

Left-to-right shunt lesions are characterized by abnormal connections between the left and right sides of the heart and/or great arteries, such as ASD, VSD, or patent ductus arteriosus (PDA). They may occur as isolated abnormalities or in combination. Atrioventricular septal defects (AVSD) include ASD and VSD components in association with abnormal mitral and tricuspid valves, often a common atrioventricular valve. The magnitude of left-to-right shunting is determined by the relationship between systemic and pulmonary vascular resistance: A low pulmonary vascular resistance compared with the normally higher systemic resistance promotes left-to-right shunting. Pulmonary vascular resistance in the fetus is normally higher than the systemic resistance. After birth, affected infants often manifest few symptoms during the first 1 to 2 months because pulmonary vascular resistance remains somewhat elevated. However, with the gradual decline in pulmonary resistance, the magnitude of the left-to-right shunt progressively increases, and babies begin to show signs and symptoms of congestive heart failure due to volume overload. Obstructive lesions, most commonly involving the outflow of the heart, include pulmonic stenosis, aortic stenosis, and coarctation of the aorta. Severe obstruction may manifest with signs of cardiac failure early in the neonatal period, whereas mild to moderate obstruction may remain asymptomatic.

### Cyanotic Congenital Heart Defects

Cardiac malformations that produce cyanosis are often characterized by either diminished pulmonary blood flow or TGA. The former usually consists of some combination of obstruction to pulmonary outflow, such as pulmonary stenosis or atresia, with VSD (tetralogy of Fallot) or ASD. Consequently, poorly oxygenated venous blood is shunted from the right to the left side of the heart, bypassing the lungs. In contrast, pulmonary blood flow in TGA is usually normal to increased. The aorta arises from the right ventricle instead of the left, and the pulmonary artery arises from the left ventricle rather than the right. Poorly oxygenated blood returning to the heart from the systemic veins is directed to the aorta, whereas highly oxygenated pulmonary venous blood is pumped back to the lungs. TGA is incompatible with postnatal survival without admixture of blood across an intracardiac communication such as an ASD.

### Medical and Surgical Management

Infants with critical obstruction to right or left ventricular outflow or with TGA have profound cyanosis or poor systemic perfusion in the immediate neonatal period due to postnatal closure of the ductus arteriosus. Administration of prostaglandin $E_1$ reopens the ductus and allows immediate stabilization of a life-threatening condition. During the past 25 years, the arterial switch operation for surgical correction of TGA in the neonate has become routine. Critical aortic or pulmonic valve stenosis may be relieved by balloon valvuloplasty in the cardiac catheterization laboratory or by surgical valvotomy. Infants with severe tetralogy of Fallot may undergo an initial palliative procedure, such as a modified Blalock-Taussig shunt to augment pulmonary blood flow, or may proceed directly to definitive intracardiac repair. The Norwood procedure for hypoplastic left heart syndrome is the primary palliative approach to this uniformly lethal, complex malformation, but it continues to be associated with significant early and late morbidity and mortality.[5]

Congestive heart failure due to volume overload develops in babies with VSD as pulmonary vascular resistance declines after birth. Medical management includes use of diuretics such as furosemide or chlorothiazide and an angiotensin-converting enzyme inhibitor such as captopril or enalapril. Because hypokalemia may result from diuretic-induced potassium losses, the addition of a potassium-sparing diuretic such as spironolactone may be helpful in maintaining electrolyte balance. Timing of the surgical intervention is based on control of heart failure symptoms, the presence of pulmonary hypertension, adequacy of systemic perfusion, and the ability to maintain normal growth. Most infants with large left-to-right shunts undergo surgical repair at 3 to 12 months of age.

### Factors To Be Considered in Nutrition Evaluation

Multiple factors contribute to the nutrition status of infants and children with CHD. Prenatal conditions such as intrauterine growth retardation, chromosomal abnormalities such as trisomy 18 or 21, and other noncardiac malformations such as cleft palate can have a major impact on nutrition, growth, and development. Cardiac factors mainly involve the hemodynamic burden of large left-to-right shunts and congestive heart failure.

The degree of hypoxemia in patients with cyanotic CHD does not correlate well with growth delay[6,7] except to the extent that there may be decreased nutritional intake due to hypoxemia-induced fatigue with feeding. Congestive heart failure may restrict growth by reducing nutritional intake as a result of tachypnea, dyspnea, and increased fatigability.[8] Reduced systemic perfusion, particularly to the splanchnic circulation and bowel, may limit gastric emptying, intestinal mobility, and nutrient uptake. Respiratory distress may also promote gastroesophageal reflux.

Balanced against the decrease in nutritional intake is the increased caloric expenditure associated with increased cardiac and respiratory work.[9,10] A portion of this increase in basal metabolic rate has been attributed to the greater proportion of metabolically active lean body mass.[11]

**Table 32–1.** Common Congenital Heart Anomalies*

| Acyanotic Defects | | Cyanotic Defects |
|---|---|---|
| Left-to-Right Shunts | Obstructive Lesions | |
| Atrial septal defect (ASD) (10%) | Valvar pulmonic stenosis (8%) | Transposition of the great arteries (TGA) (4%) |
| Ventricular septal defects (VSD) (40%) | Valvar aortic stenosis (4%) | Tetralogy of Fallot (5%) |
| Patent ductus arteriosus (PDA) (7%) | Coarctation of the aorta (5%) | Hypoplastic left heart (3%) |
| Atrioventricular septal defects (AVSD) (4%) | | Pulmonary atresia (1%) |
| | | Tricuspid atresia (1%) |

*Numbers in parentheses represent the percentage of all congenital heart anomalies and exclude bicuspid nonstenotic aortic valves.

### Nutritional Assessment

Nutritional assessment of patients with CHD includes both anthropometric analysis and clinical evaluation. Weight-for-age and rate of growth are often lower in CHD patients than in age-matched controls.[12] Height and weight may be plotted on the World Health Organization (WHO) growth charts. However, growth in patients with chromosomal anomalies, such as Down or Turner syndrome, may be affected independently. Weight gain is impacted earlier than linear growth, particularly in infants with congestive heart failure.[13–15] Weight gain goals should be determined by careful assessment of overall nutrition status, age, diagnosis, and daily intake. An average weight gain of more than 50 g/day in infants is most likely caused by fluid retention. Z score, midarm circumference, and triceps skinfold measurements can also be used as parameters for growth evaluation.

### Clinical Assessment

Clinical assessment should include a home feeding history, tolerance of enteral nutrition, oral feeding ability, and fluid and respiratory status. Medications should be evaluated for potential drug-nutrient interactions. Total fluid allowance is often restricted, particularly in infants with recent surgery. Sodium intake should be monitored carefully to prevent fluid retention. Low serum sodium and potassium levels may result from aggressive diuretic therapy, although hyponatremia may also occur secondary to fluid retention due to congestive heart failure. Serum albumin and prealbumin values in the presence of a normal C-reactive protein level[16] are useful in assessing protein status. Blood urea nitrogen also may be used as an indicator of protein intake if renal function is normal.

### Dietary and Nutrition Management

To promote optimal growth in weight and stature, restore homeostasis, and replenish tissue deficits, nutrition intervention is important to achieve an optimal medical, physical, and psychological outcome.[17] Higher calorie and moderate protein supplementation is needed in children with CHD, compared with healthy age-matched children, for postoperative wound healing and long-term catch-up growth. Parenteral nutrition should be used in acute settings when patients are not able to receive sufficient enteral nutrition. If medically indicated, a transition to nasogastric or nasojejunal tube feeding is helpful in shortening the duration of parenteral support because prolonged use of parenteral nutrition may lead to complications such as line infection, cholestasis, and hyperglycemia.

Fluid status is one of the major factors affecting the medical and nutritional condition of CHD patients. Insensible fluid loss can be as high as 10% to 15% above normal due to tachypnea or fever.[18,19] Conversely, fluids may need to be restricted (to as little as 60 to 80 mL/kg) and diuretics administered in patients with congestive heart failure to prevent fluid overload. Strict fluid limits make adequate nutritional support extremely challenging, particularly in view of the increased energy requirements. The caloric intake needed to achieve adequate growth in CHD patients may be as high as 120 to 170 kcal/kg/day.[15,20–22]

Breast milk and standard infant formulas have a caloric density of 20 kcal/oz. However, because of oral intake limitations, fluid restrictions, and higher caloric requirements, standard concentrations often cannot meet nutritional goals. A formula with higher caloric density (24, 27, or 30 kcal/oz) is usually required. However, these formulas also result in increased renal solute load and may increase the risk of dehydration, particularly in patients receiving diuretics. In hospitalized patients, total fluid intake, output, and urine specific gravity should be monitored closely to ensure proper fluid balance and normal renal function. High-solute formulas may worsen gastrointestinal function and promote diarrhea. Carbohydrate supplementation with Solcarb (Solace Nutrition, Pawcatuck, CT) and fat supplementation with Liquigen or MCT Oil (Nestle Healthcare Nutrition, Florham Park, NJ) are recommended as fortifiers when a formula with more than 27 kcal/oz or breast milk is fed.

Breast-feeding should be encouraged whenever it is medically feasible. Breast-feeding provides highly absorbable nutrients and abundant amounts of immunoglobulins and establishes vital bonding between mother and child. However, strict breast-feeding may not suffice for many infants with serious CHD. Supplemental higher-calorie formulas or fortified breast milk may be used in combination with breast-feeding to achieve desired growth. Infants with complex left-sided obstructive lesions, particularly hypoplastic left heart syndrome, may have decreased gastrointestinal perfusion both preoperatively and postoperatively and are at increased risk for development of necrotizing enterocolitis.[23] At our institution, breast milk, the semielemental formula Alimentum (Abbott Nutrition, Columbus, OH), and the elemental formula Neocate (Nutricia, Gaithersburg, MD) are used in these infants to minimize the risk of necrotizing enterocolitis. For older infants and toddlers, age-appropriate solids may be introduced along with higher-caloric-density formulas or breast milk to achieve nutritional goals.

Oral feeding skills and cognitive development may be delayed in many infants due to prolonged hospitalization and cardiorespiratory compromise. Multidisciplinary teamwork, involving the physical therapist, occupational therapist, and dietitian, is important to achieve catch-up growth and development.

In summary, nutritional management in CHD patients is challenging because of fluid restriction, higher calorie requirements, and a high prevalence of feeding intolerance. Thorough assessment, close follow-up, and creative feeding methods are essential to achieve optimal medical, nutritional, and psychosocial outcomes.

## LIPID DISORDERS IN CHILDREN

Coronary heart disease remains a major public health issue and the leading cause of mortality in the United States. More than 100 million American adults have total cholesterol (TC) levels higher than 200 mg/dL, and more than 30 million have levels in excess of 240 mg/dL.[2] Coronary artery disease (CAD) is present in 12 million adults, 1.1 million of whom have an acute event (i.e., angina, myocardial infarction, or death) each year. Approximately 1 of every 6 deaths in the United States is attributable to CAD. It is estimated that the total cost of coronary heart disease to US society is in the range of $150 billion per year, with more than $50 billion in direct medical costs alone.[2]

Numerous epidemiological studies have established overwhelming evidence linking elevated serum cholesterol levels to the development of CAD. The Framingham Heart Study, begun more than 50 years ago, showed that low serum cholesterol levels were associated with low rates of CAD and that high levels were associated with high CAD rates.[24] Other noteworthy studies have included the Multiple Risk Factor Intervention Trial (MRFIT),[25] the Coronary Primary Prevention Trial,[26] and the Helsinki Heart Study.[27] These studies showed that a 1% reduction in serum TC produces a 2% to 3% decrease in the risk of CAD.[11]

**Table 32–2.** Serum Cholesterol Levels by Gender in U.S. Children and Adolescents 4–19 Years of Age NHANES III, 1988–1994

| Lipid/Lipoprotein (mg/dL) | Percentiles | | | | | | | |
|---|---|---|---|---|---|---|---|---|
| | 50 | | 75 | | 90 | | 95 | |
| | M | F | M | F | M | F | M | F |
| Total cholesterol | 161 | 163 | 179 | 184 | 198 | 202 | 212 | 220 |
| Low-density Lipoprotein | 88 | 92 | 103 | 115 | 126 | 139 | 149 | 161 |
| High-density Lipoprotein | 48 | 50 | 57 | 58 | 65 | 65 | 71 | 70 |
| Triglyceride | 74 | 77 | 107 | 115 | 150 | 171 | 196 | 208 |

Hickman TB, Briefel RR, Carroll MD, et al. Distributions and trends of serum lipid levels among United States children and adolescents ages 4–19 years: Data from the Third National Health and Nutrition Examination Survey. Prev Medicine. 1998; 27:879–1998.

Epidemiological studies have also established the links between diet, serum cholesterol levels, and subsequent CAD risk. The Seven Countries Study[28] and the Japan-Honolulu-San Francisco Study[29] demonstrated that diets high in saturated fatty acids increased the risk of CAD and that, over time, consumption of saturated fats correlated with total mortality rates. According to these and many other studies, three diet-related factors contribute to an individual's risk of CAD: high intake of saturated fatty acids, high cholesterol levels, and obesity.[30]

Important as these data are in establishing the relationships between diet, serum cholesterol, and CAD in adults, we should recognize that the precursors for CAD are established during childhood. Pathological studies from the Korean and Vietnam wars documented the presence of atherosclerosis in young soldiers. Perhaps even more alarming was the report by Stary that 50% of children 10 to 14 years of age had fatty streaks in the left coronary artery and that more advanced lesions similar to atherosclerotic plaques were present in 8%.[31] Another study using intravascular ultrasound reported that 17% of subjects younger than 20 years of age had evidence of coronary atherosclerosis.[32] Increased public awareness of the importance of diet in influencing serum cholesterol levels, and ultimately CAD, has resulted in a fall in mean serum TC levels over the past 4 decades. Mean serum TC levels in youths aged 12 to 17 years have declined by an average of 9 to 10 mg/dL among white males and females and by 12 to 14 mg/dL among black males and females, respectively.[2] Table 32–2 summarizes the percentile distribution of lipid levels by gender in children and adolescents.[33]

## Factors To Be Considered in Nutrition and Biochemical Evaluation

Free cholesterol is a simple lipid that is used for many essential cellular functions, including cell membrane synthesis, steroid production, and bile acid formation. Although the body can produce all of the cholesterol it requires, approximately 20% to 40% of cholesterol is obtained exogenously from the diet. The liver is the primary processor of exogenous dietary cholesterol and the primary producer of endogenous cholesterol. The latter is derived from acetate by the enzymatic conversion of 3-hydroxy-3-methylglutaryl coenzyme A (HMG-CoA) to mevalonic acid by HMG-CoA reductase and finally to cholesterol.

The principal lipoproteins are chylomicrons, very-low-density lipoprotein (VLDL), intermediate-density lipoprotein (IDL), low-density lipoprotein (LDL), and high-density lipoprotein (HDL). LDL (i.e., "bad" cholesterol), IDL, and VLDL are highly atherogenic, whereas HDL (i.e., "good" cholesterol) is protective through a mechanism of reverse cholesterol transport back to the liver. In 1991, the National Cholesterol Education Program (NCEP) Expert Panel on High Blood Cholesterol in Children and Adolescents reported the cutoff points used to identify children and adolescents with abnormal serum lipids[34] (Table 32–3). The single cutoff values do not address age, gender, or racial differences in lipid or lipoprotein values. No revisions have been made in the guidelines for children and adolescents since 1991.

## Familial Hypercholesterolemia

In a landmark work that led to the award of the Nobel Prize in Physiology or Medicine in 1985, Brown et al. established that the severely elevated cholesterol level in persons with familial hypercholesterolemia (FH) was the result of a genetic defect in the cellular LDL receptor, predominantly on hepatocytes.[35] Consequently, affected individuals have markedly elevated TC and LDL levels with normal to decreased HDL and normal TG levels. The prevalence of heterozygous FH is approximately 1 in 500, whereas homozygous FH, with its extremely elevated TC and LDL plasma concentrations, is present in only 1 in 1 million people.[36] The risk of coronary heart disease in heterozygous FH reaches approximately 50% by age 50 years for men and by age 60 years for women. Homozygous individuals develop symptomatic CAD by the late second or early third decade of life.

## Cholesterol Modification in Children

To decrease the risk of CHD in adults, the NCEP Expert Panel on Blood Cholesterol in Children and Adolescents recommended a dual strategy that combines a *population* approach and an *individualized* approach.[34,37] The population approach is the principal means to lower cholesterol levels in all American children through population-wide

**Table 32–3.** Percentile Cutoff Points for Serum Total Cholesterol, LDL, Triglycerides, and HDL in Children and Adolescents

| Category | Percentile | Total Cholesterol (mg/dL) | LDL (mg/dL) | Triglycerides (mg/dL) | HDL (mg/dL) |
|---|---|---|---|---|---|
| Acceptable | <75 | <170 | <110 | <75 | >45 |
| Borderline | 75–95 | 170–199 | 110–129 | 75–129 | 40–45 |
| Elevated | >95 | >200 | >130 | >130 | Low <40 |

HDL = high-density lipoprotein; LDL = low-density lipoprotein.
Adapted from National Cholesterol Education Program. *Report of the Expert Panel on Blood Cholesterol Levels in Children and Adolescents.* NIH publication 91-2732. Washington, DC: US Department of Health and Human Services, National Institutes of Health; September 1991; National Heart, Lung, and Blood Institute. Expert Panel on Integrated Guidelines for Cardiovascular Health and Risk Reduction in Children and Adolescents: summary report. *Pediatrics.* 2011; 128(Suppl 6):S213.

**Table 32–4.** Foods to Choose

| Food Group | Recommendations |
|---|---|
| Poultry, fish, meat | Skinless white-meat chicken and turkey; fish such as salmon and other fatty fishes; lean red meat |
| Dairy products | Nonfat or low-fat (1–2%) milk; low-fat cheese |
| Fats and oils | Olive, canola, safflower, peanut, corn, or soybean oil; encourage foods high in omega-3 fatty acids (e.g., salmon, flaxseed, fish oils), nuts, peanuts (legumes), and avocado containing monounsaturated fatty acids. Avoid coconut, palm, and palm kernel oil (high in saturated fatty acids), animal fats (lard or butter), and *trans*-fatty acids. |
| Breads, grains, cereals | Whole-grain breads, pasta, and cereals; starchy vegetables; dry beans |
| Fruits and vegetables | Encourage five or more servings per day (high in vitamins, minerals, and fiber) |
| Eggs | Limit whole eggs to three per week, but egg whites may be eaten as often as desired. |

modifications of nutrition in all children 2 years of age and older. Nutritional adequacy should be achieved by eating a wide variety of foods with sufficient calories to support normal growth and development and to reach and maintain desirable body weight. The Expert Panel recommended a nutrient intake pattern in which total fat constitutes 25% to 30% of total calories, with 8% to 10% of total calories from saturated fat, up to 10% from polyunsaturated fat, and the remainder from monounsaturated fat. Dietary cholesterol should be limited to less than 300 mg/day. With up to 30% of total calories from fat, the remaining 70% should include 15% to 20% from protein and 50% to 55% from carbohydrates.

Current American Heart Association recommendations[38] emphasize the importance of eating more than five servings of fruits and vegetables and more than six servings of whole grains and cereals daily; increasing consumption of foods high in omega-3 fatty acids such as salmon, nuts, and canola, soybean, or flaxseed oil; and avoiding *trans*-fatty acids (Table 32–4). A randomized clinical trial enrolling adults showed that daily intake of 1.5 ounces of almonds, compared with a calorically equal carbohydrate snack, significantly lowered TC, LDL, TG, and abdominal adiposity.[39] These favorable results were attributed to the high unsaturated fatty acid content and perhaps also to phytosterols. Consumption of at least two fish servings per week is recommended. Numerous studies have demonstrated that such a diet does not adversely affect normal growth of children and adolescents between the ages of 3 and 19 years.[40–42] The American Academy of Pediatrics (AAP) has cautioned against overzealous adherence to an extremely low-fat diet (<20% of calories) for children. Such diets may result in deficiencies in essential fatty acids; fat-soluble vitamins A, D, E, and K; and other nutrients.

## Dietary and Drug Management

### Nutrition Therapy

The individualized approach aims to identify and treat children and adolescents who are at increased risk of having high blood cholesterol and developing CAD as adults. The revised AAP guidelines[37] recommended selective serum cholesterol screening of children between 2 and 8 years of age who have a family history of premature cardiovascular disease (adults <55 years of age) or at least one parent with elevated cholesterol levels (TC >240 mg/dL). Universal screening was recommended for children between 9 and 11 years of age and once again between 17 and 21 years.

Dietary intervention is the primary approach for children with elevated cholesterol (Table 32–5). A registered dietitian should be consulted. The NCEP Adult Treatment Panel III recommendations[43] also encourage the use of plant stanols/sterols and soluble fiber as therapeutic dietary options to enhance lowering of LDL. Dietary recommendations for the treatment of severe hypertriglyceridemia usually include a low-fat diet with at least partial substitution of dietary fat with medium-chain fatty acids. Careful follow-up is needed because low-fat, high-carbohydrate diets may increase triglyceride (TG) formation and reduce HDL.[44] Omega-3 fatty acids reduce TG and fatty acid synthesis in the liver and increase fatty acid oxidation. Administration of marine-based omega-3 polyunsaturated fatty acids, eicosapentaenoic acid (EPA), and docosahexaenoic acid (DHA) in children with severe hypertriglyceridemia for whom conventional therapy has failed was shown to reduce TG and TC significantly.[44,45]

### Drug Therapy

The Expert Panel on Blood Cholesterol Levels in Children and Adolescents recommended consideration of drug therapy in children older than 10 years of age if, after 6 to 12 months of dietary therapy, LDL remains higher than 190 mg/dL (or >160 mg/dL in children with a positive family history of premature CAD or two or more other risk factors). In selected cases, drug therapy may be considered in younger patients in whom cholesterol levels are extremely elevated. Until recently, only bile acid sequestrants such as cholestyramine and colesevelam were recommended for use in children. These nonabsorbable agents act by binding bile acids in the intestinal lumen, with eventual excretion. They have proven efficacy, are relatively free from side effects, and have an excellent safety profile. However, compliance with the long-term treatment regimen is generally poor. Niacin (nicotinic acid) has been used effectively in adults for many years to lower LDL and TG. Flushing and pruritus are common side effects that limit its tolerability in children.

Statins (HMG-CoA-reductase inhibitors) such as lovastatin, fluvastatin, simvastatin, atorvastatin, and rosuvastatin are highly effective agents for lowering LDL.[46] The US Food and Drug Administration has approved the use of statins in children 10 to 17 years of age who have FH and marked elevations in LDL. The safety and efficacy of these agents in children appear to be similar to those in adults.[47] Elevations in serum transaminases and muscle enzymes (more than three times the upper limit of normal) occur in fewer than 1% of patients but require close monitoring. Rhabdomyolysis is an extremely rare but potentially fatal complication. Of particular interest to the pediatric population, steroidogenesis is dependent on cholesterol biosynthesis. Studies in adults and children have shown that statin treatment does not affect hormone levels.[48,49] Growth and sexual maturation were no different in adolescent boys treated with lovastatin compared with placebo.[50] Nevertheless, long-term safety studies of statins are warranted before their use in children is expanded beyond those with FH and severe elevations in LDL.

Ezetimibe inhibits the intestinal absorption of dietary and biliary cholesterol by blocking the transport of cholesterol across the

**Table 32–5.** Guidelines for Dietary Management in Children and Adolescents Aged 2 to 21 Years with Elevated Cholesterol or Triglyceride Levels

| Condition | Recommendation |
|---|---|
| *Elevated LDL cholesterol* | |
| Total Fat | 25–30% of total calories |
| Saturated Fat | ≤7% of calories |
| Monounsaturated Fat | ~10% of calories |
| Dietary cholesterol | <200 mg/day |
| Trans fats | Avoid as much as possible |
| Elevated TG or non-HDL cholesterol | All of the above, plus decrease sugar intake and avoid sugar-sweetened beverages; replace simple with complex carbohydrates; increase dietary fish intake; and increase intake of omega-3 fatty acids |

HDL = high-density lipoprotein; LDL = low-density lipoprotein; TG = triglycerides.
From Marks D, Thorogood M, Neil HA, Humphries SE. A review on the diagnosis, natural history, and treatment of familial hypercholesterolaemia. *Atherosclerosis*. 2003; 168:1.

intestinal wall. It does not interfere with the absorption of bile acids, fatty acids, fat-soluble vitamins, or TG. Systemic absorption of ezetimibe is minimal, but safety and efficacy studies have yet to be performed in pediatric patients. When used alone, ezetimibe lowers LDL by approximately 18%. In combination with statins, it may lower LDL by an additional 25% to 30%.[51]

The fibrates (e.g., gemfibrozil, fenofibrate) are useful for reducing extremely elevated TG levels in children at risk for acute pancreatitis. However, experience in children is almost entirely lacking. It is therefore prudent to refer the use of fibrates and most other drugs, except for bile acid sequestrants, to lipid specialists with experience in managing hyperlipidemia in children.

## References


1. Montana E, Khoury MJ, Cragan JD, Sharma S, Dhar P, Fyfe D. Trends and outcomes after prenatal diagnosis of congenital cardiac malformations by fetal echocardiography in a well defined birth population, Atlanta, Georgia, 1990–1994. *J Am Coll Cardiol.* 1996; 28:1805.
2. Go AS, Mozaffarian D, Roger VL, et al. Executive summary: heart and stroke statistics—2014 update. A report from the American Heart Association. *Circulation.* 2014; 129:e28.
3. Hoffman JI, Kaplan S. The incidence of congenital heart disease. *J Am Coll Cardiol.* 2002; 39:1890.
4. Moller JH. Prevalence and incidence of cardiac malformations. In: Moller JH, ed. *Perspectives in Pediatric Cardiology: Surgery of Congenital Heart Disease*, vol 6. Pediatric Cardiac Care Consortium 1984–1995. Armonk, NY: Futura; 1998.
5. Ohye RG, Tabbutt S, Sleeper LA, et al. Comparison of shunt types in the Norwood procedure for single-ventricle lesions. *N Engl J Med.* 2010; 362:1980.
6. Feldt RH, Strickle GL, Weidman WH. Growth of children with heart disease. *Am J Dis Child.* 1969; 117:573.
7. Gingell RL, Hornung MG. Growth problems associated with congenital heart disease in infancy. In: Lebenthal E, ed. *Textbook of Gastroenterology and Nutrition in Infancy.* New York: Raven Press; 1989.
8. Sinden AA, Sutphen J. Growth and nutrition. In: Emmanouilides GC, Allen HD, Riemenschneider TA, Gutgesell HP, eds. *Moss and Adams' Heart Disease in Infants, Children, and Adolescents Including the Fetus and Young Adult.* Baltimore: Williams & Wilkins; 1995.
9. Lees MH, Bristow JB, Griswold HE, et al. Relative hyper-metabolism in infants with congenital heart disease and undernutrition. *Pediatrics.* 1965; 36:183.
10. Krause AN, Auld PA. Metabolic rate of neonates with congenital heart disease. *Arch Dis Child.* 1975; 50:539.
11. Heymsfield SB, Andrews JS, Hood R, Williams PJ, Bagatell CJ. Nutrition and the heart. In: Grand RJ, Sutphen JL, Dietz WH, eds. *Pediatric Nutrition.* Stoneham, MA: Butterworth; 1987.
12. Menon G, Poskitt EME. Why does congenital heart disease cause failure to thrive? *Arch Dis Child.* 1985; 60:1134.
13. Mehrizi A, Drash A. Growth disturbance in congenital heart disease. *J Pediatr.* 1962; 61:418.
14. Forchielli ML, McColl R, Walker WA, Lo C. Children with congenital heart disease: a nutrition challenge. *Nutr Rev.* 1994; 52:348.
15. Wessel JJ. Cardiology. In: Samour PQ, Helm KK, Lang CE, eds. *Handbook of Pediatric Nutrition.* Baltimore: American Society for Parenteral and Enteral Nutrition; 1999.
16. Bahn L. Serum proteins as markers of nutrition: what are we treating? Nutrition Issues in Gastroenterology, Series #43. *Practical Gastroenterol.* 2006; 30:46.
17. Gervasio MR, Bunchanan CN. Malnutrition in the pediatric cardiology patient. *Crit Care Q.* 1985; 8:49.
18. Heymsfield SB, Andrews JS, Hood R, et al. Nutrition and the heart. In: Grand RJ, Sutphen JL, Dietz WH, eds. *Pediatric Nutrition.* Stoneham, MA: Butterworth; 1987.
19. Fomon SJ, Ziegler EE. Nutritional management of infants with congenital heart disease. *Am Heart J.* 1972; 83:581.
20. Bougle D, Iselin M, Kahyat A, Duhamel JF. Nutrition treatment of congenital heart disease. *Arch Dis Child.* 1986; 61:799.
21. Schwarz SM, Gewitz MH, See CC, et al. Enteral nutrition in infants with congenital heart disease and growth failure. *Pediatrics.* 1990; 86:368.
22. Vanderhoof JA, Hofschire PJ, Baluff MA, et al. Continuous enteral feedings: an important adjunct to the management of complex congenital heart disease. *Am J Dis Child.* 1982; 136:825.
23. Booker PD, Romer H, Franks R. Gut mucosal perfusion in neonates undergoing cardiopulmonary bypass. *Br J Anaesth.* 1996; 77:597.
24. Kannel WB, Castelli WP, Gordon T, McNamara PM. Serum cholesterol, lipoproteins, and the risk of coronary heart disease. The Framingham Study. *Ann Intern Med.* 1971; 74:1.
25. Multiple Risk Factor Intervention Trial Research Group. Multiple risk factor intervention trial: risk factor changes and mortality results. *JAMA.* 1982; 248:1465.
26. The Lipid Research Clinics Program. The Lipid Research Clinics Coronary Primary Prevention Trial results: I. Reduction in incidence of coronary heart disease. *JAMA* 1984; 251:351.
27. Frick MH, Elo O, Haapa K, et al. Helsinki Heart Study. Primary-prevention trial with gemfibrozil in middle-aged men with dyslipidemia: safety in treatment, changes in risk factors, and incidence of coronary heart disease. *N Engl J Med.* 1987; 317:1237.
28. Keys A, Menotti A, Karvonen MJ, et al. The diet and 15-year death rate in the seven countries study. *Am J Epidemiol.* 1986; 124:903.
29. Kagan A, Harris BR, Winkelstein W Jr, et al. Epidemiologic studies of coronary heart disease and stroke in Japanese men living in Japan, Hawaii, and California: demographic, physical, dietary and biochemical characteristics. *J Chronic Dis.* 1974; 27:345.
30. Gotto AM Jr, LaRosa JC, Hunninghake D, et al. The cholesterol facts: a summary of the evidence relating dietary fats, serum cholesterol and coronary heart disease. A joint statement by the American Heart Association and the National Heart, Lung and Blood Institute. *Circulation.* 1990; 81:1721.
31. Stary HC. Evolution and progression of atherosclerotic lesions in coronary arteries of children and young adults. *Arteriosclerosis* 1989; 9(Suppl):I19.
32. Tuzcu EM, Kapadia SR, Tutar E, et al. High prevalence of coronary atherosclerosis in asymptomatic teenagers and young adults: evidence from intravascular ultrasound. *Circulation.* 2001; 103:2705.
33. Hickman TB, Briefel RR, Carroll MD, et al. Distributions and trends of serum lipid levels among United States children and adolescents ages 4-19 years: Data from the Third National Health and Nutrition Examination Survey. Prev Medicine. 1998; 27:879-1998
34. National Cholesterol Education Program. *Report of the Expert Panel on Blood Cholesterol Levels in Children and Adolescents.* NIH publication 91-2732. Washington, DC: US Department of Health and Human Services, National Institutes of Health; September 1991.
35. Brown MS, Kovanen PT, Goldstein JL. Regulation of plasma cholesterol by lipoprotein receptors. *Science.* 1981; 212:628.
36. Marks D, Thorogood M, Neil HA, Humphries SE. A review on the diagnosis, natural history, and treatment of familial hypercholesterolaemia. *Atherosclerosis.* 2003; 168:1.
37. National Heart, Lung, and Blood Institute. Expert Panel on Integrated Guidelines for Cardiovascular Health and Risk Reduction in Children and Adolescents: summary report. *Pediatrics.* 2011; 128(Suppl 6):S213.
38. Krauss RM, Eckel RH, Howard B, et al. AHA dietary guidelines: revision 2000. A statement for health-care professionals from the Nutrition Committee of the American Heart Association. *Circulation.* 2000; 102:2284.
39. Berryman CE, West SG, Fleming JA, Bordi PL, Kris-Etherton PM. Effects of daily almond consumption on cardiometabolic risk and abdominal adiposity in health adults with elevated LDL-cholesterol: a randomized controlled trial. *J Am Heart Assoc.* 2015; 4:e000993.
40. Obarzanek E, Hunsberger SA, Van Horn L, et al. Safety of a fat-reduced diet: the Dietary Intervention Study in Children (DISC). *Pediatrics.* 1997; 100:51.
41. Jacobson MS. Heart healthy diets for all children: no longer controversial. *J Pediatr.* 1998; 133:1.
42. Tershakovec AM, Jawad AF, Stallings VA, et al. Growth of hypercholesterolemic children completing physician-initiated low-fat dietary intervention. *J Pediatr.* 1998; 133:28.
43. Expert Panel on Detection, Evaluation, and Treatment of High Blood Cholesterol in Adults. Executive summary of the third report of the National Cholesterol Education Program (NCEP) expert panel on detection, evaluation, and treatment of high blood cholesterol in adults (Adult Treatment Panel III). *JAMA.* 2001; 285:2486.
44. Abbas IM, McLaughlin T, Lamendola C, et al. High carbohydrate diets, triglyceride-rich lipoproteins and coronary heart disease risk. *Am J Cardiol.* 2000; 85:45.
45. Volti L, Bianca S, Simone ML, Calandra S, Bertolini S. Effects of T-3 fatty acids in children with severe hypertriglyceridemia. *Pediatr Res.* 2001; 50:296.
46. Newman CB, Palmer G, Silbershatz H, Szarek M. Safety of atorvastatin derived from analysis of 44 completed trials in 9,416 patients. *Am J Cardiol.* 2003; 92:670.
47. Napoli C, Sica V. Statin treatment and the natural history of atherosclerotic-related diseases: pathogenic mechanisms and the risk-benefit profile. *Curr Pharm Des.* 2004; 10:425.
48. Jay RH, Sturley RH, Stirling C, et al. Effects of pravastatin and cholestyramine on gonadal and adrenal steroid production in familial hypercholesterolaemia. *Br J Clin Pharmacol.* 1991; 32:417.
49. Purvis K, Tollefsrud A, Rui H, et al. Short-term effects of treatment with simvastatin on testicular function in patients with heterozygous familial hypercholesterolaemia. *Eur J Clin Pharmacol.* 1992; 42:61.
50. Stein EA, Illingworth DR, Kwiterovich PO Jr, et al. Efficacy and safety of lovastatin in adolescent males with heterozygous familial hypercholesterolemia: a randomized controlled trial. *JAMA* 1999; 281:137.
51. Gagne C, Bays HE, Weiss SR, et al Efficacy and safety of ezetimibe added to ongoing statin therapy for treatment of patients with primary hypercholesterolemia. *Am J Cardiol.* 2002; 90:1084.

# 33 Chronic Kidney Disease in Children and Adults

JUDITH BETO AND VINOD BANSAL

The kidney is an excretory organ that filters, reabsorbs, and excretes electrolytes, protein byproducts, glucose, amino acids, and toxic substances. Through nephron filtration and urine production, all these substances are removed from the body. The kidney also functions as an endocrine gland, producing hormones involved in growth (i.e., human growth factor), blood pressure regulation (i.e., renin), red blood cell production (i.e., erythropoietin), and the absorption of calcium (i.e., 1,25-dihydroxycholecalciferol). Chronic renal disease involves a progressive decline in the number of functioning nephrons that may result ultimately in kidney failure. The rate of progression is fastest in children with glomerulonephropathies, followed by hereditary nephropathies and renal dysplasia; it is slowest in children with urinary tract malformations.[1]

The National Kidney Foundation (NKF) has established the Kidney Disease Outcomes Quality Initiative (K/DOQI), which convenes work groups to develop clinical practice guidelines, primarily focused on the adult population, for the management of chronic kidney disease (CKD) and kidney failure. An extensive 2008 revision concentrated on the nutritional care of children across the spectrum of CKD. The revision also emphasized the reduction in chronic morbidities and mortality risk as more children survive CKD and kidney transplantation into adulthood.[2]

The Kidney Disease Improving Global Outcomes (K/DIGO) initiative of the NKF created terminology for the international classification of stages of kidney disease based on stratifications of the estimated glomerular filtration rate (GFR), a measure of kidney function, integrated with levels of albuminuria.[3] These stages are listed in Table 33–1.

GFR is most accurately estimated with the use of formulas specifically developed for children. Two of these, the Schwartz formula:

$$\text{Creatinine clearance (mL/min)} = 0.55 \times \text{Length (cm)}/\text{Serum creatinine (mg/dL)}$$

and the Counahan-Barratt formula:

$$\text{GFR (mL/min/1.73 m2)} = 0.43 \times \text{Length (cm)}/\text{Serum creatinine (mg/dL)}$$

have been recommended for their clinical usefulness. Both are based on relationships between height and serum creatinine ratio but are sensitive to low serum creatinine levels that may be detected in persons with malnutrition and low muscle mass.[2] The progression between stages is unique to each individual based on concomitant medical factors and the etiology of kidney failure.[2,3]

The number of children in CKD stages 1 through 4 is unknown. The incidence and prevalence rates of stage 5 (i.e., kidney failure) among children are reported annually by the United States Renal Data System (USRDS) database. The incidence of pediatric kidney failure decreased between 2003 and 2008 and dropped 5.8% in 2012. The 2012 USRDS report listed 7522 patients with stage 5 disease and 5475 who were being followed as kidney transplant recipients (doubling the number from 1988 to 2012), reinforcing the growing number of children transitioning into adults with CKD. Between 2008 and 2013, 43.6% of children with CKD underwent transplantations within the first year of kidney failure, and overall 72.9% received a transplant.[4] An organ waiting list is maintained by the United Network of Organ Sharing (UNOS).[5] The 5-year survival rate was 89% for children initiating care between 2003 and 2007. Death primarily results from complications related to vascular access or peritoneal catheter infection.[4]

## BIOCHEMICAL ABNORMALITIES

Proteinuria is often found in children with kidney damage. Children without diabetes should be screened using a spot urine sample to estimate total urine protein with a standard urine dipstick or a total protein-to-creatinine ratio. Positive random sample testing should be reconfirmed with a first morning specimen to exclude orthostatic proteinuria. Microalbuminuria is not used as an early detection device, as is done in adults, because of the low incidence of diabetes and hypertension in children. Children with diabetes and more than a 5-year history of proteinuria after puberty should be monitored under the adult guidelines, which include assessing proteinuria as albumin.[1,2,6]

Renal replacement therapy (hemodialysis or peritoneal dialysis) tends to be initiated in children at lower GFR levels than in adults. This typically occurs because of the more rapid and greater changes in serum values of creatinine and blood urea nitrogen (BUN) relative to body size. Children with CKD typically have shorter stature and lower body mass index (BMI) than non-CKD children. Elevated serum creatinine and BUN can produce uremic symptoms of nausea, vomiting, poor appetite, and general malaise. These symptoms often adversely affect dietary intake.

Urea kinetic modeling measures the adequacy of the dialysis treatment by mathematically calculating the ratio between pretreatment and posttreatment solute removal. The minimal target goal for effective treatment is a urea reduction ratio of more than 65% or a Kt/V value greater than 1.2, in which K is the dialyzer clearance of urea, t is the dialysis time, and V is the volume of distribution of urea (approximately equal to the patient's total body water). Unlike measurements in adults, the use of the protein catabolic rate or protein equivalent of total nitrogen appearance (nPNA or PNA) is not recommended. Children are in an active anabolic state, with dietary protein being used both for creation maintenance of body protein.[2,6,7] Adults are typically in steady nitrogen balance unless dramatically obese or malnourished.[8]

Anemia is relatively common in stages 1 through 4. Pediatric patients are treated similar to adults with synthetic erythropoietin injections to help maintain hemoglobin levels within narrow ranges.[1,2]

Growth and nutrition status are negatively correlated with abnormal acid-base status in children. It is postulated that growth hormone secretion is interrupted, changed, and/or suppressed in multiple metabolic pathways in CKD, most of which are poorly understood. Approximately 50% of the children between 5 and 17 years of age on hemodialysis have metabolic acidosis (i.e., total venous $CO_2$ <20 mmol/L). Peritoneal dialysis produces more normal serum bicarbonate levels. Serum bicarbonate levels less than 22 mmol/L should be corrected with oral administration of alkali therapy or an appropriate sodium bicarbonate additive in the hemodialysis dialysate solution.[2,6]

Abnormal lipid profiles may include elevated triglyceride and cholesterol levels, particularly in disease stages 1 through 4 that include proteinuria. Abnormalities in electrolytes, particularly serum phosphorus and potassium, are more likely to occur near or in stage 5 as a result of nonexcretion by the failing kidney. Therapy includes dietary and drug interventions that are individually adjusted and monitored continually because of the fluctuating status of children with growth and intake.[2,6,7]

## FACTORS TO BE CONSIDERED IN NUTRITION EVALUATION

The assessment of children with CKD uses the same standard growth and evaluation parameters that are used with non-CKD children. The

**Table 33–1.** Stages of Chronic Kidney Disease as modified from K/DIGO International Terminology Using GFR and Persistent Albuminuria Groupings

| Kidney Damage Stage and Description | GFR (mL/min/1.73 m²) |
|---|---|
| G1 Normal or increased GFR | ≥90 |
| G2 Mild decreased GFR | 60–89 |
| G3a Mild to moderate decreased GFR | 45–59 |
| G3b Moderate to severely decreased GFR | 30–44 |
| G4 Severe decreased GFR | 15–29 |
| G5 Kidney failure | <15 or dialysis |
| *Categories of Persistent Albuminuria* | *Range of Albuminuria* |
| A1 Normal/mildly increased | <30 mg/g (or <3 mg/mmol) |
| A2 Moderately increased | 30–300 mg/g (or 3–30 mg/mmol) |
| A3 Severely increased | >300 mg/g (or >30 mg/mmol) |

GFR = glomerular filtration rate; K/DIGO = Kidney Disease Improving Global Outcomes.
From Kidney Disease Improving Global Outcomes. Chapter 1: Definition and Classification of CKD. http://kdigo.org/clinical_practice_guidelines/PDF/CKD/KDIGO_2012_CKD_GL.pdf

K/DOQI guidelines recommend that the following measures be collected: dietary interview/food diary, serum albumin, height/length, estimated dry weight, weight/height index, and anthropometric measures (skinfold thickness, head circumference). Actual and optimal dietary intake should be calculated with the use of computer software; the calculated standard deviation score for height and weight based on normal growth should be estimated from available growth charts. It is recommended that this basic assessment be completed at baseline, with repeated evaluation every month or more frequently if a change in risk occurs.[2,6,7]

A subjective global nutrition assessment for children has been published that aims to provide a basis on which to track changes over time as well as a baseline.[9] Periodic nutrition assessment for children progressing to adult parameters is also outlined in detail in both the K/DOQI clinical practice guidelines and the Standards of Practice and Standards of Practice Performance for practitioners specializing in renal nutrition.[2,8,10]

Additional data should be collected for use in the long-term evaluation and planning phase. This includes the medical history, blood pressure, body losses (e.g., urine, stool, emesis, ostomy), medications, consumption of nonfood items, physical and developmental eating and oral skills, physical signs of nutritional status (e.g., eyesight, hearing, condition of the tongue and teeth), and other applicable information.[2,6,7]

## DIETARY MANAGEMENT

The major challenge in pediatrics is maintaining sufficient oral intake to promote normal growth. Because each child has unique energy and nutritional needs based on multiple factors, growth progression from baseline is used as an individual benchmark of success. As a child with CKD continues into adulthood, particularly after transplantation, suitable oral intake is necessary to maintain appropriate body weight and nutrition status.

Table 33–2 illustrates general recommendations for protein and energy intake for this population at initiation of maintenance dialysis therapy in stage 5. Protein intake is higher for peritoneal dialysis because of the constant loss of amino acids through the peritoneal membrane barrier. Data suggest that age and body size influence protein loss. Smaller and younger children may have higher losses, whereas older children may require more median levels, so diet prescriptions need to be continually evaluated.[2,6,7] Stages 1 through 4 require more individualization based on growth and illness parameters. Protein guidelines require greater sensitivity to a balance between metabolic losses, needs within the context of disease progression, and control of hyperphosphatemia.

The calorie levels listed in Table 33–2 are appropriate for initial assessment of all stages (1 through 5) because they are based on Dietary Reference Intakes (DRIs). No specific caloric intake data are available for children with CKD, and the DRIs provide a generous intake margin. Children receiving peritoneal dialysis absorb significant amounts of calories from the dialysate glucose-based solution, approximately 7 to 10 kcal/kg.[2,6,7] The K/DOQI recommendations focus on short stature for chronological age as a better marker than formulas based on weight age. These recommendations are guidelines only; each child must be assessed on a regular basis to provide ongoing intervention for the nonstatic anabolic growth challenges of CKD.[2]

Dietary restrictions of calcium, phosphorus, sodium, and potassium are typically provided for adults.[8,11] Children, however, are best managed with highly individualized counseling based on clinical parameters. This philosophy restricts only those nutrients that are necessary for safety while promoting the use of adequate calories and protein for growth.[2,6–8]

The K/DOQI guidelines recommend vitamin and mineral requirements of 100% of the DRI based on age categories for thiamine, riboflavin, pyridoxine, vitamin $B_{12}$, folic acid, copper, zinc, and vitamins A, C, E, and K. Oral iron supplementation needs to be individually assessed; iron supplementation is often given intravenously in conjunction with dialysis therapy. Many studies have documented that nutritional support and supplementation is a key factor because children tend to eat poorly when not healthy. Children are often suitable candidates for nocturnal nutritional supplementation using an appropriate individualized chronic feeding tube route. This strategy maintains optimal intake while providing greater flexibility in daily oral intake.[2,6,7]

## SUMMARY AND FOLLOW-UP

The nutritional support of children with CKD requires ongoing innovative intervention to achieve optimal growth. Intensive nutrition assessment and counseling is a cornerstone of effective treatment. A large portion of the data available is extrapolated from clinical studies of adults and were adapted in practice to pediatric use. The K/DOQI

**Table 33–2.** Guidelines for Dietary Protein and Energy for Children and Adults with Emphasis on Individualization and Stage of Chronic Kidney Disease*

| Group | Age (yr) | DRI for Non-CKD (g/kg/day) | Protein Intake for Hemodialysis (g/kg/day) | Protein Intake for Peritoneal Dialysis (g/kg/day) | Energy Intake (kcal/kg/day) |
|---|---|---|---|---|---|
| Infants | 0–0.5 | 1.50 | 1.60 | 1.80 | 108 |
| | 0.6–1.0 | 1.20 | 1.30 | 1.50 | 98 |
| Children | 1–3 | 1.05 | 1.15 | 1.30 | 102 |
| | 4–13 | 0.95 | 1.05 | 1.10 | 90 |
| | 14–18 | 0.85 | 0.95 | 1.00 | 70 |
| Adults | >18 | 0.80 | 1.20 | 1.30 | 25–35 |

*Protein and energy should be adjusted to promote adequate growth and maintain nutrition status while controlling for hyperphosphatemia and individual metabolic losses; protein sources are derived at a minimum of 50% from high-biological-value sources with phosphate content awareness.
CKD = chronic kidney disease; DRI = Dietary Reference Intake.
Modified from references 2, 6, 7, 8, and 10.

guidelines are updated regularly and provide the basis for nutritional and medical practice recommendations for CKD.[2]

## References


1. Avner ED, Harmon WE, Niavdet P, Yoshikawa N, eds. *Pediatric Nephrology,* 6th ed. New York: Springer, 2009.
2. National Kidney Foundation. Kidney Disease Outcomes Quality Initiative clinical practice guidelines for nutrition in children with chronic kidney disease: 2008 update. *Am J Kidney Dis.* 2009; 53(Suppl 2):S1.
3. Kidney Disease Improving Global Outcomes. Definition and classification of chronic kidney disease. *Kidney Int.* 2013:3(suppl 3):5.
4. National Institutes of Health, National Institute of Diabetes and Digestive and Kidney Diseases. *United States Renal Data System, 2014 Annual Data Report: Epidemiology of Kidney Disease in the United States.* Bethesda, MD: National Institutes of Health, National Institute of Diabetes and Digestive and Kidney Diseases; 2014.
5. Matas AJ, Smith JM, Skeans MA, et al. OPTN/SRTR 2013 annual data report: kidney. *Am J Transplant.* 2015; 15(Suppl 2):1.
6. Secker D. Nutrition management of chronic kidney disease in the pediatric patient. In: Byham-Gray L, Stover J, Wiesen K, eds. *A Clinical Guide to Nutrition Care in Kidney Disease*, 2nd ed. Chicago IL: Academy of Nutrition and Dietetics, 2013.
7. McCann L, ed. *Pocket Guide to Nutrition Assessment of the Patient with Kidney Disease: A Project of the Council on Renal Nutrition of the National Kidney Foundation*, 5th ed. New York: National Kidney Foundation; 2015.
8. National Kidney Foundation. *Kidney Disease Outcomes Quality Initiative Clinical Practice Guidelines for Nutrition in Chronic Renal Failure.* http://www2.kidney.org/professionals/kdoqi/guidelines_nutrition/doqi/nut.html. Accessed June 21, 2016.
9. Secker D, Jeejeebhoy K. Subjective global nutritional assessment in children. *Am J Clin Nutr.* 2007; 85:1083.
10. Academy of Nutrition and Dietetics and National Kidney Foundation. Revised 2014 standards of practice and standards of professional performance for registered dietitian nutritionists (competent, proficient, and expert) in nephrology nutrition. *J Acad Nutr Diet.* 2014; 114:1448.e45.
11. Beto JA, Ramirez WE, Bansal VK. Medical nutrition therapy in adults with chronic kidney disease: integrating evidence and consensus into practice for the generalist registered dietitian nutritionist. *J Acad Nutr Diet.* 2014; 114:1077.

# 34 Sickle Cell Disease

OMAR NISS AND RUSSELL E. WARE

Sickle cell disease (SCD) is a group of genetic disorders characterized by the predominance of sickle hemoglobin (Hb S) in red blood cells (RBC). The most common and most severe form of SCD, homozygous Hb SS, occurs when the patient inherits one Hb S gene from each parent. Persons with sickle cell trait (Hb AS) carry the sickle gene but are asymptomatic. Other compound heterozygous conditions occur when a patient inherits an Hb S with an additional β-globin gene mutation (e.g., Hb SC, or Hb Sβ thalassemia).

The sickle gene is prevalent among people of African, Italian, Sicilian, Egyptian, Turkish, Arabian, and Asiatic Indian background. In the United States, SCD is found predominantly in African Americans. About 1 of every 12 African Americans has sickle cell trait and is an asymptomatic carriers, and approximately 1 of 400 African-American newborns have the disease.[1] Millions are estimated to have SCD worldwide.[2]

## BIOCHEMICAL, PATHOLOGICAL, AND CLINICAL ABNORMALITIES

Hb S results from a single amino acid substitution of valine for glutamic acid in the sixth position of the β-globin chain. In contrast to the usual adult hemoglobin (Hb A), the sickle hemoglobin polymerizes on deoxygenation. This process alters the RBC membrane and changes the cell shape into a sickled form. These sickled RBC have shorter life span, leading to hemolytic anemia. Sickling alters the normal properties and deformability of the RBC, causing vaso-occlusion and vascular dysfunction.

The two primary manifestations of SCD are severe hemolytic anemia and widespread vaso-occlusion and infarction of various organs and tissues. The hemolytic anemia results from the markedly shortened lifespan of the sickled RBC which survive in the circulation for only 10 to 20 days, compared with 120 days for normal RBC. The clinical manifestations that reflect this ongoing hemolytic process include jaundice, pallor, weakness, and fatigue.

The widespread vaso-occlusion results from adherence of the sickled RBC to the lining of blood vessels, which plugs up the small vessels and obstructs blood flow to organs and tissues, leading to infarction and tissue death. Decreased oxygen supply to the bones and bone marrow causes the pain that is characteristic of SCD. The initial pain episode may occur in an infant or toddler, who presents with painful swelling of the hands and feet (dactylitis); in older patients, vaso-occlusion affects the sternum and ribs and the long bones of the arms and legs. Certain factors can trigger a painful episode (i.e., sickle cell crisis), including infection, hypoxia, extremes of temperature, and acidosis. Frequently, there is no obvious precipitating factor.

Other vaso-occlusive complications in SCD include acute chest syndrome and splenic involvement. Acute chest syndrome, which results from pulmonary vaso-occlusion and infarction, can be rapidly progressive or fatal if not treated aggressively.[3] Sudden massive trapping of RBC in the spleen leads to acute splenic sequestration in infants and toddlers, which is characterized by a sudden decrease in hemoglobin and can cause hemodynamic instability. Repeated splenic vaso-occlusion leads to autoinfarction of the spleen very early in life, leaving the patient with a markedly increased susceptibility to infections, especially sepsis caused by *Streptococcus pneumoniae*. The incidence of overwhelming pneumococcal sepsis is 400 times greater in children younger than 5 years of age with SCD than in healthy children.[4] A transient aplastic episode can occur when the bone marrow temporarily stops making red blood cells, typically as a result of a viral infection such as parvovirus B19, which causes severe anemia that frequently requires blood transfusion.

Chronic organ damage can affect virtually every organ of the body in SCD. Stroke caused by cerebral vascular occlusion is a devastating complication of SCD.[5] Progressive impairment of renal function can be seen in teens and adult patients.[6] Chronic leg ulcers resulting from chronic vascular insufficiency are less frequently seen, but they can be debilitating.[7] Eye involvement with sickle cell retinopathy can be progressive and may lead to blindness in older patients.[8]

Growth can also be affected in SCD. Many studies have demonstrated impairment in height and weight in children with SCD compared with healthy age-matched children. The Cooperative Study of Sickle Cell Disease (CSSCD), a national, multicenter, longitudinal study, showed that children with homozygous SCD (Hb SS) had the most severe deficits in growth compared with children with other SCD genotypes.[9] Approximately one-third of patients with SCD are below the 5th percentile for height or weight or both, and many have an associated delay in onset of puberty[10] and sexual maturation.[11,12]

## FACTORS TO BE CONSIDERED IN NUTRITION EVALUATION

### Growth and Nutrition Status in SCD

Early studies documented growth retardation and hypogonadism in children with SCD.[9] Patients with SCD have decreased weight-for-age, height-for-age, and growth velocity.[13] Other measurements such as weight-for-height, sitting height, bony breadths, and limb circumferences are also abnormal.[14] SCD patients are born with normal weight and height,[15] suggesting that fetal growth is not impaired; however, growth alteration is seen as early as 6 months of age.[13] Growth retardation affects boys more than girls and worsens with age.[13] SCD patients have significantly lower upper arm fat mass and lower muscle areas, indicating deficient energy stores and protein wasting, respectively.[16]

### Pubertal and Skeletal Maturation in SCD

Delayed pubertal and skeletal maturation are well recognized in SCD[9,16–18] and are associated with growth retardation.[19] The mean age of menarche is delayed in girls with SCD by more than 2 years.[11,20] Peak height velocity and skeletal age are also delayed.[19,21] Bone mineral density and skeletal maturation are diminished.[22–24]

Despite these abnormalities, the role of endocrine dysfunction in SCD-related growth failure is unclear. Although the hypothalamic-pituitary axis responds appropriately to pharmacological stimuli, decreased testosterone production is not uncommon in adolescents with SCD.[25] This indicates that gonadal dysfunction, when present, is more likely to be primary in nature rather than secondary to pituitary dysfunction.[12,26] Alterations in the growth hormone (GH)/insulin-like growth factor 1 (IGF-1) axis have been described in SCD. Patients with SCD have low IGF-1 and IGFBP-3 regardless of their growth pattern.[27] Similar to people with other chronic diseases, SCD patients have resistance to intrinsic GH,[21] but their response to GH therapy varies. In a small study, five SCD patients who received GH therapy demonstrated significant improvement in height.[28] Thyroid function is normal in SCD, even when growth is impaired.[29,30]

## DIETARY MANAGEMENT

### Protein and Caloric Needs

Unmet nutritional needs in SCD can result from decreased dietary intake or increased energy requirements. Although SCD patients may have decreased dietary intake temporarily around the time of acute illnesses,[31] their intake at baseline is usually comparable to that in the normal population or only minimally decreased.[32,33] Nonetheless, their growth is significantly affected. SCD patients have increased metabolic needs, as evidenced by their increased resting energy expenditure (REE), compared with matched controls.[32,34–36] The increased REE in SCD reflects a state of hypermetabolism that is caused by multiple factors, including increased myocardial energy demand due to chronic anemia,[37] increased cytokine release due to ongoing inflammation,[34,38] increased bone turnover and bone remodeling due to recurrent sickling,[39] and increased erythropoiesis due to chronic hemolysis.[37,40] Together, these factors increase metabolic demands, primarily by increasing protein turnover,[41] which contributes to about 50% of the observed increase in REE. Impaired nitrogen economy and increased REE produce a state of undernutrition despite apparently normal dietary intake in SCD.

The optimal dietary management in SCD is not known, and studies that address macronutrient and micronutrient replacement in SCD are limited. Because SCD is a multisystem disease, implementing a comprehensive care program early in life can be the most beneficial approach, even in resource-limited settings.[42] One small study demonstrated that increasing the caloric intake with nighttime nasogastric feedings produced dramatic increases in height and weight compared with no significant changes in those patients supplemented orally. In addition, there was a decrease in the number of pain episodes and number of hospitalizations among those who recived nasogastric feeding.[43] Other therapies that target the severity and complications of SCD may improve growth and development.

### Vitamins and Minerals

Several studies have reported micronutrient deficiencies in SCD. Increased vitamin and micronutrient requirements in SCD can be explained by the increased RBC turnover and nutrient losses through increased renal excretion.[44] Zinc is the most extensively studied mineral deficiency in SCD.

#### Zinc

Zinc is an essential trace mineral that is important for physical growth, gonadal development, and immune function. Zinc deficiency is considered a contributing factor to growth failure in SCD. Zinc levels have been associated with decreased liner growth and impaired sexual and skeletal maturation.[13,45] Other studies, however, did not find a correlation between plasma zinc levels and linear growth.[46]

Zinc is primarily found intracellularly and is replete in RBCs, platelets, and neutrophils. The plasma zinc level may not reflect true zinc deficiency in SCD, and patients receiving zinc supplements may have improved linear growth without significant change in their plasma levels.[46] Zinc supplementation has a small but significant positive effect on physical growth in otherwise normal children with impaired growth (i.e., non-SCD).[47] Similarly, prepubertal children with SCD demonstrated an increase in mean height and arm circumference after zinc supplementation for 12 months, but no difference was seen in weight or body mass index (BMI).[48] In one study, SCD patients who did not receive zinc supplements had decreased height and weight for age, whereas patients taking supplements did not.[48]

In a Cochrane review about the effects of zinc supplementation in SCD, patients who received zinc supplementation showed increases in serum zinc levels and had fewer infections than control groups.[49] However, zinc supplements did not appear to influence hemoglobin levels, and there were mixed results regarding the influence of zinc on the frequency of pain crises. More studies are needed to determine the optimal dose, the duration, and the long-term effects of zinc on sexual and skeletal maturation in children with SCD.[49]

#### Iron

Iron deficiency is not a common problem in SCD patients, who often have increased body iron due to transfused blood. Similar to other minerals in SCD, iron can become deficient in selected groups of patients, especially nontransfused patients with poor dietary intake. The prevalence of iron deficiency among nontransfused SCD patients ranged from 9% to 20%.[50–52] The effects of iron deficiency can be severe, especially in growing children.

Early detection and correction of iron deficiency is important, especially in high-risk children who live in poor socioeconomic conditions and have limited access to iron-rich food. The diagnosis of iron deficiency in SCD can be difficult because conventional indices of iron deficiency, such as ferritin and mean corpuscular volume (MCV), can be abnormal in SCD due to inflammation and/or reticulocytosis unrelated to iron deficiency. Children with SCD who have never received a transfusion should be screened for iron deficiency by dietary history and a complete blood count. Nontransfused infants should receive iron-fortified formula or, if breast-fed, vitamin supplementation with iron similar to the recommendations for normal infants. If iron deficiency is documented, a therapeutic trial of iron should be initiated.

#### Other Trace Minerals

Other trace elements investigated in SCD include copper and magnesium. Copper competes with zinc for similar binding sites in the body, and data confirm a mild increase in plasma copper in SCD patients who are zinc deficient.[53,54]

Changes in plasma and erythrocyte magnesium levels have also been observed in SCD patients,[54] although they were likely a result of a redistribution phenomenon. Plasma selenium levels are significantly lower in SCD patients compared with controls. This finding is consistent with the increased oxidative stress reported in SCD.[55,56]

#### Vitamin A

Vitamin A is a fat-soluble vitamin that is essential for growth, development, immune function, and vision. Suboptimal vitamin A status (defined by a retinol level <30 μg/dL) and vitamin A deficiency (retinol <20 μg/dL) are prevalent in children with SCD.[57,58] Low vitamin A levels in SCD have been associated with increased hospitalizations, poor growth, and abnormal hematological indices.[58] However, in a randomized, placebo-controlled trial, 12 months of vitamin A supplementation at the RDA dose did not improve vitamin A status in children with SCD.[57]

Zinc is also involved in absorption, transport, and metabolism of vitamin A, primarily by affecting the synthesis of retinol-binding protein. Vitamin A status did not improve even when zinc was supplemented with vitamin A, suggesting that SCD patients may require higher doses of vitamin A.[57]

In developing countries, vitamin A deficiency is more common and is associated with increased mortality and severe infections even in children without SCD;[59] vitamin A deficiency may have worse impact on children with SCD. More studies are needed to determine the optimal treatment of vitamin A deficiency in SCD.

#### Vitamin D

Vitamin D deficiency is seen in many populations, including breastfed infants, the elderly people, African Americans, and patients with chronic diseases.[60] The serum level of 25-hydroxyvitamin D (25-OHD) is considered a reliable marker of vitamin D status because it represents a summation of cutaneous vitamin D synthesis and dietary intake of vitamin D. Low 25-OHD levels are prevalent among children with SCD compared with healthy African-American children.[61–63]

Decreased oral intake of vitamin D appears to be the most common risk factor for vitamin D deficiency in SCD,[61] which contributes to the decreased bone mineral density observed in these children.[64] Vitamin D supplementation improves bone mineral density and decreases bone resorption in healthy girls.[65] Adult patients who were treated with vitamin $D_2$ and calcium for 12 months had normalization of 25-OHD levels and improvement in bone mass density, although the markers of bone resorption remained abnormal.[66]

There is a correlation between vitamin D deficiency and the prevalence of vaso-occlusive complications in children with SCD.[67] Although high doses of vitamin D supplementation may help to improve chronic pain in SCD,[68] it is unclear whether vitamin D supplements have a role in the management of acute vaso-occlusive crises.

### B Vitamins: Folate, $B_6$, and $B_{12}$

Previous studies suggested that SCD patients are at risk for folate and $B_{12}$ deficiency due to accelerated hematopoiesis.[69,70] Kennedy and colleagues found that 15% and 3% of SCD patients had low levels of RBC folate and serum $B_{12}$, respectively, despite folate supplementation.[71] The role of these deficiencies in SCD remains undetermined. In a placebo-controlled, randomized trial of folate supplementation in children with SCD, there was no difference in growth, hemoglobin, or SCD-related complications between the two groups.[72] In countries such as the United States, where folate fortification of food is common, folate supplementation is not routinely recommended for SCD patients.

Serum folate and $B_{12}$ levels are determinants of the homocysteine level, and increased homocysteine is associated with increased risk of vascular disease and thrombosis.[73] Stroke is a devastating complication of SCD, occurring in 11% of nontransfused Hb SS patients by the age of 20 years.[74] Stroke in SCD is primarily caused by cerebrovascular disease, but other factors may contribute to increasing the risk of stroke in some patients. Hyperhomocysteinemia is prevalent among patients with SCD, but its role in the development of stroke is unclear.[75] Although there is no correlation between folate and homocysteine levels in SCD,[75,76] plasma pyridoxine levels are significantly lower[77] and correlate negatively with homocysteine levels,[75] suggesting a potential role for pyridoxine deficiency in hyperhomocysteinemia in SCD.

Certain genetic polymorphisms influence folate metabolism and homocysteine status in SCD, adding to the complexity of hyperhomocysteinemia and its possible contribution to thrombosis.[78] Further studies are needed to clarify the impact of these metabolic pathways on growth and on development of SCD complications such as stroke and whether there is a role for nutritional supplementation designed to mitigate complications.

### Effects of SCD Therapies on Growth and Development

Newborn screening programs allow for early detection of SCD and early interventions with potential beneficial effects on growth and development. Medical interventions that target the symptoms and complications of SCD can ameliorate the cause of nutritional deficiencies and improve growth.

Despite significant progress in understanding the molecular pathophysiology of SCD, therapeutic options remain limited. Stem cell transplantation provides a cure for the disease, but its use is limited by the availability of suitable donors and the significant toxicity associated with the transplantation process. The only clinically available disease-modifying treatment modalities are the oral agent hydroxyurea and blood transfusions.

### Hydroxyurea

Hydroxyurea is the only agent approved by the US Food and Drug Administration (FDA) for treatment of adults with SCD. It is an oral medication with proven benefits in decreasing many acute and chronic complications of SCD, including pain episodes, acute chest syndrome, hospitalizations, and the need for blood transfusions.[79] Hydroxyurea may also have effect in preserving organ function[80] and decreasing mortality.[81]

Current guidelines recommend starting SCD patients on hydroxyurea as early as 9 months of age.[82] Hydroxyurea use in children did not have harmful effects on growth parameters.[83,84] On the contrary, infants with SCD who took hydroxyurea in the Hydroxyurea Safety and Organ Toxicity (HUSOFT) study demonstrated significant improvement in growth, especially the boys.[85] Other studies have shown that hydroxyurea use in children is associated with improvement in weight, height, body fat, fat-free mass, and a subjective increase in appetite.[86] Growth improvement in SCD patients taking hydroxyurea is at least partially mediated by a decrease in REE.[86] The effect of hydroxyurea on SCD patients in developing countries, where growth and nutritional deficiencies are more prevalent and advanced, has not been studied.

### Blood Transfusion

Although transfusion of donor RBCs can ameliorate many SCD complications, blood transfusions are associated with many complications, including iron overload and alloimmunization. Blood transfusion is limited to certain indications such as secondary stroke prophylaxis and cannot be routinely used in all patients. SCD patients who received regular blood transfusions in the Stroke Prevention (STOP) Trial for Sickle Cell Anemia had significant improvements in weight, height, and BMI.[87] This positive effect possibly resulted from amelioration of anemia, which is a major contributor to the increased energy expenditure in SCD. REE increased in five SCD patients who received a single blood transfusion,[88] although the exact mechanisms by which blood transfusions improve growth in SCD remain unclear.

## FOLLOW-UP AND SUMMARY

The clinical manifestations of SCD involve chronic hemolytic anemia and recurrent, unpredictable bouts of pain related primarily to vaso-occlusion and bone infarction. Patients also experience increased numbers of infections and frequent hospitalizations. All of these factors contribute to hypermetabolism, increased protein and bone turnover, and enhanced REE. Despite their increased caloric needs, many children with SCD have poor dietary intake, especially when ill. These factors contribute to the progressive growth delay in SCD that starts as early as 6 months of age.

The significance of the various micronutrients that are low in SCD patients and their relationship to growth and complications such as stroke are not completely understood. More studies are needed to define these relationships more precisely and to determine the benefit of micronutrient supplementation. Treatments that minimize the anemia and vaso-occlusive episodes, such as hydroxyurea or blood transfusions, allow for growth improvement, especially if initiated early in life. As more infants are started on hydroxyurea early in life, the growth patterns in SCD may change. Additional nutrition interventions in SCD therapy are under investigation. The effect of these interventions in the developing countries, where SCD is common and nutritional deficiencies are prevalent, is unknown and needs to be studied.

### References


1. Ashley-Koch A, Yang Q, Olney RS. Sickle hemoglobin (HbS) allele and sickle cell disease: a HuGE review. *Am J Epidemiol.* 2000; 151:839.
2. Odame I. Developing a global agenda for sickle cell disease: report of an international symposium and workshop in Cotonou, Republic of Benin. *Am J Prev Med.* 2010; 38(4 Suppl):S571.
3. Vichinsky EP, Styles LA, Colangelo LH, Wright EC, Castro O, Nickerson B. Acute chest syndrome in sickle cell disease: clinical presentation and course. Cooperative Study of Sickle Cell Disease. *Blood.* 1997; 89:1787.
4. Wong WY, Overturf GD, Powars DR. Infection caused by *Streptococcus pneumoniae* in children with sickle cell disease: epidemiology, immunologic mechanisms, prophylaxis, and vaccination. *Clin Infect Dis.* 1992; 14:1124.
5. Adams R, McKie V, Nichols F, et al. The use of transcranial ultrasonography to predict stroke in sickle cell disease. *N Engl J Med.* 1992; 326:605.
6. Nath KA, Hebbel RP. Sickle cell disease: renal manifestations and mechanisms. *Nat Rev Nephrol.* 2015; 11:161.
7. Minniti CP, Delaney KM, Gorbach AM, et al. Vasculopathy, inflammation, and blood flow in leg ulcers of patients with sickle cell anemia. *Am J Hematol.* 2014; 89:1.
8. Fadugbagbe AO, Gurgel RQ, Mendonca CQ, Cipolotti R, dos Santos AM, Cuevas LE. Ocular manifestations of sickle cell disease. *Ann Trop Paediatr.* 2010; 30:19.
9. Platt OS, Rosenstock W, Espeland MA. Influence of sickle hemoglobinopathies on growth and development. *N Engl J Med.* 1984; 311:7.
10. Henderson RA, Saavedra JM, Dover GJ. Prevalence of impaired growth in children with homozygous sickle cell anemia. *Am J Med Sci.* 1994; 307:405.
11. Serjeant GR, Singhal A, Hambleton IR. Sickle cell disease and age at menarche in Jamaican girls: observations from a cohort study. *Arch Dis Child.* 2001; 85:375.
12. Abbasi AA, Prasad AS, Ortega J, Congco E, Oberleas D. Gonadal function abnormalities in sickle cell anemia: studies in adult male patients. *Ann Intern Med.* 1976; 85:601.
13. Phebus CK, Gloninger MF, Maciak BJ. Growth patterns by age and sex in children with sickle cell disease. *J Pediatr.* 1984; 105:28.

14. McCormack MK, Dicker L, Katz SH, et al. Growth patterns of children with sickle-cell disease. *Hum Biol.* 1976; 48:429.
15. Kramer MS, Rooks Y, Washington LA, Pearson HA. Pre- and postnatal growth and development in sickle cell anemia. *J Pediatr.* 1980; 96:857.
16. Barden EM, Kawchak DA, Ohene-Frempong K, Stallings VA, Zemel BS. Body composition in children with sickle cell disease. *Am J Clin Nutr.* 2002; 76:218.
17. Stevens MC, Maude GH, Cupidore L, Jackson H, Hayes RJ, Serjeant GR. Prepubertal growth and skeletal maturation in children with sickle cell disease. *Pediatrics.* 1986; 78:124.
18. Serjeant GR, Ashcroft MT. Delayed skeletal maturation in sickle cell anemia in Jamaica. *Johns Hopkins Med J.* 1973; 132:95.
19. Zemel BS, Kawchak DA, Ohene-Frempong K, Schall JI, Stallings VA. Effects of delayed pubertal development, nutritional status, and disease severity on longitudinal patterns of growth failure in children with sickle cell disease. *Pediatr Res.* 2007; 61(Pt 1):607.
20. Singhal A, Thomas P, Cook R, Wierenga K, Serjeant G. Delayed adolescent growth in homozygous sickle cell disease. *Arch Dis Child.* 1994; 71:404.
21. Olambiwonnu NO, Penny R, Frasier SD. Sexual maturation in subjects with sickle cell anemia: studies of serum gonadotropin concentration, height, weight, and skeletal age. *J Pediatr.* 1975; 87:459.
22. Buison AM, Kawchak DA, Schall JI, et al. Bone area and bone mineral content deficits in children with sickle cell disease. *Pediatrics.* 2005; 116:943.
23. Meeuwes M, Souza de Carvalho TF, Cipolotti R, et al. Bone mineral density, growth, pubertal development and other parameters in Brazilian children and young adults with sickle cell anaemia. *Trop Med Int Health.* 2013; 18:1539.
24. Nelson DA, Rizvi S, Bhattacharyya T, Ortega J, Lachant N, Swerdlow P. Trabecular and integral bone density in adults with sickle cell disease. *J Clin Densitom.* 2003; 6:125.
25. Singhal A, Gabay L, Serjeant GR. Testosterone deficiency and extreme retardation of puberty in homozygous sickle-cell disease. *West Indian Med J.* 1995; 44:20.
26. Parshad O, Stevens MC, Preece MA, Thomas PW, Serjeant GR. The mechanism of low testosterone levels in homozygous sickle-cell disease. *West Indian Med J.* 1994; 43:12.
27. Collett-Solberg PF, Fleenor D, Schultz WH, Ware RE. Short stature in children with sickle cell anemia correlates with alterations in the IGF-I axis. *J Pediatr Endocrinol Metab.* 2007; 20:211.
28. Nunlee-Bland G, Rana SR, Houston-Yu PE, Odonkor W. Growth hormone deficiency in patients with sickle cell disease and growth failure. *J Pediatr Endocrinol Metab.* 2004; 17:601.
29. el-Hazmi MA, Bahakim HM, al-Fawaz I. Endocrine functions in sickle cell anaemia patients. *J Trop Pediatr.* 1992; 38:307.
30. Evliyaoglu N, Kilinc Y, Sargin O. Thyroid functions in mild and severe forms of sickle cell anemia. *Acta Paediatr Jpn.* 1996; 38:460.
31. Malinauskas BM, Gropper SS, Kawchak DA, Zemel BS, Ohene-Frempong K, Stallings VA. Impact of acute illness on nutritional status of infants and young children with sickle cell disease. *J Am Diet Assoc.* 2000; 100:330.
32. Singhal A, Parker S, Linsell L, Serjeant G. Energy intake and resting metabolic rate in preschool Jamaican children with homozygous sickle cell disease. *Am J Clin Nutr.* 2002; 75:1093.
33. Gray NT, Bartlett JM, Kolasa KM, Marcuard SP, Holbrook CT, Horner RD. Nutritional status and dietary intake of children with sickle cell anemia. *Am J Pediatr Hematol Oncol.* 1992; 14:57.
34. Akohoue SA, Shankar S, Milne GL, et al. Energy expenditure, inflammation, and oxidative stress in steady-state adolescents with sickle cell anemia. *Pediatr Res.* 2007; 61:233.
35. Kopp-Hoolihan LE, van Loan MD, Mentzer WC, Heyman MB. Elevated resting energy expenditure in adolescents with sickle cell anemia. *J Am Diet Assoc.* 1999; 99:195.
36. Williams R, Olivi S, Li CS, et al. Oral glutamine supplementation decreases resting energy expenditure in children and adolescents with sickle cell anemia. *J Pediatr Hematol Oncol.* 2004; 26:619.
37. Hibbert JM, Creary MS, Gee BE, Buchanan ID, Quarshie A, Hsu LL. Erythropoiesis and myocardial energy requirements contribute to the hypermetabolism of childhood sickle cell anemia. *J Pediatr Gastroenterol Nutr.* 2006; 43:680.
38. Hibbert JM, Hsu LL, Bhathena SJ, et al. Proinflammatory cytokines and the hypermetabolism of children with sickle cell disease. *Exp Biol Med (Maywood).* 2005; 230:68.
39. Buchowski MS, de la Fuente FA, Flakoll PJ, Chen KY, Turner EA. Increased bone turnover is associated with protein and energy metabolism in adolescents with sickle cell anemia. *Am J Physiol Endocrinol Metab.* 2001; 280:E518.
40. Salman EK, Haymond MW, Bayne E, et al. Protein and energy metabolism in prepubertal children with sickle cell anemia. *Pediatr Res.* 1996; 40:34.
41. Borel MJ, Buchowski MS, Turner EA, Goldstein RE, Flakoll PJ. Protein turnover and energy expenditure increase during exogenous nutrient availability in sickle cell disease. *Am J Clin Nutr.* 1998; 68:607.
42. Rahimy MC, Gangbo A, Ahouignan G, et al. Effect of a comprehensive clinical care program on disease course in severely ill children with sickle cell anemia in a sub-Saharan African setting. *Blood.* 2003; 102:834.
43. Heyman MB, Vichinsky E, Katz R, et al. Growth retardation in sickle-cell disease treated by nutritional support. *Lancet.* 1985; 1(8434):903.
44. VanderJagt DJ, Kanellis GJ, Isichei C, Patuszyn A, Glew RH. Serum and urinary amino acid levels in sickle cell disease. *J Trop Pediatr.* 1997; 43:220.
45. Leonard MB, Zemel BS, Kawchak DA, Ohene-Frempong K, Stallings VA. Plasma zinc status, growth, and maturation in children with sickle cell disease. *J Pediatr.* 1998; 132( Pt 1):467.
46. Fung EB, Kawchak DA, Zemel BS, Ohene-Frempong K, Stallings VA. Plasma zinc is an insensitive predictor of zinc status: use of plasma zinc in children with sickle cell disease. *Nutr Clin Pract.* 2002; 17:365.
47. Brown KH, Peerson JM, Rivera J, Allen LH. Effect of supplemental zinc on the growth and serum zinc concentrations of prepubertal children: a meta-analysis of randomized controlled trials. *Am J Clin Nutr.* 2002; 75:1062.
48. Zemel BS, Kawchak DA, Fung EB, Ohene-Frempong K, Stallings VA. Effect of zinc supplementation on growth and body composition in children with sickle cell disease. *Am J Clin Nutr.* 2002; 75:300.
49. Swe KM, Abas AB, Bhardwaj A, Barua A, Nair NS. Zinc supplements for treating thalassaemia and sickle cell disease. *Cochrane Database Syst Rev.* 2013; (6):CD009415.
50. Vichinsky E, Kleman K, Embury S, Lubin B. The diagnosis of iron deficiency anemia in sickle cell disease. *Blood.* 1981; 58:963.
51. Rodrigues PC, Norton RC, Murao M, Januario JN, Viana MB. Iron deficiency in Brazilian infants with sickle cell disease. *J Pediatr (Rio J).* 2011; 87:405.
52. Kassim A, Thabet S, Al-Kabban M, Al-Nihari K. Iron deficiency in Yemeni patients with sickle-cell disease. *East Mediterr Health J.* 2012; 18:241.
53. Pellegrini Braga JA, Kerbauy J, Fisberg M. Zinc, copper and iron and their interrelations in the growth of sickle cell patients. *Arch Latinoam Nutr.* 1995; 45:198.
54. Prasad AS, Ortega J, Brewer GJ, Oberleas D, Schoomaker EB. Trace elements in sickle cell disease. *JAMA.* 1976; 235:2396.
55. Natta CL, Chen LC, Chow CK. Selenium and glutathione peroxidase levels in sickle cell anemia. *Acta Haematol.* 1990; 83:130.
56. Kilinc Y. Plasma, erythrocyte and urinary selenium levels in sickle cell homozygotes and traits. *Turk J Pediatr.* 1993; 35:105.
57. Dougherty KA, Schall JI, Kawchak DA, et al. No improvement in suboptimal vitamin A status with a randomized, double-blind, placebo-controlled trial of vitamin A supplementation in children with sickle cell disease. *Am J Clin Nutr.* 2012; 96:932.
58. Schall JI, Zemel BS, Kawchak DA, Ohene-Frempong K, Stallings VA. Vitamin A status, hospitalizations, and other outcomes in young children with sickle cell disease. *J Pediatr.* 2004; 145:99.
59. Villamor E, Fawzi WW. Vitamin A supplementation: implications for morbidity and mortality in children. *J Infect Dis.* 2000; 182(Suppl 1):S122.
60. Spiro A, Buttriss JL. Vitamin D: an overview of vitamin D status and intake in Europe. *Nutr Bull.* 2014; 39:322.
61. Buison AM, Kawchak DA, Schall J, Ohene-Frempong K, Stallings VA, Zemel BS. Low vitamin D status in children with sickle cell disease. *J Pediatr.* 2004; 145:622.
62. Rovner AJ, Stallings VA, Kawchak DA, Schall JI, Ohene-Frempong K, Zemel BS. High risk of vitamin D deficiency in children with sickle cell disease. *J Am Diet Assoc.* 2008; 108:1512.
63. Tayo BO, Akingbola TS, Salako BL, et al. Vitamin D levels are low in adult patients with sickle cell disease in Jamaica and West Africa. *BMC Hematol.* 2014; 14:12.
64. Lal A, Fung EB, Pakbaz Z, Hackney-Stephens E, Vichinsky EP. Bone mineral density in children with sickle cell anemia. *Pediatr Blood Cancer.* 2006; 47:901.
65. El-Hajj Fuleihan G, Nabulsi M, Tamim H, et al. Effect of vitamin D replacement on musculoskeletal parameters in school children: a randomized controlled trial. *J Clin Endocrinol Metab.* 2006; 91:405.
66. Adewoye AH, Chen TC, Ma Q, et al. Sickle cell bone disease: response to vitamin D and calcium. *Am J Hematol.* 2008; 83:271.
67. Lee MT, Licursi M, McMahon DJ. Vitamin D deficiency and acute vaso-occlusive complications in children with sickle cell disease. *Pediatr Blood Cancer.* 2015; 62:643.
68. Osunkwo I, Ziegler TR, Alvarez J, et al. High dose vitamin D therapy for chronic pain in children and adolescents with sickle cell disease: results of a randomized double blind pilot study. *Br J Haematol.* 2012; 159:211.
69. Lopez R, Shimizu N, Cooperman JM. Recurrent folic acid deficiency in sickle cell disease. *Am J Dis Child.* 1973; 125:544.
70. al-Momen AK. Diminished vitamin B12 levels in patients with severe sickle cell disease. *J Intern Med.* 1995; 237:551.
71. Kennedy TS, Fung EB, Kawchak DA, Zemel BS, Ohene-Frempong K, Stallings VA. Red blood cell folate and serum vitamin B12 status in children with sickle cell disease. *J Pediatr Hematol Oncol.* 2001; 23:165.
72. Rabb LM, Grandison Y, Mason K, Hayes RJ, Serjeant B, Serjeant GR. A trial of folate supplementation in children with homozygous sickle cell disease. *Br J Haematol.* 1983; 54:589.
73. D'Angelo A, Selhub J. Homocysteine and thrombotic disease. *Blood.* 1997; 90:1.
74. Ohene-Frempong K, Weiner SJ, Sleeper LA, et al. Cerebrovascular accidents in sickle cell disease: rates and risk factors. *Blood.* 1998; 91:288.
75. Balasa VV, Kalinyak KA, Bean JA, Stroop D, Gruppo RA. Hyperhomocysteinemia is associated with low plasma pyridoxine levels in children with sickle cell disease. *J Pediatr Hematol Oncol.* 2002; 24:374.
76. Rodriguez-Cortes HM, Griener JC, Hyland K, et al. Plasma homocysteine levels and folate status in children with sickle cell anemia. *J Pediatr Hematol Oncol.* 1999; 21:219.
77. Nelson MC, Zemel BS, Kawchak DA, et al. Vitamin B6 status of children with sickle cell disease. *J Pediatr Hematol Oncol.* 2002; 24:463.
78. Zimmerman SA, Ware RE. Inherited DNA mutations contributing to thrombotic complications in patients with sickle cell disease. *Am J Hematol.* 1998; 59:267.
79. Charache S, Terrin ML, Moore RD, et al. Effect of hydroxyurea on the frequency of painful crises in sickle cell anemia. Investigators of the Multicenter Study of Hydroxyurea in Sickle Cell Anemia. *N Engl J Med.* 1995; 332:1317.
80. Hankins JS, Helton KJ, McCarville MB, Li CS, Wang WC, Ware RE. Preservation of spleen and brain function in children with sickle cell anemia treated with hydroxyurea. *Pediatr Blood Cancer.* 2008; 50:293.
81. Voskaridou E, Christoulas D, Bilalis A, et al. The effect of prolonged administration of hydroxyurea on morbidity and mortality in adult patients with sickle cell syndromes: results of a 17-year, single-center trial (LaSHS). *Blood.* 2010; 115:2354.

82. Yawn BP, Buchanan GR, Afenyi-Annan AN, et al. Management of sickle cell disease: summary of the 2014 evidence-based report by expert panel members. *JAMA*. 2014; 312:1033.
83. Wang WC, Helms RW, Lynn HS, et al. Effect of hydroxyurea on growth in children with sickle cell anemia: results of the HUG-KIDS Study. *J Pediatr.* 2002; 140:225.
84. Rana S, Houston PE, Wang WC, et al. Hydroxyurea and growth in young children with sickle cell disease. *Pediatrics*. 2014; 134:465.
85. Hankins JS, Ware RE, Rogers ZR, et al. Long-term hydroxyurea therapy for infants with sickle cell anemia: the HUSOFT extension study. *Blood*. 2005; 106:2269.
86. Fung EB, Barden EM, Kawchak DA, Zemel BS, Ohene-Frempong K, Stallings VA. Effect of hydroxyurea therapy on resting energy expenditure in children with sickle cell disease. *J Pediatr Hematol Oncol.* 2001; 23:604.
87. Wang WC, Morales KH, Scher CD, et al. Effect of long-term transfusion on growth in children with sickle cell anemia: results of the STOP trial. *J Pediatr.* 2005; 147:244.
88. Harmatz P, Heyman MB, Cunningham J, et al. Effects of red blood cell transfusion on resting energy expenditure in adolescents with sickle cell anemia. *J Pediatr Gastroenterol Nutr.* 1999; 29:127.

# 35 Gastrointestinal Disorders of Infancy and Childhood

MICHAEL FARRELL, ALISON CASSIN, AND REBECCA WILHELM

For a child to grow and develop normally, food must be ingested, digested, and absorbed. The gastrointestinal (GI) tract is crucial in this process. This chapter describes primary and secondary conditions that interfere with the normal digestive and absorptive functions of the GI tract. The past decade has seen the development of a variety of nutritional support modalities that allow children with any type of gastroenterological dysfunction to develop normally. An understanding of the physiology of digestion and the pathophysiology of GI diseases allows selection of the appropriate method of nutritional support.

Nutritional problems are common in children with neuromotor disorders and other chronic conditions. The most frequent nutritional problems are inadequate nutrient intake, obesity, constipation, nutrient-drug interactions, and inadequate standards with which to evaluate the growth and adequacy of nutrient intake.[1] Adequate nutrition begins with ingestion of the appropriate amounts and types of calories. Infants with chronic medical and developmental disorders often have difficulty ingesting adequate nutrients. This may be related to oral-motor dysfunction, a decreased level of consciousness, or spasticity (see Chapter 24). The practitioner must remember that feeding difficulties may be the initial manifestation of a chronic condition, neurological or otherwise. Regardless of the etiology, malnutrition adversely affects the quality of life of children and adults with cerebral palsy and other chronic neurological conditions.[2]

## GASTROESOPHAGEAL REFLUX

After ingestion, food must be processed through the stomach and propelled into the intestine, where digestion and absorption take place. Vomiting is a common pediatric problem and must be considered a symptom, not a diagnosis. The differential diagnosis of vomiting is vast and encompasses many serious disorders. Gastroesophageal reflux (GER), the spontaneous passage of gastric contents from the stomach into the esophagus, is the most common cause of vomiting in infants.[3] In most infants, it is a benign disorder; in infants and children with underlying neurological dysfunction, however, it is often a major problem that interferes with adequate nutrition and the quality of life.

### Biochemical and Clinical Abnormalities

Certain signs and symptoms warn of potentially serious conditions. Vomiting in the neonate must always be investigated. Bilious or projectile vomiting mandates the exclusion of anatomic disorders such as malrotation or pyloric stenosis. Failure to thrive and fluid and electrolyte disturbances such as metabolic alkalosis or metabolic acidosis are worrisome and warrant further evaluation. Prolonged vomiting demands the exclusion of intracranial disorders, anatomic abnormalities, and other systemic disorders such as cardiac or renal failure. However, most infants have GER, the effortless postprandial spitting or regurgitation of feedings with no associated symptoms. In several studies, up to 50% of infants 2 months of age vomited more than two times per day. Regurgitation tends to peak at about 4 months of age and begins to improve spontaneously at 6 to 7 months of age; most cases resolve by the second year of life.[4,5] The regurgitation is the result of an immature lower esophageal sphincter and inappropriate transient relaxation of the sphincter.[6,7]

Carré[8] was one of the first to study the natural history of GER; 60% of infants were found to improve spontaneously by 18 months of age, and only 10% developed severe complications. Numerous subsequent studies have confirmed the benign nature of infantile GER.[4,9–11] Simple advice regarding formula selection, feeding techniques, thickened feedings, avoidance of tobacco smoke, and proper positioning can improve symptoms in a substantial number of infants.[12]

### Factors To Be Considered in Nutrition Evaluation

When vomiting persists, food allergy may be considered, and a cow's milk formula may be changed to a soy-based formula. Approximately 10% to 15% of GER has been attributed to protein allergy. Risk factors for the presence of allergy include multisystem involvement and a personal or family history of atopy. The emphasis should be on changing the protein content of the formula because this is the allergenic component. A hydrolyzed protein or, very rarely, an elemental formula may be necessary.[13–15] A definite response should be noted within 1 to 2 weeks; if vomiting persists after several appropriate formula changes, other causes should be sought (see Chapter 3). During the time of formula manipulation, adequate nutrition must be maintained. Prolonged hypocaloric or clear liquid intake is never appropriate for an infant.[16–23]

### Management

A detailed feeding history must be obtained. The volume and frequency of feeding and the formula concentration must be examined. There is a tendency, particularly among young mothers, to overfeed infants, which results in postprandial vomiting. The primary treatments for GER are timing and positioning; in 90% of infants, symptoms resolve within the first year.

After feeding, the child should be placed in the supine position, not in an infant seat, because the sitting position increases intra-abdominal pressure and reflux.[24–26] Although the prone position may decrease the amount of reflux, this sleeping position is not recommended because of concern about sudden infant death syndrome.[27]

The use of thickened feedings is controversial; studies have yielded conflicting results. In one study, there was less vomiting, but another found delayed gastric emptying and increased reflux. Commercially thickened formulas are available and may be beneficial.[26,28–32]

Medical therapy for GER is usually expectant and supportive. No data support the routine use of prokinetic agents. Histamine 2 receptor ($H_2$) antagonists or proton pump inhibitors may be used if esophagitis is suspected. Published guidelines outline the approach to the treatment of GER.[33]

The crying, irritable infant presents unique challenges. Crying may or may not be related to esophagitis. An empirical trial of formula change or acid-blocking therapy may be appropriate. A response should occur within 2 weeks.[34–38] It is critical that adequate nutrition for growth and development be provided at all times. However, the child who is *neurologically impaired* presents a different set of problems. Approximately 15% of severely handicapped, institutionalized children have chronic vomiting; 80% have significant GER.[39,40] These children may have myriad symptoms—vomiting, pain, anemia, hypoalbuminemia, malnutrition, and bizarre contortions (i.e., Sandifer syndrome) have been reported[41,42]—and are often at great nutritional risk.[1,43,44] Any neurologically impaired child with anemia should be investigated for iron deficiency. If iron deficiency is documented, it is likely that blood loss from esophagitis is the source. The neurologically impaired child is also at risk for aspiration and pneumonia from oropharyngeal incoordination and from GER.[45] Factors that increase the risk of severe GER include scoliosis, severe impairment, nonambulatory status, and intractable seizures.

Medical therapy may not be very effective for these children. In one study, there was a mortality rate of approximately 20% associated with medical therapy and a poor response by the remaining patients.[46] These studies were performed before proton pump inhibitors became available.

Surgery frequently is the only method for controlling severe GER.[47] The preferred surgical procedure is fundoplication, with or without a gastrostomy. The most common techniques in the United States are the Nissen or Thal fundoplications; they may be performed by an open or a laparoscopic approach.[48–54] However, before a child undergoes an antireflux procedure, there should be a vigorous trial of aggressive medical therapy, and the nutrition status must be assessed and improved. The esophagitis is controlled with $H_2$ blockers or proton pump inhibitors. Emerging data indicate that proton pump inhibitors are the preferred therapy for esophagitis.[55–60] If gastric emptying is delayed or other motility disturbances are present, metoclopramide or low-dose erythromycin may improve motility.[60,61] Cisapride is no longer available in the United States; it was withdrawn from the market because of concerns about cardiac arrhythmias.[62,63]

Short-term nasojejunal feedings have been used to promote positive nitrogen balance and weight gain and to correct the iron deficiency anemia and hypoalbuminemia so often found in these patients before surgery. Long-term nasojejunal feedings are not practical; the tubes become dislodged and must be replaced radiologically. If fundoplication is not an option, a surgically placed jejunostomy will allow adequate nutritional support; intensive acid suppression therapy should continue. Fundoplication is effective in approximately 90% of patients; for those requiring a second operation, the success rate is 72%.[50] The laparoscopic approach has decreased complications and the length of the postoperative recovery period. The most common complications are retching and gagging and dumping syndrome.[64] These can be treated by continuous feedings with a low-carbohydrate formula.[65,66]

Children who are *neurologically impaired* are often referred for gastrostomy because of feeding difficulty. The gastrostomy tube may be placed surgically, endoscopically, or radiologically. Consideration must be given to excluding GER. If the child has a history of vomiting or other symptoms suggestive of chronic reflux, a pH study should be performed to exclude significant reflux. In the patient with minimal reflux, the placement of a gastrostomy tube by any means may reduce the symptoms of reflux. If necessary, a fundoplication can be done at a later date. The decision to place a gastrostomy tube in a neurologically impaired child is complex and should involve the nutritionist, the physician, the surgeon, and the child's primary caregivers.

### Follow-up

With intensive medical care and nutritional support, symptoms improve in approximately 85% of neurologically impaired children. Children with chronic esophagitis are at risk for development of Barrett's esophagus, a premalignant condition.[67,68] There is increasing evidence that long-term esophagitis is a causative factor in the development of adenocarcinoma of the esophagus. Affected children should undergo periodic endoscopic surveillance.[69,70]

## LIVER DISEASE

Chronic liver disease is relatively rare in the pediatric age group. The estimated incidence of neonatal cholestatic liver diseases—neonatal hepatitis, biliary atresia, biliary hypoplasia, and various metabolic disorders—is 1 case in 8000 to 10,000 live births. However, liver transplantation has extended the lives of many of these children, and the practitioner may encounter them before or after transplantation. Growth failure is a frequent complication of chronic liver disease.[71] There are very few medical therapies for these disorders, and liver transplantation has become the major treatment.[72] Donor availability is a major limitation and is a function of recipient weight; maintaining an optimal nutritional status is therefore crucial. Despite the use of techniques such as splitting the donor liver and those of living related donors, donor availability remains the major limiting factor.[73,74]

### Biochemical and Clinical Abnormalities

Liver diseases encountered in infants and children usually have a significant cholestatic component.[75] Serum total and direct bilirubin are elevated, as are the aminotransferases. Bile flow is obstructed from the hepatocyte into the biliary system and hence into the intestine; there is a marked decrease in the concentration of intraluminal bile acids, often below the critical concentration necessary for micelle formation and fat absorption.[76] The result is malabsorption of fat and fat-soluble vitamins. These patients, like many infants with chronic disease, may also have anorexia, which results in protein-calorie malnutrition, as well as specific nutrient deficiencies.

The infant with biliary atresia is usually normal at birth. The disease is the result of postnatal obliteration of extrahepatic and intrahepatic ducts. Symptoms usually begin at 3 to 4 weeks of age; hence, jaundice in any infant at that age, even if breast-fed, mandates a fractionated bilirubin test. Hepatic portoenterostomy (the Kasai procedure) attempts to restore bile flow in the infant with biliary atresia.[77] It is successful in approximately 35% of cases. The earlier the procedure is performed, the greater the chance for success.[78] However, even if bile drainage is established, cholestasis often persists despite declining serum bilirubin concentrations. The natural history of these disorders is progression to cirrhosis and end-stage liver disease. As the seriousness of the liver disease increases, ascites develops. The child becomes very sensitive to fluid and sodium. The ongoing destruction of functioning liver cells makes processing of nutrients difficult. Glycogen stores are limited, and glyconeogenesis may be impaired; hypoglycemia is a serious risk. Production of coagulation factors is decreased, and this is compounded by vitamin K deficiency. Nutrition intervention must occur as soon as possible.

### Factors To Be Considered in Nutrition Evaluation

The long-chain fatty acids are poorly absorbed in the absence of bile acids. Medium-chain triglycerides (MCT) do not require micelle formation and are absorbed into the portal system directly. Any formula used in cholestatic liver disease should contain sufficient long-chain fats to prevent essential fatty acid deficiency and should use MCT as a caloric source. Portagen, a milk-based powder with MCT, has been used frequently but has several limitations. Its linoleic acid content is suboptimal, and essential fatty deficiency has been reported in infants with cholestatic liver disease.[79] Hepatic conversion of essential precursor fatty acids into their long-chain metabolites may be impaired with increasing severity of liver disease.[80,81] Pediatric patients with cholestatic diseases often have increased energy needs due to both malabsorption and the underlying disease; however the mechanisms are not well understood.[71,82] A formula containing approximately half MCT oil and half long-chain fats, with 10% to 12% of the total calories as linoleic acid (e.g., Pregestimil, Alimentum), is preferable. No controlled studies support the superiority of high-branched-chain amino acid diets. They may be useful in the treatment of acute decompensation and/or encephalopathy, but the lack of data on their efficacy and their cost preclude routine use for children with chronic liver disease.

Nutrition and growth must be monitored carefully; any deviation from established percentiles must be investigated promptly. Nutrition status is difficult to assess because weight may be affected by edema, ascites, and organomegaly. Anthropometric measurements may be unreliable because of fluid retention. Linear growth and growth velocity are the best indicators.

### Management

Breast-feeding should be encouraged and allowed as long as the infant is gaining weight appropriately. If weight gain decreases, supplementation with an MCT-containing formula should be initiated. The caloric intake of any infant who is failing to gain weight appropriately should be assessed; if it is inadequate, supplementation should be begun. Although a gastrostomy tube may be placed, in the face of portal hypertension there frequently is peristomal variceal bleeding. We prefer nasogastric feeding, in which small-bore Silastic or polyurethane tubes are inserted and the formula is delivered continuously throughout a specified portion of the day to provide the needed calories. The use of small, soft tubes decreases the chances of variceal bleeding. Oral feedings should continue during the tube feeding. Ascites and organomegaly may limit the gastric capacity and the respiratory effort; hence, smaller feeds may be better tolerated. If weight gain does not occur on the 20 cal/oz formula, caloric density may be increased by the addition of Polycose or MCT. The formula may be concentrated, but adequate free water must be provided. Most infants can tolerate a protein concentration of 2.5 to 3 g/kg/day. If necessary, concentration of the formula to 30 cal/oz is possible. Because a balanced diet for growth is essential, close dietary follow-up is mandatory.

Specific metabolic disorders such as galactosemia (see Chapter 49) and tyrosinemia (see Chapter 40) require strict dietary control and elimination of the offending nutrient. Tyrosinemia is a recessively inherited metabolic liver and kidney disease that results from fumarylacetoacetate deficiency. It is a prime example of a metabolic disorder that can be successfully treated by a combined nutritional and pharmacological approach. Dietary restriction alone is not very successful; infants often develop liver failure. Older children are at risk for the development of cirrhosis and hepatocellular carcinoma. Nitisinone (Orfadin) is an inhibitor of tyrosine degradation at the 4-hydroxyphenylpyruvate dioxygenase step. Its use has resulted in normalization of liver abnormalities and a decreased incidence of liver failure.[83]

## Vitamins

### Vitamin A

Malabsorption results in a fat-soluble vitamin A deficiency. If cholestyramine is being administered in an attempt to control pruritus, further vitamin malabsorption may occur.[84] The usual supplement is 5000 to 15,000 units per day of water-miscible compound (Aquasol A). Clinical vitamin A deficiency also occurs despite supplementation if a zinc deficiency is present.[85] However, because vitamin A toxicity may occur, the serum concentration should be monitored; the goal is 400 to 500 μg/mL. If cholestasis resolves, supplementation should be promptly discontinued because of the risk of vitamin A toxicosis.

### Vitamin D

Vitamin D is essential for bone formation and for calcium and phosphorus homeostasis. Deficiency of vitamin D results in osteopenia, rickets, and fractures. Exposure to sunshine should be encouraged as a major source of vitamin D because orally administered vitamin $D_2$ is poorly absorbed in cholestasis. The vitamin D metabolites, 25-hydroxyvitamin D (25-OHD) and 1,25-dihydroxyvitamin D, are more polar compounds and are therefore are better absorbed. The serum concentration of 25-OHD level is the best indicator of total vitamin D status. If there is no response to sunlight exposure or vitamin D supplementation, 25-OHD should be administered at a dose of 5 to 7 μg/kg/day. The serum concentration should be monitored. A bone radiograph or an assessment of bone mineral density also provides an adequate indication of mineralization.

### Vitamin E

Vitamin E requires bile for absorption.[86] A vitamin E deficiency syndrome of peripheral neuropathy, ataxia, and ophthalmoplegia has been described in cholestatic patients.[87,88] The early neurological findings are reversible, but as the deficiency progresses they become irreversible. Vitamin E deficiency occurs before any clinical symptoms are detectable and may develop by 18 months of age. The initial clinical findings are loss of deep tendon reflexes and loss of vibratory sense.

Vitamin E supplementation should be initiated when cholestasis is diagnosed. The patient's ability to absorb vitamin E can be determined by an oral vitamin E tolerance test. Vitamin E levels should be determined at 3-month intervals rather than waiting for clinical deficiency states to develop. Because vitamin E is transported in serum by the lipid fraction, the ratio of serum vitamin E to total lipid should be determined.[87] A ratio of less than 0.8 indicates deficiency, and supplementation should be given with intramuscular vitamin E or oral tocopherol polyethylene glycol-1000 succinate (15 to 25 IU/kg/day).[88] This may also improve vitamin D absorption.

### Vitamin K

Hemorrhage due to vitamin D deficiency may be the initial sign of cholestatic liver disease and can be devastating.[89] Hence, any infant with suspected liver disease should receive supplemental vitamin K.[90,91] Children with cholestasis are particularly at risk for bleeding due to portal hypertension, gastroesophageal varices, and exteriorized conduits. Absorption of either dietary vitamin K or the vitamin K synthesized by intestinal bacteria requires bile acid–containing micelles. The coagulation status should be monitored carefully by measurements of prothrombin time, and vitamin K supplementation should be provided. The initial dose is 2.5 to 5 mg orally every 1 to 3 days. Vitamin $K_1$ has minimal side effects compared with other forms. If no absorption occurs or if intraluminal bile acid concentrations are very low, synthetic water-soluble vitamin $K_3$ (Synkavite) may be necessary. Parenteral vitamin K may be necessary to reverse prolonged prothrombin times in the face of bleeding and in the child who does not improve with oral therapy.

### Water-Soluble Vitamins

Deficiencies of water-soluble vitamins have been reported in adults with liver disease[92]; no data are available for children. It is reasonable to provide a daily dose of a standard multivitamin preparation.

## Minerals

### Iron

Malabsorption of iron, as well as ongoing bleeding, may result in iron deficiency. However, the judicious use of iron supplementation is warranted because iron overload may injure the liver. Early in iron deficiency, the serum ferritin level decreases, followed by an increase in transferrin. The mean corpuscular volume (MCV) decreases as the intracellular iron content decreases. Cirrhosis itself increases serum ferritin concentrations. MCV, the serum iron concentration, and the saturation index should be examined; the saturation index should be kept above 16%.

### Calcium

Calcium is malabsorbed in infants with cholestasis.[92] The exact mechanisms remain to be elucidated, but calcium malabsorption is believed to be caused by binding of calcium in fatty acids, which results in insoluble soaps. Osteopenia is common in children; it is aggravated by corticosteroid therapy. Calcium and vitamin D supplementation should be provided. A dual energy X-ray absorptiometry (DEXA) scan should be obtained to quantitate bone density and tailor therapy.

### Zinc

Zinc deficiency accompanies chronic malnutrition, cirrhosis, and any stress state. However, identification of zinc deficiency is difficult. The serum zinc concentration is at best an imprecise measure of total body zinc status. This concentration is directly correlated with the serum albumin concentration, which is frequently lowered in chronic liver disease. If persistent vitamin A deficiency, poor growth, or persistent anorexia is present, zinc supplementation at 1 mg/kg/day should be begun.[93]

### Copper and Manganese

Copper and manganese accumulate in the liver during cholestasis and may further injure hepatic tissue. Intake should be limited. Chronic liver disease in infants is difficult to manage. Because of fat malabsorption, these infants should be started on formulas containing MCT. Fat-soluble vitamin supplementation should be initiated immediately and should be monitored both clinically and biochemically at 3-month intervals.

## Follow-up

Growth parameters, including height, weight, and anthropometric measurements, should be followed serially. Aggressive intervention is warranted at the first indication of growth failure. With appropriate medical, surgical, and nutritional intervention, children with liver disease can lead normal lives.

## INFLAMMATORY BOWEL DISEASE

The incidence and prevalence of inflammatory bowel disease or IBD (i.e., Crohn's disease and ulcerative colitis) vary widely, depending on the population studied, but appear to be increasing.[94–96] The peak period of onset is the second and third decades of life; approximately 20% of patients are younger than 21 years of age.[97]

### Biochemical and Clinical Abnormalities

A common misconception is that patients with IBD must have overt GI symptoms. In fact, they may present with a variety of extraintestinal problems such as arthritis, fever of unknown origin, uveitis, and cholangitis. In the pediatric population, malnutrition and growth failure frequently complicate IBD. Delayed sexual maturation and decreased linear growth are present in 20% to 30% of affected children.[98–100] Delayed pubarche is caused by both inadequate nutrition and the presence of inflammatory mediators.[101]

Ulcerative colitis often begins with the acute or semiacute onset of bloody diarrhea, which then persists. Often, fever, abdominal pain and cramps, and tenesmus occur. There may be extraintestinal manifestations. Characteristically, mucosal involvement begins at the anal verge and spreads continuously to involve varying amounts of the colon. The diagnosis of ulcerative colitis is established by excluding infectious etiologies and demonstrating the typical endoscopic and histological features.[102]

Crohn's disease, in contrast, usually has an insidious onset and follows a chronic course of relapses and exacerbations. Any portion of the GI tract, from the mouth to the anus, may be involved. Abdominal pain and/or diarrhea are not necessary for the diagnosis, and they are frequently absent initially. Presenting symptoms may include unexplained fever, anemia, growth failure, delayed sexual maturation, amenorrhea, and joint symptoms; perianal disease is frequently a problem, and its presence in a child or adolescent should prompt a search for IBD.[103] The cause of growth failure is multifactorial and includes enteric losses of blood and protein, malabsorption of carbohydrate and fat (depending on the area and length of small bowel involvement), and increased needs due to poor growth.[104] The most common etiology is inadequate caloric intake; several studies have shown that the usual intake in these patients is 60% to 70% of the recommended intake for age.[105] Inappropriate dietary restrictions, postprandial pain, and trace metal deficiencies (especially zinc), along with anorexia, contribute to the reduced nutrient intake.[100] Proinflammatory cytokines also contribute to the anorexia.[106]

### Factors To Be Considered in Nutrition Evaluation

The adolescent or child with suspected IBD should have a detailed nutrition evaluation. Serial height and weight data are invaluable and should be plotted on standard growth charts, with any deviation noted. Growth velocity (in centimeters per year) should be determined and compared with standards because a decline is frequently the initial nutritional indicator; linear growth of less than 4 cm/year in a preadolescent patient is a red flag. The degree of sexual development in adolescents should be estimated and expressed as Tanner ratings (see Appendix 9).

Anthropometric measurements may show decreased subcutaneous fat and depleted somatic protein stores. Useful biochemical determinations include a blood count (looking for evidence of iron deficiency) and measurements of serum albumin and prealbumin to estimate the visceral protein status. Specific nutrient deficiencies may include vitamin $B_{12}$ deficiency if there is extensive ileal involvement. Folic acid depletion results from the rapid turnover of mucosal cells (and sulfasalazine interferes with folate metabolism). Calcium and magnesium deficiencies may occur as a result of malabsorption and the formation of soaps with fatty acids within the intestinal lumen. Zinc deficiency frequently develops as a result of stress, protein losses, and use of corticosteroids, which increase the urinary excretion of zinc. Osteopenia is common both at the time of diagnosis and during therapy; a measure of bone density guides its treatment. Osteopenia correlates with steroid use and nutrition status.[107–109] Depletion of vitamins $B_1$, $B_2$, and $B_6$ may occur, depending on disease activity.[110]

Dietary intake should be evaluated by a 7-day food recall. It frequently is inadequate, but concrete data increase support for nutritional intervention. Energy needs should be estimated; the dietary reference intake (DRI) provides an approximate estimate. Although there may be increased energy requirements due to fever and inflammation, a hypermetabolic state is uncommon. Calories may be used inefficiently because of circulating inflammatory cytokines such as interleukin 1β and tumor necrosis factor-α. If there is no response to what appears to be adequate caloric intake, indirect calorimetry may be used to determine actual energy needs.

### Dietary and Nutrition Management

Management begins with the recognition that nutrition is crucial for patients with IBD.[111] Because no specific foods have been implicated in this disease, no food should be excluded unless there is evidence that it causes problems in a particular patient. Up to two-thirds of patients with IBD report food intolerance; a wide variety of foods are implicated.[112] Lactose intolerance may occur with small bowel inflammation, but it is not more common than in the general population. Lactose should not be restricted unless there is evidence of intolerance.[113,114] If lactose is restricted, adequate calcium and vitamin D intake should be provided. Inappropriate dietary restrictions further compound the nutritional deficits.

There is little specific nutritional therapy for ulcerative colitis.[115] Therapy is medical or surgical, and adequate nutrition should be provided. Chronic steroid therapy hampers normal growth and should be minimized. Patients are at risk for iron deficiency due to chronic bleeding, and sulfasalazine therapy increases the folic acid requirement. Parenteral nutrition has not been shown to be effective in ulcerative colitis and should not be used as a primary therapy. Fish oil has been successful in treating ulcerative colitis; the increased omega-3 fatty acids decrease the production of proinflammatory cytokines.[116] Similar benefits have been reported in Crohn's disease.[117,118]

Crohn's disease has a significant nutritional component. Every attempt should be made to maximize the nutritional intake.[119] If counseling is not effective, supplementation should be considered. The most effective means is nocturnal (10–12 hours) nasogastric feedings.[113] The patient is taught to insert the nasogastric tube nightly, and the formula is infused at a constant rate by means of a pump. The rate of the enteral feedings should be adjusted according to the patient's needs and the average daily oral intake. Intervention must be prompt to maximize growth. The choice of enteral product is controversial. In most cases, a specialized formula is not required. Some patients have lactose intolerance due to small bowel disease and benefit from a nonlactose formula.[120] Studies suggest that an elemental formula may induce remission; the theory is that absorption of intact proteins aggravates inflammation. However, these studies did not compare the effects of improved nutrition alone.[121,122] Studies also have demonstrated that hydrolyzed protein may be as effective as amino acids; the fat content may also be important.[123,124]

There appears to be a better response to nutritional therapy in patients with new-onset disease than in those with frequent relapses. Patients with severe colitis respond less well. Although nutrition therapy alone may induce remission, there is a high dropout rate. A combined nutritional and pharmacological approach is most successful. Newer pharmacological treatments have emphasized steroid sparing and thereby remove the confounding problem of steroid-suppressed growth. A standard formula for caloric supplementation may be used, with the semielemental formulas reserved for refractory situations. If necessary, a gastrostomy tube can be inserted.[125] Additional calories will be needed for catch-up growth.

Total parenteral nutrition (TPN) should be reserved for patients with extensive intestinal resection, those who are obstructed, and postoperative patients. It should not be used as a primary therapy unless the GI tract is nonfunctional. Long-term nutritional needs can be met by nocturnal enteral feedings at home.[126] Severely affected patients who cannot tolerate enteral feedings can be treated with home parenteral nutrition.[127]

### Follow-up

Regardless of which nutrition modality is used, there must be close follow-up; particular attention must be paid to linear growth and sexual maturation. The potential for growth decreases as puberty advances, especially in girls. Close attention must be paid to the adolescent female with growth retardation to maximize adult height before the epiphyses close. If adequate nutrition is provided, most patients with IBD can grow and lead useful, functional lives.

## SHORT BOWEL SYNDROME

The short bowel syndrome is a malabsorptive disorder caused by extensive small bowel resection. Modern surgical techniques and advances in nutritional support have allowed infants to survive previously lethal resections.[128] Loss of absorptive surface is the primary problem, but motility disturbances, bile acid deficiency, and bacterial overgrowth are additional complications. A precise anatomic definition is difficult because measurements are notoriously inaccurate. A useful functional definition is that "the gut is short when it acts short."

The most common etiologies of short gut in infants are congenital anomalies, necrotizing enterocolitis, and congenital vascular malformations. In older children, Crohn's disease is the major cause. Factors affecting outcome include the extent and site of resection, presence or absence of the ileocecal valve, the absorptive capacity of the remaining bowel, and the potential for adaptation as well as the functional state of organs involved in digestion. Abnormalities in the remaining bowel, especially motility dysfunctions, also affect the outcome. Most neonatal intestinal growth occurs in the last trimester, so premature infants have a greater capacity to lengthen their bowel than do older children and adults.[129] The overall survival of these infants is 85% with meticulous nutritional support and carefully planned secondary surgical interventions.[130] The major complications of therapy are those of parenteral nutrition; namely, infection and cholestatic liver disease.

### Biochemical and Clinical Abnormalities

Infants and children with short bowel syndrome are susceptible to dehydration due to massive fluid and electrolyte losses. Specific nutrients are lost depending on the portion of the bowel involved. Anemia occurs as a result of poor iron intake and absorption as well as chronic blood loss. Major complications are cholestasis and progressive liver failure.

### Factors To Be Considered in Nutrition Evaluation

Major factors to be determined include the site and extent of involvement and/or resection because each portion of the bowel has distinct functions. The colon absorbs water and electrolytes and acts as a scavenger, absorbing the fatty acid byproducts of carbohydrate digestion and fermentation. The ileum specifically absorbs vitamin $B_{12}$ and bile acids; these functions cannot be assumed by the jejunum. The jejunum is the major source of carbohydrate and fat absorption, but the ileum can partially adapt to perform these functions. Small bowel involvement results in carbohydrate malabsorption and osmotic diarrhea.[131] Steatorrhea is common; its causes include insufficient mucosal surface area, bacterial overgrowth, and bile acid deficiency due to the lack of ileal absorption and/or hepatic dysfunction. If the colon is absent, there may be excessive loss of cations.[132,133] Losses of sodium (90 to 120 mEq/L) and zinc (8 to 12 mg/L) are the most common problems, but increased losses of magnesium, calcium, and phosphorus also occur.

The infant's nutritional status must be assessed and growth and weight gain closely monitored. The goals of therapy are normal weight gain and growth and adaptation of the remaining bowel. Adaptation is the process by which the remaining intestine compensates for the reduced mucosal absorptive area. Adaptation is proportional to the length of intestine lost and results in taller villi, deeper crypts, and greater bowel caliber.[134,135] The major stimulus to mucosal adaptation is intraluminal nutrients, mediated by a variety of trophic factors.[136–138]

### Nutrition Management

Management is based on the phase of the infant's response and the clinical factors in each phase.

#### Phase 1

Immediately after resection, the major goal is replacement of ongoing fluid and electrolyte losses, which may be extensive. There may be gastric hypersecretion. TPN should be started within the first few postoperative days. Usually, a central venous catheter is required to deliver the necessary volume. Caloric needs should be determined based on age, losses, and nutrition status. Serum electrolyte, urea nitrogen, glucose, and phosphorus concentrations should be monitored frequently. Hepatic status should be evaluated weekly to detect cholestasis. Elevation of serum bile acids may be the first indicator of cholestasis before an increase in serum direct bilirubin or aminotransferase concentration occurs.[139]

#### Phase 2

After initial stabilization has occurred and GI motility returns, enteral feedings must begin. It is critical to begin enteral feeding as soon as possible, even in minuscule amounts because this is a major factor in preventing TPN-associated cholestasis. These feedings are best delivered by continuous infusion through a nasogastric tube, gastrostomy, or jejunostomy, depending on the clinical indications. Stool volume, pH, and reducing substances must be monitored. A stool pH of less than 5 or reducing substances greater than 1% indicates carbohydrate malabsorption and requires adjustment of the feedings. This phase may last for months. The choice of formula is controversial. A hydrolyzed protein, consisting of dipeptides and tripeptides, allows easier absorption and avoids sensitization from absorption of intact protein. Peptides are reabsorbed more efficiently than amino acids. Many patients have lactose intolerance, so lactose should be avoided (see Chapter 50). Formulas containing glucose polymers and sucrose are preferred. The choice of fat is problematic: MCTs are absorbed more efficiently, especially if there is bile acid deficiency. However, long-chain triglycerides appear to provide better mucosal hyperplasia in animal studies.[140] The best approach is to use a formula that contains both fat sources. The preferred formula is semielemental; it should be started at 3% to 5% of caloric needs. Enteral feedings are increased as tolerated, and parenteral nutrition is reduced isocalorically. After 1 or 2 months, if TPN is still required, home therapy should be considered.[141] Intestinal continuity should be reestablished as soon as possible.

#### Phase 3

There are long-term problems associated with treatment of the short bowel syndrome. One complication is feeding refusal after prolonged TPN.[142] The best therapy appears to be prevention of this problem by early introduction of small oral feedings and encouragement of nonnutritive sucking. Patients who make limited progress in weaning from TPN may be candidates for surgical interventions such as tapering enteroplasties or a lengthening procedure.[130] When the patient is gaining weight on enteral feedings and all his or her nutrition needs are met, the central line can be removed. Solid feedings can then begin. Bolus feedings should be gradually introduced as the continuous feedings are decreased. During this phase, the major problems encountered are deficiencies of trace metals and vitamins. If there has been extensive ileal resection, vitamin $B_{12}$ supplementation may be necessary. Fat-soluble vitamin malabsorption resulting in rickets, osteopenia, and other clinical symptoms may be present.[143] Intermittent parenteral supplementation may be necessary. Patients who have steatorrhea and an intact colon are at risk for renal oxalate stone formation and should avoid high-oxalate foods. Medication-nutrient interactions should also be identified. A subset of patients continue to be dependent on TPN; they are at risk for developing end-stage liver disease. Combined liver and small bowel or isolated small bowel transplantation has become feasible. The 1-year survival rate is approximately a 60%, but survival rates are constantly improving. A major limitation is the availability of donors: These patients are more likely to die while waiting than are patients awaiting other solid organ transplants.[144–147]

### Follow-up

With attention to detail and the use of a multidisciplinary team, children can survive their intestinal resection and lead normal lives.

## ENTERAL AND PARENTERAL NUTRITION

Parenteral nutrition provides adequate nutrition to patients who cannot or will not eat. Many patients have a functioning GI tract, but anorexia, weakness, or neurological impairments prevent adequate oral intake. The primary stimulus for gut health and repair is nutrition, specifically intraluminal nutrients. A variety of methods to obtain access to the GI tract and formulas have been developed to provide optimal nutrition regardless of the underlying disease process. However, there is a tendency to view parenteral and enteral nutrition as exclusive rather than complementary therapies. What matters most is that the child receives adequate *total* nutrition and that some of it is administered enterally.

Parenteral nutrition should be initiated only if the child's caloric needs cannot be met through enteral or oral feedings. It may be administered via peripheral or central veins (see Chapter 3). The peripheral route can be started quickly; however, peripheral veins tolerate hyperosmolar fluids poorly, and total caloric support is difficult to achieve. The maximum dextrose concentration that can be administered through a peripheral vein is 10%; use of lipid emulsions is mandatory to achieve reasonable caloric intake. For example, 10% dextrose parenteral fluid provides 0.34 kcal/mL, and 20% lipid emulsion provides 2 kcal/mL. The central venous route should be used for those patients who require prolonged support (Table 35–1). Many complications have been reported, such as infection, thrombosis, pneumothorax, and metabolic derangements. Catheters should be placed only by experienced physicians. Several studies have shown that institutions with nutrition support teams that carefully follow protocols have much lower complication rates.[148]

Nutritional support is begun as soon as the child is identified as being at risk. Methods of nutritional support include oral supplementation, increasing the caloric density of formula, enteral feedings, and parenteral nutrition. Enteral feedings can be nasogastric (continuous or bolus) or nasojejunal, and parenteral nutrition can be total or partial, peripheral or central (see Appendix 6). Risk factors necessitating nutritional intervention include present nutrition status, disease process, anticipated medical or surgical therapy, current caloric intake, and past history. If possible, oral supplementation is recommended as the initial step, either with specific supplements or by increasing the caloric density of the formula. If the caloric density is increased, care must be taken to provide adequate free water to excrete the increased renal solute load.

If oral supplementation is unsuccessful and the GI tract is functional, a nasoenteric tube is placed. Small-bore (5.8-French), soft Silastic catheters are easily inserted and well tolerated; they may be placed in the stomach or jejunum. Nasogastric feedings are simple to administer, and the tube can be placed by the child or by caregivers. Placement in the stomach allows normal digestive processes and a hormonal response. Nasogastric feedings allow greater freedom and mobility for the child; they can be administered as a bolus or continuously. An intact gag reflex is an absolute requirement for intragastric feedings to prevent aspiration.

If prolonged gastric feedings are required, a gastrostomy tube can be placed. The percutaneous endoscopic approach has simplified the placement procedure. Transpyloric feedings are indicated for patients with GER, impaired gag reflex, vocal cord paralysis, gastric motor abnormalities, or intractable vomiting. A weighted tube may be allowed to pass out of the stomach into the small bowel, with its position verified radiographically. Alternatively, the tube may be passed through the pylorus under fluoroscopic or endoscopic guidance. If a gastrostomy tube is in place and jejunal feedings are necessary, the tube can be passed through the gastrostomy tube into the jejunum under fluoroscopy. Jejunal feedings usually are administered continuously for a specified period to meet caloric needs. Oral stimulation is needed during enteral and parenteral feedings (see Chapter 24).

**Table 35–1.** Daily Electrolyte and Mineral Requirements in Total Parental Nutrition

| | Infant | Child or Adult |
|---|---|---|
| Sodium | 2–4 mEq/kg | 1–2 mEq/kg |
| Potassium | 2–3 mEq/kg | 0.5–1.0 mEq/kg |
| Calcium | 3–4 mEq/kg | 1–2 mEq/kg |
| Phosphate | 1–2 mmol/kg | 0.3–1 mmol/kg |
| Magnesium | 0.25–0.5 mEq/kg | 0.25–0.5 mEq/kg |
| Chloride | 2–5 mEq/kg | 2–3 mEq/kg |
| Zinc* | 400 μg/kg (premature)<br>100 μg/kg (term) | 2.5–4 mg*† |
| Copper‡ | 20 μg | 0.5–1.5 μg† |
| Chromium | 0.14–0.2 μg | 10–15 μg† |
| Manganese | 2–10 μg (total) | 0.05–0.2 mg |
| Molybdenum | 0.25 μg/kg | |
| Selenium | 2.0 μg/kg | |

*Increase zinc if there is excessive gastrointestinal loss (8–12 mg/L intestinal fluid).
†Maximum recommended adult concentration.
‡Decrease copper (10 μg/kg) if liver disease is present.

### Follow-up

If nutritional therapy is chosen appropriately and the child's needs are met, children with a wide variety of GI disorders can be discharged from the hospital, grow normally, and lead normal lives. An interdisciplinary team including a nutritionist, nurse, parent, and special educator can facilitate the transition of a child fed by gastrostomy tube to school. Growth, nutrients, oral feeding skills, gastrostomy feeding, behavior, constipation, and positioning should continue to be evaluated as the child matures and develops.[149]

## GUT MICROBIOME

The ecology of the GI tract is rich and complex. The GI tract is sterile at birth but is rapidly colonized with a microbiota that evolves with age and diet changes. Once established, it is difficult to modify but may be altered negatively, through the use of antibiotics, or positively, through the introduction of desirable species (probiotics) or diet modifications providing fuel (prebiotics) for intestinal flora. The intestinal flora contains a wide variety of microorganisms, up to 1000 bacterial species.[150] There is increasing realization that imbalances in the microbiota, or *dysbiosis*, may cause or perpetuate GI illnesses. Evidence suggests a role for the bacterial microbiota in the pathogenesis of certain GI disorders, such as Crohn's disease or irritable bowel syndrome, and in the treatment of others, such as diarrhea and *Clostridium difficile* infection.[151,152]

### Dietary Prebiotics

Certain dietary patterns, such as high-fat and high-sugar diets, may alter GI flora and contribute to chronic illness, including GI disorders. Consumption of prebiotics—nutritional compounds that feed and promote the growth of favorable bacteria—may confer health benefits to the individual. A prebiotic is a selectively fermented ingredient, usually an oligomer such as the soluble fiber inulin, that occurs naturally in plant-based foods or can be taken as a supplement.[153]

### Probiotics as Treatment

Specific organisms may be useful in treating GI illnesses. *Lactobacillus* has been successful in reducing the duration and shedding of organisms in acute infectious diarrhea and in decreasing the effects of *Clostridium difficile* infection.[154,155] Probiotic therapy might be useful in the management of IBD because decreased bacterial diversity is often observed in patients with Crohn's disease and ulcerative colitis.[156,157] Antibiotics have been successful in treating both Crohn's disease and ulcerative colitis, suggesting imbalance of the fecal flora.[158] Remission in ulcerative colitis has been maintained with probiotic therapy. Probiotic bacteria may be antagonistic to *Helicobacter pylori*.[159] There are suggestions that fecal flora imbalances may be responsible in part for the exaggerated acute phase reactions seen in some critically ill patients.[160] Probiotic therapy shows great promise as both a primary and a complementary therapy for a variety of GI ailments, but more research needs to be done.

## References


1. Greecher CP, Cohen IT, Ballantine TV. Survey of nutritional problems encountered in children with neuromotor disorders. *JPEN J Parenter Enteral Nutr.* 1980; 4:490.
2. Sampson-Fang L, Stallings VA, Conaway M, et al. Relationship of nutritional status to health and societal participation in children with cerebral palsy. *J Pediatr.* 2002; 141:637.
3. Sondheimer J. Vomiting. In: Walker WA, Hamilton J, Walker-Smith J, Watkins J, eds. *Pediatric Gastrointestinal Disease: Pathophysiology, Diagnosis, Management.* Hamilton: BC: Decker; 2000.
4. Nelson SP, Chen EH, Syniar GM, Christoffel KK. Prevalence of symptoms of gastroesophageal reflux during infancy: a pediatric practice-based survey. Pediatric Practice Research Group. *Arch Pediatr Adolesc Med.* 1997; 151:569.
5. Miyazawa R, Tomomasa T, Kaneko H, Tachibana A, Ogawa T, Morikawa A. Prevalence of gastro-esophageal reflux–related symptoms in Japanese infants. *Pediatr Int.* 2002; 44:513.
6. Boix-Ochoa J, Canals J. Maturation of the lower esophagus. *J Pediatr Surg.* 1976; 11:749.
7. Vargas JH. Gastroesophageal reflux: mechanisms in infants. *J Pediatr Gastroenterol Nutr.* 1995; 21:479.
8. Carré, J. The natural history of the partial thoracic stomach ("hiatus hernia") in children. *Arch Dis Child.* 1960; 35:481.
9. Martin AJ, Pratt N, Kennedy JD, Ryan P, Ruffin RE, Miles H. Natural history and familial relationships of infant spilling to 9 years of age. *Pediatrics.* 2002; 109:1061.
10. Nelson SP, Chen EH, Syniar GM, Christoffel KK. One-year follow-up of symptoms of gastroesophageal reflux during infancy. Pediatric Practice Research Group. *Pediatrics.* 1998; 102:E67.
11. Osatakul S, Sriplung H, Puetpaiboon A, Junjana CO, Chamnongpakdi S. Prevalence and natural course of gastroesophageal reflux symptoms: a 1-year cohort study in Thai infants. *J Pediatr Gastroenterol Nutr.* 2002; 34:63.
12. Shalaby TM, Orenstein SR. Efficacy of telephone teaching of conservative therapy for infants with symptomatic gastroesophageal reflux referred by pediatricians to pediatric gastroenterologists. *J Pediatr.* 2003; 142:57.
13. American Academy of Pediatrics Committee on Nutrition. Hypoallergenic infant formulas. *Pediatrics.* 2000; 106:346.
14. deBoissieu D, Dupont C. Allergy to extensively hydrolyzed cow's milk proteins in infants: safety and duration of amino acid–based formula. *J Pediatr.* 2002; 141:271.
15. Sicherer S, Noone S, Koerner C, Christie L, Burks A, Sampson HA. Hypoallergenicity and efficacy of an amino acid–based formula in children with cow's milk and multiple food hypersensitivities. *J Pediatr.* 2001; 138:688.
16. Cavataio F, Iacono G, Montalto G, et al. Gastroesophageal reflux associated with cow's milk allergy in infants: which diagnostic examinations are useful? *Am. J Gastroenterol.* 1996; 91:1215.
17. Host A. Cow's milk protein allergy and intolerance in infancy: some clinical, epidemiological and immunological aspects. *Pediatr Allergy Immunol.* 1994; 5(Suppl 5):1.
18. Iacono G, Carroccio A, Cavataio F, et al. Gastroesophageal reflux and cow's milk allergy in infancts: a prospective study. *J Allergy Clin. Immunol.* 1996; 97:822.
19. Kamer B, Chilarski A, Lange A, Piaseczna-Piotrowska A. Gastroesophageal reflux in infants with food allergy. *Med Sci Monit.* 2000; 6:348.
20. Maguzzu G, Scoglio R. Gastrointestinal manifestations of cow's milk allergy. *Ann Allergy Asthma Immunol.* 2002; 89:65.
21. Milocco C, Torre G, Ventura A. Gastro-oesophageal reflux and cows' milk protein allergy. *Arch Dis Child.* 1997; 77:183.
22. Ravelli AM, Tobanelli P, Volpi S, Ugazio AG. Vomiting and gastric motility in infants with cow's milk allergy. *J Pediatr Gastroenterol Nutr.* 2001; 32:59.
23. Salvatore S, Vandenplas Y. Gastroesophageal reflux and cow milk allergy: is there a link? *Pediatrics.* 2002; 110:972.
24. Orenstein SR, Whitington PF. Positioning for prevention of infant gastroesophageal reflux. *J Pediatr.* 1983; 103:534.
25. Orenstein SR, Whitington PF, Orenstein DM. The infant seat as treatment for gastroesophageal reflux. *N Engl J Med.* 1983; 309:760.
26. Orenstein SR, Magill HL, Brooks P. Thickening of infant feedings for therapy of gastroesophageal reflux. *J Pediatr.* 1987; 110:181.
27. American Academy of Pediatrics. Changing concepts of sudden infant death syndrome: implications for infant sleeping environment and sleep position (RE9946). *Pediatrics.* 2000; 105:650.
28. Bailey DJ, Andres JM, Danek GD, Pineiro-Carrero VM. Lack of efficacy of thickened feeding as treatment for gastroesophageal reflux. *J Pediatr.* 1987; 110:187.
29. Iacono G, Vetrano S, Cataldo F, et al. Clinical trial with thickened feeding for treatment of regurgitation in infants. *Dig Liver Dis.* 2002; 34:532.
30. Khoshoo V, Ross G, Brown S, Edell D. Smaller volume, thickened formulas in the management of gastroesophageal reflux in thriving infants. *J Pediatr Gastroenterol Nutr.* 2000; 31:554.
31. Orenstein SR, Shalaby TM, Putnam PE. Thickened feedings as a cause of increased coughing when used as therapy for gastroesophageal reflux in infants. *J Pediatr.* 1992; 121:913.
32. Ramierez-Mayans J, Palacio-del Carmen L, Cervantes-Bustamante R, et al. Nutritional management of children with gastrosophageal reflux: a comparison of two different formulas. *Int Pediatr.* 2003; 18:78.
33. Colletti RB, Christie DL, Orenstein SR. Statement of the North American Society for Pediatric Gastroenterology and Nutrition (NASPGN): indications for pediatric esophageal pH monitoring. *J Pediatr Gastroenterol Nutr.* 1995; 21:253.
34. Sutphen JL. Is it colic or is it gastroesophageal reflux? *J Pediatr Gastroenterol Nutr.* 2001; 33:110.
35. Armstrong K, Previtera N, McCallum R. Medicalizing normality?: banagement of irritability in babies. *J Paediatr Child Health.* 2000; 36:301.
36. Berkowitz D, Naveh Y, Berant M. "Infantile colic" as the sole manifestation of gastroesophageal reflux. *J Pediatr Gastroenterol Nutr.* 1997; 24:231.
37. Heine RG, Jaquiery A, Lubitz L, Cameron DJ, Catto-Smith AG. Role of gastrooesophageal reflux in infant irritability. *Arch Dis Child.* 1995; 73:121.
38. Putnam PE. GERD and crying: cause and effect or unhappy coexistence? *J Pediatr.* 2002; 140:3.
39. Sondheimer JM., Morris BA. Gastroesophageal reflux among severely retarded children. *J Pediatr.* 1979; 94:710.
40. Gangil A, Patwari AK, Bajaj P, Kashyap R, Anand VK. Gastroesophageal reflux disease in children with cerebral palsy. *Indian Pediatr.* 2001; 38:766.
41. Herbst JJ, Johnson DG, Oliveros MA. Gastroesophageal reflux with protein-losing enteropathy and finger clubbing. *Am J Dis Child.* 1976; 130:1256.
42. Sullivan PB. Gastrointestinal problems in the neurologically impaired child. *Baillieres Clin Gastroenterol.* 1997; 11:529.
43. Couriel JM, Bisset R, Miller R, Thomas A, Clarke M. Assessment of feeding problems in neurodevelopmental handicap: a team approach. *Arch Dis Child.* 1993; 69:609.
44. Gisel EG, Patrick J. Identification of children with cerebral palsy unable to maintain a normal nutritional state. *Lancet* 1988; 1:283.
45. Guill MF. Respiratory manifestations of gastroesophageal reflux in children. *J Asthma.* 1995; 32:173.
46. Wilkinson JD, Dudgeon DL, Sondheimer JM. A comparison of medical and surgical treatment of gastroesophageal reflux in severely retarded children. *J Pediatr.* 1981; 99:202.
47. Vane DW, Harmel RP, King DR, Boles ET. The effectiveness of Nissen fundoplication in neurologically impaired children with gastroesophageal reflux. *Surgery.* 1985; 98:662.
48. Bergmeijer JH, Tibboel D, Hazebroek FW. Nissen fundoplication in the management of gastroesophageal reflux occurring after repair of esophageal atresia. *J Pediatr Surg.* 2000; 35:573.
49. Ceriati E, Guarino N, Zaccara A, et al. Gastroesophageal reflux in neurologically impaired children: partial or total fundoplication? *Langenbecks Arch Surg.* 1998; 383:317.
50. Dalla Vecchia LK, Grosfeld JL, West KW, Rescorla FJ, Scherer LR, Engum SA. Reoperation after Nissen fundoplication in children with gastroesophageal reflux: experience with 130 patients. *Ann Surg.* 1997; 226:315.
51. Gatti C, diAbriola GF, Villa M, et al. Esophagogastric dissociation versus fundoplication: which is best for severely neurologically impaired children? *J Pediatr Surg.* 2001; 36:677.
52. Mira-Navarro J, Bayle-Bastos F, Frieyro-Segui M, Garramone N, Gambarini A. Long-term follow-up of Nissen fundoplication. *Eur J Pediatr Surg.* 1994; 4:7.
53. Ostlie DJ, Miller KA, Holcomb GW. Effective Nissen fundoplication length and bougie diameter size in young children undergoing laparoscopic Nissen fundoplication. *J Pediatr Surg.* 2002; 37:1664.
54. Ostlie DJ, Holcomb GW. Laparoscopic fundoplication and gastrostomy. *Semin Laparosc Surg.* 2002; 11:196.
55. Alliet P, Raes M, Gillis P, Zimmermann A. Optimal dose of omeprazole in infants and children. *J Pediatr.* 1994; 124:332.
56. Bohmer C, Niezen-de Boer R, Klinkenberg-Knol E, Meuwissen S. Omeprazole: therapy of choice in intellectually disabled children. *Arch Pediatr Adolesc Med.* 1998; 152:1113.
57. Hassall E, Israel D, Shepherd R, Radke M, Dalvag A, Skold B. Omeprazole for treatment of chronic erosive esophagitis in children: a multicenter study of efficacy, safety, tolerability and dose requirements. International Pediatric Omeprazole Study Group. *J Pediatr.* 2000; 137:800.
58. Pashankar D, Blair GK, Israel DM. Omeprazole maintenance therapy for gastroesophageal reflux disease after failure of fundoplication. *J Pediatr Gastroenterol Nutr.* 2001; 32:145.
59. Varughese LA, Mazur LJ. Is omeprazole helpful in the management of children with reflux oesophagitis? *Arch Dis Child.* 2002; 87:78.
60. Zimmermann AE, Walters JK, Katona BG, Souney PE, Levine D. A review of omeprazole in the treatment of acid-related disorders in children. *Clin Ther.* 2001; 23:660.
61. Hillemeier AC, Lange R, McCallum R, Seashore J, Gryboski J. Delayed gastric emptying in infants with gastroesophageal reflux. *J Pediatr.* 1981; 1981:190.
62. Vandenplas Y. (In)efficacy of cisapride. *J Pediatr.* 2000; 137:288.
63. Bourke B, Drumm B. Cochrane's epitaph for cisapride in childhood gastroesophageal reflux. *Arch Dis Child.* 2002; 86:71.
64. Richards CA, Milla PJ, Andrews PL, Spitz L. Retching and vomiting in neurologically impaired children after fundoplication: predictive preoperative factors. *J Pediatr Surg.* 2001; 36:1401.
65. Khoshoo V, Roberts PL, Loe WA, Golladay ES, Pencharz PB. Nutritional management of dumping syndrome associated with antireflux surgery. *J Pediatr Surg.* 1994; 29:1452.
66. Samuk I, Afriat R, Horne T, Bistritzer T, Barr J, Vinograd I. Dumping syndrome following Nissen fundoplication, diagnosis, and treatment. *J Pediatr Gastroenterol Nutr.* 1996; 23:235.
67. Beddow EC, Wilcox DT, Drake DP, Pierro A, Kiely EM, Spitz L. Surveillance of Barrett's esophagus in children. *J Pediatr Surg.* 1999; 34:88.
68. Roberts IM, Curtis RL, Madara JL. Gastroesophageal reflux and Barrett's esophagus in developmentally disabled patients. *Am J Gastroenterol.* 1986; 81:519.
69. Hoeffel JC, Nihoul-Fekete C, Schmitt M. Esophageal adenocarcinoma after gastroesophageal reflux in children. *Clin Lab Observ.* 1989; 115:259.
70. Lagergren J, Bergsgtrom R, Lindgren A, Nyren O. Symptomatic gastroesophageal reflux as a risk factor for esophageal adenocarcinoma. *N Engl J Med.* 1999; 340:825.
71. Heubi J, Heyman M, Shulman R. The impact of liver disease on growth and nutrition. *J Pediatr Gastroenterol Nutr.* 2002; 35:S55.

72. Shaw BW, Wood RP, Kaufman SS, et al. Liver transplantation therapy for children. *J Pediatr Gastroenterol Nutr.* 1988; 7:157.
73. Spada M, Gridelli B, Colledan M, et al. Extensive use of split liver for pediatric liver transplantation: a single center experience. *Liver Transplant.* 2000; 6:415.
74. Emre S, Schwartz ME, Shneider B, et al. Living related liver transplantation for acute liver failure in children. *Liver Transplant.* 1999; 5:161.
75. Balistreri WF. Pediatric hepatology: a half-century of progress. *Clin. Liver Dis.* 2000; 4:191.
76. Weber A, Roy CC. The malabsorption associated with chronic liver disease in children. *Pediatrics.* 1972; 50:73.
77. Kasai M. Treatment of biliary atresia with special reference to hepatic portoenterostomy and its modifications. *Prog Pediatr Surg.* 1974; 6:5.
78. Chardot C, Carton M, Spire-Bendelac N, et al. Is the Kasai operation still indicated in children older than 3 months diagnosed with biliary atresia? *J Pediatr.* 2001; 138:224.
79. Gourley GR, Farrell P, O'Dell GB. Essential fatty acid deficiency after hepatic portoenterostomy for biliary atresia. *Am J Clin Nutr.* 1982; 36:194.
80. Socha P, Koletzko B, Pawlowska J, Socha J. Essential fatty acid status in children with cholestasis, in relation to serum bilirubin concentration. *J Pediatr.* 1997; 131:700.
81. Socha J, Koletzko B, Swiakowska E, Pawlowska J, Stolarczyk A. Essential fatty acid metabolism in infants with cholestasis. *Acta Paediatr.* 1998; 87:278.
82. Greer R, Lehnert M, Lewindon P, Cleghorn G, Shepherd R. Body composition and components of energy expenditure in children with end-stage liver disease. *J Pediatr Gastroenterol Nutr.* 2003; 36:358.
83. Holme E, Lindstedt S. Nontransplant treatment of tyrosinemia. *Clin Liver Dis.* 2000; 4:805.
84. Ramaccioni V, Soriano HE, Arumugam R, Klish WJ. Nutritional aspects of chronic liver disease and liver transplantation in children. *J Pediatr Gastroenterol Nutr.* 2000; 30:361.
85. Smith JC. The vitamin A-zinc connection. *Ann N Y Acad Sci.* 1980; 355:62.
86. Guggenheim M, Ringel S, Silverman A, Grabert B. Progressive neuromuscular disease in children with chronic cholestasis and vitamin E deficiency: diagnosis and treatment with alpha tocopherol. *J Pediatr.* 1982; 100:51.
87. Sokol RJ, Guggenheim MA, Iannaccone ST, et al. Improved neurologic function after long-term correction of vitamin E deficiency in children with chronic cholestasis. *N Engl J Med.* 1985; 313:1580.
88. Sokol RJ, Butler-Simoin NA, Bettis D, Smith DJ, Silverman A. Tocopherol polyethylene glycol 1000 succinate therapy for vitamin E deficiency during chronic childhood cholestasis: neurologic outcome. *J Pediatr.* 1987; 111:830.
89. Payne NR, Hasegawa DK. Vitamin K deficiency in a newborn: a case report in alpha-1-antitrypsin deficiency and a review of factors predisposing to hemorrhage. *Pediatrics.* 1984; 73:712.
90. Suttie JW. Recent advances in hepatic vitamin K metabolism and function. *Hepatology.* 1987; 7:367.
91. Rossourn J, Labadarios D, Davis M, Williams R. Water soluble vitamins in severe liver disease. *S Afr Med J.* 1979; 54:183.
92. Bengoa JM, Setrin MD, Meredith S, Kelly SE, Shak N, Baker AL. Intestinal calcium absorption and vitamin D status in chronic cholestatic liver disease. *Hepatology.* 1984; 4:261.
93. Barness LA, Mauer AM, Anderson AS. Zinc. *Pediatrics.* 1978; 62:408.
94. Kanof ME, Lake AM, Bayless TM. Decreased height velocity in children and adolescents before the diagnosis of Crohn's disease. *Gastroenterology.* 1988; 95:1523.
95. Kirsner JB. The historical basis of the idiopathic inflammatory bowel disease. *Inflamm Bowel Dis.* 1995; 1:2.
96. Barton JR, Gillon S, Ferguson A. Incidence of Crohn's disease in Scottish children between 1968 and 1983. *Gut.* 1989; 30:618.
97. Whelan G. Epidemiology of inflammatory bowel disease. *Med Clin North Am.* 1990; 74:1.
98. Michner WM, Wyllie R. Management of children and adolescents with inflammatory bowel disease. *Med Clin North Am.* 1990; 74:103.
99. Cezard JP, Touati G, Alberti C, Hugot JP, Brinon C, Czernichow P. Growth in paediatric Crohn's disease. *Horm Res.* 2002; 58(Suppl 1):11.
100. Oliva MM, Lake AM. Nutritional considerations and management of the child with inflammatory bowel disease. *Nutrition.* 1996; 12:151.
101. Ballinger AB, Savage MO, Sanderson IR. Delayed puberty associated with inflammatory bowel disease. *Pediatr Res.* 2002; 53:205.
102. Markowitz J, Daum F, Aiges H, Kahn E, Silverberg M, Fisher SE. Perianal disease in children and adolescents with Crohn's disease. *Gastroenterology.* 1984; 86:829.
103. Kirschner BS. Nutritional consequences of inflammatory bowel disease on growth. *J Am Coll Nutr.* 1988; 7:301.
104. Kelts DG, Grand RJ, Shen G, Watkins JB, Werlin SL, Boehme C. Nutritional basis of growth failure in children and adolescents with Crohn's disease. *Gastroenterology.* 1979; 76:720.
105. Nishi Y, Lifshitz F, Bayne MA, Daum F, Silverberg M, Aiges H. Zinc status and its relation to growth retardation in children with chronic inflammatory bowel disease. *Am J Clin Nutr.* 1980; 33:2613.
106. Grimble RF. Nutrition and cytokine action. *Nutr Res Rev.* 1990; 2:193.
107. Boot AM, Bouquet J, Krenning EP, de Muinick Keizer-Scharma SM. Bone mineral density and nutritional status in children with chronic inflammatory bowel disease. *Gut.* 1998; 42:188.
108. von Westarp C, Thomson ABR, Overton TR, et al. Disorders of mineral and bone metabolism in patients with Crohn's disease. *Can J Gastroenterol.* 1987; 1:11.
109. Cowan FJ, Warner JT, Dunstan FDJ, Evans WD, Gregory JW, Jenkins HR. Inflammatory bowel disease and predisposition to osteopenia. *Arch Dis Child.* 1997; 76:325.
110. Kuroki F, Iida M, Tominaga M, et al. Multiple vitamin status in Crohn's disease: correlation with disease activity. *Dig Dis Sci.* 1993; 38:1614.
111. McIntyre PB, Powell-Tuck J, Lennard-Jones JE, et al. Controlled trial of bowel rest in the treatment of severe acute colitis. *Gut.* 1986; 27:481.
112. Ballegaard M, Bjiergstrom A, Brondum S, et al. Self-reported food intolerance in chronic inflammatory bowel disease. *Scand J Gastroenterol.* 1997; 32:569.
113. Kirschner BS, DeFavaro MV, Jensen W. Lactose malabsorption in adolescents with inflammatory bowel disease. *Gastroenterology.* 1981; 81:829.
114. Mishkin S. Dairy sensitivity, lactose malabsorption, and elimination diets in inflammatory bowel disease. *Am J Clin Nutr.* 1997; 65:564.
115. Kleinman RE, Balistreri WF, Heyman MB, et al. Nutritional support of pediatric patients with inflammatory bowel disease. *J Pediatr Gastroenterol Nutr.* 1989; 8:8.
116. Stenson WF, Cort D, Rodgers J, et al. Dietary supplementation with fish oil in ulcerative colitis. *Ann Intern Med.* 1992; 116:609.
117. Kim Y. Can fish oil maintain Crohn's disease in remission? *Nutr Rev.* 1996; 54:248.
118. Belluzzi A. N-3 fatty acids for the treatment of inflammatory bowel disease. *Proc Nutr Soc.* 2002; 61:391.
119. Morin CL, Roulet M, Roy CC, Weber A. Continuous elemental enteral alimentation in children with Crohn's disease and growth failure. *Gastroenterology.* 1980; 79:1205.
120. Belli DC, Seidman E, Bouthillier L, et al. Chronic intermittent elemental diet improves growth failure in children with Crohn's disease. *Gastroenterology.* 1988; 94:603.
121. Sanderson IR, Udeen S, Davies PSW, Savage MO, Walker-Smith J. Remission induced by an elemental diet in small bowel Crohn's disease. *Arch Dis Child.* 1987; 61:123.
122. Aiges H, Markowitz J, Rosa J, Daum F. Home nocturnal supplemental nasogastric feedings in growth-retarded adolescents with Crohn's disease. *Gastroenterology.* 1989; 97:905.
123. Griffiths AM, Ohlsson A, Sherman PM, Sutherland LR. Meta-analysis of enteral nutrition as a primary treatment of active Crohn's disease. *Gastroenterology.* 1995; 108:1056.
124. Gassull M, Frenandez-Banares F, Cabre E, et al. Fat composition may be a clue to explain the primary therapeutic effect of enteral nutrition in Crohn's disease: results of a double blind randomised multicentre European trial. *Gut.* 2002; 52:164.
125. Cosgrove M, Jenkins HR. Experience of percutaneous endoscopic gastrostomy in children with Crohn's disease. *Arch Dis Child.* 1997; 76:141.
126. Strobel CT, Byrne WJ, Ament ME. Home parenteral nutrition in children with Crohn's disease: an effective management alternative. *Gastroenterology.* 1979; 77:272.
127. Dorney SFA, Ament ME, Berquist WE, Vargas JH, Hassall E. Improved survival in very short small bowel of infancy with use of long term parenteral nutrition. *J Pediatr.* 1985; 107:521.
128. Caniano DA, Starr BS, Ginn-Pease ME. Extensive short-bowel syndrome in neonates in the 1980's. *Surgery.* 1989; 105:119.
129. Touloukian RJ, Walker Smith GJ. Normal intestinal length in preterm infants. *J Pediatr Surg.* 1983; 18:720.
130. Chaet M, Farrell M, Ziegler M, Warner B. Intensive nutritional support and remedial surgical intervention for extreme short bowel syndrome. *J Pediatr Gastroenterol Nutr.* 1994; 19:295.
131. Ameen VZ, Powell GK, Jones VZ. Quantitation of fecal carbohydrate excretion in patients with short bowel syndrome. *Gastroenterology.* 1987; 92:493.
132. Ladefoged K, Olgaard K. Fluid and electrolyte absorption and rennin-angiotensin-aldosterone axis in patients with severe short bowel syndrome. *Scand J Gastroenterol.* 1979; 14:729.
133. Naveh Y, Lightman A, Zinder O. Effect of diarrhea on serum zinc concentrations in infants and children. *J Pediatr.* 1982; 101:730.
134. Warner B. GLP-2 as therapy for the short bowel syndrome. *Gastroenterology.* 2001; 120:1041.
135. O'Brien D, Nelson L, Huang F, Warner B. Intestinal adaptation: structure, function and regulation. *Semin Pediatr Surg.* 2001; 10:56.
136. Lentze MJ. Intestinal adaptation in short-bowel syndrome. *Eur J Pediatr.* 1989; 148:294.
137. Stern L, Erwin C, O'Brien D, Huang F, Warner B. Epidermal growth factor is critical for intestinal adaptation following small bowel resection. *Microsc Res Tech.* 2000; 15:138.
138. Jeppesen PB, Hartmann B, Thulesen J, et al. Glucagon-like peptide 2 improves nutrient absorption and nutritional status in short-bowel patients with no colon. *Gastroenterology.* 2001; 120:806.
139. Balistreri WF, Suchy FJ, Farrell MK, Heubi JE. Pathologic versus physiologic cholestasis: elevated serum concentration of a secondary bile acid occurs only in the presence of hepatobiliary disease. *J Pediatr.* 1981; 98:399.
140. Vanderhoof JA, Grandjean CJ, Kaufman SS, Burkley KT, Antonson DL. Effect of high percentage medium chain triglyceride diet on mucosal adaptation following massive bowel resection in rats. *JPEN J Parenter Enteral Nutr.* 1984; 8:685.
141. Nuty SFA, Byrne WJ, Ament ME. Case of congenital short small intestine: survival with use of long term parenteral feedings. *Pediatrics.* 1986; 77:386.
142. Tinscheid TR, Tarnowski KJ, Rasnake LK, Brams JS. Behavioral treatment of food refusal in a child with short-gut syndrome. *J Pediatr Psychol.* 1987; 12:451.
143. Markestad T, Akones L, Finne PH, Aarskog D. Decreased vitamin D absorption after limited jejunal resection in a premature infant. *J Pediatr.* 1982; 101:1001.
144. Buchman AL, Scolapio J, Fryer J. AGA technical review on short bowel syndrome and intestinal transplantation. *Gastroenterology.* 2003; 124:1111.
145. Fishbein T, Gondolesi G, Kaufman S. Intestinal transplantation for gut failure. *Gastroenterology.* 2003; 124:1615.

146. Fryer J, Pellar S, Ormond D, Koffron A, Abecassis M. Mortality in candidates waiting for combined liver-intestine transplants exceeds that for other candidates waiting for liver transplants. *Liver Transplant.* 2003; 9:748.
147. Fishbein TM, Kaufman SS, Florman SS, et al. Isolated small bowel transplantation: proof of clinical efficacy. *Transplantation.* 2003; 76:636.
148. Nehme AE. Nutritional support of the hospitalized patient: the team concept. *JAMA.* 1980; 243:1906.
149. Isaacs J, Davis B, Montagne M. Transitioning the child fed by gastrostomy into school. *J Am Diet Assoc.* 1990; 90:982.
150. Qin J, Li R, Raes J, et al. A human gut microbial gene catalogue established by metagenomics sequencing. *Nature.* 2010. 464:59.
151. Markowitz JE, Bengmark S. Probiotics in health and disease in the pediatric patient. *Pediatr Clin North Am.* 2002; 49:127.
152. Guinane CM, Cotter PD. Role of the gut microbiota in heath and chronic gastrointestinal disease: understanding the hidden metabolic organ. *Therap Adv Gastroenterol.* 2013; 6:295.
153. Gibson GR, Scott KP, Rastall RA, et al. Dietary prebiotics: current status and new definition. *Food Sci Tech Bull.* 2010: 1:1.
154. Oberhelman RA, Gilman RH, Sheen P, et al. A placebo-controlled trial of *Lactobacillus* GG to prevent diarrhea in undernourished Peruvian children. *J Pediatr.* 1999; 134:15.
155. Vanderhoof JA, Young RJ. Use of probiotics in childhood gastrointestinal disorders. *J Pediatr Gastroenterol Nutr.* 1998; 27:323.
156. Lepage P, Hasler R, Spelmann M, et al. Twin study indicates loss of interaction between microbiota and mucosa of patients with ulcerative colitis. *Gastroenterology.* 2011; 141:227.
157. Manichanh C, Borruel N, Casellas F, Guarner F. The gut microbiota in IBD. *Nat Rev Gastroenterol Hepatol.* 2012: 9:599.
158. Gitnick G. Antibiotics and inflammatory bowel disease [review]. *Gastroenterol Clin. North Am.* 1989; 18:51.
159. Canducci F, Armuzzi A, Cremonini F, et al. A lyophilized and inactivated culture of *Lactobacillus acidophilus* increases *Helicobacter pylori* eradication rates. *Aliment Pharmacol Ther.* 2000; 14:1625.
160. Bengmark S. Immunonutrition: role of biosurfactants, fiber and probiotic bacteria. *Nutrition.* 1998; 14:585.

# 36 Constipation and Fiber

SHIRLEY W. EKVALL

As many as one-fourth of pediatric patients report constipation as a complaint. Di Lorenzo[1] stated that "immobilization, abnormal colonic motility, inability to contract the abdominal muscles, and inadequate fiber intake contribute to the high prevalence of constipation in children with neurological impairments." Typically, formula-fed infants have only one bowel movement daily, whereas breast-fed infants have two or three. Constipation exists only when the stools are hard, dry, and eliminated with difficulty. Gabriel et al.[2] divided the causes of constipation into five categories:

1. *Local organic problems:* Anorectal malformations, anal fissure, and external rectal compression by an abscess or neoplasm are some of the conditions included in this category.
2. *Conditions causing a change in stool character:* Undernutrition, cystic fibrosis, and insufficient dietary fiber and/or fluid may cause scanty, viscid, or hard stools.
3. *Intrinsic motility disorders:* Metabolic and endocrine disorders, including hyperkalemia, hyperthyroidism, and hyperparathyroidism. Pharmacological agents such as phenothiazines and opiates may temporarily affect intestinal motility and cause constipation.
4. *Extrinsic neurological or muscular disorders:* Myelomeningocele, spastic quadriplegia, myotonic dystrophy, epilepsy, Down syndrome, spinal injury, or tumor may interfere with extrinsic intestinal innervation. Abdominal wall or diaphragmatic muscular weakness or paresis prevents the voluntary increase in intra-abdominal pressure that is necessary for defecation.
5. *Functional constipation:* Habitual inhibition of the defecation reflexes is the most common cause of childhood constipation. In time, delayed elimination weakens normal peristalsis, and the stools become dry, hard, and difficult to eliminate.

Anal irritation or parents' references to stools as "dirty" may also lead to constipation.[3]

The North American Society for Pediatric Gastroenterology and Nutrition has developed a plan for evaluation and treatment by clinical practitioners.[4] A personal history and physical examination are the main components of the evaluation. Treatment includes education, behavior modification, and possibly medication.

## BIOCHEMICAL, ANATOMIC, AND OTHER ABNORMALITIES

The average stool weighs approximately 25 g, depending on diet and fiber intake, and has a transit time of 33 hours. Emptying of the rectum occurs when there is increased abdominal pressure caused by peristalsis in the rectal wall. This increased pressure is generated through synchronization of autonomic and voluntary muscles and sensory fibers.[1] As the infant matures, the rectum length increases, and rectal valves develop. By 39 weeks of functional age, the internal anal sphincter reflex appears. Infants who have chronic constipation tend to have increased tonus in the distal colon, with delay in storage passages and dryness in the intraluminal contents. At 1 to 2 years of age, a change in diet such as from breast milk to cow's milk, which has a higher ratio of phosphorus to calcium ratio, may produce constipation.[5] At 2.5 years of age, these muscles and fibers are mature, so that is a good time for toilet training.[1] Staiano et al.[6] found that glucomannan increases the number of bowel movements; however, it does not increase colonic motility.

Studies of identical versus fraternal twins indicate that chronic constipation may have a major genetic component. Boys tend to be more constipated than girls. The age at peak incidence is 2 to 4 years, although the problem often begins at 1 year of age.[7] Functional idiopathic constipation without an associated abnormality is the most frequent type. Some children do not understand how to defecate, some have a maturational abnormality,[7] and more have a painful experience with dry, hard stools. One study found significant increases in dietary fiber, energy intake, and triceps skinfolds with treatment over a period of 45 to 90 days. Mineral oil was used, but this is not recommended for more than a few days because it leads to loss of fat soluble vitamins.[8]

## FACTORS TO BE CONSIDERED IN NUTRITIONAL EVALUATION

Understanding the cause of constipation is important for proper treatment. Poor muscle tone, as in myelomeningocele or Down syndrome, or increased muscle tone, as in cerebral palsy, can cause the problem. A thorough dietary, medical, and social history is needed. A combination dietary intake and bowel movement or stool evaluation can delineate the personal elimination pattern. Dietary intake, fluid and fiber intake, and bowel movement frequency and consistency should be assessed with a 7-day food, fluid, bowel movement, and physical activity list (e.g., 7-day, 24-hour recalls of bowel movement size, amount, consistency, passage, and physical activity).[9]

## DIETARY MANAGEMENT

Physical activity, fiber, and fluid are three major modes of treatment for constipation.[6]

### Fiber

A variety of foods, including whole grains, fruits, vegetables, nuts, legumes, and various parts of these foods,[9] supply significant amounts of dietary fiber. The following foods are recommended[1]:

- Vegetables that retain a crunchy texture when properly cooked—broccoli, carrots, cabbage, corn, cauliflower, and others
- Whole grains and whole-grain products
- Tuberous root vegetables—beets, carrots, white potatoes (and skins), sweet potatoes, and turnips
- Tough-skinned fresh fruits, vegetables, and/or those containing seeds; dried fruits, such as prunes, plums, and apricots
- Pod vegetables—peas and green beans, dried peas and beans, and lima beans
- Nuts of all kinds; crunchy peanut butter
- Miscellaneous—tortilla chips (if made with whole corn and water), popcorn, sunflower seeds, pumpkin seeds, and toasted soybeans

Lettuce, celery, and other salad greens are not as high in fiber as the aforementioned foods. Rice-based cereals are especially low in fiber but represent a substantial portion of the solid content. Potatoes and starchy vegetables supply significant amounts of fiber if consumed in fairly large quantities.

The physiological effects of fiber are not uniform and depend on its capacity to dissolve in aqueous solutions. Fiber in food comes in two forms: dietary (soluble or insoluble) and crude. All components of plants that are resistant to human digestive enzymes are dietary fiber.

The small fraction of the plant that remains after exposure to alkali or acid is crude fiber. Dietary fiber is the edible portion of carbohydrates in plants that resists digestion and absorption in the small intestine; it is the more helpful form in constipation management.[10] Intake of approximately 5 to 8 g/day of crude fiber[11] (although not as important today) or 25 to 30 g/day of dietary fiber is recommended after 20 years of age.[12] In young children aged 3 years or older, daily consumption of 5 g per year of age is recommended, but more research is needed. The addition of sufficient bran to muffins increases stool volume and decreases the total intestinal transit time. Fruits and vegetables have a similar effect of increasing the fecal output, but bran appears to be the most popular food product.[13]

Objections have been raised to increased fiber intake for children.[12,14] First, because children have a small stomach capacity and the caloric density of high-fiber foods is low, a high-fiber diet may not provide sufficient calories. To avoid this problem, particularly for those on highly restricted vegetarian diets, nuts and legumes, which are relatively high in protein and fat, should be added to the diet. Second, dietary fiber may influence adversely the absorption of certain essential minerals such as calcium, iron, copper, magnesium, phosphorus, and zinc. Many foods that are good sources of fiber—primarily whole-grain products—are also high in phytate. Phytate may form insoluble compounds with these minerals, rendering them unavailable. If intake of these minerals is low and the small amounts consumed are chelated, a deficiency may occur. Using large amounts of fiber for its laxative effect may also reduce vitamin and mineral levels in children.[13] However, high-fiber diets are often enriched in minerals.[15,16]

The major constituents of dietary fiber are structural materials of plant cell walls: cellulose, hemicellulose, pectin, mucilages, lignin, and gums. These fibers can be classified as highly fermentable, with low indigestible residue, or less fermentable, with high indigestible residue[17] (Table 36–1). The fiber constituents of fruits and vegetables are much more fermentable than those of cereal brans, which have thicker cell walls and a high degree of lignification. Crude fiber is composed primarily of lignin and cellulose. Dietary fiber contains soluble and insoluble fiber fractions. Current methods permit more precise definition of the amounts and types of dietary fiber polymers in various foodstuffs and of those that may be used for experimental studies.

The extent of fiber degradation in the colon depends on the bacterial flora, the transit time through the colon, and the physical and chemical composition of the fiber. Digestion of polysaccharides varies from 30% to more than 90%. Pectin, mucilages, gums, and hemicellulose are almost completely lost during passage through the stool; cellulose is digested somewhat less completely. Lignin, by virtue of its polymeric cross-linked structure, is resistant to bacterial degradation and is almost completely recovered in the stool.[17] The physical structure of the plant fiber also determines access to bacterial enzymes. Polysaccharides from older, highly lignified plant tissues are less well digested because physical encrustation and chemical bonding to lignin occur.

*Fiber may affect the water-holding capacity* and has important physiological effects in the upper and lower intestines. Hydration of fiber occurs by absorption to the surface of the macromolecules and by entrapment within the interstices of the fibrous or gel matrix. The fiber saturation capacity is determined by the chemistry and morphology of the macromolecules and by the pH and electrolyte concentration of the surrounding medium.[17]

*Adsorption* occurs at the surface of the fiber when substances are taken from the surrounding medium.[17] The forces that bind the adsorbed layer to the surface may be physical or chemical in nature. In addition to fiber's ability to adsorb water, a number of organic materials, such as bile acid, other steroids, various toxic compounds, and bacteria, may be reversibly bound to fiber as it passes along the gastrointestinal tract.

The existence of *cation-exchange properties* of dietary fiber is well established.[17] Their effect is related to the number of free carboxyl groups on the sugar residues. Formation of cation complexes with acid polysaccharides affects mineral balance, electrolyte absorption, and heavy metal toxicity[15] against the intestinal walls.

**Table 36–1.** Comparison of Soluble and Insoluble Dietary Fiber in Certain Foods

| | Dietary Fiber (g/dL) | | |
|---|---|---|---|
| | Total | Soluble | Insoluble |
| *Breads and Cereals* | | | |
| White bread | 3.22 | 1.58 | 3.08 |
| Whole wheat bread | 9.26 | 2.03 | 8.15 |
| All Bran cereal (Kellogg Co.) | 31.60 | 5.24 | 28.43 |
| Cornflakes (Kellogg Co.) | 1.65 | 0.48 | 1.06 |
| Puffed wheat | 7.20 | 3.40 | 6.68 |
| Rice Krispies (Kellogg Co.) | 1.21 | 0.32 | 0.81 |
| Fiber 1 (General Mills) | 44.02 | 3.10 | 40.98 |
| Rolled oats | 10.51 | 5.53 | 9.47 |
| Graham crackers | 2.47 | 1.22 | 2.29 |
| *Vegetables* | | | |
| Broccoli, frozen | 30.40 | 13.63 | 28.94 |
| Beets, canned | 24.27 | 7.50 | 23.67 |
| Carrots, raw | 23.76 | 11.32 | 22.75 |
| Lettuce, raw | 21.02 | 4.70 | 19.00 |
| Sweet corn, cooked | 9.43 | 1.24 | 8.88 |
| Potatoes, white, raw | 9.48 | 4.91 | 8.58 |
| Tomatoes, raw | 13.13 | 2.13 | 11.44 |
| *Fruits* | | | |
| Apple, raw | 12.73 | 4.48 | 10.50 |
| Banana, raw | 7.35 | 2.14 | 4.13 |
| Orange, raw, seedless, California navel | 11.45 | 6.70 | 11.14 |
| Peach, canned | 18.80 | 7.60 | 17.06 |
| Pear, canned | 32.18 | 6.89 | 27.24 |
| Pineapple, canned | 9.54 | 1.22 | 9.33 |
| Plums, purple, canned | 22.81 | 9.9 | 19.71 |
| *Legumes* | | | |
| Green beans, canned | 33.97 | 8.13 | 31.42 |
| Kidney beans, canned | 20.90 | 5.2 | 17.53 |
| Pinto beans, canned | 24.10 | 7.52 | 21.42 |
| Pork and beans, canned | 15.67 | 7.70 | 14.88 |
| White beans, dried, cooked | 18.16 | 5.2 | 17.21 |
| Lentils, dried, cooked | 12.71 | 1.32 | 10.61 |
| Green peas, canned | 21.30 | 3.00 | 20.40 |

Modified from Anderson JW, Bridges SR. Dietary fiber content of selected foods. *Am J Clin Nutr*. 1988; 47:440.

The *bulkier* or larger the stool, the greater the pressure against the intestinal wall. This pressure activates the peristaltic motion, resulting in a more rapid movement of the stool. As the stool moves down the intestine, water is reabsorbed into the body. If the stool moves too slowly, then more water is absorbed and the stool becomes hard, impacted, and difficult to eliminate.

Stephen and Cummings[18] demonstrated that 48% of the increase in stool bulk and water content in subjects fed wheat fiber could be accounted for by the water-holding capacity of the hydrated fiber. Only 36% of the wheat fiber fed was bacterially degraded. By contrast, when an almost completely (92%) digestible fiber (cabbage) was fed, stool bulk and water content also increased, but much of this increase (35%) resulted from enhanced bacterial output. Although large amounts of fermentable fibers enhance fecal bulk and water content, they are somewhat less effective than less fermentable types. Stasse-Wolthuis et al.[19] demonstrated in a carefully controlled study that the mean increase in stool weight was 4.1 g per 1 g of added fiber for coarse wheat bran, compared with 1.9 g per 1 g of added fiber when fruits and vegetables were used as fiber sources. The total fiber, polysaccharide, and lignin components and the sugar constituents of selected foods were measured by Anderson and Bridges,[20] who reported that soluble fiber content as a percentage of total fiber averaged 32% for cereal products, 32% for vegetables, 25% for dried beans, and 38% for fruits[20] (see Table 36–1), and by Marlett and Cheung,[21] found the soluble fiber content to be 23% for refined grains, 3% for nuts, and 13% to 20% for other food groups. The pectin content was 15% to 30% in fruits, vegetables, legumes, and nuts and 0% in grains, whereas hemicellulose content was 50% in grains and 30% in other foods. Cellulose content was 30% in most foods and 50% in legumes.

## Fiber and Diseases or Disorders

*Diverticular disease* of the sigmoid colon is characterized by thickening of the circular muscle and contraction of the teniae coli, resulting in the formation of pouches (diverticula). This condition is often accompanied by pain on the lower left side, alternating diarrhea and constipation, and flatulence. A diet that provides little colonic residue results in a small, hard stool that requires vigorous segmentation for propulsion along the colon, eventually culminating in circular muscle hypertrophy, high colonic pressure, and production of diverticula. In contrast, populations that ingest a diet high in fiber have bulky stools and low colonic pressure, and the disease incidence is low. Diverticulosis is frequently treated with a high-fiber diet, with good results.[22] A key factor in reducing the symptoms of irritable bowel syndrome (IBS) is dietary manipulation.

*Esophageal reflux* symptoms can be reduced by eliminating foods that lower the esophageal sphincter pressure, such as chocolate, alcohol, peppermint, and coffee. Esophageal mucosal irritants such as tomatoes, citrus juices, and sharp condiments also may need to be limited. Treatment with rapid or delayed gastric emptying or gastric acid secretions might be useful in gastroduodenal IBS; however, diabetes mellitus, anorexia nervosa, and collagen diseases may be confused with IBS. Gastric emptying and small bowel motility appear to be slowed by soluble dietary fiber (pectin, gum, psyllium, and oat bran, which ferment) and by fatty foods. Insoluble fiber (lignin, cellulose, and hemicellulose, such as in cereals and whole grains) may be helpful by increasing distention and peristalsis. Metoclopramide, domperidone, and cisapride also may be used to alleviate delayed gastric emptying. Small bowel problems may be exaggerated by the ingestion of lactose, sorbitol, and fructose. Complex carbohydrates or soluble fiber may relieve symptoms that originate in the small bowel.[23]

Fiber and other nutrients may reduce the incidence of *colon cancer*.[24] The mechanisms that inhibit mutagenesis and carcinogenesis at the *extracellular level* in the gastrointestinal tract include deactivation of mutagens, modification of metabolism during enterohepatic circulation, protection of the mucosal barrier, inhibition of transepithelial absorption, dilution and complexation of mutagens and carcinogens, acceleration of transit time, maintenance of optimal pH, inhibition of nitrosation, increased production of short bowel fatty acids, inhibition of metabolic activation by gut-colonizing bacteria, and decreased fecal pH. At the *cellular level*, mechanisms that inhibit mutagenesis and carcinogenesis include favoring sequestration in nontarget cells; inhibiting uptake and metabolic activation by target cells; stimulating detoxification; reacting with electrophiles; scavenging reactive oxygen species; protecting nucleophilic sites of DNA; inhibiting cell proliferation before DNA repair and favoring repair of DNA damage; inhibiting error-prone repair pathways; increasing fidelity of DNA replication; and controlling gene expression.[25] Examples of these mechanisms in disease states are discussed later.

Dietary fiber can *decrease cardiovascular disease (CVD)* and *lower blood lipid levels* by reducing the transit time through the gastrointestinal tract, resulting in decreased absorption of dietary lipids.[26] There is also a widespread conviction that the effect of dietary fiber on serum lipids may be largely mediated by enhanced fecal excretion of bile acids. In a long-term study in humans, legumes (which are high in guar gum) enhanced fecal bile output in accordance with bile acid adsorption observed in vitro. Wheat bran demonstrated moderate bile acid affinity in vitro, but few human studies have indicated an effect on fecal bile acid excretion. Oat bran, however, did significantly increase fecal bile acid loss.

Compared with wheat bran, oat bran is more mucilaginous because of its high content of β-glucans. Other mucilaginous fibers, such as pectin, guar gum, and psyllium seed colloid, have consistently been shown to increase bile acid excretion by 33% to 300%.[15,27] Overall, mucilaginous fibers appear to have the greatest effect in decreasing total serum cholesterol concentrations. Beet and psyillium fiber (i.e., soluble dietary fiber) produced the greatest reduction in low-density lipoprotein (LDL)-cholesterol and serum glucose in healthy men aged 18 to 55 years.[28] The use of 2.5 g of psyllium fiber twice daily in a diet for children from 3 to 7 years of age (3.5 g twice daily for children older than 7 years of age) with 8 oz water was found to be safe and effective in reducing total cholesterol and LDL-cholesterol in type II A hyercholesterolemia.[29] Antioxidants found in vegetables and fruits may also be beneficial in CVD.[30]

Dietary fiber shortens the transit time and may lower the concentration of fecal carcinogens or change the bacterial flora by modifying bile acids, thus reducing the incidence of *colorectal cancer*.[31] Fermentable fiber may alter the production of secondary sterols through its effects on colonic pH because most bacterial enzymes acting on acidic and neutral sterols have pH optima of 6.5 or greater. Bacterial modification of fecal steroids is apparently reduced in individuals consuming high-fiber diets.[32] Some reports indicate specific benefits for pentose sugars in reducing colon cancer; the sugar components of the polysaccharides are being determined.[20,21] In wheat products, pentose sugars were the major component of the soluble fractions, whereas in all cereals, pentose sugars were the major component of the insoluble fractions.[20] The wise choice of using high-antioxidant foods in reducing colon cancer should also be considered. Several plant phenolic compounds have been shown to have anticancer properties in experimental cancer models.[33] The lignin fraction of dietary fiber may be responsible for the anticarcinogenic activity in fiber.[21] Indoles, plant sterols, thiols, and protease inhibitors may also have anticarcinogenic activity.

Several studies have found that normal adults and persons with mild cases of *diabetes mellitus* (i.e., those taking only oral hypoglycemic agents or <20 U of insulin per day) may benefit from a higher-fiber diet because it improves their glucose tolerance.[34] Soluble dietary fibers appear to have the greatest glycemic effect.[20,35] The glycemic index for several foods can be found in chapters on diabetes or on the Internet (www.diabetesnet.com/food-diabetes/glycemic-index).

The hypothesis linking *obesity* with ingestion of an excessive proportion of fiber-depleted carbohydrates is supported by several arguments.[36] First, fiber-depleted food is calorically more concentrated than fiber-intact food. Second, food fiber promotes chewing, thereby increasing the effort required to eat and retarding the rate of food ingestion. Third, diets rich in fiber tend to decrease absorptive efficiency.[37] Fourth, fiber-depleted food is less satiating than a calorically equivalent amount of high-fiber food. These arguments appear to have validity, but more research is required before firm conclusions can be drawn. Research on modification of fiber by processing or cooking is also being developed.[38]

The use of fiber in *enteral nutrition* has been studied on an international basis. In the United States, the effect of dietary soy polysaccharide (18–24 g/day) fiber and vitamin D on 11 profoundly retarded institutionalized youth who were fed by gastrostomy tube and received anticonvulsants for 1 year was assessed by determining the plasma levels and balances of zinc, magnesium, calcium, and phosphorus. Nitrogen and phosphorus levels increased, but zinc and calcium levels were reduced or equal to 150% of the Dietary Reference Intakes (DRA).[39] In England, the use of a pectin-supplemented, predigested diet in animals with short bowel syndrome maintained body weight and serum albumin, although the mineral content was reduced and supplementation was required.[40] The diet liberated acetate, propionate, and butyrate during colonic fiber digestion and enhanced intestinal adaptation. A single-blind crossover study in Denmark used a nongelling water-insoluble fiber (30 g/day of plant cellulose) to treat marked obesity, along with a very-low-calorie nutrition powder formula (388 cal for women and 466 cal for men) that was adequate in protein, vitamins, and minerals. This diet produced an increased number of bowel movements and reduced hunger without impairing absorption of calcium, magnesium, or iron. However, it did not increase weight loss or decrease the levels of plasma cholesterol, triglycerides, or glucose.[36,41] Fiber may be used as part of a standard tube-feeding regimen to provide gut mucosal integrity but not specifically to treat constipation or diarrhea.[42] Soy polysaccharides (i.e., hemicellulose, cellulose, and pectin) are frequently used as fiber sources. More research is needed on the administration of soluble versus insoluble fibers.[43]

Glycerin suppositories and stool softeners should be used in infants younger than 1 year of age. Some children aged 2 years or older who are developmentally delayed and have diminished stool reflexes may need ½ tsp/day of bran or Metamucil (a natural vegetable source high in psyllium) with 6 oz water, with frequent medical assessments to assess intestinal blockage and obtain height and weight measurements. Eating high-fiber snacks is a good way to relieve constipation. When solid foods are introduced into the diet of an older child, care should be taken to include whole-grain cereals, breads, fruits, and vegetables. If whole grains are used for breads or cereals, raw fruits and vegetables are consumed and nuts (if tolerated) or legumes are used one time each day as a meat source, adequate fiber should be obtained.

Raw wheat bran, a concentrated source of dietary fiber, should be used (along with plenty of water) to promote further stool bulk.[44] The bran should be gradually incorporated into the diet. If excessive amounts are given initially, they may irritate a sensitive alimentary tract and cause flatulence, loose stools, or intestinal blockage. Children between 3 and 5 years of age with constipation need about ½ tsp/day, whereas children between 5 and13 years of age with constipation may need ½ tsp two or three times daily. The bran can be included in the diet in several ways, such as sprinkling it on cereal, pudding, or mashed fruit; mixing it with peanut butter and jelly; or adding it to pancakes, hamburgers, casseroles, or other cooked foods during preparation.

Prunes and prune juice have been found to stimulate intestinal motility. The laxative substance found in prunes is dihydrophenylisatin. Other foods may have this same ability, but data on the pharmacological laxative properties of food are limited.[45,46]

Diet plays an important role in the treatment of *chronic constipation*. In a study of 60 cases, control by diet alone was found to be more effective than other treatment plans. The anticonstipation diet should include enough bulk (i.e., vegetables, fruits, and whole-grain products) so that the fiber residue left in the bowel after digestion will encourage the movement of the intestinal contents and stimulate periodic evacuation. Daily consumption of 6 to 8 servings from the fruit and vegetable group and 6 to 11 servings from the whole-grain bread and cereal group will add a significant amount of fiber to the stool. Certain foods implicated in the delay of stool passage, such as applesauce, bananas, rice cereal, and tea, should be restricted until the constipation resolves.

Constipation is a common problem in children with developmental disabilities. Increasing the fiber intake to 17 to 21 g/day was found to relieve constipation and significantly reduced the use of laxatives in immobilized patients.[47] A sample high-fiber diet is presented in Table 36–2.

## Fluid

Because water is absorbed by the colon, intake of 6 to 8 glasses each day is necessary to form a soft, bulky stool. This amount includes beverages and the water present in foods such as soups, cereal with milk, fruits, and raw vegetables. Ingesting adequate amounts of fluid is also important when using bran to prevent impaction.

## Physical Activity and Regimen

Physical activity can be effective in relieving constipation, particularly for the child with a handicap; exercise increases intestinal motility. Establishment of regular mealtimes and sleep patterns is also helpful.

**Table 36–2.** Sample Menu for a High-Fiber Diet

| | Sunday | Monday | Tuesday | Wednesday | Thursday | Friday | Saturday |
|---|---|---|---|---|---|---|---|
| Breakfast | Orange juice<br>Pancakes with bran and blueberries in the batter<br>Margarine<br>Milk | Tomato juice<br>Poached egg<br>WW toast<br>Milk | Orange sections<br>Oatmeal sprinkled with bran and raisins<br>Milk | Prune juice<br>Hard-cooked egg<br>WW toast<br>Milk | Orange juice<br>Bran cereal<br>Milk | Tomato juice<br>Scrambled egg<br>WW toast<br>Milk | Orange juice<br>WW French toast<br>Strawberries<br>Milk |
| Midmorning snack | Pineapple juice | Grape juice | Apple juice | Water | Pineapple juice | Orange juice | Cranberry juice |
| Lunch | Roast beef<br>Baked potato with skin<br>Squash<br>Peas | Crunchy peanut butter on WW bread<br>Carrot and celery strips<br>Diced peaches, canned or fresh<br>Milk | Turkey sandwich on WW bread<br>Fresh or canned pear<br>Milk | Bean soup<br>Hamburger<br>WW roll<br>Tomato (optional) | Potato soup<br>Crunchy peanut butter on WW bread<br>Tomato wedges<br>Carrot strips | Vegetable soup<br>Ry-Krisp<br>Pineapple rings<br>Milk | Egg salad sandwich on WW bread<br>Celery strips<br>Fruit cocktail with bran<br>Milk |
| Canned or fresh | Orange sections and pineapple salad<br>Oatmeal cookie<br>Milk | | | Fruit cocktail<br>Milk | Milk | | |
| Midafternoon snack | Apple juice | Orange juice<br>Raisins | Lemonade<br>Dried apricots | Cranberry juice<br>Walnuts | Water<br>Dates | Grape juice<br>Sunflower seeds | Water<br>Prunes |
| Dinner | Fish sandwich<br>Corn on the cob or canned corn<br>Cole slaw<br>½ Apple w/skin<br>Milk | Tomato soup<br>Meatloaf on WW bread<br>Grapes<br>Milk | Chili with beans<br>Carrot and raisin salad<br>Baked or fresh apple<br>Milk | Chicken noodle casserole<br>Broccoli<br>Bran muffin<br>Lettuce salad with dressing<br>Strawberries<br>Milk | Pork chop<br>Brown rice<br>Brussels sprouts<br>Apple Brown Betty made with bran<br>Milk | Chicken<br>Spinach<br>Waldorf salad<br>Bran muffin<br>Milk | Meatloaf with bran<br>Mashed potatoes<br>Peas and carrots<br>Fresh or canned plums<br>Milk |
| Evening snack | Water<br>½ Apple | Cranberry juice<br>Popcorn | Pineapple juice<br>Mixed nuts | Lemonade | Cranberry juice<br>Peanuts | Pear juice | Grape juice |
| Dietary fiber | 30 | 34 | 49 | 30 | 47 | 24 | 24 |
| Crude fiber | 10 | 11 | 13 | 13 | 16 | 11 | 9 |

WW = whole wheat.

For example, times may be designated each day for the child to rise, drink fluid, use the bathroom, eat breakfast with fluid, use the bathroom, drink fluid, eat lunch with fluid, use the bathroom, drink fluid, exercise, use the bathroom, eat supper with fluid, use the bathroom, drink fluid, and retire to bed.

## Other Treatments

A variety of treatment programs, including medical, behavioral, pharmacological, dietary, and surgical approaches, have been used in the treatment of *encopresis bowel incontinence*. Treatment of most encopretic children should consist of counseling and education about the medical treatment, retraining, monitoring, and follow-up. Explaining to the parents the physiological abnormalities found in the child (if applicable) helps decrease guilt and blame. Retraining should include frequent toilet use after meals and regulation of bowel habits with the use of high-fiber foods and laxatives when indicated by a physician. With this interdisciplinary approach, a marked decrease of soiling episodes can be achieved in every child. Disappearance of irritability, moodiness, and abdominal pain, and often improvement of behavioral symptoms, also have been observed.[48] Biofeedback control over function also may be used to treat fecal incontinence. The decreased ability of the anal sphincter to relax helps to reduce the risk of recurrence of constipation.[49]

A study by Voderholzer et al.[50] found that dietary fiber therapy is not useful for patients with slow gastrointestinal transit time and/or a disorder of defecation. Most physicians agree that the colon must be cleaned out initially with enemas, fiber, laxatives, or surgical treatment (in extreme cases) before any regimen is established to manage chronic constipation. Treatment for constipation should begin with relieving any impactions. Then a course of fiber supplementation of at least 20 g/day can be started, depending on the child's age (after 3 years of age, 5 g times per year of age is given daily).[51] Other treatments include lactulose, polyethylene glycol solution, and stimulants. Surgical procedures are the last resort. Physicians often prescribe Metamucil or psyllium. Long-term management is usually necessary, comprising all forms of therapy including dietary fiber.[52] Occasionally, mineral oil is used but it is not recommended because it appears to decrease the absorption of fat-soluble vitamins (i.e., vitamins A, D, E, and K), which are excreted in the feces.[53] Cisapride appears to improve gastrointestinal motility and bowel habits in children with chronic idiopathic constipation.[54]

Information on an effective program called Smart Choice, which significantly decreased dietary fat by increasing fiber in the diets of schoolchildren in Connecticut, is available from the State of Connecticut Department of Health.[55] American children need more information regarding low-fat and high-fiber foods.[56]

Any of the following can provide a convenient natural constipation remedy:

1. 8 oz glass of hot water with lemon
2. 8 oz glass of warm prune juice
3. Equal amounts of unprocessed bran (1–2 T), vegetable fiber, and stewed prunes (taken with an 8-oz glass of water)

## Follow-up

A dietary, physical activity, fluid, and bowel movement record is recommended weekly or for 1 month if constipation is severe. The 7-day food list is a good tool to use in evaluating the beneficial effects of the diet. Increased physical activity, consumption of fresh produce, and fluid intake should increase bowel movement frequency, volume, or both. A natural vegetable source high in psyllium may also be needed.[57]

### References


1. Di Lorenzo C. Childhood constipation: finally some hard data about hard stools! *J Pediatr.* 2000; 136:4.
2. Dinari G, Rosenbach Y, Zahavi I, Nitzan M. Constipation as a presenting symptom in childhood: a diagnostic problem. *Am J Proctol Gastroenterol Colon Rectal Surg.* 1981; 32:16.
3. Levine MJ. Colic, constipation and diarrhea: old symptoms, new approaches. *Pediatr Ann.* 1987; 16:765.
4. Morais M, Vitolo M, Aguirre A, Fagundes-Neto U. Measurement of low dietary fiber intake as a risk factor for chronic constipation. *J Pediatr Gastroenterol Nutr.* 1999; 29:132.
5. Pettei MJ. Chronic constipation. *Pediatr Ann.* 1987; 16:796.
6. Staiano A, Simeone D, Giudice ED, Miele E, Tozzi A, Toraldo C. Effect of the dietary fiber glucomannan on chronic constipation in neurologically impaired children. *J Pediatr.* 2000; 136:41.
7. Wald A, Chandra R, Chiponis D, Gabel D. Anorectal function and continence mechanisms in childhood encopresis. *J Pediatr Gastroenterol Nutr.* 1986; 5:346.
8. Speridiao PG, Tahan S, Fagundes-Neto U, Morais MB. Dietary fiber, energy intake and nutritional status during the treatment of children with chronic constipation. *Braz J Med Biol Res.* 2003; 36:753.
9. Ekvall S. Constipation and fiber. In: Ekvall S, ed. *Pediatric Nutrition in Chronic Diseases and Developmental Disorders.* New York: Oxford University Press; 1993.
10. American Association of Cereal Chemists, Dietary Fiber Definition Committee. The definition of dietary fiber. Publication no. W-2001-0222-010. *Cereal Foods World.* 2001; 46:112.
11. Williams CL, Bollella M, Wynder EL. A new recommendation for dietary intake in childhood. *Pediatrics.* 1995; 96(Suppl S):985.
12. Food and Nutrition Board of the Institute of Medicine. *Dietary Reference Intakes: Proposed Definition of Dietary Fiber.* Washington, DC: National Academy Press; 2001.
13. Floch MG. The pharmacology of dietary fiber for laxation. *Am J Gastroenterol.* 1987; 82:1259.
14. American Academy of Pediatrics Committee on Nutrition. Plant fiber intake in the pediatric diet. *Pediatrics.* 1981; 67:574.
15. Kay RM. Dietary fiber. *J Lipid Res.* 1982; 23:221.
16. Hanson CF, Kopel BH, Hermann JR. Intake of trace minerals and fiber by healthy elderly people. *J Am Diet Assoc.* 1991; 91:A118.
17. Spiro HM. Medical aspects of dietary fiber. In: Spiller GA, Kay RM, eds. *Dietary Fiber.* New York: Plenum; 1980.
18. Stephen AM, Cummings JH. Mechanism of action of dietary fiber in the human colon. *Nature.* 1980; 284:283.
19. Stasse-Wolthuis M, Albers HF, van Jevesen JG, et al. Influence of dietary fiber from vegetables and fruits, bran or citrus pectin on serum lipids, fecal lipids, and colon function. *Am J Clin Nutr.* 1980; 33:1745.
20. Anderson JW, Bridges SR. Dietary fiber content of selected foods. *Am J Clin Nutr.* 1988; 47:440.
21. Marlett, JA, Cheung TF. Database and quick methods of assessing typical dietary fiber intake using data for 228 commonly consumed foods. *J Am Diet. Assoc.* 1997; 97:1139.
22. Brodribb AJM. Treatment of symptomatic diverticular disease with a high fiber diet. *Lancet.* 1977; 1:665.
23. Friedman G. Diet and the irritable bowel syndrome. *Gastroenterol Clin North Am.* 1991; 20:313.
24. Ben Q, Sun Y, Chai R, Quan A, Xu B, Yuan Y. Dietary fiber intake reduces risk for colorectal adenoma: a meta-analysis. *Gastroenterology.* 2014;146:689
25. Hayatsu H. *Mutagens in Food: Detection and Prevention.* Boca Raton, FL: CRC Press; 1990.
26. Threapleton DE, Greenwood DC, Evans CE, et al. Dietary fibre intake and risk of cardiovascular disease: systematic review and meta-analysis. *BMJ.* 2013; 347;f6879.
27. Kritchevsky D. Dietary fiber in health and disease. In: Bonfield C, Kritchevsky D, eds. *Dietary Fiber.* New York: Kluwer Academic; 1997.
28. Spiller GA, Freeman HJ. Recent advances in dietary fiber and colorectal disease. *Am J Clin Nutr.* 1981; 34:1145.
29. Spark A, Glassman MS, Newman LJ. A psyllium-supplemented simplified diet for treatment of primary type II-A hypercholesterolemia in children. *J Am Diet Assoc.* 1990; 91:A112.
30. Kritchevsky D. Antioxidant vitamins in the prevention of cardiovascular disease. *Nutr. Today.* 1992; 27:30.
31. Sugerman SB, Bowen PE, Tiongson BB, Tan NT. Physiological effects of four types of dietary fiber in healthy subjects. *J Am Diet. Assoc.* 1990; 91:A112.
32. Augerinos GC, Fuchs HM, Floch MH. Increased cholesterol and bile acid excretion during a high fiber diet. *Gastroenterology.* 1977; 72:1026.
33. Newmark H. Plant phenolics as inhibitors of mutational and pre-carcinogenic events. *Can J Physiol Pharmacol.* 1987; 65:461.
34. Trowell H. Diabetes mellitus and dietary fiber of starchy foods. *Am J Clin Nutr.* 1978; 31:553.
35. Bhupathirahu SN, Tobias DK, Malik VS. Glycemic index, glycemic load, and risk of type 2 diabetes: results from 3 large US cohorts and an updated meta-analysis. *Am J Clin Nutr.* 2014; 100:218.
36. Van Itallie TB. Dietary fiber and obesity. *Am J Clin Nutr.* 1978; 31:S45.
37. Wanders AJ, van den Borne JJ, de Graaf C, et al. Effects of dietary fibre on subjective appetite, energy intake and body weight: a systematic review of randomized controlled trials. *Obes Rev.* 2011; 12:724.
38. Eastwood M, Morris E. Physical properties of dietary fiber that influence physiological function: a model for polymers along the gastrointestinal tract. *Am J Clin Nutr.* 1992; 55:346.
39. Liebl BH, Fischer MH, Van Calcar SC, Marlett JA. Dietary fiber and long-term large bowel response in enterally nourished nonambulatory profoundly retarded youth. *JPEN J Parenter Enteral Nutr.* 1990; 14:371.
40. Progress report, fibre and enteral nutrition. *Gut.* 1989; 30:246.
41. Astrup A, Vrist E, Quaade F. Dietary fibre added to very low calorie diet reduces hunger and alleviates constipation. *Int J Obes.* 1990; 14:105.
42. David LA, Maurice DF, Carmody RN, et al. Diet rapidly and reproducibly alters the human guy microbiome. *Nature.* 2014; 505;559.
43. Frankenfield DC, Beyer PL. Dietary fiber and bowel function in tube-fed patients. *Perspect Pract.* 1991; 91:590.
44. Stewart ML, Schroeder NM. Dietary treatments for childhood constipation: efficacy of dietary fiber and whole grains. *Nutr Rev.* 2013; 71:98.

45. Olness K, Tobin J. Chronic constipation in children: can it be managed by diet alone? *Postgrad Med.* 1982; 72:149.
46. Hongisto SM, Paajanen L, Saxelin M, Korpela R. A combination of fibre-rich rye bread and yogurt containing *Lactobacillus* GG improves bowel function in women with self-reported constipation. *Eur J Clin Nutr.* 2006; 60:319.
47. Nair P, Mayberry J. Vegetarianism, dietary fibre and gastrointestinal disease. *Dig Dis.* 1994; 12:177.
48. Loening-Baucke V, Cruikshank B, Savage C. Defecation dynamics and behavior profiles in encopretic children. *Pediatrics.* 1987; 80:672.
49. Weber J, Ducrotte PH, Touchais JY, Roussignol C, Denis P. Biofeedback training for constipation in adults and children. *Dis Colon Rectum.* 1987; 30:844.
50. Voderholzer WA, Schatke W, Muhldorfer BE, Klauser AG, Birkner B, Muller-Lissner SA. Clinical response to dietary fiber treatment of chronic constipation. *Am J Gastroenterol.* 1997; 92:95.
51. Grant L, Wanger L, Neill K. Fiber-fortified feedings in immobile patients. *Clin Nurs Res.* 1994; 3:166.
52. Katz C, Drongowski RA, Coran AG. Long-term management of chronic constipation in children. *J Pediatr Surg.* 1987; 22:976.
53. Clark JH, Russell GJ, Fitzgerald JF, Nagamori KE. Serum carotene, retinol, and tocopherol levels during mineral oil therapy for constipation. *Am J Dis Child.* 1987; 141:1210.
54. Staiamo A, Salatore C, Andreotti MR, Raffaele M, Manzi G. Effect of cisapride on chronic idiopathic constipation in children. *Dig Dis Sci.* 1991; 36:733.
55. Cobb KF, Berger NE, Zamore PR, Gebo SC. Smart Choice: effective program to decrease fat and increase fiber in school meals. *J Am Diet. Assoc.* 1991; 91:A76.
56. Resnicow K, Reinhardt J. What do children know about fat, fiber, and cholesterol: a survey of 5116 primary and secondary school students. *J Nutr Educ.* 1991; 23:65.
57. Bliss DZ, Jung HJ, Savik K, et al. Supplementation with dietary fiber improves fecal incontinence. *Nurs Res.* 2001; 50:203.

# PART III

# HEREDITARY METABOLIC DISORDERS

*Harvey Levy*

The discovery of phenylketonuria (PKU) as a biochemical cause of mental retardation had an enormous impact on the perception of mental disability.[1] When the urine ferric chloride test was used to test people who were institutionalized because of mental retardation, it was revealed that at least 0.5% excreted phenylpyruvic acid and hence had PKU.[2] Therefore, it was no longer sufficient to simply assume that the cause of the mental retardation was cerebral palsy or congenital encephalopathy. It was now evident that there could be a definable cause that illustrated an inborn error of metabolism, as first described by Garrod.[3]

But what truly launched the interest in hereditary metabolic disorders was the demonstration by Bickel et al.[4] that nutritional reduction of phenylalanine in individuals with PKU corrected the biochemical abnormalities and improved the neurological features of the condition, and especially the subsequent demonstrations that dietary treatment beginning within the first few days after birth prevented mental retardation.[5] Very soon thereafter, Guthrie developed newborn screening in the belief that, when used in combination with early nutritional therapy, it would eliminate mental retardation in children with PKU.[6]

From almost the beginning of newborn screening, it was evident that mental retardation from PKU was likely to be eliminated. Excitement concerning the benefit of nutritional treatment for an inborn error led to interest in developing nutrition therapies for other metabolic disorders analogous to PKU—that is, those in which the mental defect develops postnatally, in which an increased concentration of a specific amino acid is presumed to be the toxic factor, and in which the amino acid is essential and its level therefore is controllable by diet. Thus were developed methionine restriction to treat homocystinuria,[7] restriction of leucine and other branched-chain amino acids to treat maple syrup urine disease,[8] and restriction of tyrosine and phenylalanine in the treatment of tyrosinemia type I.[9] With rare exceptions,[9] these nutrition therapies also corrected the observed biochemical phenotypes and prevented or modified the clinical phenotypes.

Much has occurred since those early days. As a result of better understanding of the biochemical alterations in metabolic disorders and of nutritional needs in general, as well as the interest in developing proprietary products by industry, therapies have been greatly improved. This is especially so since the first edition of this book. For instance, much more is now known about essential fatty acids in treated PKU.[10] Breast milk alternating with the phenylalanine-free formula for infants with PKU has become accepted and even preferred in the dietary treatment of homocystinuria,[11,12] and megadoses of tetrahydrobiopterin (BH4) cofactor for some children with PKU[13] have become prominent, expanding the concept of nutrition to the border of drug therapy.

Although nondietary therapies are appearing for the metabolic disorders, nutrition will continue to be very important in the care of these patients. For instance, 2-(2-nitro-4-trifluoromethylbenzoyl)-1,3-cyclohexanedione (NTBC) prevents liver failure and hepatocellular carcinoma in tyrosinemia type I,[14,15] but dietary therapy to control the elevated level of tyrosine produced by this therapy remains a vital component of treatment in this disorder.[16] A new alternative enzyme therapy for PKU is under development and may soon be available for the treatment of patients.[17] Because this therapy requires subcutaneous injection, many patients will likely prefer to continue nutrition therapy, but even those who adopt the enzyme therapy may still require some degree of nutritional treatment, and all patients will need tyrosine supplementation. Chaperone therapy for homocystinuria may not be far away but may apply only to those affected individuals with specific mutations. Even those who respond to this new approach are likely to require a degree of nutritional treatment.[18]

Accordingly, the new information provided in this section by experts in the treatment of metabolic disorders is critical to providing not only current optimal therapy but nutritional therapy well into the future.

## References


1. Fölling A. Über ausscheidung von phenylbrenztraubensäure in den harn also stoffwechselanomalie in verbindung mit imbezillitat. *Hoppe-Seyl Z.* 1934; 227:169.
2. Jervis GA. Phenylpyruvic oligophrenia. *Arch Neurol Psychiatry.* 1937; 37:944.
3. Garrod AE. Inborn errors of metabolism. Croonian lectures. *Lancet* 1908: 2:1, 73,142, 214.
4. Bickel H, Gerrard J, Hickmans EM. The influence of phenylalanine intake on the chemistry and behavior of a phenylketonuric child. *Acta Paediatr.* 1954; 43:64.
5. Hornelr FA, Streamer CW. Effect of a phenylalanine-restricted diet on patients with phenylketonuria. *JAMA.* 1956; 161:1628.
6. Guthrie R, Susi A. A simple phenylalanine method for detecting phenylketonuria in large populations of newborn infants. *Pediatrics.* 1963; 32:338.
7. Perry TL, Dunn HG, Hansen S, MacDougall L, Warrington PD. Early diagnosis and treatment of homocystinuria. *Pediatrics.* 1966; 37:502.
8. Snyderman SE, Norton PM, Roitman E, Holt LE Jr. Maple syrup urine disease, with particular reference to dietotherapy. *Pediatrics.* 1964; 34:454.
9. Bodegård G, Gentz J, Lindbland B, Lindstedt S, Zetterström R. Hereditary tyrosinemia: III. On the differential diagnosis and the lack of effect of early dietary treatment. *Acta Paediatr Scand.* 1969; 58:37.
10. Acosta PB, Yannicelli S, Singh R, et al. Intake and blood levels of fatty acids in treated patients with phenylketonuria. *J Pediatr Gastroenteronal Nutr.* 2001; 33:253.
11. Riva E, Agostoni C, Biasucci G, et al. Early breastfeeding is linked to higher intelligence quotient scores in dietary treated phenylketonuric children. *Acta Paediatr.* 1996; 85:56.
12. Singh RH, Kruger WD, Wang L, Pasquali M, Elsas LJ II. Cystathionine B-synthase deficiency: effects of betaine supplementation after methionine restriction in B6-nonrepsonsive homocystinuria. *Genet Med.* 2004; 6:90.
13. Shintaku H, Kure S, Ohura T, et al. Long-term treatment and diagnosis of tetrahydrobiopterin-responsive hydroxylase gene. *Pediatr Res.* 2004; 55:425.

14. Lindstedt S, Holme E, Lock EA, Hjalmarson O, Strandvik B. Treatment of hereditary tyrosinaemia type I by inhibition of 4-hydroxyphenylpyruvate dioxygenase. *Lancet.* 1992; 340:813.
15. Larochelle J, Alvarez F, Bussières JF, et al. Effect of nitisinone (NTBC) treatment on the clinical course of hepatorenal tyrosinemia in Québec. *Molec Genet Metab.* 2012; 107:49.
16. de Laet C, Dionisi-Vici C, Leonard JV, et al. Recommendations for the management of tyrosinaemia type 1. *Orphan J Rare Dis.* 2013; 8:1.
17. Gámez A, Sarkissian CN, Wang L, et al. Development of pegylated forms of recombinant *Rhodosporidium toruloides* phenylalanine ammonia-lyase for the treatment of classical phenylketonuria. *Molec Ther.* 2005; 11:986.
18. Melenovská P, Kopecká J, Krijt J, et al. Chaperone therapy for homocystinuria: the rescue of CBS mutations by heme arginate. *J Inherit Metab Dis.* 2015; 38:287.

# A.

# DISORDERS OF AMINO ACID METABOLISM

## 37 Homocystinuria

RANI H. SINGH AND TERESA D. DOUGLAS

Homocystinuria can result from hereditary or acquired enzymatic deficiencies in either the remethylation pathway of homocysteine to methionine or the transsulfuration of homocysteine to cysteine.[1,2] Homocysteine occupies a central position in methyl metabolism, specifically methyl cycling involving methionine, homocysteine, and cysteine (Fig. 37–1). One fate of homocysteine is remethylation to synthesize methionine using the methyl donor from 5-methyl-tetrahydrofolate (THF), with methyl cobalamin as coenzyme, or the methyl donor from betaine, which is catalyzed by betaine-homocysteine methyl transferase. The other fate, transsulfuration of homocysteine, includes synthesis of S-adenosyl methionine (SAM), catalyzed by methionine-S-adenosyltransferase to produce S-adenosylhomocysteine. S-adenosylhomocysteine is further hydrolyzed to homocysteine and adenosine. Most homocysteine is irreversibly converted to cysteine by cystathionine β-synthase (CBS) using pyridoxal phosphate as a coenzyme.[1]

In conditions of excessive homocysteine accumulation, such as homocystinuria, increased formation of the disulfide form, homocystine, can be detected in plasma. Less common hereditary defects of metabolism cause homocystinuria due to impairment of 5-methyltetrahydrofolate homocysteine methyltransferase, also known as methionine synthase.[3,4] This defect may be indirectly related to insufficient synthesis of methylcobalamin from vitamin $B_{12}$ or to reduced activity of either 5,10-methylenetetrahydrofolate reductase (MTHFR)[3] or methionine synthase reductase[5–7] (see Fig. 37–1).

CBS deficiency, the most common cause of homocystinuria, is inherited as an autosomal recessive trait.[8] A wide range of genetic heterogeneity is observed, with wide expression of the CBS enzyme, from none to small residual activity. The human gene that encodes this enzyme, *CBS*, has been cloned and is located on chromosome 21; more than 160 pathogenic mutations have been identified.[8] The true incidence of homocystinuria is unknown; however, worldwide estimates vary from 1 in 1800 people in Qatar to 1 in 800,000 people in Japan.[9,10] Overall prevalence numbers are believed to be underestimated.[8] The defect in CBS results in the accumulation of plasma homocysteine and methionine and decreased levels of cysteine. Elevated levels of plasma methionine may be quantitated by tandem mass spectrometry (MS/MS), and this forms the basis of newborn screening. A positive newborn screen is followed by plasma amino acid analysis, enzyme activity assay, or genetic analysis to confirm the diagnosis.[8]

### DIAGNOSIS

Homocystinuria caused by CBS deficiency is characterized biochemically by elevated levels of plasma total homocysteine (tHcy), homocystine, and methionine. However, in cases of decreased activity in

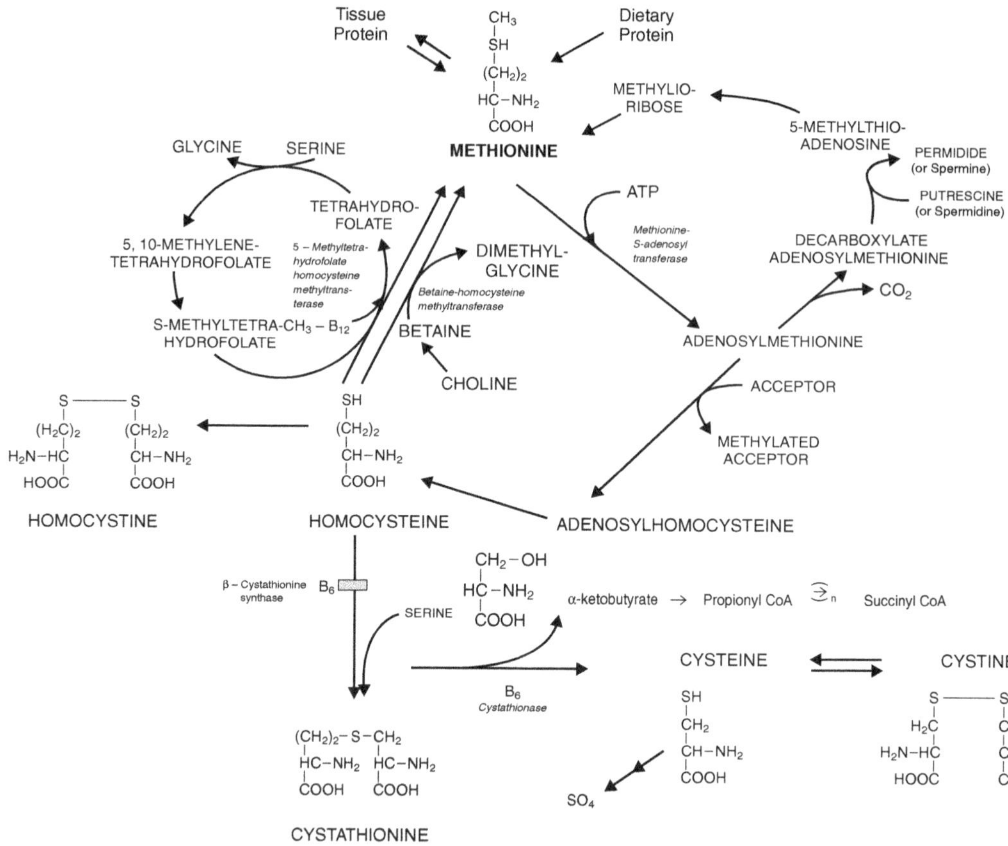


**Figure 37–1.** Methionine metabolism. (Adapted from Acosta P. *The Ross Metabolic Formula System Nutrition Support Protocols*, 4th ed. Columbus, OH: Ross Products Division; 2001.)

the remethylation pathway that catalyzes homocysteine methylation to methionine (e.g., isolated or comorbid MTHFR deficiency), plasma methionine levels may be normal to low.[11] Elevated plasma methionine levels in the absence of high homocysteine levels may be indicative of neonatal transient liver disease or of defects in S-adenosylmethionine methyltransferase, also known as methionine adenosyltransferase I (MAT I), MAT II, or MAT III. In the case of MAT deficiencies, the prognosis is benign with rare exceptions.[12–14] Thus, it is necessary to differentiate the cause of high methionine levels (i.e., remethylation versus transsulfuration defects) in order to prescribe the appropriate therapy.

The diagnosis of CBS deficiency can also be confirmed in cultured fibroblasts by direct enzyme assay or through genetic analysis. Once the diagnosis of CBS deficiency is established, it can be further characterized as $B_6$-responsive or $B_6$-nonresponsive based on the patient's biochemical profile in response to a pyridoxine ($B_6$) challenge. In previous reports, this vitamin was given at doses ranging from 100 to 750 mg/day for periods of 3 days to 6 weeks.[15,16] Current recommendations are to start patients at an oral dose of 100 mg/day while on normal diet; if there is no response, the dose is increased to 300 mg/day and then to 500 mg/day orally, although infants should not receive more than 300 mg/day. Patients in whom plasma homocysteine and/or methionine decreases by at least 30% during the pyridoxine challenge test are classified as $B_6$-responsive.[8] Some correlation between CBS genotype and the biochemical and clinical phenotypes is now becoming apparent based on vitamin $B_6$ responsivity.[17] A handful of mutant alleles are known to be predictive of B6-response outcome, although the predictive status of most alleles and allele combinations remains undetermined. Enzyme activity assays are not considered to be reliable enough to determine $B_6$ responsivity without pyridoxine challenge.[8] For prenatal diagnosis, a direct enzyme assay for CBS activity can be performed on cultured amniocytes,[18] or direct mutation analysis of the *CBS* gene can be performed if the mutation in a family is known.

## CLINICAL ABNORMALITIES

Newborn infants with homocystinuria appear normal and may exhibit no early symptoms. If not treated, most progressively deteriorate and develop clinical symptoms associated with the metabolic derangements. Considerable diversity in symptoms exists, spanning the central nervous, ocular, skeletal, and vascular systems. One or all of these systems may be affected.[8] Typical symptoms include mild delayed development or failure to thrive in the early stages, gradually progressing to impaired vision associated with dislocated lenses, more significant developmental delay with intellectual disability, high risk of thromboembolism, and marfanoid-like features (i.e., tall, thin build with long limbs, arachnodactyly, and pectus excavatum or deformity of the chest). Presentation of ectopia lentis is variable and can occur at any time during early childhood. Other ocular abnormalities secondary to homocystinuria are myopia, glaucoma, cataracts, and retinal detachment. Osteoporosis is also common(found in half of all patients by their teen years[8]), as are pes cavus, dental abnormalities,[19] knock-knees or genu valgum, and scoliosis.[20] Mental status varies from normal to mild or moderate neurocognitive disability. Increasing severity of neurocognitive impairment is associated with increasingly aggressive behavior and other disturbances in behavioral conduct.[21] Seizures and dystonia have also been reported to affect some individuals with homocystinuria. An increased risk of psychiatric disorders has been observed, with more than half of cases consisting of episodic depression, chronic disorders of behavior, chronic obsessive-compulsive disorder, and personality disorders, presenting even in adolescence.[8]

The most serious complications that prove fatal result largely from thromboembolytic events. Premature vascular disease is also associated with mild elevations of plasma homocysteine.[22–24] Early, progressive cardiovascular disease and atherothrombosis are proposed to be related to increased fragility of the connective tissue and endothelial cell dysfunction.[23,24] However, abnormal lipid metabolism,[25–27] oxidative stress, and inflammation as consequences of elevated homocysteine may also contribute to the atherothrombotic risk.[28,29]

## Treatment

Management of homocystinuria varies according to the specific genetic defect and the extent of CBS enzyme activity. Major goals for management of CBS deficiency include, first, normalization of accumulated metabolites to reduce their toxic effects, and second, supportive treatment for complications that are irreversible, such as ocular changes and thrombosis.

Many patients with CBS deficiency respond to relatively supraphysiological doses of pyridoxine, usually 200 mg/day but up to 1000 mg/day in adults.[8] The mechanism involves stabilization of the CBS enzyme with vitamin $B_6$ as a cofactor; therefore, the greater the residual enzyme activity present, the greater the anticipated response with pyridoxine supplementation. The pyridoxine supplement should be titrated to the lowest dose needed to obtain the maximal response. Chronic use of high doses of pyridoxine has been associated with peripheral neuropathy and rhabdomyolysis, so caution with higher doses is essential.[30] Vitamin $B_6$-nonresponsive patients usually show minimal or no residual CBS activity in cultured fibroblasts.[31]

The treatment of vitamin $B_6$–nonresponsive patients is aimed at lowering homocysteine and its disulfide derivatives by administering a methionine-restricted diet supplemented with L-cysteine, which becomes a conditionally essential amino acid.[32] Several synthetic methionine-free amino acid formulas known as medical foods are now available. When provided immediately to infants who are diagnosed presymptomatically on newborn screening, medical foods use can lead to an improved clinical outcome and better prognosis. In addition to administering a low-methionine diet and supplementing with L-cysteine, one must evaluate the diet for optimal therapeutic provision of energy, protein, folate, vitamins $B_6$ and $B_{12}$, betaine, and fluids.

Methionine restriction is accomplished by simultaneous dietary restriction of intact protein and supplementation with methionine-free medical foods to achieve protein requirements for the growing infant and lifelong through adulthood. The methionine requirement can vary from 5 to 30 mg/kg/day based on age and amount of enzyme activity.[31] Because of the low methionine requirement and the moderate amounts of methionine available inintact protein (zero to <5%), only small amounts of foods containing protein are allowed, making dietary compliance difficult. Several brands of specialty modified low-protein foods are available to improve the palatability and quality of the diet and the quality of life for these patients. In addition to maintaining the vitamin and mineral content of the diet, supplementation with folate and possibly with vitamin $B_{12}$ has been recommended.[33,34] Low plasma folate levels in these patients have been attributed to their increased use of homocysteine for remethylation to methionine. Doses of folate ranging from 500 µg/day to 5 mg/day have been used. If red blood cell folate is depleted, oral folate at 5 mg/day is recommended.[8] Clinical practice with regard to vitamin $B_{12}$ supplementation varies in both dose and frequency, from administration of hydroxycobalamin twice yearly to supplementation only when the plasma levels fall below normal limits.[16,35] If plasma $B_{12}$ does fall below normal, 1 mg monthly is recommended.[8]

The use of oral betaine at doses ranging from 150 mg/kg/day in infants to 6 to 9 g/day in children and adults (often divided into two doses) has been reported to be effective for improving metabolic control in patients with CBS deficiency.[8] Patients on betaine treatment have achieved decreased plasma homocysteine in both plasma and cerebrospinal fluid.[36] Because betaine (*N,N,N*-trimethylglycine) is a natural product of choline catabolism, it serves as an additional methyl donor for homocysteine to synthesize methionine through betaine-homocysteine S-methyl transferase activity (see Fig. 37–1). Betaine lowers free and total homocysteine levels, although it also simultaneously increases methionine levels. Normalization of plasma homocysteine levels may not be achieved in patients with vitamin $B_6$–nonresponsive CBS deficiency using the methionine-restricted diet alone, especially because of the varying compliance observed, reportedly because of the poor taste of the formula. Betaine has also been found to reduce risk of thrombosis in these patients.[8]

Betaine is also recommended as treatment for variant forms of homocystinuria, such as MTHFR deficiency. In such cases, betaine should be initiated as early in life as possible and has been shown to dramatically decrease morbidity and mortality.[37] Riboflavin treatment also has been shown to lower homocysteine and, in one case study, to decrease the body odor sometimes associated with betaine treatment.[38–40] As with CBS deficiency, variant homocystinuria may require folate supplementation.

It has been reported that the ratio of plasma methionine to tHcy increased when betaine was administered in conjunction with dietary methionine restriction in patients with vitamin B6–nonresponsive CBS deficiency.[41] Elevated methionine levels appear to contribute less to the pathophysiology of the disease, and methionine can be metabolized by pathways other than transsulfuration, although methionine levels should still be routinely checked in patients taking betaine.[8] The importance of a low-methionine diet to betaine's therapeutic effect has been acknowledged.[41,42]

Dietary treatment for life is recommended by most clinicians because increased protein intake results in elevated homocysteine levels that are potentially harmful at any age. Despite variable compliance, dietary intervention initiated early in life is known to improve IQ, reduce eye complications, prevent seizures, and decrease osteoporosis and thromboembolism. Other supportive medical therapies aimed mainly at reducing thrombolic events by improving the decreased platelet survival time—dipyridamole (100 mg daily), either alone or together with acetyl-salicylic acid (1 g daily)—have been used.[16] Newer anticoagulants that work by inhibiting clotting factors Xa (apixaban) or thrombin (dabigatran) may be an option for patients with CBS deficiency. However, no case reports or published studies are available at this time regarding the efficacy of newer-generation anticoagulants in reducing thrombotic events for patients with CBS deficiency.

Estrogen-based contraceptive use or hormone treatment is typically discouraged in women with CBS deficiency because of their increased risk of thrombotic events.[8] Contraceptives with only progesterone or progestin typically have a lower thrombotic risk than their estrogen counterparts. However risks should still be discussed between patient and doctor before prescribing.[43,44] Pregnancies in women with CBS deficiency appear to have minimal complications but a slightly higher incidence of spontaneous abortion. There is also a higher risk of thromboembolism in the third trimester and postpartum. Homocystinuria is not teratogenic, and pregnancy outcomes are usually good.[8] No effect of the degree of metabolic control or the type of medical intervention on pregnancy complications or offspring has been reported. However, continuous intervention (i.e., diet and/or $B_6$ supplementation) during pregnancy is recommended.[45] Published case reports have indicated that betaine is safe during pregnancy with no teratogenic effect.[8] Anticoagulation therapy, usually in the form of low-molecular-weight heparin, during the third trimester and the postpartum recovery period is recommended to reduce the risk of thromboemobolic complications. Low-dose aspirin throughout pregnancy has also been used.[44]

Increases in homocysteine and homocystine after surgery or trauma can place patients at risk. In such situations, intravenous fluids and monitoring for thrombotic complications is recommended.[8]

Liver transplantation in homocystinuria is infrequently reported. In the existing case studies, patients recovered from surgery and were able to maintain metabolic control with no need for dietary intervention.[45,46] The role of liver transplantation and its risks and benefits for homocystinuria patients warrant further attention.

## Follow-up

Plasma amino acids are monitored to evaluate the efficacy of nutritional support. The frequency of monitoring decreases with age, from weekly during infancy or shortly after diagnosis to monthly after stabilization and every 3 to 6 months thereafter. The goal of the therapy is to maintain fasting plasma methionine levels between 15 and 45 µmol/L; free plasma homocysteine concentrations should be minimized to attain levels as close as possible to zero.

The level of tHcy has been acknowledged as a critical indicator of metabolic control in response to the diet, and it is routinely evaluated throughout the individual's early life. Levels of tHcy in control subjects are less than 15 μmol/L; in untreated children and adults with homocystinuria, they can exceed 100 μmol/L.[8] Patients with variable compliance can attain levels lower than 30 μmol/L and can further reduce concentrations to 5 to 10 μmol/L with the addition of betaine therapy.[47] Some vitamin $B_6$–responsive patients may require dietary methionine restriction to achieve optimal reductions in plasma tHcy. Assessments of growth and development along with routine clinical cardiac, ophthalmological, and neurological evaluations are recommended.

Regardless of the diagnosis-specific treatment strategies used for the management of homocystinuria, it is possible to attain therapeutic levels of metabolites in only a few lifelong compliant patients. There is a need for development of methods, programs, and strategies to improve compliance in this population. However, accumulating evidence indicates that early interventions that decrease plasma tHcy result in more favorable outcomes.[32,48] Along with compliance with dietary restrictions, early establishment of diet therapy is key to effectively minimizing complications.

## References


1. Stipanuk MH. Metabolism of sulfur-containing amino acid. *Annu Rev Nutr.* 1986; 6:179.
2. Mudd SH, Finkelstein JD, Ireverre F, Laster L. Homocystinuria: an enzymatic defect. *Science.* 1964; 143:1433.
3. Schiff M, Blom HJ. Treatment of inherited homocystinurias. *Neuropediatrics.* 2012; 43:295.
4. Banerjee RV, Matthews RG. Cobalamin-dependent methionine synthase. *FASEB J.* 1990; 4:1450.
5. García-Minguillán CJ, Fernandez-Ballart JD, Ceruelo S, et al. Riboflavin status modifies the effects of methylenetetrahydrofolate reductase (MTHFR) and methionine synthase reductase (MTRR) polymorphisms on homocysteine. *Genes Nutr.* 2014; 9:435.
6. Gherasim CG, Zaman U, Raza A, Banerjee R. Impeded electron transfer from a pathogenic FMN domain mutant of methionine synthase reductase and its responsiveness to flavin supplementation. *Biochemistry.* 2008; 47:12515.
7. Baumgartner ER, Wick H, Linnell JC, et al. Congenital defects in intracellular cobalamin metabolism resulting in homocystinuria and methylmalonic aciduria: II. Biochemcial investigations. *Helv Paediatr Acta.* 1979; 34:483.
8. Picker JD, Levy HL. Homocystinuria caused by cystathionine beta-synthase deficiency. 2004; last updated November 2014. In: Pagon RA, Adam MP, Ardinger HH, et al., eds. *GeneReviews.* Seattle, WA: University of Washington; 1993–2016. http://www.ncbi.nlm.nih.gov/books/NBK1524/. Accessed June 25, 2016.
9. Elsas LJ 2nd, Acosta PB. Nutrition support of inherited metabolic disorders. In: Shils ME, Young VR, eds. *Modern Nutrition in Health and Disease,* 7th ed. Philadelphia: Lea & Febiger; 1988.
10. Gaustadnes M, Ingerslev J, Rutiger N. Prevalence of congenital homocystinuria in Denmark. *N Engl J Med.* 1999; 34:1513.
11. Carrillo-Carrasco N, Adams D, Venditti CP. Disorders of intracellular cobalamin metabolism. 2008; last updated November 2013. In: Pagon RA, Adam MP, Ardinger HH, et al., eds. *GeneReviews.* Seattle, WA: University of Washington, 1993–2016. http://www.ncbi.nlm.nih.gov/books/NBK1328/. Accessed June 25, 2016.
12. Guo DC, Gong L, Regalado ES, et al. MAT2A mutations predispose individuals to thoracic aortic aneurysms. *Am J Hum Genet.* 2015; 96:170.
13. Chadwick S, Fitzgerald K, Weiss B, Ficicioglu C. Thirteen patients with MAT1A mutations detected through newborn screening: 13 years' experience. *JIMD Rep.* 2014; 14:71.
14. Nagao M, Tanaka T, Furujo M. Spectrum of mutations associated with methionine adenosyltransferase I/III deficiency among individuals identified during newborn screening in Japan. *Mol Genet Metab.* 2013; 110:460.
15. Kluijtmans LAJ, Boers GHJ, Kraus JP, et al. The molecular basis of cystathionine β-synthase deficiency in Dutch patients with homocystinuria: effect of CBS genotype on biochemical and clinical phenotype, and on response to treatment. *Am J Hum Genet.* 1999; 65:69.
16. Yap S, Naughten E. Homocystinuria due to cystathionine β-synthase deficiency in Ireland: 25 years experience of a newborn screened and treated population with reference to clinical outcome and biochemical control. *J Inherit Metab Dis.* 1998; 21:738.
17. Kruger WD, Wang L, Jhee KH, Singh RH, Elsas LJ 2nd. Cystathionine β-synthase deficiency in Georgia (USA): correlation of clinical and biochemical phenotype with genotype. *Hum Mutat.* 2003; 22:434.
18. Fowler B, Borresen AI, Boman N. Prenatal diagnosis of homocystinuria. *Lancet.* 1982; 2:875.
19. Björksved M, Arnrup K. Homocystinuria and oral health: a report of 14 cases. *Swed Dent J.* 2012; 36:101.
20. Generoso A, Fowler B, Sebas G. Disorder of sulfur amino acid metabolism. In: Fernandes J, Saudubray JM, Van den Berghe G, eds. *Inborn Metabolic Diseases: Diagnosis and Treatment,* 3rd ed. New York: Springer; 2000.
21. Abbott MH, Folstein SE, Abbey H, Pyeritz RE. Psychiatric manifestations of homocystinuria due to cystathionine β-synthase deficiency: prevalence, natural history, and relationship to neurologic impairment and vitamin B6-responsiveness. *Am J Med Genet.* 1987; 26:959.
22. Cattaneo M. Hyperhomocysteinemia and venous thromboembolism. *Semin Thromb Hemost.* 2006; 32:716.
23. Kang S-S, Wong PWK, Malinow MR. Hyperhomocyst(e)inemia as a risk factor for occlusive vascular disease. *Annu Rev Nutr.* 1992; 12:279.
24. Stamler JS, Slivka A. Biological chemistry of thiols in the vasculature and in vascular-related disease. *Nutr Rev.* 1996; 54:1.
25. Poloni S, Leistner-Segal S, Bandeira IC, et al. Body composition in patients with classical homocystinuria: body mass relates to homocysteine and choline metabolism. *Gene.* 2014; 546:443.
26. Jiang H, Stabler SP, Allen RH, Maclean KN. Altered expression of apoA-I, apoA-IV and PON-1 activity in CBS deficient homocystinuria in the presence and absence of treatment: possible implications for cardiovascular outcomes. *Mol Genet Metab.* 2012; 107:55.
27. Nuño-Ayala M, Guillén N, Navarro MA, et al. Cysteinemia, rather than homocysteinemia, is associated with plasma apolipoprotein A-I levels in hyperhomocysteinemia: lipid metabolism in cystathionine beta-synthase deficiency. *Atherosclerosis.* 2010; 212:268.
28. Keating AK, Freehauf C, Jiang H, et al. Constitutive induction of pro-inflammatory and chemotactic cytokines in cystathionine beta-synthase deficient homocystinuria. *Mol Genet Metab.* 2011; 103:330.
29. Vanzin CS, Biancini GB, Sitta A, et al. Experimental evidence of oxidative stress in plasma of homocystinuric patients: a possible role for homocysteine. *Mol Genet Metab.* 2011; 104:112.
30. Schaumburg HH, Berger A. Pyridoxine neurotoxicity. In: Leklem JE, Reynolds RD, eds. *Clinical and Physiological Applications of Vitamin B6.* New York: Alan Liss; 1988.
31. Acosta PB, Elsas LJ 2nd. Nutrition support of vitamin $B_6$–nonresponsive homocystinuria. *Metab Currents.* 1992; 15:13.
32. Acosta P. *The Ross Metabolic Formula System Nutrition Support Protocols,* 4th ed. Columbus, OH: Ross Products Division; 2001.
33. Carey MC, Fennelly JJ, Fitzgerald O. Homocystinuria: II. Subnormal serum folate levels, increased folate clearance and effects of folic acid therapy. *Am J Med.* 1968; 45:26.
34. Wilcken DEL, Wilcken B. The natural history of vascular disease in homocystinuria and the effects of treatment. *J Inher Metab Dis.* 1997; 20:295.
35. Walter JH, Wraith JE, White FJ, Bridge C, Till J. Strategies for the treatment of cystathionine β-synthase deficiency: the experience of the Willink Biochemical Genetics Unit over the past 30 years. *Eur J Pediatr.* 1998; 157(Suppl 2):S71.
36. Huemer M, Kožich V, Rinaldo P, et al. Newborn screening for homocystinurias and methylation disorders: systematic review and proposed guidelines. *J Inherit Metab Dis.* 2015; 38:1007.
37. Diekman EF, de Koning TJ, Verhoeven-Duif NM, et al. Survival and psychomotor development with early betaine treatment in patients with severe methylenetetrahydrofolate reductase deficiency. *JAMA Neurol.* 2014; 71:188.
38. García-Minguillán CJ, Fernandez-Ballart JD, Ceruelo S, et al. Riboflavin status modifies the effects of methylenetetrahydrofolate reductase (MTHFR) and methionine synthase reductase (MTRR) polymorphisms on homocysteine. *Genes Nutr.* 2014; 9:435.
39. Manning NJ, Allen EK, Kirk RJ, Sharrard MJ, Smith EJ. Riboflavin-responsive trimethylaminuria in a patient with homocystinuria on betaine therapy. *JIMD Rep.* 2012; 5:71.
40. Surtees R, Bowron A, Reonard J. Cerebrospinal fluid and total homocysteine and related metabolites in children with cystathionine β-synthase deficiency: the effect of treatment. *Pediatr Res.* 1997; 42:577.
41. Steele RD, Benevenga NJ. Identification of 3-methylthiopropionic acid as an intermediate in mammalian methionine metabolism in vitro. *J Biol Chem.* 1978; 253:7844.
42. Lidegaard Ø. Hormonal contraception, thrombosis and age. *Expert Opin Drug Saf.* 2014; 13:1353.
43. Levy HL, Vargas SE, Waisbren SE, et al. Reproductive fitness in maternal homocystinuria due to cystathionine β-synthase deficiency. *J Inherit Metab Dis.* 2002; 25:299.
44. Plu-Bureau G, Maitrot-Mantelet L, Hugon-Rodin J, Canonico M. Hormonal contraceptives and venous thromboembolism: an epidemiological update. *Best Pract Res Clin Endocrinol Metab.* 2013; 27:25.
45. Lin NC, Niu DM, Loong CC, et al. Liver transplantation for a patient with homocystinuria. *Pediatr Transplant.* 2012; 16:E311.
46. Snyderman SE. Liver failure and neurologic disease in a patient with homocystinuria. *Mol Genet Metab.* 2006; 87:210.
47. Singh RH, Kruger WD, Wang L, Pasquali M, Elsas LJ 2nd. Cystathionine β-synthase deficiency: effects of betaine supplementation following methionine restriction in B6-nonresponsive homocystinuria. *Genet Med.* 2004; 6:90.
48. Mudd SH, Skouvy F, Levy HL, et al. The natural history of homocystinuria due to cystathionine β-synthase deficiency. *Am J Hum Genet.* 1985; 37:1.

# 38 Maple Syrup Urine Disease

RANI H. SINGH AND TERESA D. DOUGLAS

Maple syrup urine disease (MSUD), also known as branched-chain α-ketoacid dehydrogenase (BCKD) deficiency, is a heterogeneous genetic disorder that can result from more than 50 known mutations that impair the mitochondrial BCKD complex.[1] The components of the BCKD complex include E1, a decarboxylase; E2, an acyl transferase; and E3, a lipomide dehydrogenase (dihydrolipoamide dehydrogenase). The defect in this multienzyme complex results in abnormal accumulation of the branched-chain amino acids (BCAAs) leucine, isoleucine, and valine and their respective α-ketoacids (BCKAs) in body fluids (Fig. 38–1).

MSUD is inherited as an autosomal recessive trait. The greatest incidence occurs within Mennonite groups in the northeastern and midwestern United States, approximately 1 of every 380 live births.[2,3] However, in most populations the incidence is more rare, approximating 1 in 185,000 live births.[2,4] Three primary genotypic variants are reported for MSUD: type IA, caused by *BCKDHA* mutations; type IB, caused by *BCKDHB* mutations; and type II, caused by *DBT* mutations.[2] In general, patients with MSUD type IA have a more classic or severe phenotype compared with patients affected by either type IB or type II;[5] however, phenotypic outcome is highly variable even among similar or identical genotypes.[2] *PPM1K* mutation leading to an intermediate MSUD phenotype has been reported in a single case study,[6] but this is not a typical gene variant of MSUD. Mutations in the *DLD* gene that affect the E3 segment of the BCKD complex are occasionally referred to as MSUD type III; however, this condition has an overlapping but distinct phenotype from MSUD that responds poorly to treatment.[7,8] Dihydrolipoamide dehydrogenase (DLD) deficiency, as it is most commonly called, is not be covered in detail in this chapter, but information on the condition can be found in *GeneReviews*.[9]

The spectrum of enzyme activity in MSUD has been reported to range from less than 3% to 40%, and it is one of many factors that contribute to the metabolic phenotype of someone with MSUD. Ex vivo enzymatic assay is not considered a reliable predictor for determining actual residual BCKD complex activity or clinical outcome.[2] Clinical outcome is associated with additional factors such as the age at diagnosis, the time at which diet therapy is begun, growth, energy intake, degree of metabolic control, and rapid intervention for metabolic disturbances caused by catabolic episodes such as injury or illness.[2,10]

The disease was first described in 1954 by Menkes, Hurst, and Craig, who observed four infants with progressive neurological disease associated with a maple syrup odor of the urine in the first weeks of life.[11] In 1960, Dancis et al. demonstrated that the defect was at the enzymatic level of BCAA decarboxylation.[12] Infants with MSUD may appear normal after birth, but within a few hours to days, elevations in leucine can be observed and are associated with progressive neurological deterioration and possibly with a maple syrup odor of the urine and sweet earwax. The clinical symptoms may include poor sucking, irregular respiration, irritability, rigidity alternating with periods of flaccidity, opisthotonos, progressive loss of Moro reflex, and seizures. Symptoms can progress to apnea and coma. Death ensues unless rigorous treatment is implemented. Early diagnosis and treatment may prevent complications and may result in normal or near-normal growth and development.[2]

## CLINICAL AND BIOCHEMICAL ABNORMALITIES

Four clinical and biochemical phenotype classes exist based on clinical presentation and observed therapeutic responses to thiamine.[2,7,13] Classifications of the heterogeneous forms of MSUD have been based on clinical manifestations of the three forms that exhibit varying degrees of partial BCKD enzyme activity (i.e., classic, intermediate, and intermittent) and a thiamine-responsive fourth form[2,13] (Table 38–1).

## FACTORS TO BE CONSIDERED IN NUTRITION EVALUATION

In classic MSUD, BCKAs are derived mainly from leucine, and the activity of the BCKD complex in skin fibroblasts or lymphoblast cultures is usually less than 3% of normal. Clinical symptoms such as lethargy, poor sucking, neurological signs of alternating hypertonia and hypotonia, dystonia, seizures, and encephalopathy develop and progress rapidly within the first few days of life. Dietary BCAA tolerance is usually very low in this group, and symptoms typically develop between 5 and 7 days of age.[2,7] Early diagnosis and initiation of treatment prior to development of neurological symptoms in infants has been associated with lower risk of mental illness and neurocognitive delay later in life.[2,14] Because of newborn screening and diagnostic advances and improvements to enteral and parenteral nutrition for MSUD, neurological outcomes have improved significantly for patients with the classic form. Even so, the possibility of neurological damage, and even death, remains a lifelong concern for these patients, particularly in situations of metabolic intoxication.[2,14]

Even with treatment, the outcome of patients in this group is less than satisfactory with regard to normal neonatal growth and development.[15–17] Impaired bone mineral density affects 90% of patients with classic MSUD by the time they reach adolescence. Improvements in the essential fatty acid and micronutrient content of MSUD enteral formulas have lowered the risk of both nutrient deficiencies and pancreatitis in classic MSUD. Nevertheless, pancreatitis is still a risk during instances of metabolic intoxication, and the patient's nutrition status still needs routine monitoring.[2,18,19] Several studies have found oxidative stress measures to be higher in MSUD, partially accounting for the neurological damage that occurs with the disease.[20–22] L-Carnitine appears to be a useful antioxidant supplement in reducing oxidative stress in MSUD patients.[20,23]

Patients with the intermediate form of MSUD have greater residual enzyme activity than those with the classic form (3% to 30% of normal). Patients with intermediate MSUD have persistent elevations of BCAA, although they may be asymptomatic during the neonatal period. BCAA tolerance is generally higher than that of patients with classic MSUD. Although such patients typically tolerate greater amounts of dietary leucine, dietary management similar to that for classic MSUD is required. Like patients with classic MSUD, those with intermediate MSUD are vulnerable to metabolic decompensations and have the same acute and chronic neurological risks.[2] The onset of symptoms is variable and is usually precipitated by the stress of infection, surgery, or trauma, which can lead to catabolism, or by excessive protein intake. Some patients have shown larger excretion of isoleucine BCKA derivatives compared with the leucine BCKA seen in classic MSUD.[24,25] Mental delays and spasticity have been reported as clinical features, often as a result of delayed diagnosis and management.[2,24,26]

Patients with intermittent forms of MSUD usually demonstrate normal early growth and development and typically can tolerate normal

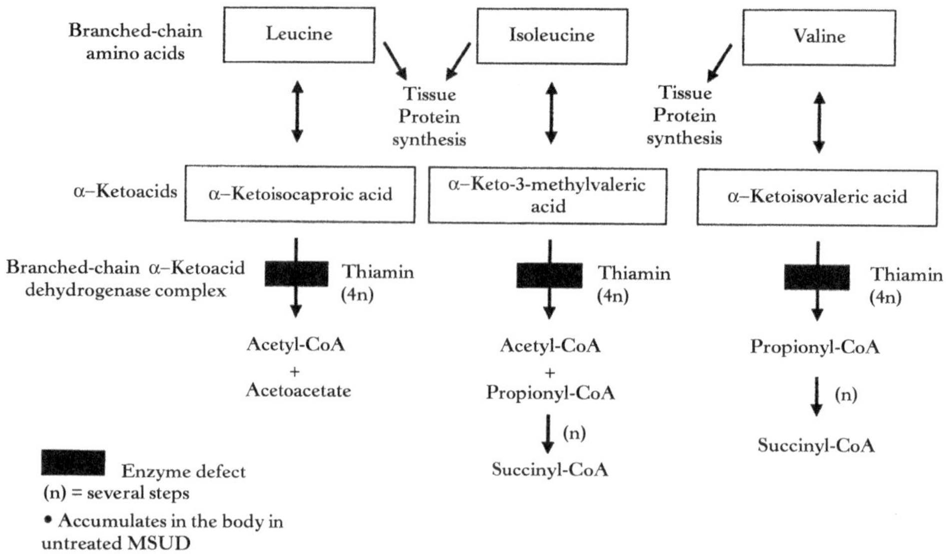


**Figure 38–1.** Metabolic pathways in the catabolism of leucine, isoleucine, and valine demonstrating the site of the defect in maple syrup urine disease (MSUD). CoA = coenzyme A.

amounts of dietary leucine. The BCKD complex enzyme activity is reportedly 5% to 20% of normal. The BCAAs and urine organic acids are within the normal range, or only slightly elevated, when the patient is asymptomatic.[2,13] However, during metabolic decompensation—associated with catabolic shocks or illness, fasting, infections, or surgery—the patient may display clinical symptoms akin to classic MSUD, including elevated BCAAs, increased urine organic acids, and neurological sequelae. These episodes may be associated with progressive changes including acute behavioral changes and unsteady gait progressing to seizures, coma, and even death.[2,27]

Patients with the thiamine-responsive form of MSUD usually have a clinical presentation similar to that of patients with the intermediate form, albeit with the absence of acute neonatal illness. Enzyme activity can be up to 40% of normal, and research attributethe thiamine response to mutations to *BCKDHB*.[2,28] Thiamine response has not been curative of MSUD but has been used adjunctively with typical MSUD nutrition therapy.[2,29,30] Lack of controlled clinical trials evaluating thiamine administration has limited the establishment of clear criteria for thiamin-responsive MSUD. Pharmacological doses of 10 to 1000 mg , have been used to reduce BCKA excretion and plasma BCAA and BCKA concentrations, maximally after approximately 4 weeks. Recent recommendations include 50-200mgms per day.(31) Because dietary changes during a thiamine trial can confound response conclusions, the diet should remain consistent throughout the trial period.[2] All patients with this form of MSUD require thiamine treatment in conjunction with the diet therapy to normalize plasma BCAA levels.[31]

In the past, newborn diagnosis or screening for MSUD was not mandatory in all US states; therefore, infants were frequently diagnosed after they became symptomatic. However, according to the National Newborn Screening Status Report,[32] MSUD is now included in the newborn screening program of every US state. Diagnosis is confirmed by evaluating urine BCKAs, which produce a yellow precipitate with 2,4-dinitrophenylhydrazine (DNPH), and by quantitating plasma BCAAs (leucine, isoleucine, and valine) using ion-exchange chromatography. With elevated BCAA levels, the presence in the plasma of alloisoleucine, a metabolite of isoleucine, is pathognomonic for MSUD.[33] Even if other BCAA levels are normal, leucine and alloisoleucine will still be increased.[2]

The enzyme activity can be measured in lymphocytes or cultured fibroblasts when deemed necessary to confirm the diagnosis, although the reliability of the enzyme activity assay for MSUD has been called into question.[2] Identification of mutations in MSUD patients, and of unaffected carrier status, is best established by molecular genetic analysis. Prenatal diagnosis with molecular genetic testing can be performed using cultured amniotic fluid cells or chorion villus cells.[2,34]

## Dietary Treatment

Dietary interventions to achieve and maintain normal plasma amino acid levels appear to be best correlated with a good outcome in patients with MSUD.[2,35] Nutritional support should be initiated promptly to promote anabolism and to reduce BCAA levels and accumulation of toxic metabolites. Overall, the MSUD diet involves dietary leucine

**Table 38–1.** Clinical and Biochemical Phenotypes in Maple Syrup Urine Disease (MSUD)

| Clinical Phenotype | Prominent Clinical Features | Biochemical Features | Decarboxylation Activity (% of Normal)* |
|---|---|---|---|
| Classic | Neonatal onset, poor feeding, lethargy, increased/decreased tone, ketoacidosis, seizures, "fencing" or "bicycling" movements | Markedly increased alloisoleucine, BCAA, and BCKA | 0–2 |
| Intermediate | Irritability, failure to thrive, often no ketoacidosis, developmental delay | Persistently increased alloisoleucine, BCAA, and BCKA | 3–30 |
| Intermittent | Normal early development, episodic ataxia/ketoacidosis precipitated by infection or stress; episodes can be fatal; usually intellect is normal | Normal BCAA when asymptomatic | 5–20 |
| Thiamine-responsive | Similar to intermediate MSUD | Decreased BCKA and/or BCAA with thiamine therapy | 2–40 |

*Most commonly measured in intact peripheral blood leukocytes or cultured fibroblasts or lymphoblasts with $[1\text{-}^{14}C]$-labeled BCAA or BCKA as substrate.
BCAA = branched-chain amino acids; BCKA = branched-chain α-ketoacids.
Data from Danner DJ, Doering CB. Human mutations affecting branched chain alphaketoacid dehydrogenase. *Front Biosci.* 1998; 3:517.

restriction, BCAA-free medical foods (formula), careful supplementation with essential amino acids valine and isoleucine, and lifelong monitoring of biochemical and clinical status.[2] Management criteria for newborns newly diagnosed with MSUD includes stabilizing plasma BCAA; determining leucine, isoleucine, and valine tolerance according to age, growth, and phenotype; avoiding micronutrient and macronutrient deficiencies; and working to achieve normal growth and neurocognitive development through appropriate treatment and monitoring. For asymptomatic newborns and young children with MSUD, dietary management involves prescribing a BCAA-free medical food that helps to achieve normal caloric intake and protein intake at 2.0 to 3.0 g/kg/day.[2,31] If medical food is deficient in alanine, glutamine, micronutrients, or essential fatty acids, these can be supplemented along with appropriate amounts of leucine, isoleucine, and valine according to patient tolerance. Tolerance of leucine decreases with age and growth stabilization: typically, 65 to 85 mg/kg/day is tolerated in infants, 20 to 40 mg/kg/day in children, and 10 to 15 mg/kg/day in adults.[2]

Long-term treatment of MSUD involves lifelong dietary therapy to maintain plasma BCAAs within the therapeutic range while promoting normal growth and development. This involves careful titration by a registered dietitian of protein from several commercial BCAA-free medical foods and of essential BCAA from standard formulas for infants and natural foods in older patients with MSUD. The daily BCAA requirements vary with age, severity of the enzyme defect, and growth rate.[2,13] The suggested range of intake of these nutrients for individuals with MSUD is outlined in Table 38–2. Frequent adjustments of the dietary prescription, along with lifelong monitoring of plasma BCAA and urinary BCAA and BCKA, are necessary.

Adequate protein and calorie intake is possible through the use of medical foods and a wide variety of specialized low-protein foods. Medical foods with different nutrient compositions and forms are available, including BCAA-free modules only or in combination with carbohydrates or fats. Medical foods are available in the form of powders, capsules, or bars. A complete diet analysis to assess adequate nutrient intake is essential. Docosahexaenoic acid (DHA) deficiency, despite adequate intake of α-linolenic acid (ALA), has been reported in MSUD patients.[36,37] Therefore, DHA should be supplemented if not incorporated into the medical food. MSUD food lists for counting leucine and protein content of foods are available to both clinicians and patients.[38] With the help of registered dietitians and other clinical personnel, parents are instructed in the tasks of recording and monitoring amino acid and energy intake of their infant or child with MSUD and submitting dried blood spots to a nearby laboratory for routine BCAA analysis.[2] Over time, these responsibilities should be taken on by the growing child, adolescent, or adult with MSUD.

Having a sick-day dietary protocol in place can allow for outpatient treatment of catabolic events (e.g., illness, injury) while avoiding metabolic decompensation. This typically involves a leucine-free diet with additional amounts of isoleucine, valine, medical food, and calories. Immediate and frequent monitoring of BCAA in the blood is likewise critical until the catabolic event is resolved (i.e., recovery from the illness or injury).[2,31] If common illnesses, infections, or surgeries are left untreated in MSUD, serious consequences such as coma and death may occur. Acute episodes, which are usually associated with ketoacidosis, require large amounts of parenteral fluids and electrolytes to prevent catabolism. In the symptomatic infant, nutritional support should be initiated promptly to promote anabolism and to reduce levels of BCAA and toxic metabolites. Initiation of a BCAA-free hypercaloric diet providing a minimum of 1.25 times the estimated energy requirement (up to 3 times the requirement for older children and adults), and protein at 2.0 to 3.5 g/kg/day may achieve net body protein accretion and the resolution of clinical symptoms.[2] It is essential to decrease leucine and increase calorie and fluid intake to prevent catabolism. Orogastric feedings are usually preferred for infants; however, if necessary, parenteral nutrition by itself or simultaneously with BCAA-free orogastric feeds may be used to achieve anabolism. If a child or adult cannot tolerate oral feedings during illness, hospitalization may be necessary to provide nutritional support intravenously.

Intravenous solutions without BCAAs are available and have been shown to be rapidly effective in correcting BCAA elevations and the related symptoms.[39] Immediate and short-term infusion of glucose to achieve hypercaloric status, as well as insulin to manage hyperglycemia and replenish glycogen stores, has been shown to help reduce catabolism, produce anabolism, and normalize BCAAs.[2,31,40] However, prolonged exclusion, overrestriction, or imbalance of BCAAs leads to anemia, desquamation of the skin, diarrhea, and failure to thrive.[41-43] Emergency treatment with hemodialysis, in combination with nutrition therapy, may be effective in rapidly lowering plasma BCAA and BCKA concentrations,[2,44,45] but it is not without risks.[46] Whether or not hemodialysis is used, aggressive nutrition intervention involving an energy-dense diet is the key therapeutic method to normalizing BCAAs and resolving a metabolic crisis.

The declination rate of elevated amino acids may vary as a result of several factors, including genotype and the amount or source of the amino acid calories. Leucine declination appears to be accelerated in patients provided BCAA-free essential and nonessential amino acids with supplemental isoleucine, valine, alanine, glutamine, and tyrosine.[2] In general, plasma concentrations of isoleucine and valine may decrease more rapidly than leucine concentrations, possibly declining to subnormal levels while leucine levels remain high.[47] In these conditions, addition of L-isoleucine and L-valine to medical foods prevents catabolism and normalizes all plasma amino acids, possibly, in part, by restoring the limited amino acid substrate required for normal rates of protein synthesis.[2]

**Table 38–2.** Recommended Daily Nutrient Intakes for Infants and Children with Maple Syrup Urine Disease

| | Age | | | | | | |
|---|---|---|---|---|---|---|---|
| Nutrient* | <6 mo | 6–12 mo | 1–3 yr | 4–8 yr | 9–13 yr | 14–18 yr | 19+ yr |
| **Energy** (kcal/kg) | 95–145 | 80–135 | 80–130 | 50–120 | 40–90 | 35–70 | 35–45 |
| **Protein** (g/kg) | 2.5–3.5 | 2.5–3.0 | 1.5–2.5 | 1.3–2.0 | 1.2–1.8 | 1.2–1.8 | 1.1–1.7 |
| **Carbohydrate** (% of kcal) | 35 | 35 | 35 | 50 | 50 | 50 | 50 |
| **Fat** (% of kcal) | 40–50 | 40–50 | 40–50 | 30–35 | 30–35 | 33–35 | 30–35 |
| **Isoleucine**† | | | | | | | |
| (mg/kg/day) | 30–90 | 30–70 | 20–70 | 20–30 | 20–30 | 10–30 | 10–30 |
| *(mg/day)* | | | *165–325* | *215–420* | *245–470* | *325–345* | *330–570* |
| **Leucine** | | | | | | | |
| (mg/kg/day) | 40–100 | 40–75 | 40–70 | 35–65 | 30–60 | 15–50 | 15–50 |
| *(mg/day)* | | | *275–535* | *360–695* | *410–785* | *540–740* | *550–945* |
| **Valine**‡ | | | | | | | |
| (mg/kg/day) | 40–95 | 30–80 | 30–70 | 30–50 | 25–40 | 15–30 | 15–30 |
| *(mg/day)* | | | *190–400* | *250–490* | *285–550* | *375–520* | *385–665* |

*Adapted from Frazier DM, Allgeier C, Homer C, et al. Nutrition management guideline for maple syrup urine disease: an evidence- and consensus-based approach. *Mol Genet Metab.* 2014; 112:210.

There are a several published case studies indicating that appropriate nutrition management during pregnancy in women with MSUD can result in successful pregnancy outcomes.[48–51] As with phenylalanine in phenylketonuria (PKU), high levels of leucine may not be teratogenic. Additionally, catabolic stress during critical times of the pregnancy (e.g., sickness and vomiting, labor and delivery) and and after delivery can place the mother at risk of metabolic decompensation.[2,31] The available data suggest that a critical aspect of nutrition intervention is preserving maternal anabolism for an optimal outcome. This can be accomplished through rigorous monitoring of maternal BCAA status throughout the pregnancy, meeting increased protein and BCAA needs as the pregnancy progresses, and being proactive in reducing catabolic stress during the pregnancy and after delivery.[2,31]

The role of exercise and physical activity levels in MSUD is unstudied at this time, as is MSUD management in the geriatric patient group. Presumably, caution must be taken to prevent metabolic decompensation in either case.

Liver transplantation has become more frequent in the amelioration of MSUD in affected patients. There are some case studies of unsuccessful liver transplantation in MSUD, although mostly successful cases are found in the literature.[52] The option of transplantation is most often provided in cases of classic MSUD and has been successfully accomplished in ages ranging from infant to adult.[2,53,54] Long-term follow-up of patients across several years indicates success, with complete normalization of plasma BCAA and protein tolerance typical of the background population, eliminating need for specialized diet.[2,52,54] Additionally, liver transplantation, although unable to reverse neurological damage in MSUD, does result in arrest of further damage,[14,55] so there is no progression of brain injury or risk of future metabolic decompensation.[2,52,54] The risks are typical of those for any patient receiving a liver transplant, including the need for lifelong immunosuppression.[2,56] However, patients ideally should be in good metabolic status on diet therapy at the time of transplantation to reduce risk of complications. Metabolic decompensation can still occur during the perioperative period, so precautions are necessary.[31] After transplantation, the patient's metabolic status should be monitored carefully for at least 1 year to ensure healthy BCAA status and acceptance of the graft.

Psychosocial issues for families and MSUD-affected individuals are common. Living with MSUD has been shown to increase life stress, decrease quality of life,[57,58] and affect social functioning of the MSUD patient well into the adult years.[59,60] Additionally, MSUD patients are at greater risk of developing attention-deficit hyperactivity disorder (ADHD), anxiety, depression, and other psychiatric disturbances.[2,14] Therefore, intervention in the form of counseling, support networks, occupational therapy, and psychiatric expertise is typically a part of treatment for the patient with MSUD.

## References


1. Danner DJ, Doering CB. Human mutations affecting branched chain alphaketoacid dehydrogenase. *Front Biosci.* 1998; 3:517.
2. Strauss KA, Puffenberger EG, Morton DH. Maple syrup urine disease. 2006; last updated May 2013. In: Pagon RA, Adam MP, Ardinger HH, et al., eds. *GeneReviews.* Seattle, WA: University of Washington; 1993–2015. Available from: http://www.ncbi.nlm.nih.gov/books/NBK1319/. Accessed June 25, 2016.
3. Puffenberger EG. Genetic heritage of the Old Order Mennonites of southeastern Pennsylvania. *Am J Med Genet C Semin Med Genet.* 2003; 121C(1):18.
4. Nellis MM, Kasinski A, Carlson M, et al. Relationship of causative genetic mutations in maple syrup urine disease with their clinical expression. *Mol Genet Metab.* 2003; 80(1–2):189.
5. Flaschker N, Feyen O, Fend S, Simon E, Schadewaldt P, Wendel U. Description of the mutations in 15 subjects with variant forms of maple syrup urine disease. *J Inherit Metab Dis.* 2007; 30:903.
6. Oyarzabal A, Martínez-Pardo M, Merinero B, et al. . A novel regulatory defect in the branched-chain α-keto acid dehydrogenase complex due to a mutation in the *PPM1K* gene causes a mild variant phenotype of maple syrup urine disease. *Hum Mutat.* 2013; 34:355.
7. Online Mendelian Inheritance in Man. *Maple syrup urine disease.* OMIM entry # 248600. Last edited 3/31/2013. Baltimore, MD: Johns Hopkins University.
8. Online Mendelian Inheritance in Man. *Dihydrolipoamide dehydrogenase deficiency.* OMIM # 246900: Last edited 6/23/2016. Baltimore, MD: Johns Hopkins University.
9. Quinonez SC, Thoene JG. Dihydrolipoamide dehydrogenase deficiency. 2014. In: Pagon RA, Adam MP, Ardinger HH, et al., eds. *GeneReviews.* Seattle, WA: University of Washington; 1993–2016. http://www.ncbi.nlm.nih.gov/books/NBK220444/. Accessed June 25, 2016.
10. Danner DJ, Elsas LJ 2nd. Disorders of branched chain amino and keto-acid metabolism. In: Scirver CR, Beaudet AL, Sly WS, Vallee D, eds. *The Metabolic Basis of Inherited Disease*, 6th ed. New York: McGraw-Hill; 1988.
11. Menkes JH, Hurst PL, Craig JM. A new syndrome: progressive familial infantile cerebral dysfunction associated with an unusual urinary substance. *Pediatrics.* 1954; 14:462.
12. Dancis J, Hutzler J, Levitz M. Metabolism of the white blood cells in maple syrup urine disease. *Biochim Biophys Acta.* 1960; 43:342.
13. Chuang DT, Shih VE. Maple syrup urine disease (branched-chain ketoaciduria). In: Scriver CR, Beaudet AL, Sly WS, Vallee D, eds. *The Metabolic and Molecular Basis of Inherited Disease*, 8th ed. New York: McGraw-Hill; 2001.
14. Muelly ER, Moore GJ, Bunce SC, et al. Biochemical correlates of neuropsychiatric illness in maple syrup urine disease. *J Clin Invest.* 2013; 123:1809.
15. Knerr I, Weinhold N, Vockley J, Gibson KM. Advances and challenges in the treatment of branched-chain amino/keto acid metabolic defects. *J Inherit Metab Dis.* 2012; 35:29.
16. Treacy E, Clow CL, Reade TR, Chitayat D, Mamer OA, Scriver CR. Maple syrup urine disease: interrelations between branched-chain amino-, oxo- and hydroxyacids; implications for treatment; associations with CNS dysmyelination. *J Inherit Metab Dis.* 1992; 15:121.
17. Riviello JJ, Rezvani I, Digeorge AM, Foley CM. Cerebral edema causing death in children with maple syrup urine disease. *J Pediatr.* 1991; 119:42.
18. Kahler SG, Woolf DA, Leonard JV, Zaritsky A, Lawless ST, Sherwood WG. *Pancreatitis and Organic Acidurias: An Under-recognized Association?* (abstract). Presented at the Fifth International Congress on Inborn Errors of Metabolism, Pacific Grove, CA, June 1–5, 1990.
19. Friedrich CA, Marble M, Maher J, Valle D. Successful control of branched-chain amino acids (BCAA) in maple syrup urine disease using elemental amino acids in total parenteral nutrition during acute pancreatitis. *Am J Hum Genet.* 1992; 51:A350.
20. Guerreiro G, Mescka CP, Sitta A, et al. Urinary biomarkers of oxidative damage in maple syrup urine disease: the L-carnitine role. *Int J Dev Neurosci.* 2015; 42:10.
21. Sitta A, Ribas GS, Mescka CP, Barschak AG, Wajner M, Vargas CR. Neurological damage in MSUD: the role of oxidative stress. *Cell Mol Neurobiol.* 2014; 34:157.
22. Mescka CP, Wayhs CA, Vanzin CS, et al. Protein and lipid damage in maple syrup urine disease patients: L-carnitine effect. *Int J Dev Neurosci.* 2013; 31:21.
23. Ribas GS, Vargas CR, Wajner M. L-Carnitine supplementation as a potential antioxidant therapy for inherited neurometabolic disorders. *Gene.* 2014; 533:469.
24. Fischer MH, Gerritsen T. Biochemical studies on a variant of branched chain ketoaciduria in a 19-year-old female. *Pediatrics.* 1971; 48:795.
25. Duran M, Tielens AG, Wadman SK, Stigter JC, Kleijer WJ. Effects of thiamine in a patient with a variant form of branched-chain ketoaciduria. *Acta Paediatr Scand.* 1987; 60:594.
26. Gonzalez-Rios MC, Chuang DT, Cox RP, Schmidt K, Knopf K, Packman S. A distinct variant of intermediate maple syrup urine disease. *Clin Genet.* 1985; 27:153.
27. Dancis J, Levitz M, Westall RG. Intermittent branched-chain ketonuria: variant of maple-syrup-urine-disease. *N Engl J Med.* 1967; 276:84.
28. Chuang DT, Chuang JL, Wynn RM. Lessons from genetic disorders of branched-chain amino acid metabolism. *J Nutr.* 2006; 136(1 Suppl):243S.
29. Elsas LJ 2nd, Danner DJ. The role of thiamin in maple syrup urine disease. *Ann N Y Acad Sci.* 1982; 378:404.
30. Fernhoff PM, Lubitz D, Danner DJ, et al. Thiamin response in maple urine disease. *Pediatr Res.* 1985; 19:1011.
31. Frazier DM, Allgeier C, Homer C, et al. Nutrition management guideline for maple syrup urine disease: an evidence- and consensus-based approach. *Mol Genet Metab.* 2014; 112:210.
32. National Newborn Screening and Genetics Resource Center, University of Texas Health Science Center, San Antonio. *National Newborn Screening Status Report.* November 2, 2014. https://genes-r-us.uthscsa.edu/sites/genes-r-us/files/nbsdisorders.pdf. Accessed June 25, 2016.
33. Schadewaldt P, Bodner-Leidecker A, Hammen HW, Wendel U. Significance of L-alloisoleucine in plasma for diagnosis of maple syrup urine disease. *Clin Chem.* 1999; 45:1734.
34. Borden M. Methodology: screening for metabolic diseases. In: Nyhan WL, ed. *Abnormalities in Amino Acid Metabolism in Clinical Medicine.* Norwalk, CT: Appleton-Century-Crofts; 1984.
35. Hilliges C, Awiszus D, Wendel U. Intellectual performance of children with maple syrup urine disease. *Eur J Pediatr.* 1993; 152:144.
36. Mazer LM, Yi SH, Singh RH. Docosahexaenoic acid status in females of reproductive age with maple syrup urine disease. *J Inherit Metab Dis.* 2010; 33:121.
37. Strauss KA, Wardley B, Robinson D, et al. Classical maple syrup urine disease and brain development: principles of management and formula design. *Mol Genet Metab.* 2010; 99:333.
38. Singh RH, Lesperance E. *MSUD Food List: Keeping Track of the Foods You Eat.* Atlanta: Emory University, Department of Human Genetics; 2002.
39. Berry GT, Heidenreich R, Kaplan P, et al. Branched-chain amino acid-free parenteral nutrition in the treatment of acute metabolic decompensation in patients with maple syrup urine disease. *N Engl J Med.* 1991; 324:175.
40. Biggeman B, Zass R, Wendel U. Postoperative metabolic decompensation in maple syrup urine disease is completely prevented by insulin. *J Inherit Metab Dis.* 1993; 16:912.
41. Giacoia GP, Berry GT. Acrodermatitis enteropathica-like syndrome secondary to isoleucine deficiency during treatment of maple syrup urine disease. *Am J Dis Child.* 1993; 147:954.
42. Koch SE, Packman S, Koch TK, Williams ML. Dermatitis in treated maple syrup urine disease. *J Am Acad Dermatol.* 1993; 28:289.

43. Northrup H, Sigman ES, Herbert AA. Exfoliative erythroderma resulting from inadequate intake of branched-chain amino acids in infants with MSUD. *Arch Dermatol.* 1993; 129:385.
44. Puliyanda DP, Harmon WE, Peterschmitt MJ, Irons M, Somers MJ. Utility of hemodialysis in maple syrup urine disease. *Pediatr Nephrol.* 2002; 17:239.
45. Jouvet P, Jugie M, Rabier D, et al. Combined nutritional support and continuous extracorporeal removal therapy in the severe acute phase of maple syrup urine disease. *Intensive Care Med.* 2001; 27:1798.
46. Schaefer F, Straube E, Oh J, Mehls O, Mayatepek E. Dialysis in neonates with inborn errors of metabolism. *Nephrol Dial Transplant.* 1999; 14:910.
47. Naglak M, Elsas LJ 2nd. Nutrition support of maple syrup urine disease. *Metab Currents.* 1988; 1:15.
48. Heiber S, Zulewski H, Zaugg M, Kiss C, Baumgartner M. Successful pregnancy in a woman with maple syrup urine disease: case report. *JIMD Rep.* 2015; 21:103.
49. Wessel AE, Mogensen KM, Rohr F, et al. Management of a woman with maple syrup urine disease during pregnancy, delivery, and lactation. *JPEN J Parenter Enteral Nutr.* 2015; 39:875.
50. Tchan M, Westbrook M, Wilcox G, et al. The management of pregnancy in maple syrup urine disease: experience with two patients. *JIMD Rep.* 2013; 10:113.
51. Van Calcar SC, Harding CO, Davidson SR, Barness LA, Wolff JA. Case reports of successful pregnancy in women with maple syrup urine disease and proprionic acidemia. *Am J Med Genet.* 1992; 4:641.
52. Díaz VM, Camarena C, de la Vega Á, et al. Liver transplantation for classical maple syrup urine disease: long-term follow-up. *J Pediatr Gastroenterol Nutr.* 2014; 59:636.
53. McLaughlin PM, Hinshaw J, Stringer AY. Maple syrup urine disease (MSUD): a case with long-term follow-up after liver transplantation. *Clin Neuropsychol.* 2013; 27:1199.
54. Mazariegos GV, Morton DH, Sindhi R, et al. Liver transplantation for classical maple syrup urine disease: long-term follow-up in 37 patients and comparative United Network for Organ Sharing experience. *J Pediatr.* 2012; 160:116.
55. Shellmer DA, DeVito Dabbs A, Dew MA, et al. Cognitive and adaptive functioning after liver transplantation for maple syrup urine disease: a case series. *Pediatr Transplant.* 2011; 15:58.
56. Strauss KA, Mazariegos GV, Sindhi R, et al. Elective liver transplantation for the treatment of classical maple syrup urine disease. *Am J Transplant.* 2006; 6:557.
57. Fabre A, Baumstarck K, Cano A, et al. Assessment of quality of life of the children and parents affected by inborn errors of metabolism with restricted diet: preliminary results of a cross-sectional study. *Health Qual Life Outcomes.* 2013; 11:158.
58. Packman W, Henderson SL, Mehta I, et al. Psychosocial issues in families affected by maple syrup urine disease. *J Genet Couns.* 2007; 16:799.
59. Packman W, Mehta I, Rafie S, Mehta J, Naldi M, Mooney KH. Young adults with MSUD and their transition to adulthood: psychosocial issues. *J Genet Couns.* 2012; 21:692.
60. Simon E, Schwarz M, Wendel U. Social outcome in adults with maple syrup urine disease (MSUD). *J Inherit Metab Dis.* 2007; 30:264.

# 39 Phenylketonuria and Maternal Phenylketonuria

SUSAN A. BERRY, DOROTHY MARKOWITZ, AND NANCY D. LESLIE

Phenylketonuria (PKU), now known to be caused by a deficiency in phenylalanine hydroxylase (PAH), was first described by Asbjörn Fölling in 1934, after a persistent and observant mother asked him to determine the cause of intellectual disability in her two children. He noted a peculiar clinging odor about the children and suspected that it might be a clue to their challenges. He tested their urine with a ferric chloride solution, expecting to find the red-brown color characteristic of ketones. Instead, he observed a dark green color now known to be caused by phenylpyruvic acid,[1] a metabolite of phenylalanine. Phenylketonuria remained a somewhat obscure biochemical curiosity for almost 20 years until 1951, when Woolf and Vulliamy suggested that there might be a relationship between excess phenylalanine and brain damage.[2] Soon afterward, Bickel et al.[3] published the first report describing marked clinical improvement after use of a phenylalanine-restricted diet. However, these initial attempts at therapy also showed that initiation of treatment after recognition of developmental delay was futile in reversing established cognitive damage. In contrast, initiation of therapy in affected newborns born into families known to be at high risk for PKU established the principle that diet could prevent intellectual disability.[4]

The need for an effective means of testing newborns on a population basis led to programs initially testing urine at the time of the 6-week well-child visit, using the ferric chloride indicator used by Fölling. Although this program was logistically more feasible in the late 1950s than can be imagined today, it was far from ideal. Simple, cost-effective mass screening for PKU became a reality in 1963 after Robert Guthrie devised the bacterial inhibition method for testing phenylalanine levels in dried blood collected on filter paper.[5] Routine screening of newborns now makes late diagnosis of PKU rare (Fig. 39–1).

Classical PKU, or severe PAH deficiency, is inherited in an autosomal recessive manner and has an incidence of 1 in 11,400 live births in the United States.[6] In Western Europe and North America, most elevations in phenylalanine on newborn screening are caused by mutations in the gene, *PAH*.[7] Defects in genes coding for enzymes involved in the synthesis or recycling of the required biopterin cofactor are responsible for a minority of positive newborn screens for phenylalanine. Cofactor-dependent PKU affects neurotransmitter synthesis in a more global manner than PAH-deficient PKU and requires a complex medical regimen in addition to a phenylalanine-restricted diet.

Characteristic features of untreated individuals with severe PAH deficiency include mental retardation, diminished pigmentation, eczema, hypertonicity, seizures, and an unusual body odor. Untreated adults with PAH deficiency may also develop behavioral problems such as hyperactivity, aggressiveness, self-inflicted injury, and negative mood swings.[8] However, many individuals with elevated phenylalanine levels have mild or no cognitive or behavioral manifestations, so the disease spectrum of PAH deficiency includes individuals with mild or benign hyperphenylalaninemia.

The current treatment regimen for severe PAH deficiency, as established by new guidelines from the American College of Medical Genetics and Genomics (ACMG), recommends that all affected persons with PAH deficiency, including adolescents, adults, and pregnant women, maintain phenylalanine levels between 60 and 360 μmol/L.[9] It is unknown whether levels up to 600 μmol/L in individuals on an ambient diet (i.e., those previously categorized as having benign hyperphenylalaninemia) might be improved by additional therapy.

## PHENYLALANINE EMBRYOPATHY: A CONSEQUENCE OF MATERNAL PHENYLKETONURIA

The teratogenic consequences of elevated maternal phenylalanine during pregnancy were recognized and described first by C. E. Dent in 1956.[10] In 1980, Lenke and Levy described the full spectrum of effects of maternal hyperphenylalaninemia on the fetus.[11] This retrospective survey of the literature reviewed 524 pregnancies in 155 women with PKU or hyperphenylalaninemia who had 423 offspring and 101 spontaneous abortions. It revealed an increased incidence of intellectual disability, microcephaly, and congenital heart disease in offspring of women with untreated PKU during pregnancy that was correlated with elevated maternal serum phenylalanine levels. Other features in these infants included thin upper lip, upturned nose, short nasal bridge, and/or epicanthal folds.[11] In 1984, the National Institutes of Health funded a multicenter collaborative study to evaluate the efficacy of a phenylalanine-restricted diet during pregnancy. The study, which enrolled subjects from 1984 to 1995, conclusively showed that women who achieved phenylalanine levels lower than 600 μmol/L by 8 to 10 weeks of gestation[12] and maintained those levels throughout pregnancy had very good physical and fetal outcomes.[13] Based on these findings, it is recommended that women with PKU maintain phenylalanine levels below 360 μmol/L before conception and throughout pregnancy.

## BIOCHEMICAL ABNORMALITY

The biochemical defect in PKU is a functional deficiency of the liver enzyme PAH, which catalyzes the parahydroxylation of phenylalanine to yield tyrosine.[12] The hydroxylase system requires a cofactor, tetrahydrobiopterin (BH4). A second enzyme, dihydropteridine reductase, recycles the pterin cofactor back to the active state. In individuals with two null mutations in the PAH gene, serum or plasma phenylalanine concentrations on an unrestricted diet are greater than 1200 μmol/L, and the characteristic metabolites of phenylalanine (i.e., phenylpyruvic acid, phenylacetic acid, phenyllactic acid, 2-hydroxphenylacetic acid, and phenylethylamine) are excreted in the urine.[14] Phenylacetic acid is responsible for the odor associated with untreated or poorly controlled PKU.[1] In untreated individuals, pigment dilution in hair and skin is the consequence of defective transport of tyrosine, a precursor of melanin.

Accumulation of phenylalanine results in a series of direct and indirect biochemical changes that occur during early stages of development of the central nervous system and contribute to a pathogenic pattern that, without treatment, usually results in intellectual disability by a still unknown mechanism. Among the hypothesized pathogenic mechanisms are monoamine depletion and impairment of brain protein synthesis through inhibition by phenylalanine or one of its byproducts or through a relative deficiency of other essential amino acids. It is generally agreed that excess phenylalanine exerts a permanent deleterious effect on the brain during development and a reversible toxic effect subsequently.[14] Pathogenesis of the cognitive defect is probably the same whether infants are exposed to excess phenylalanine in utero or after birth, but the actual mechanism remains unclear. Possible explanations include competition for transport of large neutral amino acids (LNAA), inhibition of protein synthesis, interference with *N*-methyl-D-aspartic acid (NMDA) receptors, disturbance of myelin structure, and inhibition of neurotransmitter synthesis.[14] Active

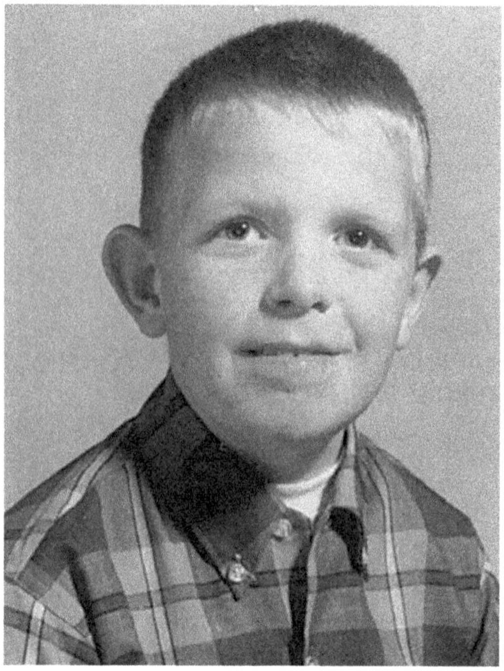

**Figure 39–1.** Phenylketonuria in this boy was recognized at age 3 years, when developmental delay was noted. At age 8 years, he remained moderately intellectually disabled. (Courtesy of Cincinnati Children's Hospital Medical Center, Division of Genetics. Used with permission.)

transport systems that carry phenylalanine across membranes also carry other LNAA,[15] and when the transport system is overloaded by a single amino acid, the others are excluded from transport. This exclusion within the transport system can result in a disruption of growth and other processes.

## FACTORS TO BE CONSIDERED IN NUTRITION EVALUATION

### Specific Nutrients

The dietary treatment of PKU consists of providing a nutritionally balanced diet that contains enough phenylalanine to meet the needs of an infant or growing child or to maintain the needs of an older child, adolescent, or adult without vastly exceeding that individual's limited capacity to utilize phenylalanine. As an essential amino acid, phenylalanine must be included in the diet in sufficient amounts to allow for protein synthesis. However, a safe and practical PKU diet almost never returns the serum phenylalanine to normal levels. The diet includes a special-purpose medical food (i.e., a protein substitute, often referred to as a *formula*), natural foods to provide the requirement for phenylalanine, and low-protein modified foods to provide additional calories and variety. The objective of treatment is to reduce serum phenylalanine to a control range of 120 to 360 μmol/L to promote normal growth and development during childhood and healthy neuropsychological function in all age groups.[9,16]

*Phenylalanine* requirements (per kilogram body weight) are greatest during infancy and diminish significantly with age.[9,17] Specific recommendations regarding phenylalanine requirements are shown in Table 39–1.[9,17] Limited amounts of natural foods and modified low-protein foods provide phenylalanine, calories, and variety in the diet. Sufficient calories must be obtained from the diet to prevent catabolism of protein and weight loss.

The *protein requirement* is provided by medical foods that are phenylalanine-free or with very low phenylalanine that provide close to 85% of the nitrogen requirement in most prescriptions.[18,19] These products are composed of L-amino acids[19] or a whole protein derived from milk, glycomacropeptide (GMP).[18] When L-amino acids are the source of protein in PKU medical foods, the absorption and rise in serum amino acid concentration is more rapid than with the usual digestion of whole protein, and the utilization of L-amino acids is different from that in whole protein.[19] When dietary phenylalanine is restricted, tyrosine becomes an essential amino acid, and other essential amino acids must be present simultaneously. Commercial PKU formulas are well fortified with L-tyrosine, and typical formula prescriptions should meet the tyrosine requirement. Occasionally, supplemental L-tyrosine is required to maintain serum tyrosine levels within an acceptable range. Recommendations for tyrosine supplementation are included in Table 39–1.[9,17]

*Energy* needs of an individual patient may not be met by the formula and the limited amounts of natural foods permitted. Modified low-protein foods and free foods such as sugar and fats may be used to provide needed calories. Part of the fat should be in the form of safflower, corn, or canola oil because they are sources of the essential fatty acid, linoleic acid.

*Vitamins and trace elements* can be limiting factors in nutrition if they are not carefully considered in management. Requirements for thiamine, riboflavin, niacin, and folic acid increase significantly during times of rapid growth; vitamins A, C, and E are needed for development of the structural and functional properties of new cells; and vitamin D is needed for skeletal growth. Because foods of animal origin are seldom used, intake of vitamin $B_{12}$, iron, calcium, copper, selenium, zinc, and cholesterol may be inadequate. However, in most cases, if the formula is consumed in an amount appropriate for the age of the individual, these nutrients, with the exception of cholesterol, should be adequately provided and a vitamin/mineral supplement should not be needed. As more novel products have been developed to improve dietary compliance, there are now a variety of formulas that do not contain a full complement of nutrients. There are formulas that do not contain fat, formulas that are free of or low in vitamins and minerals, and many that are protein-dense and lack sufficient calories. Careful consideration of nutrient composition must be made when planning individual diets.

A phenylalanine-restricted diet for *pregnant women* with PKU is similar to that prescribed for infants, children, adolescents, and adults. The diet adopted during pregnancy should continue the control of

**Table 39–1.** Recommended Daily Intakes for Individuals with Phenylalanine Hydroxylase (PAH) Deficiency

| Age | Phenylalanine (mg/day) | Tyrosine (mg/day) | Protein[a] (g/kg) |
|---|---|---|---|
| 0–3 mo[b] | 130–430 | 1100–1300 | 3–3.5 |
| 3–6 mo | 135–400 | 1400–2100 | 3–3.5 |
| 6–9 mo | 145–370 | 2500–3000 | 2.5–3 |
| 9–12 mo | 135–330 | 2500–3000 | 2.5–3 |
| 1–4 yr[c] | 200–320 | 2800–3500 | ≥30 g/day |
| 4 yr to adult[d] | 200–1100 | 4000–6000 | 120–140% of DRI for age[e] |
| Pregnancy/Lactation[f] | | | |
| Trimester 1 | 265–770 | 6000–7600 | ≥70 |
| Trimester 2 | 400–1650 | 6000–7600 | ≥70 |
| Trimester 3 | 700–2275 | 6000–7600 | ≥70 |
| Lactation | 700–2275 | 6000–7600 | ≥ 70 |

[a]Protein recommendations for individuals consuming phenylalanine-free amino acid–based medical foods as part of their protein source. Recommended intakes for infants and children <4 yr are for individuals with a severe form of PAH deficiency treated with phenylalanine-restricted diet alone. Recommendations for energy and fluid intakes do not differ from those for the normal population.

[b]Phenylalanine requirements for premature infants with PAH deficiency may be higher.

[c]Phenylalanine tolerance is usually stable by 2–5 yr; phenylalanine requirements are based on a combination of size (increasing with age) and rate of growth (decreasing with age). For any individual, phenylalanine intake is adjusted based on frequent blood monitoring.

[d]Range of phenylalanine intake is for the entire spectrum of PAH deficiency (mild to severe).

[e]Recommended protein intake greater than required daily recommended intake (DRI) is necessary to support normal growth in PAH deficiency.

[f]Recommendations are slightly higher for pregnant women ≥19 yr.

From Vockley J, Andersson HC, Antshel KM, et al. Phenylalanine hydroxylase deficiency: diagnosis and management guideline. *Genet Med.* 2014; 16:188; Singh RH, Rohr F, Frazier D, et al. Recommendations for the nutrition management of phenylalanine hydroxylase deficiency. *Genet Med.* 2014; 16:121.

serum phenylalanine begun before conception. The goal of treatment is to maintain serum phenylalanine levels between 60 and 360 μmol/L while providing adequate prenatal nutrition. The amount of phenylalanine needed during pregnancy increases with each trimester.[17] At all times, the amount of dietary phenylalanine recommended is determined by serum phenylalanine levels and fetal growth. Supplemental L-tyrosine may be needed if serum tyrosine levels cannot be maintained within an acceptable control range. Pregnant women and those contemplating pregnancy should have an appropriate phenylalanine-restricted diet (including formula and multivitamins) as well as supplemental folic acid and vitamin $B_{12}$.

In summary, requirements for essential amino acids, including phenylalanine and tyrosine, must be met for protein to be synthesized. For optimal utilization of other amino acids, phenylalanine and formula intake should be distributed evenly throughout the waking hours. Calories in the form of fat and carbohydrate must be provided in sufficient amount to ensure that protein is not used as a source of energy. During pregnancy, care must be taken to ensure intake of sufficient calories to promote good fetal growth. An inadequate intake of essential amino acids from the formula or an inadequate amount of phenylalanine and tyrosine from food can cause low weight gain. Optimal serum phenylalanine and tyrosine levels are maintained by adjusting the intake of natural foods.

## Components of the Diet

The phenylalanine-free or very-low-phenylalanine medical food is the most important part of the dietary treatment for PKU. If an inadequate amount of formula is consumed, serum phenylalanine concentrations may increase as a result of tissue catabolism, growth will be inhibited, and mental development may be impaired.

A wide variety of medical foods is available. Each product is designed to meet nutritional needs and provides varying amounts of amino acids (no phenylalanine) or GMP protein (which contains a small amount of phenylalanine), along with carbohydrate, fat, vitamins, and minerals. Most appropriate formulas used for treatment of PKU contain L-amino acids, simple sugars, and other nutrients. These products may have a high osmolarity if insufficiently diluted, and the practice of concentrating them to increase consumption exacerbates this problem. To compensate, the individual is encouraged to drink additional water or other fluids, which will also help to eliminate phenylalanine metabolites and may prevent symptoms associated with an overly concentrated formula, such as diarrhea, vomiting, and abdominal cramping.

Natural foods include all edible foods except formula; they provide essential amounts of phenylalanine, calories, vitamins, minerals, bulk, and a variety of textures and flavors. The formula and other foods should be offered within the same time frame for optimal use of all essential amino acids. Fruits and vegetables are important foods in the diet. Legumes, grains, and potatoes may be used but in limited amounts because of their relatively high phenylalanine content. High-phenylalanine foods—meat, dairy products, and eggs—should be omitted or severely restricted. No food is strictly forbidden, but all foods are restricted to some degree. Only pure sugar and pure fat contain no phenylalanine.

Commercially available low-protein or protein-free products make the phenylalanine-restricted diet more palatable and interesting. Nutricia North America, CamBrooke Foods, Ener-G Foods, PKU Perspectives, and Dietary Specialties are among the companies that provide specially designed foods modified to be low in protein. Low-protein recipes and phenylalanine food lists have been compiled into cookbooks, handbooks, Web applications, and blogs. These resources are an invaluable aid in managing a phenylalanine-restricted diet. Low-calorie foods warrant attention because many contain *aspartame* (trade names Equal and NutraSweet). Aspartame is a dipeptide, L-aspartyl-L-phenylalanyl methyl ester that is metabolized to aspartic acid and phenylalanine. Individuals who have PKU should avoid any product that contains this sweetener.

## DIETARY MANAGEMENT

An individualized prescription for phenylalanine, protein, and other nutrients is determined by the metabolic treatment team (i.e., metabolic dietitian and metabolic physician). The phenylalanine prescription may be expressed by one of several available exchange systems or by counting milligrams of phenylalanine. Each method requires that the selection of desired foods remain within the specific prescription. A description of the general strategy for diet prescription is provided in Box 39–1. Patients should be monitored frequently, and adjustments should be made when necessary. Elevated or depressed serum phenylalanine levels may reflect an imbalance between the essential amino acids in the formula and the phenylalanine obtained from natural foods or insufficient protein and calories. An imbalance may result from inadequate intake of formula, excessive intake of phenylalanine from natural foods, or illness.

### Infancy

Early initiation of the diet is crucial if serum phenylalanine levels are to be lowered before irreversible brain damage occurs. Although one study showed no effect on adult IQ if treatment was initiated within the first 30 days of life, it is recommended that phenylalanine be lowered to desired levels as quickly as possible once the diagnosis is confirmed. Infants with no residual PAH activity can have phenylalanine levels of greater than 1200 μmol/L at the time of diagnosis. If this is found, a brief *washout* can be undertaken during which phenylalanine-free formula is given with no supplemental

**Box 39–1.** Method for Determining the Amount of Formula and Supplemental Phenylalanine Needed to Provide for Growth and Development

1. Based on the age of the child or adult, or the age and weight of the infant, determine the individual's protein needs as established by the Dietary Reference Intakes (DRI) (see Table 39–1). *Note:* Acosta and Yannicelli (Ross system)[28] recommend significantly more protein per day than the DRI because of rapid absorption and metabolism of amino acids with most PKU supplements; if a PKU supplement containing whole protein is used (i.e., glytactin-containing products), protein needs may be adjusted downward and more in line with the DRI.
2. Based on the age and weight of the infant or the age of an individual older than 12 months of age, determine the amount of phenylalanine required. *Note:* The amount permitted will ultimately be determined by the individual's serum phenylalanine level.
3. Based on the age and weight of the infant or individual older than 12 months of age, determine calorie needs as established by the DRI.
4. Phenylalanine-free foods (sugars or oils) may be added to the formula or diet (specialty low-protein foods) to adjust calories as necessary.
5. Calculation of *formula:*
   *Example 1*: A child aged 2 years has a daily protein requirement (Ross system) of 30 g. The prescribed amount of phenylalanine* is ~200 mg, or ~4 g of protein. Subtract this amount of protein from the total for the day; the remainder is provided from the PKU supplement or formula.
   *Formula prescription:* 93 g powder PKU Periflex Junior Plus provides 358 calories, 26 g protein, and 0 mg phenylalanine.
   *Food:* Provides the allowed amount of phenylalanine, calories, and variety in the diet.
   *Example 2:* An adult woman in the second trimester of pregnancy has a daily protein requirement (Ross system) of 70 g. The prescribed amount of phenylalanine* is ~500 mg, or ~10 g protein. Subtract this amount of protein from the total for the day; the remainder is provided from the PKU supplement or formula.
   *Formula prescription:* 4 pouches PKU CAMINO PRO 15 (140 mL each) provides 560 calories, 60 g protein, and 0 mg phenylalanine.
   *Food:* Provides the allowed amount of phenylalanine, calories, and variety in the diet.

*Phenylalanine tolerance determines the prescribed amount of phenylalanine from food, breast milk, or regular infant formula. The amount of protein coming from these items is usually 15% to 25% of daily recommended needs. The remaining protein comes from the PKU supplement.

phenylalanine. However, most babies identified by newborn screening do not have levels requiring such an initial phase of treatment, despite having severe PAH deficiency. At the end of the washout period, as serum phenylalanine levels approach 360 µmol/L, phenylalanine in the form of standard infant formula or breast milk *must* be added. The amount of regular formula or breast milk added depends on residual phenylalanine activity. An initial amount of 25 to 70 mg phenylalanine per kilogram body weight can be provided using the initial serum phenylalanine level as a surrogate marker of residual phenylalanine activity to guide the initial prescription: The higher the diagnostic level, the lower the phenylalanine prescription. As growth slows in the latter months of infancy, the phenylalanine allowance decreases to 10 to 35 mg/kg at 9 to 12 months of age.[17] Prematurity and the associated increased protein requirement modify these recommendations toward the high side.

The infant with PKU should be considered normal and healthy unless there is a reason to think otherwise. He or she will go through the same developmental stages as any other infant. As the infant grows, baby foods will be offered, and the phenylalanine in these foods will gradually replace the phenylalanine in the regular infant formula or breast milk. As the infant approaches 1 year of age, table foods will begin to replace baby foods. A sample menu for an older infant is provided in Table 39–2. The infant should be encouraged to drink from a cup and to self-feed. However, the formula continues to be the most important element in the diet, and consideration must be given to its importance. The number of bottles and the volume of formula taken by the infant gradually decrease during the first year of life. This decrease in fluid intake is most prominent when the infant is weaned from bottle to cup feeding. Unless the formula is made more concentrated or changed to a variety with a higher ratio of protein to calories, an insufficient amount of formula is likely to be consumed, leading to a corresponding rise in serum phenylalanine. Regardless of the child's age, inadequate formula consumption requires a more concentrated formula plus supplemental fluids in the form of water, juice, or other beverages.

## Childhood

Each phase of development has its own idiosyncrasies. The toddler has expanded horizons beyond the highchair and often is more interested in things other than food. This becomes a challenge for the parent or caregiver who knows the importance of providing a specific amount of phenylalanine from natural foods and the importance of getting the child to take the prescribed amount of formula. Children learn at a very early age how to manipulate a parent, particularly where food is concerned. The preschooler and the young school-age child are relatively easy to manage. They are still within the confines of the home, and because their growth velocity is slower, it is not difficult to satisfy their hunger. It is at this age that they are learning which foods they may eat, the amount allowed, and which foods should be avoided altogether. This is also the time when families should include in their own diets the kinds of foods (i.e., fruits and vegetables) that are beneficial to the child with PKU.

**Table 39–2.** Sample Menu for an Older Infant To Provide 215 mg Phenylalanine (PHE)

| Food | PHE Content |
|---|---|
| Breakfast | |
| ¼ cup Infant Rice Cereal, single grain | 54 mg |
| ¼ cup Earth's Best Peaches | 9 mg |
| *Formula as prescribed* | |
| Snack | |
| 14 pieces Happy Baby Broccoli, Kale and Cheddar Cheese Munchies | 11 mg |
| Lunch | |
| 1 jar (4 oz) Beechnut Stage 2 Tender Sweet Carrots | 25 mg |
| 1 container Gerber 2nd Food Smart Nourish Banana Mango | 47 mg |
| *Formula as prescribed* | |
| Snack | |
| ½ cup Gerber Graduate Puffs, Peach | 27 mg |
| Dinner | |
| ¼ cup Earth's Best 2nd Foods Green Beans and Brown Rice | 36 mg |
| 1 pouch Plum Organics Just Apples | 6 mg |
| *Formula as prescribed* | |
| **DAILY TOTAL:** | **215 mg** |

From http://pkunews.org/diet/BabyFoodsList.htm.

## Late Childhood and Adolescence

Hunger is a significant problem for patients in late childhood and adolescence. During the pubertal growth spurt, increased calorie and protein needs outstrip the small increase in phenylalanine allowance expected for body mass accretion. The result is a significant decrease in prescribed phenylalanine per kilogram of body weight. In addition, busy school and extracurricular schedules, as well as a desire to blend in with peers, make dietary compliance challenging. The many modified low-protein foods that are now available have been a tremendous boon to those on a phenylalanine-restricted diet, but they are expensive, frequently inaccessible to the individual, and high in calories. Paradoxically, adolescence may reveal the first hints of obesity, especially in girls. At either end of the spectrum, nutrition goals can be achieved, but flexibility in the nutrition plan and significant patient motivation are required.

## Adults

Adults should continue to take a prescribed amount of medical foods (e.g., formula, bars) to meet their needs for protein and other nutrients. The intake of phenylalanine from natural foods should continue to be restricted, with the goal of maintaining serum phenylalanine in the control range of 120 to 360 µmol/L. The occasional personal decision to abstain from formula while restricting natural protein intake has resulted in significant nutrient deficiencies as well as poor serum phenylalanine control. Elevated levels of serum phenylalanine affect individuals differently. Among the more common consequences of high phenylalanine levels are obesity, headaches, emotional instability, and fatigue.[20] A sample menu for an adult is provided in Table 39–3.

## Pregnancy

During the early years of treating PKU, it was a common practice to discontinue the diet in childhood. Consequently, many women of child-bearing age have been off the diet for years. These women need to be identified and the diet resumed if they are contemplating pregnancy or are pregnant. The woman with PKU who becomes pregnant must restrict her intake of phenylalanine from natural foods and must achieve and maintain serum phenylalanine levels between 60 and 360 µmol/L. An excess of phenylalanine from natural foods will cause serum phenylalanine levels to increase, and the gradient of placental transfer exposes the fetus to even higher levels of phenylalanine than those reflected in maternal serum. Because of fetal growth and maternal physical changes, phenylalanine tolerance may increase during the second and third trimesters. Serum phenylalanine levels may rise if there are inadequate calories, inadequate total protein, or insufficient phenylalanine in the diet.

## Return to Diet

Termination of the diet is no longer recommended at any age,[9] and reinstating the diet can be difficult. The underlying motivation for return to the diet has a significant effect on success, particularly over the long term. Women who are pregnant or contemplating pregnancy are usually motivated to follow the diet. Other adults may anticipate a significant improvement in physical or mental well-being. To return to the diet means that one must take a prescribed amount of formula, restrict the intake of phenylalanine from natural foods, and sustain this effort indefinitely. Implementation of a phenylalanine-restricted diet in a late-treated or never-treated individual can be difficult and requires considerable structure in the environment. Several groups have reported significant benefit in terms of improved behavior after implementation.[8]

**Table 39–3.** Sample Menu for an Adult To Provide 500 to 550 mg Phenylalanine (PHE)

| *Food* | *PHE Content* |
|---|---|
| Breakfast | |
| ¾ cup Post Honey Bunches of Oats | 110 mg |
| 8 oz Original Rice Milk | 21 mg |
| ½ cup Blueberries | 18 mg |
| 1 slice Low-Protein Toast | 5 mg |
| 2 tsp Butter | 12 mg |
| *Formula as prescribed* | |
| Lunch | |
| 1 Camburger (Cambrooke Foods) | 51 mg |
| 1 low-protein Hamburger Bun | 6 mg |
| 2 slices Tomato | 15 mg |
| ½ cup Lettuce | 10 mg |
| 10 Grapes (red or green) | 9 mg |
| *Formula as prescribed* | |
| Snack: | |
| 2 Fun Size Milky Way candy bars | 74 mg |
| Dinner: | |
| ¾ cup dry LoProFin Pasta | 7 mg |
| 3 Tbsp dry low-protein Alfredo Sauce Mix | 39 mg |
| ½ cup Broccoli Florets | 45 mg |
| 1 slice Maddy's Low-Protein Yellow Cake | 4 mg |
| *Formula as prescribed* | |
| Snack: | |
| 1 oz SunChips, original flavor | 95 mg |
| **DAILY TOTAL** | **521 mg** |

From Schuett VE. *Low Protein Food List for PKU*, 3d Edition. CreateSpace; 2010.

## Illness

Illness and infections elevate phenylalanine levels because of protein catabolism. Colds, sore throat, ear infections, fever, vomiting, and diarrhea are common illnesses that may result in a temporary biochemical imbalance. Appetite and formula consumption are affected by illness, and diet alterations may be required. Although it is possible to design appropriate short-term solutions, as a practical matter departure from the diet for 2 to 3 days after a gastrointestinal illness or minor surgical procedure is not likely to cause harm. For significant illness, the metabolic dietitian should be consulted. An appropriate enteral nutrition plan can be constructed using conventional PKU products and appropriate whole-protein nutritional supplements, and custom intravenous amino acid mixtures are available for individuals who cannot be fed enterally for a prolonged period. An increasing number of medications, particularly suspensions and chewable tablets, are sweetened with aspartame. The quantity of phenylalanine in these products varies and can be appreciable, but in most cases the benefit of the medication outweighs the increase in phenylalanine consumption, particularly for short-term courses of medication.

## Follow-up and Outcome

Anthropometric measurements (linear growth and weight gain), periodic determination of serum amino acid levels (specifically phenylalanine and tyrosine), review of nutrient intake (formula and natural foods), and physical examination are key components in the long-term management of PKU. Clinical well-being, adequate height and weight parameters, normal hemoglobin values, and appropriate serum amino acid levels indicate that nutritional requirements are being met. Periodic psychological assessments aid in assessing the overall development of the child or young adult and are recommended as a part of standard care for the condition.[9]

Nutritional progress is monitored by determining serum phenylalanine levels and, as possible, the levels of other amino acids, especially tyrosine. The frequency of monitoring depends on the individual's needs and feasibility. However, the following recommendations were provided by the ACMG guidelines[9]: weekly monitoring during the first year of life; twice monthly for children 1 to 12 years of age; monthly for adolescents, adults, and nonpregnant women; and twice weekly during pregnancy. The desired control range for serum phenylalanine is 120 to 360 μmol/L. The metabolic dietitian must frequently evaluate the individual diet prescription to ensure that protein, phenylalanine, and calorie requirements are being met. The low-phenylalanine diet is fairly easy to maintain during periods of rapid growth in infancy and early childhood. However, dietary restriction of phenylalanine as a means of achieving and maintaining low serum phenylalanine concentrations becomes very difficult for the adolescent and adult because of significantly lower phenylalanine requirements and a declining growth rate. Termination of the low-phenylalanine diet is not recommended at any age.[9]

# ADDITIONAL THERAPIES

The severe restriction of natural protein and the poor organoleptic properties of formula are barriers to long-term achievement of ideal PKU control. As a consequence, efforts have been made to develop new therapies for managing PKU.

## Large Neutral Amino Acids

The LNAA—phenylalanine, tyrosine, leucine, isoleucine, methionine, tryptophan, histidine, valine, and threonine—are known to share a common receptor for transport across the blood–brain barrier. The presence in plasma of high levels of any one amino acid with appreciable affinity for the carrier reduces the rate of transport for the other amino acids using the same carrier. Thus, high phenylalanine in serum reduces the uptake by brain of other LNAA and may increase sequestration of these amino acids in peripheral tissues. Conversely, increasing the concentration of LNAA should decrease the number of sites available for phenylalanine transport and reduce entry of phenylalanine into brain. Although LNAA may reduce plasma phenylalanine levels by inhibiting phenylalanine transport at the gut–blood barrier, the use of LNAA to replace standard dietary restriction is unlikely to reduce plasma phenylalanine levels to the optimal goal range.[21,22]

## Sapropterin (Cofactor)

Sapropterin (BH4) is the cofactor used to treat some forms of cofactor-dependent PKU, a genetically distinct variant of hyperphenylalaninemia.[23] It has biological effects in enhancing residual PAH activity and reducing phenylalanine levels in individuals with responsive genotypes. Sapropterin was approved for use in children and adults with PKU who demonstrate an empirical response, either reduction of phenylalanine levels or enhancement of phenylalanine tolerance. The percentage of individuals who demonstrate the requisite 20% to 30% reduction in phenylalanine levels varies from study to study, but most have genotypes predicting some residual PAH activity.[24] The use of sapropterin has been extended into infant age groups, and long-term safety data are being collected in the PKU-DOS registry.[25] In a double-blind, placebo-controlled trial, children and adults with self- or parent-reported symptoms of attention-deficit hyperactivity disorder (ADHD) who responded to sapropterin administration with a reduction in phenylalanine levels were found to have improvement in ADHD symptoms and global function.[26]

## Phenylalanine Ammonia Lyase

Phenylalanine ammonia lyase (PAL) is a bacterial enzyme that converts phenylalanine to transcinnamic acid. Unlike PAH, it requires no cofactor and can be modified for long biological half-life with polyethylene glycol. Recombinant AvPAL-PEG, produced in *Escherichia coli*, is in clinical trials as of 2015. A phase I dose-finding study in adults showed that doses of 0.1 mg/kg/day, administered by subcutaneous injection, could reduce phenylalanine levels for several days.[27] A phase III trial in adults is in progress. PAL is likely to have broader efficacy than sapropterin, particularly in individuals with no residual PAH activity.

### References

1. Centerwall SA, Centerwall WR. The discovery of phenylketonuria: the story of a young couple, two retarded children, and a scientist. *Pediatrics*. 2000; 105(1 Pt 1):89.

2. Woolf LI, Vulliamy DG. Phenylketonuria with a study of the effect upon it of glutamic acid. *Arch Dis Child.* 1951; 26:487.
3. Bickel H, Gerrard J, Hickmans EM. Preliminary communication: influence of phenylalanine intake on phenylketonuria. *Lancet.* 1953; 262:812.
4. Horner FA, Streamer CW. Effect of a phenylalanine-restricted diet on patients with phenylketonuria: clinical observations in three cases. *JAMA.* 1956; 161:1628.
5. Guthrie R, Susi A. A simple phenylalanine method for detecting phenylketonuria in large populations of newborn infants. *Pediatrics.* 1963; 32:338.
6. Hertzberg VS, Hinton CF, Therrell BL, Shapira SK. Birth prevalence rates of newborn screening disorders in relation to screening practices in the United States. *J Pediatr.* 2011; 159:555.
7. Blau N, Hennermann JB, Langenbeck U, Lichter-Konecki U. Diagnosis, classification, and genetics of phenylketonuria and tetrahydrobiopterin (BH4) deficiencies. *Mol Genet Metab.* 2011; 104(Suppl):S2.
8. Yannicelli S, Ryan A. Improvements in behaviour and physical manifestations in previously untreated adults with phenylketonuria using a phenylalanine-restricted diet: a national survey. *J Inherit Metab Dis.* 1995; 18:131.
9. Vockley J, Andersson HC, Antshel KM, et al. Phenylalanine hydroxylase deficiency: diagnosis and management guideline. *Genet Med.* 2014; 16:188.
10. Dent CE. Discussion of Armstrong MD: The relation of biochemical abnormality to the development of mental defect in phenylketonuria. In: *Etiologic Factors in Mental Retardation: Report for the Twenty-Third Ross Pediatric Research Conference.* Columbus, OH: Ross Laboratories; 1957:32.
11. Lenke RR, Levy HL. Maternal phenylketonuria and hyperphenylalaninemia: an international survey of the outcome of untreated and treated pregnancies. *N Engl J Med.* 1980; 303:1202.
12. Heintz C, Cotton RG, Blau N. Tetrahydrobiopterin, its mode of action on phenylalanine hydroxylase, and importance of genotypes for pharmacological therapy of phenylketonuria. *Hum Mutat.* 2013; 34:927.
13. Platt LD, Koch R, Hanley WB, et al. The international study of pregnancy outcome in women with maternal phenylketonuria: report of a 12-year study. *Am J Obstet Gynecol.* 2000; 182:326.
14. Donlon J, Sarkissian C, Levy H, Scriver CR. Hyperphenylalaninemia: phenylalanine hydroxylase deficiency. In: Beaudet AL, Vogelstein B, Kinzler KW, et al., eds. *The Online Metabolic and Molecular Bases of Inherited Disease.* New York: McGraw-Hill; 2014. http://ommbid.mhmedical.com/book.aspx?bookid=971. Accessed June 27, 2016.
15. Pietz J, Kreis R, Rupp A, et al. Large neutral amino acids block phenylalanine transport into brain tissue in patients with phenylketonuria. *J Clin Invest.* 1999; 103:1169.
16. Ris MD, Weber AM, Hunt MM, Berry HK, Williams SE, Leslie N. Adult psychosocial outcome in early-treated phenylketonuria. *J Inherit Metab Dis.* 1997; 20:499.
17. Singh RH, Rohr F, Frazier D, et al. Recommendations for the nutrition management of phenylalanine hydroxylase deficiency. *Genet Med.* 2014; 16:121.
18. Ney DM, Gleason ST, van Calcar SC, et al. Nutritional management of PKU with glycomacropeptide from cheese whey. *J Inherit Metab Dis.* 2009; 32:32.
19. Gropper SS, Gropper DM, Acosta PB. Plasma amino acid response to ingestion of L-amino acids and whole protein. *J Pediatr Gastroenterol Nutr.* 1993; 16:143.
20. Koch R, Azen C, Friedman EG, Fishler K, Baumann-Frischling C, Lin T. Care of the adult with phenylketonuria. *Eur J Pediatr.* 1996; 155(Suppl 1):S90.
21. de Groot MJ, Hoeksma M, Blau N, Reijngoud DJ, van Spronsen FJ. Pathogenesis of cognitive dysfunction in phenylketonuria: review of hypotheses. *Mol Genet Metab.* 2010; 99(Suppl 1):S86.
22. Lindegren ML, Krishnaswami S, Fonnesbeck C, et al. Adjuvant treatment for phenylketonuria (PKU). Comparative Effectiveness Review No. 56. AHRQ Publication No. 12-EHC035-EF. Rockville, MD: Agency for Healthcare Research and Quality; February 2012.
23. Blau N, Trefz FK. Tetrahydrobiopterin-responsive phenylalanine hydroxylase deficiency: possible regulation of gene expression in a patient with the homozygous L48S mutation. *Mol Genet Metab.* 2002; 75:186.
24. Quirk ME, Dobrowolski SF, Nelson BE, Coffee B, Singh RH. Utility of phenylalanine hydroxylase genotype for tetrahydrobiopterin responsiveness classification in patients with phenylketonuria. *Mol Genet Metab.* 2012; 107:31.
25. Somaraju UR, Merrin M. Sapropterin dihydrochloride for phenylketonuria. *Cochrane Database Syst Rev.* 2012; (12):CD008005.
26. Burton B, Grant M, Feigenbaum A, et al. A randomized, placebo-controlled, double-blind study of sapropterin to treat ADHD symptoms and executive function impairment in children and adults with sapropterin-responsive phenylketonuria. *Mol Genet Metab.* 2015; 114:415.
27. Longo N, Harding CO, Burton BK, et al. Single-dose, subcutaneous recombinant phenylalanine ammonia lyase conjugated with polyethylene glycol in adult patients with phenylketonuria: an open-label, multicentre, phase 1 dose-escalation trial. *Lancet.* 2014; 384:37.
28. Acosta PB, Yannicelli S. Protocol 1: Phenylketonuria (PKU). In: Acosta PB, Yannicelli S, eds. *The Ross Metabolic Formula System: Nutrition Support Protocols*, 4th ed. Columbus, OH: Ross Products Division; 2001.

# 40 Tyrosinemia

FRANCJAN VAN SPRONSEN AND MARGREET VAN RIJN

There are various causes of high tyrosine concentrations. First, five defects in the catabolic pathway of tyrosine metabolism have been described (Fig. 40–1).[1] Apart from the well-known tyrosinemia types I, II, and III and alkaptonuria, maleylacetoacetate isomerase deficiency has been described. However, only two patients have been reported, and their problems clinically corresponded with those of tyrosinemia type I. Therefore, this chapter does not address maleylacetoacetate isomerase deficiency. Mutations in the gene encoding 4-phenylpyruvate dioxygenase may also cause hawkinsinuria, which is inherited in an autosomal dominant fashion.[2]

Second, tyrosine may be increased in cases of liver disease, usually together with high phenylalanine and methionine without clear relation to a special disease. Third, it may be increased in very young children, especially premature infants, owing to a temporary deficiency of 4-phenylpyruvate dioxygenase. Fourth, it may be increased in citrin deficiency, a transporter defect of citrulline at the border of cytoplasm and mitochondria.

## BIOCHEMICAL AND CLINICAL ABNORMALITIES

### Tyrosinemia Type I

Clinically, hereditary tyrosinemia type I (HT1; OMIM 276700), also known as hereditary tyrosinemia or hepatorenal tyrosinemia,[3] is characterized by severe liver disease (e.g., liver failure, liver cancer), renal tubulopathy, porphyria-like syndrome, and cardiomyopathy in infants and children. Biochemically, the hallmark is the pathognomonic elevation of succinylacetone in plasma and urine. The final diagnosis is usually based on DNA analysis. Enzyme studies on lymphocytes or fibroblasts are not necessary. The succinylacetone reflects the increase of fumarylacetoacetate and maleylacetoacetate, which are hepatotoxic and are considered to lead to tubulopathy by succinylacetone. Because of the liver disease and liver regeneration, phenylalanine, tyrosine, methionine, and alpha-1-fetoprotein (AFP) are increased in blood; synthesis functions are largely affected, rather than liver cell injury or decreased detoxification, especially with clotting abnormalities, low glucose, and low albumin. Increasing bilirubin or ammonia is considered a sign of end-stage liver failure and is a poor sign if not responding to treatment with 2-(2-nitro-4-trifluoromethyl-benzyl)-1,3 cyclohexanedione (NTBC). Urinary excretion of tyrosine and tyrosine compounds is increased, as is excretion of delta-aminolevulinic acid (due to inhibition by succinylacetone on porphobilinogen synthase). The tubulopathy results in increased excretion of amino acids, phosphate, bicarbonate, and glucose, and as a consequence low concentrations of especially phosphate and bicarbonate are found in blood. The incidence of HT1 is about 1 in 100,000 in most populations3 but is much higher in the Chicoutine–Lac St. Jean region in Quebec of Canada.

Clinically, the disorder can be divided into three forms based on age at presentation: a very early presenting form (<2 months of age), an early presenting form (2–6 months of age), and a late presenting form (>6 months of age).[4] In the very early presenting form, symptoms include vomiting, sometimes jaundice, failure to thrive, and abdominal enlargement, together with a peculiar (methionine- or cabbage-like) odor. Liver failure may range from failure to thrive to profound bleeding tendency, ascites and edema. Jaundice does not need to be present. Death, usually from liver failure, occurs in 70% to 90% of these patients by 1 year of age if treated only by diet. Patients with the late presenting form may present with liver disease, hepatocellular carcinoma (HCC), hepatomegaly, porphyria-like syndrome including symptoms similar to those of Guillain Barré syndrome, motor developmental problems, acute abdominal pain, hypertension, or hypophosphatemic (vitamin D–resistant) rickets caused by renal tubulopathy. The presentation of patients with the early form is somewhat in between. In all patients treated with diet only and surviving the acute period, HCC is a frequent complication.[4]

Until 1992, the outcome for patients with HT1 was very poor as described above. At that time, the question was when, rather than whether, liver transplantation was necessary. In 1992, it was reported that NTBC could block the activity of the enzyme 4-hydroxyphenylpyruvate dioxygenase (HPPD) upstream from the primary enzyme defect and thereby prevent production of the toxic compounds.[5] The introduction of NTBC seemed to diminish all these problems, but if a patient presents with liver failure, NTBC may not be started in time, so sometimes liver transplantation is still necessary.[6,7] Increasing bilirubin and ammonia levels after 1 week of NTBC therapy suggests that liver transplantation is needed.[8] It is also needed for patients with increasing AFP or new nodules after NTBC has been started. A slow decrease in AFP or a level that does not decrease to normal concentrations suggests a risk of developing HCC.[9]

It seems important to start NTBC within the first months of life to prevent HCC development.[7] However, NTBC gives rise to high tyrosine concentrations that may be related to the finding of neurocognitive delay in these patients, necessitating a diet that restricts phenylalanine and tyrosine, with the goal of reducing tyrosine concentrations to between 200 and 400 μmol/L keeping phenylalanine at normal levels.[10,11] Special tyrosine-free, phenylalanine-free medical foods, in addition to a low-tyrosine, low-phenylalanine diet, are needed to meet the restrictions and provide adequate nutrition. NTBC itself seems to be responsible for the eye problems sometimes observed in these patients.[12] Further improvement is seen by the introduction of neonatal screening using blood succinylacetone rather than tyrosine as the marker for the disease.[6,7]

### Tyrosinemia Type II

Hereditary tyrosinemia type II (HT2; OMIM 276600), also known as Richner-Hanhart syndrome or oculocutaneous tyrosinemia), is a rare disease that has most frequently been reported in Italy. The cornerstones of the clinical entity are corneal erosions and plaques, palm and sole erosions, and hyperkeratosis, as well as a delay in mental development. The eye and skin problems may occur during the first month of life.[1,13] Eye lesions include lacrimation, photophobia, microfollicular conjunctivitis, and dendritic keratosis. It has been postulated that keratosis results from tyrosine crystal formation within the cell due to elevated tyrosine levels. Long-term effects include corneal scarring, nystagmus, and glaucoma. Skin lesions are more variable, occurring with or after eye lesions. Initial blister-like lesions form on the hands and feet, become crusty, and finally become hyperkeratotic. These painful lesions can hinder mobility. The mental retardation occurs in about half of the patients, some of whom experience microcephaly and convulsions.[13,14]

The site of the defect in HT2 is hepatic tyrosine aminotransferase (see Fig. 40–1). Diagnosis is based on increased tyrosine in blood and urine with increased excretion of tyrosine metabolites (i.e., p-HPLA,

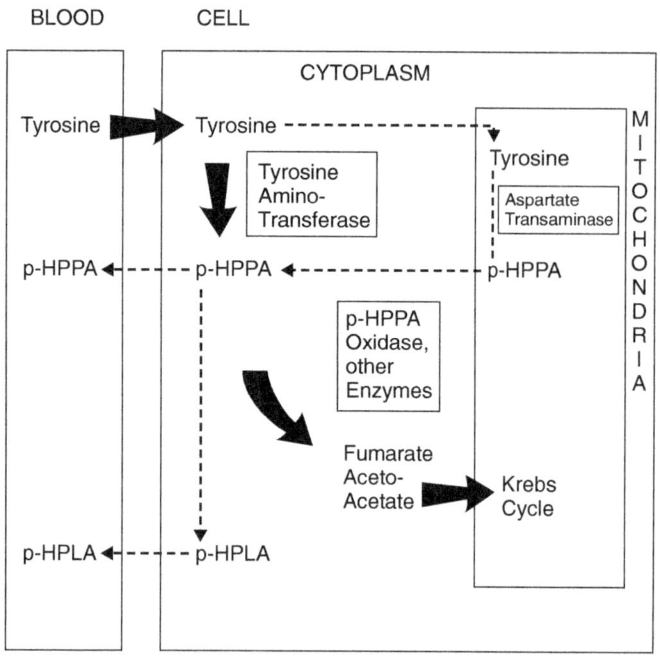


**Figure 40–1.** Tyrosine metabolism.

p-HPPA, and N-acetyl tyrosine), as well as tyramine. These findings are usually followed by genotyping and enzyme measurement necessitating a liver biopsy. For some reason, younger patients have higher plasma tyrosine levels than adults do. Older patients develop eye and skin lesions at blood tyrosine levels that produce no symptoms in younger patients.

Dietary treatment is necessary to resolve the eye and skin lesions and keep tyrosine levels below 10 mg/dL (600 µmol/L). Special tyrosine-free, phenylalanine-free medical foods, in addition to a low-tyrosine, low-phenylalanine diet, are needed to meet the restrictions and provide adequate nutrition. As can be concluded from this discussion, at present the clinical entity, especially the occurrence of mental retardation, is not clear for a variety of reasons, including the difficulty of diagnosis.

### Tyrosinemia Type III and Hawkinsinuria

As discussed earlier, giving NTBC to patients with HT1 results in a more or less complete deficiency of the enzyme HPPD. Deficiency of this enzyme has also been related to two genetic causes.[2,15]

Tyrosinemia type III is an extremely rare condition caused by a deficiency of the enzyme HPPD that is characterized by elevated levels of blood tyrosine and massive urinary excretion of tyrosine and tyrosyluria. Patients with this disorder have been described as having mild mental retardation and/or seizures,[15] although clinical problems are not always present. Therefore, it is difficult to advise families on the need for dietary treatment. We would advocate a diet that is not very strict to continue for the first 4 to 6 years.

Hawkinsinuria is reported only in a few families.[2,15] Consequently, it is unclear whether the clinical entity with metabolic acidosis and failure to thrive is related to the biochemical abnormalities—increased levels of tyrosine in blood and the finding of hawkinsin in urine as well as tyrosyluria. If treatment with a mild protein-restricted diet is considered, this diet may stop after infancy, because no clinical problems are known after this period.

## ALKAPTONURIA

Alkaptonuria (AKU; OMIM 203500), is a very rare disease, occurring in 1 of every 250,000 to 1,000,000 people. Strictly speaking, there is no hypertyrosinemia in AKU, but this is a genetic disorder within the catabolic pathway of tyrosine. It was the first metabolic disease to be described, reported as early as the Egyptian period, and it was the first inherited metabolic disorder described in the original work of Garrod in 1908.[16] Clinically, the first and only sign often is the darkening of urine when exposed to oxygen. Patients may remain without clinical symptoms until well into adulthood. The sclerae and the shell of the ear may become gray. After that, the skin may become gray at locations where the bones are just below the skin. The deposition of the pathological compounds produced in this disease not only causes the coloration but also leads to inflammation processes within joints (usually the hip and knee) and on the inner sides of large vessels, sometimes causing cardiovascular problems.

The diagnosis is easy when urine is analyzed for organic acids. The influence of treatment is unclear. Vitamin C and protein restriction are prescribed, but the effect is unclear. The use of NTBC has been suggested,[17] but it remains to be established whether this therapy will prevent symptoms later.

## FACTORS TO BE CONSIDERED IN NUTRITION INTERVENTION

Notwithstanding the advice given, it is not completely clear to what level tyrosine may rise in children with HT1 treated with NTBC or in those with HT2. Dietary therapy consists of restriction of both tyrosine and phenylalanine, effectively lowering the tyrosine concentration in body fluids, but it is not known whether this might lead to a problem with low phenylalanine concentrations, at least in HT1.[12]

## ENERGY REQUIREMENTS

During the first few months of life, some clinically presenting children with HT1 may have severe vomiting and diarrhea. These children require additional energy for catch-up growth. The additional energy should come from foods that are low in protein. Special protein-free modules provide energy without tyrosine or its precursor, phenylalanine. Small, frequent feedings are indicated to help alleviate severe vomiting and diarrhea if they occur. Patients identified as having HT1 on newborn screening are still normal and just need NTBC and a diet restricting phenylalanine and tyrosine, without other special issues.

## LOW-PHENYLALANINE, LOW-TYROSINE DIET

The regimen calls for a restricted intake of phenylalanine and tyrosine. The dietary principles applied to phenylketonuria should be followed (see Chapter 39). Commercial products with mixtures of l-amino acids (omitting phenylalanine and tyrosine), supplemented with vitamins and minerals, are used to provide the necessary amino acids and micronutrients in the diet. Today, the range of medical food (tyrosine- and phenylalanine-free amino acid mixtures) available for dietary treatment offers many possibilities for planning age-related dietary prescriptions. Table 40–1 shows age-related product ranges of metabolic formulas with and without energy produced by different manufacturers. The availability and reimbursement systems differ from country to country (Table 40–2).

## VITAMIN C AND VITAMIN D

Vitamin C is important in the oxidation of p-HPPA but is of no benefit in the treatment of hereditary tyrosinemias. Since the introduction of NTBC treatment, most patients no longer show evidence of renal damage. Therefore, prophylactic administration of active vitamin D to prevent rickets or promote normal growth is probably no longer needed unless intake is inadequate or other special circumstances occur.

## DIETARY MANAGEMENT AND FOLLOW-UP

The objective of dietary therapy for the hereditary tyrosinemias is to provide adequate nutrition for normal growth and development while strictly controlling the intake of tyrosine and its precursor, phenylalanine.

**Table 40–1.** Special Dietary Products (Metabolic Formula) for Tyrosinemia Available in the United States and Canada, 2015*

| Product | Protein Equivalent (g) | Energy (kcal) | Age Indication | Flavored | Micronutrients Added |
|---|---|---|---|---|---|
| *Powdered (400–500g cans; details shown for 100-g)* | | | | | |
| TYR Anamix Early Years | 13.5 | 473 | Infants, children <3 yr | − | + |
| TYR Anamix Next | 28 | 385 | >1 yr | − | + |
| XPhe, XTyr Maxamaid | 25 | 324 | Young children | + | + |
| XPhe, XTyr Analog | 13 | 475 | Infants, children <3 yr | − | + |
| XPHEN, TYR Maxamaid | 25 | 309 | Young children | − | + |
| XPHEN, TYR Maxamum | 39 | 297 | Older children and adults | − | + |
| Tyrex-1 (Abbott) | 15 | 480 | 0–12 mo | − | + |
| Tyrex-2 (Abbott) | 30 | 410 | >1 yr | − | + |
| Comida-TYRo A | 11.8 | 506 | 0–12 mo | − | + |
| Comida-TYRo B | 31.1 | 420 | 1–14 yr | − | + |
| Tyros 1 (Enfamil) | 16.7 | 500 | Infants, toddlers | − | + |
| Tyros 2 (Enfamil) | 22 | 410 | Children, adults | + | + |
| *Prepacked portions* | | | | | |
| Tyr Gel (Vitaflo) | 10 | 81 | >1 yr | −S | + |
| Tyr Express 15 (Vitaflo) | 15 | 74 | >3 yr | −S | + |
| Tyr Express 20 (Vitaflo) | 20 | 99 | >3 yr | −S | + |
| *Ready to use* | | | | | |
| Cooler 10 (Vitaflo) | 10 | 62 | >3 yr | + | + |
| Cooler 15 (Vitaflo) | 15 | 92 | >3 yr | + | + |
| Cooler 20 (Vitaflo) | 20 | 124 | >3 yr | + | + |
| Tylactin RTD (Cambrooke) | 15 | 200 | Children, adults | + | + |
| Tylactin restore (Cambrooke) | 10 | 170 | Children, adults | + | + |
| TYR Lophlex LQ | 20 | 120 | >4 yr | + | + |

*Worldwide, different products and other manufacturers are available; see country details on websites.
+ = Yes; − = No; S = separate flavoring.

**Table 40–2.** Contact Information for Manufacturers of Tyrosine- and Phenylalanine-Free Medical Foods

| Manufacturer and Website Address | Contact Details |
|---|---|
| Abbott Nutrition www.abbottnutrition.com | 3300 Stelzer Road, Columbus, OH 43219 Office Phone: 614-624-4416, Toll Free: 800-986-8755 Cell: 614-264-4388, Fax: 614-727-4416 |
| Vitaflo www.vitaflousa.com | Distributed by Vitaflo USA 211 N. Union St. Suite 100, Alexandria, VA 22314 Phone: 1-888-VITAFLO (1-888-848-2356), Fax: 1-631-693-2002 Email: vitaflo@vitaflousa.com |
| Mead Johnson (Enfamil) www.meadjohnson.com/pediatrics/us-en/product-information/products | Phone: 1-812-429-6399 Email: mjmedicalaffairs@mjn.com |
| Cambrooke www.cambrooke.com | 4 Copeland Drive, Ayer, MA 01432 Phone: 866 456 9776, Fax: 978 443 1318 Mail: info@cambrooke.com |
| Nutricia-NA USA www.medicalfood.com | Phone: 301-795-2300 or 1-800-365-7354 Fax: 301-795-2301 |
| Nutricia-NA Canada www.Nutricia-NA.com | Phone: 877-636-2283 Fax: 514-745-6625 |
| Comida www.comidamed.de | Phone: 888-8-SOLACE or 888-876-5223 Fax: 401-633-6066 Email: info@solacenutrition.com |
| MetaX www.metax.org/EN/Products/Metabolics.aspx | Email: info@metax.org |

There have been many questions about the phenylalanine requirements for healthy individuals, as reviewed by Pencharz et al.[18] Such studies are necessary for all different age groups and are very laborious. Initial data suggested that phenylalanine and tyrosine intake (in total for both) should be somewhere between 15 and 39 mg/kg/day with a ratio of 60:40. However, later studies have shown that phenylalanine intake, by itself should be between 38 and 48 mg/kg/day.[18] Therefore, the maximum phenylalanine requirement (if no tyrosine is given) is considered to be 42 mg/kg/day, while about 9 mg/kg/day is needed when enough tyrosine is given.[18]

Some children with HT1 on the phenylalanine/tyrosine -restricted diet have been found to have low phenylalanine levels.[12,19] There has been concern that these low levels could be detrimental to the child, and it was thought that the addition of phenylalanine to the diet would increase levels in blood and tissues without increasing the tyrosine level. An initial study found that supplementing the diet with an additional 20 to 40 mg/kg/day phenylalanine increased the blood phenylalanine concentration while maintaining the tyrosine level.[19] Therefore, supplementation with phenylalanine may be beneficial, but the risk of hypertyrosinemia should be considered. Further studies must be performed over an extended period before a recommendation for standard supplementation can be made. Because of the important risk of development of liver cancer, careful evaluation should be performed, with AFP measurement and ultrasound or magnetic resonance imaging studies.[3,6,9]

## References

1. Scott CR. The genetic tyrosinemias. Am J Med Genet C Semin Med Genet. 2006; 142C:121.
2. Item CB, Mihalek I, Lichtarge O, et al. Manifestation of hawkinsinuria in a patient compound heterozygous for hawkinsinuria and tyrosinemia III. Mol Genet Metab. 2007; 91:379.
3. de Laet C, Dionisi-Vici C, Leonard JV, et al. Recommendations for the management of tyrosinaemia type 1. Orphan J Rare Dis 2013; 8:8.
4. van Spronsen FJ, Thomasse Y, Smit GPA, et al. Hereditary tyrosinaemia type I: a new classification with difference in prognosis on dietary management. Hepatology. 1994; 20:1187.

5. Lindstedt S, Holme E, Lock EA, Hjalmarson O, Strandvik B. Treatment of hereditary tyrosinemia type I by inhibition of 4-hydroxyphenylpyruvate dioxygenase. Lancet. 1992; 340:813.
6. Mayorandan S, Meyer U, Gokcay G, et al. Cross-sectional study of 168 patients with hepatorenal tyrosinaemia and implications for clinical practice. Orphan J Rare Dis. 2014; 9:107.
7. Larochelle J, Alvarez F, Bussières JF, et al. Effect of nitisinone (NTBC) treatment on the clinical course of hepatorenal tyrosinemia in Québec. Mol Genet Metab. 2012; 107:49.
8. McKiernan PJ, Lindstedt S, Holme E, Robinson PH, Kelly DA. Effect of NTBC in acute liver failure due to tyrosinemia type I. J Inherit Metab Dis. 1997; 20(Suppl 1):2.
9. Koelink CJ, van Hasselt P, van der Ploeg A, et al. Tyrosinemia type I treated by NTBC: how does AFP predict liver cancer? Mol Genet Metab. 2006; 89:310.
10. Bendadi F, de Koning TJ, Visser G, et al. Impaired cognitive functioning in patients with tyrosinemia type I receiving nitisinone. J Pediatr. 2014; 164:398.
11. van Vliet D, van Dam E, van Rijn M, et al. Infants with tyrosinemia type 1: should phenylalanine be supplemented? JIMD Rep. 2015; 18:117.
12. Schauwvlieghe PP, Jaeken J, Kestelyn P, Claerhout I. Confocal microscopy of corneal crystals in a patient with hereditary tyrosinemia type I, treated with NTBC. Cornea. 2013; 32:91.
13. Tsai CP, Lin PY, Lee NC, Niu DM, Lee SM, Hsu WM. Corneal lesion as the initial manifestation of tyrosinemia type II. J Chin Med Assoc. 2006; 69:286.
14. Charfeddine C, Monastiri K, Mokni M, et al. Clinical and mutational investigations of tyrosinemia type II in northern Tunisia: identification and structural characterization of two novel TAT mutations. Mol Genet Metab. 2006; 88:184.
15. Tomoeda K, Awata H, Matsuura T, et al. Mutations in the 4-hydroxyphenylpyruvic acid dioxygenase gene are responsible for tyrosinemia type III and hawkinsinuria. Mol Genet Metab. 2000; 71:506.
16. Garrod, AE. The Croonian lectures on inborn errors of metabolism. Delivered before the Royal College of Physicians of London on June 18th, 23rd, 25th, and 30th, 1908; Lancet. 1908; 172:1.
17. Keenan CM, Preston AJ, Sutherland H, et al. Nitisinone arrests but does not reverse ochronosis in alkaptonuric mice. JIMD Rep. 2015; 24:45.
18. Pencharz PB, Hsu JW, Ball RO. Aromatic amino acid requirements in healthy human subjects. J Nutr. 2007; 137(Suppl 1):1576S.
19. Wilson CJ, Van Wyk KG, Leonard JV, Clayton PT. Phenylalanine supplementation improves the phenylalanine profile in tyrosinemia. J Inherit Metab Dis. 2000; 23:677.

# 41 Urea Cycle Pathway

SANDY VAN CALCAR

The function of the urea cycle is twofold: to convert waste nitrogen into urea and to synthesize the amino acid arginine. Waste nitrogen in the form of ammonia is derived from dietary protein and the breakdown of protein in the tissues. It is transported in the blood to the liver, where it is converted to urea (Fig. 41–1). The urea cycle operates primarily in the liver and is compartmentalized between the cystolic and mitochondrial components of the cell. At each of the six steps of the pathway, enzyme deficiencies have been identified that lead to the accumulation of ammonia and associated toxicity[1,2] (Table 41–1). Collectively, urea cycle disorders (UCD) are relatively common, with an incidence of approximately 1 in 35,000 births.[3] Additionally, inherited disorders of dibasic amino acid transport (lysinuric protein intolerance), mitochondrial ornithine transport (HHH syndrome), and the mitochondrial aspartate/glutamate carrier (citrullinemia type II) also result in hyperammonemia and are often included under the umbrella of UCD.[1,2]

The first enzyme of the urea cycle, *carbamyl phosphate synthetase* (CPS), combines ammonia ($NH_3$) and $CO_2$ to form carbamoyl phosphate. This enzyme is located in the mitochondrion and is allosterically activated by *N*-acetylglutamate, a metabolite that is generated from acetyl-coenzyme A (CoA) and glutamate by *N-acetylglutamate synthetase* (NAGS). The level of *N*-acetylglutamate reflects the cellular level of glutamate and glutamine, which are affected by the level of ammonia. It is thought that the concentration of ammonia indirectly controls the activity of the urea cycle by its effect on the level of *N*-acetylglutamate. Carbamyl phosphate is then combined with ornithine by *ornithine transcarbamylase* (OTC), forming citrulline, which is exported to the cytosol and reacts with aspartate to form argininosuccinate, a reaction catalyzed by *argininosuccinate synthetase* (ASS). Argininosuccinate is cleaved into arginine and fumarate, a tricarboxylic cycle acid intermediate, by *argininosuccinate lyase* (ASL). *Arginase* then liberates a molecule of urea from arginine, a process that regenerates ornithine. The ornithine formed in the cytosol is transported back into the mitochondrion, where it can serve as a substrate for another round of the urea cycle. The urea exits the hepatic cells, is transported to the kidneys in the blood, and is excreted in the urine, resulting in a net loss of two molecules of $NH_3$.[1,2]

Ammonia is neurotoxic, and its elevation can lead to an encephalopathy primarily affecting white matter tissue. The mechanism for ammonia toxicity is unclear, but alterations in amino acid pathways, neurotransmitter systems, and cerebral energy metabolism have been proposed.[4,5] The likelihood of hyperammonemia in an individual is primarily related to the degree of enzyme deficiency caused by the severity of mutations in the gene for that enzyme. There is considerable genetic and phenotypic heterogeneity in UCD disorders; patients who present in the neonatal period or early infancy have mutations causing the greatest reductions in enzyme activity and are at the greatest risk for lethal hyperammonemia.[6,7] However, severe clinical manifestations and even death can also occur in patients who present at later stages of life. The neonatal presentation typically involves seizure activity, hyperpnea, lethargy, vomiting, poor feeding, and coma. Late-onset presentations can include a variety of symptoms, including stroke-like episodes, hepatitis-like liver dysfunction, confusion, disorientation, combativeness, irritability, ataxia, headaches, and focal neurological signs.[6–9]

Treatment for UCD involves three interventions: (1) reduction of waste nitrogen production through restriction of dietary protein; (2) supplementation of arginine, which becomes a conditionally essential amino acid in all UCD except for arginase deficiency and; (3) utilization of alternative pathways of waste nitrogen excretion through the use of medications.[6,7,10–14] With improvements in treatment strategies, strides have been made in reducing the mortality of UCD.[2,6] For those with intractable ammonia elevations that do not adequately respond to conventional treatment, liver transplantation is increasingly becoming the treatment of choice.[15]

## NUTRITIONAL THERAPY

The overall goal for medical nutritional therapy is to provide adequate but not excessive protein, energy, and other essential nutrients to support normal growth and development.[7,10,11,13,14] Inherent in protein-restricted diets is the risk of potential deficiencies for both macronutrients and micronutrients. A protein-restricted diet makes the provision of adequate energy, vitamins, and minerals difficult without the use of fortified medical foods and, often, additional supplements.[10,11]

### Protein Restriction

Dietary therapy needs to provide sufficient protein for normal growth and protein maintenance while preventing excessive protein (nitrogen) intake, which can contribute to hyperammonemia in an individual with a defective urea cycle. Unlike dietary treatment for most other inborn errors of amino acid metabolism that require restriction of only one to four amino acids, the diet for UCD requires restriction of total protein intake. Protein tolerance for some patients may be below the intake for age established by the Institute of Medicine (IOM) and the World Health Organization (WHO).[11,16–18]

Variations in protein tolerance are dynamic and are determined by an individual's age and state of health; protein tolerance for weight is greatest during the rapid growth period of infancy.[16,17] Any febrile illness or other catabolic conditions such as dental infections, sunburn, dehydration, and menses can increase waste nitrogen metabolism.[20,21] In women with UCD, for instance, restriction of typical protein intake may be required up to 7 days before menstruation begins to prevent metabolic decompensation (S. van Calcar, personal observation).

Table 41–2 details a suggested range of adequate total protein for individuals with UCD of various ages.[11,18] Typically, medical formulas that contain only the essential amino acids (EAA) as the source of protein equivalents are included in dietary management of UCD (Table 41–3). Use of these products allows for a greater restriction of total protein because excess intake of nitrogen from nonessential amino acids can be limited. Although practices vary widely,[22] 50% of an infant's total protein requirement is often provided from an EAA-based medical formula and the remaining 50% is from intact (dietary) protein sources.[7,10,11] In older children, a greater proportion of intact protein is often possible, with only 20% to 30% of total protein provided by an EAA medical food.[22] However, controlled studies to evaluate the efficacy of various treatment modalities, including protein and overall diet composition, are lacking.[22,23]

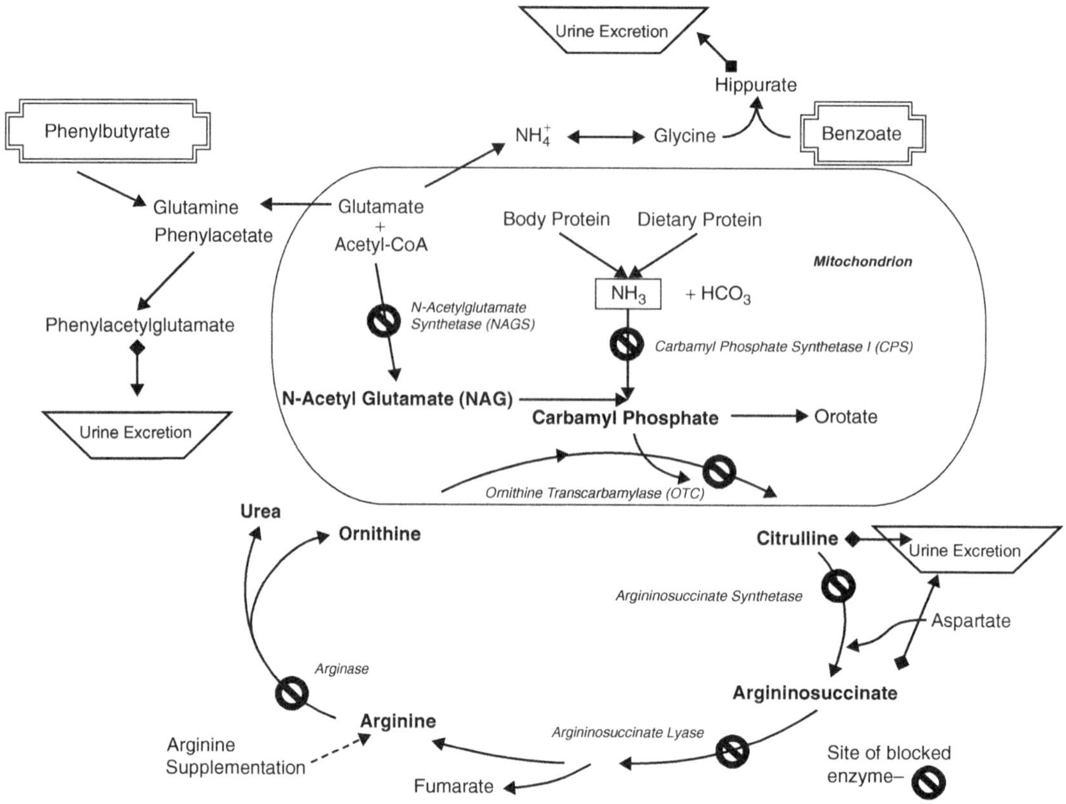


**Figure 41–1.** Urea cycle pathway and alternative nitrogen excretion pathways using nitrogen scavengers.

For infants, the intact protein source includes expressed breast milk or a standard infant formula. Allowing an infant to feed from the breast to meet intact protein needs may be possible if the child has a mild phenotype, but poor feeding is common in this population, and close monitoring of weight gain is required.[24,25] However, because breast milk has a lower protein content than standard infant formulas, it is often possible to incorporate expressed breast milk into the diet prescription[25] (Table 41–4).

Depending on the feeding capabilities of the older child, intact protein sources often include grain products, fruits, and vegetables. Modified low-protein products, many made from wheat starch, are commercially available (Table 41–5). These products contain negligible protein compared to standard grain products and allow for a greater variety of foods without exceeding dietary protein limits.[11] For older individuals and those with a milder phenotype, a high biological protein source (e.g., milk, egg) rather than a medical food may be appropriate to provide a source of EAA[13] (see Table 41–4). Given the minimal protein tolerance of many individuals with UCD, it can be difficult to meet EAA needs using only plant-based protein sources.[21]

## Providing Sufficient Nonprotein Energy

Restricting natural protein to reduce waste nitrogen accumulation must be accompanied by supplying sufficient energy intake from dietary sources that contain negligible protein. Deficits in energy intake can result in catabolism, which places demands on muscle protein to supply the main sources of carbon for glucose production.[1,2,26] As a result of this gluconeogenic response, the concentrations of alanine and glutamine in the plasma are increased, particularly in the fasting state. These two amino acids, along with citrulline, are taken up by the liver and used for the synthesis of glucose and ketones. The utilization of these amino acids (and relatively smaller amounts of others) for energy results in hepatic production of ammonia that then must be converted to urea.[26]

**Table 41–1.** Enzymes of the Urea Cycle, Their Associated Disorders, and Corresponding Laboratory Findings*

| Enzyme | Disorder | Ammonia Concentration | Citrulline Concentration | Arginine Concentration |
|---|---|---|---|---|
| *N*-Acetylglutamate synthetase | NAGS deficiency | Markedly elevated | Absent to low | Absent to low |
| Carbamoyl phosphate synthetase | CPS deficiency | Markedly elevated | Absent to low | Absent to low |
| Ornithine transcarbamylase | OTC deficiency† | Markedly elevated | Absent to low | Absent to low |
| Argininosuccinic acid synthetase | ASS deficiency; citrulinemia I | Elevated | Elevated | Low |
| Argininosuccinic acid lyase | ASL deficiency‡; argininosuccinic aciduria (ASA) | Elevated | Elevated | Low |
| Arginase | Arginase deficiency; argininemia | Rarely elevated | Normal | Elevated |

Adapted from Wijburg FA, Nassogne M. Disorders of the urea cycle and related enzymes. In: Saudubray JM, van den Berghe G, Walter JH, et al., eds. *Inborn Metabolic Diseases: Diagnosis and Treatment*, 5th ed. Heidelberg, Germany: Springer-Verlag; 2012; Ah Mew N, Lanpher BC, Gropman A, et al. Urea cycle disorders overview. 2003; last revision April 2015. In: Pagon RA, Adam MP, Ardinger HH, et al., eds. *GeneReviews* Seattle, WA: University of Washington, 1993–2016. http://www.ncbi.nlm.nih.gov/books/NBK1217. Accessed June 26, 2016; Rohr F. Nutrition management of urea cycle disorders. In: Bernstein LE, Rohr F, Helm JR, eds. *Nutrition Management of Inherited Metabolic Diseases: Lessons from Metabolic University.* Cham, Switzerland: Springer International Publishing; 2015: 159.

*Laboratory findings indicate blood concentrations that are found at time of diagnosis, before treatment is initiated.

†Urine orotic acid is also present in OTC deficiency.

‡Urine and plasma argininosuccinic acid are elevated in ASL deficiency.

**Table 41–2.** Recommended Dietary Intakes for Patients with Inherited Metabolic Disorders of the Urea Cycle

| Age | Total Protein*† (g/kg) | Energy*‡ (kcal/day after 12 mo of age) | Fluid (mL/kcal) |
|---|---|---|---|
| *Infants (mo)* | | | |
| 0–1 | 2.5–1.7 | 145–120 kcal/kg | 1.5 |
| 1–2 | 2.1–1.7 | 140–115 kcal/kg | 1.5 |
| 2–3 | 2.1–1.6 | 135–115 kcal/kg | 1.5 |
| 3–4 | 2.1–1.0 | 130–110 kcal/kg | 1.5 |
| 4–5 | 2.0–1.0 | 125–105 kcal/kg | 1.5 |
| 5–6 | 1.9–1.0 | 120–100 kcal/kg | 1.5 |
| 6–9 | 1.6–1.0 | 115–95 kcal/kg | 1.5 |
| 9–12 | 1.6–1.0 | 110–90 kcal/kg | 1.5 |
| *Children (yr)* | | | |
| 1–4 | 1.8–0.7 | 900–1800 | 1.0 |
| 4–7 | 1.3–0.7 | 1300–2300 | 1.0 |
| 7–11 | 1.7–0.9 | 1650–3300 | 1.0 |
| *Females (yr)* | | | |
| 11–15 | 1.0–0.6 | 1650–2450 | 1.0 |
| 15–19 | 0.9–0.6 | 1500–3000 | 1.0 |
| ≥19 | 0.8–0.6 | 1200–3000 | 1.0 |
| *Males (yr)* | | | |
| 11–15 | 1.4–1.0 | 2000–3700 | 1.0 |
| 15–19 | 1.2–0.8 | 2100–3900 | 1.0 |
| ≥19 | 1.2–0.8 | 2300–3300 | 1.0 |

Adapted from Singh R.H. Nutrition management of patients with inherited disorders of the urea cycle enzymes. In: Acosta P.B. eds. *Nutrition Management of Patients with Inherited Metabolic Disorders*. Sudbury, MA: Jones and Bartlett Publishers, 2009: 405.

*Based on ideal body weight for height and age. Amount per kilogram body weight declines with age.

†The usual distribution of total protein is 50% from essential amino acids provided by a medical formula and 50% from intact protein, but it can vary depending on age, severity of disease, and other factors.

‡Use estimated energy requirement (EER) equations that consider sex, age, and activity level to determine more specific energy prescriptions.

Assurance of adequate energy intake improves total protein tolerance and facilitates a normal growth pattern in those with UCD.[10,11,21] Calorie recommendations for those affected by UCD may exceed standard recommendations, especially during illness or other catabolic events.[17,10,11,27] Protein-free medical foods containing carbohydrate with or without added fat (e.g., Prophree, Abbott Nutrition; DuoCal, Nutricia North America) are often added to EAA-based medical foods to increase the energy content of the formula feedings (see Table 41–5). Use of these medical foods, along with modified low-protein products, increases the variety of foods allowed in the diet and provides more flexibility in menu planning.[10,11,18,28]

## Feeding Difficulties

The dietary management of UCD in children and adults is complicated by chronic anorexia and food avoidance.[24] The physiology behind anorexia in this population is unclear, although elevated brain glutamine concentrations or abnormal levels of satiety hormones may play a role.[29,30] Avoidance of protein-containing foods is common and is often noted in dietary patterns of those diagnosed with UCD after infancy. Placement of a gastrostomy tube should be considered for patients with poor growth, frequent episodes of hyperammonemia, and/or a neurological impairment that affects food intake.[10] Even if not required on a routine basis, a gastrostomy tube is often helpful for administering sources of nonprotein calories that may prevent hyperammonemic episodes during intercurrent illnesses and for administering nitrogen-scavenging medications or other pharmacological treatments that are often poorly tolerated orally.[12,31]

Parental anxiety regarding excess protein can interfere with a relaxed atmosphere at mealtime and, if excessive, can lead to behavioral feeding disorders.[24,32] This anxiety, along with a child's poor oral intake, can also lead to intake of protein and calories that is chronically lower than prescribed.[22,23] Clinicians need to recognize this pattern because it can lead to chronically compromised metabolic control and poor growth.

## Acute Management

Acute management is often necessary at the time of initial presentation, particularly with neonatal- or infant-onset UCD, and during any intercurrent illness, injury, or surgical procedure.[7,11,14,33,34] The goal of acute management for UCD is to slow protein catabolism and reduce ammonia production by providing a nonprotein, high-calorie nutrition source via enteral and/or parenteral nutrition. Total energy goals during acute events are often 100% to 120% of recommended needs.[7,22] However, a source of EAA, either as an enteral medical food or as a total parenteral nutrition (TPN) solution, needs to be introduced within 24 to 48 hours after discontinuation of protein intake to prevent further protein catabolism.[7,11,33,34] Protocols vary, but recent studies suggest that earlier introduction of EAA could be of benefit, especially for those with several days of poor oral intake and low plasma EAA concentrations at the time of admission.[22,23] Typically, reintroduction

**Table 41–3.** Protein Equivalents and Essential Amino Acid Content (g) of Medical Protein Options for Urea Cycle Disorders (in 100 g powder)

| Amount* | Cyclinex 1† | Cyclinex 2† | Essential Amino Acid Mix‡ | WND-1* | UCD Anamix Junior‡ | UCD Trio§ | EAA Supplement§ |
|---|---|---|---|---|---|---|---|
| Protein | 7.5 | 15 | 79 | 6.5 | 12 | 15 | 40 |
| Calories | 510 | 440 | 316 | 500 | 385 | 393 | 288 |
| Carbohydrate | 57 | 45 | 0 | 60 | 46 | 51 | 31.8 |
| Fat | 24.6 | 17.0 | 0 | 26 | 17 | 14.3 | 0.1 |
| Tryptophan | 0.28 | 0.56 | 2.36 | 0.38 | 0.48 | 0.49 | 1.3 |
| Threonine | 0.75 | 1.50 | 11.35 | 0.85 | 1.59 | 1.55 | 4.1 |
| Isoleucine | 1.28 | 2.56 | 10.4 | 0.99 | 2.26 | 2.71 | 5.7 |
| Leucine | 2.17 | 4.34 | 16.17 | 1.93 | 3.82 | 4.52 | 9.8 |
| Lysine | 1.11 | 2.22 | 13.25 | 1.23 | 1.92 | 2.48 | 6.6 |
| Methionine | 0.34 | 0.68 | 3.78 | 0.24 | 0.4 | 0.71 | 1.8 |
| Cystine | 0.30 | 0.60 | 3.78 | 0.2 | 0.43 | 0.56 | 1.8 |
| Phenylalanine | 0.75 | 1.50 | 5.67 | 0.67 | 0.67 | 0.85 | 3.4 |
| Tyrosine | 0.88 | 1.76 | 9.46 | 0.8 | 1.23 | 1.47 | 4.7 |
| Valine | 1.43 | 2.86 | 14.56 | 0.99 | 2.29 | 2.71 | 7.2 |
| Arginine | 0 | 0 | 0 | 0 | 0 | 0 | 0 |
| Histidine | 0.36 | 0.72 | 3.78 | 0.43 | 0.51 | 0.68 | 1.8 |
| Vitamins and Minerals | Yes | Yes | No | Yes | Yes | Yes | Yes |

*Data collected in July 2016; check manufacturers' websites for the most current medical food composition data.

†Abbott Nutrition; Columbus, OH

‡Nutricia North America, Gaithersburg, MD

*Mead Johnson, Evansville, IN

§Vitaflo, Alexandria, VA

**Table 41–4.** Macronutrient Composition of Milk Protein Sources and Milk Beverage Substitutes*

| Amount | Breast Milk (1 fl oz/30 mL) | Infant Formula (milk based)† (1 fl oz/30 mL) | Cow's Milk 3.25% Fat (1 fl oz/30 mL) | Evaporated Milk (1 fl oz/30 mL) | Nonfat Dry Milk (1/3 cup/23 g) | Rice Milk (1 fl oz/30 mL) | Soy Milk (1 fl oz/30 mL) |
|---|---|---|---|---|---|---|---|
| Protein (g) | 0.3 | 0.4 | 1.0 | 2.1 | 8.3 | 0.1 | 1.0 |
| Calories (kcal) | 21.6 | 20 | 18.6 | 42.5 | 83 | 14.0 | 16.5 |
| Carbohydrate (g) | 2.1 | 2.1 | 1.5 | 3.2 | 12 | 2.8 | 1.9 |
| Fat (g) | 1.3 | 1.1 | 1.0 | 2.4 | 0.2 | 0.3 | 0.5 |

*Data from Metabolic Pro, Genetic Metabolic Dietitians International. https://metabolicpro.org. Accessed July 2016.
†Values based on Similac Advance with Iron, Ready to Feed.

of a protein source is initiated at 50% of the patient's total protein needs.[11,23] Acute medical management may also include use of oral or intravenous (IV) nitrogen-scavenger drugs and supplementation with an oral or IV source of L-arginine, as discussed later.[7,12,33] Treatment at a medical center with access to a metabolic team including a biochemical geneticist and a dietitian specializing in the treatment of inborn errors of metabolism, as well as emergent access to biochemical laboratory studies and hemodialysis, is essential for the best clinical outcomes.

To manage less severe illnesses, patients with UCD may be prescribed a home sick-day diet regimen that reduces total protein but maintains or increases caloric intake using nonprotein calorie sources. Sick-day diets should not be used for longer than 24 to 48 hours,[10,11] and there should be a low threshold for emergency care. All individuals with UCD should be provided with an emergency protocol that outlines acute management and provides contact information for the on-call metabolic team.

## ARGININE AND OTHER SUPPLEMENTS

Except for those with arginase deficiency, arginine becomes an EAA in patients with UCD, and supplementation with a source of arginine is required to normalize plasma arginine concentrations.[7,11,35] The appropriate dose of L-arginine depends on the patient's weight and the severity of the enzyme deficiency.[1,18,35] Typical doses for L-arginine supplementation range from 400 to 700 mg/kg/day[14,25] (Table 41–6). However, newer studies suggest that a lower dose of L-arginine (100 mg/kg) may be needed in cases of ASL deficiency to reduce production of argininosuccinic acid, which contributes to liver and neurological disease in this disorder.[36] L-Citrulline, which is converted to arginine via the urea cycle, can be used in place of L-arginine in patients with OTC or CPS deficiency. Supplementation with L-citrulline (100–170 mg/kg) in these two disorders results in elimination of one additional nitrogen molecule compared with supplementation with L-arginine.[1,2] Table 41–5 lists suppliers of single amino acids.

## WASTE NITROGEN CONJUGATION AND ADJUNCT THERAPIES

Dietary protein restriction with arginine or citrulline supplementation alone does not always provide complete protection against the complications of UCD. Therefore, pharmacological agents to augment alternative pathways of waste nitrogen disposal are frequently prescribed. Alternative pathway therapy with sodium benzoate and/or sodium phenylacetate remains a therapeutic cornerstone for both acute and long-term treatment.[12] Sodium benzoate combines with the amino group of glycine to form hippurate via an enzymatic reaction in the liver. Hippurate is excreted into the urine, resulting in the loss

**Table 41–5.** Distributors and Manufacturers of Medical Formula, Modified Low-Protein Products, and Single Amino Acids for Treatment of Urea Cycle Disorders

| Company | Website | EAA Medical Formulas* | Carbohydrate ± Fat Modules† | Low-Protein Foods‡ | Amino Acids§ |
|---|---|---|---|---|---|
| *Abbott Nutrition* Columbus, OH | www.abbottnutrition.com | X | X | | |
| *Ajinomato North America* Fort Lee, NJ | www.ajinomoto-usa.com | | | | X |
| *Cambrooke Foods* Framingham, MA | www.cambrookefoods.com | | | X | |
| *Dietary Specialties* Randolph, NJ | www.dietspec.com | | | X | |
| *Ener-G-Foods* Seattle, WA | www.ener-g.com | | | X | |
| *Glutino* Laval, Quebec | www.glutino.com | | | X | |
| *Jo-Mar Labs* Scotts Valley, CA | www.jomarlabs.com | | | | X |
| *Kingsmill Foods* Scarborough, ON | www.kingsmillfoods.com | | | X | |
| *Liv-N-Well Distributors* Richmond, British Columbia | www.liv-n-well.com | | | X | |
| *Mead Johnson* Evansville, IN | www.meadjohnson.com | X | X | | |
| *Nutricia North America* Gaithersburg, MD | www.nutricia-na.com | X | X | X | X |
| *Vitaflo* Alexandria, VA | www.vitaflousa.com | X | X | X | X |

*Medical formulas containing essential amino acids (EAA) as the source of protein equivalents. See Table 41–3 for the composition of these products.
†Medical formulas that are protein-free, containing either carbohydrate alone or carbohydrate and fat. These may or may not contain vitamins and minerals.
‡Modified low-protein products containing minimal protein. Products vary greatly by company but can include baking mixes, breads, pasta, baked goods, and milk or meat substitutes.
§Single amino acids used for treatment of urea cycle disorders include L-citrulline and L-arginine.

**Table 41–6.** Suggested Ranges for Supplementation of Amino Acids for the Treatment of Urea Cycle Disorders*

| Disorder | L-Arginine (mg/kg) | L-Citrulline (mg/kg) |
|---|---|---|
| **CPS1 and OTC deficiency** | 100–170 | 100–170 |
| **ASS and ASL deficiency** | 400–700† | — |

Adapted from Haberle J, Boddaert N, Burlina A, et al. Suggested guidelines for the diagnosis and management of urea cycle disorders. *Orphan J Rare Dis.* 2012; 7:32; Singh RH. Nutritional management of patients with urea cycle disorders. *J Inherit Metab Dis.* 2007; 30:880; Singh RH. *Nutritional management of urea cycle disorders: a practical reference for clinicians.* 2006. Decatur, GA: Emory University.http://genetics.emory.edu/clinical/index/index.php?assetID=309. Accessed June 26, 2016.
*L-arginine or L-citrulline is not indicated for arginase deficiency.
†Recent studies suggest that a lower dose of L-arginine (100 mg/kg) may be more appropriate for ASL deficiency.
ASL, argininosuccinic acid lyase; ASS, argininosuccinic acid synthetase; CPS1, carbamoyl phosphate synthetase; OTC, ornithine transcarbamylase.

of 1 mole of waste nitrogen for each mole of benzoate administered. Sodium phenylacetate combines with glutamine to form phenylacetylglutamine via a reaction that occurs in both the liver and the kidney. Excretion of phenylacetylglutamine results in the removal of 2 moles of nitrogen for each mole of sodium phenylacetate administered[12] (see Fig. 41–1).

The offensive odor of sodium phenylacetate makes oral administration difficult, and this prompted the development of sodium phenylbutyrate (Buphenyl, Hyperion Pharmaceuticals), which is converted to phenylacetate after ingestion. The half-lives of these drugs are only 2 to 4 hours, requiring dosing three to four times per day. Some children experience side effects with sodium phenylbutyrate, including gastrointestinal distress, abnormal liver function tests, and rashes, among other clinical symptoms.[12] A newer nitrogen scavenger medication, glycerol phenylbutyrate (Ravicti, Hyperion Pharmaceuticals) has recently been approved.[37,38] Like sodium phenylbutyrate, glycerol phenylbutyrate is converted to sodium phenylacetate in the liver; however, less frequent administration, fewer side effects, and improved chronic metabolic control have been observed with this newer agent.[37,38] For acute episodes of hyperammonemia, an IV source of sodium benzoate and sodium phenylacetate (Ammunol, Hyperion Pharmaceuticals) is administered together with IV arginine.[18,39]

Low plasma concentrations of the branched-chain amino acids (i.e., leucine, valine and isoleucine) have been measured in those chronically treated with phenylbutyrate.[40] Additional protein, either as EAA or as intact protein, may not correct these abnormalities without adversely affecting metabolic control; for some, supplementation with a source of branched-chain amino acids may become necessary.[11] Some of the EAA-based medical foods now include additional branched chain amino acids.

Another medication, *N*-carbamylglutamate (Carbaglu, Orphan Europe SARL) is indicated to treat hyperammonemia caused by NAGS deficiency or partial CPS-1 deficiency. *N*-Carbamylglutamate is not a nitrogen scavenger but an analog of *N*-acetylglutamate, which is required to activate CPS-1.[41]

## MONITORING TREATMENT EFFICACY

During infancy and childhood, frequent growth measurements and laboratory assessments are required to determine the adequacy of treatment (see Table 41–6). Appropriate growth velocity indicates protein adequacy; low velocity may reflect inadequate intake of calories and/or protein. The goal of treatment is to normalize the ammonia concentration; a level lower than 80 µmol/L is recommended, although this can vary depending on reference ranges for the laboratory used.[42] Ammonia levels can be affected by exertion, and a multitude of effects can be caused by improper sampling techniques, storage, handling, or timing of the analysis.[43]

Quantitative amino acids analysis should be completed on samples taken 2 to 4 hours postprandially.[35] Plasma glutamine levels lower than 800 to 1000 µmol/L are recommended and may be a better marker than ammonia for assessment of treatment efficacy.[44] However, because of clinical variance, high glutamine levels may not reflect

**Table 41–7.** Laboratory Monitoring in Urea Cycle Disorders*

| Parameter | Notes/Goal Ranges |
|---|---|
| Ammonia ($NH_3$) | Goal: < 80 µmol/L |
| *UCD-specific amino acids (plasma)* | |
| Glutamine | Goal: 800 (to 1000) µmol/L |
| Citrulline | Normal if supplementing with L-citrulline; minimize in argininosuccinic acid synthase deficiency |
| Arginine | Normal if supplementing L-citrulline or L-arginine; minimize in arginase deficiency |
| Argininosuccinic acid | Minimize in argininosuccinic acid lyase deficiency |
| Branched-chain amino acids | May be low with nitrogen-scavenger medications |
| *Markers of protein sufficiency* | |
| Albumin | Long-term marker: 20-day half-life |
| Preabumin | Short-term marker: 48-hr half-life |
| Essential amino acids | Goal: normal concentrations |
| *General nutrition status* | |
| Nutritional anemia | Hemoglobin, hematocrit, ferritin, MCV, total iron binding capacity, methylmalonic acid, total homocysteine, folate |
| Vitamin and mineral status | Total 25-OH vitamin D, zinc, other trace minerals |
| Others to consider | Essential fatty acid profile |

Adapted from Rohr F. Nutrition management of urea cycle disorders. In: Bernstein LE, Rohr F, Helm JR, eds. *Nutrition Management of Inherited Metabolic Diseases: Lessons from Metabolic University.* Cham, Switzerland: Springer International Publishing; 2015; Yannicelli S. Protein requirements in inherited metabolic disorders In: Bernstein LE, Rohr F, Helm JR, eds. *Nutrition Management of Inherited Metabolic Diseases: Lessons from Metabolic University.* Cham, Switzerland: Springer International Publishing; 2015; Zschocke J, Hoffmann GF. Urea cycle disorders and inherited hyperammonaemias. In: Zschocke J, Hoffmann GF, eds. *Vademecum Metabolicum: Diagnosis and Treatment of Inborn Errors of Metabolism,* 3rd ed. Stuttgart, Germany: Schattauer; 2011; Bolann BJ, Solli JD, Schneede J, et al. Evaluation of indicators of cobalamin deficiency defined as cobalamin-induced reduction in increased serum methylmalonic acid. *Clin Chem.* 2000; 46:1744.
*Reference ranges vary among laboratories and need to considered in monitoring goals.; MCV, mean corpuscular volume; UCD, urea cycle disorders.

excessive protein or inadequate dosing of medication. Low concentrations of EAA and of standard markers of short- and long-term protein adequacy (e.g., albumin, prealbumin) suggest inadequate intake of protein.[11,21]

Iron and vitamin $B_{12}$ status should be checked yearly[10]; measurement of serum methylmalonic acid is the preferred method for determining vitamin $B_{12}$ status.[45] Potassium should be monitored because of urinary losses associated with sodium phenylbutyrate and sodium benzoate therapy.[12] Other markers of nutrition status are suggested in Table 41–7.[10]

## CONCLUSION

Outcomes for those with UCD have improved with advances in diet treatment and medication regimens, although there continues to be significant morbidity and mortality, especially in those with severe neonatal presentations. Further research is needed to determine optimal diet composition and improve monitoring regimens for both acute and chronic nutrition management.

### References

1. Wijburg FA, Nassogne M. Disorders of the urea cycle and related enzymes. In: Saudubray JM, van den Berghe G, Walter JH, et al., eds. *Inborn Metabolic Diseases: Diagnosis and Treatment,* 5th ed. Heidelberg, Germany: Springer-Verlag; 2012: 297.
2. Ah Mew N, Lanpher BC, Gropman A, et al. Urea cycle disorders overview. 2003; last revision April 2015. In: Pagon RA, Adam MP, Ardinger HH, et al., eds. *GeneReviews* Seattle, WA: University of Washington, 1993–2016. http://www.ncbi.nlm.nih.gov/books/NBK1217. Accessed June 26, 2016.
3. Summar ML, Koelker S, Freedenberg D, et al. The incidence of urea cycle disorders. *Mol Genet Metab.* 2013; 110:179.

4. Albrecht J, Zielinska M, Norenberg MD. Glutamine as a mediator of ammonia neurotoxicity: a critical appraisal. *Biochem Pharmacol.* 2010; 80:1303.
5. Braissant O, McLin VA, Cudalbu C. Ammonia toxicity to the brain. *J Inherit Metab Dis.* 2013; 36:595.
6. Batshaw ML, Tuchman M, Summar M, et al. A longitudinal study of urea cycle disorders. *Mol Genet Metab.* 2014; 113:127.
7. Haberle J, Boddaert N, Burlina A, et al. Suggested guidelines for the diagnosis and management of urea cycle disorders. *Orphan J Rare Dis.* 2012; 7:32.
8. Ahrens-Nicklas RC, Slap G, Ficicioglu C. Adolescent presentations of inborn errors of metabolism. *J Adolesc Health.* 2015; 56:477.
9. Demily C, Sedel F. Psychiatric manifestations of treatable hereditary metabolic disorders in adults. *Ann Gen Psychiatry.* 2014; 13:27.
10. Rohr F. Nutrition management of urea cycle disorders. In: Bernstein LE, Rohr F, Helm JR, eds. *Nutrition Management of Inherited Metabolic Diseases: Lessons from Metabolic University.* Cham, Switzerland: Springer International Publishing; 2015: 159.
11. Singh RH. Nutritional management of patients with urea cycle disorders. *J Inherit Metab Dis.* 2007; 30:880.
12. Batshaw ML, MacArthur RB, Tuchman M. Alternative pathway therapy for urea cycle disorders: twenty years later. *J Pediatr.* 2001; 138(Suppl 1):S46.
13. Adam S, Almeida MF, Assoun M, et al. Dietary management of urea cycle disorders: European practice. *Mol Genet Metab.* 2013; 110:439.
14. Summar M. Current strategies for the management of neonatal urea cycle disorders. *J Pediatr.* 2001; 138(Suppl 1):S30.
15. Perito ER, Rhee S, Roberts JP, Rosenthal P. Pediatric liver transplantation for urea cycle disorders and organic acidemias: United Network for Organ Sharing data for 2002–2012. *Liver Transpl.* 2014; 20:89.
16. Institute of Medicine Panel on Macronutrients, Standing Committee on the Scientific Evaluation of Dietary Reference Intakes. *Dietary Reference Intakes for Energy, Carbohydrate, Fiber, Fat, Fatty Acids, Cholesterol, Protein and Amino Acids.* Washington, DC: National Academies Press, 2005.
17. World Health Organization, Food and Agriculture Organization of the United Nations, United Nations University. Protein and amino acid requirements in human nutrition: report of a Joint FAO/WHO/UNU Expert Consultation. WHO Technical Report Series 935. Geneva: World Health Organization; 2007.
18. Singh RH. Nutritional management of urea cycle disorders: a practical reference for clinicians. Crit Care Clin 2005;21(4 Suppl):S27. Accessed June 26, 2016.
19. Elongo R, Ball RO, Pencharz PB. Recent advances in determining protein and amino acid requirements in humans. *Br J Nutr.* 2012; 108(Suppl):S22.
20. Mehta NM, Compher C, A.S.P.E.N. Board of Directors. A.S.P.E.N. clinical guidelines: nutrition support of the critically ill child. *J Parenter Enteral Nutr.* 2009; 33:260.
21. Yannicelli S. Protein requirements in inherited metabolic disorders In: Bernstein LE, Rohr F, Helm JR, eds. *Nutrition Management of Inherited Metabolic Diseases: Lessons from Metabolic University.* Cham, Switzerland: Springer International Publishing; 2015: 63.
22. Boneh A. Dietary protein in urea cycle disorders: how much? which? how? *Mol Genet Metab.* 2014; 113:109.
23. Humphrey M, Truby H, Boneh A. New ways of defining protein and energy relationships in inborn errors of metabolism. *Mol Genet Metab.* 2014; 112:247.
24. Gardeitchik T, Humphrey M, Nation J, Boneh A. Early clinical manifestations and eating patterns in patients with urea cycle disorders. *J Pediatr.* 2012; 161:328.
25. Huner G, Baykal T, Dernir F, Demirkol M. Breastfeeding experience in inborn errors of metabolism other than phenylketonuria. *J Inherit Metab Dis.* 2005; 28:457.
26. Barrett KE, Bortano S, Barman SM, Brooks HL. Amino acids and proteins. In: Barrett KE, Bortano S, Barman SM, Brooks HL, eds. *Ganong's Review of Medical Physiology*, 24th ed. New York: McGraw-Hill Education, 2012.
27. Acosta PB. Evaluation of nutrition status. In: Acosta PB, ed. *Nutrition Management of Patients with Inherited Metabolic Disorders.* Boston: Jones and Bartlett; 2009: 67.
28. MacDonald A, van Rijn M, Feillet F, et al. Adherence issues in inherited metabolic disease treated by low natural protein diets. *Ann Nutr Metab.* 2012; 61:289.
29. Delgado TC. Glutamate and GABA in appetite regulation. *Front Endocrinol (Lausanne).* 2013; 4:103.
30. Mitchell S, Welch-Burke T, Dumitresai L, et al. Peptide tyrosine tyrosine (PYY) levels are increased in patients with urea cycle disorders. *Mol Genet Metab.* 2012; 161:39.
31. Glycerol phenylbutyrate (Ravicti) for urea cycle disorders. *Med Lett Drugs Ther.* 2014; 56:77.
32. Hatzmann J, Valstar MJ, Bosch AM, Wijburg FA, Heymans HS, Grootenhuis MA. Predicting health-related quality of life of parents of children with inherited metabolic disease. *Acta Paediatr.* 2009; 98:1205.
33. New England Consortium of Metabolic Programs. *Acute Illness Protocols: Urea Cycle Disorders.* 2013. newenglandconsortium.org/for-professionals/acute-illness-protocols/urea-cycle-disorders. Accessed June 26, 2016.
34. Prietsch V, Lindner M, Zschocke J, Nyhan WL, Hoffmann GF. Emergency management of inherited metabolic diseases. *J Inherit Metab Dis.* 2002; 25:531.
35. Berry GT, Steiner RD. Long-term management of patients with urea cycle disorders. *J Pediatr.* 2001; 138:556.
36. Nagamani SC, Shchelochkoy OA, Mullins MA, et al. A randomized controlled trial to evaluate the effects of high-dose versus low-dose of arginine therapy on hepatic function tests in argininosuccinic aciduria. *Mol Genet Metab.* 2012; 107:315.
37. Diaz GA, Krivitzky LS, Mokhtarani M, et al. Ammonia control and neurocognitive outcome among urea cycle disorder patients treated with glycerol phenylbutyrate. *Hepatology.* 2013; 57:2171.
38. Berry SA, Lichter-Konecki U, Diaz GA, et al. Glycerol phenylbutyrate treatment in children with urea cycle disorders: pooled analysis of short and long-term ammonia control and outcomes. *Mol Genet Metab.* 2014; 112:17.
39. Enns GM. Nitrogen-sparing therapy revisited 2009. *Mol Genet Metab.* 2010; 100:565.
40. Burrage LC, Jain M, Gandolfo L, et al. Sodium phenylbutyrate decreases plasma amino acids in patients with urea cycle disorders. *Mol Genet Metab.* 2014; 113:131.
41. Daniotti M, LaMarca G, Florini P, Filippi L. New developments in the treatment of hyperammonemia: emerging use of carglumic acid. *Int J Gen Med.* 2011; 4:21.
42. Zschocke J, Hoffmann GF. Urea cycle disorders and inherited hyperammonaemias. In: Zschocke J, Hoffmann GF, eds. *Vademecum Metabolicum: Diagnosis and Treatment of Inborn Errors of Metabolism,* 3rd ed. Stuttgart, Germany: Schattauer; 2011: 57.
43. Barsotti RJ. Measurement of ammonia in blood. *J Pediatr.* 2001; 138(Suppl):S11.
44. Serrano M, Ormazabal A, Vilaseca N, et al. Assessment of plasma ammonia and glutamine concentrations in urea cycle disorders. *Clin Biochem.* 2011; 44:742.
45. Bolann BJ, Solli JD, Schneede J, et al. Evaluation of indicators of cobalamin deficiency defined as cobalamin-induced reduction in increased serum methylmalonic acid. *Clin Chem.* 2000; 46:1744.

# B.

# ORGANIC ACIDEMIAS

## 42 Methylmalonic Acidemia and Propionic Acidemia

DIANNE FRAZIER

The organic acidemias are a class of autosomal recessive inborn errors of metabolism sharing the characteristic of having a block in a specific step of amino acid catabolism that results in the excretion of abnormally high concentrations of non-amino organic acids.[1,2] This chapter discusses two of these disorders, propionic acidemia (PROP) and methylmalonic acidemia (MMA). The disorders 3-methylcrotonyl-CoA carboxylase deficiency (3MCCD), isovaleryl-CoA dehydrogenase deficiency (IVA), and glutaric acidemia type I (GAI), are described in later chapters.

### CLINICAL FEATURES

In 1961, Childs et al.[3] published the first description of an infant with a condition referred to as *ketotic hyperglycinemia*. Extensive studies of this infant and similar patients[4] found the disorder to be a defect of propionate rather than glycine metabolism. In 1967, Oberholzer et al.[5] described a series of patients who had a clinical picture almost identical to that of the individuals with PROP except that they excreted huge amounts of methylmalonic acid. It was then realized that PROP and MMA, although clinically similar, were different disorders.

Individuals with either PROP or MMA may present with a wide range of clinical symptoms, from life-threatening disease in the neonatal period to milder symptoms apparent only during intercurrent episodes of illness or other catabolic events. Presenting symptoms of the severe forms may include vomiting, poor feeding, lethargy, metabolic ketoacidosis, dehydration, hypoglycemia, hyperammonemia, hyperglycinemia, seizures, and coma. The presence of methylmalonic acid in the blood and urine can distinguish between the two disorders, both of which may have propionic acid, 3-OH propionic acid, methylcitric acid, and propionyl glycine in the urine and propionyl carnitine and increased glycine in the blood. Elevated propionyl carnitine is the analyte used in tandem mass spectrometry newborn screening MS/MS NBS for these disorders.[6] Rapid and efficient screening programs may be able to detect PROP and MMA in infants presymptomatically. The false-positive rate can be lowered by looking at the ratio of propionyl carnitine to acetyl carnitine (C3/C2) in addition to the isolated propionyl carnitine (C3) value.[7] Infants born to mothers who are vitamin $B_{12}$ deficient may also have a positive screening result. Confirmatory testing after a positive screen is necessary to distinguish between the two disorders. False-negative newborn screening results are possible in infants with the milder variants of these disorders. These infants may come to medical attention only after a period of poor growth, developmental delays, neutropenia and pancytopenia, or onset of metabolic decompensation with a catabolic illness.

The worldwide incidence of PROP is estimated to be 1:100,000 to 1:150,000 live births, with exceptions, such as in Saudi Arabia, where it is reported to be as high as 1:2000 to 1:5000 live births. The worldwide incidence of MMA has been estimated to be 1:50,000; again, there are exceptions in areas where consanguinity is common.[8]

### BIOCHEMICAL ABNORMALITIES

Both PROP and MMA result from blocks in the catabolic pathway of the essential amino acids isoleucine (ILE), valine (VAL), methionine

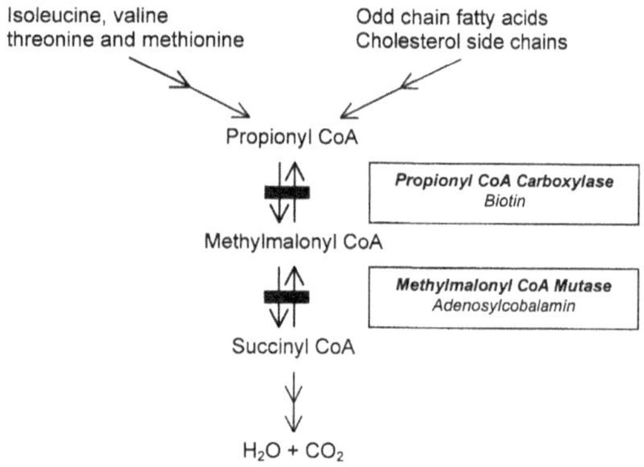


**Figure 42–1.** Blocks in the catabolic pathway of the propiogenic amino acids that cause propionic academia or methymalonic acidemia. CoA: coenzyme A.

(MET), and threonine (THR), and of the odd-chain fatty acids and cholesterol side chain (Fig. 42–1). The primary pathway for propionyl coenzyme A (CoA) degradation is by conversion to methylmalonyl CoAthat is then isomerized to succinyl CoA and further metabolized via the citric acid (tricarboxylic acid or TCA) cycle.

The first step is catalyzed by propionyl CoA carboxylase (E.C. 6.4.1.3). The enzyme is a complex of six αβ dimers and requires biotin as a cofactor. Patients with primary propionyl carboxylase deficiency have been shown to have mutations in either the α subunits (gene locus 13q32) or the β subunits (gene locus 3q13.3–22).[9,10] Propionyl CoA carboxylase activity is also compromised by defects in the biotin utilization pathway, as in biotinidase or holocarboxylase synthetase deficiency.

Methylmalonyl CoA mutase (E.C. 5.4.66.2) is a dimer with two identical subunits (gene locus 6p21).[11] It requires the cofactor adenosylcobalamin (a vitamin $B_{12}$ derivative). Isolated MMA results from either partial ($mut^-$) or complete ($mut^0$) mutase deficiency, or from cobalamin reductase (cblA) or cobalamin adenosyltransferase (cblB) deficiency. Individuals with $mut^0$ deficiency usually present earlier and have more significant disease than those with $mut^-$, cblA, or cblB deficiency. Other defects of cobalamin metabolism (cblC, cblD, and cblF) cause MMA with homocystinuria.[12] The remainder of this chapter focuses on the isolated forms of PROP and MMA.

## FACTORS TO BE CONSIDERED IN NUTRITION EVALUATION AND TREATMENT

Treatment of the acutely ill neonate is directed at correcting the metabolic acidosis and catabolism by stopping all protein feedings in the short term (24–36 hours), increasing energy intake, and initiating rehydration and electrolyte replacement. Severe neonatal hyperammonemia may require hemodialysis and/or temporary treatment with nitrogen scavengers (sodium benzoate/sodium phenylacetate and/or *N*-carbamylglutamate).[8,13]

Older children who come to the attention of the medical community with late onset of symptoms may require similar initial treatment, as do known patients in metabolic crisis during an intercurrent illness. If the newly diagnosed patient has MMA, the response to pharmacological doses of cyanocobalamin or hydroxycobalamin (1 mg/day for 5–7 days)[12] should be evaluated. If the methylmalonic acid level begins to fall within 24 hours, the patient has either a cobalamin defect or acquired vitamin $B_{12}$ deficiency and may not need severe dietary protein restriction.[12,13]

## DIETARY MANAGEMENT

The aim of dietary management of PROP and MMA is to minimize the endogenous production of propionic and methylmalonic acids by decreasing their precursors. The propiogenic amino acids, ILE, VAL, THR, and MET, can be decreased by limiting intact protein intake. The availability of medical foods (metabolic formulas)[14], that are prepared from amino acid mixtures essentially devoid of these amino acids, has made it possible to provide a diet with adequate, even liberal, protein while limiting the intake of propiogenic amino acids to that required for endogenous protein synthesis. Medical foods appropriate for individuals with PROP or MMA are listed in Table 42–1. The individualized prescription for infants is created by combining precise amounts of regular infant formula or breast milk containing intact protein (and the propiogenic amino acids) with the medical food. The ratio of the medical food to intact protein is determined by first meeting the propiogenic amino acid requirement, based on age and weight, with the intact protein. Then the ratio is adjusted based on the concentration of plasma propiogenic amino acids, which should be in the low-normal to normal range (Table 42–2), and measurements of appropriate growth and clinical status. When patients are unable to raise the propiogenic amino acids into the desired range, it has recently been suggested that additional intact protein, rather than supplemental amino acids be given.[15] It is important to avoid iatrogenic amino acid deficiencies by overzealous restriction.

After infancy, the intact protein provided from infant formula or breast milk is gradually replaced by solid foods having an equivalent amount of protein while continuing the age- and size-appropriate intake of medical food. Assessing and planning the diet based on its VAL content is a more precise method preferred by some clinicians. Of the four propiogenic amino acids, VAL is found in the highest concentration (approximately 4.5%) in natural proteins. To keep intact protein within the tolerated limits, most patients must avoid all high-protein foods and may need to use modified low-protein baked goods and pastas to meet their energy demands. The protein (or VAL) content of meals can be calculated with the use of food lists that provide the protein content per gram or volume of food[16,17] or its VAL content[17,18] or with the use of food analysis programs (e.g., MetabolicPro[19]) designed specifically for inborn errors of amino acid and organic acid metabolism.

Small amounts of propionate may come from other exogenous sources. Sodium and calcium propionate are often added to baked products to increase their shelf life. Careful label reading is important. Acosta and Yannicelli[18] recommended avoiding excessive intake of dietary fats known to contain varying amounts of odd-chain fatty acids, that are broken down to the three-carbon propionate. These fats include butter, cream, lard, and olive oil. However, there has not been good evidence that this impacts outcomes. The single greatest source of propionate is that which accumulates during catabolism. It comes from breakdown of odd-chain fatty acids stored in adipose tissue[20] and the catabolism of endogenous protein to meet increased energy requirements.

As much as 25% of the accumulated propionate may come from its production by anaerobic bacteria in the gastrointestinal tract.[21] Elimination or reduction of this source, through the use of continuous or intermittent administration of oral antibiotics, is another aim of the treatment.[8,22] Metronidazole therapy has been successfully used in patients to decrease gut bacteria. Using suggested dosages of 10 to 20 mg/kg/day of this antibiotic for 1 to 3 weeks, patients have reportedly shown significant improvements in appetite and decreases in both acidotic events and episodes of vomiting.[8,22] However, some patients do not tolerate the alteration in intestinal flora.

Providing adequate calories is a challenge when patients with PROP or MMA have poor appetites, neurological deficits that impair normal feeding, or compromised immune systems that lead to frequent illnesses. Many patients require feeding by nasogastric tube or direct gastric access. Some children need these alternative feeding strategies only during illness, some need them to supplement their limited oral intake, and others rely on them for their complete nutritional intake.

Aggressive treatment during illness is essential to prevent further complications of PROP and MMA.[8,20,21] If there is a lingering gastrointestinal intolerance to enteral feeds after treatment in the acute phase of the illness (as described earlier), parenteral amino acid solutions that are limited in propiogenic amino acids are available to be used in combination with regular parenteral amino acid solutions, intravenous lipids, and glucose. Fluid and electrolyte requirements need to

**Table 42–1.** Comparison of Medical Foods for Methylmalonic Acidemia and Propionic Acidemia Content (per 100 g Product)**

| | OA-1* | OA-2* | Propimex-1† | Propimex-2† | XMTVI Analog‡ | XMTVI Maxamaid‡ | XMTVI Maxamum‡ | Milupa OS-2‡ | MMA/ PA Gel§ per 24 g | MMA/PA Express 15§ per 100 g | MMA/PA Cooler 15§ per 100 mL |
|---|---|---|---|---|---|---|---|---|---|---|---|
| *Energy (kcal)* | 500 | 420 | 480 | 410 | 475 | 324 | 305 | 300 | 338 | 297 | 79 |
| *Protein equivalent (g)* | 15.7 | 21 | 15 | 30 | 13 | 25 | 40 | 56 | 41.7 | 60 | 11.5 |
| *Amino acids* | | | | | | | | | | | |
| Alanine (mg) | 4600 | 6100 | 2560 | 5120 | 1480 | 2890 | 4600 | 3100 | 4105 | 5920 | 1290 |
| Arginine (mg) | 1000 | 1340 | 1550 | 3100 | 1330 | 2590 | 4100 | 2700 | 4300 | 6140 | 1330 |
| Aspartic acid (mg) | 1320 | 1760 | 1590 | 3180 | 1170 | 2300 | 3600 | 7600 | 7460 | 10640 | 2310 |
| Carnitine (mg) | 50 | 49 | 900 | 1800 | 1.01 | 20 | 39 | NA | 46 | 64 | 13 |
| Cystine (mg) | 290 | 420 | 450 | 900 | 490 | 950 | 1500 | 1800 | 1770 | 2530 | 560 |
| Glutamic acid (mg) | 0 | 0 | 2450 | 4900 | 1470 | 0 | 4500 | 16,000 | NA | NA | NA |
| Glutamine (mg) | NA | NA | 0 | 0 | 100 | 1500 | 320 | NA | 5060 | 7220 | 0 |
| Glycine (mg) | 1000 | 1340 | 495 | 1000 | 590 | 1160 | 1800 | 1800 | 1950 | 2790 | 610 |
| Histidine (mg) | 470 | 650 | 420 | 840 | 900 | 1750 | 2800 | 1800 | 2780 | 3970 | 870 |
| Isoleucine (mg) | 0 | 0 | 120 | 240 | 0 | <70 | <140 | 0 | 150 | 220 | 40 |
| Leucine (mg) | 2400 | 3400 | 1380 | 2760 | 2000 | 3900 | 6200 | 7600 | 6580 | 9390 | 1820 |
| Lysine (mg) | 1510 | 2100 | 1000 | 2000 | 1360 | 2650 | 4200 | 5400 | 4580 | 6540 | 1420 |
| Methionine (mg) | 0 | 0 | 0 | 0 | 0 | 0 | 0 | 0 | 0 | 0 | 0 |
| Phenylalanine (mg) | 790 | 1100 | 880 | 1760 | 880 | 1720 | 2710 | 3200 | 2780 | 3970 | 870 |
| Proline (mg) | 1320 | 1760 | 2160 | 3200 | 590 | 1160 | 1900 | 7100 | 2020 | 2890 | 640 |
| Serine (mg) | 690 | 920 | 1150 | 1700 | 830 | 1620 | 2600 | 4000 | 2930 | 4190 | 960 |
| Taurine (mg) | 30 | 49 | 40 | 50 | 20 | 140 | 140 | NA | 92 | 132 | 25 |
| Threonine (mg) | 0 | 0 | 100 | 200 | 0 | 0 | 0 | 0 | 0 | 0 | 0 |
| Tryptophan (mg) | 350 | 480 | 170 | 340 | 390 | 760 | 1200 | 1400 | 1100 | 1590 | 360 |
| Tyrosine (mg) | 790 | 1100 | 890 | 1780 | 880 | 1720 | 2700 | 3900 | 2780 | 3970 | 870 |
| Valine (mg) | 0 | 0 | 0 | 0 | 0 | 0 | 0 | 0 | 0 | 0 | 0 |
| *Fat* | | | | | | | | | | | |
| Total (g) | 26 | 9 | 21.7 | 13 | 20.9 | <0.1 | <1.0 | 0 | 50 | 0.2 | 1.3 |
| Linoleic/α-linolenic (g) | 4.5/0.4 | 4.4/0.6 | 3.5/0.35 | 2.2/0.23 | 3.03/0.2 | 0 | 0 | 0 | NA | NA | NA |
| *Carbohydrate* | | | | | | | | | | | |
| Total (g) | 51 | 59 | 53 | 35 | 59 | 56 | 34 | 18.9 | 42.9 | 13.7 | 5.4 |
| *Minerals* | | | | | | | | | | | |
| Calcium (mg) | 660 | 760 | 575 | 880 | 600 | 810 | 1183 | 1310 | 1083 | 1196 | 230 |
| Chloride (mg) | 410 | 480 | 1160 | 290 | 290 | 450 | 560 | 990 | 583 | 728 | 140 |
| Chromium (μg) | 11 | NA | 27 | 15 | 15 | 21.5 | 26 | NA | 71 | 88 | 17 |
| Copper (mg) | 0.86 | 1.2 | 1.1 | 1 | 0.45 | 1.0 | 0.82 | 2.0 | 0.8 | 2.2 | 0.45 |
| Iodine (μg) | 76 | 66 | 65 | 47 | 47 | 144 | 131 | 120 | 138 | 252 | 49 |
| Iron (mg) | 9.6 | 12.3 | 9 | 10 | 10 | 14 | 14.7 | 15 | 14 | 21.6 | 4.2 |
| Magnesium (mg) | 50 | 177 | 50 | 225 | 40 | 128 | 306 | 156 | 167 | 376 | 72 |
| Manganese (mg) | 0.38 | 1.35 | 0.5 | 0.80 | 0.6 | 1.9 | 1.8 | 0.7 | 1.7 | 3.2 | 0.6 |
| Molybdenum (μg) | NA | 37 | 12 | 30 | 15 | 33 | 37 | 32 | 50 | 144 | 28 |
| Phosphorous (mg) | 440 | 760 | 400 | 760 | 500 | 810 | 1137 | 1010 | 825 | 1068 | 205 |
| Potassium (mg) | 560 | 1160 | 675 | 1370 | 420 | 840 | 700 | 1330 | 938 | 940 | 181 |
| Selenium (μg) | 14.1 | 27 | 20 | 35 | 15 | 40 | 58 | NA | 35 | 88 | 17 |
| Sodium (mg) | 240 | 610 | 190 | 880 | 120 | 580 | 560 | 640 | 379 | 508 | 98 |
| Zinc (mg) | 8.6 | 12.3 | 8.0 | 13 | 8 | 11 | 9 | 7.8 | 11 | 21.6 | 4.2 |
| *Vitamins* | | | | | | | | | | | |
| Vitamin A (IU) | 1520 | 1430 | 1400 | 2200 | 1760 | 1665 | 2228 | 5200 | 2000 | 2773 | 533 |
| Vitamin D (IU) | 380 | 290 | 300 | 300 | 340 | 480 | 332 | 1310 | 584 | 528 | 231 |
| Vitamin E, α-TE (mg) | 6.7 | 10.3 | 10.1 | 12.1 | 3.3 | 9.6 | 12.3 | 12 | 9 | 15.6 | 4.5 |
| Vitamin K (μg) | 40 | 41 | 50 | 60 | 21 | 48 | 82 | 167 | 41 | 100 | 19 |
| Vitamin C (mg) | 60 | 49 | 50 | 60 | 40 | 62.5 | 62 | 80 | 63 | 108 | 21 |
| Thiamine (mg) | 1.0 | 1.2 | 1.9 | 3.3 | 0.5 | 0.8 | 0.91 | 1.4 | 1 | 2 | 0.4 |
| Riboflavin (mg) | 1.0 | 1.0 | 0.9 | 1.8 | 0.6 | 0.8 | 0.97 | 2.0 | 1.2 | 2.3 | 0.44 |
| Vitamin $B_6$ (mg) | 1.0 | 1.0 | 0.75 | 1.3 | 0.52 | 0.8 | 1.6 | 1.5 | 1.1 | 2.8 | 0.5 |
| Vitamin $B_{12}$ (μg) | 2.0 | 2.4 | 4.9 | 5.0 | 1.25 | 2.0 | 3.1 | 3 | 2 | 4.8 | 0.9 |
| Niacin (mg) | 12.8 | 22 | 10 | 4.5 | 4.5 | 5.0 | 24 | 24 | 14 | 24.8 | 4.8 |
| Folic acid (μg) | 100 | 350 | 230 | 38 | 38 | 240 | 400 | 400 | 208 | 400 | 77 |
| Pantothenic acid (mg) | 3.8 | 4.8 | 6.9 | 8.0 | 2.6 | 3.2 | 4.9 | 11 | 5 | 8 | 1.5 |
| Biotin (μg) | 38 | 49 | 65 | 100 | 26 | 18 | 24.5 | 300 | 25 | 188 | 36 |
| Choline (mg) | 124 | 102 | 80 | 100 | 50 | 250 | 430 | 260 | 279 | 600 | 115 |
| Inositol (mg) | 40 | 86 | 70 | 100 | 100 | 56 | 80 | 300 | NA | NA | 0 |

*Mead Johnson, Evansville, IN 47712 @ http://www.meadjohnson.com.
**Data as of 1/2015
†Ross Products Division, Abbott Laboratories, Columbus, OH 43215-1724 @ http://www.abbott.com.
‡Nutricia North America, Gaithersburg, MD 20884 @ http://www.nutricia-na.com.
§Vitaflo USA Alexandria, VA 22314 @ http://www.VitafloUSA.com
NA = information not available.

**Table 42–2.** Recommended Daily Nutrient Intakes for Infants with Methylmalonic Acidemia or Propionic Acidemia

| Age (mo) | ILE* (mg/kg) | MET* (mg/kg) | THR* (mg/kg) | VAL* (mg/kg) | Protein† (g/kg) | kcal† (per kg) |
|---|---|---|---|---|---|---|
| 0–3 | 75–120 | 30–50 | 75–135 | 75–105 | 2.5–3.5 | 90–140 |
| 3–6 | 65–100 | 20–45 | 60–100 | 65–90 | 2.5–3.5 | 85–135 |
| 6–9 | 50–90 | 10–40 | 40–75 | 35–75 | 2.5–3.0 | 80–125 |
| 9–12 | 40–80 | 10–30 | 20–40 | 30–60 | 2.0–3.0 | 80–125 |
| Plasma amino acid‡ range (µmol/L) | 26–94 | 3–45 | 37–235 | 57–305 | | |

*From Acosta PB, Yannicelli S. *The Ross Metabolic Formula System Nutrition Support Protocols*, 4th ed. Columbus, OH: Ross Products Division; 2001.†Guidelines used at the University of North Carolina Division of Genetics and Metabolism Clinic for patients who are on a combination of intact protein and medical food; see text for modifications during illness.

‡Ranges used for plasma amino acid analysis in the University of North Carolina at Chapel Hill Biochemical Genetics Laboratory; the goal for patients with methylmalonic acidemia or propionic acidemia is to have plasma values for ILE, MET, THR, and VAL in the low-normal range.

Note: An individual's requirements may vary depending on genotype, growth, and intercurrent illnesses; close monitoring of biochemical status, growth, and development are necessary.

be more carefully monitored for a subgroup of MMA patients who develop chronic renal failure.[8,13]

In these disorders, free carnitine becomes depleted as it replaces the CoA moiety in accumulated propionyl and methylmalonyl CoA, resulting in elevated tissue levels of the organic acid carnitine adjunct.[13,20] The recommended carnitine supplementation for most individuals is in the range of 50 to 200 mg/kg/day, given in divided doses. A few medical foods (see Table 42–1) contain supplemental carnitine, that may be sufficient for some patients to maintain the plasma level of free carnitine at 30 µmol/L plasma or higher. Intravenous carnitine (100 mg/kg) may be used during acute illness.[8] Excessive carnitine supplementation can cause a fishy odor and loose stools.

## MONITORING AND FOLLOW-UP

Monitoring of individuals with PROP or MMA is an integral part of disease management.[8] Caregivers should measure urinary ketones at home whenever they have any concerns about possible illness. They should contact the clinic with abnormal results so that the appropriate intervention can begin immediately. Quantitative plasma amino acid monitoring should be done at regular intervals, along with anthropometric measurements. In addition, at regularly scheduled clinic visits (at least every 3 months during the first 2 years of life), the following should be ordered: complete blood count with differential; urine organic acids; electrolytes; iron status; blood carnitine; albumin and total protein; and, for MMA, plasma methylmalonic acid or a megaloblastic anemia panel. Other tests may be appropriate for certain individuals or under particular circumstances.

Resources for MMA and PROP information and supplies are listed in Box 42–1.

**Box 42–1.** Resources for MMA and PROP

National Library of Medicine Genetics Home Reference (propionic academia and methylmalonic academia):
http://ghr.nlm.nih.gov/condition/propionic-acidemia
http://ghr.nlm.nih.gov/condition/methylmalonic-acidemia

Propionic Acidemia Foundation:
www.pafoundation.com

Organic Acidemia Association:
www.oaanews.org

Save Babies Through Screening Foundation, Inc.:
http://www.savebabies.org

STAR-G: Expanded Newborn Screening Using New Technologies—Financial, Ethical, Legal and Social Issues (FELSI) (organic acid disorders):
http://www.newbornscreening.info/Parents/organicaciddisorders/MMA.html

CLIMB (Children Living with Inherited Metabolic Diseases):
http://www.climb.org.uk

Genetic Alliance:
http://www.geneticalliance.org/

Source of L-carnitine:
http://www.sigmatau.com

Sources of L-amino acids:
http://www.ajinomoto-usa.com
http://www.fishersci.com
http://www.vitaflousa.com
http://www.jomarlabs.com

Information and links on low-protein foods:
https:pkunews.org
http://www.GMDI.org

Source of parenteral amino acid mixtures (Coram CVS/Specialty Infusion Services: phone 800-423-1411):
http://www.coramhc.com

## OTHER TREATMENTS

Organ transplantation has been implemented in some individuals with PROP or MMA. In PROP, reports indicate that liver transplantation decreases the number of metabolic decompensation episodes, feeding issues, neurological sequelae, and cardiomyopathies.[20] However, the limited case reports also suggest that some continued protein restriction and carnitine supplementation may be necessary. Combined liver/kidney transplantation has been considered a treatment option for individuals with MMA.[13] In all patients, the decision to transplant must be individualized based on a consideration of the benefits versus the risks.

## LONG-TERM OUTCOMES

Despite greater knowledge of the underlying pathology of these disorders and the possibility of earlier diagnosis and initiation of treatment with the adoption of MS/MS NBS, both PROP and MMA (especially mut° and cblB subtypes) still result in high morbidity and mortality rates.[24] The manifestations include intellectual disability, neurological findings including metabolic stroke, pancreatitis, growth failure, functional immune impairment, and optic nerve atrophy.[13,20] In addition, there is a higher prevalence of cardiomyopathy and cardiac rhythm abnormalities in PROP and renal insufficiency often developing into end-stage renal disease in MMA.[13,20]

### References


1. Seashore MR. The organic acidemias: an overview. 2009. In: Pagon RA, Adam MP, Ardinger HH, et al., eds. *GeneReviews*. Seattle, WA: University of Washington; 1993–2016. http://www.ncbi.nlm.nih.gov/books/n/gene/oa-overview/
2. Knerr I, Weinhold N, Vockley J, Gibson KM. Advances and challenges in the treatment of branched-chain amino/keto acid metabolic defects. *J Inherit Metab Dis.* 2012: 35:29.
3. Childs B, Nyhan WL, Borden M, Bard L, Cooke RE. Idiopathic hyperglycinemia and hyperglycinuria: new disorder of amino acid metabolism I. *Pediatrics.* 1961; 27:522.
4. Hsia YE, Scully KJ, Rosenberg LE. Defective propionate carboxylation in ketotic hyperglycinaemia. *Lancet.* 1969; 1:757.
5. Oberholzer VC, Levin B, Burgess EA, Young WF. Methylmalonic aciduria: an inborn error of metabolism leading to chronic metabolic acidosis. *Arch Dis Child.* 1967; 42:492.
6. Charrow J, Goodman S, McCabe E, Rinaldo P. Tandem mass spectrometry in newborn screening. *Genet Med.* 2000; 2:267.

7. Frazier DM, Millington, DS, McCandless SE, Koeberl DD, Weavil SD, Muenzer, J. The tandem mass spectrometry newborn screening experience in North Carolina: 1997–2005. *J Inherit Metab Dis.* 2006; 29:76.
8. Baumgartner MR, Horster F, Dionisi-Vici C, et al. Proposed guidelines for the diagnosis and management of methylmalonic and propionic academia. *Orphan J Rare Dis.* 2014; 9:130.
9. Lamhonwah AM, Barankiewics TJ, Willard HF, Mahuran DJ, Quan F, Gravel RA. Isolation of cDNA clones coding for the α and β chains of human propionyl-CoA carboxylase: chromosomal assignments and DNA polymorphisms associated with *PCCA* and *PCCB* genes. *Proc Natl Acad Sci U S A.* 1986; 83:4864.
10. Kraus JP, Williamson CL, Firgaira FA, et al. Cloning and screening with nanogram amounts of immunopurified messenger RNAs: cDNA cloning and chromosomal mapping of cystathionine β-synthetase and the β-subunit of propionyl CoA carboxylase. *Proc Natl Acad Sci U S A.* 1986; 83:2047.
11. Fenton WA, Hack AM, Willard HF, Gertler A, Rosenberg LE. Purification and properties of methylmalonyl CoA mutase from human liver. *Arch Biochem Biophys.* 1982; 214:815.
12. Fenton WA, Gravel RA, Rosenblatt DS. Disorders of propionate and methylmalonate metabolism. In: Scriver CR, Beaudet AL, Sly WS, Valle D, eds. *The Metabolic and Molecular Bases of Inherited Disease*, 8th ed. New York: McGraw-Hill; 2001; 2165.
13. Manoli I, Sloan JL, Venditti CP. Isolated methylmalonic academia. 2005; last updated 2016. In: Pagon RA, Adam MP, Ardinger HH, et al., eds. *GeneReviews.* 2009. Seattle, WA: University of Washington; 1993–2016. http://www.ncbi.nlm.nih.gov/books/NBK1231/?report. Accessed June 29, 2016.
14. Camp KM, Lloyd-Puryear MA, Huntington KL. Nutritional treatment of inborn errors of metabolism: indications, regulations, and availability of medical foods and dietary supplements using phenylketonuria as an example. *Mol Genet Metab.* 2012; 107:3.
15. Manoli I, Myles JG, Sloan JL, Shchelochkov OA, Venditti CP. A critical reappraisal of dietary practices in methylmalonic acidemia raises concerns about the safety of medical foods. Part 1: isolated methylmalonic acidemias. *Genet Med.* 2016 Apr;18(4):386–95.
16. Shuett VE. *Low Protein Food List for PKU*, 3rd ed. CreateSpace; 2010. Available at by mail at pkubooks@shsna.com.
17. Pennington J. *Bowes and Church's Food Values of Portions Commonly Used*, 17th ed. New York: Lippincott; 1998.
18. Acosta PB, Yannicelli S. *The Ross Metabolic Formula System Nutrition Support Protocols*, 4th ed. Columbus, OH: Ross Products Division; 2001.
19. Metabolicpro: Web-based nutrient analysis software program designed specifically for metabolic nutritionists. https://www.metabolicpro.org/. Accessed June 29, 2016.
20. Carrillo-Carrasco N, Venditti C. Propionic academia. 2012. In: Pagon RA, Adam MP, Ardinger HH, et al., eds. *GeneReviews.* 2009. Seattle, WA: University of Washington; 1993–2016. http://www.ncbi.nlm.nih.gov/books/NBK92946/?report. Accessed June 29, 2016.
21. Thompson GN, Walter JH, Bresson J-L, et al. Sources of propionate in inborn errors of propionate metabolism. *Metabolism.* 1990; 39:1133.
22. Koletzko B, Bachmann C, Wendel U. Antibiotic therapy for improvement of metabolic control in methylmalonic aciduria. *J Pediatr.* 1990; 117:99.
23. Chapman KA, Gropman A, MacLeod E, et al. Acute management of propionic acidemia. *Mol Genet Metab.* 2012; 105:16.
24. deBaulny HO, Benoist JF, Rigal O, et al. Methylmalonic and propionic acidaemias: management and outcome. *J Inherited Metab Dis.* 2005; 28:415.

# 43 Isovaleric Acidemia and 3-Methylcrotonyl Glycinuria

DIANNE FRAZIER

The essential branched-chain amino acids, leucine (LEU), isoleucine (ILE), and valine (VAL), are catabolized by separate but similar pathways that involve two steps: transamination and oxidative decarboxylation. The coenzyme A (CoA) thioesters formed by the latter step are metabolized to simple organic acid intermediates that can then enter the general metabolic pathway. In this chapter, two organic acidemias that result from impaired LEU catabolism are discussed: isovaleryl CoA dehydrogenase deficiency (isovaleric acidemia, or IVA) and 3-methylcrotonyl-CoA carboxylase deficiency (3-MCCD). Both of these disorders respond to dietary intervention. Normal outcomes are possible, especially in infants who are diagnosed and treated presymptomatically after newborn screening by tandem mass spectrometry (MS/MS NBS). This technology can detect abnormal concentrations of the carnitine adjuncts, isovaleryl carnitine (C5) in IVA and 5-OH-isovaleryl carnitine (C5OH) in 3-MCCD, in blood spotted on filter paper.[1]

## CLINICAL FEATURES OF IVA

IVA has often been described as occurring in two forms, an acute neonatal form and a chronic intermittent form.[2] As both forms have appeared within single sibships, the phenotype of the disorder is influenced by the timing of concurrent catabolic stress,[3] adherence to management recommendations,[4] and other factors beyond mutational differences in the isovaleryl CoA dehydrogenase (IVD) gene.[5] With the acute form, infants appear normal at birth. They soon begin to refuse feedings, vomit, and become dehydrated and lethargic. Metabolic acidosis with mild to moderate ketosis and lactic acidemia follow. The initial presentation in some undiagnosed individuals has been severe pancreatitis[6,7]; others have had symptoms similar to diabetic ketoacidosis.[8,9] Affected individuals may also have hyperammonemia, thrombocytopenia, neutropenia, pancytopenia, and hypocalcemia. Before MS/MS NBS, approximately half of the reported infants with acute neonatal IVA became cyanotic comatose and died with their first episode.[5] At the other end of the spectrum are healthy adults, some of whom have reported that they have had a lifetime aversion to high-protein meals.

The incidence of IVA was recently estimated to be 1: 70,000–250,000, based on MS/MS NBS data from several European, Australian, and US studies.[10] Using the MS/MS screening methodology, the analyte, isovalerylcarnitine (C5OH), is indistinguishable from two other markers, 2-methylbutyrylcarnitine and 2,2-dimethylpropinylcarnitine, that are present, respectively, in individuals with 3-methylbutryl CoA deficiency[11] and in those using antibiotics and unguents containing pivalic acid or its derivatives.[10,12] Confirmatory testing of all newborns who have an apparent elevation of isovalerylcarnitine on MS/MS NBS is imperative. Studies suggest that MS/MS NBS can detect a mild phenotype of IVA in individuals with a 932C>T mutation in the *IVD* gene.[13]

## BIOCHEMICAL ABNORMALITIES IN IVA

IVA is an autosomal recessive disorder that was first described by Tanaka et al. in 1966.[14] The gene for isovaleryl CoA dehydrogenase (E.C. 1.3.99.10) is located on chromosome 15q14–15.[15] The normal enzyme is a complex of four identical subunits,[16] but disease-causing mutations fall into three classes: those causing normal-sized proteins with missense mutations, those causing truncated proteins, and those causing no detectable protein synthesis.[17] In the absence of the dehydrogenase step, LEU is converted to isovaleryl CoA but cannot be further metabolized to 3-methylcrotonyl CoA (Fig. 43–1). This results in an accumulation of isovaleryl conjugates and other products formed from normally minor degradative pathways. Analysis of urine for isovalerylglycine and blood for isovaleryl carnitine forms part of the diagnostic testing for IVA. It is also possible to detect isovaleryl carnitine in the amniotic fluid of pregnant women when the fetus has IVA.[18] During illness, there is a characteristic pungent odor from the accumulated isovalerylglycine in the sweat and urine, described as a "sweaty feet" or ripe cheese odor. A similar odor may be detected in individuals with glutaric acidemia type II.

## CLINICAL FEATURES OF MCCD

3-MCCD has a highly variable clinical phenotype. There are reports of infants who presented in the neonatal period with acute metabolic decompensation, lethargy, hypotonia, coma, seizures, and death. At the other end of the spectrum are healthy adults who were diagnosed only after studies in families with an affected proband.[19] More typically, patients have normal growth and development. However, they may present acutely with an intercurrent catabolic illness in childhood. The presentation is similar to that of Reye syndrome, with feeding difficulty, vomiting, lethargy, apnea, hypotonia, or hyperflexia. The typical laboratory findings during such a rare acute episode are hypoglycemia, hyperammonemia, elevated liver function test values, mild metabolic acidosis, and moderate ketonuria. The metabolic phenotype includes an organic aciduria with abnormally high excretion of 3-methylcrotonyl glycine and 3-hydroxy (3-OH)-isovaleric acid, often in combination with a severe secondary carnitine deficiency. An elevated blood level of 3-OH-isovalerylcarnitine is the basis for MS/MS NBS for this disorder.

The incidence of 3-MCCD, calculated from presymptomatic MS/MS NBS , suggests that it may be the most common inherited organic acidemia.[19] Estimates from several publications place the incidence at 1: 40,000 - 80,000 individuals.[20–22] The mothers of infants who have an initial elevated 3-OH-isovalerylcarnitine level on NBS which then decreases or normalizes on repeat testing should themselves be evaluated for 3-MCCD.[23] We, and others, have found maternal 3-MCCD to be the cause of an abnormal NBS in approximately 10% of cases.[20,24] Also, breast milk from a woman with 3-MCCD may cause elevated 3-OH-isovalerylcarnitine in her unaffected infant.[25] Some of these late-diagnosed women report some self-limiting of high-protein foods and more severe symptoms than expected during intercurrent illness.[24] However, the apparent higher incidence of this disorder since MS/MS NBS became available suggests that 3-MCCD is not life-threatening for most individuals, and many may be symptom-free.[24,26,27] Germany has decided to exclude 3-MCCD from its MS/MS NBS panel because a positive result has a low ratio of benefit (i.e., treatment for a mild disorder) to harm (i.e., psychological burden for families and financial burden for the health care system).[28]

## BIOCHEMICAL ABNORMALITIES OF 3-MCCD

Isolated 3-MCCD is another autosomal recessive disorder of LEU catabolism. As can be seen in Figure 43–1, the compound,

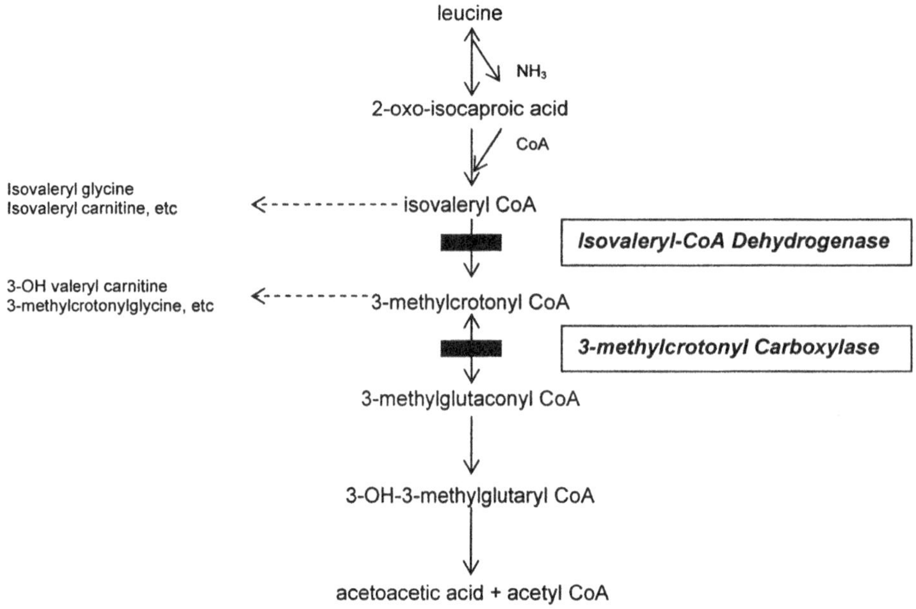


**Figure 43–1.** Leucine catabolic pathway. CoA= coenzyme A; 3-OH = 3-hydroxy.

3-methyl-crotonyl CoA is normally converted to 3-methylglutaconyl CoA by 3-methylcrotonyl-coenzyme A carboxylase (E.C. 6.4.1.4), also called 3-MCC, a biotin-dependent carboxylase. 3-MCCD must be distinguished from multiple carboxylase deficiency, in which an inability to utilize biotin affects all four of the human biotin-dependent carboxylases. The 3-MCC enzyme does, however, share some structural features with the three other enzymes. They all have three functional domains: a biotin carboxyl carrier and biotin carboxylation and carboxy-transferase domains.[29] 3-MCC is made up of six αβ heterodimers. The α subunit gene maps to chromosome 3q25–27 and the β subunit gene to chromosome 5q12–q13. Disease-causing mutations have been identified in both subunits, but no phenotype-genotype correlations have been established.[29–32]

## FACTORS TO BE CONSIDERED IN NUTRITION EVALUATION AND TREATMENT

Like all the inherited organic acidemias, 3-MCCD and IVA may manifest with overwhelming illness, whether the patient is a newborn or an older patient with catabolic stress. It is important to correct the metabolic acidosis, reverse the catabolism, and treat dehydration and possible hyperammonemia immediately. Many patients are carnitine-depleted at presentation. A 24- to 36-hour suspension of all LEU sources, with adequate calories obtained from parenteral LEU-free amino acids, glucose, and lipids, may be necessary in the short term if oral feeding is not possible. Prompt biochemical analysis of blood and urine should give a probable diagnosis and allow the choice of an appropriate amino acid–based medical food to be used when enteral feeds are resumed. The initiation of dietary treatment, when appropriate, for presymptomatically diagnosed infants should occur as soon as confirmatory testing is complete.[23]

## DIETARY MANAGEMENT

The goal of dietary treatment of IVA and 3-MCCD is to limit the precursor to the accumulated intermediates (isovaleryl CoA and 3-methylcrotonyl CoA, respectively) and to provide alternative pathways for their removal.

The availability of a number of medical foods (Table 43–1) prepared with amino acid mixtures devoid of LEU has made it possible to limit the precursor of the toxic intermediates without risk of iatrogenic protein deficiency. However, care must be taken to avoid overrestriction of LEU itself. Characteristics of LEU deficiency include decreased plasma LEU with increased ILE, VAL, methionine (MET), serine (SER), and threonine (THR) as well as loss of appetite, apathy or irritability, poor growth, hair loss, and skin lesions.[33] During infancy, the recommended intake (Table 43–2) of LEU needed for growth and maintenance can be met with the use of a combination of carefully measured, regular infant formula or breast milk and a LEU -free medical food. Feeding at the breast is also possible based on an individualized schedule, with alternate or partial feedings being measured amounts of medical food.[34,35]

As an infant becomes developmentally ready for solid foods, the breast milk or infant formula is slowly replaced by foods with an equivalent amount of LEU. With careful monitoring (discussed later), it is also possible to manage the IVA or 3-MCCD diet by "counting protein." This presumes that the individual is eating a wide variety of fruits, vegetables, and grain products so that the mean content of LEU per gram of protein is approximately 6%. This food protein (containing the prescribed LEU) usually provides 50% or more of the total recommended protein intake, with the medical food completing the recommendation. Food labeling information can be used as a rough guide to the protein composition of the contents.

The LEU and/or protein content of foods can be obtained from a variety of print and online sources.[36–40] Other resources are the lists and recipes made available for persons with maple syrup urine disease. In patients requiring severe restriction of LEU, the use of special low-protein modified baked goods and pasta products makes the diet more palatable and varied. Resources for information and support are listed in Box 43–1.

As the toxic intermediates accumulate in these disorders, both CoA and carnitine can become limiting. Supplemental carnitine can replace the CoA moiety of the acyl CoA intermediates and can augment the endogenously produced carnitine. A supplemental carnitine dosage of 50 to 100 mg/kg for infants and young children is usually sufficient. Those individuals using certain LEU-restricted medical foods that contain substantial carnitine (see Table 43–1) may be able to meet part or all of their requirement without further supplementation. The carnitine supplement should be prescription grade; products sold as dietary supplements may not be of consistent potency to allow accurate dosing.

Patients with IVA have long been successfully treated with supplemental glycine[41] in conjunction with their low-LEU/low-protein diets.[42] Glycine conjugates with isovaleric acid to form isovalerylglycine, which is readily excreted. The recommended glycine intake is 150 to 300 mg/kg

**Table 43–1.** Comparison of Medical Foods for Individuals with IVA and 3-MCCD (per 100 g of Product)

| | I-Valex-1* | I-Valex-2* | XLeu Analog† | XLeu Maxamaid† | XLeu Maxamum† | LMD |
|---|---|---|---|---|---|---|
| *Energy (kcal)* | 480 | 410 | 475 | 350 | 340 | 500 |
| *Protein Equivalent (g)* | 15 | 30 | 13 | 25 | 39 | 16.2 |
| *Amino acids (mg)* | | | | | | |
| Alanine | 2540 | 5080 | 600 | 1360 | 2200 | 4900 |
| Arginine | 1350 | 3100 | 1000 | 2220 | 3600 | 1100 |
| Aspartic acid | 1590 | 3180 | 800 | 1870 | 3000 | 1430 |
| Carnitine | 900 | 1800 | 10 | 20 | 39 | 50 |
| Cystine | 150 | 300 | 420 | 820 | 1300 | 290 |
| Glutamic acid | 2450 | 3550 | 1000 | 2390 | 3900 | 0 |
| Glutamine | 0 | 0 | 100 | 220 | 32 | NA |
| Glycine | 1000 | 2000 | 2050 | 3990 | 6300 | 1100 |
| Histidine | 420 | 840 | 660 | 1280 | 2100 | 470 |
| Isoleucine | 430 | 860 | 490 | 780 | 1200 | 580 |
| Leucine | Trace | Trace | 0 | 0 | 0 | 0 |
| Lysine | 1000 | 2000 | 1180 | 1950 | 3000 | 1510 |
| Methionine | 300 | 600 | 280 | 540 | 860 | 410 |
| Phenylalanine | 880 | 1760 | 770 | 1500 | 2300 | 780 |
| Proline | 1440 | 2880 | 2000 | 4010 | 6300 | 1430 |
| Serine | 760 | 1520 | 600 | 1240 | 1900 | 750 |
| Taurine | 400 | 400 | 20 | 140 | 140 | 30 |
| Threonine | 700 | 1400 | 860 | 1320 | 2100 | 870 |
| Tryptophan | 170 | 340 | 340 | 500 | 790 | 340 |
| Tyrosine | 890 | 1780 | 770 | 1450 | 2300 | 780 |
| Valine | 480 | 960 | 550 | 870 | 1400 | 630 |
| *Fat* | | | | | | |
| Total (g) | 21.7 | 13 | 20.9 | < 0.5 | < 1 | 26 |
| Linoleic/α-linolenic (g) | 2.00/0.36 | 1.50/0.17 | 3.025/0 | 0 | 0 | 4.5/0.36 |
| *Carbohydrate* | | | | | | |
| Total (g) | 53.0 | 35 | 59 | 62 | 45 | 51 |
| *Minerals* | | | | | | |
| Calcium (mg) | 576 | 880 | 600 | 810 | 670 | 660 |
| Chloride (mg) | 325 | 940 | 290 | 450 | 560 | 480 |
| Chromium (μg) | 11 | 27 | 15 | 45 | 50 | NA |
| Copper (mg) | 1.1 | 1 | 450 | 2.0 | 1.4 | 0.86 |
| Iodine (μg) | 65 | 100 | 47 | 90 | 107 | 76 |
| Iron (mg) | 9.0 | 13 | 10 | 12 | 23.5 | 9.6 |
| Magnesium (mg) | 50 | 225 | 40 | 200 | 285 | 66 |
| Manganese (mg) | 0.50 | 0.80 | 600 | 1.3 | 1.7 | 0.38 |
| Molybdenum (μg) | 12 | 30 | 15 | 45 | 100 | NA |
| Phosphorous (mg) | 400 | 760 | 500 | 810 | 670 | 440 |
| Potassium (mg) | 675 | 1,370 | 420 | 840 | 700 | 580 |
| Selenium (μg) | 20 | 35 | 15 | 40 | 50 | 14.1 |
| Sodium (mg) | 190 | 880 | 120 | 580 | 560 | 240 |
| Zinc (mg) | 8 | 13.0 | 8 | 13 | 13.6 | 8.6 |
| *Vitamins* | | | | | | |
| Vitamin A (IU) | 1400 | 2200 | 1760 | 1664 | 2228 | 1520 |
| Vitamin D (IU) | 300 | 300 | 340 | 480 | 332 | 380 |
| Vitamin E, α-TE (mg) | 10.1 | 12.1 | 3.3 | 5.2 | 5.2 | 6.7 |
| Vitamin K (μg) | 50 | 60 | 21 | 70 | 70 | 40 |
| Vitamin C (mg) | 50 | 60 | 40 | 135 | 90 | 60 |
| Thiamine (mg) | 1.90 | 3.25 | 0.5 | 1.4 | 1.4 | 1.0 |
| Riboflavin (mg) | 0.90 | 1.80 | 0.6 | 1.4 | 1.4 | 1.0 |
| Vitamin $B_6$ (mg) | 0.75 | 1.30 | 0.52 | 2.1 | 2.1 | 1.0 |
| Vitamin $B_{12}$ (μg) | 4.90 | 5.0 | 1.25 | 4 | 1.4 | 2.0 |
| Niacin (mg) | 12.8 | 21.7 | 4.5 | 12 | 13.6 | 10 |
| Folic acid (μg) | 230 | 430 | 38 | 150 | 500 | 100 |
| Pantothenic acid (mg) | 6.90 | 8.0 | 2.6 | 3.7 | 5 | 3.8 |
| Biotin (μg) | 65 | 100 | 26 | 120 | 140 | 38 |
| Choline (mg) | 80 | 100 | 50 | 110 | 320 | 124 |
| Inositol (mg) | 40 | 70 | 100 | 56 | 86 | 86 |

Information current as of December 2014.
IVA = isovaleryl coenzyme A dehydrogenase deficiency ; 3-MCCD = 3-methylcrotonyl coenzyme A carboxylase deficiency ; NA = information not available.
*Ross Products Division, Abbott Laboratories, Columbus, OH 43215-1724 @ http://www.abbott.com.
†Nutricia North America, Gaithersburg, MD 20884 @ http://www.nutricia-na.com.
⁺Mead Johnson, Evansville, IN 47712 @ http://www.meadjohnson.com.

**Table 43–2.** Nutrient Intake Recommendations for Infants with IVA and 3-MCCD

| | LEU* (mg/kg) | Protein† (g/kg) | kcal† (per kg) |
|---|---|---|---|
| Age (mo) | | | |
| 0–3 | 80–150 | 2.5–3.5 | 90–140 |
| 3–6 | 70–140 | 2.5–3.5 | 85–135 |
| 6–9 | 60–130 | 2.5–3.0 | 80–125 |
| 9–12 | 50–120 | 2.0–3.0 | 80–125 |
| Plasma amino acid range‡ in μmol/L | 45–161 | | |

*Adapted from Acosta PB, Yannicelli S. *The Ross Metabolic Formula System Nutrition Support Protocols*, 4th ed. Columbus, OH: Ross Products Division; 2001.
†Guidelines used at the University of North Carolina (UNC) Division of Genetics and Metabolism Clinic for patients who are on a combination of intact protein and medical food; see text for modifications during illness.
‡Ranges used in the University of North Carolina-Chapel Hill Biochemical Genetics Laboratory; the goal for individuals with isovaleryl coenzyme A dehydrogenase deficiency (IVA) and 3-methylcrotonyl coenzyme A carboxylase deficiency (3-MCCD) is to have plasma values for leucine (LEU) in the low-normal range.

of body weight in IVA with glycine from a 100 mg/mL solution used to supplement other intake. We and others[43] have successfully treated individuals with IVA using a low-LEU diet and supplemental carnitine without supplemental glycine. Plasma glycine levels should be monitored during catabolic stress to ensure that the loss of glycine through excretion of isovalerylglycine does not surpass the body's glycine production.

Some older individuals may need only a mild dietary protein restriction (1–1.5 g/kg of body weight), with carnitine supplementation only if their plasma free carnitine level falls below 30 μmol/L (or the monitoring laboratory's lower limit of normal). However, it is important not to become complacent because treatment may be necessary during intercurrent illness. The goal is as for all individuals with IVA or 3-MCCD: to prevent the accumulation of LEU metabolites from endogenous protein catabolism. High-calorie, low-LEU feeding should be initiated, and carnitine supplementation should be used.

Some infants with IVA or 3-MCCD who are detected presymptomatically by MS/MS NBS may be found, on diagnostic testing, to have partial enzyme activity and very mild disease.[20,13] Daily dietary intervention may not be required for these individuals, but families should be counseled about the potential metabolic decompensation that may occur during either intercurrent illness or the fasting period required before a medical procedure. Like all metabolic patients, they should be provided with an emergency letter describing their disorder, emergency treatment during illness (as discussed earlier), and means to access their metabolic physician.[23]

**Box 43–1.** Resources for Isovaleryl Coenzyme A Dehydrogenase Deficiency and 3-Methylcrotonyl-Coenzyme A Carboxylase Deficiency

Support groups:
Organic Acidemia Association, Inc. (13210 35th Avenue North, Plymouth, MN 55441):
http://www.oaanews.org
Maple Syrup Urine Disease Family Support Group:
http://www.msud-support.org
*MSUD Newsletter*: MSUD Family Support Group, 24806 SR 119, Goshen, IN 46526
Source of L-carnitine (Carnitor, Sigma-Tau Pharmaceuticals, Inc., 800 South Frederick Ave., Suite 300, Gaithersburg, MD 20877):
http://www.sigmatau.com
Information and links to low-protein foods:
https://pkunews.org
http://www.GMDI.org
Pocket leucine food list:
MSUD food list:
http://genetics.emory.edu/documents/Nutrition/MSUDorderform 9-29-05.pdf

## MONITORING AND FOLLOW-UP

Monitoring is an essential part of the treatment regimen for individuals with IVA or 3-MCCD. Because LEU is not the immediate substrate of the defective enzymes, elevated plasma LEU concentrations are not a hallmark of these disorders. However, plasma amino acid analyses are necessary to ascertain that plasma LEU is within the lower limits of the normal range (see Table 43–2) and to ensure that total protein intake is adequate. For individuals with IVA who are receiving glycine supplementation, plasma glycine concentrations should not exceed the upper limit of the normal range. Daily amino acid analyses are necessary when the diet is being initiated and during serious intercurrent illness. Monthly values are usually adequate in the first year when frequent dietary changes are made. Urine organic acids, a plasma carnitine profile, blood carnitine (free and total), complete blood count with differential, anthropometric measurements, and dietary analysis, along with plasma amino acid monitoring, should be done at each metabolic clinic visit.

With early diagnosis, avoidance of the accumulation of LEU metabolites, frequent monitoring, and prompt intervention during illness, patients with IVA and 3-MCCD can achieve very successful outcomes.

### References


1. Charrow J, Goodman S, McCabe E, Rinaldo P. Tandem mass spectrometry in newborn screening. *Genet Med.* 2000; 2:267.
2. Vockley J, Ensenauer R. Isovaleric acidemia: new aspects of genetic and phenotypic heterogeneity. *Am J Med C Semin Med Genet.* 2006; 142C:95.
3. Grunert C, Wendel U, Linder M, et al. Clinical and neurocognitive outcome in symptomatic isovaleric academia. *Orphan J Rare Dis.* 2012; 7:9.
4. Castorina M, Rigante D, Antuzzi D. Differennt outcome in isovaleric acidemia might be related to unsatisfactory diet compliance. *J Gastroenterol.* 2008; 43:767.
5. Sweetman L, Williams JC. Branched chain organic acidurias. In: Scriver CR, Beaudet AL, Sly WS, Valle P, eds. *The Metabolic and Molecular Bases of Inherited Disease*, 8th ed. New York: McGraw-Hill; 2001.
6. Mantadakis E, Chrysafis I, Tsouvala E, et al. Acute pancreatitis with rapid clinical improvement in a child with isovaleric academia. *Case Reports in Pediatr.* 2013; Article ID 721871. http://dx.doi.org/10.1155/2013/721871. Accessed July 1, 2016.
7. Kahler SG, Sherwood G, Woolf D, et al. Pancreatitis in patients with organic acidemias. *J Pediatr.* 1994; 124: 239.
8. Erdem E, Cayonu N, Uysalol E, Yildirmak ZY. Chronic intermittent form of isovaleric academia mimicking diabetic ketoacidosis. *J Pediatr Endocrinol Metab* 2010; 23:503.
9. Kilic M, Kaymaz N, Ozgul RK. Isovaleria academia presenting as diabetic ketoacidosis: a case report. *J Clin Pediatr Endocrinol.* 2014; 6:59.
10. Ensenauer R, Fingerhut R, Maier EM, et al. Newborn screening for isovaleric academia using tandem mass spectrometry: data from 1.6 million newborns. *Clin Chem.* 2011; 57:623.
11. van Calcar SC, Baker MW, Williams P, Jones SA, et al. Prevalence and mutation analysis of short/branched chain acyl-CoA dehydrogenase deficiency (SBCADD) detected on newborn screening in Wisconsin. *Mol Genet Metab.* 2013; 110:111.
12. Boemer F, Schoos R, deHalleaus V, et al. Surprising causes of C5-carnitine false positive results in newborn screening. *Mol Genet Metab.* 2014; 111: 52.
13. Ensenauer R, Vockley J, Willard J-M. A common mutation is associated with a mild, potentially asymptomatic phenotype in patients with isovaleric academia diagnosed by newborn screening. *Am J Hum Genet.* 2004; 75:1136.
14. Tanaka K, Budd MA, Efron ML, et al. Isovaleric acidemia: a new genetic defect of leucine metabolism. *Proc Natl Acad Sci U S A.* 1966; 56:236.
15. Kraus JP, Matsubara Y, Barton D, et al. Isolating cDNA clones coding for rat isovaleryl-CoA dehydrogenase and assignment of the gene to human chromosome 15. *Genomics.* 1987; 1:264.
16. Ikeda Y, Tanaka K. Purification and characterization of isovaleryl coenzyme A dehydrogenase from rat liver mitochondria. *J Biol Chem.* 1983; 258:1077.
17. Ikeda Y, Keese SM, Tanaka K. Molecular heterogeneity of variant isovaleryl-CoA dehydrogenase from cultured isovaleric acidemia fibroblasts. *Proc Natl Acad Sci U S A.* 1985; 82:7081.
18. Shigematsu Y, Hata I, Nakai A, et al. Prenatal diagnosis of organic acidemias based on amniotic fluid levels of acylcarnitines. *Pediatr Res.* 1996; 39:680.
19. Gibson HM, Bennett MJ, Naylor EW, Morton DH. 3-Methyl-crotonyl-coenzyme A carboxylase deficiency in Amish/Mennonite adults identified by detection of increased acylcarnitines in blood spots of their children. *J Pediatr.* 1998; 132:519.
20. Frazier DM, Millington, DS, McCandless SE, Koeberl DD, Weavil SD, Muenzer, J, The tandem mass spectrometry newborn screening experience in North Carolina: 1997–2005. *J Inherit Metab Dis.* 2006; 29:76.
21. Koeberl DD, Millington DS, Smith WE, et al. Evaluation of 3-methylcrotonyl-CoA carboxylase deficiency detected by tandem mass spectrometry newborn screening. *J Inherit Metab Dis.* 2003; 26:25.
22. Lam C, Carter JM, Cederbaum SD, et al. Analysis of cases of 3-methylcrotonyl CoA carboxylase deficiency (3-MCCD) in the California newborn screening program reported in the state database. *Mol Genet Metab.* 2013; 110:477.
23. Arnold GL, Koeberl DD, Matern D, et al. A Delphi-based consensus clinical practice protocol for the diagnosis and management of 3-methylcrotonyl CoA carboxylase deficiency. *Mol Genet Metab.* 2008; 93:363.

24. Frazier DM, Wood T. Maternal 3-MCC deficiency as a model for long term outcome. *Mol Genet Metab.* 2012; 105:282.
25. Eichhorst J, Alcorn J, LePage J, et al. Elevated neonatal 3-OH isovalerylcarnitine due to breast milk sources in maternal 3-MCC deficiency. *Mol Genet Metab.* 2010; 101:84.
26. Arnold GL, Salazar D, Neidich JA. Outcome of infants diagnosed with 3-methylcrotonyl-CoA carboxylase deficiency by newborn screening. *Mol Genet Metab.* 2012; 106:439.
27. Grunert SC, Stucki M, Morscher RJ, et al. 3-Methylcrotonyl-CoA carboxylase deficiency: clinical, biochemical, enzymatic and molecular studies in 88 individuals. *Orphan J Rare Dis.* 2012; 7:31.
28. Stadler SC, Polanetz R, Maier EM, et al. Newborn screening for 3-methylcrotonyl-CoA carboxylase deficiency: population heterogeneity of MCCA and MCCB mutations and impact on risk assessment. *Hum Mut.* 2006; 27:748.
29. Shih VE, Aubry RH, DeGrande G, Gursky SF, Tanaka K. Maternal isovaleric acidemia. *J Pediatr.* 1984; 105:77.
30. Gallardo ME, Desviat LR, Rodriguez JM, et al. The molecular basis of 3-methylcrotonyl glycinuria, a disorder of leucine catabolism. *Am J Hum Genet.* 2001; 68:334.
31. Baumgartner MR, Almashanu S, Suormala T, et al. The molecular basis of human 3-methycrotonyl-CoA carboxylase deficiency. *J Clin Invest.* 2001; 107:495.
32. Morscher RJ, Grunert SC, Burer C, et al. A single mutation in MCCC1 or MCCC2 a potential cause of positive screening for 3-methylcrotonyl-CoA carboxylase deficiency. *Mol Genet Metab.* 2012; 105;602.
33. Snyderman SE, Roitman EL, Boyer A, et al. The essential amino acid requirements of infants: leucine. *Am J Dis Child.* 1961; 102:157.
34. Huner G, Baykal T, Demir T, Demirkol M. Breastfeeding experience in inborn errors of metabolism other than phenylketonuria. *J Inherit Metab Dis.* 2005; 28:457.
35. MacDonald, A. Depondt E, Evans S, et al. Breast feeding in IMD. *J Inherit Metab Dis.* 2006; 29:299.
36. Acosta PB, Yannicelli S. *The Ross Metabolic Formula System Nutrition Support Protocols*, 4th ed. Columbus, OH: Ross Products Division; 2001.
37. Pennington JAT, Spungen J. *Bowes and Church's Food Values of Portions Commonly Used*, 19th ed. Philadelphia: Wolters Kluwar; 2010.
38. US Department of Agriculture, Agricultural Research Service, Nutrient Data Laboratory. *USDA National Nutrient Database for Standard Reference Dataset for What We Eat in America*, NHANES (Survey-SR). October 2015. https://ndb.nal.usda.gov/. Accessed July 1, 2016.
39. MetabolicPro: Web-based nutrient analysis software program designed specifically for metabolic nutritionists. https://www.metabolicpro.org/. Accessed July 1, 2016.
40. Schuett VE. *Low Protein Food List for PKU*, 3rd ed. CreateSpace; 2010. Searchable database is available at https://howmuchphe.org/site/demo. Accessed July 1, 2016.
41. Cohn RM, Yudkoff R, Rothman R, Segal S. Isovaleric acidemia: use of glycine therapy in neonates. *N Engl J Med.* 1978; 299:996.
42. Naglak M, Salvo R, Madsen K, Dembure P, Elsas L. The treatment of isovaleric acidemia with glycine supplement. *Pediatr Res.* 1988; 24:9.
43. Mayatapek E, Kurczynski TW, Hoppel CL. Long-term L-carnitine treatment in isovaleric acidaemea. *Pediatr Neurol.* 1991; 7:137.

# 44 Glutaric Acidemia Type I

DIANNE FRAZIER

Glutaric acidemia type I (GAI), first described in 1975 by Goodman et al.,[1] is one of several rare autosomal recessive organic acidemias caused by a defect in the pathways of amino acid catabolism. It was designated "type I" to distinguish it from glutaric acidemia type II, or multiple acyl-coenzyme A (CoA) dehydrogenase deficiency, that is a defect of the mitochondrial respiratory chain affecting fatty acid oxidation as well as amino acid catabolism.

## CLINICAL FEATURES

A significant number of infants with GAI have an enlarged head circumference at birth,[2] but otherwise they appear healthy and grow and develop normally throughout the first few months of life. Symptoms may gradually appear or may occur suddenly as an encephalopathic crisis during a catabolic intercurrent illness or mild head trauma. The symptoms include hypotonia, loss of head control, seizures, tongue thrusting, rigidity, athetosis, and/or dystonia. Clinically, GAI is described as an extrapyramidal movement disorder. Pathologically, it is characterized by fibrous gliosis and neuronal loss in the basal ganglia.[3,4] Recovery from the neurological disease is rarely complete, although in many instances the intellect remains relatively intact.[2,5] Current experience with presymptomatic treatment has been very promising.

Because the phenotype of GAI is extremely varied and because the clinical course can be confused with that of cerebral palsy, true incidence figures have been unavailable. This is changing since the implementation of tandem mass spectrometry newborn screening (MS/MS NBS). The presence of increased concentrations of glutaryl carnitine (C5DC) in blood spots from a newborn indicates the need for diagnostic testing for GAI. The concentration of glutaryl carnitine may start to fall several days after birth in the asymptomatic infant with GAI, so it is important not to depend solely on a repeat NBS to rule out this disorder.

The worldwide incidence of GAI is estimated to be 1:100,000.[6] The incidence of GAI in North Carolina is approximately 1:80,000 as determined through the North Carolina MS/MS NBS Program and confirmation testing since 1998.[7,8] The incidence is much higher in certain isolated groups such as the Old Order Amish of Pennsylvania,[9] the Saulteaux/Ojibway native peoples of Canada,[10] the Lumbee native Americans in North Carolina,[11] and Black South Africans.[12]

## BIOCHEMICAL ABNORMALITIES

The catabolic pathway for the amino acids lysine (LYS), hydroxylysine (HYL), and tryptophan (TRP) can be seen in Figure 44–1. A deficiency of glutaryl CoA dehydrogenase (E.C. 1.3.99.7) in GAI prevents the conversion of glutaryl CoA to crotonyl CoA. The enzyme is found in the mitochondrial matrix and is composed of four identical subunits, each binding one molecule of flavin adenine dinucleotide (FAD). Almost 200 mutations[13] of glutaryl CoA dehydrogenase (gene location 19p13.2)[14] have been described. There does not appear to be a correlation between the genotype and the clinical phenotype.[15,16]

When the formation of crotonyl CoA is blocked, glutaryl CoA must be converted to alternative metabolites. Without treatment, large amounts of glutaric acid and lesser amounts of 3-hydroxyglutaric acid and glutaconic acid are typically excreted in the urine. There are increased concentrations of glutaryl carnitine in blood and urine and a relative deficiency of free carnitine. Glutaric acid is also elevated in the blood and cerebrospinal fluid, but detection may be possible only with isotope dilution methods[17] and/or during acute illness. The

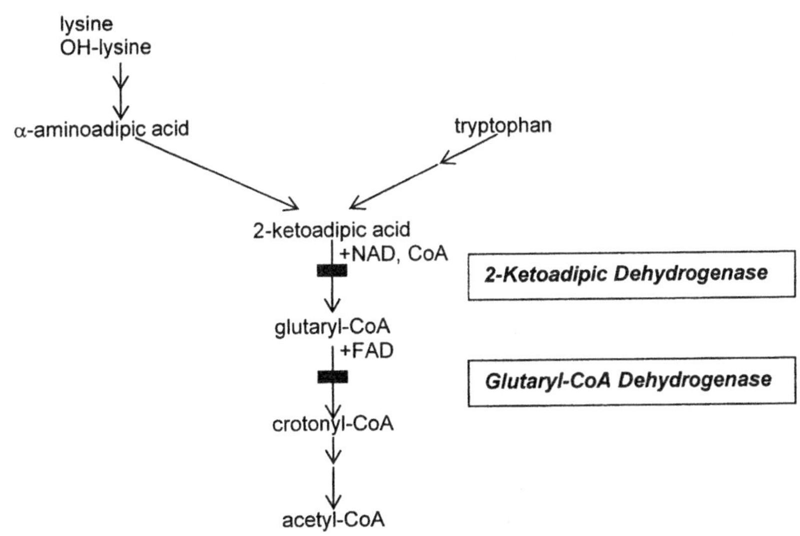


**Figure 44–1.** Catabolic pathway for the amino acids lysine, hydroxylysine, and tryptophan. CoA = coenzyme A; FAD = flavin adenine dinucleotide; NAD = nicotine adenine dinucleotide.

**Table 44–1.** Comparison of Medical Foods for Glutaric Acidemia Type I (per 100 g Powder)**

| | Glutarex-1[*] | XLYS, TRP Analog[†] | Glutarex-2[*] | XLYS, TRP Maxamaid[†] | XLYS, TRP Maxamum[†] | Glutar Ade Junior[†] | Glutar Ade Essential[†] | Glutar Ade AA Blend[†] | GA Gel[‡] | GA Express 15[‡] | GA[§] |
|---|---|---|---|---|---|---|---|---|---|---|---|
| *Energy (kcal)* | 480 | 475 | 410 | 350 | 340 | 410 | 385 | 324 | 338 | 297 | 500 |
| *Protein Equivalent (g)* | 15 | 13 | 30 | 25 | 39 | 10 | 25 | 81 | 41.7 | 60 | 15.1 |
| *L-Amino Acids (mg)* | | | | | | | | | | | |
| Alanine | 1170 | 610 | 2340 | 1280 | 2000 | 480 | 1200 | 3860 | 4070 | 5780 | 3600 |
| Arginine | 1550 | 1100 | 3100 | 2230 | 3400 | 1080 | 2700 | 8690 | 3460 | 4910 | 1040 |
| Aspartic acid | 1590 | 900 | 3180 | 1860 | 2900 | NA | NA | NA | 2640 | 3750 | 1360 |
| Asparagine | NA | NA | NA | NA | NA | 720 | 1800 | 5790 | NA | NA | NA |
| Carnitine | 900 | 10 | 1800 | 20 | 40 | 30 | 40 | 200 | 46 | 64 | 50 |
| Cystine | 150 | 430 | 300 | 830 | 1300 | 180 | 450 | 1450 | 1530 | 2170 | 260 |
| Glutamic acid | 245 | 1100 | 4900 | NA | NA | 360 | 900 | 2900 | NA | NA | 0 |
| Glutamine | NA | 100 | NA | 1500 | 3200 | 1800 | 4510 | 14480 | 3010 | 4280 | NA |
| Glycine | 1000 | 1000 | 2000 | 2000 | 3100 | 240 | 600 | 1930 | 2540 | 3610 | 1040 |
| Histidine | 420 | 650 | 840 | 1270 | 2000 | 360 | 900 | 2900 | 1780 | 2530 | 420 |
| Isoleucine | 1080 | 1030 | 2160 | 2000 | 3100 | 840 | 2100 | 6760 | 3660 | 5200 | 1210 |
| Leucine | 1680 | 1750 | 3360 | 3420 | 5300 | 1380 | 3460 | 11100 | 6360 | 9030 | 2200 |
| Lysine | Trace | 0 | Trace | 0 | 0 | 0 | 0 | 0 | 0 | 0 | 0 |
| Methionine | 300 | 270 | 600 | 530 | 82 | 410 | 1020 | 3280 | 1120 | 1590 | 360 |
| Ornithine | NA | NA | NA | NA | NA | 240 | 600 | 1930 | NA | 0 | NA |
| Phenylalanine | 880 | 770 | 1760 | 1510 | 2300 | 640 | 1590 | 5120 | 3050 | 4330 | 710 |
| Proline | 1620 | 1240 | 3240 | 2420 | 370 | 600 | 1500 | 4830 | 3560 | 5060 | 1360 |
| Serine | 800 | 770 | 1600 | 1490 | 2300 | 240 | 600 | 1930 | 2800 | 3970 | 710 |
| Taurine | 40 | 20 | 40 | 140 | 140 | 60 | 150 | 480 | 92. | 132 | 30 |
| Threonine | 700 | 860 | 1400 | 1680 | 2600 | 640 | 1590 | 5120 | 3050 | 433 | 790 |
| Tryptophan | Trace | 0 | Trace | 0 | 0 | 60 | 150 | 480 | 270 | 380 | 0 |
| Tyrosine | 890 | 770 | 1780 | 1510 | 2300 | 720 | 1800 | 5790 | 3560 | 5060 | 710 |
| Valine | 1220 | 1120 | 2440 | 2180 | 3400 | 960 | 2400 | 7720 | 4070 | 5780 | 1310 |
| *Fat* | | | | | | | | | | | |
| Total (g) | 21.7 | 20.9 | 13 | <0.5 | <1 | 10 | 13 | 0 | 0.05 | 0.20 | 26 |
| Linoleic/α-linolenic (g) | 2.0/0.36 | 3.03/NA | 1.50/0.17 | NA | NA | 1.9/0.72 | 2.2/0.68 | 0 | NA | NA | 4.5/0.38 |
| *Carbohydrate* | | | | | | | | | | | |
| Total(g) | 53 | 59 | 35 | 62 | 45 | 69 | 45 | 0 | 42.9 | 13.7 | 52 |
| *Minerals* | | | | | | | | | | | |
| Calcium (mg) | 575 | 600 | 880 | 810 | 670 | 460 | 1257 | NA | 1083 | 1196 | 660 |
| Chloride (mg) | 325 | 290 | 940 | 810 | 560 | 332 | 475 | NA | 583 | 728 | NA |
| Chromium (μg) | 11 | 15 | 27 | 45 | 50 | 12 | 21 | NA | 71 | 88 | NA |
| Copper (mg) | 1.1 | 0.45 | 1.00 | 2.0 | 1.4 | 5 | 1 | NA | 0.8 | 2.2 | 0.86 |
| Iodine (μg) | 65 | 47 | 100 | 90 | 107 | 90 | 115 | NA | 138 | 252 | 76 |
| Iron (mg) | 9.0 | 10 | 13 | 12 | 23.5 | 8 | 11.3 | NA | 14 | 21.6 | 9.6 |
| Magnesium (mg) | 50 | 40 | 225 | 200 | 285 | 60 | 201 | NA | 167 | 376 | 66 |
| Manganese (mg) | 0.50 | 0.60 | 0.80 | 1.3 | 1.7 | 0.43 | 1.9 | NA | 1.7 | 3.2 | 0.38 |
| Molybdenum (μg) | 12 | 15 | 30 | 45 | 100 | 18 | 31 | NA | 50 | 144 | NA |
| Phosphorus (mg) | 400 | 500 | 760 | 810 | 670 | 400 | 787 | NA | 825 | 1068 | 440 |
| Potassium (mg) | 675 | 420 | 1,370 | 840 | 700 | 589 | 874 | NA | 938 | 940 | 800 |
| Selenium (μg) | 20 | 15 | 35 | 40 | 50 | 40 | 63 | NA | 35 | 88 | 14.1 |
| Sodium (mg) | 190 | 120 | 880 | 580 | 560 | 221 | 384 | 115 | 379 | 508 | 240 |
| Zinc (mg) | 8.0 | 8 | 13 | 13 | 13.6 | 7 | 10 | NA | 11 | 21.6 | 8.6 |
| *Vitamins* | | | | | | | | | | | |
| Vitamin A, RE (μg) | 420 | 528 | 660 | 500 | 705 | 412 | 637 | NA | 600 | 832 | 460 |
| Vitamin D (μg) | 7.50 | 8.5 | 7.50 | 12 | 8 | 13.1 | 15 | NA | 14.6 | 13.2 | 9.5 |
| Vitamin E, α-TE (mg) | 10.1 | 3.3 | 12.10 | 4.4 | 5.2 | 5.7 | 12.8 | NA | 9.0 | 15.6 | 6.7 |
| Vitamin K (μg) | 50 | 21 | 60 | 35 | 70 | 34 | 70 | NA | 41 | 100 | 40 |
| Vitamin C (mg) | 50 | 40 | 60 | 135 | 90 | 56 | 60 | NA | 63 | 108 | 60 |
| Thiamine (mg) | 1.90 | 0.5 | 3.25 | 1.1 | 1.4 | 0.83 | 1.5 | NA | 1.0 | 2.0 | 1 |
| Riboflavin (mg) | 0.90 | 0.60 | 1.80 | 1.2 | 1.4 | 0.69 | 1.5 | NA | 1.2 | 2.3 | 1 |
| Vitamin $B_6$ (mg) | 0.75 | 0.52 | 1.30 | 1.0 | 2.1 | 0.66 | 1.4 | NA | 1.1 | 2.8 | 1 |
| Vitamin $B_{12}$ (μg) | 4.90 | 1.25 | 5.00 | 2.0 | 4.0 | 1.4 | 3 | NA | 2.0 | 4.8 | 2 |
| Niacin (mg) | 10.0 | 4.5 | 16.0 | 12 | 13.6 | 6.6 | 15.5 | NA | 14 | 24.8 | 10 |
| Folic acid (μg) | 230 | 38 | 430 | 150 | 500 | 150 | 300 | NA | 208 | 400 | 100 |
| Pantothenic acid (mg) | 6.90 | 2.60 | 8.00 | 3.7 | 5 | 6 | 7.5 | NA | 5.0 | 8.0 | 3.8 |
| Biotin (μg) | 65 | 26 | 100 | 120 | 140 | 31 | 30 | NA | 25 | 188 | 38 |
| Choline (mg) | 80 | 50 | 100 | 110 | 320 | 213 | 313 | NA | 279 | 600 | 124 |
| Inositol (mg) | 40 | 100 | 70 | 56 | 86 | 125 | 50 | NA | NA | NA | NA |

NA = data not available.
[*]Ross Products Division, Abbott Laboratories, Columbus, OH 43215-1724 @ http://www.abbott.com.
**Data current as of 1/2015.
[†]Nutricia North America, Gaithersburg, MD 20884 @ http://www.nutricia-na.com.
[‡]Vitaflo USA Alexandria, VA 22314 @ http://www.VitafloUSA.com
[§] Mead Johnson, Evansville, IN 47712 @ http://www.meadjohnson.com.

exact molecular mechanism of the neurotoxicity of glutaric acid and its metabolites on the developing striatum is a matter of intense study.[18]

## FACTORS TO BE CONSIDERED IN NUTRITION EVALUATION AND TREATMENT

Diagnosis of GAI may follow a positive MS/MS NBS , prenatal or neonatal diagnosis in the sibling of a known GAI patient, or the appearance of clinical symptoms, either gradually or with an intercurrent catabolic illness. In the last case, rapid treatment of the intercurrent illness and acute symptoms of acidosis, hypoglycemia, ketonuria, and possible hyperammonemia will help prevent further catabolism and accumulation of glutaric acid and its toxic metabolites. Goodman et al.[1] were the first to show that by decreasing intake of dietary protein, the glutaric acid production could be greatly decreased. Later reports indicated that decreasing the intake of only LYS and TRP can improve the biochemical status of individuals with GAI. Improvement of neurological status has been mixed.[3,4] We and others have seen preservation of normal neurological status in presymptomatically treated individuals.[19–21]

## DIETARY TREATMENT

The main objective of the dietary management of GAI is to decrease the production of glutaric acid and its metabolites. In addition, aggressive intervention during intercurrent illness or trauma is essential to prevent glutaric acid production from endogenous protein catabolism. Originally, individuals with GAI were given low-protein diets to limit intake of the offending amino acids. The availability of medical foods that use amino acid mixtures devoid of TRP and LYS (Table 44–1) has allowed more flexibility and improved the nutrient profile in the dietary management of GAI. For an infant, the recommended intake of TRP and LYS for optimal growth and maintenance (Table 44–2) is provided by intact protein from precisely measured amounts of regular infant formula or breast milk. The remainder of the protein and energy requirement is provided by the GAI-specific medical food. When the infant is ready for the introduction of solids, low-protein foods, given in carefully measured serving sizes, gradually replace the infant formula or breast milk as the source of limited TRP and LYS. HLY is found mainly in animal collagen and is not a concern in diets that contain no meats or meat byproducts.

Menus for the GAI diet can be planned and evaluated using either the LYS content or the protein content of food items. The LYS content of foods can be found in several excellent print and online sources.[22–25] Similarly, data listing accurate protein content of foods are also available.[22–26] As with any of the metabolic disorders requiring dietary intervention, it is important not to overrestrict the essential amino acids. Inadequate LYS or TRP can cause poor weight gain and increased urinary nitrogen loss.[22,27] In addition, TRP deficiency can cause decreased plasma cholesterol, irritability, sleeplessness, and anorexia.[4] Because adequate TRP is required for endogenous niacin production, the daily recommended intake of this vitamin may need to be supplied by preformed niacin (as in found in most GAI-specific medical foods).

Studies are ongoing to investigate the benefits of increased arginine (ARG) intake and a decreased dietary LYS-to-ARG ratio on neurological outcome. The rationale is that ARG is both a precursor of nitrous oxide and a competitor of LYS for transport across the blood–brain barrier.[28]

In addition to a LYS- and TYR-restricted diet, individuals with GAI need adequate carnitine to free the CoA moiety bound in glutaryl CoA. Some GAI-specific medical foods may have sufficient added carnitine so that further supplementation is unnecessary. Ideally, the daily dosage should be approximately 100 mg/kg given in divided doses to establish a plasma-free carnitine level of 30 μmol/L or higher. Certain medications such as the anticonvulsant, valproic acid, can cause a secondary carnitine deficiency.

Because riboflavin is the precursor of the FAD cofactor for glutaryl-CoA dehydrogenase, its addition to the treatment regimen has been found to be helpful in a few individuals with certain mutations.[29] At a dosage of 100 mg/day, a trial may be considered in all individuals with GAI.

Sufficient calories are necessary to prevent endogenous protein catabolism and to replace the energy used in symptomatic individuals as a result of extraneous movement, hypertonia, or occasional hyperthermia and during intercurrent illness or trauma.[30,31] If adequate energy and fluid intake is not possible orally, either nasogastric or direct gastric access should be considered. If enteral feedings must be stopped for any period, appropriate amino acid mixtures are available for parenteral use. Nonambulatory patients may have chronic constipation. A gradual increase in the fiber content of the diet or use of a fiber supplement, along with adequate fluids, may be preferable to long-term laxative or mineral oil use.

## MONITORING

Continuous monitoring of the adequacy of the LYS- and TRP-restricted diet is essential.[32] Anthropometric measurements should be obtained monthly in the first year, with less frequent measurements as good growth is established in childhood. Ideally, plasma amino acids levels should be monitored daily until the LYS and TRP requirements are established, then monthly throughout the first year of life and at regular clinic visits thereafter. The iron status, complete blood count and differential, urine/plasma glutaric acid, free carnitine, and protein status should be assessed at each visit to the metabolism clinic. A regular schedule of evaluating nutrient intake from diet records should be established.

**Table 44–2.** Nutrient Requirements for Infants with Glutaric Acidemia Type I

| | LYS* (mg/kg) | TRP* (g/kg) | Protein† (g/kg) | kcal† (per kg) |
|---|---|---|---|---|
| *Age (mo)* | | | | |
| 0–3 | 80–100 | 10–12 | 2.5–3.5 | 90–140 |
| 3–6 | 70–90 | 10–15 | 2.5–3.5 | 85–135 |
| 6–9 | 60–80 | 10–12 | 2.5–3.0 | 80–125 |
| 9–12 | 50–70 | 10–12 | 2.0–3.0 | 80–125 |
| Plasma AAA range‡ in μmol/L | 110–290 | 24–81 | | |

*From Acosta PB, Yannicelli S. *The Ross Metabolic Formula System Nutrition Support Protocols*, 4th ed. Columbus, OH; Ross Products Division; 2001.

†Guidelines used at the University of North Carolina (UNC) Division of Genetics and Metabolism Clinic, for patients who are on a combination of intact protein and metabolic formula; see the text for modifications during illness.

‡Ranges used in the McClendon Clinical Laboratory of the UNC-Chapel Hill Hospitals, Chapel Hill, NC; the goal for these patients is to have plasma values for lysine (LYS) and tryptophan (TRP) in the low-normal range.

**Box 44–1.** Resources for Glutaric Acidemia Type I

Support groups:
- Organic Acidemia Association, Inc. (13210 35th Ave. North, Plymouth, MN 55441):
  www.oaanews.org
- The International Organization of Glutaric Acidemia
  www.glutaricacidemia.org

Source of L-carnitine (Carnitor, Sigma-Tau Pharmaceuticals, Inc., 800 South Frederick Ave., Suite 300, Gaithersburg, MD 20877):
- www.sigmatau.com
- Information and links to low-protein foods:
  https://pkunews.org
  https://www.gmdi.org/Resources

Source of parenteral amino acid mixtures:
- PharmaTherma, 1785 Nonconnah Boulevard, Suite 118, Memphis, TN 88132; phone 1-800-767-8-6714

Source of oral riboflavin (Nature's Bounty, Inc., 90 Orville Drive, Bohemia, NY 11716; phone 1-800-645-5412):
- www.naturesbounty.com

Although the LYS- and TRP-restricted diet cannot reverse neurological insults once they have occurred, it has been shown to be effective in preventing these insults in presymptomatically diagnosed individuals.[20,21] When appropriately prescribed and adequately monitored, this dietary intervention should be an effective and safe way to limit the formation of toxic intermediates in individuals with GAI.

Resources for GAI information and supplies are listed in Box 42–1.

## References


1. Goodman SI, Dratz LE, Moe PG, Miles BS, Teng CC. Glutaric aciduria: a "new" disorder of amino acid metabolism. *Biochem Med.* 1975; 12:12.
2. Online Mendelian Inheritance in Man. *Glutaric acidemia I.* OMIM entry # 231670. Last edited 04/02/2012.Baltimore, MD: Johns Hopkins University.
3. Hoffman GF, Zschocke J. Glutaric aciduria type 1: from clinical, biochemical and molecular diversity to successful therapy. *J Inherit Metab Dis.* 1999; 22:381.
4. Barić I, Zschocke J, Christainsen E, et al. Diagnosis and management of glutaric aciduria type 1. *J Inherit Metab Dis.* 1998; 21:326.
5. Hoffman GF, Bohles HJ, Burlina A, et al. Early signs and course of disease of glutaryl-CoA dehydrogenase deficiency. *J Inherit Metab Dis.* 1995; 18:173.
6. Lindner M, Kölker S, Schulze A, et al. Neonatal screening for glutaryl-CoA dehydrogenase deficiency. *J Inherit Metab Dis* 2004; 27:851.
7. *North Carolina MS/MS Newborn Screening Follow-up Reports, 1997–2014.* Unpublished report to the North Carolina Newborn Screening Advisory Board, Raleigh, NC February 2015.
8. Frazier DM, Millington DS, McCandless SE, Koeberl DD, Weavil SD, Muenzer J. The tandem mass spectrometry newborn screening experience in North Carolina: 1997-2005. *J Inherit Metab Dis.* 2006; 29:76.
9. Mortan DH, Bennett MJ, Seargeant LE, Nichter CA, Kelley RI. Glutaric aciduria type 1: a common cause of episodic encephalopathy and spastic paralysis in the Amish of Lancaster County, Pennsylvania. *Am J Med Genet.* 1991; 41:89.
10. Greenberg CR, Prasad AN, Dilling LA, Thompson JR, Haworth JC, Martin B, Wood-Steiman P, Seargeant LE, Seifert B, Booth FA, Prasad C. Outcome of the first 3-years of a DNA-based neonatal screening program for glutaric acidemia type 1 in Manitoba and northwestern Ontario, Canada. *Mol Genet Metab.* 2002 Jan;75(1):70–8.
11. Bassinger AA, Booker JK, Frazier DM, Koeberl DD, Sullivan JA, Muenzer J. Gluaric acidemia type 1 in patients of Lumbee heritage from North Carolina. *Mol Genet Metab.* 2006; 88:90.
12. van der Watt G, Owen EP, Berman P, et al. Gluatric aciduria type 1 in South Africa: high incidence of glutaryl-CoA dehydrogenase deficiency in black South Africa. *Mol Genet Metab.*2010; 101:178.
13. *Known Mutations of the Glutaryl-CoA Dehydrogenase Gene.* Denver: University of Colorado; 2015. https://www.childrenscolorado.org/contentassets/495918f523604a17bff808533e253d65/gcdh_mutations.pdf
14. Greenberg CR, Duncan AMV, Gregory CA, Singal R, Goodman SI. Assignment of human glutaryl-CoA dehydrogenase gene (GCDH) to the short arm of chromosome 19 (19p 13.2) by in situ hybridization and somatic cell hybrid analysis. *Genomics* 1994; 21:289.
15. Goodman SI, Stein DE, Schlesinger S, et al. Glutaryl-CoA dehydrogenase mutations in glutaric acidemia (type 1): review and report of thirty novel mutations. *Hum Mutat.* 1998; 12:141.
16. Sen S, Pillay RS. Striatal necrosis in type 1 glutaric aciduria: different stages in two siblings. *J Pediatr Neurosci.* 2011; 6:146.
17. Barić I, Wagner L, Buckel W, Hoffman GF. Sensitivity of free and total glutaric and 3-OH-glutaric acid measurements by stable isotope dilution: assays from the diagnosis of glutaric aciduria type 1. *J Inherit Metab Dis.* 1997; 20:34.
18. Ullrich K, Flott-Rahmel B, Schluff P, et al. Glutaric aciduria type 1: pathomechanisms of neurodegeneration. *J Inherit Metab Dis.* 1999; 22:392.
19. Superti-Furga A. Glutaric aciduria type 1 and neonatal screening: time to proceed—with caution. *Eur J Pediatr.* 2003; 162:S17.
20. Couce ML, Lopez-Suarez O, Boveda MD, et al. Glutaric aciduria type 1: outcome of patients with early-versus late-diagnosis. *Eur J Pediatr Neurol.* 2013; 17:383.
21. Viau K, Ernst SL, Vanzo RJ, et al. Glutaric acidemia type 1: outcomes before and after expanded newborn screening. *Mol Genet Metab.* 2012; 106:430.
22. Acosta PB, Yannicelli S. *The Ross Metabolic Formula System Nutrition Support Protocols*, 4th ed. Columbus, OH: Ross Products Division; 2001.
23. Pennington JAT, Spungen J. *Bowes and Church's Food Values of Portions Commonly Used*, 19th ed. Philadelphia: Wolters Kluwar; 2010.
24. US Department of Agriculture, Agricultural Research Service, Nutrient Data Laboratory. *USDA National Nutrient Database for Standard Reference Dataset for What We Eat in America*, NHANES (Survey-SR). October 2015. http://www.ars.usda.gov/Services/docs.htm?docid=25662. Accessed July 1, 2016.
25. MetabolicPro: Web-based nutrient analysis software program designed specifically for metabolic nutritionists. https://www.metabolicpro.org/. Accessed July 1, 2016.
26. Schuett VE. *Low Protein Food List for PKU*, 3rd ed. CreateSpace; 2010. Searchable database is available at https://howmuchphe.org/site/demo. Accessed July 1, 2016.
27. Ma K, Savory S, Agim NG. Acquired protein-energy malnutrition in glutaric academia. *Pediatr Dermatol.* 2013; 30:502.
28. Kölker S, Nikolas Boy SP, Heringer J, et al. Complementary dietary treatment using lysine-free, tryptophan-free, arginine-fortified amino acid supplements in glutaric aciduria type 1: a decade of experience. *Mol Genet Metab.* 2012; 107:72.
29. Chalmers RA, Bain MD, Zschocke J. Riboflavin-responsive glutaryl-CoA dehydrogenase deficiency. *Mol Genet Metab.* 2006; 29:162.
30. Kölker S, Christensen E, Leonard JV, et al. Diagnosis and management of glutaric aciduria type 1: revised recommendations. *J Inherit Metab Dis.* 2011; 34:677.
31. Gokmen-Ozel H, MacDonald A, Daly A, et al. Dietary practices in glutaric aciduria type 1 over 16 years. *J Hum Nutr Diet.* 2012; 25:514.
32. Boy N. Haege G, Heringer J, et al. Low lysine diet in glutaric aciduria type 1: effect on anthropometric and biochemical follow-up parameters. *J Inherit Metab Dis.* 2013; 36:525.

# C.

# FATTY ACID OXIDATION DISORDERS

## 45 Adrenoleukodystrophy and Other Peroxisomal Disorders

NGA HONG BRERETON, ANN B. MOSER, AND GERALD V. RAYMOND

### THE PEROXISOMAL DISORDERS

Genetically determined peroxisomal disorders are divided into two major categories: (1) disorders of peroxisome biogenesis, in which the organelle is not formed normally, and (2) disorders that involve a single peroxisomal enzyme[1] (Table 45–1). Nutrition intervention is particularly relevant in the management of X-linked adrenoleukodystrophy and adult Refsum disease, the entities covered in this chapter.

### X-LINKED ADRENOLEUKODYSTROPHY

X-linked adrenoleukodystrophy (X-ALD) is the most common peroxisomal disorder. Its frequency is estimated to be 1:17,000. The gene defect involves *ABCD1*, a gene that has been mapped to chromosome Xq28 and codes for a transporter, ALDP. The principal biochemical abnormality is the accumulation of saturated very-long-chain fatty acids (VLCFA), mainly hexacosanoic acid (C26:0) and tetracosanoic acid (C24:0), in tissues and plasma.[2]

#### Genetic and Clinical Abnormalities

X-ALD affects the adrenal glands and nervous system. Because it is an X-linked disorder, affected males (hemizygotes), who have only one X chromosome, are more severely affected than females. Affected females who have one abnormal X chromosome, are referred to as *heterozygotes* and are protected to a varying extent by their other X chromosome, which is almost always normal.

Early neurological and mental development is entirely normal. Approximately 40% of affected boys develop the most serious form of the illness, the childhood cerebral adrenoleukodystrophy (CCALD). This manifests most commonly between 4 and 8 years of age and often is misdiagnosed initially as attention deficit disorder or another neuropsychiatric condition. However, the initial symptoms are followed by rapidly progressive cognitive, visual, and motor deficits that lead to total disability within 2 years and death at varying intervals. Another 40% of males with X-ALD develop the adult variant, referred to as *adrenomyeloneuropathy* (AMN), which manifests with progressive stiffness and weakness of the legs (paraparesis). Beginning typically in early adulthood, it progresses over decades. Approximately 50% of heterozygous women develop a slowly progressive AMN-like syndrome in middle age or later.

Cerebral disease is characterized by inflammatory demyelination, whereas patients with AMN have slowly progressive degenerative changes that involve mainly the spinal cord without the inflammatory reaction. It is postulated that the accumulation of VLCFA causes cellular injury with reactive oxidative compounds resulting in varying degrees of inflammation. For unknown reasons, the severe and milder forms often co-occur in the same family. It is not uncommon for one brother to have died of the severe childhood form while his sibling is an adult with AMN who is raising a family and gainfully employed.

Diagnosis of X-ALD depends on the demonstration of abnormally high VLCFA levels in plasma or pathogenic mutations in *ABCD1*. More than 1000 different *ABCD1* mutations have been described in X-ALD patients; these are listed and updated on the website http://

**Table 45–1.** Peroxisomal Disorders

| Disorders of Peroxisome Biogenesis | Single Peroxisomal Protein Defects |
|---|---|
| Zellweger syndrome | X-linked adrenoleukodystrophy |
| Neonatal adrenoleukodystrophy | Acyl-CoA oxidase deficiency |
| Infantile Refsum disease | Bifunctional enzyme deficiency |
| Rhizomelic chondrodysplasia punctata | DHAPAT deficiency |
| | Alkyl-CoA synthase deficiency |
| | Racemase deficiency |
| | Adult Refsum disease |

CoA = coenzyme A; DHAPAT = dihydroxyacetone-phosphate acyltransferase.

www.x-ald.nl.[3] Mutations are often unique to a family and do not correlate with the severity of the clinical expression. It is not possible to predict whether an asymptomatic male will later develop the severe childhood form or the adult form of the illness.

Treatment of X-ALD focuses on the adrenal and neurological aspects of the condition. The primary adrenal insufficiency requires steroid replacement therapy. This is mandatory and life-saving for patients with impaired adrenal function and is highly effective in correcting this condition, but it does not alter neurological progression. Hematopoietic stem cell transplantation, sometimes referred to as bone marrow transplantation, can arrest the progression of neurological disease and may be of lasting benefit, but it is recommended only in patients with early evidence of the progressive demyelinating disease. This may be detected at an early stage by magnetic resonance imaging (MRI) of the brain.[2]

## Nutrition Management of X-ALD

### Biological Basis and Clinical Experience

The nutrition therapy for X-ALD is based on the hypothesis that VLCFA are involved in the pathogenesis and that reduction of VLCFA could be of therapeutic benefit. VLCFA are derived partially from the diet but primarily by endogenous synthesis from C16 and C18 fatty acids via a microsomal fatty acid elongating system. Therapeutic trials in X-ALD patients suggest that endogenous synthesis is quantitatively more significant: Plasma VLCFA levels remain unchanged even with a diet that greatly reduces VLCFA intake but are normalized rapidly by monounsaturated fatty acids, such as erucic acid, that inhibit endogenous synthesis of saturated VLCFA. This observation forms the basis of current nutrition therapy.[4]

The oral administration of a 4:1 mixture of glyceryl trioleate (GTO) and glyceryl trierucate (GTE), often referred to as *Lorenzo's oil* (LO), when combined with moderate reduction of fat intake, normalized plasma VLCFA levels within 4 weeks. Although this was a striking biochemical effect, there did not appear to be a clinical effect in boys with CCALD, and limited studies in AMN have not produced a definitive answer. Even though all studies to date have been uncontrolled, have involved variable study populations, and have provided limited information on compliance and effective reduction of VLCFA levels, these disappointing results led to the widespread view that this dietary therapy is not effective.

Between 1989 and 2002, an open prevention trial in asymptomatic boys with X-ALD was carried out at the Kennedy Krieger Institute (Baltimore, MD). Boys were neurologically asymptomatic with normal MRI findings at enrollment and were treated with LO and monitored for the primary outcome of development of MRI changes. It was found that those subjects who lowered their mean plasma C26:0 levels to the normal range for 2 or more years reduced by 70% their risk of developing neurological abnormalities during a mean 3-year follow-up period, compared with subjects who failed to lower their levels to this extent and duration. The difference was highly statistically significant. However, this study suffered from limitations in that it was not randomized and the follow-up period was short.[5]

### Details of Nutrition Management

The role of LO and the modified diet remain under study.[6] LO is available in the United States under an investigational new drug permit from the US Food and Drug Administration (FDA). Individuals who are interested in using the oil should consult with their physicians and review the available clinical studies (www.clinicaltrials.gov). The source of LO in the United States is Nutricia NA (Gaithersburg, MD). Outside of the United States, availability and costs are determined by local regulations and suppliers. GTO, which previously was used in certain circumstances, is no longer readily available in the United States.

At this time, we recommend the consideration of LO for boys with proven X-ALD who are neurologically asymptomatic and have a normal result on brain MRI. This recommendation is based on the preventive trial experience, recognizing the limitations of that information. The use of this therapy requires the full participation of a multidisciplinary team that includes a registered dietitian.

Nutrition management of X-ALD has three elements (Fig. 45–1): (1) oral administration of LO; (2) reduction of fat intake from other sources, with the general aim of limiting it to no more than 10% of total calories; and (3) assurance of adequate essential fatty acids and fat-soluble vitamins. The more rigorous fat restriction that was recommended in the past is not required. However, combined use of the oil and the fat restriction is required to achieve the reduction in plasma VLCFA levels. Use of the oil without fat restriction does not achieve this end and exposes the patient to inconvenience and risk with little or no benefit. Likewise, dietary restriction of fat without the oil does not alter VLCFA levels and is not recommended. The results of the prevention trial suggest that a preventive effect occurs only when plasma VLCFA levels are lowered substantially for 2 years or longer. VLCFA levels must be actively monitored if the theoretical benefit is to be achieved.

We estimate the patient's energy need from the Dietary Reference Intakes (DRI). Caloric intake and fat content are provided by both LO and the other foods consumed. LO, which contains only fat (Table 45–2), is administered orally in a dosage that provides approximately 20% of the total caloric intake. This is usually accomplished with a daily intake of 2 to 3 mL/kg. (Table 45–3 shows a typical worksheet). It can be taken alone or mixed with foods in a single daily dose or in multiple doses in accordance with the patient's preference.

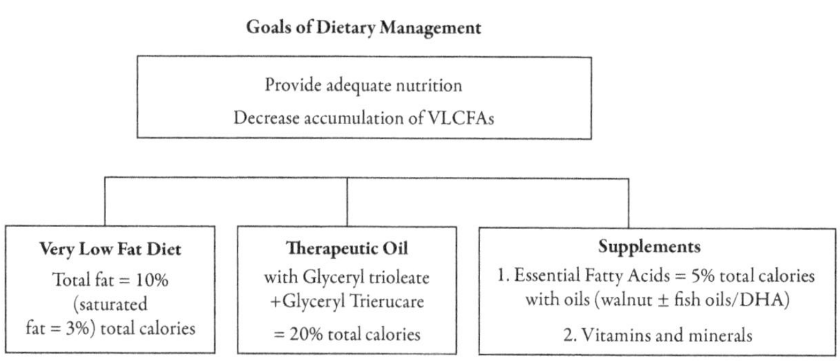


**Figure 45–1.** Elements of nutrition management of X-linked adrenoleukodystrophy. DHA = docosahexaenoic acid; VLCFAs = very-long-chain fatty acids.

**Table 45–2.** Fatty Acid Composition of Lorenzo's Oil

| | Fatty Acid | Percentage Present | |
|---|---|---|---|
| | | GTO | GTE |
| C12:0 | Lauric | 1.25 | 0 |
| C16:0 | Palmitic | 1.07 | 0 |
| C18:0 | Stearic | 3.02 | 0.5 |
| C18:1 | Oleic | 87.45 | 0.5 |
| C18:2 | Linoleic | 4.79 | 0.5 |
| C18:3 | Linolenic | 0 | 0.5 |
| C20:1 | Eicosenoic | 0 | 1.0–3.5 |
| C22:1 | Erucic | 0 | 91.5–94.0 |
| C24:0 | Lignoceric | 0 | 0 |
| C24:1 | Nervonic | 0 | 1.0–3.5 |
| C26:0 | Hexacosanoic | Trace | 0 |

GTE = glycerol trierucate; GTO = glycerol trioleate.
EER = estimated energy requirement; GTE = glycerol trierucate; GTO = glycerol trioleate; VLCFA = very-long-chain fatty acids.

The challenge is to design the patient's diet so that its fat content is limited to no more than 10% of total calories and with other needed supplements. Our studies indicate that normal growth can be achieved with this regimen. Foods are chosen to meet these needs and in accord with patient preferences. A sample menu is provided in Table 45–4. In order to keep to this low-fat diet, families are instructed to shop for low-fat and fat-free dairy products, low-fat cuts of meat, Fresh fruits, vegetables, and whole grains are encouraged, as well as the use of cooking spray and nonstick cookware. The preferred methods of cooking are boiling, steaming, grilling, and microwaving; frying is avoided. We limit foods that contain high levels of saturated VLCFA, such as C24:0 and C26:0, including peanut butter and beef fat; their intake should be less than 3% of total calories.

In order to limit total dietary fat intake (other than from LO) to less than 10% of calories, families must read food labels. In calculating fat intake, it is important to count the grams of fat instead of relying on the percentage of fat in the caloric intake. Both food information and low-fat recipes can be found on the Internet, and families should be provided with reliable sources. Care must be taken when eating out because restaurants are not transparent in their ingredients and cooking methods. The fat content of various fast foods are reported by the US Department of Agriculture at http://ndb.nal.usda.gov/ndb/nutrients/.

## Potential Medical Problems

Because of the restriction of fats, there has been concern for a potential deficiency in essential fatty acids and fat-soluble vitamins. We suggest the use of walnuts or walnut oil, which are rich in both linoleic acid (omega-6) and α-linolenic acid (omega-3) at a 5:1 ratio, amounting to 5% of estimated caloric need. In addition, we recommend that participants take a multivitamin supplement to cover their fat-soluble vitamins needs.

Moderate reduction of the platelet count is the main medical concern associated with LO therapy.[7] It occurs in approximately 30% to 50% of patients. It has not been associated with bleeding diathesis. The reduction appears to be caused by the presence of erucic acid in the platelet membrane. We monitor platelet counts at 3-month intervals. If the count falls below 80,000 platelets per microliter of blood, the LO is discontinued and replaced by an oil that is high in monounsaturated fats and low in saturated fats, such as olive oil. This usually maintains some degree of lowered VLCFA, although not as much as with LO. Platelet counts will increase within a few weeks, permitting titration of LO. With this strategy, it is usually possible to maintain VLCFA and platelet counts at desired levels.

Transient mild increases in liver enzymes (alanine transaminase [ALT], aspartate transaminase [AST]) may be seen without other evidence of liver disease. Initially there was concern about possible cardiac toxicity, because rodents fed large amounts of erucic acid developed cardiac lipidosis. However, this does not appear to occur in human beings. None of the patients treated with LO have developed cardiac abnormalities, and there were no changes in their electrocardiogram or echocardiogram in initial studies.

## Potential Nutritional Problems

At the start of the low-fat diet and with the inclusion of LO, a loss of appetite may occur, resulting in failure to gain weight. Most children gain weight adequately because LO is given in addition to the low-fat diet. One may reduce the fat in the diet gradually, starting with preferred food patterns. The LO dose is increased in small increments weekly until the final dose is reached, both to avoid a rapid drop in platelet count and also to allow individuals to adapt to taking the therapeutic oils and enable them to consume adequate energy for their growth and activities. Children should be encouraged to make low-fat food choices before they set out for school. School staff should be informed of the importance of compliance with the fat restriction. This, of course, requires communication between the family, the dietitian, and the physician.

Patients who take LO in combination with a reduced fat intake could develop reduced plasma levels of essential fatty acids. This is a particular concern when limited food choices are made or when the supplemental oils are not provided. We have used a variety of approaches to compensate for this effect, but the focus is on supplementing with food oils such as safflower, fish oil capsules, and other sources. If deficiency is a concern after the introduction of dietary therapy, the essential fatty acids should be monitored.

Fat-soluble vitamins (vitamins A, D, E, and K), as well as calcium and zinc, may be inadequate due to the avoidance of dietary products and the reduction of red meat intake. Fat-free milk, cheese, yogurt, and ice cream; low-fat soy-based milk; or skinless lean chicken and turkey

**Table 45–3.** Worksheet to Calculate Individualized Doses of Dietary Fat, GTO:GTE, and Walnut Oil

| Nutrient | Calculate Amount Based on Total Caloric Need | Daily Dosage |
|---|---|---|
| Energy | 100% of total caloric need, estimated from<br>• EER at different activity levels<br>• Current diet and oil intake<br>• Latest laboratory results (platelets, VLCFAs) | Total energy amount = ____ kcal/day |
| Total fat<br>Saturated fat | 10% of Energy, of which 3% of Energy may be from saturated fat | Total fat g = total fat cal ÷ 9 cal/g = ____ g/day<br>Total saturated fat g = total saturated fat cal ÷ 9 cal/g = ____ g/day |
| Lorenzo's oil (LO), a 4:1 GTO:GTE mixture<br>Substitute olive oil (OO) for some or all of LO if thrombocytopenia is present | 20% of Energy | LO volume = LO cal ÷ 8 cal/ml = _____ mL/day<br>OO volume = OO cal ÷ 8 cal/ml = _____ mL/day |
| Walnut oil (WO)<br>Walnut halves or walnut pieces may be substituted | 5% of Energy | WO volume = WO cal ÷ 8 cal/ml = _____ mL/day<br>_Walnut halves = walnut cal ÷ 13.2 (average cal of one walnut half) = ______ walnut halves/day<br>_Walnut pieces' weight = WO cal × 0.15 (calculate from 100 g walnut has 654 cal) = ____ g walnut pieces/day. |

**Table 45–4.** Sample Diet Prescription and Daily Menu*

| Item | Calories | Total Fat (g) | Saturated Fat (g) |
|---|---|---|---|
| 1 cup Rice Krispies | 87 | 0.06 | 0.02 |
| 1 cup Skim milk | 85 | 0.44 | 0.29 |
| Scrambled egg (2 egg whites + 2 tsp Promise Ultra Fat-Free margarine) | 36 | 0.14 | 0.02 |
| 1 slice Whole wheat toast | 80 | 0.99 | 0.21 |
| 1 cup Orange juice (calcium fortified) | 112 | 0.00 | 0.00 |
| Low-fat grilled cheese sandwich (2 slices bread + 2 tsp Promise Ultra Fat-Free Margarine + 2 slices fat-free American cheese) | 190 | 0.30 | 0.20 |
| 1 oz Baked potato chips | 110 | 1.5 | 0.4 |
| 1 Apple | 62 | 0 | 0 |
| 2 Fat-free oatmeal cookies | 103 | 1.48 | 0.15 |
| 1 cup Watermelon | 51 | 0 | 0 |
| ½ cup Cranberry juice | 72 | 0.13 | 0.01 |
| 3 oz Chicken tenders, low-fat recipe (boneless, skinless, cooked in 2 tsp olive oil) | 237 | 12.84 | 2.32 |
| ½ cup Mashed potatoes (with skim milk) | 70 | 0.3 | 0.3 |
| ¼ cup String beans | 10 | 0.03 | 0.01 |
| ¼ cup Corn | 41 | 0.2 | 0.03 |
| *TOTAL from Foods* | 1266 cal | 18.41 g | 3.96 g |

*Prescription is for 1500 cal/day, including approximately 20% from Lorenzo's oil (38 mL/day), 5% from walnut oil (9 mL/day), and 10% from dietary fats (16–17 g total fat/day).

breast meat can replace high-fat and red meat. Intake of calcium-fortified juice, skim milk, and fat-free foods and snacks should be encouraged to meet micronutrient needs.

Children with X-ALD who have food allergies, especially to nuts, require a careful plan. The currently used low-fat diet does not limit fresh fruits, vegetables including green vegetables, or, to some extent, high-fiber breads and cereals, so constipation is usually not a concern.

LO is not recommended for individuals with CCALD, but in rare circumstances may be used on a compassionate basis. If there are severe swallowing disturbances, tube feeding can be instituted to meet fluid and nutritional needs. Low-fat formulas range from 0.6 to 7 g total fat per serving (2% to 28% of calories). Tolerex elemental powder has 0.6 g fat per packet; Pediasure SideKicks has 5.3 g fat; and Promote has 6.2 g of fat per can (8 fluid oz.) Benefiber, supplied by Resource, is a powder fiber made from partially hydrogenated guar gum that can be added to a nonfiber formula. Adequate free water needs to be supplied.

## ADULT REFSUM DISEASE

Phytanic acid (4,7,11,15-tetramethylhexadecanoic acid) is degraded exclusively in the peroxisome and accumulates in several peroxisomal disorders, including Refsum disease and the disorders of peroxisome biogenesis (see Table 45–1). Because it is not synthesized in human beings, it is of dietary origin only in these patients, and its level can be modified by dietary manipulation. Dietary restriction of phytanic acid has been the main therapeutic strategy in the treatment of Refsum disease and has been quite effective, particularly if begun early.[8]

It has been suggested that dietary restriction of phytanic acid may also have a place in management of the other peroxisomal disorders, but in those cases there are other biochemical abnormalities that overshadow the consequences of phytanic acid accumulation. The more severe peroxisome assembly disorders are sometimes referred to as infantile Refsum disease. They are more common than adult Refsum disease and often manifest in infancy or early childhood. However, the two conditions should not be confused, because children with infantile Refsum disease are not likely to benefit from diet.

### Biochemical and Clinical Abnormalities

Refsum disease is a rare autosomal recessive disorder that is associated with phytanic acid accumulation due to deficiency of the enzyme phytanoyl-coenzyme A hydroxylase or mild alterations in peroxisomal biogenesis factor 7 (PEX7).[8] The clinical manifestations are progressive pigmentary degeneration of the retina (which may lead to blindness), polyneuropathy, ataxia, hearing loss, ichthyosis, and loss of the sense of smell. These conditions vary in severity and may manifest in childhood, adolescence, or young adulthood. Cardiomyopathy with heart failure and conduction defects often occur and may be the cause of sudden death. Half of the untreated patients die before the age of 30 years.

Plasma levels of phytanic acid can be reduced or normalized by dietary reduction of phytanic acid intake. This can improve the polyneuropathy, and it appears to arrest the progression of hearing loss and retinal abnormalities and improve the cardiomyopathy, indicating that phytanic acid plays a role in the pathogenesis of the disease. The normal plasma level of phytanic acid in our laboratory is 0.54 ± 0.29 μg/mL. In untreated patients with Refsum disease, the level may exceed 100 μg/mL, and this can be life-threatening due to cardiac disturbances or tetraparesis. Carefully controlled dietary therapy in patients with Refsum disease can maintain the level at less than 10 μg/mL, and this represents the main therapy. Plasma exchange can bring about a rapid reduction in plasma phytanic acid levels and is indicated as an emergency therapy when the plasma levels are markedly increased.

It is important to diagnose Refsum disease as early as possible because it represents a treatable form of retinal degeneration and of polyneuropathy and also because of its potential cardiac complications. Refsum disease may be difficult to differentiate clinically from other causes of retinal degeneration and polyneuropathy, and it is recommended that all patients with such disorders be screened for the disease. The most effective method is to test a plasma sample simultaneously for phytanic acid, pristanic acid, and VLCFA. This not only permits the identification of patients with Refsum disease (in whom phytanic acid is the only one of these substances that is present in excess) but also facilitates its differentiation from other disorders in which phytanic acid levels are increased, such as the disorders of peroxisome biogenesis (see Table 45–1). The diagnosis of Refsum disease can be confirmed by more specialized techniques such as DNA mutation analysis.

### Nutrition Management in Refsum Disease

Detailed information is available on the phytanic acid content of common foods.[9] The main dietary sources of phytanic acid are dairy products of all kinds. Ruminant fat and ruminant meat must be avoided. Fish and fish products contain phytanic acid, which is increased in proportion to the fat content of the fish. Poultry meat, such as chicken, turkey, or duck, is free of phytanic acid, as are dairy products from which fat has been removed, nondairy ice cream, and all vegetables and fruits. Contrary to what was recommended in the past, phytol- and chlorophyll-containing vegetables need not be restricted. The dietary regimen permits reduction of phytanic acid intake to less than 10 mg/day; if followed, it will reduce plasma phytanic acid levels substantially. It is essential that caloric intake be maintained. Before initiation of therapy, large amounts of phytanic acid are stored in tissues, particularly adipose tissue. During periods of reduced caloric intake associated with stress, infections, or surgical or dental procedures, the patient's tissue fat with its high phytanic acid content may be mobilized. There may also be a paradoxical increase in the plasma phytanic acid level during initiation of the diet, when total caloric intake may be reduced as the patient eliminates forbidden foods from the diet. This highlights the importance of careful supervision and good communication between the patient and the nutritionist.

Infants born with Refsum disease can be breast-fed.[10] Breast milk phytanic acid levels were measured from 30 women of mixed ethnic background and were found to be 1.63 ± 0.95 µg/mL. When infants consume 750 to 960 mL breast milk daily, they get 0.5 to 2.5 mg phytanic acid per day. These values fall within the low phytanic acid diet guidelines.

## References


1. Braverman NE, D'Agostino MD, Maclean GE. Peroxisome biogenesis disorders: biological, clinical and pathophysiological perspectives. *Dev Disabil Res Rev.* 2013; 17:187.
2. Moser HW, Mahmood A, Raymond GV. X-linked adrenoleukodystrophy. *Nat Clin Pract Neurol.* 2007; 3:140.
3. Kemp S, Pujol A, Waterham HR, et al. ABCD1 mutations and the X-linked adrenoleukodystrophy mutation database: role in diagnosis and clinical correlations. *Hum Mutat.* 2001; 18:499.
4. Moser HW, Raymond GV, Koehler W, et al. Evaluation of the preventive effect of glyceryl trioleate-trierucate ("Lorenzo's oil") therapy in X-linked adrenoleukodystrophy: results of two concurrent trials. *Adv Exp Med Biol.* 2003; 544:369.
5. Moser HW, Raymond GV, Lu SE, et al. Follow-up of 89 asymptomatic patients with adrenoleukodystrophy treated with Lorenzo's oil. *Arch Neurol.* 2005; 62:1073.
6. Moser HW, Moser AB, Hollandsworth K, Brereton NH, Raymond GV. "Lorenzo's oil" therapy for X-linked adrenoleukodystrophy: rationale and current assessment of efficacy. *J Mol Neurosci.* 2007; 33:105.
7. Zinkham WH, Kickler T, Borel J, Moser HW. Lorenzo's oil and thrombocytopenia in patients with adrenoleukodystrophy. *N Engl J Med.* 1993; 328:1126.
8. Wanders RJA, Waterham HR, Leroy BP. Refsum disease. 2006; last updated 2015. In: Pagon RA, Adam MP, Ardinger HH, et al., eds. *GeneReviews*. Seattle, WA: University of Washington; 1993–2015. http://www.ncbi.nlm.nih.gov/pubmed/20301527. Accessed July 1, 2016.
9. Masters-Thomas A, Bailes J, Billimoria JD, Clemens ME, Gibberd FB, Page NG. Heredopathia atactica polyneuritiformis (Refsum's disease): 2. Estimation of phytanic acid in foods. *J Hum Nutr.* 1980; 34:251.
10. Brereton NH, Raymond GV, Moser AB, Vogelhut J. Phytanic, Pristanic, and DHA levls of Human Breast Milk. National Association fo GCRC Bionutritionists, Nutrition Research fNews Fall 2003 @ http://nabconnection.org/forum/Newsletters/03Fall.pdf.

# 46 Mitochondrial Fatty Acid Oxidation Defects

MELANIE GILLINGHAM AND SANDY VAN CALCAR

Fatty acid oxidation (FAO) disorders are a family of 22 different genetic disorders in the mitochondrial FAO pathway. All are inherited in an autosomal recessive manner, and specific gene defects have been identified for most of the disorders. FAO disorders have an increasingly broad range of recognized phenotypes from mild to severe.[1–4] Severe phenotypes typically manifest in infancy with catastrophic episodes of fasting- or illness-induced hypoketotic hypoglycemia. The most common clinical presentation of FAO disorders in childhood includes nausea, vomiting, somnolence, and hepatic encephalopathy, similar to Reye syndrome, which can progress to coma and death if untreated.[5,6] Cardiomyopathy can be a life-threatening complication of acute metabolic decompensation in long-chain FAO defects.[7] These defects may also manifest as sudden infant death syndrome (SIDS); before the introduction of expanded newborn screening (NBS) for these disorders, as many as one-third of the initial episodes were fatal.[6]

Children who present symptomatically and survive an initial metabolic crisis may suffer recurrent decompensation episodes and develop chronic disabilities including muscular hypotonia and developmental delay. NBS has dramatically reduced the number of infants who present with catastrophic metabolic crisis and allowed initiation of early treatment. However, it has not eliminated these episodes, and some patients still suffer from intermittent metabolic decompensation with hypoglycemia during infancy. Alternatively, mild phenotypes of FAO deficiency may not manifest until adolescence or adulthood; as presentation, these patients have exercise intolerance with recurrent episodes of rhabdomyolysis and myoglobinuria. Patients with milder phenotypes presenting later in life typically do not develop hypoglycemia during fasting or illness.[3] In some cases, individuals have known gene mutations believed to be disease causing but never develop symptoms. Collectively, FAO defects are relatively common; the estimated incidence in reports from Germany, Australia, and the United States is 1 per 9300 births.[8]

## FATTY ACID OXIDATION

The process of mitochondrial fatty acid beta-oxidation is depicted in Figure 46–1. Transport of long-chain fatty acids (LCFA), which are those 12 to 18 carbons in length, into the mitochondria requires L-carnitine. Transport of medium-chain fatty acids (6 to 10 carbons) and short-chain fatty acids (4 to 6 carbons) into the mitochondria does not absolutely require L-carnitine, although the carnitine shuttle system may contribute to mitochondrial uptake of these substrates. Carnitine palmitoyl transferase-1 (CPT-1) forms fatty acylcarnitine conjugates (step 1 in Fig. 46–1) that are then transported into the mitochondria by a translocase (step 2). Once inside the matrix, the conjugation reaction is reversed by CPT-2, yielding free carnitine and long-chain fatty acyl-coenzyme A (CoA) (step 3).

Beta-oxidation of fatty acyl-CoAs occurs in a repeating four-enzyme cycle, each "spiral" of the cycle releasing one molecule of acetyl-CoA (steps 4–7). The first reaction is performed by an acyl-CoA dehydrogenase; the choice of enzyme depends on the structure and chain length of the fatty acid substrate. Straight-chain LCFAs (C12–C18) are metabolized by very-long-chain acyl-CoA dehydrogenase (VLCAD), an enzyme that is bound to the inner mitochondrial membrane. Long-chain branched or desaturated fatty acids are likely substrates for long-chain acyl-CoA dehydrogenase (LCAD), an enzyme found within the mitochondrial matrix. Chain-shortened fatty acids become substrates for either medium-chain acyl-CoA dehydrogenase (MCAD; C6–C12) or short-chain acyl-CoA dehydrogenase (SCAD; C4–C6). All of these reactions provide reducing equivalents ($FADH^+$) that are coupled through electron transfer flavoprotein (ETF) and ETF:CoQ oxidoreductase (ETF:QO) to coenzyme Q of the electron transport chain. Three further enzymatic steps (steps 5–7) complete one cycle, leaving a fatty acyl-CoA two carbons shorter for further beta-oxidation. For LCFAs, steps 5 through 7 are catalyzed by a single membrane-bound enzyme complex called the *trifunctional protein* (TFP). For shorter fatty acids, distinct mitochondrial matrix proteins catalyze the three remaining steps of the beta-oxidation cycle; they include crotonase or short-chain enoyl-CoA hydratase, hydroxyacyl-CoA dehydrogenase (HAD), medium 3-ketoacyl-CoA thiolase, and β-ketothiolase.

Reducing equivalents ($NADH^+$) generated in step 6 (3-hydroxyacyl-CoA dehydrogenase) are coupled to complex I of the electron transport chain and used to generate adenosine triphosphate (ATP). Acetyl-CoA generated through FAO is a substrate for the citric acid cycle, sparing glycogen in liver and muscle and preventing glucose depletion. In the liver, acetyl-CoA from FAO is also used to generate ketone bodies that are released into the systemic circulation to be used as an alternative energy substrate for some tissues such as the central nervous system.

## METABOLIC ABNORMALITIES

### Fatty Acid Oxidation Disorders

The primary FAO disorders are listed in Table 46–1 along with the biochemical abnormalities observed in these conditions. FAO does not play a major role in energy production under nonfasting conditions. Therefore, defects in FAO may be clinically silent until relatively late in fasting or during an intercurrent illness or other significant environmental stress. The episodic nature and variable presentation of the FAO disorders can make them difficult to identify and correctly diagnosis. The following descriptions provide the key clinical features of the FAO disorders.

*CPT-1A deficiency* causes symptomatic fasting hypoketotic hypoglycemia and occasionally hepatocellular damage. The heart and muscle are rarely involved because CPT-1A is the liver isoform of the enzyme. In CPT-1A deficiency, total and free plasma carnitine are characteristically elevated; this observation is unique among all known FAO defects and is otherwise seen only in association with carnitine supplementation or renal insufficiency.[7]

In *CPT-2 deficiency*, an infantile form manifests with severe hypoglycemia, myopathy, and cardiomyopathy often resulting in death.[9] Plasma free carnitine is low and acylcarnitines are elevated. A milder form causes myopathy, recurrent rhabdomyolysis, and myoglobinuria in young adults. *Carnitine/acylcarnitine translocase deficiency* is clinically similar to infantile CPT-2 deficiency. Patients often present in the neonatal or infancy period with severe hypoketotic hypoglycemia, hyperammonemia probably due to liver failure, and elevated acylcarnitines associated with intercurrent illness.[10]

*VLCAD deficiency* manifests with three main phenotypes: the severe infantile presentation with cardiomyopathy, the childhood/adolescent form with hypoketotic hypoglycemia and recurrent rhabdomyolysis, and the adult-onset form with only recurrent rhabdomyolysis.[11] The severe phenotype is characterized by dilated or hypertrophic cardiomyopathy very early in life.[12,13] The cardiomyopathy may be severe

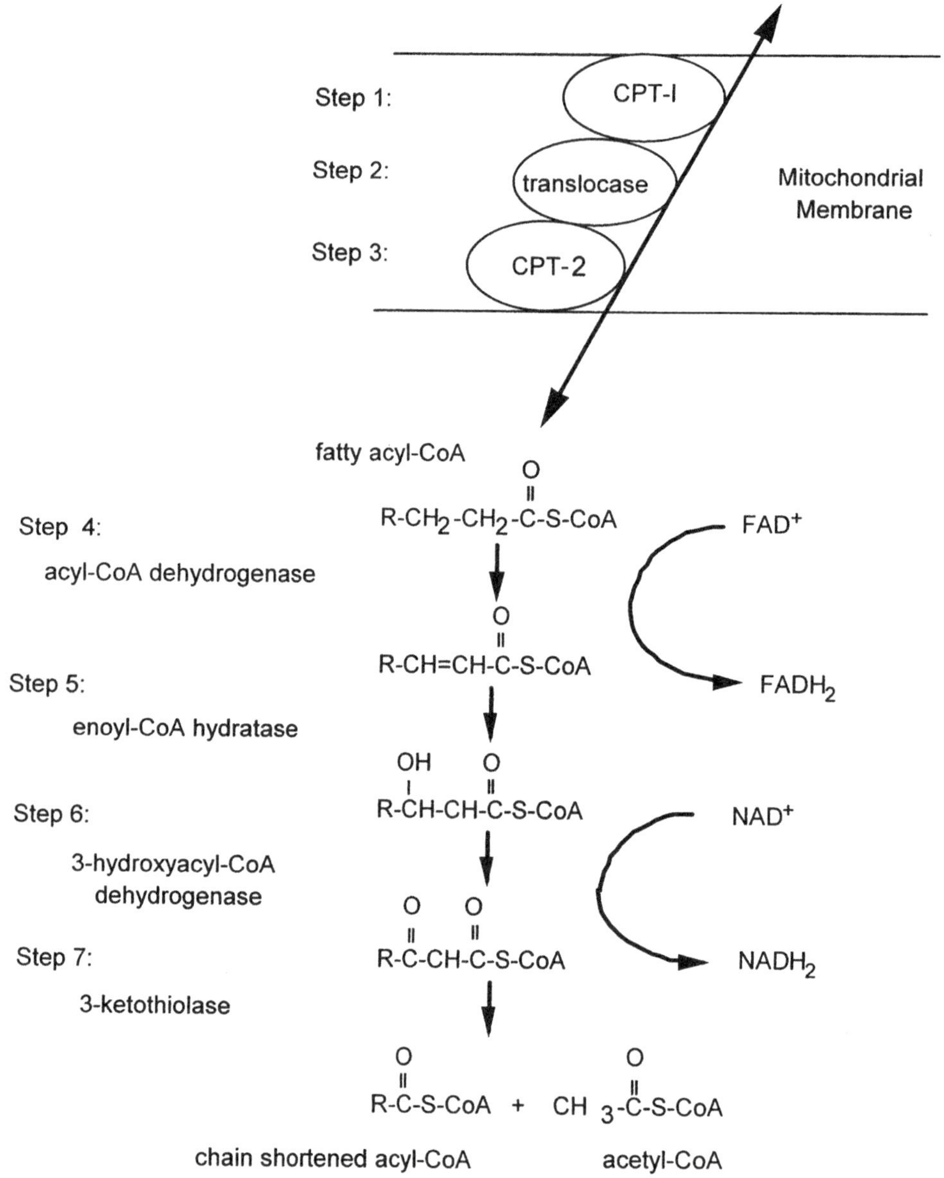


**Figure 46–1.** Fatty acid beta-oxidation. CoA = coenzyme A; CPT = carnitine palmitoyltransferase; $FAD^+$ = flavin adenine dinucleotide; $FADH_2$ = reduced FAD; $NAD^+$ = nicotinamide adenine dinucleotide; $NADH_2$ = reduced nicotinamide adenine dinucleotide.

and results in early demise in up to 44% of patients.[12] The presentation can also be characterized by hypoketotic hypoglycemia and hepatic steatosis.[14]

The intermediate phenotype often manifests as hypoketotic hypoglycemia in childhood, similar to MCAD deficiency, along with myopathy or rhabdomyolysis. During acute illness, there are characteristic increases in plasma long-chain acylcarnitines including C14:0, C14:1, C16:0, C16:1, C18:0, C18:1, and C18:2 acylcarnitine esters but especially in C14:1.[15] Rhabdomyolysis and myoglobinuria are often related to a bout of prolonged exercise, an illness with fever or poor oral

**Table 46–1.** Metabolic Abnormalities Detected in Fatty Acid Oxidation Disorders

| Fatty Acid Oxidation Disorder | Plasma Acylcarnitine | Urine Organic Acids |
|---|---|---|
| Carnitine palmitoyltranferase 1A (CPT1A) deficiency | ↑ C0, ↓ long-chain acylcarnitines | Normal |
| Carnitine palmitoyltransferase 2 (CPT-2) deficiency | ↑ C16, C18:1, C14 | Normal |
| Carnitine acylcarnitine translocase (CACT) deficiency | ↑ C16, C18:1, C14 | Normal or ↑ dicarboxylic acids |
| Very-long-chain acyl-CoA dehydrogenase (VLCAD) deficiency | ↑ C14:1, C14, C14:1/C12 ratio | ↑ Dicarboxylic acids |
| Long-chain 3-hydroxyacyl-CoA dehydrogenase (LCHAD)/mitochondrial trifunctonal protein (TFP) deficiency | ↑ C14OH, C16OH, C18:1OH, C18:2OH | ↑ Dicarboxylic acids |
| Medium-chain acyl-CoA dehydrogenase (MCAD) deficiency | ↑ C8, C10, C10:1 | ↑ Dicarboxylic acids, acylgylcines |
| Medium/Short-chain 3-hydroxyacyl-CoA dehydrogenase (SCHAD) deficiency | ↑ C4OH | ↑ Dicarboxylic acids |
| Short-chain acyl-CoA dehydrogenase (SCAD) deficiency | ↑ C4 | ↑ Ethylmalonic acid |

CoA = coenzyme A.

intake, cold temperatures, or a combination of these factors. Creatine phosphokinase levels can be extremely elevated, and rhabdomyolysis/myoglobinuria can cause renal failure requiring hemodialysis.[16]

The mild adult-onset form is most often associated with exercise intolerance and myoglobinuria. Adult patients have presented with a history of recurrent rhabdomyolysis, muscle pain, and weakness that begins in adolescence and may continue intermittently for decades before a diagnosis of VLCAD deficiency is made.[17] Conversely, adult patients may present with an acute rhabdomyolysis event with no prior history of muscle disease.[16,18]

*Long-chain 3-hydroxyacyl-CoA dehydrogenase (LCHAD) deficiency* (selective loss of the LCHAD activity within TFP) and *mitochondrial TFP deficiency* (loss of all three enzymatic functions) have very similar presentations and clinical courses. Children typically present with hypoketotic hypoglycemia associated with metabolic acidosis, hepatocellular dysfunction, and sometimes cardiomyopathy. Elevated plasma long-chain hydroxyacylcarnitines including C16:0-OH, C16:1-OH, C18:0-OH, C18:1-OH, C18:2-OH are diagnostic of *LCHAD or TFP deficiency*. Pigmentary retinopathy with vision loss during childhood and progressive peripheral neuropathy are complications specific to LCHAD/TFP deficiency that are not observed in the other FAO disorders.[19] Not all patients experience all complications of the disease. The underlying etiology of the hypoketotic hypoglycemia appears to be a deficiency of energy from depleted carbohydrate stores, but the etiology of the other complications is not completely understood. A depletion of energy or the toxic effects of the accumulation of metabolic products are thought to be causative.[20,21]

*MCAD deficiency* is the most common defect in FAO, with an incidence of approximately 1 in 12,000 live births.[22] The typical acute clinical presentation includes fasting- or illness-induced hypoketotic hypoglycemia, often associated with metabolic acidosis and hepatomegaly.[23] The most severe presentation is of sudden unexpected death in infancy.[24] Sudden unexpected death has been reported in the first few days after birth, almost exclusively in breast-fed infants, presumably due to the relative fasting status in nursing infants.[25–28] On the other hand, some MCAD-deficient individuals never become symptomatic[29,30]; the reason is unknown, but it is hypothesized that they never develop carnitine depletion coincident with sufficient stress to induce a metabolic crisis or because they carry mutations with relatively mild physiological effects.

Since the advent of NBS for MCAD deficiency, many infants have been identified and treated with excellent outcome.[22,31,32] Most of these patients who are treated are completely healthy, although they may need to receive intravenous fluids containing glucose when ill or fasting, to prevent metabolic crisis. Rarely, some neurological impairment has been observed later in life among people with MCAD-deficiency, particularly in unscreened populations, but the evidence for neurological impairment in treated patients who have avoided metabolic crisis is scant. Deficits in learning and speech/language communication were reported in symptomatic individuals before the advent of NBS, but further study is needed to determine the prevalence of these complications in screened populations and in affected individuals who are identified early and effectively treated.[33,34]

*HAD deficiency* has a similar presentation to other FAO disorders, including hypoglycemia, hypotonia, and seizures. Approximately five patients with HAD deficiency have been described in the literature, so the phenotype is likely incompletely characterized. What sets this condition apart from other FAO disorders is hyperinsulinemia with mild elevations in ammonia associated with postprandial hypoglycemia in those with null mutations, despite dietary therapy.[35,36] HAD protein forms a complex and can inhibit glutamate dehydrogenase in the pancreatic beta cell.[37]

In HAD knockout mice, the absence of HAD protein permits activation of glutamate dehydrogenase, resulting in increased ATP synthesis and insulin release. The hyperinsulinemia was further stimulated in the mice after an oral protein load containing leucine. Subsequently, oral protein loads induced hyperinsulinemia with hypoglycemia in three human patients with HAD deficiency.[38] The data suggest that in some patients, a leucine-restricted diet may help decrease the hyperinsulinemia. Diagnosis and metabolic status of HAD deficiency is evaluated with the use of plasma free 3-hydroxy fatty acid profiles because short- and medium-chain 3-hydroxy fatty acids do not readily form acylcarnitine conjugates and therefore cannot be detected by current NBS technology.[39,40]

*SCAD deficiency* can cause failure to thrive, recurrent vomiting with or without hypoglycemia and/or ketosis, hypotonia, marked developmental delay, seizures, and early demise.[41] However, two common *SCAD* gene polymorphisms observed in the general population are typically not associated with disease and probably do not require treatment. It is controversial whether SCAD deficiency alone is sufficient to cause human disease.[42]

### Sudden Infant Death

The most severe presentation of an FAO disorder is SIDS.[43–51] Retrospective studies of siblings of individuals known to have SIDS diagnosed in postmortem studies suggest that about 5% of SIDS cases could be caused by an FAO disorder.[52–55] Many cases occur during intercurrent illness or after prolonged fasting. The advent of screening for FAO disorders has decreased the incidence of SIDS in screened populations.[22,33,56,57] However, no screening program can completely eliminate the possibility of sudden death in affected individuals. Some infants die 2 to 4 days after birth, for example, which is too early for NBS to be preventive.

## FACTORS TO BE CONSIDERED IN DIAGNOSIS

Since the advent of expanded NBS utilizing tandem mass spectrometry (MS/MS), most FAO patients are diagnosed after identification by NBS. Each specific FAO defect is associated with a unique profile of acylcarnitines that can be measured in filter paper blood spots collected 24 to 48 hours after birth. All states in the United States and most developed countries include acylcarnitine profiling for FAO disorders and organic acid disorders in their NBS program. MS/MS NBS can detect affected children presymptomatically and, with proper dietary and medical treatment, prevent catastrophic illness and death. However, these programs cannot prevent death within the first 2 to 4 days of life, which can occur in some FAO disorders.[58–61] For this and other reasons, postmortem screening for FAO disorders in cases of unexplained death can be useful, and many states in the United States routinely pursue such testing in cases of unexplained childhood or infant death.

Once an FAO defect has been suggested by NBS or in symptomatic patients by initial laboratory testing, further specific tests are usually necessary to confirm the diagnosis. Confirmatory tests may include plasma acylcarnitine profiles, fibroblast in-vitro FAO probes, direct enzymatic assays in peripheral blood lymphocytes or cultured skin fibroblasts, and/or mutation analysis, typically from blood, saliva, or buccal cells.

Some affected infants may be missed by NBS and present symptomatically later in life, making it important to pursue diagnostic testing in patients with suggestive symptoms of an FAO defect even if they had a normal NBS result. Diagnostic testing for patients presenting symptomatically typically includes plasma acylcarnitine profiling as the first step, followed, as indicated, by additional confirmatory testing as described for those identified by NBS.

FAO disorders should be considered in patients who present with Reye-like syndrome, myopathy, rhabdomyolysis/myoglobinuria, cardiomyopathy, unexplained liver disease, and/or hypoglycemia (especially when hypoketotic). Prenatal diagnostic testing is available routinely for many of the FAO disorders and is theoretically possible for all of those for which the gene defect has been identified. Most families of a child with a very treatable FAO disorder such as MCAD deficiency choose not to undergo prenatal diagnostic testing in subsequent pregnancies but rather to treat the infant presumptively until postnatal diagnostic testing results are available.

## NUTRITION MANAGEMENT

The goal of treatment for all FAO defects is to minimize FAO by avoiding fasting and providing adequate nonfat calories via enteral or parenteral routes during stresses such as intercurrent illness. Provision of adequate energy and frequent feedings sufficient to avoid fasting should be initiated in infants with a suspected FAO disorder before confirmation of the diagnosis. Additional treatment modalities have been incompletely studied; they include carnitine supplementation, dietary fat restriction, and medium-chain triglyceride (MCT) supplementation, which is indicated for long-chain defects only (contraindicated in medium-chain defects). Most treatments are based primarily on anecdotal report and expert opinion; these treatments can vary widely across metabolic centers around the world.[62–64] The major components of medical nutrition therapy and the evidence to support these therapies are described in the following sections.

## Avoidance of Fasting

Healthy infants and children adapt to fasting by sequentially turning on glycogenolysis, increasing hepatic gluconeogenesis, and mobilizing fat stores for ketogenesis in order to maintain adequate blood levels of substrates for systemic energy production. Glycogenolysis can supply glucose only for a matter of hours before glycogen supplies are depleted, and gluconeogenesis can prevent hypoglycemia for a maximum of approximately 24 hours in older children and adults, less in infants. Therefore, mobilization of fat stores and FAO for ketogenesis and energy production is the main alternative to glucose oxidation in most infants who are fasting and in older children and adults who fast for prolonged periods. An FAO disorder reduces the capacity to utilize free fatty acids for energy and ketone production. This is compounded by the increased systemic need for glucose resulting from the lack of ketones under fasting conditions and ultimately leads to hypoglycemia. Controlled fasting studies have been used in the development of guidelines for the treatment of known FAO disorders. However, such studies should be carried out only after routine confirmatory testing has been completed and under the supervision of specialists experienced in the treatment of FAO disorders, because fasting in individuals with FAO defects can be dangerous.[65]

Several fasting studies in patients with MCAD deficiency, the most common of the FAO disorders, have been published.[23,65–67] Based on an analysis of 35 fasting studies involving 31 patients with MCAD deficiency, a maximum duration of fasting of 8 hours in infants between 6 and 12 months of age, 10 hours during the second year of life, and 12 hours thereafter has been recommended.[66] The authors of these studies defined a safe duration of fasting as that period during which no clinical symptoms (e.g., lethargy, vomiting, sweating, tachycardia) or hypoglycemia (i.e., glucose <47 mg/dL) was observed. In 6 of the 35 fasting tests in patients with MCAD deficiency, clinical symptoms were observed before hypoglycemia was noted, consistent with the generally held belief that blood glucose levels are a poor indicator of metabolic status in patients with FAO disorders. For these reasons, blood glucose monitoring is usually not helpful in the management of these disorders and may provide a false sense of security to families.

Other fasting studies have measured abnormal metabolites, such as increased plasma acylcarnitine concentrations, as an end point. Long-chain acylcarnitines rose dramatically after a 12-hour fast in a 10-year-old subject with VLCAD deficiency, and long-chain hydroxyacylcarnitines rose after 6 hours of fasting in a toddler with LCHAD deficiency.[68,69] Plasma glucose remained normal during these controlled fasts, and the effects of elevated plasma acylcarnitines on clinical outcomes are not completely understood.

In general, the results of controlled fasting studies suggest that prolonged periods of fasting (>12 hours, or less in younger children), should be avoided. The usefulness of more specific fasting guidelines is debatable; most healthy children and adults choose to eat frequently, approximately every 6 to 8 hours during waking periods. However, some metabolic centers use the following guidelines: in infants younger than 4 months of age, fasting should not exceed 4 hours; between 5 and 12 months, an additional hour of fasting can be added for each month of age.[70,71] Dietary therapy that includes avoidance of fasting and frequent high-carbohydrate meals for the routine management of all FAO disorders prevents most episodes of metabolic decompensation.[3,6]

It is important to note that all controlled fasting studies have been conducted in healthy subjects with FAO disorders. Most episodes of metabolic decompensation in patients with FAO disorders occur with intercurrent illness or prolonged exercise. The ability of patients with FAO disorders to tolerate fasting during illness or stress is significantly reduced.

## Acute Management

Illness increases energy requirements while decreasing appetite and potentially increasing energy and fluid loss from emesis and diarrhea. The result is a negative energy balance that induces increased FAO to produce ATP. Increased fluid and carbohydrate intake is essential during illness or stress. Frequent intake of sweetened beverages such as fruit juices can be used to manage an illness at home under the direction of the supervising physician. Most oral rehydration solutions contain insufficient carbohydrates to be used as the major hydration solution for those with FAO disorders.

Patients with FAO disorders are often provided with emergency treatment plans outlining the steps to be taken by the family or the emergency department, including contact information for the metabolic specialist in the event of illness. Should the patient develop alteration in mental status or hypoglycemia, emergency care should be initiated immediately. Metabolic acidosis is a common complication of metabolic decompensation in FAO disorders and is most often associated with elevated blood lactate concentrations. Acute treatment with glucose-containing intravenous fluids can resolve both the hypoglycemia and lactic acidosis if instituted sufficiently early in the illness. Aggressive treatment for the acidosis is usually unnecessary. Large boluses of concentrated glucose solutions can lead to a hyperinsulinemic response followed by rebound hypoglycemia and are to be avoided unless there is no other way to provide glucose rapidly (e.g., in the field by paramedics), but this treatment needs to be followed up immediately by constant provision of glucose until the patient's condition stabilizes. Emergency resuscitation and critical care should be instituted when necessary based on age-appropriate guidelines for non-FAO patients, with the reminder to ensure adequate provision of glucose at all times and with modifications for hepatic or cardiac disease if present, as well as monitoring for cerebral edema.

*Nighttime hypoglycemia* has been reported in some patients with FAO disorders and is a major concern for parents. The risk of nighttime hypoglycemia appears to diminish as the child ages, and most patients can safely sleep through the night by age 4 years or earlier. Overnight tube feedings have been used to provide a continuous source of carbohydrate throughout the night. Uncooked cornstarch (1 g/kg of body weight) given at bedtime has also been used successfully in patients with both long-chain and short-chain FAO disorders,[72–74] although is it not usually indicated in MCAD deficiency. Overnight tube feedings carry their own risks; for example, inadvertent disconnection of the tubing during the night can lead to hypoglycemia, and use of alarm systems or other measures need to be taken to lower the risks.

## l-Carnitine Supplementation

Carnitine is found in meat and dairy products in the diet or synthesized in vivo from lysine and methionine in the liver. Carnitine deficiency is rare but can occur in liver or kidney disease, malnutrition, vegetarian or vegan diets, and malabsorption in addition to FAO disorders. FAO disorder patients can develop secondary carnitine deficiency due to high acylcarnitine excretion in the urine that may exceed synthetic capabilities.

L-Carnitine (typically 50–300 mg/kg/day orally or cautious administration of up to 300 mg/kg/day intravenously) is often prescribed for some disorders of FAO to prevent or treat carnitine deficiency and to enhance urinary excretion of potentially toxic FAO intermediates as carnitine conjugates. However, few controlled trials of carnitine supplementation have been performed to prove its clinical efficacy.[75] In patients with MCAD deficiency, carnitine supplementation does increase the excretion of medium-chain acylcarnitine moieties, but this has not been shown to improve symptoms precipitated by fasting or acute illness.[67,75,76] Carnitine supplementation also impairs the formation of medium-chain glycine conjugates, which is the major pathway for excretion of potentially toxic medium-chain metabolites, suggesting that long-term carnitine supplementation may not be beneficial.[75] Carnitine supplementation in medium-chain FAO defects is controversial but may be useful in preventing metabolic crisis even when plasma carnitine levels are normal and is probably indicated when plasma carnitine levels are low.

Carnitine supplementation in children with long-chain FAO defects is also controversial.[77] Some clinicians are concerned that carnitine supplementation will increase plasma levels of potentially toxic acylcarnitines, whereas others believe that carnitine supplementation will improve the excretion of these abnormal metabolites. Two reports of patients with LCHAD/TFP deficiency concluded that carnitine supplementation was not associated with a decreased incidence of metabolic decompensation or lower plasma concentrations of hydroxylated acylcarnitines but did not cause obvious harm either.[6,19] However, carnitine supplementation in children with the infantile form of VLCAD deficiency complicated by severe cardiomyopathy appears to be life-saving.[78,79]

## Dietary Fat Restriction

Restricting dietary fat intake in patients with short- or medium-chain FAO disorders does not appear to be beneficial. A study of subjects with SCAD deficiency found that dietary fat restriction did not improve the clinical course.[74] To date, there has been no study examining the effects of a low-fat diet on clinical outcomes in MCAD deficiency. In practice, some metabolic centers recommend that patients with MCAD deficiency consume a moderately low-fat diet (30% of total energy from fat), similar to a heart healthy diet, but others do not recommend a specific restriction in dietary fat. There is no research establishing the clinical benefit or lack thereof of dietary fat restriction among patients with MCAD deficiency, but instruction on use of a heart-healthy diet would certainly be reasonable.

Restricting dietary fat intake decreases the accumulation of potentially toxic metabolites such as plasma acylcarnitines in patients with CPT-2, LCHAD, TFP, or VLCAD deficiency.[68,80–82] In addition, supplemental MCT provides an alternative energy source downstream of the enzymatic block and decreases oxidation of LCFA.[19,81,83–85] (MCT supplementation should not be given to patients with medium- or short-chain FAO defects.) Patients with LCHAD or TFP deficiency consuming 10% of energy from LCFA and 10% to 20% of energy from MCT have significantly lower plasma hydroxylated acylcarnitine levels than subjects consuming more LCFA or less MCT.[81] Although the relationship between increasing dietary long-chain fat intake and increasing circulating acylcarnitine concentrations is well-established, the effects of lowering acylcarnitines on long-term outcomes have not been determined for all long-chain FAO disorders.

To date, restricting dietary fat intake and lowering long-chain acylcarnitine levels in patients with VLCAD or CPT-2 deficiency has not been correlated with an improvement in clinical outcomes, such as a decreased incidence of rhabdomyolysis. However, lower hydroxyacylcarnitine levels in subjects with LCHAD or TFP deficiency is associated with improved retinal function and a slower progression of chorioretinopathy of LCHAD.[21] Subjects with LCHAD or TFP deficiency who maintained lower hydroxyacylcarnitine levels had significantly better vision and slower progression of chorioretinopathy over 5 years of follow-up. In addition, patients who had fewer episodes of metabolic decompensation and fewer hospitalizations also had better vision and slower progression of retinopathy.[86]

In contrast, feeding a very high fat can be detrimental and can precipitate metabolic decompensation. In a single case report, a young child with VLCAD was accidentally provided a ketogenic formula rather than his standard low-fat, MCT-containing formula.[87] After 2.5 days, the child presented to the emergency room with lethargy, hypoglycemia, and very elevated concentrations of long-chain acylcarnitines. It is impossible to determine whether it was the presence of the fat or the absence of carbohydrate in the diet precipitated the decompensation, but it did take several days to develop. No additional reports of continuous fat loading or high-fat diet have been published.

## Essential Fatty Acids

Biochemical essential fatty acid deficiencies have been diagnosed in treated patients with LCHAD, TFP, or VLCAD deficiency, although overt clinical symptoms of deficiency are rarely documented.[19,81,88] Patients with long-chain FAO defects on low-fat diets are at high risk for essential fatty acid deficiency, and plasma fatty acids should be regularly monitored, preferably by a quantitative method.[89] Providing 4% of energy as linoleic acid and 0.6% as α-linolenic acid normalized the plasma levels of essential fatty acids in two children with VLCADD.[88] Therefore, saturated LCFA intake from prepared foods should be minimized, and the majority of the LCFA intake should be provided by oils rich in essential fatty acids. In addition to preventing deficiency of essential fatty acids, consuming more polyunsaturated fatty acids and decreasing consumption of saturated fat may lower plasma acylcarnitine concentrations. A study in cultured fibroblasts of patients with VLCAD, LCHAD, or TFP deficiency suggested that linoleic (18:2) and linolenic (18:3) acids produced significantly fewer acylcarnitines than oleic (18:1) and palmitic (16:0) acids.[90]

A specific deficiency of docosahexaenoic acid, or DHA (C22:6n-3) has been observed in some children with LCHAD, TFP, or VLCAD deficiency.[19,88,91] DHA is an essential component of cell membranes and is necessary for normal retinal and brain function. Whether the cause of the DHA deficiency is related to the low-fat diet or to poor synthesis of DHA from its precursor, α-linolenic acid, is not known. Supplementing children who have LCHAD, TFP, or VLCAD deficiency with preformed DHA (60 mg/day for infant and toddlers; 100 mg/day for children and teenagers) normalizes plasma DHA levels and may slow progression of pigmentary retinopathy and peripheral neuropathy in LCHAD/TFP deficiency.[21,92,93]

Treated children with LCHAD, TFP, or VLCAD deficiency may also be at risk for fat-soluble vitamin deficiency because of the low-fat diet. A review of the dietary intake of 10 children with LCHAD or TFP deficiency found adequate vitamin A and D intake related to the regular consumption of 2 to 3 cups of skim milk per day.[81] Skim milk provided a low-fat source of protein, B vitamins, and vitamins A and D; however, the intake of vitamins E and K was only about 50% of the recommended daily allowance (RDA). A daily multivitamin and mineral supplement providing the RDA for vitamins A, D, and E seems prudent for patients with LCHAD, TFP, or VLCAD deficiency on fat-restricted diets. Vitamin K is not routinely found in multivitamins, but no biochemical or clinical deficiencies of this micronutrient have been reported.

## Fatty Acid Oxidation During Exercise

At rest, skeletal muscle burns free fatty acids almost exclusively to provide 85% to 90% of total energy production.[94] During exercise, muscle glycogen stores provide the majority of energy during the initial 20 minutes. Thereafter, the ratio of energy from stored carbohydrate and fatty acids is dependent on the intensity of the exercise. At low or moderate exercise intensity, fatty acids provide as much as 60% of the required energy for exercise.[95] Patients with long-chain FAO disorders including VLCAD, LCHAD, TFP, and CPT-2 deficiencies often have recurrent episodes of exercise-induced rhabdomyolysis. Rhabdomyolysis may be related to an energy deficit in skeletal muscle resulting from the inability to oxidize LCFAs. Standard treatment has been a low-fat, high-carbohydrate diet designed to maximize energy production from glucose oxidation. Subjects with CPT-2 deficiency have been shown to have a lower heart rate and lower perceived exertion (Borg scale) with increased duration of exercise when given carbohydrates intravenously or orally before exercise.[96,97] Carbohydrates before and during exercise may help prevent the onset of exercise-induced rhabdomyolysis.

Alternatively, fatty acid supplements that bypass the block in long-chain FAO may prove to be beneficial. The use of MCT as a performance-enhancing energy substrate has been studied in athletes. Trained adult athletes given MCT while exercising oxidized 72% of the MCT dose during that bout of exercise.[98] Oral MCT is rapidly absorbed into the circulatory system (<20 minutes) and preferentially oxidized by liver and muscle.[99,100] MCT given immediately before exercise improved exercise tolerance in subjects with a long-chain FAO disorder.[101,102] Patients had significantly lower heart rates with higher ketone synthesis when given MCT before a moderate-intensity treadmill exercise test. Similarly, a case report found that MCT before exercise lowered muscle pain and the incidence of rhabdomyolysis in a patient with VLCAD deficiency.[103] Oral MCT supplementation with or without carbohydrates immediately before exercise may improve exercise tolerance among patients with VLCAD, LCHAD/TFP, or CPT-2 deficiency.

### B-Vitamin Supplementation

All of the acyl-CoA dehydrogenase enzymes utilize riboflavin as a cofactor. There are reports of patients with specific SCAD mutations responding to riboflavin supplementation. High doses of riboflavin (25 mg/day) appear to improve clinical symptoms in some, but not all, genotypes.[74,104] Niacin is the required cofactor for the LCHAD function of TFP and for HAD. However, there are no reports of improved residual enzyme activity with supplemental niacin, and there are no reports of niacin deficiency in these disorders. Niacin supplementation above normal requirements does not appear to be warranted.

## LIVER DISEASE IN PREGNANCY

Mothers carrying fetuses affected by certain FAO defects have a greater propensity toward late pregnancy complications, including preeclampsia, HELLP syndrome (hemolysis, elevated liver enzymes, and low platelets), and acute fatty liver of pregnancy (AFLP), when compared with the general population.[105–110] The incidence of maternal HELLP and AFLP is particularly high in mothers carrying fetuses with LCHAD/TFP deficiency, but it also has been documented in pregnancies in which the fetus was subsequently diagnosed with other FAO defects.[111–113] The cause of the toxicity of the affected fetus to the heterozygote mother is unknown, but studies suggest that the placenta performs substantial FAO and may produce toxic metabolites that are filtered into the mother's circulation.[114–116]

## CONCLUSION

Mitochondrial FAO disorders are a family of disorders characterized by hypoketotic hypoglycemia with fasting. Since the identification of the first FAO disorder in the 1980s, more than 22 different disorders have been described. The ability to diagnose affected infants was greatly improved with the advent of expanded NBS. Maternal liver disease during pregnancy results in significant morbidity and mortality in both mother and infant. Treatment of infants and children is based on nutrition interventions designed to decrease FAO and provide adequate energy. Research is underway to develop further understanding of the natural history of these disorders and future treatments.

### References


1. Vockley J, Singh RH, Whiteman DA. Diagnosis and management of defects of mitochondrial beta-oxidation. *Curr Opin Clin Nutr Metab Care.* 2002; 5:601.
2. Vockley J, Whiteman DA. Defects of mitochondrial beta-oxidation: a growing group of disorders. *Neuromuscul Disord,* 2002; 12:235.
3. Spiekerkoetter U, Lindner M, Santer R, et al. Management and outcome in 75 individuals with long-chain fatty acid oxidation defects: results from a workshop. *J Inherit Metab Dis.* 2009; 32:488.
4. Spiekerkoetter U. Mitochondrial fatty acid oxidation disorders: clinical presentation of long-chain fatty acid oxidation defects before and after newborn screening. *J Inherit Metab Dis.* 2010; 33:527.
5. Rinaldo P, Matern D, Bennett MJ. Fatty acid oxidation disorders. *Annu Rev Physiol.* 2002; 64:477.
6. Saudubray JM, Martin D, de Lonlay P, et al. Recognition and management of fatty acid oxidation defects: a series of 107 patients. *J Inherit Metab Dis.* 1999; 22:488.
7. Bonnet D, Martin D, De Lonlay P, et al. Arrhythmias and conduction defects as presenting symptoms of fatty acid oxidation disorders in children. *Circulation.* 1999; 100:2248.
8. Lindner M, Hoffmann GF, Matern D. Newborn screening for disorders of fatty-acid oxidation: experience and recommendations from an expert meeting. *J Inherit Metab Dis.* 2010; 33:521.
9. Brivet M, Boutron A, Slama A, et al. Defects in activation and transport of fatty acids. *J Inherit Metab Dis.* 1999; 22:428.
10. Lopriore E, Gemke RJ, Verhoeven NM, et al. Carnitine-acylcarnitine translocase deficiency: phenotype, residual enzyme activity and outcome. *Eur J Pediatr.* 2001; 160:101.
11. Gregersen N, Andresen BS, Corydon MJ, et al. Mutation analysis in mitochondrial fatty acid oxidation defects: exemplified by acyl-CoA dehydrogenase deficiencies, with special focus on genotype-phenotype relationship. *Hum Mutat.* 2001; 18:169.
12. Mathur A, Sims HF, Gopalakrishnan D, et al. Molecular heterogeneity in very-long-chain acyl-CoA dehydrogenase deficiency causing pediatric cardiomyopathy and sudden death. *Circulation.* 1999; 99:1337.
13. Strauss AW, Powell CK, Hale DE, et al. Molecular basis of human mitochondrial very-long-chain acyl-CoA dehydrogenase deficiency causing cardiomyopathy and sudden death in childhood. *Proc Natl Acad Sci U S A.* 1995; 92:10496.
14. Pons R, Cavadini P, Baratta S, et al. Clinical and molecular heterogeneity in very-long-chain acyl-coenzyme A dehydrogenase deficiency. *Pediatr Neurol.* 2000; 22:98.
15. Vianey-Saban C, Divry P, Brivet M, et al. Mitochondrial very-long-chain acyl-coenzyme A dehydrogenase deficiency: clinical characteristics and diagnostic considerations in 30 patients. *Clin Chim Acta.* 1998; 269:43.
16. Kluge S, Kuhnelt P, Block A, et al. A young woman with persistent hypoglycemia, rhabdomyolysis, and coma: recognizing fatty acid oxidation defects in adults. *Crit Care Med.* 2003; 31:1273.
17. Zia A, Kolodny EH, Pastores GM. Very long chain acyl-CoA dehydrogenase deficiency in a pair of mildly affected monozygotic twin sisters in their late fifties. *J Inherit Metab Dis.* 2007; 30:817.
18. Hoffman JD, Steiner RD, Paradise L, et al. Rhabdomyolysis in the military: recognizing late-onset very long-chain acyl Co-A dehydrogenase deficiency. *Mil Med.* 2006; 171:657.
19. Gillingham M, Van Calcar S, Ney D, Wolff J, Harding C. Dietary management of long-chain 3-hydroxyacyl-CoA dehydrogenase deficiency (LCHADD): a case report and survey. *J Inherit Metab Dis.* 1999; 22:123.
20. Fletcher AL, Pennesi ME, Harding CO, Weleber RG, Gillingham MB. Observations regarding retinopathy in mitochondrial trifunctional protein deficiencies. *Mol Genet Metab.* 2012; 106:18.
21. Gillingham MB, Weleber RG, Neuringer M, et al. Effect of optimal dietary therapy upon visual function in children with long-chain 3-hydroxyacyl CoA dehydrogenase and trifunctional protein deficiency. *Mol Genet Metab.* 2005; 86:124.
22. Horvath GA, Davidson AG, Stockler-Ipsiroglu SG, Lillquist YP, et al. Newborn screening for MCAD deficiency: experience of the first three years in British Columbia, Canada. *Can J Public Health.* 2008; 99:276.
23. Stanley CA, Hale DE, Coates PM, et al. Medium-chain acyl-CoA dehydrogenase deficiency in children with non-ketotic hypoglycemia and low carnitine levels. *Pediatr Res.* 1983; 17:877.
24. Wilcox RL, CC Nelson, P Stenzel, Steiner RD. Postmortem screening for fatty acid oxidation disorders by analysis of Guthrie cards with tandem mass spectrometry in sudden unexpected death in infancy. *J Pediatr.* 2002; 141:833.
25. Bennett MJ, Hale DE, Coates PM, Stanley CA. Postmortem recognition of fatty acid oxidation disorders. *Pediatr Pathol.* 1991; 11:365.
26. Kelly DP, Hale DE, Rutledge SL, et al. Molecular basis of inherited medium-chain acyl-CoA dehydrogenase deficiency causing sudden child death. *J Inherit Metab Dis.* 1992; 15:171.
27. Perper JA, Ahdab-Barmada M. Fatty liver, encephalopathy, and sudden unexpected death in early childhood due to medium-chain acyl-coenzyme A dehydrogenase deficiency. *Am J Forensic Med Pathol.* 1992; 13:329.
28. Yusupov R, Finegold DN, Naylor EW, et al. Sudden death in medium chain acyl-coenzyme a dehydrogenase deficiency (MCADD) despite newborn screening. *Mol Genet Metab.* 2010; 101:33.
29. Arnold GL, Saavedra-Matiz CA, Galvin-Parton PA, et al. Lack of genotype-phenotype correlations and outcome in MCAD deficiency diagnosed by newborn screening in New York State. *Mol Genet Metab.* 2010; 99:263.
30. Roe CR, Millington DS, Maltby DA, Kinnebrew P. Recognition of medium-chain acyl-CoA dehydrogenase deficiency in asymptomatic siblings of children dying of sudden infant death or Reye-like syndromes. *J Pediatr.* 1986; 108:13.
31. Marsden D. Expanded newborn screening by tandem mass spectrometry: the Massachusetts and New England experience. *Southeast Asian J Trop Med Public Health.* 2003; 34(Suppl 3):111.
32. Wilcken B, Haas M, Joy P, et al. Expanded newborn screening: outcome in screened and unscreened patients at age 6 years. *Pediatrics.* 2009; 124:e241.
33. Joy P, Black C, Rocca A, Haas M, Wilcken B. Neuropsychological functioning in children with medium chain acyl coenzyme a dehydrogenase deficiency (MCADD): the impact of early diagnosis and screening on outcome. *Child Neuropsychol.* 2009; 15:8.
34. Pollitt RJ, Leonard JV. Prospective surveillance study of medium chain acyl-CoA dehydrogenase deficiency in the UK. *Arch Dis Child.* 1998; 79:116.
35. Eaton S, Chatziandreou I, Krywawych S, Pen S, Clayton PT, Hussain K. Short-chain 3-hydroxyacyl-CoA dehydrogenase deficiency associated with hyperinsulinism: a novel glucose-fatty acid cycle? *Biochem Soc Trans.* 2003; 31(Pt 6):1137.
36. Molven A, Matre GE, Duran M, et al. Familial hyperinsulinemic hypoglycemia caused by a defect in the SCHAD enzyme of mitochondrial fatty acid oxidation. *Diabetes.* 2004; 53:221.
37. Li C, Chen P, Palladino A, et al. Mechanism of hyperinsulinism in short-chain 3-hydroxyacyl-CoA dehydrogenase deficiency involves activation of glutamate dehydrogenase. *J Biol Chem.* 2010; 285:31806.
38. Kapoor RR, James C, Flanagan SE, Ellard S, Eaton S, Hussain K. 3-Hydroxyacyl-coenzyme A dehydrogenase deficiency and hyperinsulinemic hypoglycemia: characterization of a novel mutation and severe dietary protein sensitivity. *J Clin Endocrinol Metab.* 2009; 94:2221.
39. Jones PM, Burlina AB, Bennett MJ. Quantitative measurement of total and free 3-hydroxy fatty acids in serum or plasma samples: short-chain 3-hydroxy fatty acids are not esterified. *J Inherit Metab Dis.* 2000; 23:745.
40. Treacy EP, Lambert DM, Barnes R, et al. Short-chain hydroxyacyl-coenzyme A dehydrogenase deficiency presenting as unexpected infant death: a family study. *J Pediatr.* 2000; 137:257.

41. Pedersen CB, Kolvraa S, Kolvraa A, et al. The ACADS gene variation spectrum in 114 patients with short-chain acyl-CoA dehydrogenase (SCAD) deficiency is dominated by missense variations leading to protein misfolding at the cellular level. *Hum Genet.* 2008; 124:43.
42. Gallant NM, Leydiker K, Tang H, et al. Biochemical, molecular, and clinical characteristics of children with short chain acyl-CoA dehydrogenase deficiency detected by newborn screening in California. *Mol Genet Metab.* 2012; 106:55.
43. Arens R, Gozal D, Jain K, et al. Prevalence of medium-chain acyl-coenzyme A dehydrogenase deficiency in the sudden infant death syndrome. *J Pediatr.* 1993; 122(5 Pt 1):715.
44. Brooks JG. Unraveling the mysteries of sudden infant death syndrome. *Curr Opin Pediatr.* 1993; 5:266.
45. Courts C, Madea B. Genetics of the sudden infant death syndrome. *Forensic Sci Int.* 2010; 203:25.
46. Hegyi T, Ostfeld B, Gardner K. Medium chain acyl-coenzyme A dehydrogenase deficiency and SIDS. *N J Med.* 1992; 89:385.
47. Holton JB, Allen JT, Green CA, Partington S, Gilbert RE, Berry PJ. Inherited metabolic diseases in the sudden infant death syndrome. *Arch Dis Child.* 1991; 66:1315.
48. Keppen LD, Randall B. Inborn defects of fatty acid oxidation: a preventable cause of SIDS. *S D J Med.* 1999; 52:187.
49. Lundemose JB, Kolvraa S, Gregersen N, Christensen E, Gregersen M., Fatty acid oxidation disorders as primary cause of sudden and unexpected death in infants and young children: an investigation performed on cultured fibroblasts from 79 children who died aged between 0-4 years. *Mol Pathol.* 1997; 50:212.
50. Miller ME, Brooks JG, Forbes N, Insel R. Frequency of medium-chain acyl-CoA dehydrogenase deficiency G-985 mutation in sudden infant death syndrome. *Pediatr Res.* 1992; 31(4 Pt 1):305.
51. Opdal SH, Rognum TO. Gene variants predisposing to SIDS: current knowledge. *Forensic Sci Med Pathol.* 2011; 7:26.
52. Boles RG, Buck EA, Blitzer MG, et al. Retrospective biochemical screening of fatty acid oxidation disorders in postmortem livers of 418 cases of sudden death in the first year of life. *J Pediatr.* 1998; 132:924.
53. Boles RG, Martin SK, Blitzer MG, Rinaldo P. Biochemical diagnosis of fatty acid oxidation disorders by metabolite analysis of postmortem liver. *Hum Pathol.* 1994; 25:735.
54. Chace DH, DiPerna JC, Mitchell BL, Sgroi B, Hofman LF, Naylor EW. Electrospray tandem mass spectrometry for analysis of acylcarnitines in dried postmortem blood specimens collected at autopsy from infants with unexplained cause of death. *Clin Chem.* 2001; 47:1166.
55. Rinaldo P, Yoon HR, Yu C, Raymond K, Tiozzo C, Giordano G. Sudden and unexpected neonatal death: a protocol for the postmortem diagnosis of fatty acid oxidation disorders. *Semin Perinatol.* 1999; 23:204.
56. Goddard P. Newborn screening for medium chain acyl-CoA dehydrogenase deficiency (MCADD) in the UK. *J Fam Health Care.* 2004; 14:90.
57. Kennedy S, Potter BK, Wilson K, et al. The first three years of screening for medium chain acyl-CoA dehydrogenase deficiency (MCADD) by newborn screening ontario. *BMC Pediatr.* 2010; 10:82.
58. Hintz SR, Matern D, Strauss A, et al. Early neonatal diagnosis of long-chain 3-hydroxyacyl coenzyme a dehydrogenase and mitochondrial trifunctional protein deficiencies. *Mol Genet Metab.* 2002; 75:120.
59. Matern D, Strauss AW, Hillman SL, Mayatepek E, Millington DS, Trefz FK. Diagnosis of mitochondrial trifunctional protein deficiency in a blood spot from the newborn screening card by tandem mass spectrometry and DNA analysis. *Pediatr Res.* 1999; 46:45.
60. Rinaldo P, Matern D. Disorders of fatty acid transport and mitochondrial oxidation: challenges and dilemmas of metabolic evaluation. *Genet Med.* 2000; 2:338.
61. Chace DH, Hillman SL, Van Hove JL, Naylor EW. Rapid diagnosis of MCAD deficiency: quantitative analysis of octanoylcarnitine and other acylcarnitines in newborn blood spots by tandem mass spectrometry. *Clin Chem.* 1997; 43:2106.
62. Arnold GL, Van Hove J, Freedenberg D, et al. A Delphi clinical practice protocol for the management of very long chain acyl-CoA dehydrogenase deficiency. *Mol Genet Metab.* 2009; 96:85.
63. Potter BK, Little J, Chakraborty P, et al. Variability in the clinical management of fatty acid oxidation disorders: results of a survey of Canadian metabolic physicians. *J Inherit Metab Dis.* 2012; 35:115.
64. Spiekerkoetter U, Lindner M, Santer R, et al. Treatment recommendations in long-chain fatty acid oxidation defects: consensus from a workshop. *J Inherit Metab Dis.* 2009; 32:498.
65. Bonnefont JP, Specola NB, Vassault A, et al. The fasting test in paediatrics: application to the diagnosis of pathological hypo- and hyperketotic states. *Eur J Pediatr.* 1990; 150:80.
66. Derks TG, van Spronsen FJ, Rake JP, van der Hilst CS, Span MM, Smit GP. Safe and unsafe duration of fasting for children with MCAD deficiency. *Eur J Pediatr.* 2007; 166:5.
67. Treem WR, Stanley CA, Goodman SI. Medium-chain acyl-CoA dehydrogenase deficiency: metabolic effects and therapeutic efficacy of long-term L-carnitine supplementation. *J Inherit Metab Dis.* 1989; 12:112.
68. Costa CG, Dorland L, de Almeida IT, Jakobs C, Duran M, Poll-The BT. The effect of fasting, long-chain triglyceride load and carnitine load on plasma long-chain acylcarnitine levels in mitochondrial very long-chain acyl-CoA dehydrogenase deficiency. *J Inherit Metab Dis.* 1998; 21:391.
69. Halldin MU, Forslund A, von Dobeln U, Eklund C, Gustafsson J. Increased lipolysis in LCHAD deficiency. *J Inherit Metab Dis.* 2007; 30:39.
70. Frazier D. *Nutrition Guidelines: Medium Chain Acyl CoA Dehydrogenase Deficiency (MCADD) OMIM 201450.* 2008. http://www.gmdi.org/Resources/Nutrition-Guidelines/MCAD. Accessed July 1, 2016.
71. Rohr F, Van Calcar S. Nutrition Guidelines: Very Long Chain Acyl CoA Dehydrogenase Deficiency (VLCADD) OMIM 201475. 2008. http://www.gmdi.org/Resources/Nutrition-Guidelines/VLCAD. Accessed July 1, 2016.
72. Birkebaek NH, Simonsen H, Gregersen N. Hypoglycaemia and elevated urine ethylmalonic acid in a child homozygous for the short-chain acyl-CoA dehydrogenase 625G>A gene variation. *Acta Paediatr.* 2002; 91:480.
73. Clayton PT, Eaton S, Aynsley-Green A, et al. Hyperinsulinism in short-chain L-3-hydroxyacyl-CoA dehydrogenase deficiency reveals the importance of beta-oxidation in insulin secretion. *J Clin Invest.* 2001; 108:457.
74. Tein I, Haslam RH, Rhead WJ, Bennett MJ, Becker LE, Vockley J. Short-chain acyl-CoA dehydrogenase deficiency: a cause of ophthalmoplegia and multicore myopathy. *Neurology.* 1999; 52:366.
75. Rinaldo P, Schmidt-Sommerfeld E, Posca AP, Heales SJ, Woolf DA, Leonard JV. Effect of treatment with glycine and L-carnitine in medium-chain acyl-coenzyme A dehydrogenase deficiency. *J Pediatr.* 1993; 122:580.
76. Schmidt-Sommerfeld E, Penn D, Kerner J, Bieber LL, Rossi TM, Lebenthal E. Quantitation of urinary carnitine esters in a patient with medium-chain acyl-coenzyme A dehydrogenase deficiency: effect of metabolic state and L-carnitine therapy. *J Pediatr.* 1989; 115:577.
77. Spiekerkoetter U, Bastin J, Gillingham M, Morris A, Wijburg F, Wilcken B. Current issues regarding treatment of mitochondrial fatty acid oxidation disorders. *J Inherit Metab Dis.* 2010; 33:555.
78. Brown-Harrison MC, Nada MA, Sprecher H, et al. Very long chain acyl-CoA dehydrogenase deficiency: successful treatment of acute cardiomyopathy. *Biochem Mol Med.* 1996; 58:59.
79. Cox GF, Souri M, Aoyama T, et al. Reversal of severe hypertrophic cardiomyopathy and excellent neuropsychologic outcome in very-long-chain acyl-coenzyme A dehydrogenase deficiency. *J Pediatr.* 1998; 133:247.
80. Bonnefont JP, Djouadi F, Prip-Buus C, Gobin S, Munnich A, Bastin J. Carnitine palmitoyltransferases 1 and 2: biochemical, molecular and medical aspects. *Mol Aspects Med.* 2004; 25:495.
81. Gillingham MB, Connor WE, Matern D, et al. Optimal dietary therapy of long-chain 3-hydroxyacyl-CoA dehydrogenase deficiency. *Mol Genet Metab.* 2003; 79:114.
82. Spiekerkotter U, Schwahn B, Korall H, Trefz FK, Andresen BS, Wendel U. Very-long-chain acyl-coenzyme A dehydrogenase (VLCAD) deficiency: monitoring of treatment by carnitine/acylcarnitine analysis in blood spots. *Acta Paediatr.* 2000; 89:492.
83. Duran M, Wanders RJ, de Jager JP, et al. 3-Hydroxydicarboxylic aciduria due to long-chain 3-hydroxyacyl-coenzyme A dehydrogenase deficiency associated with sudden neonatal death: protective effect of medium-chain triglyceride treatment. *Eur J Pediatr.* 1991; 150:190.
84. Moore R, Glasgow JF, Bingham MA, et al. Long-chain 3-hydroxyacyl-coenzyme A dehydrogenase deficiency: diagnosis, plasma carnitine fractions and management in a further patient. *Eur J Pediatr.* 1993; 152:433.
85. Van Hove JL, Kahler SG, Feezor MD, et al. Acylcarnitines in plasma and blood spots of patients with long-chain 3-hydroxyacyl-coenzyme A dehydrogenase defiency. *J Inherit Metab Dis.* 2000; 23:571.
86. Fahnehjelm KT, Holmstrom G, Ying L, et al. Ocular characteristics in 10 children with long-chain 3-hydroxyacyl-CoA dehydrogenase deficiency: a cross-sectional study with long-term follow-up. *Acta Ophthalmol.* 2008; 86:329.
87. Ficicioglu C, Hussa D. Very long-chain acyl-CoA dehydrogenase deficiency: the effects of accidental fat loading in a patient detected through newborn screening. *J Inherit Metab Dis.* 2009; 32(Suppl 1):S187.
88. Ruiz-Sanz JI, Aldamiz-Echevarria L, Arrizabalaga J, et al. Polyunsaturated fatty acid deficiency during dietary treatment of very long-chain acyl-CoA dehydrogenase deficiency: rescue with soybean oil. *J Inherit Metab Dis.* 2001; 24:493.
89. Lagerstedt SA, Hinrichs DR, Batt SM, Magera MJ, Rinaldo P, McConnell JP. Quantitative determination of plasma C8-C26 total fatty acids for the biochemical diagnosis of nutritional and metabolic disorders. *Mol Genet Metab.* 2001; 73:38.
90. Roe CR, Roe DS, Wallace M, Garritson B. Choice of oils for essential fat supplements can enhance production of abnormal metabolites in fat oxidation disorders. *Mol Genet Metab.* 2007; 92:346.
91. Harding CO, Gillingham MB, Van Calcar SC, Wolff JA, Verhoeve JN, Mills MD. Docosahexaenoic acid (DHA) and retinal function in children with long chain 3-hydroxyacyl-CoA dehydrogenase (LCHAD) deficiency. *J Inher Met Dis.* 1999; 22:276.
92. Harding C, Gillingham M, Vancalcar S, Wolff J, Verhoeve J, Mills M. *Effects of docosahexaenoic acid (DHA) supplementation upon retinal function in children with long chain 3-hydroxyacyl-CoA dehydrogenase deficiency.* 36th Annual Symposium of the Society for the Study of Inborn Errors of Metabolism, York, England; 1998.
93. Tein I, Vajsar J, MacMillan L, Sherwood WG. Long-chain L-3-hydroxyacyl-coenzyme A dehydrogenase deficiency neuropathy: response to cod liver oil. *Neurology.* 1999; 52:640.
94. Wahren J. Glucose turnover during exercise in man. *Ann N Y Acad Sci.* 1977; 301:45.
95. Romijn JA, Coyle EF, Sidossis LS, et al. Regulation of endogenous fat and carbohydrate metabolism in relation to exercise intensity and duration. *Am J Physiol.* 1993; 265(3 Pt 1):E380.
96. Orngreen MC, Ejstrup R, Vissing J. Effect of diet on exercise tolerance in carnitine palmitoyltransferase II deficiency. *Neurology.* 2003; 61:559.
97. Orngreen MC, Olsen DB, Vissing J. Exercise tolerance in carnitine palmitoyltransferase II deficiency with IV and oral glucose. *Neurology.* 2002; 59:1046.
98. Jeukendrup AE, Thielen JJ, Wagenmakers AJ, Brouns F, Saris WH. Effect of medium-chain triacylglycerol and carbohydrate ingestion during exercise on substrate utilization and subsequent cycling performance. *Am J Clin Nutr.* 1998; 67:397.
99. Odle J. New insights into the utilization of medium-chain triglycerides by the neonate: observations from a piglet model. *J Nutr.* 1997; 127:1061.
100. Odle J, Benevenga NJ, Crenshaw TD. Utilization of medium-chain triglycerides by neonatal piglets: chain length of even- and odd-carbon fatty acids and apparent digestion/absorption and hepatic metabolism. *J Nutr.* 1991; 121:605.

101. Gillingham MB, Scott B, Elliott D, Harding CO. Metabolic control during exercise with and without medium-chain triglycerides (MCT) in children with long-chain 3-hydroxy acyl-CoA dehydrogenase (LCHAD) or trifunctional protein (TFP) deficiency. *Mol Genet Metab.* 2006; 89:58.
102. Behrend AM, Harding CO, Shoemaker JD, et al. Substrate oxidation and cardiac performance during exercise in disorders of long chain fatty acid oxidation. *Mol Genet Metab.* 2011; 105:110.
103. Salmenniemi U, Ruotsalainen E, Pihlajamaki J, et al. Multiple abnormalities in glucose and energy metabolism and coordinated changes in levels of adiponectin, cytokines, and adhesion molecules in subjects with metabolic syndrome. *Circulation.* 2004; 110:3842.
104. Kmoch S, Zeman J, Hrebicek M, Ryba L, Kristensen MJ, Gregersen N. Riboflavin-responsive epilepsy in a patient with SER209 variant form of short-chain acyl-CoA dehydrogenase. *J Inherit Metab Dis.* 1995; 18:227.
105. Ibdah JA, Bennett MJ, Rinaldo P, et al. A fetal fatty-acid oxidation disorder as a cause of liver disease in pregnant women. *N Engl J Med.* 1999; 340:1723.
106. Isaacs JD Jr, Sims HF, Powell CK, et al. Maternal acute fatty liver of pregnancy associated with fetal trifunctional protein deficiency: molecular characterization of a novel maternal mutant allele. *Pediatr Res.* 1996; 40:393.
107. Schoeman MN, Batey RG, Wilcken B. Recurrent acute fatty liver of pregnancy associated with a fatty-acid oxidation defect in the offspring. *Gastroenterology.* 1991; 100:544.
108. Treem WR, Rinaldo P, Hale DE, et al. Acute fatty liver of pregnancy and long-chain 3-hydroxyacyl-coenzyme A dehydrogenase deficiency. *Hepatology.* 1994; 19:339.
109. Treem WR, Shoup ME, Hale DE, et al. Acute fatty liver of pregnancy, hemolysis, elevated liver enzymes, and low platelets syndrome, and long chain 3-hydroxyacyl-coenzyme A dehydrogenase deficiency [see comments]. *Am J Gastroenterol.* 1996; 91:2293.
110. Wilcken B, Leung KC, Hammond J, Kamath R, Leonard JV. Pregnancy and fetal long-chain 3-hydroxyacyl coenzyme A dehydrogenase deficiency. *Lancet.* 1993; 341:407.
111. Ibdah JA, Yang Z, Bennett MJ. Liver disease in pregnancy and fetal fatty acid oxidation defects. *Mol Genet Metab.* 2000; 71:182.
112. Matern D, Hart P, Murtha AP, et al. Acute fatty liver of pregnancy associated with short-chain acyl-coenzyme A dehydrogenase deficiency. *J Pediatr.* 2001; 138:585.
113. Nelson J, Lewis B, Walters B. The HELLP syndrome associated wiht fetal medium-chain acyl-CoA dehydrogenase deficiency. *J Inherit Metab Dis.* 2000; 23:518.
114. Rakheja D, Bennett MJ, Foster BM, Domiati-Saad R, Rogers BB. Evidence for fatty acid oxidation in human placenta, and the relationship of fatty acid oxidation enzyme activities with gestational age. *Placenta.* 2002; 23:447.
115. Shekhawat PS, Bennett MJ, Sadovsky Y, Nelson DM, Rakheja D, Strauss AW. Human placenta metabolizes fatty acids: implications for fetal fatty acid oxidation disorders and maternal liver diseases. *Am J Physiol Endocrinol Metab.* 2003; 284:E1098.
116. Shekhawat PS, Matern D, Strauss AW. Fetal fatty acid oxidation disorders, their effect on maternal health and neonatal outcome: impact of expanded newborn screening on their diagnosis and management. *Pediatr Res.* 2005; 57:78R.

# 47 Mitochondrial Disorders

RICHARD BOLES AND KATHRYN MOSELEY

The mitochondrial disorders represent a very large number of distinct inborn errors of metabolism. Mitochondrial medicine is exceedingly complex. Mitochondrial disease is highly variable in terms of degree of severity, age at onset, organ or tissue involvement, and mode of inheritance. In terms of severity and age at onset, mitochondrial disease can cause every degree of illness from migraine headaches in an adult to lethal multisystem disease in an infant. In terms of organ or tissue involvement, energy is a universal cellular requirement, so essentially any organ or tissue can fail and result in disease. However, because disease manifestations occur in general when the local energy supply is inadequate to meet the local energy demand, disorders of those tissues with the highest energy requirements usually predominate (i.e., nerve, muscle, endocrine gland, and renal tubular epithelium). [1,2] Because diseases of brain and muscle often predominate, mitochondrial disorders are often referred to as *encephalomyopathies*.[1,3–5]

Mitochondrial disorders result from defects (mutations) in genes that encode proteins affecting cellular energy metabolism, including genes encoded by the nuclear DNA as well as the mitochondrial DNA (mtDNA).[1,6] Mitochondrial disorders resulting from mutations in nuclear genes can follow essentially any mode of inheritance, autosomal recessive inheritance being common in young children. Mutations in mtDNA genes are usually maternally inherited. In families with autosomal dominant and maternally inherited defects of mtDNA, intrafamilial and extrafamilial variability is usually very broad, even for the same mutation in the same gene. Some of the common and uncommon mitochondria-associated disease manifestations are listed in Table 47–1. In general, disease is more likely to strike at times of stress—that is, at times when energy demands are high, such as fasting, exercise, illness, and psychological stress.

## FACTORS TO BE CONSIDERED IN THE NUTRITION EVALUATION

The purposes of the nutrition evaluation are as follows:

- To identify and remove diet-related triggers that exacerbate clinical illness
- To provide dietary therapy for any disorders that arise secondary to the mitochondrial disease
- To prevent fasting
- To provide essential nutrition and trace nutritional needs
- To provide cofactor therapy as a potential primary mitochondrial treatment, including antioxidants

## DIETARY MANAGEMENT

Restrictive diets that are standard therapy for other metabolic diseases are rarely effective in the treatment of mitochondrial disorders. Because the metabolic block is typically at the level of the electron transport chain, essentially *all* nutrients enter the pathway before the block[7,8] (Fig. 47–1). A potential exception is pyruvate dehydrogenase deficiency, which may respond to restriction of carbohydrates.[9–13]

Families often report that certain events trigger acute episodes of increased symptomatology in their affected children. Children quickly learn to avoid foods that make them feel ill but frequently fail to communicate this need. Triggers can be diverse, including multiple dietary factors.

Fasting intolerance occurs in an undetermined proportion of children with mitochondrial disease but can be severe. By inducing a shift in several metabolic pathways toward catabolism, fasting adversely affects energy demand as well as energy supply. Fasting can result in disease manifestations in the presence or absence of hypoglycemia, and the results can be catastrophic, including stroke, cardiomyopathy, or sudden death. In practical terms, children with proven or suspected mitochondrial disease who are unable to take calories by mouth because of nausea or vomiting should be tube-fed or hospitalized for intravenous nutrition until they can demonstrate adequate caloric intake. In addition, patients undergoing a medical or surgical procedure should receive intravenous calories before, during, and after the procedure (Box 47–1).

A controversial area is the appropriate dietary fat content. Some providers prescribe an empirical trial of a low-fat and/or high-fat diet, possibly including medium-chain triglyceride (MCT) oil,[14] but

**Table 47–1.** Tissues with High and Moderate Energy Requirements and Some Specific Disease Manifestations Seen in Children with Mitochondrial Disease

| Tissue | Disease Manifestations |
|---|---|
| *High Energy Requirement* | |
| Nerve | |
| Cerebral cortex | Mental retardation, seizures |
| Cerebellum | Ataxia |
| Basal ganglia | Chorea, dystonia |
| Brain stem | Apnea, vomiting |
| Retina | Pigmentary retinopathy, optic atrophy |
| Cochlea | Sensorineural hearing loss |
| Peripheral nerve | Peripheral neuropathy |
| Autonomic nerve | Dysautonomia, gastrointestinal dysmotility |
| Muscle | |
| Large skeletal muscles | Hypotonia, weakness |
| Extraocular muscles | Eye muscle weakness, ptosis |
| Cardiac muscle | Cardiomyopathy, arrhythmia |
| Smooth muscle | Gastrointestinal dysmotility |
| Endocrine gland | |
| Thyroid | Hypothyroidism |
| Islets of Langerhans | Diabetes mellitus |
| Adrenal | Addison disease |
| Pituitary | Growth hormone deficiency, hypoglycemia |
| Kidney | |
| Tubular epithelium | Acidosis, Fanconi amino and organic aciduria |
| *Moderate Energy Requirement* | |
| Hematological | |
| Bone marrow | Anemia, neutropenia, low platelet count |
| Exocrine gland | |
| Liver parenchyma | Liver failure, hypoglycemia |
| Exocrine pancreas | Pancreatitis |
| Kidney | |
| Nephron | Renal failure |

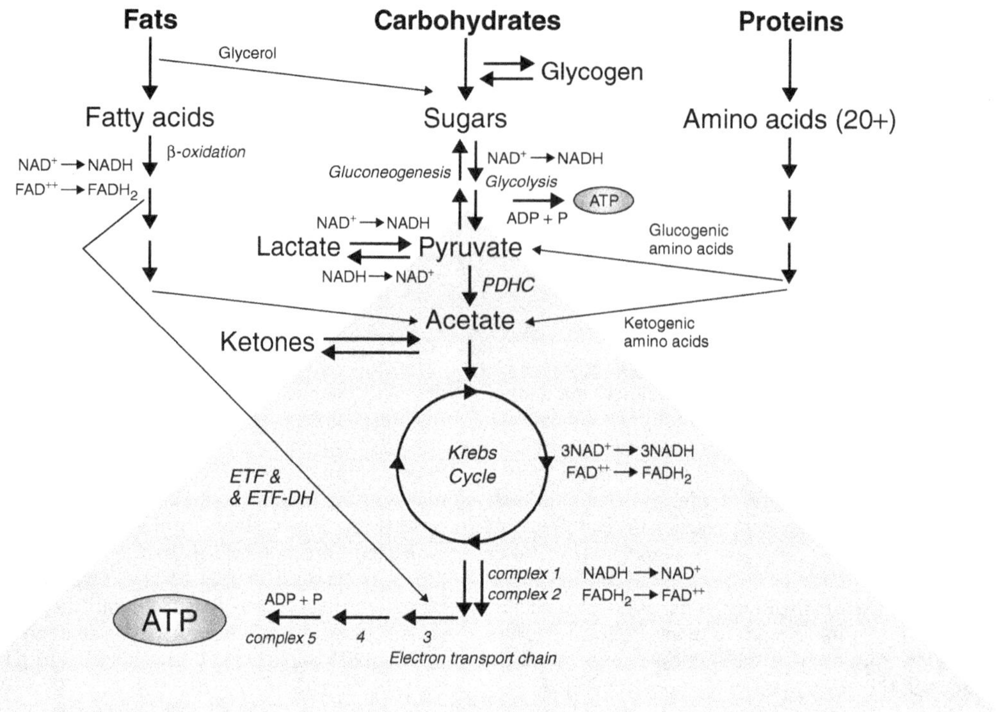


**Figure 47–1.** Simplified map of energy metabolism showing the major fates of fats, carbohydrates, and proteins as related to cellular energy metabolism. The large shaded triangle denotes metabolic steps that are affected by defects associated with the mitochondrial disorders. Mitochondrial disorders involve the final common pathway of fat, carbohydrate, and protein metabolism, and this pathway accounts for most of the cellular adenosine triphosphate (ATP) produced. ADP = adenosine diphosphate; ETF = electron transfer flavoprotein; FAD = flavin adenine dinucleotide; NAD = nictotinamide adenine dinucleotide; PDHC = pyruvate dehydrogenase complex.

in our experience, high-fat meals are often not tolerated because they worsen gastrointestinal dysmotility. Even less is known about the effect of high levels of dietary simple sugars in mitochondrial disease, although some patients report a postprandial lack of energy and other symptoms,[15] and intolerance to dietary fructose has been reported in some.[16] Some patients demonstrate persistent intolerance to all but highly elemental formulas (authors' unpublished observations).

Conditions that are common in children with mitochondrial disorders include growth retardation, obesity, gastrointestinal dysmotility, abdominal pain, and vomiting.[17–20] Each of these conditions can occur secondary to a wide range of medical and nutrition-related conditions. For example, asymmetrical growth failure can occur secondary to neurological or gastrointestinal disease, in which case it often responds to increased caloric intake and/or enteral tube placement. However, in a child with symmetrical growth retardation due to an endocrine cause or secondary to the defective energy metabolism itself, those management interventions can result in obesity, not increased linear growth.Note that low muscle mass, which is common in these patients, results in a reduced weight and a child can

**Box 47–1.** Potential Dietary Management Strategies in Children with Mitochondrial Disease Aimed at Preventing or Limiting Fasting*

If there is a history of fasting-related complications including fatigue, decreased concentration, abdominal pain, vomiting, or headache:

1. Provide low glycemic index, possibly high-protein snacks between meals and before retiring at night.
2. Provide a substantial breakfast (low-fat in the presence of gastrointestinal dysmotility).
3. Control overall calories consumed to prevent metabolic decompensation (low caloric intake) or obesity (high caloric intake).

If oral intake is severely decreased due to acute viral illness:

1. Provide snacks and juices frequently to avoid significant fasting or dehydration.
2. Perform clinical and laboratory evaluation and treatment if the patient has significant vomiting, altered mental status, a "small" or higher level of ketones on urine dipstick, or other worrisome findings or is unable to take 50% of the usual calories for 2 or more days.
   a. In the emergency department, perform rapid placement of an intravenous (IV) catheter with delivery of 10% dextrose-containing IV fluid (usually D10 0.45% saline) at 1.5 times the maintenance rate; higher dextrose infusions may cause lactic acidosis; consider fluid boluses for dehydration.
   b. Recommended laboratory tests include blood sodium, potassium, chloride, bicarbonate, urea nitrogen, glucose, and complete blood count with differential, as well as urine dipstick (mostly for ketones and specific gravity).
   c. Consider urine microscopic examination, serum lipase, liver enzymes, creatine kinase, and urine organic acids.
3. The ability to tolerate adequate feedings in order to prevent fasting is an important consideration in the decision regarding hospital admission and discharge.

For elective medical or surgical procedure requiring fasting:

1. If the patient tolerates overnight fasting without incident, it is usually acceptable to place him or her on "no oral intake" status after midnight following a late high-starch snack.
2. The patient should proceed to outpatient surgery early in the morning and have an IV catheter placed with delivery of D10 0.45% saline at 1.5 times the maintenance rate before, during, and after the procedure until the patient can tolerate oral feedings.

*This table is designed to assist the clinician after completion of a full evaluation; it is not intended to dictate clinical management or to apply to all cases. The parameters given are approximate and anecdotal; they are based on clinical experience, not experimental data. Individuals with mitochondrial disease and the situations they encounter are highly variable, and individual clinical judgment cannot be substituted.

**Table 47–2.** Cofactor and Vitamin Supplements That Have Been Advocated in the Treatment of Mitochondrial Disease

| Supplement | Empirically Recommended Dose Range Obtained from Several Sources* | Prescribed by Present Author for Age >5 Yr† |
|---|---|---|
| Coenzyme $Q_{10}$ | 30–300 mg/day; 2–15 mg/kg/day (10 mg/kg/day is an often used dose) | Frequently 200–300 mg BID or 20 mg/kg/day, and titrated until blood level is > 4 mg/L |
| Vitamin B complex | One tablet daily (often B-50 or B-100 complex) | Frequently one B-100 tablet daily; B-50 in small children |
| Carnitine | 50–200 mg/kg/day divided TID; frequently used adult dose is 1 g TID | Frequently 1000 mg BID or 100 mg/kg/day |
| Riboflavin (vitamin $B_2$) | 50–200 mg/day; in one source, up to 600 mg/day (a component of B-50 complex) | Often 100 mg by itself (often given as part of a B complex) |
| Creatine | 5–10 g/day; 0.1–0.2 g/kg/day | Occasionally as 2.5–5 g BID |
| Vitamin C | 100–500 mg/day; 25–57 mg/kg/day; divided doses often recommended | Frequently at 250–500 mg BID |
| Vitamin E | 200–400 mg/day; divided doses often recommended | Frequently at 200 mg BID |
| Thiamine (vitamin $B_1$) | 50–300 mg/day; in one source, up to 900 mg/day (a component of B-50 complex) | Rarely by itself (usually given as part of a B complex) |
| Pyridoxine (vitamin $B_6$) | 50 mg (a component of B-50 complex) | Rarely by itself |
| Cobalamin (vitamin $B_{12}$), hydroxy-vitamin $B_{12}$ | 0.05–1 mg daily; injected dose (an oral component of B-50 complex) | Rarely by itself |
| Biotin | 2.5–20 mg/day (a component of B-50 complex) | Rarely by itself |
| Folic acid | 0.4–10 mg/day (a component of B-50 complex) | Rarely by itself |
| Nicotinamide (vitamin $B_3$) | 50–100 mg/day | Occasionally |
| α-Lipoic acid | 60–200 mg divided TID; 10–12.5 mg/kg/day | Frequently at 200 mg BID; half dose in young children |
| Selenium | 25–50 μg/day | No |
| Acetyl-L-Carnitine | 250–1000 mg/day | No |
| Menadione ($K_3$) | 5–80 mg/day; 1.1–1.5 mg/kg/day | No |
| Succinate | 6 g/day | No |
| Uridine | 0.2–1.0 g/kg/day divided TID; adult dose 4–20 g; start at lower end | No |
| Idebenone (a coenzyme Q analog) | 90–225 mg/day | Not easily available in US |

*Data from Shoffner,[1] Chinnery and Turnbull,[15] Gold and Cohen,[14] Naviaux,[19] Gillis and Kaye,[20] and the authors' clinical practice. The present authors do not attest to the safety or efficacy of listed dosages, and very few data are available.

†Prescribing patterns vary widely among mitochondrial disease specialists, although coenzyme $Q_{10}$, carnitine, and a riboflavin-containing source (i.e., B-50 or B-100 complex) are widely used. The present authors assay carnitine levels in all cases of known or suspected mitochondrial disease and prescribe supplementation if the free carnitine level is low. Other supplements are often given, depending on the individual cases. In particular, dosing in infants is much lower than that listed.

falsely appear to be failure-to-thrive if fat stores are not assessed on physical examination

Because activity levels can be low in these frequently handicapped children, obesity is often encountered. Weight reduction diets are problematic in children with fasting intolerance, although mild caloric restriction coupled with moderate exercise and close follow-up is often successful. Several studies have demonstrated the benefits of endurance exercise in children with mitochondrial disease, which include increased mitochondrial content, antioxidant and muscle enzyme activity, increased oxygen uptake, and increased peripheral muscle strength, as well as lower lactate levels.[21] However, because of the common presence of neuromuscular disease and exercise intolerance, both progressive and resistance exercise should start at a low intensity level and be supervised.

For children with dysmotility, low-fat diets, frequent small meals, fruits and fiber, and/or medications are helpful in many cases. Abdominal pain may occur secondary to constipation, pancreatitis, and abdominal migraine/cyclic vomiting syndrome, all of which have prominent dietary components in their management. Cyclic vomiting consists of acute episodes of nausea, vomiting, headache, abdominal pain, lethargy, and/or diarrhea separated by periods devoid of these symptoms.[22,23] Treatment is can be highly effective and includes fasting avoidance, frequent snacks, and a moderately low-fat diet.

Empirically, many patients with a variety of mitochondrial disorders clinically improve on diets with moderate to high protein content. This is most commonly seen in hospitalized patients on dextrose only, for whom the addition of partial (or total) parental nutrition with 1.5 to 2 g protein per kilogram body weight per day is associated with improvement. Trace minerals such as magnesium, zinc, and selenium are also required for mitochondrial function, and some patients benefit from their addition either enterally or parenterally.

Although there are few to no related hard data, supplementation with various cofactors (Table 47–2) is frequently advocated in the treatment of specific mitochondrial disorders and for all patients with mitochondrial disease in general.[3,16–18] The evidence supporting the use of coenzyme $Q_{10}$ is better than that concerning the other cofactors. The presence of increased reactive oxygen species in mitochondrial disease is increasingly being recognized as a cause of pathology, and expert providers are adding antioxidant therapies to their recommendations for cofactor therapy (as part of a treatment "cocktail"). Because next-generation (high-throughput) DNA sequencing of all genes encoding mitochondrial proteins is now available, decisions regarding cofactors and other aspects of therapy are becoming less generic and more targeted to the specific genetic abnormalities in individual patients.

## References


1. Shoffner JM. Oxidative phosphorylation diseases. In: Scriver CR, Beaudet AL, Sly WS, et al., eds. *The Metabolic and Molecular Bases of Inherited Disease*, 8th ed. New York: McGraw-Hill; 2001.
2. Neiberger RE, George JC, Perkins LA, Theriaque DW, Hutson AD, Stacpoole PW. Renal manifestations of congenital lactic acidosis. *Am J Kidney Dis.* 2002; 39:12.
3. Schapira AH, Cock HR. Mitochondrial myopathies and encephalomyopathies. *Eur J Clin Invest.* 1999; 10:886.
4. DiMauro S, Bonilla E. Mitochondrial encephalomyopathies. In: Rosenberg RN, Prusiner SB, DiMauro S, Barci RI, eds. *The Molecular and Genetic Basis of Neurological Disease*. Boston: Butterworth-Heinemann, 1997.
5. Oldfors A, Tulinius M. Mitochondrial encephalomyopathies. *J Neuropathol Exp Neurol.* 2003; 62:217.
6. *MITOMAP: A Human Mitochondrial Genome Database*. Last revised June 2016. http://www.mitomap.org/MITOMAP. Accessed July 1, 2016.
7. Przyrembel H. Therapy of mitochondrial disorders. *J Inherit Metab Dis.* 1987; 10:129.
8. Gropman AL. Diagnosis and treatment of childhood mitochondrial diseases. *Curr Neurol Neurosci Rep.* 2001; 1:185.
9. Weber TA, Antognetti MR, Stacpoole PW. Caveats when considering ketogenic diets for the treatment of pyruvate dehydrogenase complex deficiency. *J Pediatr.* 2001; 138:390.
10. Wexler ID, Hemalatha SC, McConnell J, et al. Outcome of pyruvate dehydrogenase deficiency treated with ketogenic diets: studies in patients with identical mutations. *Neurology.* 1997; 49:1655.
11. Cederbaum SD, Blass JP, Minkoff N, Brown WJ, Cotton ME, Harris SH. Sensitivity to carbohydrate in a patient with familial intermittent lactic acidosis and pyruvate dehydrogenase deficiency. *Pediatr Res.* 1976; 8:713.

12. Ahmad A, Kahler SC, Kishnani PS, et al. Treatment of pyruvate carboxylase deficiency with high doses of citrate and aspartate. *Am J Med Genet.* 1999; 4:331.
13. Kerr DS, Wexler ID, Zinn AB. Disorders of pyruvate metabolism and the tricarboxylic acid cycle. In: Fernandes K, Saudubray JM, van den Berghe G, Walter JH, eds. *Inborn Metabolic Diseases: Diagnosis and Treatment.* New York: Springer-Verlag, 2000; 3:124.
14. Gold DR, Cohen BH. Treatment of mitochondrial cytopathies. *Semin Neurol.* 2001; 21:309.
15. Chinnery PF, Turnbull M. Epidemiology and treatment of mitochondrial disorders. *Am J Med Genet.* 2001; 106:94.
16. Haas RH, Barshop BA. Diet change in the management of metabolic encephalomyopathies. *Biofactors.* 1998; 7:259.
17. Cohen BH. Mitochondrial cytopathies: a primer. June 2000. Pittsburg, PA: United Mitochondrial Disease Foundatation. http://www.umdf.org/site/c.jtJWJaMMIsE/b.4090399/. Accessed July 1, 2016.
18. Pons R, De Vivo DC. Mitochondrial disease. *Curr Treat Options Neurol.* 2000; 3:271.
19. Naviaux RK. The spectrum of mitochondrial disease. In: Weber K, ed. *Mitochondrial and Metabolic Disorders: A Primary Care Physician's Guide.* Psy-Ed Corp., Oradell, NJ; 1997.
20. Gillis L, Kaye E. Diagnosis and management of mitochondrial diseases. *Pediatr Gastroenterol Nutr.* 2002; 49:203.
21. Boles RG, Adams K, Masamichi I, Li BUK. Maternal inheritance in cyclic vomiting syndrome with neuromuscular disease. *Am J Med Genet.* 2003; 120A(4): 474.
22. Parikh S, Saneto R, Falk M, et al. A modern approach to the treatment of mitochondrial disease. *Pediatr Neurol.* 2009; 11:414.
23. Li BUK. Cyclic vomiting: the pattern and syndrome paradigm. *J Pediatr Gastroenterol Nutr.* 1999; 21(Suppl 1):S6.

# D.

# DISORDERS OF CARBOHYDRATE METABOLISM

## 48 Type 1 and Type 2 Diabetes

AMY FULLER AND CYNTHIA STEGEMAN

Diabetes is the seventh leading cause of death in the United States and can be diagnosed in early childhood as well as throughout adulthood.[1] In 2012, a total of 29.1 million children and adults, or 9.3% of the US population, had diabetes, including 8.1 million who were undiagnosed. Seventy-five percent of individuals diagnosed with type 1 diabetes are 18 years and younger.[2] In addition, 79 million people had prediabetes. According to the Centers for Disease Control and Prevention, the prevalence of type 2 diabetes in those younger than 20 years of age will quadruple in the next 40 years.

The costs associated with diabetes in the United States were estimated to be $245 billion in 2012. This includes $176 billion in direct costs and $69 billion in reduced productivity. Health care costs for a person with diabetes are 2.3 times greater than those for a person without diabetes.[1]

In addition to its financial costs, diabetes has a detrimental effect on the quality of life. The undesirable effects of diabetes on health are manifold. Individuals with diabetes are almost two times more likely to have a heart attack or stroke than those without diabetes. More than 50% of nontraumatic lower-limb amputations among people aged 20 years or older occur in those with diagnosed diabetes. Diabetes is a leading cause of blindness in adults, and more than one-third of kidney failure cases are caused by diabetes.[1]

### DEFINITION

Type 1 diabetes (T1DM) involves immune-mediated destruction of functional pancreatic beta-cell mass, with serum beta-cell autoimmunity found in the majority of cases. Insulin is always indicated, even when there is residual insulin secretory capacity at the time of diagnosis. It is difficult to predict the overall dietary intake of children younger than 4 years of age. For that reason, bolus insulin may be administered after the meal is consumed. Otherwise, for both T1DM and T2DM, pharmacological treatment in children typically does not differ from that in adults.[2]

Type 2 (T2DM) diabetes is a chronic condition that involves insulin resistance and elevated blood glucose (BG) after years of reduced hepatic and skeletal muscle insulin sensitivity that is compensated by increased pancreatic insulin secretion. T2DM may be managed with diet (medical nutrition therapy [MNT]) and exercise or with MNT, exercise, and oral medication. Insulin may be needed in some patients to obtain best results. Information on exercise can be found in Chapter 7.

### TYPE 1 DIABETES

#### Clinical and Biochemical Abnormalities

T1DM manifests with the rapid clinical development of polyuria, polydipsia, polyphagia, and weight loss. Microvascular, neurological, and macrovascular complications are common as the disease progresses, although when optimal BG control is maintained, the incidence of these complications is reduced.

A classic study, The Diabetes Control and Complications Trial, reported advantages and disadvantages of tight BG control (as

**Box 48–1.** Example of Tight Blood Glucose Control

Blood glucose level before a meal: 70–120 mg/dL
Blood glucose level 2 hours after a meal: <180 mg/dL
Hemoglobin $A_{1C}$: <6.05%*

*Hemoglobin $A_{1C}$ should be measured at least twice a year, more often if blood glucose levels are not in the target range.

Adapted from The Diabetes Control and Complication Trial Research Group. The effect of intensive treatment of diabetes on the development and progression of long-term complications in insulin dependent diabetes mellitus. *N Engl J Med.* 1993; 14:977.

exemplified in Box 48–1). Tight control has been shown to delay the onset of albuminuria and some measures of diabetic retinopathy and neuropathy.[3] However, achieving these standards requires close monitoring of BG and multiple daily doses of insulin. Although newer insulins and delivery methods make BG control less labor intensive, the main risks of hypoglycemia and weight gain remain. Patients, and often their families, may find this treatment method overwhelming. Patients must work with their practitioner to best determine their own BG goals and methods of treatment.

Tight control is not recommended for children, older adults, those who struggle with frequent bouts of hypoglycemia, or those patients who have heart disease, blood vessel disease, or severe diabetes complications, because hypoglycemia may cause strokes and heart attacks.[4,5]

## Components of Treatment

All individuals with diabetes should be directed to seek comprehensive care from a multidisciplinary team of diabetes experts to incorporate therapeutic lifestyle behavior changes. This team can consist of a primary care physician, endocrinologist, nurse practitioner, physician's assistant, nurse, dietitian, pharmacist, exercise specialist, and mental health professionals. For successful ongoing management of diabetes, it is also essential for the individual with diabetes to take an active role in their own care.[6]

The treatment goal for T1DM is to maintain BG values that are near normal. This can be achieved through an insulin regimen that simulates normal physiology by combining basal and meal-related doses:

1. Most people with T1DM should be treated with multiple daily injections or with continuous subcutaneous insulin infusion.
   a. Self-monitoring of BG may need to be performed:
      - Before meals and snacks (preprandial)
      - Before the insulin injection
      - Occasional postprandial
      - Bedtime
      - Before exercise
      - Sick days
      - Travel days
      - Before potential life-threatening activities (e.g., driving)
      - Middle of the night
      - More often when there are many episodes of hypoglycemia
      - When low BG levels are suspected[2,6]
2. Most people with T1DM should be educated about how to match the prandial insulin dose to carbohydrate intake, premeal BG level, and anticipated activity.
3. Most people with T1DM should use insulin analogs to reduce hypoglycemia risk.[6]

Youth and adults with T1DM, as well as their parents or caregivers, should receive culturally sensitive and developmentally appropriate individualized knowledge, skills, and abilities as part of diabetes self-management education (DSME) to empower diabetes self-care. In addition, diabetes self-management support (DSMS) encourages application and assistance of coping skills and the behaviors needed to self-manage on an ongoing basis. Both DSME and DSMS are to be provided to patients according to national standards when their diabetes is diagnosed and routinely thereafter.[6]

The patient must be taught the mechanics of administering insulin; the action of the insulin; monitoring of BG, food composition, and food portion sizes; and the skill of assessing what specific BG readings really mean. The patient is encouraged to actively change insulin doses to match the circumstances of daily life. The health-care team empowers the patient and family to make decisions regarding insulin doses for sick days, for variable carbohydrate intake, and for times of exercise. The initial instructions include teaching the function of insulin and its interaction with carbohydrate as well as the mechanics of drawing up insulin into syringes and testing BG levels with a meter. The instruction then advances to adjusting insulin for elevated BG levels with and without ketones, for the insulin:carbohydrate ratio, and for various intensities of exercise. The patient and, if needed, the caregiver, guide the pace of skill and knowledge advancement. Certified diabetes educators (CDE) are charged with teaching therapeutic lifestyle skills, providing individualized instruction on the newest and most reliable technologies available to patients, and matching the recommendations to the ability of the patient and his or her support system.

## Factors To Be Considered in Nutrition Evaluation and Nutritional Management

The American Diabetes Association's 2015 goals for MNT for diabetes for adults are as follows[6]:

1. To promote and support healthful eating patterns, emphasizing a variety of nutrient-dense foods in appropriate portion sizes, in order to improve overall health and specifically to
   - Attain individualized glycemic, blood pressure, and lipid goals
   - Achieve and maintain body weight goals
   - Delay or prevent complications of diabetes
2. To address individual nutrition needs based on personal and cultural preferences, health literacy and numeracy, access to healthful food choices, willingness and ability to make behavioral changes, and barriers to change.
3. To maintain the pleasure of eating by providing positive messages about food choices while limiting food choices only when indicated by scientific evidence.
4. To provide the individual with diabetes with practical tools for day-to-day meal planning rather than focusing on individual macronutrients, micronutrients, or single foods.

For children, nutrition management starts with assessing the caloric needs of the patient to optimize growth. Reviewing usual food patterns that have allowed for optimal growth is usually the best way to determine the child's needs. Calorie, protein, fat, micronutrient (vitamins and minerals), fiber, and fluid needs for children with diabetes do not differ from those of other children, so formulations for nutritional needs based on age, gender, and height or weight can be used to complement the usual food patterns described by the patient to determine caloric needs. For adults, caloric needs are based on the need for weight loss, gain, or maintenance.

The patient should be taught food portion sizes to provide the best possible estimate of the carbohydrate content of foods. This instruction needs to include typical foods eaten both at home and away from home. When patients have mastered the skill of carbohydrate counting, they should be instructed to keep their calorie and carbohydrate intake consistent with respect to time for a few weeks. The meal-related bolus insulin dose is calibrated to the consistent carbohydrate intake and provides near-normal BG levels. One way of counting carbohydrate intake is the electronic food diary. Close contact via phone or personal visits is required to plan the needed changes in insulin doses to achieve the goal of near-normal BG values. BG monitoring before meals and 2-hour postprandial readings are necessary to determine the fine adjustments for meal-related insulin doses.

Once a close estimate of the insulin dose has been made, the patient can be taught how to calculate insulin:carbohydrate ratios, allowing for more flexibility in choosing meal amounts and composition. These ratios should be used only for people with T1DM. A common method for adjusting insulin is the following:

*Insulin:carbohydrate ratio* (for Humalog and Novolog): 500 divided by the total usual insulin dose = the number of grams of carbohydrate corresponding to each unit of insulin taken.

*Sensitivity factor:* 1800 divided by the total usual insulin dose = the estimated amount by which BG would be lowered by 1 unit of insulin (Lispro). Use 1500 divided by the total usual insulin dose if Regular insulin is used.

*Activity factor:* These two calculations can be fine-tuned by BG readings obtained from the patient and differ for each meal according to circadian rhythms. These readings allow the child to check the BG value, choose what to eat, and administer an insulin dose that will return the BG value to near-normal. For example, if the target BG level is 120 mg/dL, the present GB is 220 mg/dL, and the correction factor is 50, the dose of insulin needed to correct for the high BG is 2 units ([220 – 120] ÷ 50). If the insulin:carbohydrate ratio is 15 g carbohydrate for each 1 unit of insulin and the carbohydrate composition of the meal to be eaten is 60 g, then 4 units of insulin is administered (60 ÷ 15). The 2 units of insulin needed for the elevated BG value is added to the 4 units for the carbohydrate meal to achieve a near-normal blood sugar and a chosen lifestyle.

According to the American Diabetes Association position statement 2015, "carbohydrate intake from vegetables, fruits, whole grains, legumes, and dairy products should be advised over intake from other carbohydrates, especially those that contain added fats, sugars, or sodium. Substituting low glycemic-load foods for higher glycemic-load foods may modestly improve glycemic control."[6] A food's glycemic load is determined by multiplying its glycemic index (considered low if <55 out of 100) by the amount of carbohydrate per serving it contains and divided by 100. The glycemic indices are calculated on individual foods, and the glycemic effect of a food changes when combined with another food at a meal (e.g., when butter is added to yams, the glycemic index is lower than when yams are eaten alone). Harvard Health Publications, February 3, 2015, provides a list of 100+ foods and their glycemic index and glycemic load; some examples are provided in Table 48-1.[7] However, monitoring of the glycemic load of foods is a controversial topic.

## Follow-up and Summary

Management of T1DM affects the everyday life of the patient and the family, and both should receive DSME and DSMS from a health care provider with an expertise in diabetes, preferably a CDE. Controlling BG levels in relation to extra exercise, varying amounts of food, sick days, or travel days requires complex analytical skills. Cultural eating patterns and the need for children and teens to conform to their peers must be accounted for in educational sessions. Teaching how to overcome common pitfalls in achieving glycemic control can aid patients when they are facing new and difficult situations in their lives.

Nutrient intake patterns and anthropometric indices should be assessed every 3 to 6 months to ensure that adequate growth is occurring. The hemoglobin $A_{1C}$ ($HbA_{1C}$) level should also be assessed at that time. A goal of less than 7.5% $HbA_{1C}$ is recommended for all pediatric patients with diabetes.[6] If dyslipidemia is a problem, biochemical values are assessed annually.

# TYPE 2 DIABETES

## Clinical and Biochemical Abnormalities

Children with T2DM can present with polyuria, polydipsia, and polyphagia with weight loss, but they often present with fatigue and weight gain. Impaired glucose tolerance and the progression to T2DM occurs when the production of insulin can no longer control the insulin resistance occurring in the tissues. Hypertension, dyslipidemia (high levels of triglycerides and cholesterol), and menstrual irregularities are known consequences of chronic hyperinsulinemia. Polycystic ovarian syndrome can result from hyperandrogenism secondary to chronic hyperinsulinemia. Acanthosis nigricans, a dark, rough thickening of the skin on areas exposed to repeated flexion or friction (often on the neck), is recognized as a marker of hyperinsulinemia. Obstructive sleep apnea is also associated with obesity, T2DM, and hyperinsulinemia.

A systematic review of the literature published in 2011 concluded that there was no clear benefit for tight BG control in T2DM.[8] In a major study, intensive insulin therapy did not significantly reduce major cardiovascular events; however, the study participants had more long-standing T2DM and evidence of preexisting cardiovascular disease.[9] Patients need to work with their diabetes care team to determine their individual goals.

## Components of Treatment

The American Diabetes Association outlined the goals for treating T2DM as follows[6]:

1. Weight control and/or weight reduction
2. Maintenance of normal physical growth
3. Near-normal BG levels
   - Preprandial (before meals) 80–130 mg/dL
   - Postprandial (1–2 hr after the first bite of a meal) <180 mg/dL
4. Near-normal glycosylated hemoglobin ($HbA_{1C}$ <7%)
5. Effective treatment of comorbid problems (e.g., hypertension, dyslipidemia)
6. Prevention of complications
7. Maintenance of emotional well-being

Principles of management for children with type 2 diabetes include the following:

1. Diabetes self-management education (DSME) to develop therapeutic lifestyle behaviors[10]
2. Diabetes self-management support (DSMS) programs to maintain behaviors[10]
2. Medical nutrition therapy (MNT)
3. Exercise prescription
   - At least 150 min/week
   - No more than 90 consecutive minutes of sedentary activity
4. Pharmacological management
5. Psychosocial considerations

For children with T2DM, regular monitoring of BG levels to assess the quality of control is essential. Patient empowerment is critical for all patients, regardless of age, to achieve near-normal BG control. Reviewing the monitoring data with the patient is beneficial because

**Table 48–1.** Glycemic Load for Various Foods

| Food Item | Glycemic Index (Glucose = 100) | Serving Size (g) | Glycemic Load Per Serving |
|---|---|---|---|
| White bread bagel | 72 | 70 | 25 |
| Whole wheat bread slice | 71 | 30 | 9 |
| Coca-cola | 63 | 250 mL | 16 |
| Skim milk | 32 | 250 mL | 4 |
| Russet potatoes | 111 | 150 | 33 |
| Carrots | 35 | 80 | 2 |
| Chicken nuggets | 46 | 100 | 7 |
| Baked beans | 40 | 150 | 6 |
| Snickers bar | 51 | 60 | 18 |
| Microwave popcorn | 55 | 20 | 6 |

it illustrates the importance health professionals place on the data and on the effort the patient has taken to record them. Teaching the skills needed to interpret the data and make appropriate food choices and medication alterations is a major goal in DSME.

The principles for choosing a pharmacological agent for managing T2DM should include safety, effectiveness, ease of administration, and cost. Insulin therapy may be used to achieve optimal glycemic control, but it can result in weight gain. Oral medications have been effective in the treatment of pediatric diabetes. All new medications under consideration for approval by the US Food and Drug Administration (FDA) must be evaluated for their use in children. Oral medications are considerably easier to administer than insulin injections (and with less teaching required). The cost associated with reducing the prevalence and comorbidities of T2DM is significant. Added benefits of the oral hypoglycemic agents are weight loss and potential breaking of the cycle of hyperinsulinemia and obesity. The side effects of any medication should be reviewed with the patient so that any complications can be prevented. MNT is always combined with pharmacological treatment for diabetes.

## Factors To Be Considered in Nutrition Evaluation and Nutritional Management

For children, the goals of MNT are to maintain balanced nutrition and promote normal linear growth while depleting fat stores. Although caloric intake may need to be reduced in adults with T2DM, additional caloric intake may be necessary for children during the pubertal growth spurt. Frequent follow-up appointments with the registered dietitian nutritionist (RDN) to assess the goals of adequate and appropriate growth, physical activity, and regular monitoring of BG are recommended. For both children and adults, the overall emphasis should be placed on reducing excessive caloric intake and increasing physical activity rather than following a rigid weight loss program. An experienced RDN should provide MNT.

Optimal nutrition using a wide variety of foods through individualized instruction is needed. The patient and the parent or caregiver should be taught how to estimate portion sizes, the carbohydrate content of foods, consistent timing of meals, and to consume a similar amount of carbohydrate at each meal or snack. Many tools are available to teach the nutrient content of foods, and the patient's knowledge base should determine the complexity of the method chosen. Some patients may choose an intensive program of carbohydrate counting that is often taught for patients with T1DM, in addition to enjoyable methods of increasing physical activity.

In certain circumstances, it may be necessary to limit the nutrition teaching to food portion sizes using the Create Your Plate method,[11] accompanied by enjoyable methods to increase physical activity. The focus of the Create Your Plate method (see Appendices 7–7 and 7–8) is to balance nutrient intake with variety. The plate is divided in half. The first half represents nonstarchy vegetables. The second half is sectioned in half again: one section (one-fourth of the plate) for a serving of protein and a second section for a serving of a grain or starchy food (e.g., rice). A serving of fruit and one of dairy sit outside of the plate. The patient's level of metabolic control, the goals of the patient, the family support system, and the support of the health care team will determine the best method for nutrition education.

## Follow-up and Summary

Nutrition education is the cornerstone of therapy for patients with T2DM. Healthy eating habits for the whole family should be taught. An environment in which the family supports healthy eating, proper portion control, consumption of a variety of foods, and avoiding skipping meals and consuming heavy snacks will be the most successful. Incorporating physical activity on a daily basis, with acknowledgment and curtailment of excessive sedentary activities (e.g., watching television, playing video games, using a computer) is also essential for success in both children and adults.

Most successful weight management programs focus on positive and enjoyable behavior changes and deemphasize weight loss as the goal. A weight management program should start by helping patients recognize eating cues and satiety factors. Patients should learn appropriate portion sizes and model behaviors that demonstrate good nutrition principles. Parents have significant influence on their child. They provide the child's genetic makeup and serve as role models for health-related behaviors. The parent buys the food, prepares the meal, provides access to activities, and sets limits on sedentary activities. Weight maintenance programs for children need to focus on increasing general parenting skills rather than on the child's weight or growth.[12]

Because of the sensitive nature of obtaining anthropometric data in overweight individuals and the emphasis on behavior modification, monitoring should focus on quarterly assessment with the health care provider including strength improvements, biochemical parameters (especially $HbA_{1C}$), and goal achievements.

### References


1. *StatisticsAboutDiabetes: OverallNumbers, DiabetesandPrediabetes.* LastupdatedApril 2016. http://www.diabetes.org/diabetes-basics/statistics/?loc=db-slabnav. Accessed July 5, 2016.
2. Handelsman Y, Bloomgarden Z, Grunberger G, et al. American Association of Clinical Endocrinologists and American College of Endocrinology: clinical practice guidelines for developing a diabetes mellitus comprehensive care plan, 2015. *Endocr Pract.* 2014; 21(Suppl 1): 1.
3. The Diabetes Control and Complication Trial Research Group. The effect of intensive treatment of diabetes on the development and progression of long-term complications in insulin dependent diabetes mellitus. *N Engl J Med.* 1993; 14:977.
4. Mayo Clinic Staff. *Diseases and Conditions: Diabetes.* 2014. http://www.mayoclinic.org. Accessed July 5, 2016.
5. Holland K, Kinmans T. *Tight Diabetes Control.* http://www.healthline.com. Accessed July 5, 2016.
6. American Diabetes Association. Standards of medical care in diabetes—2015. Section 1: Strategies for improving care. *Diab Care.* 2015;38(suppl. 1):55.
7. *Glycemic Index and Glycemic Load for 100 Foods.* Harvard Health Publications; February 3, 2015. www.health.harvard.edu/.../glycemic_index_and_glycemic_load_for_100_foods. Accessed July 5, 2016.
8. Hemmingsen B, Lund SS, Gluud C, et al. Targeting intensive glycaemic control versus targeting conventional glycaemic control for type 2 diabetes mellitus. *Cochrane Database Syst Rev.* 2011; (6):CD008143.
9. National Heart, Lung, and Blood Institute, biologic Specimen and Data Repository Information Coordinating Center. *Action to Control Cardiovascular Risk in Diabetes (ACCORD).* August 13, 2013. https://biolincc.nhlbi.nih.gov/studies/accord. Accessed July 5, 2016.
10. Powers A, Bardsley J, Cypress M, et al. Diabetes self-management education and support in type 2 diabetes: a joint position statement of the American Diabetes Association, the American Association of Diabetes Educators, and the Academy of Nutrition and dietetics. *J Acad Nutr Diet.* 2015; 115:1323.
11. American Diabetes Association. *Create Your Plate.* http://www.diabetes.org/food-and-fitness/food/planning-meals/create-your-plate/. Accessed July 6, 2016.
12. Gurnani M, Birken C, Hamilton J. Childhood obesity: causes, consequences, and management. *Pediatr Clin North Am.* 2015; 62:821.

# 49 Galactosemia

SANDY VAN CALCAR

Galactose metabolism involves three enzymes: galactokinase, galactose-1-phosphate uridyl transferase (GALT) and uridine diphosphate-4-epimerase (Fig. 49–1). Inborn errors of metabolism (IEM) have been described for all three enzymes. The most common inborn error in galactose metabolism is deficiency of the GALT enzyme, which has an incidence in North America of approximately 1 in 48,000 births.[1] Newborn screening (NBS) can detect these disorders by measuring galactose concentrations and/or GALT activity in dried blood spots collected from infants at 24 to 48 hours of age. Infants with elevated galactose and/or decreased enzyme activity should be immediately referred to a biochemical genetics program that specializes in treatment of IEM. This chapter focuses on GALT deficiency because the classic form of the disease requires lifelong dietary treatment. In classic galactosemia, the affected individual has severe GALT deficiency with absent or barely detectable enzyme activity.[1]

## CLINICAL AND BIOCHEMICAL ABNORMALITIES

Neonates with untreated classic GALT deficiency present a few days after starting milk-based formula or breast milk feeding.[1–3] The initial symptoms include poor feeding, vomiting, and jaundice. Failure to thrive, hepatomegaly, edema, splenomegaly, and *Escherichia coli* sepsis can follow. The disease is rapidly fatal if milk feedings continue. Before the advent of NBS, intellectual disabilities and behavioral problems were common among those affected children who survived this initial episode.[2] With NBS, earlier detection is possible, and severe manifestations of untreated galactosemia can be avoided if sources of galactose are immediately removed from the infant's diet.[3]

However, despite lifelong dietary restriction of galactose, long-term complications often develop in adolescents and adults with classic galactosemia, including cognitive and psychological impairment, learning problems, speech and language delays, neurological abnormalities such as ataxia or dementia, poor bone mineralization, and premature ovarian dysfunction in females.[4–7] The specific cause of these long-term manifestations remains unknown. Prenatal exposure to galactose, endogenous galactose production, abnormal glycosylation of galactoproteins and galactolipids, and dietary indiscretions are all potential causes of these adverse developments.[8–12]

## GENETIC BACKGROUND

Galactosemia is inherited as an autosomal recessive trait. Approximately 250 genetic mutations have been identified in the *GALT* gene, which is located on the short arm of chromosome 9.[3] The most common mutation in people of European descent is Q188R. Homozygosity for this mutation always results in the classic form of the disease without any residual enzyme activity, and it is this group that is most likely to develop long-term complications associated with the disorder.[6,7] A milder phenotype, common among those of African-American descent, is caused by the S135L mutation.[13] Several other variant forms of GALT deficiency have been identified. The most common is the Duarte variant, in which approximately 25% of total enzyme activity remains.[1,2]

## FACTORS TO BE CONSIDERED IN NUTRITION EVALUATION

The most important factor affecting the length and degree of dietary treatment required for galactosemia is the amount of remaining GALT enzyme activity. The type of galactosemia is verified by direct enzyme analysis, targeted mutation analysis, or, if necessary, full gene sequencing.[1] Knowing a child's specific mutations can provide useful information about the required degree of dietary treatment and the potential long-term clinical outcome.[14] Studies have suggested that older individuals with classic galactosemia may be able to tolerate more galactose than previously thought.[14–17] This is an active area of research, and no specific recommendations are yet available; the current policy is that those diagnosed with classic galactosemia must remain on a galactose-restricted diet for life.[18–20]

It is unclear whether any dietary treatment is necessary for those with Duarte galactosemia. However, many clinics treat infants with soy-based formula and lactose-free solids for the first year of life. Long-term follow-up of those with Duarte galactosemia has revealed that some patients develop subtle developmental problems, although the research is very limited and the need for any diet treatment for this group remains unclear.[18–20]

## DIETARY MANAGEMENT

### Diet During Infancy

An infant with presumed classic galactosemia identified by NBS and/or clinical symptoms should immediately be placed on a soy-based formula to reduce galactose intake. All sources of galactose, including breast milk, need to be eliminated, and initiation of dietary treatment should not be postponed while awaiting final confirmation of the diagnosis.[3] Soy protein isolate, the protein source in soy formulas, contains a small amount of galactose; as a result, soy formula contains approximately 4 mg galactose/240 mL. However, this is substantially lower than the galactose content of breast milk or milk-based formulas, which is approximately 2200 mg/240 mL.

Galactose can be completely eliminated from the diet by giving an elemental amino acid–based formula (e.g., Elecare, Neocate), and this has been used in infants, with in slowly decreasing galactose-1-phosphate (Gal-1-P) concentrations.[21,22] However, it is unknown whether use of these formulas during infancy provides any short-term clinical benefit or helps prevent development of any of the long-term complications.[14] At this time, elemental formulas are not routinely recommended for neonates with classic galactosemia.

Soy formulas are not recommended for preterm infants because lower phosphorus and higher alkaline phosphatase concentrations can lead to an increased incidence of osteopenia in preterm infants fed soy formula compared with cow's milk formula.[23] Therefore, premature infants with suspected galactosemia should be treated with an elemental formula.[14] Casein hydrolysate formulas (e.g., Nutramigen, Pregestimil) are also appropriate for infants with galactosemia, but, like soy formulas, they do contain a small amount of galactose.

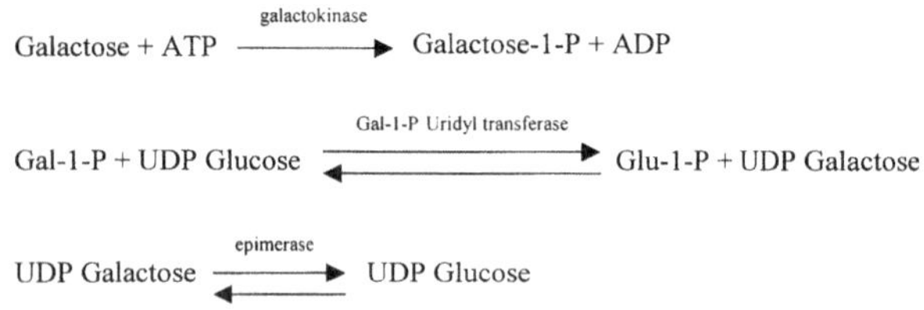


**Figure 49–1.** Enzymes involved in metabolism of galactose. ADP = adenosine diphosphate; ATP = adenosine triphosphate; Gal-1-P = galactose-1-phosphate; UDP = uridine diphosphate.

Solids are started at 4 to 6 months of age, and advances in diet follow the usual progression, except that all foods containing lactose or galactose must be eliminated.[14]

### Diet After Infancy

After infancy, most milk and dairy products are excluded from the diet, including various dairy-based ingredients such as dry milk solids and whey, which are used in many processed foods (Table 49–1). However, some products made from milk that were previously eliminated from the diet are now considered acceptable. Because of extensive processing and washing of casein proteins to produce caseinates, sodium and calcium caseinate contains approximately 35 mg of galactose per 100 g and is now allowed in the diet.[14,24] In addition, some aged cheeses contain negligible galactose, and these have now been added to the "allowed" list[14,24,25] (see Table 49–1). Because there is a high concentration of galactoproteins and other galactose-containing compounds stored in organs of animals, organ meats are excluded from the diet.

Galactose is found in plant tissues as free (unbound) galactose, galactose oligomers, and galactose conjugates with protein, lipid, and cell wall polysaccharides. Much of the bound galactose is in a form that is not available for digestion in the human gastrointestinal tract.[26–28] The amount of free galactose ranges from 0 to 77 mg in 100 g of various fruits, vegetables, and juices.[29–32]

Legumes (e.g., garbanzo beans, black beans) contain a substantial amount of bound galactose. An analysis of various commercially canned legumes found that bound galactose ranged from 294 to 1100 mg in 100 g beans and from 483 to 1170 mg in 100 mL of the canning liquid.[24] However, the free galactose content of these canned products was similar to that found in fruits and vegetables. Therefore, all legumes are now considered acceptable in the diet for people with galactosemia.

Unfermented products made from soy (e.g., soy milk, tofu) are also low in free galactose and are acceptable for those with galactosemia. However, the fermentation process that is used to produce soy sauce, miso, natto, and other fermented products releases bound galactose and substantially increases the amount of free galactose.[33] Given the small amount of these products that are typically used in foods, moderation in intake is recommended.

### Reading Food Labels

Parents, and later the affected child, are taught to read food labels and search for any excluded ingredients. Lists of acceptable and unacceptable foods and ingredients, as well as general diet guidelines, are available for professionals and parents.[14,34,35]

Some of the dietary practices observed by the Jewish culture can be helpful when looking for acceptable foods. *Kosher* is the term used to designate a food that is acceptable in the Jewish diet. Kosher foods labeled *pareve* are dairy-free and can be included in the diet for individuals with galactosemia.[36] Dairy-free cookbooks, typically recommended for those with dairy allergy or lactose intolerance, can also be introduced for galactosemia.[36] Milk substitutes (e.g., rice milk, soy milk) are often used in these recipes. However, any product that is marketed to reduce lactose in dairy products (e.g., LactAid) should not be used because foods treated with these products will still contain galactose.[14] Occasionally, food labels are unclear and the manufacturer will have to be contacted to verify whether the product contains only acceptable ingredients. Parents and individuals with galactosemia also need instruction on how to identify appropriate foods at restaurants and while pursuing various activities outside the home.[34,35]

## NUTRIENT SUPPLEMENT NEEDS

Because the diet for galactosemia is dairy free, additional calcium is always necessary and is usually started when formula intake decreases after 1 year of age.[14,37] Use of calcium-fortified milk substitutes and juices should be encouraged, and additional supplementation may be needed as well. Poor calcium intake in galactosemia has been linked to low bone density.[38] Girls are especially prone to low bone density because bone metabolism is also affected by low estrogen production associated with ovarian insufficiency.[38,39] Both adequate calcium intake and hormonal replacement therapy are necessary to prevent early osteoporosis in these young women.[39]

Low intake of vitamin D is frequently found in these patients, and supplementation is often needed. Yearly assessment of serum total 25-hydroxyvitamin D concentrations is recommended.[39] Depending on sun exposure, additional vitamin D beyond the established Dietary Reference Intake (DRI) may be necessary to ensure adequate blood concentrations.[40] Assessment of intake of other nutrients is suggested, and a vitamin/mineral supplement may be necessary. All supplements need to be lactose free.

## LACTOSE IN MEDICATIONS

Lactose is often used as an extender in prescription and over-the-counter medications and dietary supplements. Lactose will be listed on labels as an inactive ingredient[41]; if lactose is present, finding an alternative is suggested. Usually, appropriate medications can be found without added lactose; however, some classes of medications may not have lactose-free alternatives. In these cases, the necessity of the medication and the length of treatment must be weighed against the additional intake of galactose. However, the amount of galactose ingested with medications is insignificant compared with the amounts that are found in various dairy products or produced by endogenous production.[2]

## MONITORING AND FOLLOW-UP

All individuals with classic galactosemia should be followed by a clinic specializing in the treatment of IEM.[42] Clinic visits should include a physical examination, nutrition and genetic counseling, and laboratory monitoring. Referral to appropriate specialty clinics for psychological and speech evaluations is needed at an early age so that any necessary therapies can be initiated. All affected girls should be seen by an endocrinologist beginning at the age of 10 to 12 years to evaluate the need for hormone replacement.[39] Psychiatric treatment may become necessary to manage attention or behavioral issues. Routine dual-energy x-ray absorptiometry (DXA) scans are also needed given the risk for decreased bone density in this population.[39]

Laboratory tests are available to assess the degree of metabolic control in this disorder. The most common laboratory assessment is measurement of the concentration of Gal-1-P in red blood cells (RBCs); Gal-1-P is the precursor that accumulates in cells deficient in GALT activity (see Fig. 49–1). In classic galactosemia, high concentrations of RBC Gal-1-P are present at diagnosis and may take several months to decrease to the treatment range.[2] For those on dietary treatment, the goal is to maintain RBC Gal-1-P concentrations below 4 mg/dL.[42] However, RBC Gal-1-P is relatively insensitive to diet changes, and there is little correlation between Gal-1-P levels and clinical outcome.[11,43] It is unlikely that those with RBC Gal-1-P levels consistently above the treatment range will benefit from stricter diet control.

Further exploration of galactose metabolism is needed to determine more appropriate markers that reflect adequacy of diet restriction. There are promising studies showing a relationship between the glycan chains that are linked to circulating proteins and dietary galactose intake.[11]

**Table 49–1.** The Galactose-Restricted Diet*

| Foods Permitted | Foods Not Permitted | Foods Suggested in Moderation |
|---|---|---|
| *Milk Substitutes and Ingredients* | *Milk Products and Milk-Based Ingredients* | |
| Soy formulas containing soy protein isolate: Similac Isomil, Prosobee; soy milk, rice milk, other plant-based milks | Breast milk<br>Milk-based infant formulas | |
| Nondairy cream substitutes | | |
| Nondairy frozen desserts | All animal milks and milk products: buttermilk, cream, sour cream, yogurt, ice cream, ice milk, sherbet, butter | |
| Aged cheeses: Jarlsberg, Emmentaler, Swiss, Gruyere, Tilsiter, Parmesan aged >10 months (brick and grated), sharp Cheddar cheese aged > 1 year | All cheeses and cheese-based products except those aged cheeses listed as permitted | |
| Sodium and calcium caseinate | Milk-based ingredients including buttermilk solids, casein, dry milk solids, dry milk protein, hydrolyzed whey protein, hydrolyzed casein protein, lactose, lactalbumin, whey | |
| *Protein Foods* | | |
| Plain meats, fish, poultry—without added milk products | Breaded or creamed meat, fish, poultry | |
| All-meat frankfurters, sausage, cold cuts | Organ meats, meat byproducts | |
| Eggs without milk or milk products | Processed meats with added milk products | |
| Nuts, nut butters, seeds | | |
| Nonfermented soy products: tofu, meat analogs, hydrolyzed vegetable protein, etc. | | Fermented soy sauce<br>Other fermented soy products: tempeh, natto, sufu |
| Legumes (dried beans and peas): garbanzo, kidney, pinto, navy, etc. | | |
| *Fruit and Vegetables* | | |
| All fruits and vegetables—fresh, frozen, canned, dried—unless processed with lactose or milk products | Fruit with milk, cream, or any milk products | |
| Fermented vegetables: pickles, sauerkraut | Vegetables with milk, cream, or other milk products | |
| *Grains and Breads* | | |
| Cooked and dry cereals without milk, lactose, or milk products added | Cooked or dry cereals with added whey, casein, or other milk products | |
| Breads, rolls, buns without added milk, milk products, or lactose (e.g., French bread, Italian bread) | Breads, rolls, buns, cakes, cookies, crackers, or any baked products with added milk or milk products | |
| Crackers, saltines, biscuits, cookies without lactose or other milk products added | Bread or pancake mixes containing milk products | |
| Flour or corn tortillas without milk or milk products added | | |
| Macaroni, noodles, spaghetti, rice | | |
| *Fats* | | |
| All vegetable oils—soybean, corn, olive, cottonseed, safflower, peanut, canola, etc. | Butter, cream, sour cream, milk fat | |
| Margarine without milk or milk products added | Margarines with added milk or milk products | |
| Vegetable shortening, lard, suet | | |
| Mayonnaise, milk-free salad dressings | | |
| *Beverages* | | |
| Carbonated drinks | All drinks that contain a dairy product | |
| Artificial drinks without lactose or milk-based extenders | | |
| All fruit and vegetable juices | | |
| Tea, coffee | | |
| *Miscellaneous* | | |
| Sugar, corn syrup, molasses, plain carob, maple syrup | Syrups or other sweeteners with added milk. | |
| Monosodium glutamate (MSG) and any spices without added lactose or dairy-based extenders | | |
| Clear candies, gum drops, marshmallows, chewing gum, fruit pectins | All candies and sweets with milk products | |
| All natural and artificial flavorings and colorings | | |
| All cocoa/chocolate products except milk chocolate | Milk chocolate, cocoa mixes containing milk | |
| All gums: Arabic, carrageenan, guar, xanthan, etc. | | |
| Dough conditioner, modified food starch | | |
| Artificial sweeteners | | |

*A summary of galactose analyses of mature cheese, caseinates, and various plant-based foods is provided in Van Calcar SC, Bernstein LE, Rohr FJ, Scaman CH, Yannicelli S, Berry GT. A re-evaluation of life-long severe galactose restriction for the nutrition management of classic galactosemia. *Mol Genet Metab.* 2014; 112:191.

Adapted from Van Calcar SC, Bernstein LE, Rohr FJ, Scaman CH, Yannicelli S, Berry GT. A re-evaluation of life-long severe galactose restriction for the nutrition management of classic galactosemia. *Mol Genet Metab.* 2014; 112:191; Bernstein LE, Van Calcar SC, Rohr F, Yannicelli S. *Galactosemia: The Diet.* Aurora, CO: Inherited Metabolic Disease Program, Children's Hospital Colorado; 2014; Gleason L, Rasberry M, Van Calcar S. *Understanding Galactosemia: A Diet Guide.* Columbus, OH: Abbott Nutrition; 2010.

## CONCLUSION

Diagnosis by NBS and immediate elimination of lactose from feedings are life-saving for infants with classic galactosemia. However, despite a lifelong diet restricted in lactose and galactose, long-term complications frequently develop in older individuals with this disorder. Diet recommendations have evolved over the past decade, and minor sources of galactose in plant and some dairy products are no longer restricted. Research continues to better determine the etiology of complications associated with galactosemia and improve treatment recommendations.

### References


1. Berry GT. Classic galactosemia and clinical variant galactosemia. 1999; last updated April 2014. In: Pagon RA, Adam MP, Ardinger HH, et al., eds. *Gene Reviews.* Seattle, WA: University of Washington; 1993–2016. http://www.ncbi.nlm.nih.gov/books/NBK1518. Accessed July 5, 2016.
2. Berry GT, Walter JH. Disorders of galactose metabolism. In: Saudubray JM, Van der Berghe G, Walter JH, eds. *Inborn Metabolic Diseases: Diagnosis and Treatment,* 5th ed. New York: Springer-Verlag; 2012:141.
3. Berry GT. Galactosemia: when is it a newborn screening emergency? *Mol Genet Metab.* 2012; 106:7.
4. Waggoner DD, Buist NRM, Donnell GN. Long-term prognosis in galactosaemia: results of a survey of 350 cases. *J Inherit Metab Dis.* 1990; 13:802.
5. Hughes J, Ryan S, Lambert D, et al. Outcome of siblings with classical galactosemia. *J Pediatr.* 2009; 154:721.
6. Waisbren SE, Potter NL, Gordon CM et al. The adult galactosemic phenotype. *J Inherit Metab Dis.* 2011; 35:279.
7. Coss KP, Doran PP, Owoeye C, et al. Classical galactosemia in Ireland: incidence, complications and outcomes of treatment. *J Inherit Metab Dis.* 2013; 36:21.
8. Berry G, Nissim I, Gibson JB, et al. Quantitative assessment of whole body galactose metabolism in galactosemic patients. *Eur J Pediatr.* 1997; 156:S43.
9. Schadewaldt P, Kamalanathan L, Hammen HW, Wendel U. Age dependence of endogenous galactose formation in Q188R homozygous patients. *Mol Genet Metab.* 2004; 81:31.
10. Berry GT. Is prenatal myo-inositol deficiency a mechanism of CNS injury in galactosemia? *J Inherit Metab Dis.* 2011; 34:345.
11. Coss KP, Byrne JC, Coman DJ, et al. IgG N-glycans as potential biomarkers for determining galactose tolerance in classical galactosemia. *Mol Genet Metab.* 2012; 105:212.
12. Coss KP, Hawkes CP, Adamczyk B, et al. N-Glycan abnormalities in children with galactosemia. *J Proteome Res.* 2014; 13:385.
13. Lai K, Langley SD, Singh RH, Dembure LN, Hjelm LN, Elsas LJ. A prevalent mutation for galactosemia among black Americans. *J Pediatr.* 1996; 128:89.
14. Van Calcar SC, Bernstein LE, Rohr FJ, Scaman CH, Yannicelli S, Berry GT. A re-evaluation of life-long severe galactose restriction for the nutrition management of classic galactosemia. *Mol Genet Metab.* 2014; 112:191.
15. Berry GT, Elsas LJ. Introduction to the Maastricht workshop: lessons from the past and new directions in galactosemia. *J Inherit Metab Dis.* 2011; 34:249.
16. Knerr I, Coss KP, Kratzsch J, et al. Effects of temporary low-dose galactose supplements in children aged 5-12 years with classical galactosemia: a pilot study. *Pediatr Res.* 2015; 78:272.
17. Bosch A, Bakker H, Wenniger-Prick L, Wanders RJ, Wijburg FA. High tolerance for oral galactose in classical galactosemia: dietary implications. *Arch Dis Child.* 2004; 89:1034.
18. Ficicioglu C, Thomas N, Yager C, et al. Duarte (DG) galactosemia: a pilot study of biochemical and neurodevelopmental assessment in children detected by newborn screening. *Mol Genet Metab.* 2008; 95:206.
19. Powell KK, Van Naarden Braun K, Singh RH, Shapira SK, Olney RS, Yeargin-Allsopp M. Long-term speech and language developmental issues among children with Duarte galactosemia. *Genet Med.* 2009; 11:874.
20. Lynch ME, Potter NL, Coles CD, Fridovich-Keil JL. Developmental outcomes of school-age children with Duarte galactosemia: a pilot study. *JIMD Rep.* 2015; 19:75.
21. Ficicioglu C, Hussa C, Yager C, Segal S. Effect of galactose free formula on galactose-1-phosphate in two infants with classical galactosemia. *Eur J Pediatr.* 2008; 167:595.
22. Zlatunich CO, Packman S. Galactosaemia: early treatment with an elemental formula. *J Inherit Metab Dis.* 2005; 28:163.
23. Bhatia J, Greer F; American Academy of Pediatrics Committee on Nutrition. Use of soy protein-based formulas in infant feeding. *Pediatrics.* 2008; 121:1062.
24. Van Calcar SC, Bernstein LE, Rohr FJ, Yannicelli S, Berry GT, Scaman CH. Galactose content of legumes, caseinates, and some hard cheeses: implications for diet treatment of classic galactosemia. *J Agric Food Chem.* 2014; 62:1397.
25. Portnoi PA, MacDonald A. Determination of the lactose and galactose content of cheese for use in the galactosaemia diet. *J Hum Nutr Diet.* 2009; 22:400.
26. Quemener B, Brillouet J. Ciceritol, a pinitol digalactoside from seeds of chickpea, lentil and white lupin. *Phytochemistry.* 1983; 22:1745.
27. Fry SC. Cell wall polysaccharide composition and covalent crosslinking. In: Ulvskov P, ed. *Annual Plant Reviews, Vol 41: Plant Polysaccharides: Biosynthesis and Bioengineering.* Ames, IA: Wiley-Blackwell; 2011:Chapter 1.
28. Dey PM, Campillo ED. Biochemistry of the multiple forms of glycosidases in plants. In: Meister A, ed. *Advances in Enzymology and Related Areas of Molecular Biology,* vol 56. John Wiley & Sons; 2006: 141.
29. Acosta PB, Gross KC. Hidden sources of galactose in the environment. *Eur J Pediatr.* 1995; 154(Suppl 2):S87.
30. Gross K, Acosta PB. Fruits and vegetables are a source of galactose: implications in planning the diets of patients with galactosaemia. *J Inherit Metab Dis.* 1991; 14:253.
31. Gropper S, Weese J, West P, Gross KC. Free galactose content of fresh fruits and strained fruit and vegetable baby foods: more foods to consider for the galactose-restricted diet. *J Am Diet Assoc.* 2000; 100:573.
32. Kim H, Hartnett C, Scaman CH. Free galactose content in selected fresh fruits and vegetables and soy beverages. *J Agric Food Chem.* 2007; 55:8133.
33. Moy YS, Chou CC. Changes in the content of sugars and organic acids during the ripening and storage of sufu, a traditional oriental fermented product of soybean cubes. *J Agric Food Chem.* 2010; 58:12790.
34. Bernstein LE, Van Calcar SC, Rohr F, Yannicelli S. *Galactosemia: The Diet.* Aurora, CO: Inherited Metabolic Disease Program, Children's Hospital Colorado; 2014.
35. Gleason L, Rasberry M, Van Calcar S. *Understanding Galactosemia: A Diet Guide.* Columbus, OH: Abbott Nutrition; 2010.
36. Zukin J. *Dairy Free Cookbook.* Rocklin, CA: Prima Publishing and Communications; 1998.
37. Rutherford PJ, Davidson DC, Matthai SM. Dietary calcium in galactosemia. *J Hum Nutr Diet.* 2002; 15:39.
38. Kaufman FR, Loro ML, Azen C, Wenz E, Gilsanz V. Effect of hypogonadism and deficient calcium intake on bone density in patients with galactosemia. *J Pediatr.* 1993; 123:365.
39. Van Ervin B, Romers MMM, Rubio-Gozalbo ME. Revised proposal for the prevention of low bone mass in patients with classic galactosemia. *JIMD Rep.* 2014; 17:41.
40. Pramyothin P, Holick MF. Vitamin D supplementation: guidelines and evidence for subclinical deficiency. *Curr Opin Gastroenterol.* 2012; 28:139.
41. US FDA Drug Labeling Requirements. Hampton, VA: Registrar Corp, 2016. http://www.registrarcorp.com/fda-drugs/labeling/regulations.jsp?lang=en. Accessed July 5, 2016.
42. Walter JH, Collins JE, Leonard JV. Recommendations for the management of galactosaemia. *Arch Dis Child.* 1999; 80:93.
43. Hutchesson AC, Murdoch-Davis C, Green A, et al. Biochemical monitoring of treatment for galactosaemia: biological variability in metabolic correlations. *J Inherit Metab Dis.* 1999; 22:139.

# 50 Lactose Intolerance

PATRICIA J. BECKER, ALISON CASSIN, AND SCOTT PENTIUK

Food intolerances are common but often difficult to identify. Lactose maldigestion is reported to be the most common food intolerance, affecting 80% of African-Americans, 50% of Hispanic Americans, and 15% of the Caucasian-American population.[1] The true prevalence of lactose intolerance is more difficult to identify because of the limitations in diagnosis and the lack of consistent definition, standarized assessment methodology, and symptomatology.[2]

## BIOCHEMICAL ABNORMALITIES

Lactose intolerance is a type of maldigestion in which a standard dose of the sugar lactose cannot be tolerated without development of gut dysfunction. Diarrhea, abdominal pain, bloating, and flatulence are the most common symptoms.

The lactase enzyme is a membrane-bound enzyme located in the brush border or microvilli of the small bowel. The lactase enzyme hydrolyzes lactose into its constituent monosaccharides, glucose and galactose, which are then transported across the brush border of the small intestines.[3] In individuals with lactase deficiency, up to 75% of ingested lactose remains intact. The lactose that is not digested in the small bowel passes rapidly into the colon, where it is converted to short-chain fatty acids and hydrogen or methane gas by colonic bacteria. The short-chain fatty acids, butyrate, acetate, and propionate are utilized by both colonocytes and bacteria as an energy source. This lactose salvaging in the newborn gut allows for support of beneficial gut flora and increased nutrient absorption for the infant.[4,5] In the adult with lactase insufficiency or deficiency, this mechanism allows for the ingestion, digestion, and absorption of small amounts of lactose without symptoms of intolerance. It is when this mechanism becomes overwhelmed that excess gas is produced, and this is the source of hydrogen production and gastrointestinal symptoms.[6–8]

Lactose intolerance may be either primary or secondary. The disorders of primary intolerance include developmental lactase deficiency, congenital lactase deficiency (CLD), and lactase nonpersistence, with developmental and late-onset forms.[4] Secondary lactose malabsorption is the result of gut dysfunction due to mucosal injury.

## FACTORS TO BE CONSIDERED IN NUTRITION EVALUATION

The goal of therapy in secondary lactose intolerance is to treat the disease that induced the intolerance. The capacity to tolerate lactose recovers once mucosal villi regenerate; dietary restriction may not be permanent once the primary illness has improved. However, the rate of recovery is variable and may not correlate with histological recovery of the absorptive surface. Intolerance may persist for months.

Lactose Digestion and Absorption in Infants, Children, and Adults Compared with other mammalian species, human milk has the highest concentration of the disaccharide lactose. Lactose is the major carbohydrate source in the neonatal period. It is the preferred carbohydrate for infants because it enhances the absorption of minerals such as calcium and magnesium and the growth of lactobacilli and bifidobacteria in the intestinal tract.[9–11]

### Primary Lactose Intolerance: Congenital

CLD is a rare autosomal recessive disorder characterized by the absence of lactase activity in the small bowel. This condition, described by Holzel et al.[12] in 1959, manifests at birth with explosive, watery diarrhea and can, although very rarely, lasts throughout life. The symptoms occur immediately on introduction of lactose in the neonatal period due to the complete absence or severe reduction of lactase activity. Before the introduction of lactose-free infant formula, this disorder was life-threatening.[13,14]

### Primary Lactose Intolerance: Developmental

Lactase activity increases from the early months of fetal life, reaching peak activity shortly after birth. Twenty-five percent of 1-week-old term infants have lactose malabsorption.[15] Even if enzyme levels are low, colonic bacteria can salvage the lactose that is not digested in the small intestine of very small premature infants. As much as 66% of ingested lactose enters the colon in premature infants, and the low lactase activity at birth in these infants has little clinical significance. Despite the lag in development of enzyme activity, the term and even the premature infant can tolerate the levels of lactose in human milk and formulas.[4,5]

### Lactose Intolerance in Children

The 1978 American Academy of Pediatrics statement, "The Practical Significance of Lactose Intolerance in Children," and its 1990 update stated that the major concerns were (1) the prevalence of lactose intolerance at specific ages in particular populations, (2) the relationship between intolerance and the quantity of milk consumed, (3) the response to hydrolyzed lactose products, and (4) the absorption of other nutrients in the presence of lactose that has surpassed digestive capacity.[15–17]

Significant problems are not usually seen in children with lactose malabsorption due to primary late-onset lactase deficiency. Most of these children experience no adverse effects from moderate milk intake. Studies have shown that most individuals can tolerate milk and milk products in small amounts and with other foods.[7,9,18] Factors such as fat content, amount, and timing of lactose ingestion determine the tolerance and resulting symptoms. In these children, cultured and fermented dairy products such as aged cheese (e.g., cheddar, Swiss, Parmesan) and yogurt are often tolerated.

Live-culture yogurt contains *Lactobacillus bulgaricus* and *Streptococcus thermophilus*, which provide beta-galactosidase.[19,20] The degree of lactose reduction by bacteria found in yogurt can vary. Yogurt is well tolerated for other reasons. The consistency of yogurt slows gastric emptying and the fermentation process removes some of the lactose, resulting in a lower lactose content compared with nonfermented dairy products. Milk containing *Lactobacillus acidophilus* may also be tolerated and may have beneficial effects for individuals with lactose intolerance.

### Adults: Primary Lactase Persistence and Nonpersistence

The occurrence of lactose persistence and nonpersistence is genetically dictated and therefore related to ethnicity. Caucasians of European descent have a high occurrence of lactase persistence.

Lactase nonpersistence is the genetically regulated reduction of lactase activity; it is the underlying cause of primary lactose intolerance. The majority of the world's population exhibit low intestinal lactase levels after weaning before 5 years of age.[10,21,22] The diagnosis of lactose intolerance is most often suspected in this population with the presentation of abdominal distention, bloating, flatulence, and diarrhea after the ingestion of foods containing lactose.[1,23,24]

Children from Thailand and Bangladesh show decreased enzyme activity as early as 2 years of age, whereas African Americans, Asians, and Latin Americans show adult values in children after the first decade of life.[15]

### Secondary Lactose Intolerance

Secondary lactose intolerance occurs in individuals who by age or heredity have normal lactase activity; it is caused by conditions that negatively impact the intestinal mucosa. These conditions include malnutrition, acute gastroenteritis, cow's milk enteropathy, small bowel syndrome, and celiac disease.

#### Malnutrition

Inadequate nutrient intake that results in malnutrition affects all organs including the gut. Reduced villi height and villi atrophy result in diminished brush border enzymes, with decreased lactase activity in severe cases of malnutrition. The return of lactase synthesis occurs with the occurrence of adequate nutrient intake and the replenishing of nutrient stores.

#### Acute Gastroenteritis

Organisms such as viruses, parasites, and bacteria can injure the brush border. Diarrhea associated with gastroenteritis is common in infancy. In infants and children with giardiasis, the giardia adhere to the microvillus membrane, leading to overgrowth on the surface of the intestine, mucosal injury, and lactose intolerance. Rotavirus is also associated with temporary lactose intolerance.[9,15]

Breast-feeding should not be interrupted. Data suggest that for non–breast-fed infants and young children in the hospital setting, lactose-free feedings can be considered in the management of gastroenteritis. This therapy may reduce the duration and severity of diarrhea.[25,26]

#### Cow's Milk Enteropathy

Children with milk protein allergy may also have a secondary lactase deficiency. Investigations have demonstrated reduced disaccharidase activity after mucosal damage due to sensitivity to cow's milk or soy protein.[27,28] Gastrointestinal symptoms such as loose stools and abdominal distention occur in both cow's milk protein allergy and lactose intolerance. However, because milk allergy has an immunological etiology, vomiting, dermatological symptoms, and respiratory reactions occur only in milk allergy.

#### Short Bowel Syndrome

Lactose intolerance may be present in infants and children with short bowel due to damage to the intestinal mucosa, decreased absorptive surface area, and shortened transit time. A lactose-free diet may be beneficial if these conditions are present. Several studies have shown that adults with short bowel syndrome tolerate small amounts of lactose in milk or yogurt without symptoms or differences on breath hydrogen testing.[29]

### Lactose Deficiency due to Other Gastrointestinal Conditions

Patients with active Crohn's disease may also experience lactose maldigestion and malabsorption due to decreased brush border lactase levels or other mechanisms. Patients newly diagnosed with celiac disease may have temporary lactose intolerance as a result of damage to the lining of the small intestine. After ingestion of lactose, patients with celiac disease may complain of rumbling bowel sounds, distention, flatus, and osmotic diarrhea. This resolves once the intestine heals in response to the gluten-free diet.

Radiation therapy can have effects on the gastrointestinal tract in children with cancer. This can contribute to some degree of lactose intolerance. Lactose malabsorption can be a cause of diarrhea in patients with human immunodeficiency virus (HIV) infection or acquired immune deficiency syndrome (AIDS). Recurrent abdominal pain in children also may be caused by lactose maldigestion.[28,30]

### Small Intestinal Bacterial Overgrowth

In general, symptoms of lactose intolerance are produced when lactose is digested by gut bacteria. In the normal bowel, these microbes are located in the colon. For individuals with small intestinal bacterial overgrowth (SIBO), lactose intolerance occurs when undigested lactose encounters bacteria. This may result not from lactose deficiency but from premature exposure of lactose to bacteria in the small bowel, which leads to increased production of gas and short-chain fatty acids plus increased transit time and osmotic load.[31]

## SIGNS AND SYMPTOMS

Symptoms of lactose intolerance include abdominal pain, cramps, distention, nausea, flatulence, and diarrhea; they occur within 30 minutes to 2 hours after eating or drinking foods containing lactose. The severity of symptoms varies, depending on the amount of lactose each patient can tolerate (influenced by physiological and psychological factors). Symptoms depend on the level of lactase activity, the amount of lactose ingested, meal composition, and other factors.

## DIAGNOSIS OF LACTOSE INTOLERANCE

Lactose intolerance can be diagnosed by several methods, testing either for absorption or for malabsorption.

### Lactose Absorption Test

The capacity to absorb lactose can be measured by administering a dose of lactose and measuring blood glucose levels after 0, 60, and 120 minutes. A 50-g dose of lactose that results in an increase in blood glucose of 20 mg/dL along with the development of the gastrointestinal symptoms of lactose malabsorption is diagnostic. False-negative tests occur in individuals with diabetes, delayed gastric emptying, or SIBO small intestinal bacterial overgrowth.[6,17,20,21,30] This test is cumbersome and requires blood sampling to determine serum glucose levels. It has largely been replaced by the hydrogen breath test.[31–33]

### Breath Hydrogen Test

The breath hydrogen test is the most accurate test for identifying lactose malabsorption; it is simple and noninvasive. Hydrogen in breath is measured after administration of a lactose load. The lactose dose varies (usually 1–2 g/kg, with a maximum of 50 g). The physiological dose is 12 g lactose (the amount in 1 cup of milk), and this is often the dose used for testing. A positive test is indicated by a rise of 20 ppm or more in expired hydrogen above baseline. Samples are collected before administration of lactose and in 30-minute intervals for 3 hours thereafter.

A diagnosis of lactose maldigestion does not predict the occurrence of symptoms. The test is also used to determine other forms of carbohydrate maldigestion or malabsorption and SIBO.[6,18,20,21,28] In individuals with suspected SIBO, a hydrogen breath test using lactulose may be required to differentiate the two disorders.[6,31,32]

### Genetic Test

A new genetic test It detects the single nucleotide polymorphism C/T 13910 of the lactase gene (*LCT*) on chromosome 2. This DNA variant has been associated with adult-type hypolactasia. Use of this test would enable children to be diagnosed without lactose challenge.

### Stool Acidity Test

A stool acidity test can be used in infants and young children. This test measures lactic acid and other short-chain fatty acids present in the stool that are derived from undigested lactose fermented by bacteria. The test uses pH measurements (pH $\leq$5.5 is abnormal). However, this test is not specific for lactose intolerance; a positive test is also present in people with other carbohydrate malabsorption disorders.[6,18,21,27,30]

### Intestinal Biopsy

Biopsies may not always yield abnormal results, because lactase deficiency after mucosal injury may be patchy. Lactase measurement with intestinal biopsies is time-consuming and invasive. However, it may be useful if the patient is already undergoing endoscopy as part of his or her evaluation.

### Empirical Lactose Avoidance

A simple lactose avoidance test may aid in diagnosis. Patients avoid lactose for 1 to 2 weeks and their symptoms are tracked. This test is not as specific as others, but families often prefer it.

## DIETARY MANAGEMENT

### Medical Nutrition Therapy

Treatment for lactose intolerance aims to prevent the gastrointestinal symptoms associated with lactose malabsorption. Optimal diet therapy for lactose intolerance involves determination of a nonoffending, individualized diet. This can be achieved by using a combination of tolerated lactose-containing foods, enzymatically pretreated dairy products, lactase enzyme supplements taken concurrently with milk products, or plant-based milk alternatives and dietary supplementation to meet nutrient needs despite dietary restrictions.

Proper dietary management depends on the individual's diagnosis (i.e., primary versus secondary lactose intolerance). Complete avoidance of lactose, the offending carbohydrate, relieves symptoms in all cases of lactose intolerance. Because there is much variability in lactose tolerability among those with lactose nonpersistance or secondary lactose intolerance,[9] the degree of dietary lactose restriction necessary for symptom relief depends on the etiology of lactose malabsorption. Individuals with CLD require more stringent lactose restriction than, for example, those with lactose nonpersistance or secondary lactose intolerance, who preserve some lactase and therefore the ability to digest lactose in small quantities. For this reason, the degree of dietary restriction should be tailored to the individual. For those with secondary lactose intolerance, lactose restriction is no longer required once the underlying condition causing malabsorption is resolved.

Lactose restriction involves reducing or completely restricting lactose-containing foods, such as cow's milk products, from the diet. Depending on individual tolerance, avoidance of convenience foods to which whey, milk, milk solids, or lactose has been added may also be required. Other mammalian milks, such as goat, sheep, or mare's milk, are not lactose-free. Lactose is less sweet than other sugars, so it is used in commercial food products as a food thickener, to improve the appearance and texture of certain foods, or to enhance the solubility of instant drink mixes and powdered substances. Lactose can also be present in tablet medications, although the amount of lactose ingested in this form (<500 mg) rarely causes gastrointestinal symptoms.[34] Dairy products pretreated with lactase enzyme and thus rendered lactose-free are widely available in supermarkets and are well tolerated by individuals with lactose intolerance. These products are covered by the Women, Infants and Children (WIC) supplemental nutrition packages, and less expensive store brands are also available for purchase by those who do not qualify for WIC benefits.[9]

Published recommendations for dietary lactose restriction vary widely. More conservative recommendations suggest complete lactose elimination for 2t o 4 weeks to achieve symptom relief,[6] followed by gradual reintroduction of low-lactose cheeses and yogurt and progressing to other milk products as tolerated. Other studies define a low-lactose diet as one that restricts lactose to less than 6 g per meal[35] or less than 12 g per day.[36]

Because some lactose-intolerant children and adults can tolerate 4 to 8 ounces of cow's milk without developing symptoms, it has been suggested that 12 g of lactose (or 8 oz of milk) can be easily tolerated by those with lactose intolerance.[37–39] Blinded studies in adults with self-reported lactose intolerance suggest that at least 12 g lactose can be tolerated at one occasion without development of symptoms,[39,40] and up to 18 g lactose can be tolerated when taken with other foods.[41] Consumption of milk and dairy foods during meals with other foods may slow gastric emptying and promote tolerance.[42,43] Many lactose-intolerant individuals can tolerate milk chocolate[44] or fluid milk with cocoa added.[45] Plain yogurt is usually well tolerated because the active cultures in yogurt partially digest lactose before consumption.[46,47] The continuing presence of some degree of lactose in the diet may promote lactose tolerance due to adaptation of colonic flora.[9,41]

Drug therapy may alternatively improve an individual's ability to tolerate lactose-containing foods. Lactase-replacement supplements can be taken orally when consuming milk products to prevent gastrointestinal symptoms by breaking down lactose into glucose and galactose for improved intestinal absorption.[48] Supplement dosing and efficacy vary among brands.[49] Probiotics may promote tolerance via alterations in intestinal flora.[50] Some probiotics contain beta-galactosidase, which directly enzymatically digests dietary lactose. Other probiotics promote colonization of bacteria that hydrolyze lactose and prevent fermentation by other colonic bacteria, thus avoiding gastrointestinal symptoms.[51]

Milk and dairy products should not be entirely eliminated from the diet without appropriate substitution, because these foods are excellent sources of calories, protein, vitamins A and D, riboflavin, calcium, phosphorus, and other minerals. Children on milk-restricted diets have lower intake of these nutrients.[52] Although lactose itself has not been shown to directly affect calcium absorption, studies suggest that lactose-free diets prescribed to children are low in calcium and result in low bone mineral density.[53,54] Additionally, long-term data show that children on milk-restricted diets have shorter stature[55] and lower weight[55,56] than children on full diets. Nut- and grain-based milk alternatives such as rice, soy, almond, or coconut beverages are completely lactose free but often do not contain the nutrients found in milk unless fortified with calcium, riboflavin, and vitamins A, D, and $B_{12}$. Nut- and grain-based milks are hypocaloric and have lower protein and fat content compared with cow's milk. Therefore, they are not appropriate replacements for toddlers or children with low dietary protein and fat intake from other sources (Table 50–1). Soy and soy products have many health benefits and can be used in children's diets; their protein content comparable that found in standard cow's milk. Depending on diet composition and nutrient needs based on age (Table 50–2), calcium supplementation may be required if milk is eliminated from the diet and calcium-rich foods are not consumed (Table 50–3); they should be recommended judiciously, however, because excessive calcium intake in young children consuming milk alternatives and calcium supplements may promote iron deficiency.[57]

### Indications for Lactose-Free Infant Formulas

Lactose-free infant formulas have gained popularity in the United States,[58] but routine use is warranted only in certain cases. The degree and duration of lactose restriction depend on the etiology of lactase deficiency or lactose malabsorption.

**Table 50–1.** Comparison of Enriched Plant-Based Milk Alternatives to Whole Cow's Milk (per 8 oz)

| Milk | Calories | Protein (g) | Fat (g) | Vitamin D (IU) | Calcium (mg) |
|---|---|---|---|---|---|
| Whole Milk | 150 | 8 | 8 | 100 | 300 |
| Soy | 60–130 | 6 | 3.5 | 105 | 300–450 |
| Rice | 120 | 1 | 2.5 | 100 | 100–300 |
| Almond | 40–100 | 1 | 2.5 | 94 | 450 |
| Oat | 130 | 4 | 2.5 | 100 | 360 |
| Hemp | 70–170 | 2 | 6 | 100 | 300 |
| Coconut | 70–100 | 0–1 | 4 | 120 | 100–500 |

**Table 50–2.** Lactose-Free Formulas, Milk Substitutes, and Other Calcium Sources

| Lactose-Free Formulas Infant | Lactose-Free Formulas Pediatric | Milk Substitutes |
|---|---|---|
| *Cow's Milk-Based* | *Cow's Milk-Based* | *Cow's Milk-Based* |
| Similac Sensitive Spit-Up | Pediasure | Lactaid Milk |
| Parent's Choice Gentle | Kindercal | Dairy Ease Milk |
| | Boost Kids Essentials | |
| | Nutren Junior | |
| | Compleat Pediatric | |
| *Soy-Based* | *Soy-Based* | *Soy-Based* |
| Enfamil Prosobee | Bright Beginnings Soy | Silk |
| Similac Isomil | Enfagrow Toddler Soy | 8th Continent |
| Earth's Best Organic Soy | Similac Grow & Go Soy | WestSoy |
| Gerber GoodStart Soy | | Edensoy |
| *Semi-Elemental* | *Semi-Elemental* | *Other Plant-Based* |
| Nutramigen | Peptamen Junior | Rice Dream |
| Pregestimil | | Almond Breeze |
| Alimentum | | SoDelicious Coconut |
| *Elemental* | *Elemental* | Pacific Oat Milk |
| Elecare | Elecare Junior | Tempt Hemp Milk |
| Neocate Infant | Neocate Junior | Pure Almond |
| PurAmino | Vivonex Pediatric | |

Primary CLD requires prolonged adherence to a lactose-free diet, and in infancy this easily accomplished with a lactose-free, milk protein–based infant formula or a soy formula, which is naturally lactose free.[9] Developmental (neonatal) lactase deficiency resulting from prematurity can be managed by with the use of lactase-treated feeds or low-lactose formula.[59] However, human milk and standard premature infant formulas do not seem to have adverse effects in premature infants and may be used safely.[60]

The utility of lactose-free formulas in infants with secondary lactase deficiency is questionable. For infants with lactose intolerance secondary to malnutrition, provision of lactose-containing formula may promote lactose tolerance and improve growth outcomes.[61] However, the utility of lactose-free formula for infants with postinfectious diarrhea is unclear. A meta-analysis found that children with diarrheal illness can continue to safely consume human milk or standard, lactose-containing formula.[62] However, in malnourished infants or infants younger than 3 months of age with acute infectious diarrhea, a lactose-free formula may reduce the duration of diarrhea.[63] As diarrhea resolves, infants may be offered their previously tolerated, lactose-containing formula. If the infant is breast-feeding, the mother can continue nursing. All soy protein–containing formulas are lactose-free and can be used for refeeding if diarrhea is prolonged. Despite widespread use, lactose-free formulas for treatment of presumed lactose intolerance resulting from colic, fussiness, and gas may not be warranted.[64]

## SUMMARY AND FOLLOW-UP

The goal of medical nutrition therapy for lactose intolerance is to prevent gastrointestinal symptoms while continuing to provide adequate nutrition. An individualized management plan may include a combination of lactose restriction and lactase supplementation with appropriate food or nutritional supplements as needed. Achieving the least restrictive diet that does not elicit symptoms is the ultimate goal to promote optimal nutrition and quality of life.

**Table 50–3.** Lactose-Free Diet*

| Food Groups | Lactose-Free | Lactose-Containing |
|---|---|---|
| Beverages | See also milk and milk products. Milk-free cocoa, fruit juices, lactose-free carbonated beverages and fruit drinks, coffee and tea, decaffeinated coffee | Milk beverages, instant coffee and tea containing lactose, powdered soft drinks and artificial drinks containing lactose, instant chocolate drinks |
| Breads and cereals | Any that do not contain milk or milk products (Italian, Vienna, French, Jewish bread), saltine and graham crackers, rusk, Ry-Krisp and Ritz crackers, other snack chips without milk, infant cereals, cooked or dry cereals without added milk | Muffins, biscuits, waffles, sweet rolls, pancakes, cereals, bread and crackers containing milk and milk products; instant cereals containing lactose |
| Desserts | Fruit ices, popsicles, gelatin dessert, angel food cake, homemade cakes, fruit pies, cookies made without milk or milk products | Commercial cakes, cookies, and dessert mixes, custard pudding, ice cream, ice milk, sherbet, yogurt, frozen yogurt, most soufflés and mousses, desserts containing chocolate, caramel, reduced-calorie desserts made with sugar substitute containing lactose |
| Fats | Margarine and dressings that do not contain milk or milk products, vegetable oils, shortenings, mayonnaise, bacon | Margarine, butter, sauces and dressings containing milk or milk products; cream, half-and-half, whipped cream, cream cheese, sour cream; gravies made with milk, cream sauces and cheese, cheese dips |
| Fruits and juices | All unless processed with lactose | Fruits and juices containing milk, lactose, or whey |
| Meat, fish, poultry, eggs, legumes | Plain beef, chicken, fish, turkey, seafood, lamb, veal, pork, ham, plain eggs, legumes, kosher meat products, dried peas, beans, lentils | Creamed or breaded meat, fish, or poultry; lunch meats, sausages and frankfurters containing milk or milk products; creamed or scrambled eggs or omelettes prepared with milk |
| Milk, milk products, substitutes | Nutramigen and soybean milk used as milk substitutes (e.t., Prosobee, Isomil, Nursoy), Ensure, Pediasure and other lactose-free, high-calorie canned supplements; milk treated with lactase enzyme such as LactAid, Vitamite, nondairy creamers | Cow's milk–based infant formulas, low-fat milk, nonfat milk, whole milk, powdered milk, condensed and evaporated milk, buttermilk, goat milk, yogurt, cottage cheese, cheese, ice cream, ice milk, sherbet, malted milk, instant breakfast, hot chocolate, imitation milks |
| Potato, rice, pasta | White and sweet potatoes, yams, macaroni, noodles, spaghetti, rice | Any creamed or breaded potato, rice, or pasta; mashed or instant potatoes made with milk, macaroni and cheese mixes |
| Soups | Clear broth and bouillon-based soups, other soups made without milk or milk products | Cream soups, chowders, and commercial soups containing milk, cream, or cheese |
| Vegetables | All plain vegetables | Vegetables in cream or cheese sauce |
| Miscellaneous products | Flavorings, extracts, herbs, spices, salt, pepper, condiments, pickles, olives, sugar, jam, jelly, marmalade, preserves, honey, syrup, candy made without milk, popcorn, potato chips, corn chips, pretzels, coconut, nuts, peanut butter; pure cocoa powder, nondairy creamers and whipped toppings | Candies containing cream, milk, lactose, or chocolate; caramels, toffee, butterscotch, or peppermint candies, frosting; diet sugars and chewing gum containing lactose; frozen dinners, Italian dishes, quesadillas |

*Lactose is found in milk and milk products. Labels should be read carefully; any product that contains milk, milk solids, dry milk solids, lactose, or whey may need to be excluded. Lactose is also frequently used as a filler in many products, such as instant coffee and tea, and in some medicines. Individuals with lactose intolerance may be able to eat "Lactose-Containing" foods in limited amounts.

## References


1. Bailey RK, Fileti CP, Keith J, Tropez-Sims S, Allison-Ottley SD. Lactose intolerance and health disparities among African Americans and Hispanic Americans: an updated consensus statement. *J Natl Med Assoc.* 2013; 105:112.
2. Suchy FJ, Brannon PM, Carpenter PO, et al. National Institutes of Health consensus development conference: lactose intolerance and health. *Ann Intern Med.* 2010; 152:792.
3. Lomer MC, Parkes GC, Sanderson JD. Review article: lactose intoleracne in clinical practice—myths and realities. *Aliment Pharmacol Ther.* 2006; 27:93.
4. Cry T-D, Ohlsson A. Lactase treated feeds to promote growth and feeding tolerance in preterm infants. *Cochrane Database Syst. Rev.* 2013; (3):CD004591.
5. Douglas PS. Diagnosing gastro-esophageal reflux disease or lactose intolerance in babies who cry a lot in the first few months overlooks feeding problems. *J Pediatr Child Health.* 2013; 49(Suppl):E252.
6. Di Rienzo T, D'Angelo G, D'Aversa F, et al. Lactose intolerance: from diagnosis to correct management. *Eur Rev Med Pharmacol Sci.* 2013; 17(Suppl 2):18.
7. Heaney RP. Dietary intake, dietary adequacy and lactose intolerance. *Adv Nutr.* 2013; 4:151.
8. de Lacy Costello BP, Ledochowski M, Ratcliffe NM. The importance of methane breath testing: a review. *J Breath Res.* 2013; 7:1.
9. Heyman MB. Lactose intolerance in infants, children and adolsecents. *Pediatrics.* 2006; 118:1279.
10. Pereira PC. Milk nutritional composition and its role in human health. *Nutrition.* 2014; 30:619.
11. Suchy FJ, Brannon PM, Carpenter TO, et al. NIH consensus development conference statement: Lactose Intolerance and Health. *NIH Consens State Sci Statements.* 2010; 27:1.
12. Holzel A, Schwarz V, Sutcliffe KW. Defective lactose absorption causing malnutrition in infancy. *Lancet.* 1959; 1:1126.
13. Jarvela I, Torniainen S, Kolho KL. Moleculare genetics of human lactase deficiency. *Ann Med.* 2009; 41:568.
14. Kuokkanen M, Kokkonen J, Enattah NS, et al. Mutations in the translated region of the lactase gene underlie congenital lactase deficiency. *Am J Hum Genet.* 2006; 78:339.
15. Kleinman RE, Greer FR, eds. *Pediatric Nutrition Handbook*, 7th ed. Elk Grove Village, IL: American Academy of Pediatrics; 2014: 396.
16. American Academy of Pediatrics, Committee on Nutrition. The practical significance of lactose intolerance in children. *Pediatrics.* 1978; 62:240.
17. American Academy Pediatrics, Committee on Nutrition. The practical significance of lactose intolerance in children: supplement. *Pediatrics.* 1990; 86:643.
18. Misselwitz B, Pohl D, Fruhauf H, Fried M, Vavricka SR, Fox M. Lactose malabsorption and intolerance: pathogenesis, diagnosis, and treatment. *United European Gastroenterology J.* 2013; 1:151.
19. Morelli L. Yogurt, living cultures and gut health. *Am J Clin Nutr.* 2014; 99(5 Suppl):1248S.
20. Savaiano AD. Lactose digestion from yogurt: mechanism and relevance. *Am J Clin Nutr.* 2014; 99(5 Suppl):1251S.
21. Mattar R, Ferraz de Campos D, Carrilho FJ. Lactose intolerance: diagnosis, genetic and clinical factors. *Clin Exper Gastroenterol.* 2012; 5:113.
22. Leavitt M, Wilt T, Shaukat A. Clinical implications of lactose malabsorption versus lactose intolerance. *J Clin Gastroenterol.* 2013; 47:471.
23. Brussoow H. Nutrition, population growth and disease: a short history of lactose. *Environ Microbiol.* 2013; 15:2154.
24. Curry A. The milk revolution. *Nature.* 2013; 200:20.
25. Guarino A, Ashkenazi S, Gendrel D, Lo Vecchio A, Shamir R, Szajewska H. ESPGHN evidenced based guidelines for the management of acute gastroenteritis in children. *J Pediatr Gastroenterol Nutr.* 2014; 59:132.
26. Sauders N, Friedman JN. Lactose avoidance for young children with acute diarrhea. *Pediatr Child Health.* 2014; 19:529.
27. Vickerstaff Joneja J. Lactose intolerance. In: Vickerstaff Joneja J. *The Health Professional's Guide to Food Allergies and Intolerances.* Academy of Nutrition and Dietetics. 2013.
28. Wessel JJ. Gastrointestinal disorder. In: Samour PQ, Helm KK, Lang CE, eds. *Handbook of Pediatric Nutrition*, 3rd ed. Gaithersburg, MD: Aspen; 2012.
29. Sundaran A, Koutikia P, Apovian CM. Nutritional management of short bowel syndrome in adults. *J Clin Gastroenterol.* 2002; 34:207.
30. Gremse DA, Greer AS, Vacik J, DiPalma JA. Abdominal pain associated with lactose ingestion in children with lactose intolerance. *Clin Pediatr.* 2003; 42:341.
31. Law D, Conklin J, Pimentel M. Lactose intolerance and the role of lactose breath test. *Am J Gastroenterol.* 2010; 105:1726.
32. Misselwitz B. Lactose intolerance: new insights due to blinded testing? *Digestion.* 2014: 90:72.
33. Wilder-Smith CH, Materna A, Wermelinger C, Schluer J. Fructose and lactose intolerance and malabsorption testing: the relationship with symptoms in functional gastrointestinal disorders. *Aliment Pharmacol Ther.* 2013; 37:1074.
34. Montalto M, Gallo A, Santoro L, et al. Low-dose lactose in drugs neither increases breath hydrogen excretion nor causes gastrointestinal symptoms. *Aliment Pharmacol Ther.* 2008; 28:1003.
35. Hertzler SR, Huynh BC, Savaiano DA. How much lactose is low lactose? *J Am Diet Assoc.* 1996;96:243.
36. Academy of Nutrition and Dietetics. Nutrition therapy for lactose intolerance. In: *Nutrition Care Manual.* Chicago: Academy of Nutrition and Dietetics; 2014. https://www.nutritioncaremanual.org/client_ed.cfm?ncm_client_ed_id=19. Accessed July 5, 2016.
37. Johnson AO, Semenya JG, Buchowski MS, Enwonwu CO, Scrimshaw NS. Adaptation of lactose maldigesters to continued milk intake. *Am J Clin Nutr.* 1993; 58:879.
38. McBean LD, Miller GD. Allaying fears and fallacies about lactose intolerance. *J Am Diet Assoc.* 1998; 98:671.
39. Suarez FL, Savaiano D, Arbisi P, Levitt MD. Tolerance to the daily ingestion of two cups of milk by individuals claiming lactose intolerance. *Am J Clin Nutr.* 1997; 65:1502.
40. Suarez FL, Savaiano DA, Levitt MD: A comparison of symptoms after the consumption of milk or lactose-hydrolyzed milk by people with self-reported severe lactose intolerance. *N Engl J Med* 1995; 333:1.
41. Shaukat A, Levitt MD, Taylor BC, et al. Systematic review: effective management strategies for lactose intolerance. *Ann Intern Med.* 2010; 152:797.
42. Labayen I, Forga L, Gonzalez A, Lenoir-Wijnkoop I, Nutr R, Martinez JA. Relationship between lactose digestion, gastrointestinal transit time and symptoms in lactose malabsorbers after dairy consumption. *Aliment Pharmacol Ther.* 2001; 15:543.
43. Martini MC, Savaiano DA. Reduced intolerance symptoms for lactose consumed during a meal. *Am J Clin Nutr.* 1988; 47:57.
44. Järvinen RM, Loukaskorpi M, Uusitupa MI. Tolerance of symptomatic lactose malabsorbers to lactose in milk chocolate. *Eur J Clin Nutr.* 2003; 57:701.
45. Lee CM, Harvey CM. Cocoa feeding and human lactose intolerance. *Am J Clin Nutr.* 1989; 49:840.
46. Kolars JC, Levitt MD, Aouji M, Savaiano DA. Yogurt: an autodigesting source of lactose. *N Engl J Med.* 1984; 310:1.
47. Boudraa G, Benbouabdellah M, Hachelaf W, Boisset M, Desjeux JF, Touhami M. Effect of feeding yogurt versus milk in children with acute diarrhea and carbohydrate malabsorption. *J Pediatr Gastroenterol Nutr.* 2001; 33:307.
48. Medow MS, Thek KD, Newman LJ, Berezin S, Glassman MS, Schwarz SM. Beta-galactosidase tablets in the treatment of lactose intolerance in pediatrics. *Am J Dis Child.* 1990; 144:1261.
49. Ramirez FC1, Lee K, Graham DY. All lactase preparations are not the same: results of a prospective, randomized, placebo-controlled trial. *Am J Gastroenterol.* 1994; 89:566.
50. Almeida CC, Lorena SL, Pavan CR, Akasaka HM, Mesquita MA. Beneficial effects of long-term consumption of a probiotic combination of *Lactobacillus casei* Shirota and *Bifidobacterium breve* Yakult may persist after suspension of therapy in lactose-intolerant patients. *Nutr Clin Pract.* 2012; 27:247.
51. Ojetti V, Gigante G, Gariella M, et al. The effect of oral supplementation with *Lactobacillus reuteri* or tilactase in lactose intolerant patients: randomized trial. *Eur Rev Med Pharmacol Sci.* 2010; 1:163.
52. Henriksen C, Eggesbø M, Halvorsen R, Botten G. Nutrient intake among two-year-old children on cows' milk-restricted diets. *Acta Paediatr* 2000; 89:272.
53. Stallings VA, Oddleifson NW, Negrini BY, Zemel BS, Wellens R. Bone mineral content and dietary calcium intake in children prescribed a low-lactose diet. *J Pediatr Gastroenterol Nutr.* 1994; 18:440.
54. Di Stefano M, Veneto G, Malservisi S, et al. Lactose malabsorption and intolerance and peak bone mass. *Gastroenterology.* 2002; 122:1793.
55. Christie L, Hine RJ, Parker JG, Burks W. Food allergies in children affect nutrient intake and growth. *J Am Diet Assoc.* 2002; 102:1648.
56. Isolauri E1, Sütas Y, Salo MK, Isosomppi R, Kaila M. Elimination diet in cow's milk allergy: risk for impaired growth in young children. *J Pediatr.* 1998; 132:1004.
57. Carvalho NF, Kenney RD, Carrington PH, Hall DE. Severe nutritional deficiencies in toddlers resulting from health food milk alternatives. *Pediatrics.* 2001; 107:E46.
58. Abrams SA, Griffin, IJ, Davila PM. Calcium and zinc absorption from lactose-containing and lactose-free infant formulas. *Am J Clin Nutr.* 2002; 76:442.
59. Erasmus HD, Ludwig-Auser HM, Paterson PG, Sun D, Sankaran K. Enhanced weight gain in preterm infants receiving lactase-treated feeds: a randomized, double-blind, controlled trial. *J Pediatr.* 2002; 141:532.
60. Shulman RJ, Feste A, Ou C. Absorption of lactose, glucose polymers, or combination in premature infants. *J Pediatr.* 1995; 127:626.
61. Kukuruzovic RH, Brewster DR. Milk formulas in acute gastroenteritis and malnutrition: a randomized trial. *J Paediatr Child Health.* 2002; 38:571.
62. Brown KH, Peerson JM, Fontaine O. Use of nonhuman milks in the dietary management of young children with acute diarrhea: a meta-analysis of clinical trials. *Pediatrics.* 1994; 93:17.
63. Macgillivray S, Fahey T, McGuire W. Lactose avoidance for young children with acute diarrhea. *Cochrane Database Syst Rev.* 2013;(10):CD005433.
64. Sherman AL, Anderson J, Rudolph CD, Walker LS. Lactose-free milk or soy-based formulas do not improve caregivers' distress or perceptions of difficult infant behavior. *J Pediatr Gastroenterol Nutr.* 2015; 61:119.

# 51 Disorders of Fructose Metabolism

WENDY SMITH

Fructose is widely available in the typical Western diet. It is found as a naturally occurring monosacccharide in fruits and vegetables and as a component sugar of sucrose and sorbitol. Once ingested, it is absorbed unchanged by the small intestine and rapidly utilized in the liver and, to a lesser extent, in the kidneys. Intracellular fructose is phosphorylated by fructokinase into fructose-1-phosophate. This phosphorylated form is then cleaved by aldolase B into glyceraldehyde and dihydroxyacetone phosphate. Glyceraldehyde is further metabolized into either glycerol or pyruvate, eventually entering the Krebs cycle; dihydroxyacetone phosphate is further metabolized into fructose-1,6-diphosphate, which enters the glycolysis/gluconeogenesis pathway.[1–3] Eventually, ingested fructose is converted into glucose, lactate/pyruvate, and glycogen (Fig. 51–1). As with all inborn errors of metabolism, the clinical features associated with the deficiency of enzymes specific to fructose metabolism result from accumulation of substrate preceding the enzyme deficiency, production of products along alternative metabolic pathways, and reduced availability of products of the normal enzyme activity.

## BIOCHEMICAL AND OTHER FACTORS IN EVALUATION AND TREATMENT

When there is an abnormality of intracellular fructose metabolism, excessive fructose-1-phosphate accumulates. The phosphorylation process depletes intracellular phosphorus stores and reduces the available adenosine triphosphate (ATP), which is necessary for proper protein and energy metabolism. Levels of the dephosphorylated nucleotides adenosine diphosphate (ADP) and adenosine monophosphate (AMP) rise, and their catabolism increases uric acid production, resulting in hyperuricemia and uricosuria. Excessive fructose-1-phosphate also results in increased lactate production by increasing the concentration of glyceraldehyde and increasing the activity of pyruvate kinase. Hypoglycemia results from fructose-1-phosphate inhibition of glucogenolysis (specifically, phosphorylase) and glucolysis (aldolase B and glucose-6-phosphate isomerase).[1,3] These pathways of fructose-1-phosphate metabolism explain the laboratory and clinical findings in the inborn errors of fructose metabolism with excess intracellular fructose-1-phosphate accumulation (Table 51–1).

There are three recognized inborn errors of fructose metabolism: (1) essential fructosuria resulting from deficient hepatic fructokinase activity, (2) hereditary fructose intolerance (HFI) due to deficient aldolase B activity, and (3) fructose-1,6-bisphosphatase deficiency (see Fig. 51–1). The clinical features of these disorders are highly variable owing to the location of the deficient enzyme within the fructose metabolic pathway, the availability of alternative routes of fructose metabolism, and toxicity resulting from accumulated metabolites.

## ESSENTIAL FRUCTOSURIA

Essential fructosuria is the result of deficient activity of hepatic fructokinase. Reduced enzyme activity decreases the amount of ingested and absorbed fructose that is converted into fructose-1-phosphate; the remaining fructose is excreted unchanged in the urine. This fructosuria is detected, often on a routine urinalysis in an otherwise healthy individual, by the presence of non–glucose-reducing substances. Because there are no abnormalities of the intracellular fructose metabolic pathway, there are no other distinguishing clinical or biochemical features of fructokinase deficiency. The excessive fructose consumption in the typical Western diet allows appropriate intracellular accumulation of fructose-1-phosphate despite increased renal losses. Although reducing the ingestion of fructose will decrease the fructosuria, no dietary or medical management is required.[1]

## HEREDITARY FRUCTOSE INTOLERANCE

Deficiency of fructose-1-phosphate aldolase B results in HFI. This disorder is clinically apparent only with exposure to fructose, and the signs and symptoms reflect the timing, amount, and duration of fructose exposure. Symptoms include poor feeding, nausea, vomiting, failure to thrive, and abdominal pain; symptoms may be acute or chronic, depending on fructose exposure.

Because aldolase B is predominant in liver and kidney, signs of renal dysfunction and hepatic failure predominate in the clinical presentation. Liver failure may be life-threatening and is often preceded by hepatomegaly (which may be asymptomatic) and jaundice. Further evaluation may reveal elevated serum transaminases (aspartate transaminase [AST] and alanine transaminase [ALT]) and decreased hepatic synthetic function, including coagulation factors, leading to a bleeding diathesis. Renal dysfunction is characterized by a generalized tubulopathy with loss of protein and electrolytes in the urine, recognized as Fanconi syndrome.[3]

Classically, HFI manifests at the time of weaning, when infants are initially challenged with fructose-containing fruits and vegetables; however, the diagnosis should also be considered in older infants and children who have signs of gastrointestinal distress and hepatic or renal dysfunction. Some older children and adults have been diagnosed based on a history of avoidance of sweet foods; the absence of dental caries in older individuals may indicate long-term avoidance of offending foods.[4]

Diagnostic strategies rely on biochemical and/or molecular testing. Biochemical testing can document decreased aldolase B activity on liver biopsy; activity is typically 15% or less of control activity when fructose-1-phosphate is used as the test substrate.[1] Molecular diagnosis is available. Seven mutations in the aldolase B gene (A149P, A174D, N334K, Delta4E4, R59Op, A337V, and L256P) are responsible for 65% of mutant alleles in Americans and 82% of mutant alleles worldwide.[5] Use of additional genetic technologies, including single nucleotide polymorphism (SNP) arrays and whole exome sequencing, may facilitate molecular diagnosis in individuals who do not have diagnostic results with common mutation testing, especially in insular or consanguineous populations. Fructose challenge testing is no longer recommended as a diagnostic measure because of the potential for catastrophic hypoglycemia.[6]

Medical management of HFI involves treatment of the hepatic and renal dysfunction in the acute setting. Avoidance of fructose ingestion is the most important component of long-term treatment. With good dietary control, individuals with HFI can have normal growth and development. Patients often develop an aversion to sweet foods that assists in adherence to dietary requirements, although this may not be completely reliable in young children.[8]

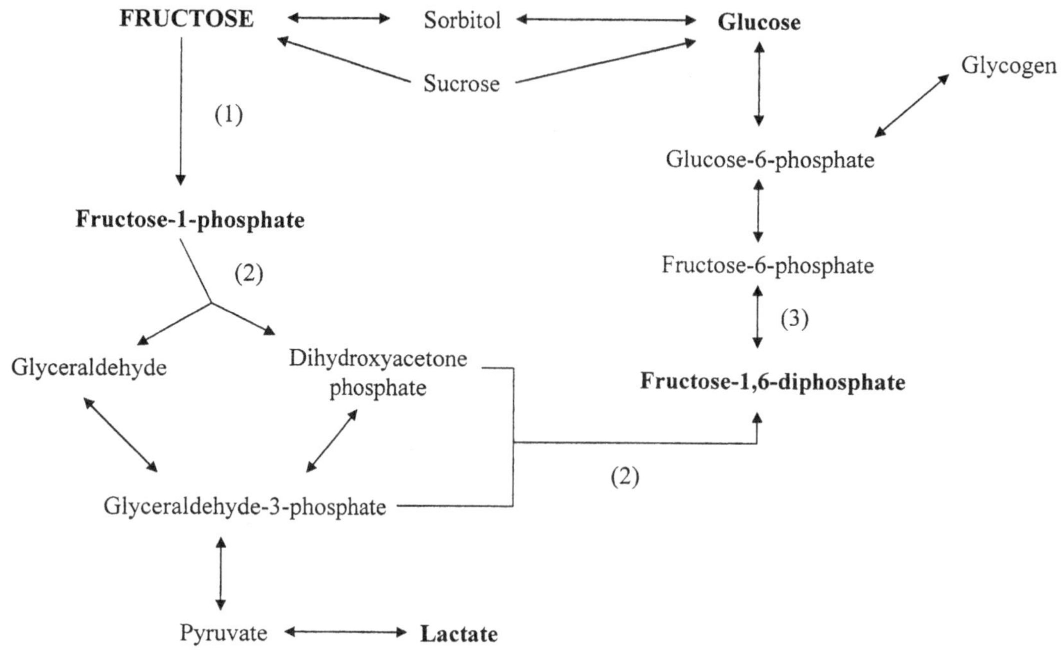


**Figure 51–1.** Fructose metabolism. The three recognized inborn errors of fructose metabolism result from deficient fructokinase (1), aldolase B (2), and fructose-1,6-bisphosphatase (3).

## FRUCTOSE-1,6-BISPHOSPHATASE DEFICIENCY

Fructose-1,6-bisphosphatase deficiency is best thought of as a disorder of gluconeogenesis rather than a disorder of fructose metabolism. In the liver, this enzyme is required for the endogenous formation of glucose from various precursors, including lactate, alanine, and glycerol. When it is deficient, patients demonstrate a significantly reduced fasting tolerance because hypoglycemia results once glycogen stores are depleted. In almost all affected individuals, symptoms begin in infancy, within the first week of life in 50%. Symptoms of hypoglycemia, including irritability, altered alertness, and changes in heart rate or muscle tone, predominate; hyperventilation as a result of profound acidosis may also be present. Initial laboratory testing reveals hypoglycemia with a variable ketotic response and a profound lactic acidosis. Signs of hepatic failure are usually absent, although there may be variable hepatomegaly. Similar episodes may occur during times of metabolic stress, such as with intercurrent infections or poor oral intake. If left untreated, these episodes can lead to respiratory or cardiac arrest and permanent neurological sequelae.

**Table 51–1.** Potential Laboratory Findings in Disorders of Intracellular Fructose Metabolism

| Serum/Plasma Values | Urine Values |
|---|---|
| Hypoglycemia | Positive reducing substances |
| Hypophosphatemia | Glucosuria |
| Hypokalemia | Proteinuria/amino aciduria |
| Hypermagnesia | Uricosuria |
| Hyperuricemia | Elevated phosphorus, potassium |
| Lactic acidosis | Acidosis |
| Hyperbilirubinemia | |
| Hypertriglyceridemia (acutely) | |
| Elevated hepatic transaminases (ALT, AST) | |
| Increased PT, PTT | |
| Abnormal tramsferrin isoelectric focusing | |

ALT, alanine transaminase; AST, aspartate transaminase; PT, prothrombin time; PTT, partial thromboplastin time.
From Quintana E, Sturiale L, Montero R, et al. Secondary disorders of glycosylation in inborn errors of fructose metabolism. *J Inherit Metab Dis.* 2009; 32(Suppl 1):S273.

The hypoglycemia associated with fructose-1,6-bisphosphatase deficiency is usually not directly related to fructose intake, as seen in HFI, although it can occur with a significant fructose load. Patients usually do not develop a dislike for sweet foods, and in fact they may learn to treat their hypoglycemia symptoms with sugar-containing foods.[1,3]

A definitive diagnosis of fructose-1,6-bisphosphatase deficiency is made by demonstrating reduced enzyme activity in a liver biopsy specimen. Molecular diagnosis is also possible. Supervised fasting studies and fructose challenge testing are not necessary and should be performed only under close observation, with prompt treatment for the non–glucagon-responsive hypoglycemia that develops.[6]

Prevention of acute episodes of acidosis and hypoglycemia is the main therapeutic goal in individuals with fructose-1,6-bisphosphatase deficiency. Avoidance of fasting and maintenance of normal blood glucose levels during periods of metabolic stress (with either intravenous or oral replenishment) can prevent most acute attacks. Treatment during an acute episode involves prompt restoration of normal blood pH and glucose levels, usually with intravenous glucose and sodium bicarbonate.

## DIETARY MANAGEMENT

Dietary management includes judicious avoidance of large amounts of fructose, which can precipitate hypoglycemia. Otherwise, avoidance of fasting by frequent feedings in infancy and use of uncooked cornstarch by older children and adults is the main therapy. In general, fasting tolerance improves with age because the liver is able to accumulate increased glycogen reserves.

## FRUCTOSE IN THE DIET

The typical Western diet includes approximately 100 g of fructose per day.[9] This fructose is ingested with the consumption of fruits, vegetables, grains, and cereals as well as sucrose, both naturally occurring and that added to prepared foods. The fructose content of fruits and vegetables varies considerably, depending on growing conditions, storage conditions, and preparation (cooking, canning,

**Table 51–2.** General Dietary Guidelines for a Fructose-Restricted Diet

| Food Category | Acceptable | Unacceptable |
|---|---|---|
| Infant feeding | Breast milk<br>Most commercial infant formulas | Some specific metabolic formulas including Portagen |
| Dairy products | Unflavored and unsweetened dairy products (including whole milk, low-fat milk, skim milk, cream, buttermilk, evaporated milk, dry milk); plain yogurt; sour cream; cottage cheese; unprocessed cheese | Sweetened dairy products including chocolate, vanilla, and fruit flavorings; sugar- or fruit-sweetened yogurts; nondairy liquid creamers; condensed milk; some processed cheeses and cheese spreads |
| Meat, fish, poultry | Plain red meats<br>Plain poultry<br>Plain fish and seafood | Sugar-cured meats; many processed meats, including flavor-injected poultry; most lunch meats; some breaded meats and fish |
| Eggs | All eggs | Sweetened prepared eggs |
| Vegetables | Greens including sprouts, cabbage, celery, endive, escarole, kale, lettuce, spinach, chard, mixed greens; root vegetables including shallots, and yams; green beans, wax beans, peas; asparagus, cauliflower; mushrooms<br>Permissible in small amounts: cucumber, green pepper, radish, summer squash, onion | All others, including carrots, leeks, and corn/maize<br>Canned or frozen vegetables with sauces |
| Fruits and juices | Lime juice | All others |
| Potatoes and starches | Fresh white potatoes<br>Some potato chips | Sweet potatoes |
| Pastas and grains | Macaroni, spaghetti, etc.<br>Egg noodles<br>Rice | Commercial pasta, rice, noodle, and potato mixes (frozen and boxed) |
| Breads and cereals | Puffed rice, puffed wheat, shredded wheat, cream of rice<br>Matzo, degermed cornmeal<br>Certain breads, crackers, pretzels, tortillas, English muffins | All sweetened cereals<br>Breads, crackers, and tortillas made with added sugar<br>Wheat germ and products containing wheat germ |
| Fats | Butter, margarine, vegetable oils, olive oil, lard, shortening; some salad dressings | Commercial salad dressings<br>Mayonnaise |
| Desserts and candy | Some gelatins<br>Some sugar-free desserts<br>Home-prepared desserts made with dextrose<br>Pixie Stix | All commercial desserts, cookies, pastries<br>All other candy<br>Chewing gum, including sugar-free (contains sorbitol) |
| Condiments | Herbs and spices<br>Gravy<br>Vinegar | Ketchup, sauces<br>Sweet pickles, relishes<br>Peanut butter, jellies, jams |
| Baking ingredients | Unsweetened cocoa, baking chocolate<br>Corn starch | Soy flour; vanilla flavoring |
| Sweeteners | Aspartame, saccharin<br>Dextrose, glucose, lactose, maltose<br>Rebaudioside A (Steviol glycoside) | Honey, syrups, molasses<br>Agave nectar, high-fructose corn syrup, hydrolyzed inulin syrup<br>Sorbitol, levulose, sucrose |
| Miscellaneous | Diet sodas<br>Sugar-free soft drinks<br>Tempeh, tofu<br>Permissible in small amounts: popcorn | Dried beans and peas<br>Coconut, nuts, seeds<br>Many alcoholic beverages, including beer, brandy, rum, vodka, sherry, vermouth, cream drinks, liquors |

and freezing). Table 51–2 provides a general guide to foods that are included and excluded in a fructose-restricted diet. The fructose content of various specific foods is available in print, on the Internet, and from manufacturers.[9–11] Common hidden dietary sources of fructose include wheat germ and whole grains.

Because fructose is considerably sweeter than glucose, it is a common component of many sweeteners and may appear on food and medication labels as sucrose, high-fructose corn syrup, sorbitol, invert sugar, hydrolyzed inulin syrup, honey, or levulose. Labels on foods, beverages, and all medications must be scrutinized carefully to avoid accidental fructose ingestion. Even foods labeled "sugar-free" are suspect. This label usually means that the foods are sucrose free, but they may not be free of all sugars (including fructose). Aspartame, saccharin, dextrose, lactose, and glucose are all safely consumed in a fructose-free diet.

Pharmaceutical companies in the United States are not required to list all inert ingredients on medication packaging, although most companies will provide such information. Prescription and over-the-counter medications should be reviewed carefully; this is especially important for liquid or syrup preparations designed to appeal to children. Several lists of the sugars and inert ingredients in medications are available; however, formulations may change over time.[12–15] Pharmacists should be notified and educated regarding the patient's diagnosis so that medications can be screened appropriately.

A fructose-restricted diet is significantly restricted in several other nutrients, most prominently vitamin C. Appropriate supplementation is recommended. Ongoing nutritional evaluation by a metabolic dietitian is necessary to ensure appropriate vitamin and mineral intake.[16] The amount of fructose restriction necessary to maintain metabolic control in individuals with HFI, and to a lesser extent in those with fructose-1,6-bisphosphatase deficiency, is unknown. Various authors have documented a wide range of potentially acceptable daily fructose intakes, from 20 to 40 mg/kg/day to less than 1.5 g/day.[8,17] Careful documentation of an individual's diet and comparison of fructose intake with growth and hepatic/renal function, can help determine the individual's fructose tolerance. Elevated uric acid can indicate excessive fructose intake despite an absence of physical symptoms.[8] Liberalization of the diet may be possible in adolescence or adulthood after growth is completed and the individual is able to determine his or her own fructose-related symptoms more accurately.

## FOLLOW-UP

The long-term prognosis for individuals with inborn errors of fructose metabolism is excellent once an accurate diagnosis is established and appropriate management is instituted. Neuropsychological development and intelligence are expected to be normal, barring any consequences of severe metabolic decompensation before diagnosis. Successful pregnancies in women with fructose-1,6-bisphosphatase deficiency and HFI have been reported.[18] Ongoing dietitian support and education are essential throughout life to maintain optimal growth and compliance with dietary therapy.

## References


1. Steinmann B, Gitzelmann R, Van den Berghe G. Disorders of fructose metabolism. In: Scriver CR, Beaudet AL, Sly WS, Valle D, eds. *The Metabolic and Molecular Bases of Inherited Disease*, 8th ed. New York: McGraw-Hill; 2001.
2. Jamar S, Evenepoel P, Kuypers D, Maes B, Vanrenterghem Y. A young patient with unexplained hepatorenal dysfunction. *Nephrol Dial Transplant*. 2003; 18:1220.
3. Van den Berghe G. Disorders of fructose metabolism. In: Fernandes J, Saudubray JM, van den Berghe G, eds. *Inborn Metabolic Diseases*, 3rd ed. Berlin: Springer-Verlag; 2000.
4. Newburn E, Hoover C, Mettraux G, Graf H. Comparison of dietary habits and dental health of subjects with hereditary fructose intolerance and control subjects. *J Am Dent Assoc*. 1980; 101:619.
5. Coffee EM, Yerkes L, Ewen EP, Zee T, Tolan DR. Increased prevalence of mutant null alleles that cause hereditary fructose intolerance in the American population. *J Inherit Metab Dis*. 2010; 33:33.
6. Hoffman GF, Nyhan WL, Zschoke J, Kahler SG, Mayatepek E, eds. *Inherited Metabolic Diseases*. Philadelphia: Lippincott Williams & Wilkins; 2002.
7. Quintana E, Sturiale L, Montero R, et al. Secondary disorders of glycosylation in inborn errors of fructose metabolism. *J Inherit Metab Dis*. 2009; 32(Suppl 1):S273.
8. Mock DM, Perman JA, Thaler MM, Morris RC. Chronic fructose intoxication after infancy in children with hereditary fructose intolerance. *N Engl J Med*. 1983; 309:764.
9. Rumessen JJ. Fructose and related food carbohydrates. *Scand J Gastroenterol*. 1992; 27:819.
10. Matthews RH, Pehrsson PR, Farhat-Sabet M. *Sugar Content of Selected Foods: Individual and Total Sugars*. USDA Home Economics Research Report Number 48. Washington, DC: US Government Printing Office; 1987. https://archive.org/details/usda-homeeconomicsresearchreport. Accessed July 7, 2016.
11. Hands ES. *Nutrients in Food*. Philadelphia: Lippincott Williams & Wilkins; 2000.
12. Kumar A, Aitas AT, Hunter AG, Beaman DC. Sweeteners, dyes and other excipients in vitamin and mineral preparations. *Clin Pediatr*. 1996; 35:443.
13. Kumar A, Rawlings RD, Beaman DC. The mystery ingredients: sweeteners, flavorings, dyes and preservatives in analgesic/antipyretic, antihistamine/decongestant, cough and cold, antidiarrheal and liquid theophylline preparations. *Pediatrics*. 1993; 91:927.
14. Kumar A, Weatherly MR, Beaman DC. Sweeteners, flavorings and dyes in antibiotic preparations. *Pediatrics*. 1991; 87:352.
15. Hill EM, Flaitz CM, Frost GR. Sweetener content of common pediatric oral liquid medications. *Am J Hosp Pharm*. 1988; 45:135.
16. Acosta PB, Yannicelli S. *Nutrition Support Protocols*, 4th ed. Columbus, OH: Ross Products Division; 2000.
17. Bell L, Sherwood WG. Current practices and important recommendations for treating hereditary fructose intolerance. *J Am Diet Assoc*. 1987; 87:721.
18. Krishnamurthy V, Eschrich K, Boney A, et al. Sullivan, J., McDonald, M., Kishnani, P.S., Koeberl, D.D. Three successful pregnancies through dietary management of fructose-1,6-bisphosphatase deficiency. *J Inherit Metab Dis*. 2007; 30:819.

# 52 Glycogen Storage Diseases

MARI MORI AND PRIYA KISHNANI

Glycogen storage diseases (GSDs) are inherited disorders that affect glycogen metabolism. The first clinical description of a patient with a defect in glycogen mobilization was published in 1928 by Snappes and Van Creveld.[1] Today, more than 16 forms of GSD have been identified, with a wide spectrum of clinical presentations and an overall frequency of approximately 1 in 20,000 to 25,000 live births.[2] The classification of GSDs is summarized in Table 52–1. Several reviews of the general and clinical aspects of GSD[2–5] and recommendations for treatment[6–8] are available. This chapter focuses on liver GSD types I and III.

## GLYCOGEN STORAGE DISEASE TYPE I

GSD type Ia was first described by von Gierke in 1929.[9] In 1952, Cori and Cori established the first metabolic disorder in which an enzyme defect was identified when they demonstrated that the absence of glucose 6-phosphatase (G6Pase) enzyme activity was the defect responsible for the disease.[10] Glucose-6-phosphatase translocase was later discovered to be deficient in GSD Ib. Comprehensive guidelines for the management of GSD I have been published by the American College of Medical Genetics and Genomics.[8]

### Biochemical Abnormalities and Manifestations

G6Pase is required for the final step of glycogenolysis and gluconeogenesis to cleave glucose from glucose 6-phosphate (Fig. 52–1). In the absence of G6Pase, hypoglycemia results, and lactic acidosis, hyperlipidemia, and hyperuricemia follow secondarily. Affected children present with hepatomegaly, enlarged kidneys, poor linear growth, and excess adipose tissue in the cheeks, which gives them doll-like facial features. GSD type Ib has additional findings of neutropenia and neutrophil dysfunction resulting in recurrent bacterial infections and, occasionally, chronic gastrointestinal inflammation.[11,12] A diagnosis of GSD I is suspected on the basis of the clinical presentation and abnormal laboratory values. A definitive diagnosis of GSD Ia or Ib is based on sequencing of the *G6PC* or *SLC37A4* gene, respectively. If snap-frozen liver tissue is available, enzyme activity can be analyzed to confirm the diagnosis of GSD Ia.[8,11,12]

### Factors To Be Considered in Nutrition Evaluation

Infants often remain asymptomatic as long as they are nursing or fed frequently; the first signs of hypoglycemia may not occur until the child begins to sleep through the night without feeding or with the onset of an illness. Early diagnosis and treatment reduces the risk of prolonged hypoglycemia, which can cause developmental and physical delay, seizures with or without cerebral damage, and even death. The initial assessment should include a complete itemized diet history, medications including supplements and herbal therapy, sleeping patterns, signs and symptoms of hypoglycemia, and gastrointestinal issues. Patients are frequently asymptomatic during hypoglycemic episodes. Ideally, a 3-day record of diet and preprandial blood glucose monitoring should be obtained to fully assess the timing and extent of hypoglycemia. The use of continuous glucose monitoring systems at home may provide trends of hypoglycemia true to the patient's life. Signs of anemia, gout, and osteopenia/osteoporosis should be assessed in adult patients. Triglycerides, cholesterol, uric acid, vitamin D, and iron storage levels should be monitored.

### Dietary Management

General dietary guidelines for the treatment of GSD I include small, frequent feedings that are high in complex carbohydrates and free of most fructose and galactose. Fructose and galactose cannot be converted to glucose owing to the deficiency of G6Pase and are restricted to varying degrees.[13–15] Because of limited fruit, juice, and dairy product intake, vitamins, minerals, and calcium are supplemented.[3,4,6] The nutrient distribution of the diet is 60% to 70% carbohydrate, 10% to 15% protein, and 20% to 30% fat. Carbohydrate calories are evenly distributed over a 24-hour period. Complex carbohydrates help maintain normoglycemia for longer periods.[16,17] A condensed list of foods allowed and not allowed on the GSD I diet is presented in Table 52–2.

Overnight tube feeding of a sucrose- and lactose-free formula or an overnight glucose drip may be used in place of frequent bottle feeds in infancy. Elemental formula with more carbohydrate or Prosobee may also be used in the older child. The rate of formula feeding should be calculated to provide glucose at a rate similar to that of normal hepatic release of glucose.[2,18,19] The rate should be[8] approximately 8 to 10 mg of glucose per kilogram body weight per minute in infancy and 4 to 8 mg/kg/min in older children. Close blood glucose monitoring is important because subclinical asymptomatic hypoglycemia is common.[8]

Uncooked cornstarch has been used in the treatment of GSD I since the early 1980s,[20–25] and it is superior to overnight glucose therapy in maintaining overnight normoglycemia.[26] Argo brand (ACH Food Companies, Summit, IL) is preferred in the United States for both taste and sustainability.[8] A small dose is typically introduced between 6 and 12 months of life.[27,28] Cornstarch is mixed in a sucrose-free, lactose-free formula, soy milk, or water. Extreme heat and acids such as ascorbic acid, sodium citrate, or lemonade break down the glucose bonds of cornstarch more readily and compromise the constant glucose supply.[21,22] Patients taking sodium citrate because of secondary hypocitraturia have become hypoglycemic when they mixed cornstarch formula with Bicitra.[8]

When introducing cornstarch, parents should watch for gastrointestinal side effects. Typically, diarrhea associated with cornstarch intake is transient, although some bloating and gas may persist.[21] Patients with GSD Ib may develop worse gastrointestinal issues reminiscent of Crohn disease.[12] A trial with pancrelipase—a combination of lipase, protease, and amylase—may be warranted for better digestion of cornstarch, especially when it is introduced at a very young age.[8]

The cornstarch goal for infants and very young children is 1.6 g/kg body weight given every 3 to 4 hours.[2,8] The school-aged child may progress to 1.7 to 2.5 g/kg every 4 to 6 hours. The postpubertal patient may be able to lengthen the time between cornstarch feedings to 6 to 8 hours, and some adults may require only a larger bedtime dose (1.7 to 2.5 g/kg).[2]

Periodic blood glucose monitoring is essential, especially when there are changes to the diet content or schedule, periods of rapid growth, puberty, or times of stress, illness, or increased activity. Recurrent (unrecognized) hypoglycemia causes poor metabolic control, hepatomegaly, and growth failure.[8] Glycosade, a modified cornstarch, has become available for overnight treatment.[17] Because data on the long-term use of Glycosade are limited, it should be used only under supervision by a metabolic team with close glucose monitoring. Medium-chain triglyceride (MCT) oil has been studied as a nutrition

**Table 52–1.** Classification of Glycogen Storage Diseases (GSDs)

| Type | Deficient Enzyme | Tissue Involved | Main Clinical Findings |
|---|---|---|---|
| Oa | Glycogen synthase | Liver | Hypoglycemia, ketosis |
| Ob | Glycogen synthase | Muscle | Exercise intolerance, cardiomyopathy |
| Ia | Glucose-6-phosphatase | Liver, kidney | Hypoglycemia, hepatomegaly, lactic acidosis, hyperlipidemia. |
| Ib | Glucose-6-phosphate translocase | Liver, kidney, gastrointestinal tract | In addition to GSD Ia: neutropenia and infections and chronic gastrointestinal inflammation |
| II | Acid alphaglucosidase (lysosomal) | Heart, muscle | Infantile form: cardiorespiratory failure<br>Later-onset forms (juvenile, childhood and adult): myopathy |
| IIIa | Debranching enzyme | Liver, muscle, heart | Hypoglycemia, hepatomegaly, myopathy |
| IIIb | Debranching enzyme | Liver | Hypoglycemia, hepatomegaly |
| IV | Branching enzyme | Liver, muscle | Hepatosplenomegaly, liver fibrosis, liver failure, myopathy, hypotonia, dilated cardiomyopathy, fetal akinesia in severe cases |
| V | Phosphorylase | Muscle | Exercise intolerance, myoglobinuria |
| VI | Phosphorylase | Liver | Hepatomegaly |
| VII | Phosphofructokinase | Muscle | Exercise intolerance |
| IX Liver Forms | Phosphorylase b kinase | Muscle | Exercise intolerance |
| IX Muscle Forms | Phosphorylase b kinase | Liver | Hepatomegaly |
| X | Phosphoglycerate mutase | Muscle | Exercise intolerance |
| XI | Lactate dehydrogenase | Muscle | Exercise intolerance, rhabdomyolysis |
| XII | Aldolase | Erythrocyte | Hemolytic anemia |
| XIII | Enolase | Muscle | Exercise intolerance |
| XV | Glycogenin 1 | Muscle, heart | Exercise intolerance, arrhythmia |
| Danon | Lysosomal-associated membrane protein 2 (LAMP2) | Heart | Cardiomyopathy, cognitive disabilities more severe in males than in females |
| PRKAG2 | Adenosine monophosphate (AMP)-activated protein kinase | Heart, muscle, kidney, testis | Cardiomyopathy, arrhythmias, myalgia, hepatomegaly, renomegaly, macroglossia |
| Fanconi Bickel | Glucose transporter 2 | Liver, pancreas | Hepatomegaly, proximal renal tubular dysfunction |

therapy to encourage ketogenesis and suppress glycolysis with inconsistent results; further studies are needed.[17,29] Care should be taken to ensure that fat intake includes sufficient essential fatty acids.[17]

Overtreatment is as detrimental as undertreatment because it can lead to several side effects, including excessive weight gain, poor oral hygiene,[30] poor development of feeding skills, and an increased risk of nutritional deficiencies.[31] Overtreatment may lead to chronic hyperinsulinism and resultant hypoglycemia when a meal or cornstarch dose is missed. Therefore, the dose of cornstarch needs to be carefully tailored to individual patient needs.

## Follow-up

The infant or child with GSD I should have lifelong follow-up in a genetic metabolic clinic. An appropriate diet should be followed to maintain normoglycemia and avoid overtreatment. Parents must be discouraged from giving excess formula or cornstarch to overcompensate for hypoglycemia. Occupational, speech, and psychological therapy should be available and used as early as possible if feeding issues are noted. Plasma calcium level should be monitored closely, especially if calcium is supplemented, because hypercalcemia can be one of the metabolic manifestations of GSD I.[32] Pump failures, occluded or disconnected feeding tubes, and alarm clock failure can lead to prolonged fasting, hypoglycemia, and even death.[33,34] Safety precautions and an emergency protocol should be in place.

With good dietary compliance, the child with GSD I can lead a productive life, possibly postponing the onset of long-term complications. However, long-term complications are still prevalent. Growth and puberty are usually delayed, with symptoms of gout starting after the onset of puberty.[35] Many patients older than 20 years of age have hypertension, renal stones, and kidney failure.[36–38] Liver adenomas should be monitored closely. One study suggested that although good metabolic control is beneficial for liver adenoma control, other

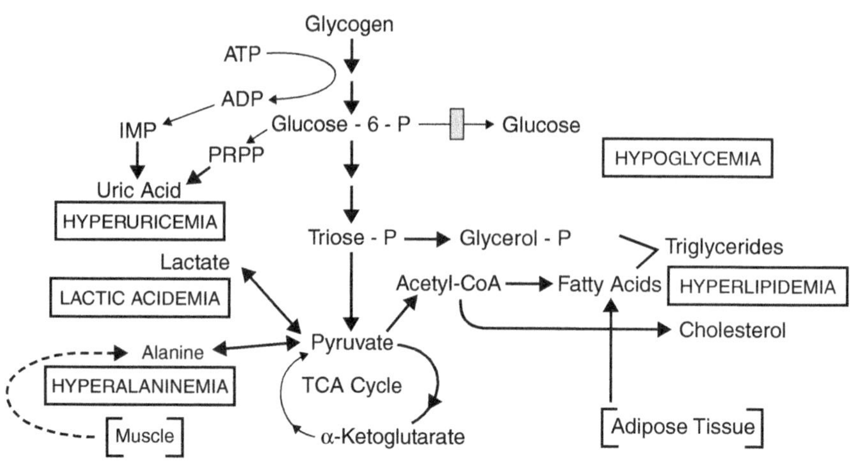


**Figure 52–1.** Metabolic consequences of glycogen storage disease type I. ADP = adenosine diphosphate; ATP = adenosine triphosphate; Acetyl-CoA = acetyl coenzyme A; IMP = inosine-5′-monophosphate; P = phosphate; PRPP = 5-phosphoribosyl-1-pyrophosphate; TCA = tricarboxylic acid.

**Table 52–2.** Selected Foods Allowed and Not Allowed on the Glycogen Storage Disease Type I Diet*

| Food Group | Foods Allowed | Foods Not Allowed |
|---|---|---|
| Dairy | Limit to 1 serving a day<br>1 cup low-fat milk<br>1 cup low-fat, sugar-free yogurt<br>1.5 oz cheese | Ice cream, sweetened yogurt with fruit, sweetened milk |
| Cereals | Dry and cooked cereals with no added sugar | Cereals with fruit or sugar added |
| Breads | White, wheat, rye bread and crackers, English muffins, dinner rolls, biscuits, pita bread, bagels | Raisin bread, muffins, sweet rolls, pies, cakes, sweet breads, waffles, and sweat pancakes |
| Starches | Brown and white rice, pasta, popcorn, tortillas, white potatoes | Any starches with sugar added, sweet potatoes |
| Vegetables | All vegetables, including asparagus, cabbage, spinach, squash, onions, green beans etc. | Any with added sugar, milk, or cheese; corn, peas, and carrots have more sugar than the others |
| Fruit | Raw limes, some lemon juice, avocados | All other fresh, canned, and dried fruits or tomatoes |
| Meat | Lean poultry, beef, pork, fish<br>Egg substitutes | Organ meats; fatty and processed meats |
| Legumes/Nuts | All beans, peas, and nuts<br>Sugar-free peanut butter | Any beans, nuts or seeds with sugar added |
| Soups | Broth soups made with allowed meat, starches, and vegetables | Creamed soups |
| Fats | Canola and olive oil<br>Corn, safflower, canola, and soybean oil–based condiments | Fats from coconut and palm oil, *trans*-fatty acids |
| Sweets | Sugar substitutes, dextrose, 100% corn syrup, sucralose, sugar-free Jell-o and pudding | All other sugars, sweets, syrups, high-fructose corn syrup, honey, molasses, sorbitol |

*This is not a complete list of foods allowed and not allowed; careful label reading is recommended.

genetic factors may play a role.[8,39] Adenomas can transform to hepatocellular carcinomas.[8] Both liver, renal, and combined liver-renal transplantations have been reported.[40–44] Hyperlipidemia associated with GSD I was not considered a cardiovascular risk factor in the past, but a few cases of patients with early coronary artery disease have been reported.[32] Because many patients are now living longer, pharmacological treatment is recommended for metabolic control.[45–49] Other complications include osteoporosis,[50–52] pulmonary arterial hypertension,[53,54] chronic anemia, and hypocitraturia.

Successful pregnancies have been reported in the literature.[55,56] Recommendations include optimal nutrition, increased cornstarch intake, adequate vitamin and mineral supplementation, blood glucose monitoring, close follow-up with a high-risk obstetrics group, and planned admission to start an intravenous glucose infusion before delivery to maintain normoglycemia and prevent bleeding complications.

## GLYCOGEN STORAGE DISEASE III

GSD III is caused by a deficiency of the debranching enzyme amylo-1,6-glucosidase, which leads to impaired glycogenolysis but intact gluconeogenesis. Therefore, a limited source of glucose is available from the outer branches of glycogen (action of phosphorylase) and from amino acids via gluconeogenesis. Figure 52–2 depicts the degradation of glycogen.

### Biochemical Abnormalities and Manifestations

Debrancher enzyme may be lacking in both liver and muscle tissue (GSD IIIa) or only in liver tissue (GSD IIIb). During infancy, the clinical signs of GSD III often mimic those of GSD I, including hypoglycemia, hyperlipidemia, hepatomegaly, and growth retardation. In contrast to individuals with GSD I, these patients have normal blood lactate and uric acid levels but markedly elevated levels of liver transaminases. Serum creatine kinase can be elevated. Hypoglycemia typically improves with age. However, progressive liver cirrhosis may occur in GSD IIIb. Those with GSD IIIa begin to show signs of progressive skeletal myopathy and cardiomyopathy at various stages of life.[2]

A diagnosis of GSD III can be suspected based on the clinical presentation and biochemical abnormalities. A definitive diagnosis can be made by mutation analysis of the *AGL* gene in blood DNA. Two mutations in exon 3—c.18_19delGA (p.Gln6Hisfs*20) and c.16C>T (p.Gln6X)—are associated with GSD IIIb, whereas private mutations scattered along the same gene have been associated with GSD IIIa. Full sequencing of the gene is clinically available.[7] If liver biopsy was performed and tissue is available, structurally abnormal glycogen

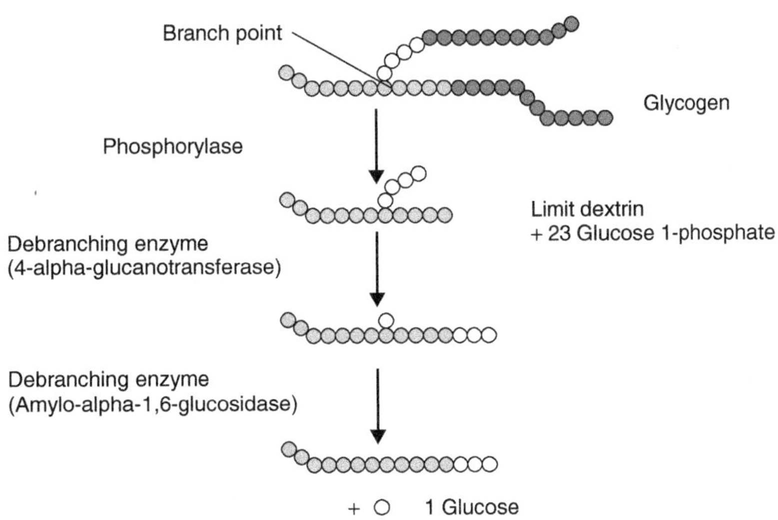


**Figure 52–2.** Degradation of glycogen.

accumulation and decreased debranching enzyme activity can confirm the diagnosis.[2]

## Factors To Be Considered in Nutrition Evaluation

Although GSD III may be almost indistinguishable from GSD I in infancy and childhood, the diet for GSD III is far less restrictive because there are no sugar restrictions. Glycogen molecules can be broken down to the point of the branched chains, and gluconeogenesis is intact, so some glucose is available and the child may fast longer, especially at older ages. Ideally, a 3-day diet record and preprandial monitoring of blood glucose and ketones should be obtained to fully assess the timing and extent of hypoglycemia and ketosis, which may be a marker of metabolic stress and may be observed before hypoglycemia. The use of continuous glucose monitoring systems at home may provide trends of hypoglycemia true to the patient's life. Preprandial glucose monitoring is important especially during intercurrent illnesses because patients may be asymptomatic. In older patients, signs of osteoporosis should be assessed, as should calcium and vitamin D intake.

## Dietary Management

The treatment goals for GSD III are to prevent both hypoglycemia and muscle damage. Distribution of calories from carbohydrates, protein, and fat should be adjusted depending on growth and myopathy symptoms. Overall, 25% to 30% protein, approximately 50% carbohydrate, and 20% to 25% fat are recommended. A high-protein diet is beneficial for patients with GSD III because it may improve muscle function, replace unnecessary carbohydrate, and reduce resultant glycogen storage, and its metabolite alanine can be a source for gluconeogenesis.[7] MCT oil may be considered because it can provide an additional form of energy that is readily utilized by the skeletal and heart muscles and provides another substrate for energy and gluconeogenesis.

As in GSD I, small, frequent feedings with avoidance of fasting are recommended to prevent hypoglycemia. Extra protein is given as an alternative source of glucose via gluconeogenesis to prevent hypoglycemia and muscle protein turnover, in the forms of breast milk, regular infant formula, or higher-protein formulas, especially in cases of GSD IIIa.[57,58] As in GSD I, some older infants and young children may require cornstarch.[59] Guidelines for cornstarch use are similar to those for GSD I with decreased doses, but the cornstarch can be mixed in regular infant formula or milk. One gram of cornstarch per kilogram of body weight may provide sufficient blood glucose for 4 hours. Overnight tube feedings may be indicated. Tailored cornstarch treatment improves growth and decreases hypoglycemic events.[60] Use of pancrelipase can be considered in younger infants who may not produce functional enzymes and experience bloating and diarrhea (as in GSD I). Adults with GSD III often outgrow the need for cornstarch therapy. As in GSD I, overtreatment should be avoided.

## Follow-Up

Food record analysis and nutrition education should be continued to ensure dietary compliance. The older patient with GSD IIIa should be monitored closely for progressive skeletal myopathy and cardiomyopathy, and the high-protein diet should be reiterated. Improvement of cardiomyopathy with high-protein diet has been reported in some case reports.[61,62] Close monitoring of the liver is also recommended in GSD III because cases of cirrhosis, adenoma formation, and HCC have been reported. Polycystic ovarian disease is also reported in female patients with GSD III.[2]

## Conclusion

Since GSD was first identified, many advances have been made in its treatment, but the current treatments remain symptomatic. Long-term consequences are not completely avoided by current therapy. Advances in the field of genetics continue to increase understanding of the pathophysiology and molecular basis of the disease. Enzyme replacement therapy and gene therapy lend much hope for the future treatment of GSD.[63,64]

### References


1. Snappes I, Van Creveld S. Un cas d'hypoglycemie avec acetonemie chez un enfant. *Bull Mem Soc Med Hop.* 1928; 52:1315.
2. Chen Y-T, Kishnani P, Koeberl D. Glycogen storage diseases. In: Valle D, Beaudert A, Vogelstein B, et al., eds. *The Online Metabolic and Molecular Basis of Inherited Disease.* New York: McGraw-Hill; 2014.
3. Heller S, Worona L, Consuelo A. Nutritional therapy for glycogen storage diseases. *J Pediatr Gastroenterol Nutr.* 2008; 47:S15.
4. Hicks J, Wartchow E, Mierau G. Glycogen storage diseases: a brief review and update on clinical features, genetic abnormalities, pathologic features, and treatment. *Ultrastruct Pathol.* 2011; 35:183.
5. Hendriksz CJ, Gissen P. Glycogen storage disease. *Paediatr Child Health.* 2011; 21:84.
6. Kishnani PS, Steiner RD, Bali D, et al. Pompe disease diagnosis and management guideline. *Genet Med.* 2006; 8:267.
7. Kishnani PS, Austin SL, Arn P, et al. Glycogen storage disease type III diagnosis and management guidelines. *Genet Med.* 2010; 12:446.
8. Kishnani PS, Austin SL, Abdenur JE, et al. Diagnosis and management of glycogen storage disease type I: a practice guideline of the American College of Medical Genetics and Genomics. *Genet Med.* 2014; 16:e1.
9. Von Gierke E. Glykogen-speicher-krankheit der Leber und Nieren. *Beitr Pathol Anat.* 1929; 82:497.
10. Cori G, Cori C. Glucose-6-phosphatase of the liver in glycogen storage disease. *J Biol Chem.* 1952; 199:661.
11. Melis D, Fulceri R, Parenti G, et al. Genotype/phenotype correlation in glycogen storage disease type 1b: a multicentre study and review of the literature. *Eur J Pediatr.* 2005; 164:501.
12. Chou JY, Jun HS, Mansfield BC. Type I glycogen storage diseases: disorders of the glucose-6-phosphatase/glucose-6-phosphate transporter complexes. *J Inherit Metab Dis.* 2014; 38:511.
13. Fernandes J, van de Kamer JH. Studies on the utilization of hexoses in liver glycogen disease. *Pediatrics.* 1965; 35:470.
14. Fernandes J. The effect of disaccharides on the hyperlactic acidemia of glucose-6-phosphatase–deficient children. *Acta Paediatr Scand.* 1974; 63:695.
15. Greene HL, Slonim AE, O'Neill JA, Burr IM. Continuous nocturnal intragastric feeding for the management of type I glycogen storage disease. *N Engl J Med.* 1976; 294:423.
16. Chen Y-T, Leinhas J, Coleman RA. Prolongation of normoglycemia in patients with type I glycogen storage disease. *J Pediatr.* 1987; 111:567.
17. Bhattacharya K. Dietary dilemmas in the management of glycogen storage disease type I. *J Inherit Metab Dis.* 2011; 34:621.
18. Tsalikian E, Simmons P, Gerich JE, Howard C, Haymond MW. Glucose production and utilization in children with glycogen storage disease type I. *Am J Physiol.* 1984; 247:E513.
19. Schwenk WF, Haymond MW. Optimal rate of enteral glucose administration in children with glycogen storage disease type I. *N Engl J Med.* 1986; 314:682.
20. Chen Y-T, Cornblath M, Sidbury JB. Cornstarch therapy in type I glycogen storage disease. *N Engl J Med.* 1984; 310:171.
21. Sidbury JB, Chen Y-T, Roe CR. The role of raw starches in the treatment of type I glycogenosis. *Arch Intern Med.* 1986; 146:370.
22. Gatti R, Galmedica G, Di Rocco M, Massocco D, Marchese N, Borrone C. Long-term cornstarch therapy in glycogen storage disease types I, Ib and III. *J Inherit Metab Dis.* 1986; 9(Suppl 2):280.
23. Wolfsdorf J, Ehrlich S, Landy H, Crigler J. Optimal daytime feeding regimen to prevent postprandial hypoglycemia in type I glycogen storage disease. *Am J Clin Nutr.* 1992; 56:587.
24. Chen Y-T, Bazzarre C, Lee M, Sidbury JB, Coleman RA. Type I glycogen storage disease: nine years of management with cornstarch. *Eur J Pediatr.* 1993; 152(Suppl 1): S56.
25. Lee PJ, Dixon MA, Leonard JV. Uncooked cornstarch: efficacy in type I glycogenosis. *Arch Dis Child.* 1996; 74:546.
26. Shah K, O'Dell S. Effect of dietary interventions in the maintenance of normoglycaemia in glycogen storage disease type 1a: a systematic review and meta-analysis. *J Hum Nutr Diet.* 2013; 26:329.
27. Vici C, Bartuli A, Mazziotta M, Sabetta G. Early introduction of uncooked cornstarch for the treatment of glycogen storage disease type I. *Acta Paediatr Scand.* 1990; 79:978.
28. Hayde M, Wildhalm K. Effects of cornstarch treatment in very young children with type I glycogen storage disease. *Eur J Pediatr.* 1990; 149:630.
29. Das AM, Lücke T, Meyer U, Hartmann H, Illsinger S. Glycogen storage disease type 1: impact of medium-chain triglycerides on metabolic control and growth. *Ann Nutr Metab.* 2010; 56:225.
30. Farrington F, Duncan L, Roth K. Looking a gift horse in the mouth: effects of cornstarch therapy and other implications of glycogen storage disease on oral hygiene and dentition. *Am Acad Pediatr Dent.* 1995; 17:311.
31. Kishnani P, Boney A, Chen Y-T. Nutritional deficiencies in a patient with glycogen storage disease type Ib. *J Inherit Metab Dis.* 1999; 22:795.
32. Kasapkara ÇS, Tümer L, Okur İ, Eminoğlu T, Ezgü FS, Hasanoğlu A. Hypercalcemia in glycogen storage disease type I patients of Turkish origin. *Turk J Pediatr.* 2012; 54:35.
33. Leonard J, Dunger D. Hypoglycemia complicating feeding regiments for glycogen storage disease. *Lancet.* 1978; 12:1203.
34. Wolfsdorf J, Keller R, Landy H, Crigler J. Glucose therapy for glycogenosis type I in infants: comparison of intermittent uncooked cornstarch and continuous overnight glucose feedings. *J Pediatr.* 1990; 117:384.
35. Mundy H, Hindmarsh P, Matthews D, Leonard J, Lee P. The regulation of growth in glycogen storage disease type I. *Clin Endocrinal.* 2003; 58:332.
36. Chen Y-T, Coleman R, Scheinman J, Kolbeck P, Sidbury JB. Renal disease in type I glycogen storage disease. *N Engl J Med.* 1988; 318:7.
37. Chen Y-T, Scheinman J, Park H, Coleman R, Roe CR. Amelioration of proximal renal tubular dysfunction in type I glycogen storage disease with dietary therapy. *N Engl J Med.* 1990; 23:590.

38. Lee P, Dalton R, Shah V, Hindmarsh P, Leonard J. Glomerular and tubular function in glycogen storage disease. *Pediatr Nephrol.* 1995; 9:705.
39. Kishnani PS, Chuang T-P, Bali D, et al. Chromosomal and genetic alterations in human hepatocellular adenomas associated with type Ia glycogen storage disease. *Hum Mol Genet.* 2009; 18:4781.
40. Parker P, Burr I, Slonim A, Ghishan F, Greene H. Regression of hepatic adenomas in type Ia glycogen storage disease with dietary therapy. *Gastroenterology.* 1981; 81:534.
41. Lee P, Mather S, Owens C, Leonard J, Dicks-Mireaux C. Hepatic ultrasound findings in the glycogen storage diseases. *Br J Radiol.* 1994; 67:1062.
42. Lee P. Glycogen storage disease type I: pathophsiology of liver adenomas. *Eur J Pediatr.* 2002; 161:S46.
43. Labrune P. Glycogen storage disease type I: indications for liver and/or kidney transplantation. *Eur J Pediatr.* 2002; 161:S53.
44. Lee P, Muiesan P, Heaton N. Successful pregnancy after combined renal-hepatic transplantation in glycogen storage disease type Ia. *J Inherit Metab Dis.* 2004; 27:537.
45. Fernandes J, Pikaar N. Hyperlipemia in children with liver glycogen disease. *Am J Clin Nutr.* 1969; 22:617.
46. Greene H, Swift L, Knapp H. Hyperlipidemia and fatty acid composition in patients treated for type 1a glycogen storage disease. *J Pediatr.* 1991; 119:398.
47. Ubels F, Rake J, Slaets J, Smit G, Smit A. Is glycogen storage disease 1a associated with atherosclerosis? *Eur J Pediatr.* 2002; 161:S62.
48. Lee P, Celermajer D, Robinson J, McCarthy S, Betteridge D, Leonard J. Hyperlipidaemia does not impair vascular endothelial function in glycogen storage disease type 1a. *Atherosclerosis.* 1994; 110:95.
49. Wierzbicki A, Watts G, Lynas J, Winder A, Wray R. Very low-density lipoprotein apolipoprotein B-100 turnover in glycogen storage disease type 1a (von Gierke disease). *J Inherit Metab Dis.* 2001; 24:527.
50. Lee PJ, Patel JS, Fewtrell M, Leonard JV, Bishop NJ. Bone mineralisation in type 1 glycogen storage disease. *Eur J Pediatr.* 1995; 154:483.
51. Schwahn B, Rauch F, Wendel U, Schönau E. Low bone mass in glycogen storage disease type 1 is associated with reduced muscle force and poor metabolic control. *J Pediatr.* 2002; 141:350.
52. Schönau E, Schwahn B, Rauch F. The muscle-bone relationship: methods and management–perspectives in glycogen storage disease. *Eur J Pediatr.* 2002; 161:S50.
53. Humbert M, Labrune P, Simonneau G. Severe pulmonary arterial hypertension in type 1 glycogen storage disease. *Eur J Pediatr.* 2002; 161:S93.
54. Humbert M, Labrune P, Sitbon O, Le Gall C, Callebert J, Hervé P, et al. Pulmonary arterial hypertension and type-I glycogen-storage disease: the serotonin hypothesis. *Eur Respir J.* 2002; 20:59.
55. Mairovitz V, Labrune P, Fernandez H, Audibert F, Frydman R. Contraception and pregnancy in women affected by glycogen storage disease. *Eur J Pediatr.* 2002; 161:S97.
56. Ferrecchia IA, Guenette G, Potocik EA, Weinstein DA. Pregnancy in women with glycogen storage disease Ia and Ib. *J Perinat Neonatal Nurs.* 2014; 28:26.
57. Slonim AE, Coleman RA, Moses WS. Myopathy and growth failure in debrancher enzyme deficiency: improvement with high-protein nocturnal enteral therapy. *J Pediatr.* 1984; 105:906.
58. Lee P, Ferguson C, Alexander F. Symptomatic hyperinsulinism reversed by dietary manipulation in glycogenosis type III. *J Inherit Metab Dis.* 1997; 20:612.
59. Gremse D, Bucuvalas JC, Balistreri WF. Efficacy of cornstarch therapy in type III glycogen-storage disease. *Am J Clin Nutr.* 1990; 52:671.
60. El-Karaksy H, El-Raziky MS, Anwar G, Mogahed E. The effect of tailoring of cornstarch intake on stature in children with glycogen storage disease type III. *J Pediatr Endocrinol Metab.* 2015; 28:195.
61. Dagli A, Zori R, McCune H, Ivsic T, Maisenbacher M, Weinstein D. Reversal of glycogen storage disease type IIIa-related cardiomyopathy with modification of diet. *J Inherit Metab Dis.* 2009; 32:103.
62. Brambilla A, Mannarino S, Pretese R, Gasperini S, Galimberti C, Parini R. Improvement of cardiomyopathy after high-fat diet in two siblings with glycogen storage disease type III. *JIMD Rep.* 2014; 17:91.
63. Chou JY, Zingone A, Pan C-J. Adenovirus-mediated gene therapy in a mouse model of glycogen storage disease type 1a. *Eur J Pediatr.* 2002; 161:S56.
64. Beaty R, Jackson M, Peterson D, et al. Delivery of glucose-6-phosphatase in a canine model for glycogen storage disease, type Ia, with adeno-associated virus (AAV) vectors. *Gene Ther.* 2002; 9:1015.

# E.

# MISCELLANEOUS GENETIC DISORDERS

## 53 Rubinstein-Taybi Syndrome

MALAI HOLLAND AND LEAH BURKE

Rubinstein-Taybi syndrome (RTS) is characterized by broad thumbs, broad big toes, distinctive facial features, short stature, and intellectual disabilities (ID). The condition was first described in 1957, and in 1963 Dr. Jack Rubinstein and Dr. Hooshang Taybi published a paper describing seven cases with similar findings that suggested a possible syndrome.[1]

### CLINICAL ABNORMALITIES

Medical issues for persons with RTS include congenital heart disease, abnormalities of the kidneys, eye problems, and hypotonia. Gastrointestinal issues are also common and can include significant gastroesophageal reflux disease (GERD), feeding difficulties, and constipation. Orthopedic problems include not only the issues related to the thumb and great toe differences but also scoliosis, spine abnormalities, and joint problems that may lead to an abnormal gait. Hypotonia in infancy and childhood can lead to difficulties in gait and balance, with impacts on ambulation, weight maintenance, and the ability to participate in physical activities. Health care guidelines for individuals with RTS Ages Birth-Adulthood can be found in article by Stevens et al.[2]

Individuals with RTS have global delays in development. Gross and fine motor skills are delayed,[3] as is speech in 90% of persons with RTS.[4] These delays in development affect nutrition status in many ways, including the ability to manage activities of daily living (ADLs) and self-help skills (e.g., self-feeding). As the child ages, the delays in gross and fine motor skills and in intellectual development can affect the child's ability to participate successfully in sports and recreational activities, which can influence weight status. Speech delays are associated with delays in the ability to safely chew and swallow foods as well as the ability to communicate about hunger, fullness, pain, or discomfort and the ability to participate in social skills that involve eating. Alternative forms of communication (e.g., sign language, communication devices) can be used to help children and adults express themselves and thereby decrease frustration and possible behavioral issues.

Most individuals with RTS have cognitive abilities that fall in the moderate range of ID. The average IQ is between 35 and 50; however, developmental outcomes vary considerably. A few individuals have been reported with IQs in the 70s. The performance IQ is usually higher than the verbal IQ.[5]

Behaviorally, children with RTS are often described by their families as loving, friendly, and happy.[4] However, short attention span, decreased tolerance for noise and crowds, impulsivity, and moodiness are frequently observed.[5] Autism-like behaviors were described by researchers in a study of 93 affected individuals,[6] and similar observations have been reported for some adults with RTS.[4]

The diagnosis of RTS is made primarily by clinical examination. The clinical findings in infants that most frequently lead to a diagnosis are the distinctive facial features and the broad thumbs and great toes. The facial features (Fig. 53–1) include eyes that slant down toward the ears, a characteristic nose that is often described as "beaked" because of the prominent bridge and a center that projects below the nares, and high-arched eyebrows. In older children, a "grimacing" smile is often recognized. Early weight gain is poor, and length or height and head

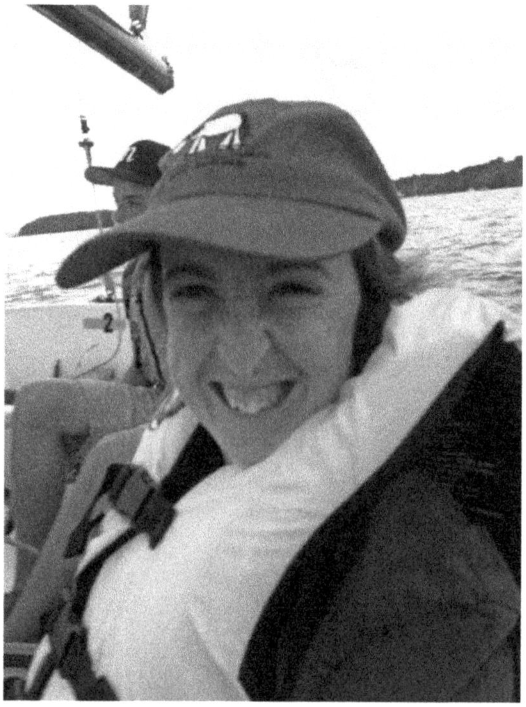

**Figure 53–1.** Adult with Rubinstein-Taybi syndrome.

circumference are below the 5th percentile. There are delays in gross and fine motor skills, language, social skills, and intellectual abilities. The diagnosis is not always quick and depends on the expertise of the examiner.

Even if the diagnosis is suspected, all individuals with presumed RTS should be evaluated by a pediatric geneticist who is knowledgeable in dysmorphology to confirm the diagnosis.

Two genes have been identified as causing RTS: *CREBBP* and *EP300*. Genetic testing is most often recommended to confirm the diagnosis when the features are atypical or very severe. Genetic testing is done in a stepwise manner with sequence analysis of *CREBBP* first, followed by duplication and deletion analysis if no pathogenic variant is detected through sequence analysis. If a pathogenic variant in *CREBBP* is not identified, sequence analysis and/or deletion and duplication analysis of *EP300* may be considered.[5]

The estimated prevalence of RTS in the Netherlands is 1 in 100,000 to 125,000 live births.[7]

## FACTORS TO BE CONSIDERED IN NUTRITION EVALUATION

A comprehensive nutritional assessment is important because patients with RTS can present with a variety of nutritional issues related to growth, dietary intake, feeding or eating problems, and gastrointestinal issues (including reflux and chronic constipation). Table 53–1 lists six assessment realms with areas of focus for a comprehensive nutritional assessment of a person diagnosed with RTS.

In early infancy, poor weight gain should be assessed in relation to expected linear growth. The evaluation for common medical problems, including GERD, chronic constipation,[7] and poor intake due to feeding or eating difficulties should be considered as a cause of poor weight gain. Delayed growth and short stature are well-recognized characteristics of persons with RTS. In early childhood, the issue of slow growth needs to be recognized so that correct interpretation of ideal weight status and body composition can be determined. Use of the World Health Organization (WHO) growth charts from birth to 2 years of age and the National Center for Health Statistics (NCHS) growth charts for older children and adolescents is recommended to assess growth and body composition.

**Table 53–1.** Areas of Focus for Comprehensive Nutritional Assessment for Person with Rubenstein-Taybi Syndrome

| Assessment Parameter | Areas of Focus |
|---|---|
| Anthropometric | Current growth and growth history especially weight for length or body mass index (BMI) |
| Biochemical and laboratory tests | Laboratory tests including iron deficiency anemia; bone age to assess growth; swallow studies (e.g., modified barium swallow, endoscopy); other radiological tests for gastrointestinal concerns |
| Clinical | History of medical conditions, surgeries, or hospitalizations that affect nutritional status (e.g., cardiac, gastrointestinal); dental issues (caries); bowel patterns; medications and nutritional side effects; degree of ambulation; language ability to express thoughts, food preferences, hunger or satiety |
| Dietary | Food intolerances and allergies; food or texture preferences; meal patterns; use of vitamin supplements or other supplements and special diets |
| Eating/Feeding | Early feeding history; choking/gagging; mealtime behaviors; sensory eating issues |
| Family | Family financial and other resources; food security; caregiver knowledge, attitudes, and beliefs about food and the child's condition |

Adopted by Holland from Cricco K, Holland M. Nutrition assessment guidelines for children with special health care needs. *Nutrition Focus.* 2007; 22:1.

Stevens et al.[8] have published RTS-specific growth charts, but they should be used as an adjunct, similar to the recommendation of the American Academy of Pediatrics for the use of Down syndrome–specific growth charts.[9]

The risk for obesity in children, adolescents, and adults with RTS should be anticipated and prevented because the prevalence of obesity in children and youth with special health care needs is almost twice that of the general population.[10] Close monitoring of weight, starting in the preschool years, is important. Encouragement of daily exercise and dietary management principles for persons with ID are described elsewhere in this book and in other references. The principles for weight management in RTS are similar to those in other genetic conditions where overweight and obesity issues are found, such as Down syndrome.[11]

Eating and feeding difficulties in early infancy include a poor, weak suck; choking and gagging on breast milk or formula; and easy fatigability. Mothers of children with RTS who attempted to breast-feed reported poor suckling, poor weight gain, swallowing difficulties, and failure to thrive (FTT).[12] Nasogastric and gastrostomy tube feedings are used with some infants. Most feeding issues related to oral motor problems resolve after 1 year of age.[7]

Because eating is both a sensory and an oral-motor experience, delays in feeding due to sensory issues must also be recognized. Sensory-related feeding difficulties can include all the sensory systems (e.g., visual, auditory, taste, smell, vestibular),[13] but for infants and children with RTS, feeding issues are mostly related to the tactile system (personal communication from MH). Tactile hypersensitivity feeding issues can lead to an unbalanced dietary intake of nutrients due to food avoidance of foods that are important for growth and development. For example, avoidance of foods that are a good source of dietary fiber (e.g., fruits, vegetables, whole grains) can contribute to chronic constipation, which is a common problem of children and adults with RTS. Addressing feeding issues, whether they are medical, oral-motor, sensory, or behavioral in nature, requires an interdisciplinary team to adequately assess and develop a realistic plan for intervention.

Gastrointestinal issues are reported by many parents and medical providers. GERD is commonly reported. Severe, untreated GERD in infancy can cause respiratory infections, aspiration pneumonia, weight loss, and chronic food refusal in toddlers. GERD can occur without vomiting and can cause esophagitis, esophageal stenosis, iron deficiency anemia, irritability, and FTT.[14,15] In cases of food refusal and FTT, it is important to rule out silent reflux. Chronic constipation in infancy, childhood, or adulthood is also frequently reported.[4] Constipation (in 40% to 74% of patients) should be aggressively managed with dietary and medical interventions.[4,7,16] Hypotonicity, which is reported with RTS, combined with preferences for foods low in dietary fiber, can easily lead to chronic constipation. Medications, dietary interventions, and adequate fluid intake are all necessary for management of chronic constipation.

Some individuals with RTS exhibit autism-like behaviors,[7]). A complementary diet that is very popular for persons with autism spectrum disorders is the gluten-free casein-free diet (GFCF), and parents of children or adults with RTS who think their child is exhibiting such behaviors may want to try it (MH, personal communication). Adherence to the GFCF diet can be difficult if the person does not like the taste or texture of the alternative foods that are used to replace gluten-containing foods. Weight loss and undesirable mealtime behaviors can occur. Providers should find out whether parents are offering any of these alternatives to their child and educate them or refer them to a nutrition professional if there are concerns.[17]

## DIETARY MANAGEMENT

The dietary management of the issues described in the previous section are addressed elsewhere in this textbook. A team approach that involves parents, teachers, and other service and care providers leads to the best results. For older children and adults, making experiences fun and engaging peers can also lead to better outcomes. For example, eating meals with peers can increase intake of a variety of foods that might not otherwise be consumed. Engaging in physical activity with peers or Special Olympics teams can increase activity and fitness levels.

## ADULTHOOD

As persons with RTS age, weight management is typically the major nutrition issue to be addressed and monitored. Overweight and obesity are common problems for many adults with ID, and they are associated with a variety of physical and environmental factors. The consequences to obesity for all adults, including persons with ID, has been well documented in the literature and includes cardiovascular disease, adult-onset diabetes, hypertension, and various orthopedic issues that can further limit ambulation.[18]

One study surveyed parents and caregivers of adults with RTS and found that the most common medical problems were short stature, obesity, visual problems, eating issues, spine curvature, and joint problems.[19] Many of these issues can directly or indirectly affect a person's weight status. Evidence-based protocols for weight management, such as those included in the Academy of Nutrition and Dietetics' Evidence Based Analysis Library, should be used.[20] These protocols should be individualized based on the person's physical abilities and the living, work, and caregiver situations.

### References


1. Rubinstein JH, Taybi H. Broad thumbs and toes and facial abnormalities: a possible mental retardation syndrome. *Am J Dis Child.* 1963; 105:588.
2. Wiley S, Swayne S, Rubinstein JH, Lanphear NE, Stevens CA. Rubinstein-Taybi syndrome medical guidelines. *Am J Med Genet A.* 2003; 119A:101.
3. Hennekam RC, Van Den Boogaard MJ, Sibbles BJ, Van Spijker HG. Rubinstein-Taybi syndrome in The Netherlands. *Am J Med Genet Suppl.* 1990; 6:17.
4. Stevens C, Carey J, Blackburn B. Rubinstein-Taybi syndrome: a natural history study. *Am J Med Genet Suppl.*1990; 6:30.
5. Stevens C. Rubinstein-Taybi syndrome. November 2014. In: Pagon RA, Adam MP, Ardinger HH, et al., eds. *GeneReviews.* Seattle, WA: University of Washington; 1993–2016. http://www.ncbi.nlm.nih.gov/books/NBK1526. Accessed July 9, 2016.
6. Schorry EK, Keddache M, Lanphear N, et al. Genotype-phenotype correlations in Rubinstein-Taybi syndrome. *Am J Med Genet A.* 2008; 146A:2512.
7. Hennekam RC. Rubinstein-Taybi syndrome. In: Cassidy S, Allanson J, eds. *Management of Genetic Syndromes,* 3rd ed. New York: John Wiley & Sons; 2010:705.
8. Stevens CA, Hennekam RC, Blackburn BL. Growth in the Rubinstein-Taybi syndrome. *Am J Med Genet Suppl.* 1990; 6:51.
9. Bull M, Committee on Genetics. Health supervision for children with Down syndrome. *Pediatrics.* 2011; 128:393.
10. Rimmer JH, Yamaki K, Lowry BM, Wang E, Vogel LC. Obesity and obesity-related secondary conditions in adolescents with intellectual/developmental disabilities. *J Intellect Disabil Res.* 2010; 54:787.
11. Wong C, Dwyer J, Holland M. Overcoming weight issues in adults with Down syndrome. *Nutr Today.* 2014; 49:109.
12. Moe JK, Holland MD, Johnson RK. Breastfeeding practices of infants with Rubinstein-Taybi syndrome. *J Hum Lact.* 1998; 14:311.
13. Pinder GL. How sensory issues impact feeding in children. *Nutr Focus.* 2008; 23:1.
14. Paton JY, Nanayakkhara CS, Simpson H. Vomiting and gastroesophageal reflux. *Arch Dis Child.* 1988; 63:837.
15. Da Dalt L, Mazzoleni S, Montini G, Donzelli F, Zachello F. Diagnostic accuracy of pH monitoring in gastrooesophageal reflux. *Arch Dis Child.* 1989; 64:1421.
16. Rubinstein JH. Broad thumb–hallux (Rubinstein-Taybi) syndrome (1957–1988). *Am J Med Genet.* 1990; 6:23.
17. Holland M. Communicating with families concerning the use of complementary or alternative nutritional therapies. *Building Blocks Life.*2000: 24; 6.
18. Melville CA, Hamilton S, Hankley CR, Miller S, Boyle S. The prevalence and determinants of obesity in adults with intellectual disabilities. *Obes Rev.* 2007; 8:223.
19. Stevens CA, Pouncey J, Knowles D. Adults with Rubinstein-Taybi syndrome. *Am J Med Genet A.* 2011;155A:1680.
20. Ptoney LT, Wittenbrook W. Position of the Academy of Nutrition and Dietetics: Nutrition Services for individuals with intellectual and developmental disabilities and special health care needs. *J Acad Nutr Diet.* 2015; 115;593.

# 54 Celiac Disease

ALISON CASSIN AND DANIEL MALLON

Celiac disease is an autoimmune disease of the small intestine. It is characterized by mucosal inflammation and blunting of intestinal villi in response to ingestion of the gliadin fraction of gluten, a protein present in wheat, barley, and rye. It was initially described by the English physician Samuel Gee in 1888, and Willem Karel-Dicke was the first to link gluten intake with gastrointestinal symptoms, in the 1940s. Since that time, a considerable body of knowledge about this condition has accumulated. Previously considered a rather unusual disease, it is now recognized to be much more common. With the development of reliable screening tests using antibodies to gliadin and tissue transglutaminase, it is now estimated that the disease may affect as many as 1 in 130 to 300 Europeans and Americans,[1] with an estimated prevalence of 1 case per 104 children.[2–4] The only treatment for celiac disease is life-long adherence to a strict gluten-free diet.

People with celiac disease may present at any age with a variety of complaints depending on the age at onset. Infants and toddlers typically present several months after the introduction of gluten-containing foods in the diet. Poor weight gain and faltering growth occur in children of all ages, and symptoms in young children may include diarrhea or pale, loose, foul-smelling stool; poor weight gain; irritability; and abdominal distention.[5] In severe cases, infants may develop "celiac crisis," in which frank watery diarrhea leads to dehydration and severe hypoproteinemia. Among older children and adolescents, complaints of abdominal pain, diarrhea, impaired linear growth, delayed puberty, and iron deficiency anemia predominate.[5] Despite the malabsorptive nature of celiac disease, constipation is a common presenting symptom in older children and adolescents.[6] Malnutrition and poor growth are common at presentation, but obesity is observed in as many as 11% of newly diagnosed individuals.[7,8] People with celiac disease may be asymptomatic, and their diagnosis may be discovered by screening programs within high-risk groups, such as people who have type 1 diabetes mellitus (T1DM) or a first-degree relative with celiac disease.[9]

## PATHOGENESIS AND ETIOLOGY

Celiac disease is an autoimmune disorder in which gluten exposure triggers an innate and adaptive immune response in genetically predisposed individuals. The predisposing genes are those that encode the human leukocyte antigen (HLA) serotypes DQ2 and DQ8 of major histocompatibility complex (MHC) class II molecules. Almost all patients with celiac disease have one or both of those serotypes.[10] Because 30% to 40% of the general population also carries the alleles for DQ2 or DQ8, other pathogenic events must occur to develop the disease. Therefore, finding these genes in a person confirms risk but not a diagnosis.[11]

Along with genetic predisposition, disease pathogenesis requires gluten ingestion. When eaten, gluten is partially digested, yielding gliadin fractions that may cross enterocyte tight junctions in the setting of increased epithelial permeability.[12] Gliadin is then deamidated by the enzyme transglutaminase (TTG) in the lamina propria and binds to MHC class II molecules (DQ2 or DQ8) on antigen-presenting cells (Fig. 54–1). Those cells present the bound gliadin or gliadin-TTG complex to $CD4^+$ T lymphocytes, which release inflammatory cytokines, and to B lymphocytes, which form autoantibodies.[13] This dysregulated immune response to gluten and the resulting inflammatory cascade lead to mucosal damage of the small intestine, including the villous atrophy and crypt hypertrophy that characterize celiac disease.[10,14] Nutrient malabsorption occurs secondary to this injury and manifests as clinical symptoms.[12,15] Contrary to prior research, more recent studies indicate that neither breast-feeding duration[16] nor timing of gluten introduction in infancy[17] affects development or prevention of celiac disease.

## BIOCHEMICAL AND CLINICAL ABNORMALITIES

Diagnosis of celiac disease is based on a combination of clinical history, serologic testing, histopathologic findings from duodenal biopsies, and clinical response to a gluten-free diet. Differential diagnoses include cow's milk or soy enteropathy, food allergies, inflammatory bowel disease, autoimmune enteropathy, irritable bowel syndrome, and nonceliac gluten sensitivity. Because removal of gluten from the diet can influence serologic and histologic findings, gluten avoidance is not recommended until after diagnosis to avoid false-negative results.[18] Diagnosis cannot be secured by the history and physical findings alone, even if symptoms resolve on a gluten-free diet.

Celiac disease should be considered in children with unexplained gastrointestinal symptoms such as diarrhea, steatorrhea, postprandial abdominal distention, and abdominal pain and for other clinical manifestations, including faltering growth, weight loss, fatigue, iron deficiency anemia, delayed puberty, and recurring bone fractures. Individuals with celiac disease may be more prone to developing neurological disorders such as chronic headache, developmental delay, and hypotonia, as well as learning disorders or attention-deficit hyperactivity disorder (ADHD).[19]

Because other autoimmune diseases can exist concurrently with celiac disease, serologic testing for celiac disease should also be done in high-risk populations, such as people who have T1DM, a first-degree relative with celiac disease, immunoglobulin A (IgA) deficiency, autoimmune thyroiditis, or other disorders such as Down syndrome, Turner syndrome, and Williams syndrome.[9] Dermatitis herpetiformis, a variant of celiac disease, manifests in adults more frequently than in children[20] and is characterized by intensely pruritic vesicular rash on extensor surfaces of the arms and legs, buttocks, trunk, neck, and scalp.[21] Celiac disease occurs in as many as 5% to 10% of children with T1DM.[22–24] Individuals with existing celiac disease have 2.4-fold increased risk of developing T1DM before 20 years of age.[25] The HLA-DQ2 and -DQ8 haplotypes are present in 80% to 90% of individuals with Down syndrome, and up to 8% of them have concurrent celiac disease.[26,27]

### Serology

Tissue transglutaminase IgA antibody (TTG) is the preferred single test for detection of celiac disease in individuals older than 2 years of age[28]; it has a sensitivity greater than 95% and specificity of about 95%.[29–31] The earliest specific autoantibody test, antigliadin antibody, has been largely replaced by TTG. Newer assays for deamidated gliadin peptide (DGP) IgA and IgG also show very high sensitivity and specificity for detecting celiac disease, and they may be more sensitive than TTG in children younger than 2 years of age.[32,33] IgA deficiency, which occurs in 2% to 10% of patients with celiac disease, can lead to a false-negative interpretation of normal (low) IgA-based testing, so a total IgA level should be obtained during initial testing.[12] These

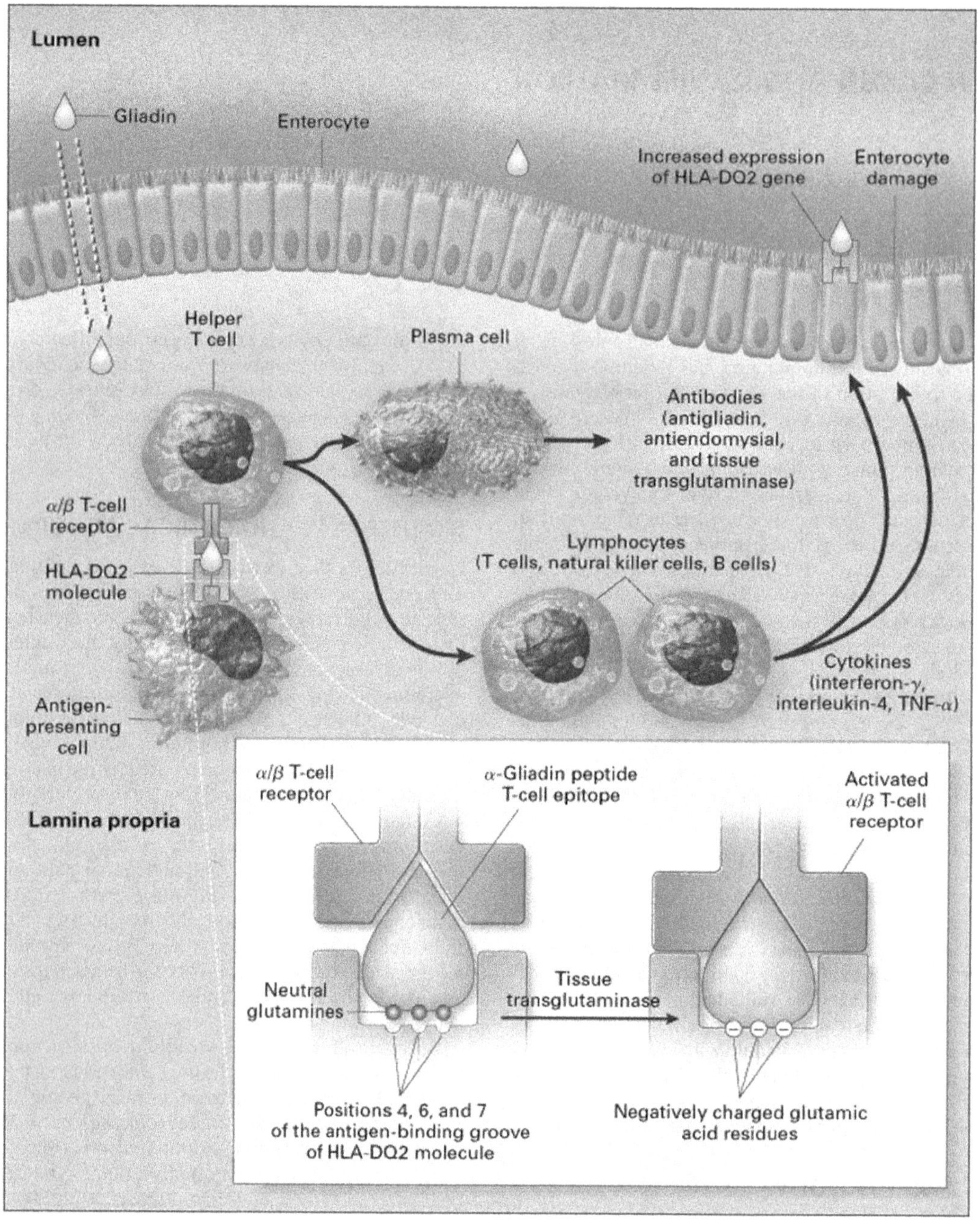


**Figure 54–1.** Pathogenesis of celiac disease. HLA = human leukocyte antigen; TNF-α = tumor necrosis factor-α. (From Green PH, Cellier C. Celiac disease. *N Engl J Med.* 2007; 357:1731. © Massachusetts Medical Society. Used with permission.)

serological tests can be used for diagnosis of suspected cases, for monitoring of compliance with the gluten-free diet, and for screening of patients with atypical manifestations of celiac disease.

Genetic testing may rule out celiac disease in individuals with negative serology results, in those with conflicting serological and histological results, and in those already following a gluten-free diet.[28] Although 40% of the general population carry either HLA-DQ2 or HLA-DQ8 coding alleles, only 1% to 3% develop celiac disease.[11] The absence of these alleles can exclude the diagnosis in almost 100% of cases.[34]

## Histopathology

If serum screening tests are positive or clinical symptoms and signs strongly suggest celiac disease, at least four biopsies of the duodenum and one to two biopsies of the duodenal bulb (9- or 12-o'clock position) should be obtained for histopathologic confirmation of the diagnosis.[28,35] Mucosal injury typically runs on a proximal-to-distal gradient, but distribution may be patchy in the duodenum, and multiple biopsy samples are preferred.[14] Villous atrophy and crypt hyperplasia are characteristic histological findings in celiac disease[36] (Figs. 54–2 and 54–3). Duodenal biopsy is recommended by the American College of Gastroenterology to secure the diagnosis. However, the European Society of Pediatric Gastroenterology, Hepatology, and Nutrition (ESPGHAN) has developed alternative criteria for diagnosis that do not include histology; they require (1) presence of typical gastrointestinal symptoms, (2) confirmation of genetic susceptibility by HLA genotype, (3) very elevated TTG IgA (>10 times the upper limit of normal), and (4) a positive anti-endomysial antibody test.

Because of the recognized high sensitivity and specificity of the serological tests, both the ESPGHAN and the North American Society

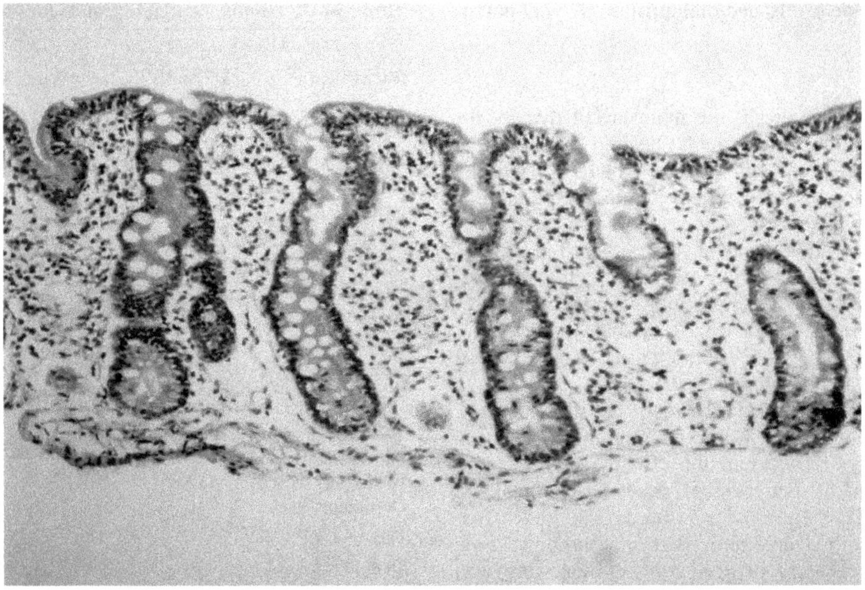

**Figure 54–2.** Duodenal mucosa in a celiac patient.

(NASPGHAN) recommend using serological testing to monitor response to therapy and do not endorse routine endoscopic follow-up to confirm the diagnosis or disease activity.[9] Follow-up small intestinal biopsy should be considered in patients who remain symptomatic or have persistently positive serology results after 6 to 12 months on a gluten-free diet.

## FACTORS TO BE CONSIDERED IN NUTRITION EVALUATION

### Pretreatment

Celiac disease affects the small intestine in a proximal-to-distal gradient, with the most severe disease activity located where the mucosa has most exposure to gluten-containing food. There are several consequences to this mucosal damage, including fluid loss and impaired fat and carbohydrate absorption from diarrhea and steatorrhea. Injury to the proximal small intestinal mucosa limits cholecystokinin secretion,[37] which can impair gallbladder contraction and pancreatic secretion, leading to further fat malabsorption. Steatorrhea with fecal calorie loss may promote subcutaneous fat loss and muscle wasting.

Destruction of villi also impairs micronutrient absorption in the small bowel, so serum iron and folate levels may be reduced at diagnosis, leading to hypochromic/microcytic anemia in the case of iron deficiency and macrocytic anemia in the case of folate deficiency.[38,39] When steatorrhea is moderate to severe, fat-soluble vitamins may also be poorly absorbed, potentially leading to neurological impairment secondary to vitamin E deficiency[40,41] or night blindness associated with vitamin A deficiency.[39,42]

As a fat-soluble vitamin, vitamin D is also susceptible to malabsorption. Vitamin D deficiency is common in patients with untreated celiac disease.[43–45] Vitamin D is an important modulator of intestinal calcium absorption and bone accretion, and its deficiency could be an important factor contributing to the low bone density commonly observed in newly diagnosed celiac patients.[46–49] However, diminished bone mass is likely multifactorial, with vitamin D and calcium

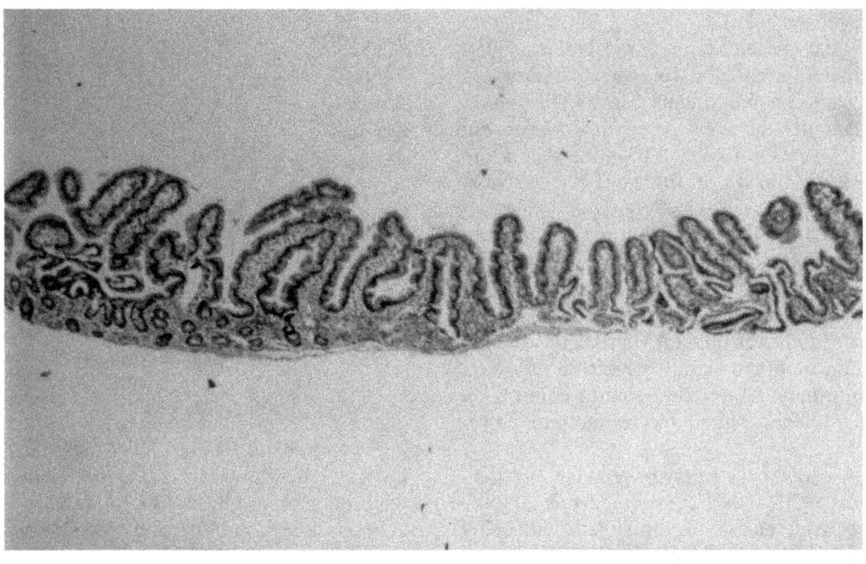

**Figure 54–3.** Duodenal mucosa in a nonceliac patient.

fecal losses, elevated cytokine levels, and malnutrition playing potential roles.[45–47,50]

## The Gluten-Free Diet

Strict adherence to a gluten free diet is the mainstay of therapy for celiac disease. Effective compliance yields healing of intestinal mucosa, symptomatic improvement, and restored growth of the child. Histological evidence of disease should regress within 6 to 12 months after implementation of the gluten-free diet.[15] When the diet is followed properly, children and adolescents have complete recovery of fat, lean body mass, and bone mass leading to normal body composition as they enter young adulthood.[51] These improvements in anthropometry do not always correspond with negative serology, which may take longer than 12 months to correct.[52] Bone density is often low at diagnosis but resolves with a gluten-free diet.[46,47]

When one is following a gluten-free diet, all forms of wheat, barley, and rye must be avoided, along with foods containing them as derivative ingredients or as traces of contamination (Table 54–1). Primary sources of gluten in a typical diet include bread, pasta, breakfast cereal, pastries, crackers, and breaded or fried foods. The gluten-free diet should mirror a well-rounded, healthy diet and should include gluten-free whole grains (e.g., brown rice, corn, quinoa, sorghum, millet), lean proteins (e.g., meat, poultry, fish, legumes), low-fat milk products, fruits, and vegetables.[53] A gluten-free diet should include a variety of these alternative grains because different grains supply various levels of essential trace minerals[54,55] and because overreliance on rice-based products can be problematic due to the high inorganic arsenic content of rice.[56] Because of the popularity of ancient grains, individuals with celiac disease should take care to identify and avoid primitive forms of wheat (e.g., triticale, farro, spelt) that are easily confused with common gluten-free grains such as millet, buckwheat, and quinoa.

Oats are naturally gluten-free, and most individuals with celiac disease can tolerate moderate amounts (1 cup cooked) in the daily diet.[57,58] Some individuals experience gastrointestinal symptoms or flares of dermatitis herpetiformis after ingestion of oats. This may be related to cross-contamination of oats with wheat and barley during commercial processing.[59] For that reason, the use of tested, certified gluten-free oats is recommended for those with celiac disease.[60]

## Label Reading

Accurate and vigilant label reading is fundamental when one is following a strict gluten-free diet. The US Food and Drug Administration (FDA) has ruled that products labeled "gluten free" must conform to specific standards, but many foods do not bear such labels, making label reading proficiency a necessary skill.

If a food product sold in the United States is not labeled gluten free, the ingredient list should be checked for wheat, barley, and rye. Wheat is easily identifiable on food labels because of mandatory disclosure requirement under the Food Allergen Labeling and Consumer Protection Act (FALCPA) of 2004.[61] If an ingredient in a packaged food contains protein from wheat, the word "wheat" must be included either in the ingredients list or in a "contains" statement. Although they are not regulated by FALCPA, barley and rye are often listed as ingredients and should be avoided. However, their derivatives, including malt and malt vinegar, may not be clearly labeled. Many commercial corn and rice cereals contain malt derived from barley or barley malt syrup.[62] Other incidental ingredients such as hydrolyzed vegetable protein, modified starch, vegetable gum, and brewer's yeast may contain gluten. Consumers should confirm the sources of these vague ingredients with the manufacturer before consumption.

Updated labeling laws now endorse the safety of products bearing a gluten-free label. As of August 5, 2014, the FDA requires that all foods labeled gluten free must be considered safe for individuals with celiac disease. Specifically, such products must not contain (1) a gluten-containing grain, (2) an ingredient derived from a gluten-containing grain (unless it has been processed to remove the gluten, as in gluten-free wheat starch), or (3) more than 20 parts per million (ppm) of

**Table 54–1.** Gluten, Nongluten, and Questionable Foods*

| *Allowed Grains and Starches* | *Not Allowed* |
|---|---|
| Buckwheat | Wheat (durum, semolina) |
| Rice | Rye |
| Corn | Barley |
| Potato | Spelt |
| Tapioca | Kamut |
| Bean | Farina |
| Sorghum | Semolina |
| Soy | Wheat germ or bran |
| Amaranth | Graham, gluten or flour |
| Arrowroot | Bulgur |
| Millet | Couscous |
| Teff | Einkorn |
| Nut flours | Emmer |
| Pea | Farro |
| Sago | Malt, malt extract, malt syrup, malt vinegar |
| Rice bran | |
| Cornmeal | |
| Flax | |
| Quinoa | |
| *Often Overlooked* | *Questionable (Verify If Derived from Gluten)* |
| Alcohol distilled from cereals (gin, vodka, whiskey, beer, ale, malts) | Brown rice syrup |
| | Caramel color |
| Breading | Canned meats |
| Broth | Dextrin (may be derived from grain) |
| Coating mixes | Commercial salad dressings |
| Commercial fruit pie fillings | Flavored or frozen yogurt |
| Communion wafers | Hydrolyzed vegetable protein |
| Condiments | Vegetable hydrolyzed plant protein |
| Creamed or breaded vegetables | Textured vegetable protein |
| Flavored instant coffee | Licorice |
| Herb tea | Modified food starch or modified starch |
| Hot cocoa mixes | Monoglycerides and diglycerides (in dry products) |
| Imitation bacon | Natural and artificial flavors |
| Imitation seafood | Soy sauce or soy sauce solids |
| Malted milk | Vegetable gum |
| Marinades | |
| Nondairy cream substitutes | |
| Pastas | |
| Prepared meats with gluten stabilizers, including some hot dogs, cold cuts | |
| Prepared soups | |
| Roux | |
| Sandwich spreads | |
| Sauces | |
| Sausages | |
| Seasonings prepared with gluten | |
| Self-basting poultry | |
| Soup base | |
| Stuffing | |
| Thickeners | |

*See the National Institute of Diabetes and Digestive and Kidney Diseases website on celiac disease (www.niddk.nih.gov/health/digest/pubs/celiac) and *CSA Cooperative Gluten Free Commercial Products Listing*, 7th ed. Omaha, NB: CSA/USA; 2002 for diet suggestions.

gluten.[63] If a product bears a gluten-free label but also has "wheat" in the ingredient list, the label must also state: "The wheat has been processed to allow this food to meet the Food and Drug Administration requirements for gluten-free foods."

Fresh meats, poultry, and eggs are regulated by the United States Department of Agriculture (USDA) and therefore are not included in the FDA labeling law. However, the USDA has adopted the regulation and confirmed that foods bearing a gluten-free label should follow the requirements set by the FDA.

**Box 54–1.** Resources for Celiac Disease

NIDDK National Digestive Diseases Information Clearinghouse www.niddk.nih.gov/health/digest/pubs/celiac

Celiac Support Association: www.csaceliacs.org

Gluten Intolerance Group of North America: www.gluten.org

Gluten-free food products: www.glutensolutions.com

Gluten-free medications and supplements: www.glutenfreedrugs.com/

American Celiac Disease Alliance: http://www.celiac.com/

National Foundation for Celiac Awareness: http://www.beyondceliac.org/

Celiac Disease Foundation: www.celiac.org

Canadian Celiac Association: www.celiac.ca

*Gluten-Free Living* magazine: www.glutenfreeliving.com

Recipes and foods: www.glutenfree.com, www.glutenfreemall.com

Cosmetics and medications fall under the jurisdiction of the FDA, but the gluten-free labeling rule does not apply to these items. Vitamin and mineral supplements are not regulated by the FDA or any government body. Because such supplements may be used to prevent nutrient deficiencies associated with gluten-free diets, products should be chosen judiciously and labels carefully checked to determine whether they contain gluten or wheat starch as fillers.

The FDA does not require routine testing of gluten-free products but instead offers recommendations to manufacturers to aid compliance with labeling standards. Recent studies found 95% to 99% of gluten-free products tested to contain less than 20 ppm of gluten despite the current lack of compulsory testing.[64,65] If there is ever concern that a product may not be gluten free, one can carefully analyze the ingredient list or call the manufacturer directly to inquire about ingredients used and manufacturing practices to ensure the safety of a given food item.

## Nutritional Implications of the Gluten-Free Diet

Wheat flour and associated products are good sources of carbohydrate, fiber, and, if fortified, thiamin, riboflavin, niacin, iron, and folate. The gluten-free diet is potentially low in these nutrients and in vitamin $B_{12}$, calcium, phosphorus, and zinc.[66] Gluten-free substitutes give individuals with celiac disease the opportunity to enjoy breads, cereals, and snack foods made from alternative grains, but many gluten-free grains are not enriched and fortified with B vitamins or iron. When following a gluten-free diet, individuals may not eat enough grain products to meet recommended intakes of fiber, thiamin, riboflavin, folate, and iron.[67] In adolescents with celiac disease, calcium and vitamin D intake is often low.[68] Multivitamin and mineral supplementation should be recommended on an individual basis.[69]

The gluten-free diet has potential to inflict unintentional weight gain for various reasons. Before diagnosis, the individual may have required more calories due to malabsorption. Once the mucosa heals with initiation of the gluten-free diet, individuals may need to adjust their calorie intake to their current needs. Gluten-free foods can be higher in fat and sugar (and therefore higher in caloric density) to increase palatability.[70] Research in food-allergic children suggests that overcompensation with allowable foods occurs when certain food groups are restricted, leading overeating and obesity.[8,71] Many gluten-free substitutes are high in carbohydrates, which may affect blood glucose control for individuals with T1DM.[72,73] For these reasons, careful follow-up with a registered dietitian is recommended.

## Dietary Compliance

As the mucosa heals, the signs and symptoms of the disease will disappear. Even if they are asymptomatic, patients with celiac disease should be counseled about the lifelong need to maintain a gluten-free diet and the health risks of consuming gliadin. Compliance to a gluten-free diet is difficult[74] and is reported to fall between 45% and 80%, depending on the population.[34] Diagnosis of celiac disease during childhood presents an opportunity for the patient to establish gluten-free dietary habits, and this is especially important considering that adults with celiac disease report low adherence, low quality of life, low satisfaction with the gluten-free diet, and a high disease burden.[75,76] Adherence to the diet is essential because patients with celiac disease are at greater risk of neoplasms, especially small intestinal lymphomas, compared with the general population.[1] However, there is evidence that maintaining a gluten-free diet reduces the risk.[77]

## Support Groups

Fellow patients with celiac disease provide a wealth of knowledge and experience to the newly diagnosed. In most metropolitan areas, support groups meet on a regular basis to share experiences and recipes using foods that are suitable for affected people. There are also a number of websites that may be useful (Box 54–1).

### References


1. Fasano A, Berti I, Gerarduzzi T, et al. Prevalence of celiac disease in at-risk and not-at-risk groups in the United States: a large multicenter study. *Arch Intern Med.* 2003; 163:286.
2. Catassi C, Fabiani E, Ratsch IM, et al. The coeliac iceberg in Italy. A multicentre antigliadin antibodies screening for coeliac disease in school-age subjects. *Acta Paediatr Suppl*, 1996; 412:29.
3. Hill ID. Celiac disease—a never-ending story? *J Pediatr*, 2003; 143:289.
4. Not T, Horvath K, Hill ID, et al. Celiac disease risk in the USA: high prevalence of antiendomysium antibodies in healthy blood donors. *Scand J Gastroenterol.* 1998; 33:494.
5. Reilly NR, Fasano A, Green PH. Presentation of celiac disease. *Gastrointest Endosc Clin North Am.* 2012; 22:613.
6. Khatib M, Baker RD, Ly EK, Kozielski R, Baker SS. The presenting pattern of pediatric celiac disease. *J Pediatr Gastroenterol Nutr.* 2016; 62:60.
7. Telega G, Bennet TR, Werlin S. Emerging new clinical patterns in the presentation of celiac disease. *Arch Pediatr Adolesc Med.* 2008; 162:164.
8. Venkatasubramani N, Telega G, Werlin SL. Obesity in pediatric celiac disease. *J Pediatr Gastroenterol Nutr.* 2010; 51:295.
9. Husby S, Koletzko S, Korponay-Szabo IR, et al. European Society for Pediatric Gastroenterology, Hepatology, and Nutrition guidelines for the diagnosis of coeliac disease. *J Pediatr Gastroenterol Nutr.* 2012; 54:136.
10. Sollid LM, Lie BA. Celiac disease genetics: current concepts and practical applications. *Clin Gastroenterol Hepatol.* 2005; 3:843.
11. Liu E, Lee HS, Aronsson CA, et al. Risk of pediatric celiac disease according to HLA haplotype and country. *N Engl J Med.* 2014; 371:42.
12. Green PH, Cellier C. Celiac disease. *N Engl J Med.* 2007; 357:1731.
13. Molberg O, McAdam SN, Korner R, et al. Tissue transglutaminase selectively modifies gliadin peptides that are recognized by gut-derived T cells in celiac disease. *Nat Med.* 1998; 4:713.
14. Oberhuber G. Histopathology of celiac disease. *Biomed Pharmacother.* 2000; 54:368.
15. Fasano A, Catassi C. Current approaches to diagnosis and treatment of celiac disease: an evolving spectrum. *Gastroenterology.* 2001; 120:636.
16. Vriezinga SL, Auricchio R, Bravi E, et al. Randomized feeding intervention in infants at high risk for celiac disease. *N Engl J Med.* 2014; 371:1304.
17. Lionetti E, Castellaneta S, Francavilla R, et al. Introduction of gluten, HLA status, and the risk of celiac disease in children. *N Engl J Med.* 2014; 371:1295.
18. Leffler D, Schuppan D, Pallav K, et al. Kinetics of the histological, serological and symptomatic responses to gluten challenge in adults with coeliac disease. *Gut.* 2013; 62:996.
19. Zelnik N, Pacht A, Obeid R, Lerner A. Range of neurologic disorders in patients with celiac disease. *Pediatrics.* 2004; 113:1672.
20. Zone JJ. Skin manifestations of celiac disease. *Gastroenterology.* 2005; 128:S87.
21. Caproni M, Antiga E, Melani L, Fabbri P, Italian Group for Cutaneous Immunopathology. Guidelines for the diagnosis and treatment of dermatitis herpetiformis. *J Eur Acad Dermatol Venereol.* 2009; 23:633.
22. Emilsson L, Wijmenga C, Murray JA, Ludvigsson JF. Autoimmune disease in first-degree relatives and spouses of individuals with celiac disease. *Clin Gastroenterol Hepatol.* 2015; 13:1271.e2.
23. Neuhausen SL, Steele L, Ryan S, et al. Co-occurrence of celiac disease and other autoimmune diseases in celiacs and their first-degree relatives. *J Autoimmun.* 2008; 31:160.
24. Holmes GK. Screening for coeliac disease in type 1 diabetes. *Arch Dis Child.* 2002; 87:495.
25. Ludvigsson JF, Ludvigsson J, Ekbom A, Montgomery SM. Celiac disease and risk of subsequent type 1 diabetes: a general population cohort study of children and adolescents. *Diabetes Care.* 2006; 29:2483.
26. Book L, Hart A, Black J, Feolo M, Zone JJ, Neuhausen SL. Prevalence and clinical characteristics of celiac disease in Downs syndrome in a US study. *Am J Med Genet.* 2001; 98:70.
27. Bonamico M, Mariani P, Danesi HM, et al. Prevalence and clinical picture of celiac disease in Italian Down syndrome patients: a multicenter study. *J Pediatr Gastroenterol Nutr.* 2001; 33:139.
28. Rubio-Tapia A, Hill ID, Kelly CP, Calderwood AH, Murray JA, American College of Gastroenterology. ACG clinical guidelines: diagnosis and management of celiac disease. *Am J Gastroenterol.* 2013; 108:656; quiz 77.
29. Troncone R, Maurano F, Rossi M, et al. IgA antibodies to tissue transglutaminase: an effective diagnostic test for celiac disease. *J Pediatr.* 1999; 134:166.
30. van der Windt DA, Jellema P, Mulder CJ, Kneepkens CM, van der Horst HE. Diagnostic testing for celiac disease among patients with abdominal symptoms: a systematic review. *JAMA.* 2010; 303:1738.

31. Sulkanen S, Halttunen T, Laurila K, et al. Tissue transglutaminase autoantibody enzyme-linked immunosorbent assay in detecting celiac disease. *Gastroenterology*. 1998; 115:1322.
32. Burgin-Wolff A, Gaze H, Hadziselimovic F, et al. Antigliadin and antiendomysium antibody determination for coeliac disease. *Arch Dis Child*. 1991; 66:941.
33. Aberg AK, Olcen P. Serologic screening for celiac disease in children: a comparison between established assays and tests with deamidated gliadin-derived peptides plus conjugates for both IgA and IgG antibodies. *APMIS*. 2009; 117:808.
34. Hill ID, Dirks MH, Liptak GS, et al. Guideline for the diagnosis and treatment of celiac disease in children: recommendations of the North American Society for Pediatric Gastroenterology, Hepatology and Nutrition. *J Pediatr Gastroenterol Nutr.* 2005; 40:1.
35. Ravelli A, Villanacci V, Monfredini C, Martinazzi S, Grassi V, Manenti S. How patchy is patchy villous atrophy? Distribution pattern of histological lesions in the duodenum of children with celiac disease. *Am J Gastroenterol*. 2010; 105:2103.
36. Marsh MN. Studies of intestinal lymphoid tissue. III. Quantitative analyses of epithelial lymphocytes in the small intestine of human control subjects and of patients with celiac sprue. *Gastroenterology*. 1980; 79:481.
37. Deprez P, Sempoux C, Van Beers BE, et al. Persistent decreased plasma cholecystokinin levels in celiac patients under gluten-free diet: respective roles of histological changes and nutrient hydrolysis. *Regul Pept*. 2002; 110:55.
38. Harper JW, Holleran SF, Ramakrishnan R, Bhagat G, Green PH. Anemia in celiac disease is multifactorial in etiology. *Am J Hematol*. 2007; 82:996.
39. Bergamaschi G, Markopoulos K, Albertini R, et al. Anemia of chronic disease and defective erythropoietin production in patients with celiac disease. *Haematologica*. 2008; 93:1785.
40. Hozyasz K, Chelchowska M. Low vitamin E level as a possible cause of complications in celiac disease. *Indian J Gastroenterol*. 2003; 22:237.
41. Henri-Bhargava A, Melmed C, Glikstein R, Schipper HM. Neurologic impairment due to vitamin E and copper deficiencies in celiac disease. *Neurology*. 2008; 71:860.
42. Alwitry A. Vitamin A deficiency in coeliac disease. *Br J Ophthalmol*. 2000; 84:1079.
43. Selby PL, Davies M, Adams JE, Mawer EB. Bone loss in celiac disease is related to secondary hyperparathyroidism. *J Bone Miner Res*. 1999; 14:652.
44. Zanchi C, Di Leo G, Ronfani L, Martelossi S, Not T, Ventura A. Bone metabolism in celiac disease. *J Pediatr*. 2008; 153:262.
45. Lerner A, Shapira Y, Agmon-Levin N, et al. The clinical significance of 25OH-vitamin D status in celiac disease. *Clin Rev Allergy Immunol*. 2012; 42:322.
46. Jatla M, Zemel BS, Bierly P, Verma R. Bone mineral content deficits of the spine and whole body in children at time of diagnosis with celiac disease. *J Pediatr Gastroenterol Nutr*. 2009; 48:175.
47. Mora S. Celiac disease in children: impact on bone health. *Rev Endocr Metab Disord*. 2008; 9:123.
48. Mustalahti K, Collin P, Sievanen H, Salmi J, Maki M. Osteopenia in patients with clinically silent coeliac disease warrants screening. *Lancet*. 1999; 354:744.
49. Turner J, Pellerin G, Mager D. Prevalence of metabolic bone disease in children with celiac disease is independent of symptoms at diagnosis. *J Pediatr Gastroenterol Nutr*. 2009; 49:589.
50. Tau C, Mautalen C, De Rosa S, Roca A, Valenzuela X. Bone mineral density in children with celiac disease. Effect of a Gluten-free diet. *Eur J Clin Nutr*. 2006; 60:358.
51. Barera G, Mora S, Brambilla P, et al. Body composition in children with celiac disease and the effects of a gluten-free diet: a prospective case-control study. *Am J Clin Nutr*. 2000; 72:71.
52. Zung A, Kori M. Lack of association between seroconversion and catch-up growth in children with celiac disease. *J Pediatr Endocrinol Metab*. 2012; 25:131.
53. Simpson S, Thompson T. Nutrition assessment in celiac disease. *Gastrointest Endosc Clin N Am*. 2012; 22:797.
54. Nascimento AC, Mota C, Coelho I, et al. Characterisation of nutrient profile of quinoa (*Chenopodium quinoa*), amaranth (*Amaranthus caudatus*), and purple corn (*Zea mays* L.) consumed in the North of Argentina: proximates, minerals and trace elements. *Food Chem*. 2014; 148:420.
55. Suliburska J, Krejpcio Z, Regula J, Grochowicz A. Evaluation of the content and the potential bioavailability of minerals from gluten-free products. *Acta Sci Pol Technol Aliment*. 2013; 12:75.
56. Munera-Picazo S, Ramirez-Gandolfo A, Burlo F, Carbonell-Barrachina AA. Inorganic and total arsenic contents in rice-based foods for children with celiac disease. *J Food Sci*. 2014; 79:T122.
57. Hoffenberg EJ, Haas J, Drescher A, et al. A trial of oats in children with newly diagnosed celiac disease. *J Pediatr*. 2000; 137:361.
58. Koskinen O, Villanen M, Korponay-Szabo I, Lindfors K, Maki M, Kaukinen K. Oats do not induce systemic or mucosal autoantibody response in children with coeliac disease. *J Pediatr Gastroenterol Nutr*. 2009; 48:559.
59. Hernando A, Mujico JR, Mena MC, Lombardia M, Mendez E. Measurement of wheat gluten and barley hordeins in contaminated oats from Europe, the United States and Canada by Sandwich R5 ELISA. *Eur J Gastroenterol Hepatol*. 2008; 20:545.
60. Thompson T. Gluten contamination of commercial oat products in the United States. *N Engl J Med*. 2004; 351:2021.
61. United States Food and Drug Administration. *Food Allergen Labeling and Consumer Protection Act of 2004 (Title II of Public Law 108e282)*. http://www.fda.gov/Food/GuidanceRegulation/GuidanceDocumentsRegulatoryInformation/Allergens/ucm106187.htm. Accessed July 9, 2016.
62. United States Food and Drug Administration. *Malt Syrup (Malt Extract)*. http://www.accessdata.fda.gov/scripts/cdrh/cfdocs/cfcfr/cfrsearch.cfm?fr=184.1445. Accessed July 9, 2016.
63. United States Food and Drug Administration. *Food Labeling: Gluten-Free Labeling of Foods*. http://www.fda.gov/food/guidanceregulation/guidancedocumentsregulatoryinformation/allergens/ucm362510.htm. Accessed July , 2016.
64. Thompson T, Simpson S. A comparison of gluten levels in labeled gluten-free and certified gluten-free foods sold in the United States. *Eur J Clin Nutr*. 2015; 69:143.
65. Sharma GM, Pereira M, Williams KM. Gluten detection in foods available in the United States—a market survey. *Food Chem*. 2015; 169:120.
66. American Dietetic Association Evidence Analysis Library. Celiac *Disease Evidence-Based Nutrition Practice Guideline*. http://www.adaevidencelibrary.com. Accessed July 9, 2016.
67. Thompson T, Dennis M, Higgins LA, Lee AR, Sharrett MK. Gluten-free diet survey: are Americans with coeliac disease consuming recommended amounts of fibre, iron, calcium and grain foods? *J Hum Nutr Diet*. 2005; 18:163.
68. Blazina S, Bratanic N, Campa AS, Blagus R, Orel R. Bone mineral density and importance of strict gluten-free diet in children and adolescents with celiac disease. *Bone*. 2010; 47:598.
69. American Dietetic Association. *Manual of Clinical Dietetics*, 6th ed. Chicago: American Dietetic Association; 2000.
70. Wu JH, Neal B, Trevena H, et al. Are gluten-free foods healthier than non-gluten-free foods? An evaluation of supermarket products in Australia. *Br J Nutr*. 2015; 114:448.
71. Meyer R, De Koker C, Dziubak R, et al. Malnutrition in children with food allergies in the UK. *J Hum Nutr Diet*. 2014; 27:227.
72. Silverstein J, Klingensmith G, Copeland K, et al. Care of children and adolescents with type 1 diabetes—a statement of the American Diabetes Association. *Diabetes Care*. 2005; 28:186.
73. Mayer M, Greco L, Troncone R, Auricchio S, Marsh MN. Compliance of adolescents with coeliac disease with a gluten free diet. *Gut*. 1991; 32:881.
74. Lee A, Newman JM. Celiac diet: its impact on quality of life. *J Am Diet Assoc*. 2003; 103:1533.
75. Barratt SM, Leeds JS, Sanders DS. Quality of life in coeliac disease is determined by perceived degree of difficulty adhering to a gluten-free diet, not the level of dietary adherence ultimately achieved. *J Gastrointest Liver Dis*. 2011; 20:241.
76. Shah S, Akbari M, Vanga R, et al. Patient perception of treatment burden is high in celiac disease compared with other common conditions. *Am J Gastroenterol*. 2014; 109:1304.
77. Corrao G, Corazza GR, Bagnardi V, et al. Mortality in patients with coeliac disease and their relatives: a cohort study. *Lancet*. 2001; 358:356.

# 55 Cystic Fibrosis and Bronchopulmonary Dysplasia

CHRISTINA C. LEWIS, GARY McPHAIL, AND ELISABETH LUDER

## CYSTIC FIBROSIS

Cystic fibrosis (CF) is the most common life-threatening genetic disease affecting whites in the United States.[1,2] It is an autosomal recessive disorder [3,4] that affects approximately 1 in 2500 to 3500 whites[5–7] and 1 in 1500 to 2000 blacks in the United States (https://www.cff.org/What-is-CF/Testing/Carrier-Testing-for-CF/). CF is caused by mutations in the *CFTR* gene which are most prevalent among northern and central Europeans and their descendants. This gene encodes a chloride and bicarbonate channel that regulates several ion transporters at the epithelial cell membrane, controlling hydration of epithelial secretions.[8] CF disease is characterized by impaired epithelial transport of electrolytes and fluid, which affects secretions of mucus, pancreatic enzymes, and digestive juices. The secretions produced in the lungs, pancreatic ducts, hepatobiliary ducts, intestinal glands, and vas deferens, are thick and viscous, and chloride reabsorption in the sweat ducts is poor.

CF is a chronic, progressive, multisystem disorder that affects the secretory glands of the body; it is characterized chiefly by chronic airway obstruction and infection, insufficiency of pancreatic digestive secretions, and gastrointestinal tract dysfunction.[1,2] The clinical sequelae reflect the multiorgan involvement and include lung disease, pancreatic insufficiency, cirrhosis, neonatal meconium ileus, CF-related diabetes (CFRD), and distal intestinal obstruction syndrome (DIOS).[9] All of these problems can interfere with the intake, assimilation, or utilization of nutrients and lead to malnutrition.

The course and severity of CF disease is highly varied, ranging from death in early infancy due to severe respiratory tract problems to an essentially asymptomatic existence for 10 to 20 years.[10] Over the past 3 decades, improved treatment modalities have dramatically increased the survival time, from a predicted median of 28 years to more than 40 years.[11] Major advances have led to discovery of the CF gene and improvements in pulmonary and nutritional care. CF is caused by mutations in *CFTR*, a gene located on the long arm of chromosome 7 that encodes a plasma membrane–associated chloride channel called the *cystic fibrosis transmembrane conductance regulator* (CFTR) protein.[12–16] More than 2000 mutations in *CFTR* have been identified.[17,18]

Because CFTR is functionally a chloride channel[19,20] and also a regulator of other ion channels,[21,22] common features of CF include abnormalities of both chloride and sodium transport by respiratory epithelium.[23] In its normal state, the CFTR protein allows chloride ions to migrate across the border of respiratory or intestinal epithelial cells; this also draws water out of the cell and into the lumen that abuts the apical border of the epithelium. These movements of chloride and water are necessary for the normal fluid homeostasis of the epithelial cells that line the airways and the gastrointestinal tract.

Most individuals affected by CF (>85%) have at least one genetic deletion of three nucleotide base pairs within the CFTR protein, which results in the loss of phenylalanine at amino acid position 508 (known as the ΔF508 mutation).[11,17,24] As a consequence, the protein is defective due to incomplete processing. Research has indicated that carriers of the ΔF508 mutation, although they do not express CF disease, are at increased risk for other disorders, including chronic rhinitis, asthma, reduced lung function, non-CF bronchiectasis, and chronic pancreatitis.

The many other mutations of the CFTR protein seem to be responsible for the remaining cases of CF, but all occur at relatively low frequencies. However, distinct mutations have specific effects on CFTR function and disease severity. Depending on the residual level of CFTR function, mutations such as ΔF508 cause a severe CF phenotype[25,26] with pancreatic insufficiency, whereas others cause only mild disease with pancreatic sufficiency.[27,28]

Improvements in pulmonary and nutritional care have dramatically reduced the mortality rate of CF. Today, many individuals with CF live into their fourth or fifth decade, with the median life expectancy being about 40.7 years.[29] As patients live longer, liver disease, glucose intolerance, CFRD, osteopenia, and osteoporosis have become more commonly recognized complications of CF.[6,9] This chapter, addresses the major clinical problems in CF, their effects on nutrition status, appropriate interventions, and management of nutrition-related complications. Stagnant mucus allows for bacteria to grow, leading to common and persistent opportunistic lung infections. Disruptions of epithelial transport in CF also causes the sweat to be salty,[30,31] leading to dehydration, abnormalities in blood pressure, and cardiovascular compensations for reduced vascular fluid.

### Factors To Be Considered in Nutritional and Clinical Evaluation

#### Pulmonary Disease and Nutrition Status

Progressive infection and inflammation in the distal airways of individuals affected by CF is very common, and once established, is rarely eradicated, limiting the length and quality of life for most patients with CF. Infection is concomitant with an active host inflammatory response that is present in CF airways from early life.[32] Airway colonization by *Staphylococcus aureus* and *Haemophilus influenzae* is often first to be detected, frequently followed by *Pseudomonas aeruginosa*, methicillin-resistant *S. aureus* (MRSA), and, rarely, *Burkholderia cepacia*. The course of the lung disease is progressive, although the rate of progression varies among patients. Evidence of airway inflammation and mucus production usually becomes prominent, with concomitant hypertrophy of submucosal glands, hyperplasia of goblet cells, and bronchiectasis—all of which are evidence of the consequences of persistent cycles of obstruction and infection.[33] Respiratory failure is the leading cause of death, and it eventually occurs in almost all patients with CF.

Pulmonary disease is related to the development of nutritional problems in CF patients. Almost one-half of CF patients have a suboptimal body mass index (BMI), and this may have a significant adverse impact on their pulmonary defenses.[34] Anorexia can occur secondary to infections or antibiotic administration, and excessive energy expenditure results from infections or chronic lung disease. In nutritionally compromised subjects, a series of infections can severely interfere with nutrient intake and metabolism.[9] A longitudinal study from a large cohort of CF patients confirmed that nutrition and lung function are codependent variables. Patients with normal weight had a significantly smaller decrease in lung function over a 2-year period, compared to patients with malnutrition.[35] Body wasting is a significant predictor of survival in patients with CF, independent of lung function, arterial blood oxygen, and carbon dioxide tension.[36]

#### Gastrointestinal Disease

A spectrum of gastrointestinal disease and malnutrition occurs in CF, with correlations between genotype and phenotype beginning to emerge. For example, homozygosity for the ΔF508 mutation almost always confers pancreatic insufficiency.[24] Many specific genotype and phenotype relationships cause problems that interfere with nutritional intake and assimilation and therefore need to be considered during investigations of the cause of malnutrition in CF. Esophagitis can produce severe symptoms of heartburn, nausea, or anorexia. Gastroesophageal reflux disease (GERD) affects up to 25% of the CF population, especially older children and adults, and up to half of them may develop esophagitis. Given this high incidence, patients with persistent anorexia should be investigated for GERD and esophagitis. Appropriate treatment with gastric acid suppression therapy, using histamine 2 ($H_2$) receptor antagonists or proton-blocking agents, can lead to dramatic improvement in symptoms and appetite.[9,37,38]

Distal intestinal obstruction syndrome (DIOS) is caused by the impaction of mucofeculent material in the distal ileum, cecum, and proximal colon. Contributing factors include abnormal intestinal mucins, undigested food residues, prolonged intestinal transit time, low-fiber diet, bowel dilatation, and abnormal intestinal electrolyte and water transport. There is often no identifiable precipitating event, but relative dehydration, inadequate enzyme supplementation, and change in diet have been implicated. DIOS manifests with significant abdominal pain and usually with decreased stool production. It has been described in CF patients of all ages but is probably more common among adolescents and adults. In the absence of complete obstruction, the treatment of choice is administration of intestinal lavage solution orally or by nasogastric tube.[39,40]

Between 10% and 15% of patients with CF present with meconium ileus in the neonatal period. It is most likely caused by a combination of abnormal pancreatic function and intestinal gland secretions. The resulting hyperviscid, relatively desiccated meconium contains high levels of calcium and undegraded serum proteins, leading to *in utero* obstruction of the distal ileum. There is evidence that meconium ileus is in part genetically determined. With rare exceptions, meconium ileus is seen only in patients who are later shown to have pancreatic insufficiency. Affected infants present within the first 48 hours of life with abdominal distention, bilious vomiting, and failure to pass meconium. In the absence of complications, these infants can be treated successfully with hyperosmolar enemas. If there are complications, management is by resection of the involved bowel. After surgery, most patients require a period of total parenteral nutrition followed by intensive enteral nutritional support.[9]

## Liver Disease

Clinically significant liver disease associated with CF is less common than other aspects of disease manifestation, affecting only an estimated 5% to 10% of individuals with CF.[11,41,42] However, with the ever-increasing life expectancy for individuals living with CF, liver disease is receiving more attention than it has in the past, and the identification, evaluation, and treatment of liver disease present increasingly important challenges. Liver disease associated with CF usually manifests in adolescence or adulthood. It is the abnormal CFTR protein in the apical surface of the biliary epithelium that causes the liver disease associated with CF. Hyperviscous bile accumulates in the biliary tree, causing cholangiocyte and hepatocyte injury and stimulating focal fibrosis. Fibrosis is thought to lead to cirrhosis over a period of years, a process that is usually asymptomatic. Steatosis and biliary tree anomalies, including cholecystitis, also occur.

Clinical signs of liver disease appear late, by which time cirrhosis may be established. Early diagnosis would allow interventions to be evaluated, but there is no gold standard for screening or treatment of CF liver disease. Regular clinical assessment, measurement of liver enzymes, ultrasound studies, and liver biopsy are all used to evaluate liver disease in CF.[43] Patients with liver disease should have close monitoring of their nutrition status to optimize caloric intake and to correct or prevent deficiencies of vitamins, minerals, and essential fatty acids.[43]

## Cystic Fibrosis–Related Diabetes

As CF patients live longer, glucose intolerance and CFRD become common complications.[9,44,45] Diabetes requiring insulin is the leading comorbidity in CF patients.[45] Approximately 20% of CF patients are reported to have CFRD, but in patients older than 18 years of age, the prevalence is 34%.[11,45] The clinical course and metabolic response seen in CFRD are different from those of type 1 or type 2 diabetes. Although CFRD begins during youth or early adulthood, it is characterized by an insidious onset, rare ketoacidosis, and normoglycemia with only intermittent periods of hyperglycemia. Reasons for the development of CFRD are not fully understood.[44,46] Patients usually are characterized by the presence of specific types of CF mutations, exocrine pancreatic insufficiency, impaired and delayed insulin secretion, impaired glucagon secretion, normal insulin sensitivity, and an increased insulin clearance rate.[44,47]

CFRD is associated with a variety of adverse consequences, including loss of calories secondary to glycosuria, muscle wasting, fatigue, impaired ability to respond to infection, renal insufficiency, and microvascular complications.[44,45] When CFRD develops in CF patients, an insidious decline in overall clinical status often occurs over several years before the CFRD is diagnosed. Body weight and BMI begin to deviate about 4 years before the diagnosis of CFRD is made, and reductions in pulmonary function may appear 1 to 3 years before the diagnosis.[18] With or without fasting hypoglycemia, CFRD can cause deterioration in body weight and pulmonary function.[44,46] An oral glucose tolerance test strongly recommended for all CF patients with poor growth. The nutrition strategy is to ensure sufficient energy intake to support adequate growth in adolescents and to maintain a normal BMI status in adults. The reader is referred to the guidelines developed by the Consensus Conference for Management of CFRD.[46]

## Cystic Fibrosis–Related Bone Disease

Bone health is of increasing interest and concern in CF as patient survival time increases. Bone disease has emerged as a common complication in long-term survivors of CF, with more than half having low bone mass and increased fracture risk.[6,48–50] Many studies have demonstrated deficits in bone mineral density resulting in premature osteopenia and osteoporosis.[6,50] The etiology of osteoporosis in CF is multifactorial, but the underlying mechanisms at play involve disturbances in the normal balance between bone formation and bone resorption. CF-related bone disease (CFBD) is characterized by impaired osteoblastic bone formation and enhanced osteoclastic bone resorption. CFTR deficiency and/or dysfunction impairs osteoblast activity and differentiation and indirectly promotes osteoclast formation.[48,51] The corticosteroid therapy and proinflammatory cytokines associated with ongoing respiratory infections during exacerbations affect bone tissue and can accelerate bone loss.[9,49,52,53] Delayed puberty, malabsorption, and reduced weight-bearing exercise in individuals with CF also contribute to inadequate bone mineral accretion in childhood and adolescence,[48,50] which are key periods in attainment of peak bone mass.

Prevention and treatment of osteopenia in children with CF are focused on general health measures, including optimizing nutrition by ensuring sufficient intake of vitamins D and K to normalize blood levels, encouraging calcium intake of 1300 mg/day for children ages 9 to 18 years, encouraging weight-bearing physical activity as tolerated, and exposure to sunlight to fulfill the vitamin D requirement.[6,9,53]

## Pancreatic Disease

The most common gastrointestinal complication in CF is pancreatic exocrine disease; in fact, only 10% to 15% of individuals with CF have sufficient exocrine function of the pancreas. The pancreas is abnormal in almost all patients with CF, and it has been found on autopsy to be almost destroyed in approximately 90% of those who have died from the disease.[9,54] Pancreatic exocrine deficiency results in fat and protein maldigestion and malabsorption, producing a distended abdomen, and bulky, greasy, foul-smelling stools. If uncorrected, pancreatic exocrine insufficiency ultimately results in failure to gain weight or undergo linear bone growth.

Approximately 85% to 90% of patients with CF have fat malabsorption and are considered to be pancreatic insufficient (PI). Between 10% and 15% of CF patients have normal fat absorption and are defined

**Table 55–1.** Pancreatic Functions and Mutations in Cystic Fibrosis (CF)

| Pancreatic-Sufficient Dominant CF Mutations | Variable Pancreatic-Sufficient CF Mutations |
|---|---|
| G551S | G85E |
| P574H | R347P |
| R117H | 3849 + 10kb C→T |
| R334W | A455E |
| R347H | 2789 5G→A |
| R352Q | |
| T3381 | |

as pancreatic sufficient (PS); that is, they have sufficient endogenous enzyme secretion to prevent malabsorption. Pancreatic functional status is a strong predictor of long-term outcome and has a direct influence on nutrition status. Among patients who are homozygous for the common ΔF508 mutation, 99% are PI. In contrast, there are some specific CFTR mutations that are associated with pancreatic sufficiency in a dominant fashion (Table 55–1), and possession of an allele from this group offers protection even in combination with an allele normally associated with PI.[2,9,18,27,28,54]

If the diagnosis of CF has been established, PI is diagnosed by the pancreatic fecal elastase test, but it can often be inferred from the clinical signs and symptoms such as frequent, malodorous, greasy stools; the presence of meconium ileus or DIOS; and rectal prolapse. In PI patients, mean fecal fat excretion is 38% of intake but may range as high as 80% in some. Clinical consequences include poor or absent weight gain, abdominal distention, abdominal pain, and reduction of subcutaneous fat and muscle tissue. Biochemical consequences include deficiencies of fat-soluble vitamins (i.e., vitamins A, D, E, and K), essential fatty acids, and albumin.[9,54–56]

Measurement of absorptive status is essential to determine whether the patient is PI or PS and thereby determine the necessity for enzyme replacement therapy. The most frequently employed test of pancreatic function is the 72-hour fecal fat excretion, expressed as the coefficient of fat absorption (CFA).[56–60] Malabsorption is diagnosed when fecal fat excretion exceeds 7% of the dietary fat ingested (15% for infants younger than 6 months of age).[61] For breast-fed infants, in whom fat intake cannot be measured, fat excretion greater than 2 g/day is indicative of PI. Patients who are PI require enzyme replacement therapy, but those who are PS do not.[9, 54,61–63]

Pancreatic enzyme replacement therapy is initiated once PI has been identified.[58,59] Enzymes are given with all foods that contain protein or fat, including predigested formulas and breast milk. Medium-chain triglycerides (MCT) require less lipase activity than long-chain fats for efficient absorption, although lipase is still needed.[9,64] There is significant individual variability in enzyme requirements. To avoid fibrosing colonopathy, it is recommended that the enzyme doses should be less than 2500 lipase units per kilogram of body weight per meal, or less than 4000 lipase units per gram of fat per day. In general, the daily dose of pancreatic enzymes should remain lower than 10,000 units of lipase per kilogram of body weight.[9,58,59,61] The adequacy of enzyme therapy can be assessed subjectively by monitoring growth parameters and stool patterns. The best objective test presently available is the 72-hour fecal fat excretion test.[9,56,58–60]

**Table 55–2.** Recommendations for Supplementation of Fat-Soluble Vitamins in Patients with Cystic Fibrosis

| Age | Vitamin A (IU) | Vitamin E (IU) | Vitamin D (IU) | Vitamin K* (mg) |
|---|---|---|---|---|
| 0–12 mo | 1500 | 40–50 | 400 | |
| 1–3 yr | 5000 | 80–150 | 400–800 | 0.3–0.5 |
| 4–8 yr | 5000–10,000 | 100–200 | 400–800 | |
| >8 yr | 10,000 | 200–400 | 400–800 | |

*Currently, commercially available products do not have ideal doses for supplementation. In a recent review, no adverse effects were reported at any dosage level of vitamin K. Clinicians should try to follow these recommendations as closely as possible until better dosage forms become available. Prothrombin time or, ideally, acarboxy prothrombin (PIVKA-II) levels should be checked in patients with liver disease, and the vitamin K dose should be titrated as indicated.

Adapted from Borowitz D, Baker RD, Stallings V. Consensus report on nutrition for pediatric patients with cystic fibrosis. *J Pediatr Gastroenterol Nutr.* 2002; 35:246.

**Table 55–3.** Laboratory Monitoring of Nutrition Status in Patients with Cystic Fibrosis*

| Nutrient | How Often to Monitor: At Diagnosis | Annually | Other | Tests |
|---|---|---|---|---|
| Beta-carotene | | | At physician's discretion | Serum levels |
| Vitamin A | X | X | | Vitamin A (retinol) |
| Vitamin D | X | X | | 25-Hydroxy vitamin D |
| Vitamin E | X | X | | α-Tocopherol |
| Vitamin K | X | X | If patient has hemoptysis or hematemesis; in patients with liver disease | PIVKA-II (preferably) or prothromin time |
| Essential fatty acids | | | Consider checking in infants or those with FTT | Triene:tetraene ratio |
| Calcium, bone status | | | At age > 8 yr if risk factors are present (see text) | Calcium, phosphorus, ionized PTH, DEXA scan |
| Iron | X | X | Consider in-depth evaluation for patients with poor appetite | Hemoglobin, hematocrit |
| Zinc | | | Consider 6-mo supplementation trial and monitor growth | No acceptable measurement |
| Sodium | | | Consider if patient is exposed to heat stress and becomes dehydrated | Serum sodium; spot urine sodium if total body sodium depletion is suspected |
| Protein stores | X | X | Check in patients with nutritional failure or those at risk | Albumin |

*Note: Patients diagnosed by neonatal screening do not need these measures.
DEXA = dual-energy x-ray absorptiometry; FTT = failure to thrive; PTH = parathyroid hormone; PIVKA-II = acarboxy prothrombin.
Adapted from Borowitz D, Baker RD, Stallings V. Consensus report on nutrition for pediatric patients with cystic fibrosis. *J Pediatr Gastroenterol Nutr.* 2002; 35:246.

## Nutrition Management

A complete overview of the nutritional care of patients with CF can be found in the Consensus Report on Nutrition for Pediatric Patients with Cystic Fibrosis.[9] The overall aim of nutrition therapy is to ensure that patients maintain normal linear growth and weight gain.[55] Most patients with CF require mealtime pancreatic enzymes and have a higher than normal caloric need because of the increased work of breathing. Nutrition management includes a high-calorie, high-fat diet; pancreatic enzyme replacement therapy; vitamin and mineral replacement; and enteric support as needed.[65] However, even with nutrition management and treatment, growth is also dependent on other parameters, such as gastrointestinal and pulmonary function and genetic potential.[9,27,28,54]

Monitoring of growth and nutrition status every 3 months is an essential part of the management; it commences at the time of diagnosis and continues throughout life. Although height, weight, and other anthropometric measurements remain a core part of the nutritional assessment, evaluation of nutrient absorption (i.e., the 72-hour fecal fat excretion test) and monitoring of laboratory values reflecting nutrition status should be performed annually (Tables 55–2 and 55–3).[9]

Nutrient requirements vary considerably with age and from one individual to another in health, and especially in disease.[55] Therefore, it is important for each patient to receive dietary counseling at regular intervals. An optional diet requires a caloric intake of 120% to 140%

(in some patients >140%) of the Recommended Daily Allowance. This can be accomplished by a well-balanced diet with 35% to 40% fat intake as a source of energy. Patients with CF who are adequately treated with pancreatic enzymes continue to malabsorb fat-soluble vitamins. Recommendations for surveillance and replacement of these substances are presented in Tables 55–2 and 55–3.[9,60]

Infants can be breast-fed, but if steatorrhea is present, they require pancreatic enzyme supplements and sodium chloride supplementation (⅛ teaspoon table salt per day or 10 mEq sodium chloride solution); the latter is especially important during the summer months, when higher temperatures result in more cutaneous salt loss in CF patients. Close monitoring of weight gain is indicated.[9] Most infants show adequate growth on standard formula feedings, which can be concentrated to maximize caloric and nutrient intake. Predigested formulas containing MCT may be recommended for infants with liver involvement, persistent steatorrhea, or short gut syndrome. MCTs require pancreatic enzymes for optimal digestion and absorption.[9,59]

Commercially available high-energy liquid dietary supplements are often prescribed for adolescents and adults with poor eating habits. However, very often oral supplements fail to improve the nutrition status significantly in patients with severe lung disease.[9,59,65] Respiratory problems usually cause restricted oral intake due to anorexia resulting from increased work of breathing, leading to acute weight loss. With improvement in respiratory symptoms, patients with mild pulmonary disease can be expected to show a rapid catch-up in weight. As the lung disease progresses, patients may not be able to consume adequate calories to maintain their nutrition status. For these patients, caloric supplementation through enteral feeding techniques (i.e., tube feeding) may be indicated.[9] The nocturnal infusion of a high-calorie formula through a nasogastric, gastrostomy, or jejunostomy tube can provide 40% to 50% of total energy needs. Nocturnal supplemental feedings, while reducing voluntary caloric intake from food by about 20%, result in a significant increase in total daily energy intake, catch-up growth, and weight gain.[9]

### Summary and Follow-up

There is no reason to accept nutritional failure or impaired growth in any individual with CF.[9,55] Achievement of normal weight gain, growth, and development requires regular surveillance, intake of adequate calories with 35% to 40% of energy from fat, and a plan for intervention if growth is suboptimal. Following this care plan, most patients grow normally in height and weight until their lung condition deteriorates significantly. Patients with advanced lung disease may not be able to consume adequate energy to prevent weight loss; for these patients, supplemental nocturnal tube feeding should be considered.[9,55]

## BRONCHOPULMONARY DYSPLASIA

The term *bronchopulmonary dysplasia* (BPD) refers to a common, long-term respiratory complication that most typically results from premature birth (<32 weeks' gestation). It affects the peripheral airways, including the small bronchi and bronchioles; it therefore involves a large cross-sectional area of lung tissue and leads to significant physiological abnormalities. BPD was originally described in newborns as infant respiratory distress syndrome (or hyaline membrane disease).[66] These early descriptions of BPD were reflective of the high concentrations of inspired oxygen and positive-pressure ventilation given to premature infants that caused cellular injury to the immature lung over time.[67] Today, the term is more commonly used to refer to a developmental arrest in an immature lung. BPD is characterized by abnormalities of the bronchioles, including significant metaplasia, obliteration, lung hyperinflation, cystic changes, and an apparent arrest of alveolarization that occurs *in utero* during the third trimester.[66,68,69] Clinical manifestations include tachypnea, wheezing, pulmonary hypertension, vascular abnormalities, and chronic respiratory insufficiency.[66,68,70,71]

School-aged children who were born prematurely with BPD exhibit detrimental effects on linear bone growth, lean muscle mass, and whole-body bone mineral mass when compared with children who were born at full term, suggesting that early nutrition may be critical to recovery.[70,72] Evidence-based nutrition recommendations do not exist for this special infant population; nutrition management depends mostly on practice-based information. Important aspects of therapy for infants with BPD include oxygen therapy; use of bronchodilators, diuretics, and anti-inflammatory agents, including corticosteroids; and special nutrition rehabilitation to achieve catch-up growth.[70]

### Factors To Be Considered in Nutrition Evaluation

Growth failure in BPD is almost universal and results from the increased caloric requirements caused by high resting energy expenditure coupled with inability to consume adequate calories because of gastroesophageal reflux (GER), emesis, acute and chronic infections, and polypharmacy, especially with exogenous steroids, as well as many adverse effects pertaining to the gastrointestinal system and bone metabolism.[73–75] Strategies for nutritional support focus on optimizing intake of calories and nutrients to meet the individual needs of each infant.[76] The energy requirements for infants may range from 120 to 160 kcal/kg/day. Infants on chronic ventilation may require less energy intake. It is important to optimize oxygen therapy and to control of GER and emesis. Concentration of formula provides increased caloric intake without an increase in fluid intake.[73]

### Dietary and Nutritional Management

In infants with growth failure, nasogastric tube feeding may be indicated for energy supplementation. However, the risk of aspiration is increased because passage of a nasogastric tube through the gastroesophageal junction can exacerbate GER. Infants who require supplemental tube feeding for a prolonged period should be considered for placement of a gastrostomy tube, either percutaneously or surgically. Because GER and aspiration can exacerbate the lung injury in BPD, the presence of reflux should be evaluated.[73–75]

Feeding dysfunction can develop in the infant with BPD as a result of behavioral feeding aversion or dysfunctional swallowing due to endotracheal intubation or tube feeding. Behavioral aversion may be prevented by early intervention with positive oral stimulation and nonnutritive sucking during tube feeding. For some infants with BPD, a behavior modification program to gradually decrease feeding resistance may be recommended. Solids are introduced slowly by spoon to promote and develop oral-motor skills, but they should not replace energy- and nutrient-dense formulas.[75,77]

Nutrient-based interventions for prevention and treatment of BPD have been investigated for inositol, intravenous fatty acids, vitamin E, and vitamin A.[74,75,77] In one study, inositol, a phospholipid that is proposed to enhance the synthesis and secretion of pulmonary surfactant and therefore could reduce the severity of lung disease, led to greater survival without BPD or neurodevelopmental handicap at 28 days of age.[78] Both intravenous fatty acids and vitamin E have been used as adjunctive antioxidant therapy in ventilated infants. In theory, these nutrients could serve as scavengers of excessive oxygen radicals produced during exposure to high oxygen toxicity that manifests as BPD.[75] Clinical trials have not proven that either polyunsaturated fatty acids or vitamin E given prophylactically promotes lung maturation or reduces the development of BPD. The available evidence only suggests a role for high-dose vitamin A in the prevention of BPD.[79]

Corticosteroids (e.g., dexamethasone) are used as therapy in very-low-birth-weight infants to promote earlier weaning from the ventilator and possible prevention of BPD. The negative effects of these potent steroids on growth, mineral metabolism, and bone metabolism must be weighed against the short-term clinical benefits.[68] Atkinson reported that dexamethasone was associated with abrupt growth restriction without recovery by term age.[79]

In a study of nutrient-enriched formula used to support catch-up growth in infants with BPD, the results showed that infants fed at the protein-to-energy ratio of the control formula (2.5 g/100 kcal) developed a greater percentage of body fat than those fed the nutrient-enriched formula (6 g/100 kcal).[77] However, sustained growth in length, lean mass, and bone mass observed at 3 months, when the intervention was completed, was not maintained at the 1-year corrected age.[77] Clearly, continuation of nutrient-enriched feeding (30 kcal/oz) to a corrected age of 1 year or older in infants with BPD may be appropriate to promote catch-up growth.[74,79,80]

## References


1. Zuelzer WW, Newton WA Jr. The pathogenesis of fibrocystic disease of the pancreas; a study of 36 cases with special reference to the pulmonary lesions. *Pediatrics.* 1949; 4:1.
2. Knowles MR, Durie PR. What is cystic fibrosis? *N Engl J Med.* 2002; 347:6.
3. Andersen DH, Hodges RG. Celiac syndrome; genetics of cystic fibrosis of the pancreas, with a consideration of etiology. *Am J Dis Child.* 1946; 72:62.
4. Zielenski J, Tsui LC. Cystic fibrosis: genotypic and phenotypic variations. *Annu Rev Genet.* 1995; 29:777.
5. Tsui LC., Buchwald M. Biochemical and molecular genetics of cystic fibrosis. *Adv Hum Genet.* 1991; 20:153.
6. Parkins MD, Parkins VM, Rendall JC, Elborn S. Changing epidemiology and clinical issues arising in an ageing cystic fibrosis population. *Ther Adv Respir Dis.* 2011; 5:2.
7. FitzSimmons SC. The changing epidemiology of cystic fibrosis. *Curr Probl Pediatr.* 1994; 24:5.
8. McPhail GL, Clancy JP. Ivacaftor: the first therapy acting on the primary cause of cystic fibrosis. *Drugs Today (Barc).* 2013; 49:4.
9. Borowitz D, Baker RD, Stallings V. Consensus report on nutrition for pediatric patients with cystic fibrosis. *J Pediatr Gastroenterol Nutr.* 2002; 35:3.
10. Stern RC, Boat TF, Doershuk CF, Tucker AS, Miller RB, Matthews LW. Cystic fibrosis diagnosed after age 13. Twenty-five teenage and adult patients including three asymptomatic men. *Ann Intern Med.* 1977; 87:2.
11. Annual Data Report of the US Organ Procurement and Transplantation Network (OPTN) and the Scientific Registry of Transplant Recipients (SRTR). Introduction. *Am J Transplant.* 2013; 13(Suppl 1):8.
12. Tsui LC, Buchwald M, Barker D, et al. Cystic fibrosis locus defined by a genetically linked polymorphic DNA marker. *Science.* 1985; 230:4729.
13. Zengerling S, Tsui LC, Grzeschik KH, Olek K, Riordan JR, Buchwald M. Mapping of DNA markers linked to the cystic fibrosis locus on the long arm of chromosome 7. *Am J Hum Genet.* 1987; 40:3.
14. White R, Woodward S, Leppert M, et al. A closely linked genetic marker for cystic fibrosis. *Nature.* 1985; 318:6044.
15. Wainwright BJ, Scambler PJ, Schmidtke J, et al. Localization of cystic fibrosis locus to human chromosome 7cen-q22. *Nature.* 1985; 318:6044.
16. Riordan JR, Rommens JM, Kerem B, et al. Identification of the cystic fibrosis gene: cloning and characterization of complementary DNA. *Science.* 1989; 245:4922.
17. Zaibak F, Williamson R. Genetics and genomics: providing new opportunities for the translation of basic research to clinical care for cystic fibrosis. *Expert Rev Respir Med.* 2008; 2:1.
18. Cystic Fibrosis Genetic Analysis Consortium. *Cystic Fibrosis Mutation Data.* http://www.genet.sickkids.on.ca/cftr. Accessed July 9, 016.
19. Anderson MP, Gregory RJ, Thompson S, et al. Demonstration that CFTR is a chloride channel by alteration of its anion selectivity. *Science.* 1991; 253:5016.
20. Bear CE, Li CH, Kartner N, et al. Purification and functional reconstitution of the cystic fibrosis transmembrane conductance regulator (CFTR). *Cell.* 1992; 68:4.
21. Egan M, Flotte T, Afione S, et al. Defective regulation of outwardly rectifying Cl- channels by protein kinase A corrected by insertion of CFTR. *Nature.* 1992; 358:6387.
22. Stutts MJ, Canessa CM, Olsen JC, et al. CFTR as a cAMP-dependent regulator of sodium channels. *Science.* 1995; 269:5225.
23. Knowles M, Gatzy J, Boucher R. Increased bioelectric potential difference across respiratory epithelia in cystic fibrosis. *N Engl J Med.* 1981; 305:25.
24. Kerem E, Corey M, Kerem BS, et al. The relation between genotype and phenotype in cystic fibrosis—analysis of the most common mutation (delta F508). *N Engl J Med.* 1990; 323:22.
25. Castellani C, Cuppens H, Macek M Jr, et al. Consensus on the use and interpretation of cystic fibrosis mutation analysis in clinical practice. *J Cyst Fibros.* 2008; 7:3.
26. Duthie A, Doherty DG, Williams C, et al. Genotype analysis for delta F508, G551D and R553X mutations in children and young adults with cystic fibrosis with and without chronic liver disease. *Hepatology.* 1992; 15:4.
27. Acton JD, Wilmott RW. Phenotype of CF and the effects of possible modifier genes. *Paediatr Respir Rev.* 2001; 2:4.
28. Kristidis P, Bozon D, Corey M, et al. Genetic determination of exocrine pancreatic function in cystic fibrosis. *Am J Hum Genet.* 1992; 50:6.
29. MacKenzie T, Gifford AH, Sabadosa KA, et al. Longevity of patients with cystic fibrosis in 2000 to 2010 and beyond: survival analysis of the Cystic Fibrosis Foundation patient registry. *Ann Intern Med.* 2014; 161:4.
30. Di Sant'Agnese PA, Darling RC, Perera GA, Shea E. Abnormal electrolyte composition of sweat in cystic fibrosis of the pancreas; clinical significance and relationship to the disease. *Pediatrics.* 1953; 12:5.
31. Gibson LE, Cooke RE. A test for concentration of electrolytes in sweat in cystic fibrosis of the pancreas utilizing pilocarpine by iontophoresis. *Pediatrics.* 1959; 23:3.
32. Cantin A. Cystic fibrosis lung inflammation: early, sustained, and severe. *Am J Respir Crit Care Med.* 1995; 151:4.
33. Sturgess J, Imrie J. Quantitative evaluation of the development of tracheal submucosal glands in infants with cystic fibrosis and control infants. *Am J Pathol.* 1982; 106:3.
34. Connett GJ. Cystic fibrosis nutrition: chewing the fat. *Paediatr Respir Rev.* 2015; 16(Suppl 1):1.
35. Steinkamp G, Wiedemann B. Relationship between nutritional status and lung function in cystic fibrosis: cross sectional and longitudinal analyses from the German CF quality assurance (CFQA) project. *Thorax.* 2002; 57:7.
36. Sharma R, Florea VG, Bolger AP, et al. Wasting as an independent predictor of mortality in patients with cystic fibrosis. *Thorax.* 2001; 56:10.
37. Rudolph CD, Mazur LJ, Liptak GS, et al. Guidelines for evaluation and treatment of gastroesophageal reflux in infants and children: recommendations of the North American Society for Pediatric Gastroenterology and Nutrition. *J Pediatr Gastroenterol Nutr.* 2001; 32(Suppl 2):S1.
38. Lee P, Rudolph C. Gastroesophageal reflux in infants and children. *Adv Pediatr.* 2001; 48:301.
39. Koletzko S, Stringer DA, Cleghorn GJ, Durie PR. Lavage treatment of distal intestinal obstruction syndrome in children with cystic fibrosis. *Pediatrics.* 1989; 83:5.
40. Stern RC, Eisenberg JD, Wagener JS, et al. A comparison of the efficacy and tolerance of pancrelipase and placebo in the treatment of steatorrhea in cystic fibrosis patients with clinical exocrine pancreatic insufficiency. *Am J Gastroenterol.* 2000; 95:8.
41. Moyer K, Balistreri W. Hepatobiliary disease in patients with cystic fibrosis. *Curr Opin Gastroenterol.* 2009; 25:3.
42. Feranchak AP. Hepatobiliary complications of cystic fibrosis. *Curr Gastroenterol Rep.* 2004; 6:3.
43. Diwakar V, Pearson L, Beath S. Liver disease in children with cystic fibrosis. *Paediatr Respir Rev.* 2001; 2:4.
44. Lek N, Acerini CL. Cystic fibrosis related diabetes mellitus—diagnostic and management challenges. *Curr Diabetes Rev.* 2010; 6:1.
45. Moran A, Becker D, Casella SJ, et al. Epidemiology, pathophysiology, and prognostic implications of cystic fibrosis-related diabetes: a technical review. *Diabetes Care.* 2010; 33:12.
46. Moran A, Brunzell C, Cohen RC, et al. Clinical care guidelines for cystic fibrosis-related diabetes: a position statement of the American Diabetes Association and a clinical practice guideline of the Cystic Fibrosis Foundation, endorsed by the Pediatric Endocrine Society. *Diabetes Care.* 2010; 33:12.
47. Costa M, Potvin S, Hammana I, et al. Increased glucose excursion in cystic fibrosis and its association with a worse clinical status. *J Cyst Fibros.* 2007; 6:6.
48. Stalvey MS, Clines GA. Cystic fibrosis-related bone disease: insights into a growing problem. *Curr Opin Endocrinol Diabetes Obes.* 2013; 20:6.
49. Aris RM, Merkel PA, Bachrach LK, et al. Guide to bone health and disease in cystic fibrosis. *J Clin Endocrinol Metab.* 2005; 90:3.
50. Ujhelyi R, Treszl A, Vasarhelyi B, et al. Bone mineral density and bone acquisition in children and young adults with cystic fibrosis: a follow-up study. *J Pediatr Gastroenterol Nutr.* 2004; 38:4.
51. Stalvey MS, Clines KL, Havasi V, et al. Osteoblast CFTR inactivation reduces differentiation and osteoprotegerin expression in a mouse model of cystic fibrosis-related bone disease. *PLoS One.* 2013; 8:11.
52. Schulze KJ, Cutchins C, Rosenstein BJ, Germain-Lee EL, O'Brien KO. Calcium acquisition rates do not support age-appropriate gains in total body bone mineral content in prepuberty and late puberty in girls with cystic fibrosis. *Osteoporos Int.* 2006; 17:5.
53. Conway SP. Impact of lung inflammation on bone metabolism in adolescents with cystic fibrosis. *Paediatr Respir Rev.* 2001; 2:4.
54. Couper R, Belli D, Durie P, Gaskin K, Sarles J, Werlin S. Pancreatic disorders and cystic fibrosis: Working Group Report of the First World Congress of Pediatric Gastroenterology, Hepatology, and Nutrition. *J Pediatr Gastroenterol Nutr.* 2002; 35(Suppl 2):S213.
55. Culhane S, George C, Pearo B, Spoede E. Malnutrition in cystic fibrosis: a review. *Nutr Clin Pract.* 2013; 28:6.
56. Palermo J, Szabo F. 50 Years ago in The Journal of Pediatrics: hypoproteinemia and edema in infants with cystic fibrosis of the pancreas. *J Pediatr.* 2014; 164:3.
57. Kutty KM, Bridger H, Vaze D, Davis AJ. A study of fat absorption in cystic fibrosis patients and controls by a rapid micro procedure: a comparison with fecal fat excretion method. *Clin Biochem.* 1983; 16:5.
58. FitzSimmons SC, Burkhart GA, Borowitz D, et al. High-dose pancreatic-enzyme supplements and fibrosing colonopathy in children with cystic fibrosis. *N Engl J Med.* 1997; 336:18.
59. Stallings VA, Stark LJ, Robinson KA, et al. Evidence-based practice recommendations for nutrition-related management of children and adults with cystic fibrosis and pancreatic insufficiency: results of a systematic review. *J Am Diet Assoc.* 2008; 108:5.
60. Feranchak AP, Sontag MK, Wagener JS, Hammond KB, Accurso FJ, Sokol RJ. Prospective, long-term study of fat-soluble vitamin status in children with cystic fibrosis identified by newborn screen. *J Pediatr.* 1999; 135:5.
61. Borowitz D. Evidence for the diagnosis of pancreatic insufficiency. *Pediatr Pulmonol.* 2000; 29:3.
62. Borowitz D. Update on the evaluation of pancreatic exocrine status in cystic fibrosis. *Curr Opin Pulm Med.* 2005; 11:6.
63. Waters DL, Dorney SF, Gaskin KJ, Gruca MA, O'Halloran M, Wilcken B. Pancreatic function in infants identified as having cystic fibrosis in a neonatal screening program. *N Engl J Med.* 1990; 322:5.
64. Caliari S, Benini L, Sembenini C, Gregori B, Carnielli V, Vantini I. Medium-chain triglyceride absorption in patients with pancreatic insufficiency. *Scand J Gastroenterol.* 1996; 31:1.
65. Schindler T, Michel S, Wilson AW. Nutrition management of cystic fibrosis in the 21st century. *Nutr Clin Pract.* 2015; 30:4.
66. Northway WH Jr, Rosan RC, Porter DY. Pulmonary disease following respirator therapy of hyaline-membrane disease. Bronchopulmonary dysplasia. *N Engl J Med.* 1967; 276:7.
67. Katz R, McWilliams B. Bronchopulmonary dysplasia in the pediatric intensive care unit. *Crit Care Clin.* 1988; 4:4.
68. Hilgendorff A, O'Reilly MA. Bronchopulmonary dysplasia early changes leading to long-term consequences. *Front Med (Lausanne).* 2015; 2:2.
69. Jobe AH, Bancalari E. Bronchopulmonary dysplasia. *Am J Respir Crit Care Med.* 2001; 163:7.
70. Niedermaier S, Hilgendorff A. Bronchopulmonary dysplasia—an overview about pathophysiologic concepts. *Mol Cell Pediatr.* 2015; 2:1.
71. Edwards DK, Dyer WM, Northway WH Jr. Twelve years' experience with bronchopulmonary dysplasia. *Pediatrics.* 1977; 59:6.

72. Giacoia GP, Venkataraman PS, West-Wilson KI, Faulkner MJ. Follow-up of school-age children with bronchopulmonary dysplasia. *J Pediatr*. 1997; 130:3.
73. Wood NS, Costeloe K, Gibson AT, et al. The EPICure study: growth and associated problems in children born at 25 weeks of gestational age or less. *Arch Dis Child Fetal Neonatal Ed*. 2003; 88:6.
74. Puangco MA, Schanler RJ. Clinical experience in enteral nutrition support for premature infants with bronchopulmonary dysplasia. *J Perinatol*. 2000; 20:2.
75. Abrams SA. Chronic pulmonary insufficiency in children and its effects on growth and development. *J Nutr*. 2001; 131:3.
76. Poindexter BB, Martin CR. Impact of nutrition on bronchopulmonary dysplasia. *Clin Perinatol*. 2015; 42:4.
77. Brunton JA, Saigal S, Atkinson SA. Growth and body composition in infants with bronchopulmonary dysplasia up to 3 months corrected age: a randomized trial of a high-energy nutrient-enriched formula fed after hospital discharge. *J Pediatr*. 1998; 133:3.
78. Hallman M, Bry K, Hoppu K, Lappi M, Pohjavuori M. Inositol supplementation in premature infants with respiratory distress syndrome. *N Engl J Med*. 1992; 326:19.
79. Atkinson SA. Special nutritional needs of infants for prevention of and recovery from bronchopulmonary dysplasia. *J Nutr*. 2001; 131:3.
80. O'Connor DL, Jacobs J, Hall R, et al. Growth and development of premature infants fed predominantly human milk, predominantly premature infant formula, or a combination of human milk and premature formula. *J Pediatr Gastroenterol Nutr*. 2003; 37:4.

# 56 Fragile X Syndrome

TORI L. SCHAEFER, DAVID L. NELSON, AND CRAIG A. ERICKSON

Fragile X syndrome (FXS) was first recognized in 1943 by Martin and Bell as an X-linked form of intellectual disability (ID).[1] The discovery in 1969[2] that affected males exhibit a folate-sensitive fragile site at Xq27.3 was followed by characterization of the site in the 1970s.[3,4] The locus containing the genetic lesion that produces the fragile site was isolated in 1991, and the affected gene was called fragile X mental retardation 1 (*FMR1*). It was found that an unstable trinucleotide repeat was massively expanded in fragile X chromosomes.[5–7] The fully expanded repeat (full mutation) inhibits expression of the *FMR1* gene,[8] and loss of function of this gene is the primary cause of FXS.

Current treatment of FXS consists of pharmacotherapy based on symptomology; for example, anxiety or irritability is treated with the same medications approved for these symptoms in non-FXS populations. Although the severity of some behavioral problems can be improved with behavioral therapy and symptom-based pharmacotherapy, the efficacy of altered nutrition or pharmacotherapy targeted to treat the underlying molecular and biochemical disruptions associated with the disorder have yet to be supported by rigorous clinical study.[9,10]

## PREVALENCE

FXS is a genetic disorder and behavioral syndrome that affects 1 in 4000 males and 1 in 4000 to 6000 females.[11–13] The frequency is roughly the same in different populations, although some isolated groups show an increased prevalence. FXS is the most common known genetic cause of autism and one of the most common forms of inherited ID. The high frequency of the disease stems from a high carrier frequency. Some populations exhibit carrier frequencies as high as 1 in 200 individuals.[14] The definition of carriers depends on the molecular genetics of the disease (see later discussion).

## PHENOTYPE AND CLINICAL ABNORMALITIES

Patients with FXS exhibit a general developmental delay that is usually apparent in the first few months of life as delayed milestones and is often accompanied by language delay. It is common for families with no history of FXS to endure many months (sometimes years) without a specific diagnosis, although this timeline is shortening as medical providers become more aware of the disorder. Males with FXS often display large head circumference, elongated faces with high foreheads, macroorchidism (enlarged testicular volume), and large, slightly dysmorphic ears. Other physical features may include mild coarsening of facial features, high arched palate, epicanthic folds, dental crowding, fine velvety skin, calluses on the hand from self-abuse, abnormal palmar creases, and mitral valve prolapse.[15] Females can also be affected by the disorder, despite the X-linked inheritance. In females, the severity of the syndrome is quite variable and depends on the expression pattern of the affected X chromosome after X inactivation. In males, ID is universal, ranging from mild to severe intellectual impairment.[14] Females are typically less affected. Approximately half of females with a full mutation express an IQ measured below 70; most of these females score in the mild to moderately affected IQ range.[16]

In addition to cognitive impairment, individuals with FXS often exhibit symptoms of attention-deficit hyperactivity disorder (ADHD) symptoms and have increased self-injurious behavior, sensitivity to sensory stimuli, anxiety (including severe social anxiety), perseverative language, aggression, and sleep issues. Approximately two of every three affected males exhibit features consistent with the broad autism spectrum.[17] However, the penetrance of these features is incomplete, and the severity of affected behavior domains is highly variable even in individuals with a full mutation.

## MOLECULAR GENETICS AND INHERITANCE

Long recognized as an X-linked form of ID, FXS received its current name with the definition of a chromosomal fragile site near the end of the long arm of the X chromosome that segregated with the disease in most affected males. Recognition of this site, along with the ability to define segregation of linked genetic markers, allowed the susceptible chromosome to be followed through families and led eventually to identification of the gene defect that causes the disease. Typically, FXS results when there is a trinucleotide CGG repeat expansion in the 5′ untranslated region of the *FMR1* gene, which also causes the fragile site. This expansion can be detected by Southern blot analysis for diagnostic purposes.[18] Increases in CGG repeat number lead to partial or full methylation of the C nucleotides of the CG pairs that extends beyond the repeat region. Coupled with compacted chromatin and alterations in histone acetylation, this results in near or complete silencing of transcription of the *FMR1* messenger RNA (mRNA) and expression the *FMR1* gene product, fragile X mental retardation protein (FMRP). Support for the loss-of-function hypothesis is provided by identification of patients with more typical loss of function point mutations in *FMR1* who exhibit an indistinguishable phenotype.

In the general population, CGG repeat lengths vary from as few as 5 triplets to as many as 50, with most X chromosomes carrying 29 or 30 repeats. In fragile X families, individuals with the full mutation carry hundreds or thousands of triplets at this location, and it appears that the threshold for clinical effects begins at approximately 200 repeats. Individuals with approximately 50 to 200 repeats, male or female, are said to be premutation carriers. These individuals were once thought to be free from any clinical effects, but it is now known that adult male (and, rarely, female) premutation carriers can suffer from fragile X–associated tremor/ataxia syndrome (FXTAS), and female premutation carriers may experience fragile X–associated primary ovarian insufficiency syndrome (FXPOI).[19] Premutation carriers may also suffer from other clinical disorders, including anxiety and mild cognitive difficulties. A maternal premutation allele may undergo further expansion, and full-mutation FXS (i.e., >200 repeats) can be transmitted from mother to child. Male premutation repeat number tends to remain in the premutation range when passed to offspring, and resulting female children are likely also to be premutation carriers. Expansion of the untranslated CGG repeats tends to occur with each subsequent generation; therefore, fragile X–associated disorders affect multiple generations, with later generations often having more affected individuals (Fig. 56–1).

## FACTORS TO BE CONSIDERED IN NUTRITION EVALUATION AND MANAGEMENT

The chromosomal fragile site can be induced in the X chromosomes of FXS patients in vitro by restricting the amount of folate in the cell culture medium. This leads to a constriction on the chromosome during

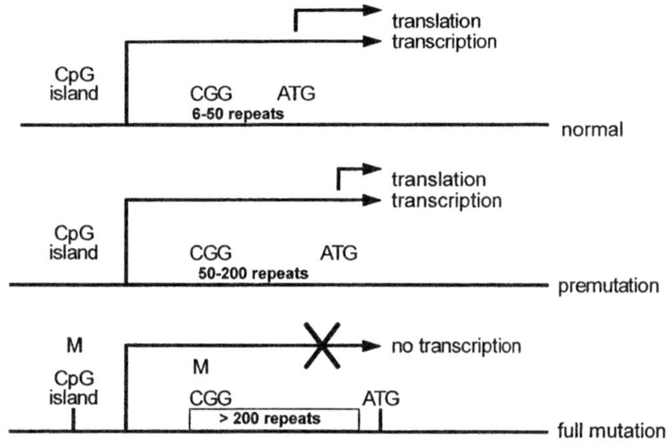


**Figure 56–1.** Size and effect of mutations in fragile X syndrome. Three situations are depicted. Normal, premutation, and full mutation alleles are drawn, indicating repeat lengths in the 5′ untranslated region of the *FMR1* gene. M indicates methylation, and arrows indicate the ability of the normal and premutation alleles to support transcription and translation.

condensation in mitosis and occasionally to breakage at the constriction (a fragile site). However, there is no indication that the fragile site manifests in patients in vivo. Nonetheless, the effect of folate on this chromosomal abnormality has led to suggestions that dietary folic acid supplementation may be beneficial. No empirical evidence currently exists to suggest any benefit of folic acid for the treatment of these patients.[20,21] However, numerous parents report decreases in hyperactivity when their children take folic acid supplements, and there is no evidence of harm from the dosages being used. These anecdotal reports are often complicated by the use of other drug therapies together with the folic acid supplements.

L-Acetylcarnitine (LAC) was suggested as a treatment for FXS because it was shown to inhibit in vitro expression of the fragile site and it effectively acetylates histones in the FMR1 promoter, although without reactivating the gene in vitro. No benefits of oral LAC treatment in FXS have been demonstrated in randomized controlled trials.[22,23] Decreased levels of choline have been reported in boys with FXS, suggesting that drugs such as donepezil, an acetylcholinesterase inhibitor, may improve cognitive-behavioral function.[24] A small controlled trial of donepezil in boys with FXS failed to show improved intelligence quotients, but the drug was safe and well tolerated.[25] Overall, no dietary adjustments or supplements have been shown to be effective in modulating any FXS phenotypes.

## *FMR1* GENE FUNCTION

Since the identification of the *FMR1* gene as the genetic defect in FXS, significant effort has been expended to determine the normal function of this gene and the consequences of its lack of function in FXS patients and to use this information to identify and test potential rational treatments. The use of model organisms such as the mouse[26–28] and the fruit fly[29–31] have greatly aided understanding of FXS. The *FMR1* gene is broadly expressed, with its product being found in most tissues at most developmental time points. The *FMR1* gene product, FMRP, is an mRNA-binding protein that binds to approximately 4% of all mRNA in the brain.[32] FMRP binding targets are involved in neuronal development and synaptic functions that underscore the cognitive and behavioral difficulties observed in FXS patients.

Over the past 20 years, it has become apparent that the actions of FMRP in the brain are complex and involve mRNA transport and localization[33] as well as positive and negative regulation of translation.[34,35] In the brain, loss of FMRP is associated with molecular and cellular signaling deficits,[36,37] morphological and electrophysiological changes,[38–40] alterations in activity-induced protein synthesis,[41] and altered expression and function of FMRP targets such as matrix metallopeptidase 9 (MMP9) and amyloid precursor protein (APP).[42,43] Immature dendritic spines have been observed in patients with FXS and in a mouse model of the disease. These findings suggest a possible mechanism for the cognitive and behavioral problems in FXS patients, although it is unclear whether correction in dendritic spine morphology will result in observable treatment response in humans. Of particular importance is the role played by FMRP in activity- and stimulus-induced neuronal activity,[44] which likely suggests that efficacious treatments will need not only to address basal deficits in brain functioning but also to augment stimulus-induced deficits.

It has been demonstrated that loss of FMRP results in an imbalance of excitatory/inhibitory signaling, with excitatory signaling being increased and exacerbated by decreases in inhibitory signaling. The mGluR5 theory of FXS, which suggests that excitatory signaling through the metabotropic glutamate receptor type 5 (mGluR5) is elevated, leading to excessive protein production and increased internalization of α-amino-3-hydroxy-5-methyl-4-isoxazolepropionic acid receptor (AMPAR), has received the most attention as a potential pathway to treatment.[45] Several large clinical trials have been completed utilizing mGluR5 antagonists in both FXS and autism, but no obvious improvements in behavior were found. Many other targeted compounds are being assessed for efficacy in FXS in humans, although the optimal treatment age, dose level, and outcome measures needed to demonstrate efficacy in this population remain unknown.[10]

## SUMMARY AND FOLLOW-UP

The past 20 years have seen significant advances in unraveling the genetics of this common form of human ID. The discovery of a novel mechanism of mutation, trinucleotide repeat expansion, led to appreciation of this process in numerous other human genetic disorders. The finding that loss of function of the *FMR1* gene is the sole determinant of FXS has allowed intense focus on the role of this gene in normal and disease states and has led to a flurry of targeted drug treatment trials in FXS. Although demonstration of clear efficacy has been challenging, it is hoped that the coming years of effort will lead to improved treatments for this most common genetic form of autism and inherited ID.

### References

1. Martin JP, Bell J. A pedigree of mental defect showing sex-linkage. *J Neurol Psychiatry.* 1943; 6:154.
2. Lubs HA. A marker X chromosome. *Am J Hum Genet.* 1969; 21:231.
3. Sutherland GR. Fragile sites on human chromosomes: demonstration of their dependence on the type of tissue culture medium. *Science.* 1977; 197:265.
4. Sutherland GR, Ashforth PL. X-linked mental retardation with macro-orchidism and the fragile site at Xq 27 or 28. *Hum Genet.* 1979; 48:117.
5. Oberle I, Rousseau F, Heitz D, et al. Instability of a 550-base pair DNA segment and abnormal methylation in fragile X syndrome. *Science.* 1991; 252:1097.
6. Verkerk AJ, Pieretti M, Sutcliffe JS, et al. Identification of a gene (FMR-1) containing a CGG repeat coincident with a breakpoint cluster region exhibiting length variation in fragile X syndrome. *Cell.* 1991; 65:905.
7. Yu S, Pritchard M, Kremer E, et al. Fragile X genotype characterized by an unstable region of DNA. *Science.* 1991; 252:1179.
8. Pieretti M, Zhang FP, Fu YH, et al. Absence of expression of the FMR-1 gene in fragile X syndrome. *Cell.* 1991; 66:817.
9. Rueda JR, Ballesteros J, Tejada MI. Systematic review of pharmacological treatments in fragile X syndrome. *BMC Neurol.* 2009; 9:53.
10. Schaefer TL, Davenport MH, Erickson CA. Emerging pharmacologic treatment options for fragile X syndrome. *Appl Clin Genet.* 2015; 8:75.
11. Turner G, Webb T, Wake S, et al. Prevalence of fragile X syndrome. *Am J Med. Genet* 1996; 64:196.
12. Song FJ, Barton P, Sleightholme V, et al. Screening for fragile X syndrome: a literature review and modelling study. *Health Technol Assess.* 2003; 7:1.
13. Coffee B, Keith K, Albizua I, et al. Incidence of fragile X syndrome by newborn screening for methylated FMR1 DNA. *Am J Hum Genet.* 2009; 85:503.
14. Tassone F, Iong KP, Tong TH, et al. FMR1 CGG allele size and prevalence ascertained through newborn screening in the United States. *Genome Med.* 2012; 4:100.
15. Garber KB, Visootsak J, Warren ST. Fragile X syndrome. *Eur J Hum Genet.* 2008; 16:666.
16. de Vries BB, Wiegers AM, Smits AP, et al. Mental status of females with an FMR1 gene full mutation. *Am J Hum Genet.* 1996; 58:1025.
17. Kaufmann WE, Cortell R, Kau AS, et al. Autism spectrum disorder in fragile X syndrome: communication, social interaction, and specific behaviors. *Am J Med Genet A.* 2004; 129A:225.
18. Curtis-Cioffi KM, Rodrigueiro DA, Rodrigues VC, et al. Comparison between the polymerase chain reaction-based screening and the Southern blot methods for identification of fragile X syndrome. *Genet Test Mol Biomarkers.* 2012; 16:1303.

19. Tassone F, Hagerman PJ, Hagerman RJ. Fragile X premutation. *J Neurodev Disord.* 2014; 6:22.
20. Hagerman RJ, Jackson AW, Levitas A, et al. Oral folic acid versus placebo in the treatment of males with the fragile X syndrome. *Am J Med Genet.* 1986; 23:241.
21. Fisch GS, Cohen IL, Gross AC, et al. Folic acid treatment of fragile X males: a further study. *Am J Med Genet.* 1988; 30:393.
22. Torrioli MG, Vernacotola S, Peruzzi L, et al. A double-blind, parallel, multicenter comparison of L-acetylcarnitine with placebo on the attention deficit hyperactivity disorder in fragile X syndrome boys. *Am J Med Genet A.* 2008; 146:803.
23. Torrioli MG VS, Mariotti P, Bianchi E, et al. Double-blind, placebo-controlled study of L-acetylcarnitine for the treatment of hyperactive behavior in fragile X syndrome. *Am J Med Genet.* 1999; 87:4.
24. Kesler SR, Lightbody AA, Reiss AL. Cholinergic dysfunction in fragile X syndrome and potential intervention: a preliminary 1H MRS study. *Am J Med Genet A.* 2009; 149A:403.
25. Sahu JK, Gulati S, Sapra S, et al. Effectiveness and safety of donepezil in boys with fragile x syndrome: a double-blind, randomized, controlled pilot study. *J Child Neurol.* 2013; 28:570.
26. The Dutch-Belgian Fragile X Consortium. Fmr1 knockout mice: a model to study fragile X mental retardation. *Cell.* 1994; 78:23.
27. Mientjes EJ, Nieuwenhuizen I, Kirkpatrick L, et al. The generation of a conditional Fmr1 knock out mouse model to study Fmrp function in vivo. *Neurobiol Dis.* 2006; 21:549.
28. Peier AM, McIlwain KL, Kenneson A, et al. (Over)correction of FMR1 deficiency with YAC transgenics: behavioral and physical features. *Hum Mol Genet.* 2000; 9:1145.
29. Wan L, Dockendorff TC, Jongens TA, et al. Characterization of dFMR1, a *Drosophila melanogaster* homolog of the fragile X mental retardation protein. *Mol Cell Biol.* 2000; 20:8536.
30. Morales J, Hiesinger PR, Schroeder AJ, et al. Drosophila fragile X protein, DFXR, regulates neuronal morphology and function in the brain. *Neuron.* 2002; 34:961.
31. Doll CA, Broadie K. Activity-dependent FMRP requirements in development of the neural circuitry of learning and memory. *Development.* 2015; 142:1346.
32. Ashley CT Jr, Wilkinson KD, Reines D, et al. FMR1 protein: conserved RNP family domains and selective RNA binding. *Science.* 1993; 262:563.
33. Feng Y, Gutekunst CA, Eberhart DE, et al. Fragile X mental retardation protein: nucleocytoplasmic shuttling and association with somatodendritic ribosomes. *J Neurosci.* 1997; 17:1539.
34. Darnell JC, Klann E. The translation of translational control by FMRP: therapeutic targets for FXS. *Nat Neurosci.* 2013; 16:1530.
35. Bechara EG, Didiot MC, Melko M, et al. A novel function for fragile X mental retardation protein in translational activation. *PLoS Biol.* 2009; 7:e16.
36. Weng N, Weiler IJ, Sumis A, et al. Early-phase ERK activation as a biomarker for metabolic status in fragile X syndrome. *Am J Med Genet B Neuropsychiatr Genet.* 2008; 147B:1253.
37. Gross C, Nakamoto M, Yao X, et al. Excess phosphoinositide 3-kinase subunit synthesis and activity as a novel therapeutic target in fragile X syndrome. *J Neurosci.* 2010; 30:10624.
38. Huber KM, Gallagher SM, Warren ST, et al. Altered synaptic plasticity in a mouse model of fragile X mental retardation. *Proc Natl Acad Sci U S A.* 2002; 99:7746.
39. Cruz-Martin A, Crespo M, Portera-Cailliau C. Delayed stabilization of dendritic spines in fragile X mice. *J Neurosci.* 2010; 30:7793.
40. Irwin SA, Galvez R, Greenough WT. Dendritic spine structural anomalies in fragile-X mental retardation syndrome. *Cereb Cortex.* 2000; 10:1038.
41. Auerbach BD, Bear MF. Loss of the fragile X mental retardation protein decouples metabotropic glutamate receptor dependent priming of long-term potentiation from protein synthesis. *J Neurophysiol.* 2010; 104:1047.
42. Westmark CJ, Westmark PR, O'Riordan KJ, et al. Reversal of fragile X phenotypes by manipulation of AbetaPP/Abeta levels in Fmr1KO mice. *PLoS One.* 2011; 6:e26549.
43. Dziembowska M, Pretto DI, Janusz A, et al. High MMP-9 activity levels in fragile X syndrome are lowered by minocycline. *Am J Med Genet A.* 2013; 161A:1897.
44. Boda B, Mendez P, Boury-Jamot B, et al. Reversal of activity-mediated spine dynamics and learning impairment in a mouse model of Fragile X syndrome. *Eur J Neurosci.* 2014; 39:1130.
45. Bear MF, Huber KM, Warren ST. The mGluR theory of fragile X mental retardation. *Trends Neurosci.* 2004; 27:370.

# 57 Hyperuricemia (Lesch-Nyhan Disease)

WILLIAM NYHAN

Lesch-Nyhan disease is an inherited disorder of purine metabolism in which there is enormous overproduction of uric acid.[1,2] It is the most common cause of hyperuricemia that is understood at the molecular level. It is caused by deficient activity of the enzyme hypoxanthine guanine phosphoribosyltransferase (HPRT). Deficiency of HPRT leads to a variety of clinical phenotypes. These range in severity from the classic Lesch-Nyhan disease, in which neurological and behavioral features are seen along with clinical manifestations of hyperuricemia that are shared with patients with gout, to patients with normal neurology and behavior, who have only manifestations directly attributable to uric acid. Among patients with HPRT deficiency, the classic Lesch-Nyhan phenotype is the most common. The variant forms are all rare.

Lesch-Nyhan disease results from a virtually total lack of HPRT activity. It is an X-linked recessive disorder that was first described in 1964.[2] It is characterized by exuberant uric acid synthesis and resultant development of uric acid nephrolithiasis, gouty arthritis, and tophaceous deposits of sodium urate in cartilage. Patients have choreoathetosis, spasticity, and mental retardation, and they cannot walk. A compulsive pattern of self-mutilation involves biting of the fingers, lips, and buccal mucosa (Fig. 57–1). In variant patients with partial HPRT deficiency, the expected clinical picture is that of severe gouty arthritis or uric acid nephropathy without neurological or behavioral abnormalities.

## BIOCHEMICAL ABNORMALITIES

A virtually complete lack of HPRT is observed in the red blood cells (RBCs) and fibroblasts of patients with classic Lesch-Nyhan disease.[3] Distinction of patients with partial activity is best made by assay of the enzyme in intact fibroblasts.[4]

The hyperuricemia in patients with HPRT deficiency is a consequence of an increased rate of purine synthesis through the de novo pathway from small molecules. Megaloblastic changes in the bone marrow and RBCs may be seen in patients with Lesch-Nyhan disease. Low levels of folic acid in plasma have also been observed.[5,6] Problems with folic acid could occur because of an increased demand for the vitamin, which is a component of the cofactor in the two formylation steps of de novo purine biosynthesis.

The mechanism responsible for the neurological problems associated with Lesch-Nyhan disease is unclear. Hypoxanthine is found in the cerebral spinal fluid in amounts four times those seen in control individuals.[7] Neurotransmitters have been implicated in the neurological and behavioral features of the disease.[8,9] Dopaminergic function is altered in the basal ganglia, and there is a reduction in dopamine transporters.

## FACTORS TO BE CONSIDERED IN DIAGNOSTIC EVALUATION

The disease is essentially a disease of males, occurring in an estimated 1 in 100,000 male births. Transmission is through female carriers. The carrier state can be detected by assay of the enzyme in individual hair follicles, which are largely clonal.[10] Prenatal diagnosis of Lesch-Nyhan disease can be achieved by directly measuring HPRT levels in cells obtained from amniocentesis or chorionic villus sampling during the first months of pregnancy. The gene, which is on the long arm of the X chromosome at Xq26, has been cloned and sequenced, and a number of mutations hasbeen identified.[11,12] This is the best method for the determination of carrier status and for prenatal diagnosis.

The diagnosis usually is not made until the appearance of self-injurious behaviors, which may begin as early as the first year of life or as late as 17 years. The average age at onset of self-mutilation is 3.3 years, and the median is 2 years. Physical restraint and extraction of the teeth are the only measures available to prevent self-mutilation.

Most males with Lesch-Nyhan disease are mentally retarded (mean IQ, 71 ± 16), but some have normal intelligence. Performance on standardized intelligence tests is limited by dysarthria, choreoathetosis, and self-destructive behavior.

Patients produce and excrete large amounts of uric acid. The serum concentration ranges from 5 to 20 mg/dL. The excretion of uric acid is always greater than 1 mg per milligram of creatinine, whereas normal individuals never excrete this much except in early infancy. The increased quantity of urinary uric acid leads to uric acid crystal formation. Orange uric acid crystals in a diaper can be the first sign of the disorder. Untreated patients develop uric acid nephrolithiasis and urate nephropathy and die from renal failure. Variants with partial HPRT deficiency may also have uric acid nephrolithiasis and may develop gout.

## MANAGEMENT

The treatment of HPRT deficiency focuses on reducing the level of uric acid. Allopurinol inhibits xanthine oxidase and reduces the accumulation of uric acid in body fluids. The enzyme xanthine oxidase is responsible for the conversion of hypoxanthine to xanthine and of xanthine to uric acid, the end product of purine metabolism. Allopurinol administration prevents uric acid stone formation, urate nephropathy, gouty arthritis, and the development of tophi. An initial daily dose of 15 to 20 mg/kg[13] may be followed by monitoring of uric acid concentrations in blood until they fall to 3 mg/dL or lower. Thereafter, the formation of xanthine stones can be minimized by monitoring urinary levels of oxypurines to produce maximum levels of hypoxanthine. There is no effective therapy for the neurological and behavioral problems.

S-Adenosylmethionine has been employed as treatment,[14] with mixed results. A small number of patients have had marked improvement in self-injurious behavior, but a similar number experienced worsening of behavior, and most were not changed.

## NUTRITIONAL CARE

Nutritional care of patients with Lesch-Nyhan disease is a component of their overall therapeutic management.[15] It is important to assess the nutrition status of all patients with handicapping conditions. Longitudinal measurements of height and weight are used to document rates of growth. Measurements of height and weight in older patients may be complicated by their nonambulatory status, spasticity, contractures, or aggressive behavior. Arm circumference and skinfold measurements can supply useful information.

Clinical examination should be used to screen for overt physical signs of nutritional deficiencies. The nutritionist should review the

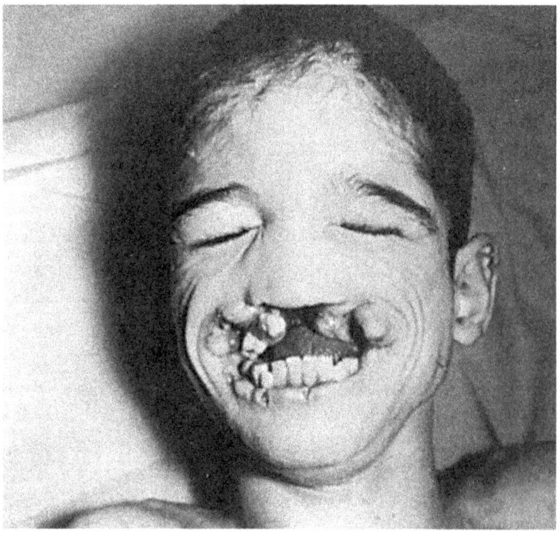

**Figure 57–1.** A 14-year-old boy illustrating an extreme degree of mutilation around the face. (From Nyhan WL, Sakati NO. *Diagnostic Recognition of Genetic Disease.* Philadelphia: Lea & Febiger; 1987. Used with permission.)

medical record to obtain information on anemia, recurrent infections, or allergies to food.

Laboratory assessment of nutrition status should be performed to determine the biochemical correlates. If undernutrition is suspected, plasma proteins should be measured. It may be helpful to measure plasma or RBC levels of folate, and RBCs should be examined for macrocytic changes, but it should be recognized that macrocytosis is the norm in this disease. An abnormal folate status could be caused by anticonvulsant drug therapy as well as an increased folic acid requirement for purine synthesis. Descriptive information about food intake, dietary patterns, feeding skills, and use of nutritional supplements are necessary to help the clinician develop a realistic nutritional care plan.

In the series reported by Christie et al.,[13] 58% of patients had feeding problems. Feeding skill development is delayed because of the motor defect and further hindered by the presence of arm restraints to prevent self-mutilation. Parents may spend large amounts of time feeding such a child. If teeth have been extracted to prevent self-injury, the texture of the food must be modified accordingly. In addition, most of these patients vomit frequently, some very frequently. Patients with partial HPRT deficiency do not have nutritional problems.

Various recommendations have been made regarding dietary management of Lesch-Nyhan disease. Some have asserted that growth retardation is a phenotypic manifestation of the disease,[15] but some patients with an otherwise complete syndrome have normal height and weight. Growth deficits appear to be secondary to energy intake that is not sufficient to the very large losses of purine and nitrogen in the urine. Dietary purines do not increase the level of uric acid found in the urine, nor does their restriction decrease the level. It appears prudent to recommend a high-protein, high-calorie diet. Fluid intake should be promoted to increase urinary volume and diminish the possibility of crystallization and stone formation. Folic acid supplementation, or at least the provision of folate-rich foods, also appears prudent.

## SUMMARY AND FOLLOW-UP

A nutritional care plan with follow-up should be an integral part of the individualized family service plan (ISFP) for boys Lesch-Nyhan disease according to the requirement of P.L. 99-457. As recommended by the American Public Health Association Maternal and Child Health Section's Committee on Children with Special Health Care Needs, respite care should also be a part of the ISFP to periodically relieve parents of the responsibilities of continuous supervision, care, and feeding of children with this disease.[16]

### References

1. Nyhan WL, Al-Aqeel AI, Barshop BA. *Atlas of Inherited Metabolic Diseases*, 3rd ed. London: Hodder Arnold; 2012.
2. Lesch M, Nyhan WL. A familial disorder of uric acid metabolism and central nervous system function. *Am J Med.* 1964; 36:561.
3. Seegmiller JE, Rosenbloom FM, Kelley WN. Enzyme defect associated with sex-linked human neurological disorder and excessive purine synthesis. *Science.* 1967; 155:1682.
4. Page T, Bakay B, Nissinen E, Nyhan WL. Hypoxanthine-guanine phosphoribosyltransferase variants: correlation of clinical phenotype with enzyme activity. *J Inherit Metab Dis.* 1981; 4:203.
5. Van Der Zee SPM, Schretlen EDAM, Monnens LAH. Megaloblastic anemia in the Lesch-Nyhan syndrome. *Lancet.* 1968; 1:1427.
6. Hernandez-Nieto L, Brito-Barraso MC, Nyhan WL. Megaloblastic anemia in Lesch-Nyhan syndrome. *Sangre.* 1988; 29:175.
7. Sweetman L. Urinary and cerebrospinal oxypurine levels and allopurinol metabolism in the Lesch-Nyhan syndrome. *Fed Proc.* 1968; 27:1055.
8. Lloyd KG, Hornykewicz OI, Davidson L, et al. Biochemical evidence of dysfunction of brain neurotransmitters in the Lesch-Nyhan syndrome. *N Engl J Med.* 1981; 305:1106.
9. Nyhan WL, Wong DF. New approaches to understanding Lesch-Nyhan disease [editorial]. *N Engl J Med.* 1996; 334:1602.
10. Page T, Bakay B, Nyhan WL. An improved procedure for the detection of hypoxanthine-guanine phosphoribosyl transferase heterozygotes. *Clin Chem.* 1982; 28:1181.
11. Jinnah HA, De Gregorio L, Harris JC, Nyhan WL, O'Neill JP. The spectrum of inherited mutations causing HPRT deficiency: 75 new cases and a review of 196 previously reported cases. *Mutat Res.* 2000; 463:309.
12. Jinnah HA, Ceballos-Picot I, Torres RJ, et al. Attenuated variants of Lesch-Nyhan disease. *Brain.* 2010; 133:671.
13. Christie R, Bay C, Kaufman I, Bakay B, Borden M, Nyhan WL. Lesch-Nyhan disease: clinical experience with nineteen patients. *Dev Med Child Neurol.* 1982; 24:293.
14. Dolcetta D, Parmigiani P, Salmaso L, et al. Quantitative evaluation of the clinical effects of S-adenosylmethionine on mood and behavior in Lesch-Nyhan patients. Nucleosides Nucleotides Nucleic Acids. 20131 32:174.
15. Thompson G, Pacy P, Watts W, Hallidy D. Protein metabolism in phenylketonuria and Lesch-Nyhan syndrome. *Pediatr Res.* 1990; 28:240.
16. American Public Health Association, Maternal and Child Health Section. *Committee Statement on Children with Special Health Care Needs.* Washington, DC: American Public Health Association; 1989.

# 58 Williams Syndrome

SHIRLEY W. EKVALL AND FLORENCE STEVENS

Williams syndrome (WS) is a neurodevelopmental disorder also known as Williams-Beuren syndrome. The complex condition involves multiple organ systems, unique personality characteristics, distinctive facial features, elastin arteriopathy, cognitive impairment (usually mild mental retardation), connective tissue abnormalities, and endocrine growth abnormalities.[1] More than 99% of individuals with a clinical diagnosis of WS have a 1.6-Mb deletion of chromosome 7q11.23 that contains the 20 contiguous genes of the critical region for WS encompassing the *elastin (ELN)* gene.[2,3] The clinical diagnostic technique is known as fluorescent in situ hybridization (FISH) confirms the diagnosis in 98% of individuals. Cardiovascular problems may be aortic and pulmonary. The prevalence of WS in Norway was reported to be 1 in 7500 births.[4]

Clinically, the pregnancy is usually described as normal, but the infants are often post term, and birth weight is low compared with the family background. At birth, an unusual facial appearance may be noted. Feeding difficulties occur early, related to hypotonia and abnormal coordination of sucking and swallowing. Vomiting due to gastroesophageal reflux is frequent, with subsequent failure to gain weight. Textural aversion often follows. Occasionally, a high serum calcium level is documented during this period. Many of the infants are described as extremely irritable and refusing to eat. Constipation is frequent, and hernias— umbilical, inguinal, and epigastric—are not uncommon. As time progresses, the feeding difficulties and failure to thrive lessen, but there are delays in motor, mental, and language development and motor coordination.[5]

Physical characteristics include microcephaly with bitemporal narrowing, a flat nasal bridge, anteverted nares, full cheeks (particularly in the lower portion), a long philtrum, full lips with frequent sagging of the lower lip, epicanthic folds, periorbital fullness, stellate irides, strabismus, micrognathia, dental malocclusion, and prominent ear lobules. As the children grow, their body build may also be quite characteristic. Many of the children continue to be small and thin. The neck and torso may be long, and pectus excavatum occurs frequently. The shoulders tend to be narrow and sloping. Clinodactyly of the fifth fingers, hallux valgus, and abnormal palmar creases may be seen. The teeth may be small, irregularly spaced, and with enamel hypoplasia and bite abnormalities (Fig. 58–1). Individuals with WS are shorter than other family members, and puberty occurs early in about 50% of affected girls.[6]

Elastic arteriopathy occurs in 75% of patients. The most frequently encountered arteriopathy is supravalvular aortic stenosis (SVAS), but there may be other associated lesions, such as pulmonary artery stenosis, aortic hypoplasia, and septal defects. Narrowing of other vessels may be seen, and systemic hypertension, at times secondary to renal artery stenosis, often is present.[7] Renal anomalies have been described, as have urinary bladder diverticula. The deep tendon reflexes are characteristically hyperactive. Hypotonia may be present, particularly during infancy[8] and childhood. Decreased flexion in the ankle joints and limitation of joint movements may occur. Some older individuals become obese and diabetic.[9]

Seventy-five percent of individuals with WS are mildly retarded (IQ, 50 to 80),[10] with poor visuomotor coordination,[11] myopia, and strabismus in 50% Other features include chronic otitis media[12] and particular strength in vocabulary and language.[13] Socially, most patients are outgoing, friendly, and very talkative.[14] However, some show behavior problems,[15] becoming easily upset, stubborn, anxious, and hyperactive.

## BIOCHEMICAL ABNORMALITIES

Idiopathic hypercalcemia is found in about 15% and hypercalciuria in 30% of children with WS. This appears to be present only during the first few months of life, and unless the diagnosis of WS is made during this period, in most cases it cannot be documented later. The vomiting, constipation, irritability, and failure to thrive seen in about 70% of infants with WS may be related to hypercalcemia, but not all children with these symptoms have a high serum calcium level. Congenital heart disease is present at the first pediatric appointment.

The etiology of the hypercalcemia and its relation to vitamin D are not yet understood, despite numerous clinical and animal studies.[16] Vitamin D has three classic forms. The dietary form and the form produced in the skin, calciferol, are converted in the liver to 25-hydroxycholecalciferol. This form is converted in the kidneys to the very potent 1,25-dihydroxycholecalciferol, which maintains the serum calcium level through absorption from the intestine. Some authors think that there may be hypersensitivity to vitamin D in the infant or in the pregnant mother. How this possible hypersensitivity affects the vitamin D regulation of calcium metabolism is unknown. Another hypothesis involves a possible disturbance in the homeostasis of calcium in utero according to Friedman and Mills.[17]

Calcitonin has been implicated as a possible cause of the hypercalcemia. Calcitonin, a hormone produced by the parafollicular cells of the thyroid gland, helps clear calcium from blood. Culler et al.[18] studied the effects of provocative infusions of calcium and parathyroid hormone in five children with WS and found delayed clearance of calcium after intravenous calcium loading. They concluded that individuals with WS may have a defect in the synthesis or release of calcitonin.

## FACTORS TO BE CONSIDERED IN NUTRITION EVALUATION

Not all children with WS have a history of feeding problems, vomiting, and failure to thrive. However, these difficulties, together with the extreme irritability, are the main causes of morbidity during the first year of life. Even later, some of the children tend to be "picky eaters."

Therapy must be directed toward the feeding difficulties, failure to thrive, hypercalcemia, constipation, obesity, and diabetes in later years. Growth in height is less than the 3rd percentile in the adult years.

## DIETARY AND OTHER MANAGEMENT

Providing dietary advice during infancy is very important to ensure that the infant receives adequate amounts of calories, fluid, and nutrients for growth and to compensate for the vomiting. In severe cases of vomiting, nasogastric or gastrointestinal tube supplementation may be provided during the night. Offering reassurance to parents is essential during this period. The infants are very difficult to feed, and the mothers frequently feel guilty and sometimes are made to feel responsible for their infant's failure to thrive, particularly in undiagnosed cases.

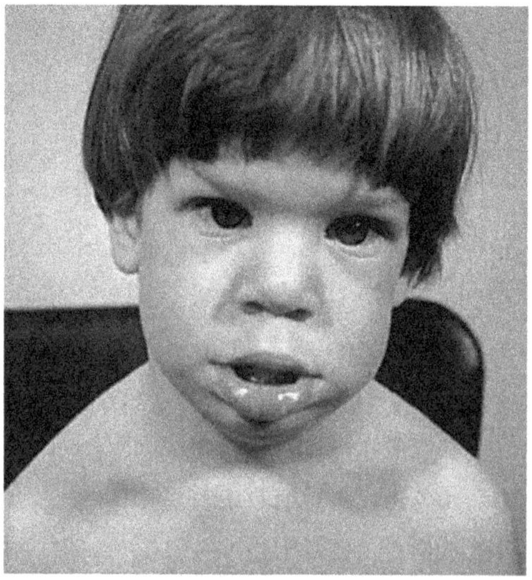

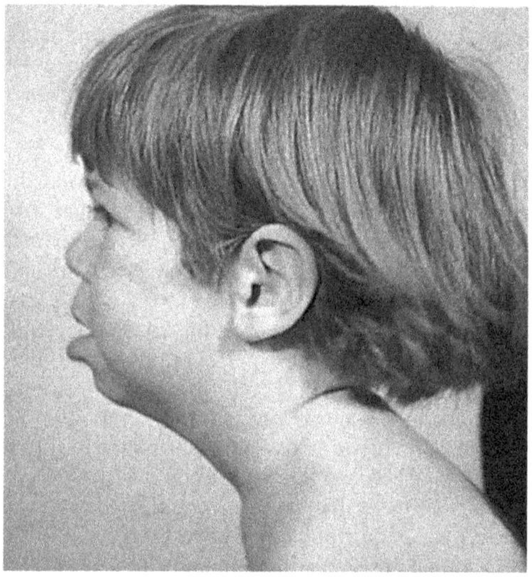

**Figure 58–1.** Front view and profile of 1-year-old child with Williams syndrome. (Courtesy of Cincinnati Children's Hospital Medical Center, Division of Developmental Disabilities.)

Some researchers think that the irritability, feeding difficulties, vomiting, and constipation occur primarily in children whose calcium level is higher than normal. Therefore, lowering the calcium level may result in an improvement in symptomatology. Martin et al.[19] investigated plasma calcium levels in children with profuse vomiting and failure to thrive in association with a heart murmur. In their survey, children were treated with a low-calcium, vitamin D–restricted diet. Some received a course of corticosteroids for 1 to 4 weeks. Noted adverse effects were hypocalcemia in 21% and iatrogenic rickets in 9%. Even on the diet, feeding problems continued, but there was some lessening of vomiting and slow weight gain. The authors advised that the therapy should be continued for no longer than 6 to 12 months. The Calcilo XD low-calcium/vitamin D infant formula may be used; however, the infant should be observed for the development of rickets. Later, a low-calcium, low–vitamin D diet may be needed. It is essential that dietary restriction of calcium and vitamin D be carefully monitored by a nutrition professional.

Constipation is seen frequently in children and adults with WS. In infants, it is believed to be related to hypercalcemia and hypotonia. A diet high in fiber and fluid probably is useful in the older child. Foods high in fiber, such as fruits, vegetables, and whole-grain cereals and breads, with adequate water, are recommended (see Chapter 36). Regular exercise should be encouraged. Obesity and diabetes should be monitored if they occur in adolescents or adults. Hypertension should be addressed with a low-sodium diet.,

Other evaluations as recommended by Morris et al.,[9,20–22] by the American Academy of Pediatrics,[23] and in our own practice, include the following:

1. A complete physical and neurological examination, plotting growth parameters on WS growth charts and typical growth charts from the Centers for Disease Control and Prevention (CDC) (see Appendix 2)
2. Evaluation by a cardiologist, including blood pressure measurements and an echocardiogram, with Doppler flow studies
3. Urinary system evaluation with urinalysis, ultrasound examination of the bladder and kidneys, and serum measurements of blood urea nitrogen and creatinine
4. Calcium status including serum concentration of calcium or ionized calcium, and calcium and creatinine determinations on a spot urine sample
5. Thyroid function tests
6. Ophthalmological evaluation
7. Genetic evaluation or consultation for individualized assessment and recommendations and discussion of clinical manifestations, natural history, and recurrence risks
8. Multidisciplinary developmental evaluation, including assessment of motor, speech, language, personal-social, general cognitive, and vocational skills and dietary management.

## FOLLOW-UP

Although most children with WS are thin or have normal weight, some tend to become obese during adolescence. Usually, children with WS should be under dietary supervision because of failure to thrive in infancy and to prevent obesity and diabetes in adolescence and adulthood (see Chapter 48). Anthropometric measurements, dietary history (particularly related to adequate growth and fiber and fluid intake), feeding history, and appropriate serum levels should be determined at each clinic visit. Growth should be plotted on WS and CDC growth charts during each visit. Genetic counseling and prenatal testing should be available to the family.

### References

1. Morris CA, Mervis CB. Williams syndrome and related disorders. *Annu Rev Genom Hum Genet.* 2000; 1:461.
2. Osborne LR, Li M, Pober B, et al. A 1.5 million base pair inversion polymorphism in families with Williams-Beuren syndrome. *Nat Genet.* 2001; 29:321.
3. Ewart AK, Morris CA, Atkinson D, et al. Hemizygosity at the elastin locus in a development disorder, Williams syndrome. *Nat Genet.* 1993; 5:11.
4. Stromme P, Bjornstad PG, Ramstad K. Prevalence estimation of Williams syndrome. *J Child Neurol.* 2002; 17:269.
5. Udwin O. A survey of adults with Williams syndrome and idiopathic infantile hypercalcemia. *Dev Med Child Neurol.* 1990; 32:129.
6. Partsch CJ, Japing I, Siebert R, et al. Central precocious puberty in girls with Williams syndrome. *J Pediatr.* 2002; 141:441.
7. Eronen M, Peippo M, Hiippala A, et al. Cardiovascular manifestations in 75 patients with Williams syndrome. *J Med Genet.* 2002; 39:554.
8. Kaplan P, Kirschner M, Watters G, Costa MT. Contractures in patients with Williams syndrome. *Pediatrics.* 1989; 84:895.
9. Morris CA, Demsey SA, Leonard CO, Dilts C, Blackburn BL. Natural history of Williams syndrome: physical characteristics. *J Pediatr.* 1988; 113:318.
10. Mervis CB, Morris CA, Bertrand J, et al. Williams syndrome: findings from an integrated program of research. In: Tager-Flusberg H, ed. *Neurodevelopmental Disorders.* Cambridge, MA: MIT Press; 1998.
11. Kapp ME, von Noorden GK, Jenkins R. Strabismus in Williams syndrome. *Am J Ophthalmol.* 1995; 119:355.
12. Van Borsel J, Curfs LM, Fryns JP. Hyperacusis in Williams syndrome: a sample survey study. *Genet Couns.* 1997; 8:121.
13. Cassidy SB, Morris CA. Behavioral phenotypes in genetic syndromes: genetic clues to human behavior. *Adv Pediatr.* 2002; 49:59.
14. Einfeld SL, Tonge BJ, Rees VW. Longitudinal course of behavioral and emotional problems in Williams syndrome. *Am J Ment Retard.* 2001; 106:73.
15. Gosch A, Pankau R. Social-emotional and behavioral adjustment in children with Williams-Beuren syndrome. *Am J Med Genet.* 1994; 53:335.
16. Kruse K, Pankau R, Gosch A, Wohlfahrt K. Calcium metabolism in Williams-Beuren syndrome. *J Speech Hear Disord.* 1992; 55:339.
17. Friedman WF, Mills LF. The relationship between vitamin D and the craniofacial dental anomalies of the supravalvular aortic stenosis syndrome. *Pediatrics.* 1969; 43:12.

18. Culler FL, Jones KJ, Deftos LN. Impaired calcitonin secretion in patients with Williams syndrome. *J Pediatr*. 1985; 107:720.
19. Martin ND, Snodgrass GJAI, Cohen RD. Idiopathic infantile hypercalcemia—a continuing enigma. *Arch Dis Child*. 1984; 59:605.
20. Martens M, Wilson SJ, Reutens DC. Research review: Williams syndrome: a critical review of the cognitive, behavioral and neuroanatomical phenotype. *J Child Psychol Psychiatry*. 2008; 49:576.
21. Cassidy SB, Allanson JE. *Management of Genetic Syndromes*. Hoboken, NJ: John Wiley & Sons; 2010.
22. Morris CA, Pober B, Wang P, Levinson M. *Medical Guidelines for Williams Syndrome*. Glawson, MI: Williams Syndrome Association; 1999.
23. American Academy of Pediatrics. Health care supervision for children with Williams syndrome. *Pediatrics*. 2002; 109:329.

# 59 Wilson Disease

FLORENCE STEVENS AND SHIRLEY W. EKVALL

In Wilson disease (WD), copper is deposited in the liver, brain, kidney, and cornea instead of forming ceruloplasmin. Copper is an essential nutrient in promoting the formation of ceruloplasmin in the liver, but chronic copper poisoning occurs with hepatolenticular degeneration.[1] The worldwide prevalence of WD is 1:30,000. This figure is higher in specific subgroups with consanguinity.[2] The gene for WD, located on the long arm of chromosome 13 (13q14), is called *ATP7B* and has a variety of mutations.[3] Affected children are identified between age 6 years and the early teens (50% before the 15 years of age). The disease onset for adults is neurological or psychiatric and occurs between the second and fourth decades of life.[4] Lack of treatment results in death by age 30.[5] The disease requires lifelong treatment.

Poor school performance may signal WD in children. A decline in school performance is accompanied by decreased coordination and fine motor ability, increased behavioral problems, decreased mental function, difficulty speaking and poor articulation, rigidity, dysphagia, deterioration in self-help skills, or spasticity. The psychiatric manifestations may include depression and schizophrenia-like symptoms. In the advanced stage of WD, cirrhosis of the liver, a Kayser-Fleischer ring in the cornea, choreoathetosis, dystonia, reduced serum ceruloplasmin, increased copper excretion, increased liver copper content, tremor, and an open-mouth grimace may occur.[6] Pancreatitis also may be associated with WD. If left untreated, WD may cause liver disease, central nervous system dysfunction, and death.

## BIOCHEMICAL ABNORMALITIES

The diagnosis is confirmed by measurements of copper in the blood, urine, and liver. As toxicity progresses, liver cells are destroyed and replaced by fibrous tissue. In liver biopsy specimens, the hepatic copper level is greater than 110 μg/g of dry weight. A renal Fanconi syndrome manifests with generalized aminoaciduria and increased glucose, uric acid, calcium, and phosphate in urine.[7] Heterozygous carriers have decreased ceruloplasmin and increased liver copper levels even though they are symptom-free. Although the patient may have no complaints, he or she may exhibit hepatomegaly or splenomegaly with mild to moderate elevations of aminotransferases.

Zinc acetate (Galvin) is given at younger ages. When treatment with D-penicillamine, a chelating agent that increases the urinary excretion of copper, is begun, activities of daily living decrease before improvement is seen. The chelator trientine dihydrochloride has been effective in cases of penicillamine-induced neutropenia, thrombocytopenia, systemic lupus erythematosus, and nephrosis in patients allergic to penicillamine. Seizures have occurred in a minority of patients using drug therapy.

Zinc acetate is an effective, nontoxic therapy for WD. In an animal model, excess dietary histidine reduced excess accumulation of liver copper and serum alanine aminotransferase levels.[8] Without drug intervention, the toxic effects of copper accumulation increase. After 2 years of treatment with chelation therapy, any symptoms that remain are permanent, and other therapeutic interventions are needed. Noncompliance produces devastating results. Liver transplantation may be the only option when liver failure occurs. Before transplantation, neurological and psychological evaluation is necessary.

## FACTORS TO BE CONSIDERED IN NUTRITION EVALUATION

Dietary restriction of foods high in copper is needed if pharmacotherapy is not enough to remedy WD. Dietary supplementation of zinc and vitamin $B_6$ is required. Patients should avoid foods that are high in copper, such as liver, organ meats, shellfish, nuts, mushrooms, chocolate, blackstrap molasses, and whole-grain cereals. Foods with a low copper content include milk and milk products, tofu, soy chicken, tomatoes, scallops, most fresh fruits, leafy vegetables, corn, and potatoes (Table 59–1).[9–11]

The nutrition status directs the development of an individualized nutritional care plan. Feeding problems need to be identified. Obesity may be a factor if mobility is limited. Underweight may indicate insufficient fluid and food consumption, requiring a fluid and food intake assessment. Motor coordination and swallowing problems make self-feeding and normal mastication of food difficult. Requirements for adaptive equipment and alterations in food textures and calories are required in advanced stages or during relapse.

Penicillamine-nutrient interactions increase excretion of zinc, iron, copper, manganese, and pyridoxine, which can cause anemias, iron deficiency, drug-induced peripheral neuropathy, and reduced white blood cell and platelet counts. Other side effects include an unpleasant taste, decreased sensation of taste for salt and sweet products, and anorexia, perhaps due to lowered zinc levels.[12]

Patients with neurological disease often worsen initially on penicillamine. Zinc acetate blocks copper absorption and acts more slowly than penicillamine. In patients without neurological disease, a period of treatment is required to induce intestinal cell production of metallothionein, a metal-binding protein with antioxidant properties. This protein interacts with copper with high affinity and prevents its serosal transfer. It is excellent for maintenance therapy and for treatment of the presymptomatic patient.

When the disease progresses, the decreased ability to perform daily functions is a result of copper intoxication. The rate of progression varies for each individual. Biochemical information is diagnostic. A 24-hour dietary recall and food frequency crosscheck should be undertaken to evaluate the copper, calorie, and protein contents of the diet.

Copper plumbing and copper cooking utensils contribute to copper ingestion. If household water contains more than 0.1 mg/L of copper, distilled water or bottled demineralized water should be used. Copper cooking utensils should not be used because copper can leach into food during cooking. Alcohol should be avoided because the liver may already be damaged from WD. A fluid intake assessment may be required.

## DIETARY MANAGEMENT

Major goals of therapy for WD are to inhibit the absorption of copper from the intestinal tract, remove copper from tissues, and prevent its reaccumulation with drug chelation. It is necessary to maintain normal levels of copper for copper balance, to prevent pyridoxine deficiency, and to provide sufficient zinc to chelate excess copper (under a physician's supervision). A lacto-ovo vegetarian diet may be useful to increase the intake of fiber and phytates and decrease copper intake. It is also important to monitor caloric intake, eating and feeding

**Table 59–1.** Copper Content of Foods

| Food | Copper Content (mg/100 g) | Food | Copper Content (mg/100 g) | Food | Copper Content (mg/100 g) |
|---|---|---|---|---|---|
| *Foods High in Copper (>1 mg/100 g)* | | | | | |
| Beef liver | 2.80 | Molasses | 1.42 | High-protein baby cereal | 1.20 |
| Calves' liver | 7.90 | Crab, canned, all varieties | 1.52 | Sunflower seeds | 1.77 |
| Oysters, all varieties | 17.14 | Lobster | 1.69 | Wheat germ | 2.39 |
| *Foods Intermediate in Copper (0.05 to 1.0 mg/100 g)* | | | | | |
| Meat, Fish, and Eggs | | Vegetables and Vegetable Products | | Nuts and Nut Products | |
| Chicken breasts, fried | 0.05 | Tomato sauce | 0.10 | Peanut butter, creamy | 0.61 |
| Tuna | 0.05 | Onion rings, breaded | 0.10 | Walnuts* | 0.66 |
| Bologna | 0.06 | Peas | 0.10 | Peanuts, dry roasted | 0.67 |
| Eggs, soft | 0.06 | Spaghetti sauce* | 0.11 | | |
| Fish sticks | 0.07 | Onion soup* | 0.13 | Legumes | |
| Beef, ground | 0.08 | French fries, commercial | 0.14 | Soy beans* | 0.10 |
| Pork cured, ham | 0.09 | Mushrooms, dry* | 0.22 | Red beans and rice* | 0.13 |
| Soy beef* | 0.10 | Mushrooms, canned* | 0.24 | Cowpeas | 0.27 |
| Veal cutlet | 0.10 | Mushrooms | 0.26 | Navy beans | 0.28 |
| Shrimp* | 0.17 | Potato chips, commercial | 0.35 | | |
| Pork chop | 0.19 | | | Desserts | |
| Mussels* | 0.47 | Fruits and Dried Fruit | | Candy bar* | 0.13 |
| Clams* | 0.60 | Avocado | 0.19 | Ice cream, chocolate | 0.14 |
| Crab* | 0.74 | Dried apple* | 0.19 | Chocolate cake | 0.23 |
| | | Dates* | 0.29 | Chocolate chip cookies | 0.23 |
| Grains and Grain Products | | Prunes | 0.29 | Chocolate cookies | 0.32 |
| Pancakes | 0.07 | Figs* | 0.31 | Milk chocolate | 0.45 |
| Macaroni | 0.08 | Raisins | 0.31 | Cocoa | 0.76 |
| Whole-wheat bread | 0.25 | Dried apricot* | 0.34 | | |
| Granola | 0.34 | Dried peach* | 0.36 | Miscellaneous | |
| Shredded Wheat cereal | 0.47 | Dried pear* | 0.37 | Super Mac* hamburger | 0.08 |
| Raisin Bran cereal | 0.48 | Mixed fruit* | 0.39 | Hash* | 0.12 |
| | | | | Tofu patties* | 0.16 |
| *Foods Low in Copper (<0.05 mg/100 g)* | | | | | |
| Milk and Milk Products | | Fruits | | Meat, Fish, and Eggs | |
| Whole milk | 0.003 | Apple juice, canned | 0.01 | Beef broth* | 0.00 |
| Yogurt | 0.004 | Applesauce* | 0.01 | Scallops* | 0.02 |
| Cheddar cheese* | 0.04 | Apples, raw | 0.02 | Chicken* | 0.03 |
| Soft cheese* | 0.04 | Orange juice, frozen, reconstituted | 0.02 | | |
| Cheese, American | 0.05 | Watermelon | 0.02 | Miscellaneous | |
| | | Orange, raw | 0.04 | Chili (vegetable)* | 0.001 |
| Beverages | | | | Tofu* | 0.02 |
| Coffee | 0.001 | Vegetables | | Soy chicken* | 0.02 |
| Tea | 0.006 | Coleslaw | 0.02 | Tetrazini* | 0.05 |
| | | Lettuce, raw | 0.03 | | |
| | | Corn, boiled, fresh | 0.04 | | |
| | | Tomato | 0.05 | | |
| | | Potatoes, mashed | 0.05 | | |

* Data from Brewer G. Copper content of various foods as measured by a laboratory by atomic absorption spectrometry. *Medicine (Baltimore)*. 1992; 71:139.
Adapted from Pennington JAT. *Bowes and Church's Food Values of Portions Commonly Used*, 17th ed. Philadelphia: Lippincott; 2009; Pennington JAT. Intakes of minerals from diet and foods: is there a need for concern? *J Nutr.* 1996; 126(Suppl):2304S.

problems, changes in the gag reflex or dysphagia, constipation, and diarrhea. Dietary intake of copper should be less than 1 mg/day.[13]

## PENICILLAMINE

Penicillamine (Cuprimine), a chelating agent that mobilizes copper from tissues and promotes its excretion, is taken 2 hours before or after meals. Potassium sulfide supplements are given during meals to absorb dietary copper and prevent its absorption in the intestinal tract. A daily pyridoxine supplement (25 mg) is necessary to prevent pyridoxine deficiency as a result of penicillamine administration. If penicillamine is not tolerated, trientine hydrochloride (Syprine) is used to increase the urinary excretion of copper. Ammonium tetrathiomolybdate has been used successfully as an initial therapy when acute neurological symptoms of WD are presented.

Pediatric patients have been treated with oral zinc and have maintained a negative or zero copper balance with no side effects or complications. Oral zinc given every 4 hours during the day and at bedtime, or zinc sulfate given three times a day, may be used as adjunctive therapy. Zinc supplementation prevents zinc deficiency caused by the chelation therapy required. Zinc acetate used alone controls the abnormal positive copper balance, blocks the uptake of orally administered copper, controls urine and plasma copper, prevents the reaccumulation of hepatic copper, and prevents the development or progression of copper toxicity in WD. If the patient is unresponsive to other therapies, dimercaptopropanol or British anti-Lewisite (BAL) may be administered by injection.

Zinc therapy is preferred in women and children because of its limited side effects. Zinc is taken 1 hour before or 2 hours after meals. The initial side effect is abdominal discomfort. Zinc acetate nutritional supplements are not bioequivalent to prescribed zinc acetate and may be ineffective.[14] Zinc intake should be decreased before and after surgical procedures. As with any medicattion, precautions are needed during pregnancy to prevent fetal toxicity. Zinc therapy for WD needs to be maintained during pregnancy, but it should be reduced to 0.5 to 0.75 g/day during the last trimester. Successful pregnancies have occurred in women taking this medication.

Foods with low levels of copper and limited amounts of food with moderate levels of copper may be consumed (see Table 59–1). In general, organ meats (e.g., liver, kidney), shellfish (e.g., oysters, lobster), nuts, mushrooms, seeds, chocolate, and dried fruits should be avoided. The copper in vegetarian diets is about 25% less bioavailable than the copper in diets that include animal products. Two patients who were noncompliant with anticopper therapy achieved adequate copper control on a vegetarian diet.[14]

With school-age children, it is important to maintain a low-copper diet and adequate fluid intake at school. Except for chocolate products, most foods that have moderate to high amounts of copper are not available on school menus. Food textures and calories require monitoring to ensure adequate intake. The school should be advised of the need for dietary therapy and the necessity of rigid compliance with the medication and mealtime sequence.

## SUMMARY AND FOLLOW-UP

Medical checkups should include nutritional care. Height, weight, skinfold measurements, and head circumference measurements (if the child is younger than 3 years of age), along with biochemical profiles, are required for children every 3 months. A 24-hour recall and a food frequency cross-check or 3-day diet diary should be used to evaluate dietary copper, zinc, pyridoxine, calories, and protein. Supplements should be added when required (multivitamin preparations must be copper-free). Management of foods and medication to be consumed in the school setting is essential. Fluid intake affects the dosage of Cuprimine. The child should drink a lot of fluids during the day, as well as at least 1 pint of fluid before bedtime and 1 pint during the night. Feeding skills are related to progression of the disease and wrequire continuous reevaluation. Although many skills deteriorate with the onset of WD, they can be improved with a variety of interventions provided by the multidisciplinary team. Most individuals with WD can live a normal lifespan.

Several approaches are required if the child has difficulty in swallowing or chewing, a decreased gag reflex, drooling, spasticity, tremors, or anorexia. One should provide foods of appropriate texture, offer milkshakes (low in copper, high in calories), check the gag reflex and swallowing ability before feeding, massage the face and neck muscles before offering foods, place the individual in an upright position during meals, feed slowly, and take weekly calorie counts and weights. For constipation and drooling, one should increase fluids, fiber, and phytates (see Chapter 36). Adaptive equipment should be provided whenever necessary to enhance self-feeding skills (see Chapter 24). These approaches should offer strategies for coping with WD. Clients who have muscle spasms and neurological symptoms may benefit from other medications such as levodopa, clonazepam, and tizanidine.

### References


1. Gitlin N. Wilson's disease: the scourge of copper. *J Hepatol.* 1998; 28:734.
2. Sternlieb I. Wilson's disease. *Clin Liver Dis.* 2000; 4:229.
3. Linder MC. The relationship of copper to DNA damage and damage prevention in humans. *Mutat Res* 2012; 733:83.
4. Sian J, Youdim MBH, Riederer P, Gerlach M. Hepatolenticular degeneration: Wilson's disease. In: Siegel GJ, Agranoff BW, Albers RW, Fisher SK, Uhler MD, eds. *Basic Neurochemistry: Molecular, Cellular and Medical Aspects. Part Six: Inherited and Neurodegenerative Diseases.* New York: Lippincott Williams & Wilkins; 1999.
5. Schilsky ML. Diagnosis and treatment of Wilson's disease. *Pediatr Transplant.* 2002; 6:15.
6. Ferenci P, Caca K, Loudianos G, et al. Diagnosis and phenotypic classification of Wilson's disease. *Liver Int.* 2003; 3:139.
7. Collins JC, Scheinberg IH, Giblin DR, Sternlieb I. Hepatic peroxisomal abnormalities in abetalipoproteinemia. *Gastroenterology.* 1989; 3:766.
8. Xu H, Sakakibara S, Morifuji M, Salamatulla Q, Aoyama Y. Excess dietary histidine decreases the liver copper level and serum alanine aminotransferase activity in Long-Evans cinnamon rats. [abstract] *Br J Nutr.* 2003; 90:593.
9. Pennington JAT. *Bowes and Church's Food Values of Portions Commonly Used*, 17th ed. Philadelphia: Lippincott; 2009.
10. Pennington JAT. Intakes of minerals from diet and foods: is there a need for concern? *J Nutr* 1996; 126(Suppl):2304S.
11. Brewer G. Copper content of various foods as measured by a laboratory by atomic absorption spectrometry. *Medicine (Baltimore).* 1992; 71:139.
12. *Physicians Desk Reference.* Oradell, NJ: Medical Economics; 2002.
13. Escott-Stump S, ed. *Nutrition and Diagnosis-Related Care*, 8th ed. Philadelphia: Williams & Wilkins; 2015.
14. Selimoglu MA, Ertekin V, Doneray H, Yildirim M. Bone mineral density of children with Wilson disease: efficacy of penicillamine and zinc therapy. *J Clin Gastroenterology*, 2008: 42:194.

# 60 Nutritional Aspects of Birth Defects

HOWARD M. SAAL

A birth defect is any anomaly, functional or structural, that manifests in infancy or later in life and is caused by events preceding birth, whether inherited or acquired.[1] Birth defects are a major cause of pediatric hospitalizations and infant mortality.[2] Birth defects are responsible for 20% of infant deaths[3] (Table 60–1). Between 3% and 5% of all children, or approximately 3.3 million children worldwide, are born with a medically significant birth defect every year.[4–6] Although several state programs exist for surveillance of birth defects in the United States, there are challenges with case ascertainment.[7]

Many causes of birth defects have been identified, the most common being single-gene disorders, chromosome disorders, environmental and teratogenic conditions, and multifactorial malformations or defects of unknown cause (Fig. 60–1). Mendelian (single-gene) disorders make up approximately 20% of all birth defects and include autosomal dominant, autosomal recessive, and X-linked disorders. Approximately 19,000 human genes encode proteins.[8] More than 7000 mendelian disorders have been described, many of which are common, such as cystic fibrosis (autosomal recessive), sickle cell disease (autosomal recessive), neurofibromatosis (autosomal dominant), and fragile X syndrome (X-linked). Because these disorders are inherited, their occurrence is dependent on the parents' carrier status. Autosomal dominant conditions have a 50% recurrence risk, and autosomal recessive and X-linked recessive disorders have a 25% recurrence risk.[7] Many autosomal dominant disorders have a high spontaneous mutation rate; in neurofibromatosis type 1, for example, approximately half of affected individuals have no prior family history. Because single-gene disorders have a specific genetic cause, maternal nutritional issues play a limited role in their occurrence and expression.

Chromosome disorders account for approximately 10% of birth defects. Most chromosome disorders are sporadic, although a small number arise from familial reciprocal chromosome translocations. The most common chromosome disorders are Down syndrome (i.e., trisomy 21), Turner syndrome (45,X), and Klinefelter syndrome (47,XXY). Trisomy 13 and trisomy 18 are much less common but well-recognized lethal chromosomal disorders.[7] As in mendelian disorders, the etiology of chromosome disorders is not related to any known nutritional concerns.

## PHYSICAL, BIOCHEMICAL, AND OTHER ABNORMALITIES

Approximately 5% of birth defects are caused by teratogens. These environmental exposures are often unintended; however, numerous licit and illicit exposures have been documented. Probably the best studied and best documented teratogen is alcohol. Significant prenatal alcohol exposure has been estimated to affect 1 in 500 live births, but the incidence may be higher in certain communities.[9] The effects of are highly variable, with the most severe presentation being fetal alcohol syndrome, characterized by intrauterine growth retardation, facial dysmorphism, microcephaly, and numerous congenital anomalies including congenital heart defects, limb anomalies, brain anomalies, hearing loss, and renal anomalies. Intellectual disability and behavior problems are seen in most cases. Milder presentations are also seen, usually including developmental disabilities and behavior disorders.[10] The effect of maternal nutritional status on the severity of signs and symptoms of fetal alcohol spectrum disorders has been studied. In a review of the effects of supplemental vitamin A, docosahexaenoic acid, folic acid, zinc, choline, vitamin E, and selenium, the investigators found that although nutritional supplementation may be important, it is only one factor in ameliorating the effects of in utero alcohol exposure.[11] Another study looked at similar issues in a population in the Western Cape Province of South Africa. They found that there was significantly lower intake of several important nutrients, including calcium, docosapentaenoic acid, riboflavin, and choline, and raised the issue that poor diet with multiple nutritional deficiencies in the setting of prenatal alcohol use may increase the risk for fetal alcohol spectrum disorder.[12]

Numerous medications have also been associated with serious birth defects. One of the best studied teratogens has been thalidomide, a medication widely used in Europe in the 1960s and known to cause multiple birth defects, including severe limb anomalies, cleft palate, and congenital heart defects.[13] Commonly prescribed antihypertensive medications, the angiotensin-converting enzyme inhibitors, are known to cause renal dysplasia and defects in skull ossification.[14] However, most teratogenic medications do not alter maternal nutrition status.

Certain maternal metabolic disorders may result in birth defects due to elevated levels of specific metabolites. A classic example is maternal phenylketonuria (PKU). Because of a deficiency of the enzyme phenylalanine hydroxylase, individuals with this autosomal recessive disorder are unable to properly metabolize the amino acid phenylalanine, resulting in elevated levels of serum phenylalanine and its metabolites. Women who are on a low-phenylalanine diet before conception are not at increased risk for having children with birth defects. However, pregnant women with untreated PKU have a greater than 80% risk of having children with congenital heart defects, microcephaly, cleft palate, and brain anomalies.[15]

Multifactorial disorders account for 65% of all birth defects. Multifactorial inheritance assumes a combination of genetic and nongenetic factors that contribute to pathogenesis. The genetic factors are thought to be the effects of several genes, probably a single predisposing gene with several modifier genes. The effects of these genes are mediated by nongenetic factors related to the fetal environment. These factors may reflect maternal nutrition, maternal exposures, external environmental exposures, or an abnormal threshold for specific nutrients and cofactors. Occasionally, physical factors play a role, such as in multiple gestation, abnormal fetal or placental blood flow, or fetal positioning.

Multifactorial disorders are usually single birth defects that may be clustered in some families. The most common multifactorial birth defects are congenital heart defects, cleft lip, cleft palate, neural tube defects, clubfoot, and congenital dysplasia of the hip. Several other conditions that are not birth defects are also inherited as multifactorial conditions. Often, the signs and symptoms develop in adulthood. These may include diabetes mellitus types 1 and 2, asthma, atherosclerosis, hypertension, rheumatoid arthritis, and glaucoma.

The recurrence risk for multifactorial disorders is different from that of autosomal recessive and autosomal dominant disorders. For multifactorial disorders, it is usually 3% to 5% because recurrence depends on the inheritance of specific genes as well as the appropriate nongenetic and environmental factors. Epidemiological studies indicate a genetic component for multifactorial disorders. For example, the incidence of cleft lip with or without cleft palate (CL/P) is 1 in 700 white people. However, when a family has a child with CL/P (or a parent

**Table 60–1.** Estimated Annual Incidence of Common Birth Defects, 2004–2006

| Birth Defect | Incidence (per 100,000 Live Births) |
|---|---|
| Heart malformations | 6136 |
| Neural tube defects | 2319 |
| Malformed genitalia | 3344 |
| Cleft lip/cleft palate | 7088 |
| Gastroschisis | 1871 |
| Down syndrome | 6037 |
| Reduction deformities of limbs | 2155 |
| Rectal and large intestine atresia/stenosis | 1952 |
| Diaphragmatic hernia | 1088 |

Adapted from Parker SE, Mai CT, Canfield MA, et al. Updated national birth prevalence estimates for selected birth defects in the United States, 2004–2006. *Birth Defects Res A Clin Mol Teratol*. 2010; 88:1008.

has CL/P), the recurrence risk is 3% to 5%, which is a 20- to 35-fold increase in risk. The more affected the first-degree relatives in a family, the greater the recurrence risk. If a family has two children with CL/P, the recurrence risk rises to 10%.[16]

Some multifactorial conditions demonstrate a higher prevalence within certain populations. This may be true because certain genes are seen more commonly in specific ethnic, racial, or cultural groups or because of specific environmental exposures or nutritional deficiencies in a particular geographic region. It is most likely a combination of these and possibly other factors. Neural tube defects (NTDs) have a higher prevalence in the British Isles, but Irish, English, and Scottish immigrants to North America have a lower risk of having a child with an NTD than do people living in the British Isles.[17,18] Similarly, individuals of Asian and Native American descent are more likely to have a child with CL/P, with a prevalence of 1 in 500, whereas the prevalence of CL/P in individuals of African or African-American descent is 1 in 2000.[16]

## NUTRITIONAL FACTORS

### Neural Tube Defects

NTDs, spina bifida, anencephaly, and encephalocele are among the most common birth defects. These are potentially preventable disorders. Research has clearly documented that dietary supplementation with folic acid before conception and continuing into pregnancy can significantly reduce the incidence of NTDs. Data collected by the US Centers for Disease Control and Prevention (CDC) documented a 23% decline in the incidence of NTDs between 1996 and 2001, coincident with fortification of all enriched cereal grain products with folic acid.[3] Later studies have clearly supported use of preconception folic acid in reducing neural tube defects, with a 50% to 70% protective effect.[19]

Most cases of NTD are multifactorial. Approximately 10% are caused by chromosome abnormalities, mostly trisomy 13 and trisomy 18.

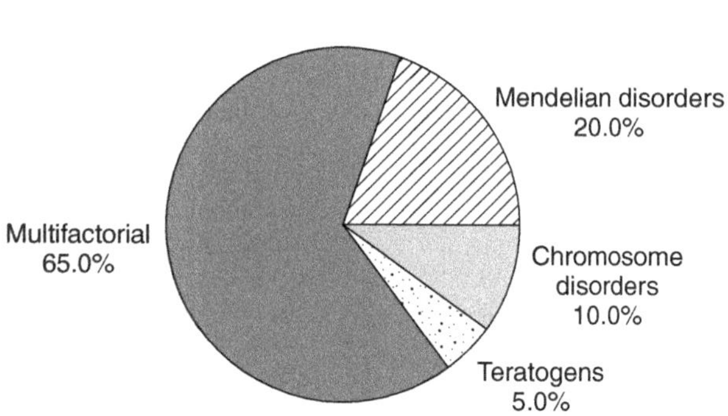


**Figure 60–1.** Causes of birth defects. Pie chart demonstrates the distribution of the etiologies of birth defects. Notice that multifactorial disorders make up the majority of birth defects, and most cases are single anomalies by definition.

A small percentage of cases are caused by the anticonvulsants valproic acid and carbamazepine. Women who take these medications before and during pregnancy have a 1% to 2% risk of having a child with an NTD.[20,21] There is no support for higher-dose folic acid to reduce risk for NTDs in women taking valproic acid.[22]

There are also geographic and racial differences with regard to the prevalence of NTDs. For example, in the United States, the prevalence is highest among Hispanics, followed by non-Hispanic whites, Native Americans, African Americans, and Asian Americans.[23] Geographic factors may also play a role. In Europe, anencephaly rates are highest in the British Isles, diminishing from west to east.[24] Although prevalence rates of anencephaly in Asia are equivalent to those in other regions of the world (except the British Isles), the prevalence of spina bifida is lower in Asia than in most other places.[24] The exception to this pattern is in northern China, where the prevalence in some regions is among the highest in the world.[25]

In the United States between 2004 and 2006, the estimated annual number of cases of spina bifida was 1460 and that of anencephaly was 859.[7] The lifetime costs associated with a typical case of spina bifida, including medical care, special education, therapy services, and loss of earnings, are formidable, and the economic burden persists throughout a person's life.[26] The benefits of preconception use of folic acid are substantial from the standpoint of personal and familial suffering and from the perspective of societal costs.

The initial approach to prevention of NTDs was screening of maternal serum alpha-fetoprotein (AFP) in the second trimester. This screening, initiated in 1972, measures AFP levels in maternal serum. If the level is significantly elevated, an amniocentesis is done, and NTDs are confirmed by elevated AFP levels in amniotic fluid and the presence of a neuronal protein called *acetylcholinesterase*, which is usually indicative of an open NTD.[27] Fetal high-resolution ultrasonography is an important adjunct in prenatal diagnosis of NTDs. Although prenatal diagnosis is helpful in identifying an NTD, it does not prevent the occurrence of an NTD in the embryo.

NTDs, especially anencephaly, have a high prevalence in the British Isles, with perhaps 1 in 200 pregnancies being affected. The birth of children with NTDs has been linked to lower socioeconomic status of the mother.[28,29] In the 1950s, there was a linkage of NTDs with poor diet. This was supported by the fact that more children appeared to be born with NTDs when conception occurred in the winter or early spring. In a landmark study, Hibbard found that megaloblastic anemia in middle to late pregnancy was associated with a defect in folate metabolism.[28] He suggested that an absolute folate deficiency was associated with a dietary inadequacy, whereas a relative deficiency was caused by a metabolic defect in the utilization of folate. Although there was a strong suspicion that folic acid was implicated in the etiology of NTDs, it took many years until the first studies confirming this relationship were completed. Laurence et al. completed a prevention study in Wales by treating women who had previously given birth to one child with an NTD with 4 mg of folic acid before conception; 60 women received folic acid and 51 women received placebo. Two recurrences of NTD were documented in the study group, both in noncompliant subjects; no recurrences were identified in compliant subjects. In the control (placebo) group, there were four recurrences.[30,31] In 1991, a multicenter study was performed in Great Britain with four study groups including 1195 pregnancies: Women received with folic acid, multivitamins with folic acid, multivitamins without folic acid, or no vitamin supplementation. There were 6 NTDs in the folic acid group and 21 in the other groups.[32]

### Gastroschisis

Gastroschisis is another disorder in which maternal nutrition may play a causative role. Gastroschisis is a ventral body wall defect, almost always located to the right of the umbilicus, that is characterized by protrusion of abdominal contents, usually intestines, and is not covered by peritoneum.[33] There is an association with low maternal age[34] and maternal nutrition.[35] One study found that higher maternal intake of fruits and vegetables during the first trimester, longer duration of folic acid supplementation, and higher body fat percentage reduced risk of fetal gastroschisis.[36]

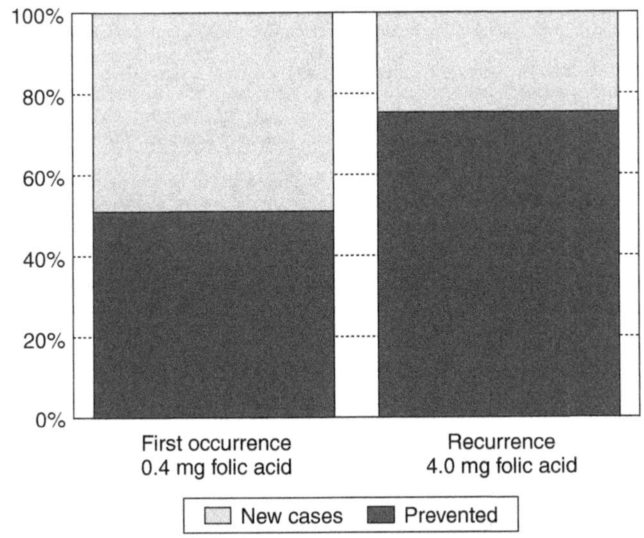


**Figure 60–2.** Prevention of neural tube defects with folic acid. Bar graphs demonstrate the estimated reduction in the number of cases of neural tube defects associated with folic acid use by women of reproductive age.

### Nutrition Management

It is now clear that adequate nutrition, especially with regard to folic acid, plays a pivotal role in the causation of certain birth defects. However, if risks for NTDs are to be diminished, adequate levels of folic acid must be present before conception. Most pregnancies are not diagnosed until at least 6 weeks' gestation and the neural tube closure is completed at 28 days' gestation. Moreover, many pregnancies are unintended. For these reasons, folic acid should be taken before conception. It is recommended in most countries and by the World Health Organization that women of child-bearing age take at least 0.4 mg (400 μg) folic acid daily to meet the Dietary Reference Intakes (DRI).[37] The US Food and Drug Administration initiated a folic acid fortification program in 1998. Food manufacturers are required to add 0.42 to 1.4 mg folic acid to each pound of enriched flour, bread, rolls, buns, farina, corn grits, corn meal, rice, masa harina, and noodle products. Each serving provides approximately 10% of the RDA for folic acid. Women with no family history of NTD who take 0.4 mg folic acid daily can reduce the risk of having a child with an NTD by 50%, and those who have an NTD or have had a child with an NTD can reduce their recurrence risk by 75% (Fig. 60–2).

## FOLIC ACID AND OTHER BIRTH DEFECTS

The first study that demonstrated a link between folic acid and vitamin $B_6$ deficiency was published by Peer and colleagues in 1958[38]; who studied a series of mothers of children with oral clefts. However, they gave no evidence from human studies to support their conclusions. The California Birth Defects Monitoring Program found some association between a possible reduced risk of CL/P and use of vitamins and fortified cereals, but the data analysis was limited by the small number of case mothers.[39] Most similar case-control studies have suffered from difficulty in data analysis due to numerous confounding issues and flaws. The efficacy of folate supplementation to prevent CL/P or other birth defects has not been supported, as reviewed in a recent meta-analysis.[40]

The American College of Medical Genetics[41] published the following recommendations for use of folic acid to prevent NTDs:

- Women with no history of a previous NTD-affected pregnancy should take at least 400 μg (0.4 mg) of folic acid daily.
- Women who have had an NTD-affected pregnancy should take 4000 μg (4 mg) folic acid daily
- Other high-risk persons, including those who have diabetes mellitus type 1 or a reproductive partner with an increased risk (i.e., family history) of NTD, should consider taking 4000 μg (4 mg) of folic acid daily starting at least 3 months before planned conception

## VITAMIN A AND VITAMIN A ANALOGS

Although most attention has been given to vitamin deficiency states, there are many known complications associated with hypervitaminosis, especially of the fat-soluble vitamins. Hypervitaminosis A is among the best-recognized and best-studied of these disorders. In the first half of the 20th century, vitamin A deficiency was found to result in growth deficiency in rats and to contribute to malformations, including skeletal, eye, renal, and urogenital anomalies in these animals.[42] Retinoic acid and other retinoids were later found to cause severe birth defects, including oral clefts, cardiac defects, and brain anomalies in animals.[43,44] In humans, there is clear evidence that excess supplementation of vitamin A leads to serious birth defects.

The DRI for vitamin A is 5000 IU daily. Birth defects have been associated with intake of more than 10,000 IU daily.[45] Women taking more than that amount have a twofold to fourfold increased risk of having a baby with a birth defect, especially cleft lip, cleft palate, congenital heart defect, and brain anomalies.[45] This has become an even more serious issue for the vitamin A analog, isotretinoin. It is an effective medication for treatment of cystic acne, but it is also a powerful teratogen that causes several birth defects, including ear anomalies and deafness, cleft palate, cardiovascular malformations, and microcephaly.[46]

## SUMMARY

There is much more to be learned about the potential associations between nutrition and birth defects. It is well known that severe nutritional deficiencies result in birth defects, severe growth retardation, and miscarriage. However, more studies must be performed that focus on the role of vitamins and nutritional supplements in the causation of structural anomalies and functional deficits. More information must be made available regarding excessive supplementation of vitamins and dietary supplements, their teratogenic potential, and their roles in causing specific birth defects.

### References

1. International Birth Defects Information Systems (IBIS). *Definitions by IBIS*. http://www.ibis-birthdefects.org/start/bd.htm. Accessed July 10, 2016.
2. Centers for Disease Control and Prevention (CDC). Hospital stays, hospital charges, and in-hospital deaths among infants with selected birth defects—United States, 2003. *MMWR Morb Mortal Wkly Rep*. 2007; 56:25.
3. Mathews TJ, MacDormand MF, Thoma ME. *Infant Mortality Statistics from the 2013 Period Linked Birth/Infant Death Data Set*. National Vital Statistics Report, 2015. http://www.cdc.gov/nchs/data/nvsr/nvsr64/nvsr64_09.pdf. Accessed July 10, 2016.
4. Holmes LB, Kleiner BC, Leppig KA, Cann CI, Munoz A, Polk BF. Predictive value of minor anomalies. II. Use in cohort studies to identify teratogens. *Teratology*. 1987; 36:291.
5. Leppig KA, Werler MM, Cann CI, Cook CA, Holmes LB. Predictive value of minor anomalies. I. Association with major malformations. *J Pediatr*. 1987; 110:531.
6. Christianson A, Howson CA, Modell B. *March of Dimes Global Report on Birth Defects: The Hidden Toll of Dying and Disabled Children*. http://www.marchofdimes.org/materials/global-report-on-birth-defects-the-hidden-toll-of-dying-and-disabled-children-full-report.pdf. Accessed July 10, 2016.
7. Parker SE, Mai CT, Canfield MA, et al. Updated national birth prevalence estimates for selected birth defects in the United States, 2004–2006. *Birth Defects Res A Clin Mol Teratol*. 2010; 88:1008.
8. Ezkurdia I, Juan D, Rodriguez JM, et al. Multiple evidence strands suggest that there may be as few as 19,000 human protein-coding genes. *Hum Mol Genet*. 2014; 23:5866.
9. May PA, Baete A, Russo J, et al. Prevalence and characteristics of fetal alcohol spectrum disorders. *Pediatrics*. 2014; 134:855.
10. O'Leary CM. Fetal alcohol syndrome: diagnosis, epidemiology, and developmental outcomes. *J Paediatr Child Health*. 2004; 40:2.
11. Young JK, Giesbrecht HE, Eskin MN, Aliani M, Suh M. Nutrition implications for fetal alcohol spectrum disorder. *Adv Nutr*. 2014; 5:675.
12. May PA, Hamrick KJ, Corbin KD, et al. Dietary intake, nutrition, and fetal alcohol spectrum disorders in the Western Cape Province of South Africa. *Reprod Toxicol*. 2014; 46:31.
13. Vargesson N. Thalidomide-induced teratogenesis: history and mechanisms. *Birth Defects Res C Embryo Today*. 2015; 105:140.
14. Walfisch A, Al-maawali A, Moretti ME, Nickel C, Koren G. Teratogenicity of angiotensin converting enzyme inhibitors or receptor blockers. *J Obstet Gynaecol*. 2011; 31:465.

15. Kesby G. Repeated adverse fetal outcome in pregnancy complicated by uncontrolled maternal phenylketonuria. *J Paediatr Child Health.* 1999; 35:499.
16. Saal HM. Classification and description of nonsyndromic oral clefts. In: Wyszinski DF, ed. *Cleft Lip and Palate: From Origin to Treatment*. New York: Oxford University Press; 2002: 47.
17. Freeman NV, Rajab A. Neural tube defects. *Trop Doct.* 1999; 29:235.
18. Gelineau-van Waes J, Finnell RH. Genetics of neural tube defects. *Semin Pediatr. Neurol.* 2001; 8:160.
19. Safi J, Joyeux L, Chalouhi GE. Periconceptional folate deficiency and implications in neural tube defects. *J Pregnancy.* 2012; 2012:295083.
20. Jentink J, Loane MA, Dolk H, et al. Valproic acid monotherapy in pregnancy and major congenital malformations. *N Engl J Med.* 2010; 362:2185.
21. Jentink J, Dolk H, Loane MA, et al. Intrauterine exposure to carbamazepine and specific congenital malformations: systematic review and case-control study. *BMJ.* 2010; 341:c6581.
22. Jentink J, Bakker MK, Nijenhuis CM, Wilffert B, de Jong-van den Berg LT. Does folic acid use decrease the risk for spina bifida after in utero exposure to valproic acid? *Pharmacoepidemiol Drug Saf.* 2010; 19:803.
23. Owen TJ, Halliday JL, Stone CA. Neural tube defects in Victoria, Australia: potential contributing factors and public health implications. *Aust N Z J Public Health.* 2000; 24:584.
24. Little LE, Elwood JM. *Epidemiology of Neural Tube Defects.* Boston: CRD Press; 1991.
25. Ren AG. Prevention of neural tube defects with folic acid: The Chinese experience. *World J Clin Pediatr.* 2015; 4:41.
26. Bowles D, Wasiak R, Kissner M, et al. Economic burden of neural tube defects in Germany. *Public Health.* 2014; 128:274.
27. Wilson RD, Audibert F, Brock JA, et al. Prenatal screening, diagnosis, and pregnancy management of fetal neural tube defects. *J Obstet Gynaecol Can.* 2014; 36:927.
28. Hibbard BM. The role of folic acid in pregnancy; with particular reference to anaemia, abruption and abortion. *J Obstet Gynaecol Br Commonw.* 1964; 71:529.
29. Hibbard BM, Hibbard ED, Jeffcoate TN. Folic acid and reproduction. *Acta Obstet Gynecol Scand.* 1965; 44:375.
30. Laurence KM, Campbell H. Trial of folate treatment to prevent recurrence of neural tube defect. *Br Med J (Clin Res Ed.)* 1981; 282:2131.
31. Laurence KM, James N, Miller MH, Tennant GB, Campbell H. Double-blind randomised controlled trial of folate treatment before conception to prevent recurrence of neural-tube defects. *Br Med J (Clin Res Ed).* 1981; 282:1509.
32. Medical Research Council Vitamin Study Research Group. Prevention of neural tube defects: results of the Medical Research Council Vitamin Study. *Lancet.* 1991; 338:131.
33. Sadler TW. The embryologic origin of ventral body wall defects. *Semin Pediatr Surg.* 2010; 19:209.
34. Emusu D, Salihu HM, Aliyu ZY, Pierre-Louis BJ, Druschel CM, Kirby RS. Gastroschisis, low maternal age, and fetal morbidity outcomes. *Birth Defects Res A Clin Mol Teratol.* 2005; 73:649.
35. Siega-Riz AM, Herring AH, Olshan AF, Smith J, Moore C. The joint effects of maternal prepregnancy body mass index and age on the risk of gastroschisis. *Paediatr Perinat Epidemiol.* 2009; 23:51.
36. Paranjothy S, Broughton H, Evans A, et al. The role of maternal nutrition in the aetiology of gastroschisis: an incident case-control study. *Int J Epidemiol.* 2012; 41:1141.
37. Gomes S, Lopes C, Pinto E. Folate and folic acid in the periconceptional period: recommendations from official health organizations in thirty-six countries worldwide and WHO. *Public Health Nutr.* 2016; 19:176.
38. Peer LA, Strean LP, Walker JC Jr, Bernhard WG, Peck GC. Study of 400 pregnancies with birth of cleft lip-palate infants; protective effect of folic acid and vitamin B6 therapy. *Plast Reconstr Surg Transplant Bull.* 1958; 22:442.
39. Shaw GM, Lammer EJ, Wasserman CR, O'Malley CD, Tolarova MM. Risks of orofacial clefts in children born to women using multivitamins containing folic acid periconceptionally. *Lancet.* 1995; 346:393.
40. De-Regil LM, Pena-Rosas JP, Fernandez-Gaxiola AC, Rayco-Solon P. Effects and safety of periconceptional oral folate supplementation for preventing birth defects. *Cochrane Database Syst Rev.* 2015; (12):CD007950.
41. Toriello HV. Policy statement on folic acid and neural tube defects. *Genet Med.* 2011; 13:593.
42. Warkany J. Congenital malformations induced in rats by maternal nutritional deficiency: IV. The preventive factor. *J Nutr* 1944; 27:477.
43. Kochhar DM. Teratogenic activity of retinoic acid. *Acta Pathol Microbiol Scand.* 1967; 70:398.
44. Fantel AG, Shepard TH, Newell-Morris LL, Moffett BC. Teratogenic effects of retinoic acid in pigtail monkeys (*Macaca nemestrina*). I. General features. *Teratology.* 1977; 15:65.
45. Rothman KJ, Moore LL, Singer MR, Nguyen US, Mannino S, Milunsky A. Teratogenicity of high vitamin A intake. *N Engl J Med.* 1995; 333:1369.
46. Lammer EJ, Chen DT, Hoar RM, et al. Retinoic acid embryopathy. *N Engl J Med.* 1985; 313:837.

# 61 Nutrition in Older Adults

AGNES M. HUBER

The elderly are the fastest growing segment of the population, and the group of aging persons with a developmental disability is growing larger. A significant factor explaining this phenomenon is the increased lifespan that has occurred. A New York review of 2752 elderly persons showed that the average lifespan at death was 70.4 years for the general population, 66.2 years for elderly people with a developmental disability, and 55.8 years for persons with Down syndrome (DS).[1] More than 210,000 people with DS are living in the United States, and this number may increase in the future. Between 1979 and 2003, the prevalence of DS increased by 31.1%, from 9 to 11.8 cases per 10,000 births, because women are having babies later in life (i.e., after the age of 35 years).[2]

Aging is determined by three major factors: genetic makeup, pathology, and lifestyle. Genetically determined premature aging, particularly in progeria and Werner syndrome, is being studied. In both cases, genetic mutations are associated with abnormalities in metabolic functions[3] and diminished DNA repair.[4] The role of trisomy 21 of DS in relation to premature aging is not well understood. Some persons with DS are living into their late 60s and 70s without showing pathology. Trisomy 21 seems to have a causal effect on intellectual disability, and Alzheimer's disease (AD) is identified in 20% to 30% of elderly people with DS.[2] Brown identified 13 pathological changes in DS that are directly related to the aging process, including premature graying, redistribution of adipose tissue, degenerative vascular changes, and possibly the senile dementia of AD.[5]

In normative aging, physical, sensory, and behavioral changes occur, some of which have direct or indirect effects on health. Some problems are related to pathology (e.g., diabetes, heart disease) or to lifestyle factors (e.g., diet, smoking, physical activity). It is not difficult to see that a person's health status is the result of multiple factors. To identify underlying pathology that can directly or indirectly cause anorexia with subsequent malnutrition, as well as other problems, elderly people should get regular medical check-ups.

## PHYSIOLOGICAL CHANGES DURING AGING

One of the most significant health-related changes during aging is the effect on muscle and fat composition of the body. Whereas muscle mass decreases, fat increases over time. The loss of muscle decreases isometric and isokinetic strength, and with progression, this has significant effects on daily activities. Walking is slower, and the person becomes tired easily. Stair climbing becomes cumbersome, and endurance for activities decreases.

With this decrease in muscle strength, the jaw muscles are also affected, and chewing food becomes more difficult and takes longer. Even if food is cut into small pieces or is pureed, eating may still be slow because elderly individuals easily tired, even too tired to hold a spoon. If food selection is poor and food intake is low, nutritional deficiencies may result.[6]

In a series of studies, Evans and colleagues showed that strength training in the elderly can attenuate or arrest the loss of muscle mass and even reverse it. High-intensity physical resistance strength training and walking, in combination with social activities, was shown in nursing homes and assisted living residences to protect muscle mass and was also beneficial in that it induced better sleep.[7]

Oral health is determined by other factors in addition to the effects of aging on muscle. To evaluate dental health, 4732 adults with intellectual and developmental disabilities were studied. Over a period of 1 year, 32.2% were identified with untreated caries, 80.3% with periodontitis, and 10.9% with edentulism, indicating that tooth decay posed a significant challenge.[8] Another study related chewing ability to diet status in elderly persons living in the community. The number of teeth was significantly related to chewing ability. A significant association was found between low chewing ability and depression and lower cognitive function. Retention of dentition into the later years of life is favorable for eating, speech, and self-esteem.[9]

## EFFECT OF AGING ON ADIPOSE TISSUE

Because activity often decreases during aging, the elderly are prone to obesity. The many excellent weight reduction programs for the younger population do not seem appropriate for the elderly. Several factors pose limitations, such as functional activity, polypharmacy, comorbidity, and social issues. The goal of weight management is preferable to that of aggressive weight reduction. Obesity in the elderly is becoming a major health problem, and prevention at earlier ages in people with developmental disability is the best goal to prevent later obesity.[10]

## NUTRITION ASSESSMENT

Nutrition assessment for optimal care of older people with developmental disabilities should be routinely carried out, whether they live independently or in a care setting. Because these elderly are a varied group with age differences, a variety of problems, and different needs, the assessment must be tailored for the specific conditions. It is assumed that dietitians who carry out these assessments are familiar with the methods and procedures. The following is a reminder of the many factors that are important in the final health outcomes.

One of the pressing issues is the prevention of malnutrition. Malnutrition has been observed in 12% to 50% of hospitalized elderly patients; among the institutionalized elderly, the rate was 23% to 60%.[11,12] The causes of malnutrition are many. It can be traced to inadequate food intake, problems with gastrointestinal absorption, nutrient losses, and the interference of medications and loss of appetite. Many physiological and socioeconomic factors can influence a person's eating habits. In some cases, a person's monthly allowance for food must instead be spent on medicines. Elderly individuals may have problems with cognition or psychiatric problems, or they may forget to eat, or may eat a limited diet that is not adequate. It is very helpful if a caretaker or a family member can provide the crucial information necessary to develop recommendations because it is difficult to tease out the relevant factors that need to be changed or altered. It is also helpful when the elderly person has had optimal care previously and can understand the recommendations he or she needs to follow.

For the nutritionist working with elderly persons, and specifically those with developmental disabilities, dietary concerns and issues around eating are important to evaluate when looking for the reasons why inadequate diets are consumed. As elderly persons gradually become weaker, their diminished strength interferes with preparing and eating food. Mastication is slower, resulting in longer meal completion times. Evans et al. concluded that the decreased muscle strength in the elderly is a major cause of disability.[13] They suggested that aging might be nothing more than a lifetime accumulation of inactivity and poor nutrition.

Regular activity, even in very old and frail individuals, has positive effects on functional status. Keeping active increases functional independence and has a beneficial effect on insulin levels, bone density, hypertension, coronary artery disease, and energy metabolism.[13]

Reducing or preventing the oropharyngeal dysphagia by preserving muscle mass helps the elderly preserve independence in eating. This is highly desirable because the anticipation of preparing for each bite, eating at one's own pace, and interacting with others at the table implies competency and gives a sense of pleasure and satisfaction. Often, simple adaptations of the elderly person's environment during a meal are very helpful. Limiting the noise level, consistency in table partner, better lighting, or having a limited number of foods so as not overwhelm the person may make a meal more enjoyable. An elderly person, even one with well-fitting dentures, will take longer to eat because he or she will chew with less force. It is important to prevent the vicious cycle of decreased food intake, borderline malnutrition, and reduced appetite that results in even less food intake. Besides assessment of food intake, the adaptations that are most helpful for achieving independence in eating need to be assessed.

The benefits of adequate nutrition in the elderly can be summarized as follows:

1. Adequate nutrition helps maintain independent living in the community and even plays a role in helping people who are chronically or terminally ill.
2. Adequate nutrition helps older people avoid premature nursing home placement.
3. Adequate nutrition helps older people avoiding use of expensive health care devices and reduces the incidence of hospitalization.
4. Appropriate nutrition promotes health.

## SARCOPENIA

As elderly people become frail and exceedingly weak, and their muscle mass moves toward exhaustion, and their health becomes seriously compromised. This syndrome, known as sarcopenia, is characterized by loss of skeletal muscle performance and endurance. This loss is associated with exhaustion and has effects on metabolism, hormones, and inflammatory functions. Dysregulation makes the elderly vulnerable to adverse health outcomes. The Society for Sarcopenia, Cachexia, and Wasting Disease has published nutrition recommendations for the prevention and management of sarcopenia. Gentle exercise (resistance and aerobic) with adequate protein intake enriched with leucine and balanced in amino acids, is recommended. Supplements are recommended for low levels of creatine and 25-hydroxyvitamin D.[14]

## GERIATRIC FAILURE TO THRIVE

Geriatric failure to thrive (GFTT) is a multifactorial condition with functional impairment, chronic ailments, weight loss, inactivity, and poor nutrition.[15] Others have defined it as the presence of weight loss, decreased appetite, poor nutrition, and inactivity. Whereas failure to thrive in the pediatric population is characterized by failure to grow, for geriatric patients, it is failure to maintain weight. As predictors of GFTT, four syndromes have been used: impaired function, malnutrition, depression, and cognitive impairment.[16]

GFTT has been also described as a spiral leading down with characteristic changes: loss of weight, gradual decline in physical and cognitive function, loss of appetite, social withdrawal, and eventually death. Causes for this spiral have been thought include such factors as disease, anorexia-producing medications, dementia, consumption of alcohol or drugs, dysphagia, and deafness or blindness. Any of these alone may be relatively unimportant, but a combination of several, together with malnutrition and aging, can cause GFTT. The seriousness of the condition and the progressive decline of the patient make premature institutionalization necessary and require a team effort to care for the patient.[17] The physician, nurses, therapists, and social service professionals are important components of the treatment team. The dietitian is foremost involved in the assessment of nutrient status and the treatment of malnutrition.[18]

The assessment should provide information about the following:

- Severity of weight loss
- Living situation of the patient
- Mobility and independence
- Mental status and possible dementia
- Food intake and medical problems that interfere
- Use of anorexic medicines

Treatment goals may include the following

- Diet modification; no restrictions
- Use of supplements
- Treatment of depression
- Replacement of anorexic medication with other agents
- Provision of food with eye and taste appeal

Healthy aging requires a healthy environment in which the elderly person can feel safe, get daily needs met, and avoid feeling lonely. Such a congenial environment not only benefits the elderly, because they are less sick and have fewer hospitalizations, but also benefits caretakers and families, because have fewer expenses.

One of the significant concerns of parents, siblings, and professionals is that adults with developmental disabilities do not have educational and vocational activities. Under these conditions, the elderly suffer significantly with depressive symptoms.[19] In a study on health promotion involving physical activity, health education, and health care screening, reduced disparities were observed, the elderly subjects were more fit, and they had some success in reducing obesity. A more holistic approach, including health and nutrition education and counseling about health behaviors and attitudes, provides greater long-term benefit.[20] Elderly people who are developmentally disabled, are underserved, and are not involved in any programs appear to do less well, and they report worse health and serious depressive symptoms. It is also of concern that this group have limited opportunities to work and be employed and that their incomes from earnings and government resources are low.[21]

The Disability Advisory Committee on Aging, which convened almost 20 years ago, adapted as a goal the intent that Americans with disability and Americans who are aging should be able to live with the greatest degree of independence and dignity. This goal is still admirable to pursue today. Over the years, policy makers have discussed equitable access to health care, but shrinking resources have often prevented progress. Research has shown that encouragement of healthy living by the elderly improves their lives and saves money. They have fewer chronic diseases and require fewer hospital admissions.

Although much still can be and should be improved, changes are slowly occurring. There are new positive attitudes among physicians, influenced by parents, advocacy groups, court decisions, and research. It has been shown that the intellectual and social skills of children with DS are greater than formerly thought and that they are able to learn healthy ways of living over an extended lifespan.[22] Such changes also have improved health and wellness among the disabled elderly[23] and others.[24]

National goals are being set for the health, retirement, and later life of older adults with intellectual and developmental disabilities.[25] Reviews of current research, practices, and policies are informing decisions about these critical issues for older people with intellectual and developmental disabilities.[26]

### References


1. Janicki MP, Mortality data provides interesting insight. *Aging MR/IG Newsletter*. 1995; p. 9.
2. Zigman WB, Atypical aging in Down syndrome. *Dev Disabil Res Rev*. 2013; 18:51.
3. Coppede F. The epidemiology of premature aging and associated comorbidities. *Clin Interv Aging*. 2013; 8:1023.
4. Weirich-Schwaiger H, Weirich HG, Gruber B, et al. Correlation between senescence and DNA repair in cells from young and old individuals and in premature aging syndromes. *Mutat Res*. 1994; 316:37.
5. Brown WT. Genetics of aging. In: Janicki MP, Wisnieski HM, eds. *Aging and Developmental Disability*. Baltimore, MD: PH Brookes; 1985: 185.

6. Kimura Y, Ogawa H, Yoshihara A, et al. Evaluation of chewing ability and its relationship with activities of daily living, depression, cognitive status and food intake in the community dwelling elderly. *Geriatr Gerontol Int*. 2013; 13:718.
7. Richards KC, Lambert C, Beck CK, et al. Strength training, walking, and social activity improve sleep in nursing home and assisted living residence: randomized control trial. *J Am Geriatr Soc*. 2011; 59:214.
8. Morgan JP, Minihan PM, Stark PC, et.al. The oral health status of 4,732 adults with intellectual and developmental disabilities. *J Am Dent Assoc*. 2012; 143:838.
9. Waldman HB, Perlman SP, Ensuring oral health for older individuals with intellectual and developmental disabilities. *J Clin Nurs*. 2012; 21:909.
10. Chau D, Cho LM, Jani P, St Jeor ST. Individualizing recommendations for weight management in the elderly. *Curr Opin Clin Nutr Metab Care*. 2008; 11:27.
11. Wallace JL. Malnutrition and enteral/parenteral alimentation. In: Hazzard WR, Blass JP, Ettinger WH Jr, Halter JB, Ouslander JG, eds. *Principles of Geriatric Medicine and Gerontology*, 4th ed. New York. McGraw-Hill. 1999;1455.
12. Endoy MP, Anorexia among older adults. *Am J Nurse Practic*. 2005; 9:31.
13. Evans WJ, Paolisso G, Abbatecola AM, et. all, Frailty and muscle metabolism dysregulation in the elderly. *Biogerontology*. 2010; 11:527.
14. Morley JE, Argiles JM, Evans WJ, et.al. Nutritional recommendations for the management of sarcopenia. *J Am Med Dir Assoc*. 2010; 11:391.
15. Robertson RG, Montagnini M. Geriatric failure to thrive. *Am Fam Physician*. 2004; 70:343.
16. Anderson K, Baraldi C, Supiano M. Identifying failure to thrive in the long term care setting. *J Am Med Dir Assoc*. 2012; 13:665.
17. Rocchiccioli JT, Sanford JT. Revisiting geriatric failure to thrive: a complex and compelling clinical condition. *J Gerontol Nurs*. 2009; 35:18.
18. Schreiber S, Lerer B, "Failure to thrive" in elderly depressed patients: a new concept or a different name for an old problem? *Isr J Psychiatry Relat Sci*. 1997; 34:108.
19. Taylor JL, Hodapp RM. Doing nothing: adults with disabilities with no daily activities and their siblings. *Am J Intellect Disabil*. 2012; 117:67.
20. Heller T, Sorensen A. Promoting healthy aging in adults with developmental disabilities. *Dev Disabil Res Rev*. 2013; 18:22.
21. Havercamp SM, Scandlin D, Roth M. Health disparities among adults with developmental disabilities, adults with other disabilities, and adults not reporting disability in North Carolina. *Publ Health Rep*. 2004; 119:418.
22. Haslam RH, Miner R. The physician and Down's syndrome: are attitudes changing? *J Child Neurol*. 1992; 7:304.
23. Hahn JE. Using NIC in an APRN-led preventive model for adults aging with developmental disabilities. *J Nurs Scholarship*. 2014; 46:304.
24. Marks B, Sisirak J, Chang YC. Efficacy of the Health Matters program train-the-trainer model. *J Appl Res Intellect Disabil*. 2013; 26:319.
25. Hahn JE, Fox S, Janicki MP. Aging among older adults with intellectual and developmental disabilities: setting national goals to address transitions in health, retirement, and late-life. *Inclusion*. 2015; 3:250.
26. Hahn JE, Gray J, McCallion P, et al. Transitions in aging: health, retirement, and later life: review of research, practice, and policy. In: *Critical Issues in Intellectual and Developmental Disabilities: Contemporary Research, Practice, and Policy*. Washington, DC: American Association on Intellectual and Developmental Disabilities; 2016.

# APPENDIX 1
## Dietary Reference Intakes



Footnotes to Appendixes 1–7:
+ = analyses performed by Research 900 Laboratories, St. Louis, MO.
N = Nonmeasurable: values are below minimum levels found by AOAC methods (40 mg riboflavin, 12 mg ascorbic acid, 50 IU vitamin A per 100 g of spice).
Mg = milligrams (0.001 g).
Mcg = micrograms (0.000001 g).
Research Committee, American Spice Trade Association, 580 Sylvan Avenue, Englewood Cliffs, NJ 07632.

**1–1** Dietary Reference Intakes (DRIs): Recommended Intakes for Individuals, Vitamins Food and Nutrition Board, Institute of Medicine, National Academies

| Life Stage Group | Vitamin A (μg/d)[a] | Vitamin C (mg/d) | Vitamin D (μg/d)[b,c] | Vitamin E (mg/d)[d] | Vitamin K (μg/d) | Thiamin (mg/d) | Riboflavin (mg/d) | Niacin (mg/d)[e] | Vitamin $B_6$ (mg/d) | Folate (μg/d)[f] | Vitamin $B_{12}$ (μg/d) | Pantothenic Acid (mg/d) | Biotin (μg/d) | Choline[g] (mg/d) |
|---|---|---|---|---|---|---|---|---|---|---|---|---|---|---|
| Infants | | | | | | | | | | | | | | |
| 0-6 mo | 400* | 40* | 5* | 4* | 2.0* | 0.2* | 0.3* | 2* | 0.1* | 65* | 0.4* | 1.7* | 5* | 125* |
| 7-12 mo | 500* | 50* | 5* | 5* | 2.5* | 0.3* | 0.4* | 4* | 0.3* | 80* | 0.5* | 1.8* | 6* | 150* |
| Children | | | | | | | | | | | | | | |
| 1-3 y | **300** | **15** | 5* | **6** | 30* | **0.5** | **0.5** | **6** | **0.5** | **150** | **0.9** | 2* | 8* | 200* |
| 4-8 y | **400** | **25** | 5* | **7** | 55* | **0.6** | **0.6** | **8** | **0.6** | **200** | **1.2** | 3* | 12* | 250* |
| Males | | | | | | | | | | | | | | |
| 9-13 y | **600** | **45** | 5* | **11** | 60* | **0.9** | **0.9** | **12** | **1.0** | **300** | **1.8** | 4* | 20* | 375* |
| 14-18 y | **900** | **75** | 5* | **15** | 75* | **1.2** | **1.3** | **16** | **1.3** | **400** | **2.4** | 5* | 25* | 550* |
| 19-30 y | **900** | **90** | 5* | **15** | 120* | **1.2** | **1.3** | **16** | **1.3** | **400** | **2.4** | 5* | 30* | 550* |
| 31-50 y | **900** | **90** | 5* | **15** | 120* | **1.2** | **1.3** | **16** | **1.3** | **400** | **2.4** | 5* | 30* | 550* |
| 51-70 y | **900** | **90** | 10* | **15** | 120* | **1.2** | **1.3** | **16** | **1.7** | **400** | **2.4**[h] | 5* | 30* | 550* |
| >70 y | **900** | **90** | 15* | **15** | 120* | **1.2** | **1.3** | **16** | **1.7** | **400** | **2.4**[h] | 5* | 30* | 550* |
| Females | | | | | | | | | | | | | | |
| 9-13 y | **600** | **45** | 5* | **11** | 60* | **0.9** | **0.9** | **12** | **1.0** | **300** | **1.8** | 4* | 20* | 375* |
| 14-18 y | **700** | **65** | 5* | **15** | 75* | **1.0** | **1.0** | **14** | **1.2** | **400**[i] | **2.4** | 5* | 25* | 400* |
| 19-30 y | **700** | **75** | 5* | **15** | 90* | **1.1** | **1.1** | **14** | **1.3** | **400**[i] | **2.4** | 5* | 30* | 425* |
| 31-50 y | **700** | **75** | 5* | **15** | 90* | **1.1** | **1.1** | **14** | **1.3** | **400**[i] | **2.4** | 5* | 30* | 425* |
| 51-70 y | **700** | **75** | 10* | **15** | 90* | **1.1** | **1.1** | **14** | **1.5** | **400** | **2.4**[h] | 5* | 30* | 425* |
| >70 y | **700** | **75** | 15* | **15** | 90* | **1.1** | **1.1** | **14** | **1.5** | **400** | **2.4**[h] | 5* | 30* | 425* |
| Pregnancy | | | | | | | | | | | | | | |
| ≤18 y | **750** | **80** | 5* | **15** | 75* | **1.4** | **1.4** | **18** | **1.9** | **600**[j] | **2.6** | 6* | 30* | 450* |
| 19-30 y | **770** | **85** | 5* | **15** | 90* | **1.4** | **1.4** | **18** | **1.9** | **600**[j] | **2.6** | 6* | 30* | 450* |
| 31-50 y | **770** | **85** | 5* | **15** | 90* | **1.4** | **1.4** | **18** | **1.9** | **600**[j] | **2.6** | 6* | 30* | 450* |
| Lactation | | | | | | | | | | | | | | |
| ≤18 y | **1,200** | **115** | 5* | **19** | 75* | **1.4** | **1.6** | **17** | **2.0** | **500** | **2.8** | 7* | 35* | 550* |
| 19-30 y | **1,300** | **120** | 5* | **19** | 90* | **1.4** | **1.6** | **17** | **2.0** | **500** | **2.8** | 7* | 35* | 550* |
| 31-50 y | **1,300** | **120** | 5* | **19** | 90* | **1.4** | **1.6** | **17** | **2.0** | **500** | **2.8** | 7* | 35* | 550* |

NOTE: This table (taken from the DRI reports, see www.nap.edu) presents Recommended Dietary Allowances (RDAs) in **bold type** and Adequate Intakes (AIs) in ordinary type followed by an asterisk (*). RDAs and AIs may both be used as goals for individual intake. RDAs are set to meet the needs of almost all (97 to 98 percent) individuals in a group. For healthy breastfed infants, the AI is the mean intake. The AI for other life stage and gender groups is believed to cover needs of all individuals in the group, but lack of data or uncertainty in the data prevent being able to specify with confidence the percentage of individuals covered by this intake.

[a]As retinol activity equivalents (RAEs). 1 RAE=1 μg retinol, 12 μg β-carotene, 24 μg α-carotene, or 24 μg β-cryptoxanthin. The RAE for dietary provitamin A carotenoids is two-fold greater than retinol equivalents (RE), whereas the RAE for preformed vitamin A is the same as RE.

[b]Cholecalciferol. 1 μg cholecalciferol=40 IU vitamin D.

[c]In the absence of adequate exposure to sunlight.

[d]As α-tocopherol. α-Tocopherol includes RRR-α-tocopherol, the only form of α-tocopherol that occurs naturally in foods, and the 2R-stereoisomeric forms of α-tocopherol (RRR-, RSR-, RRS-, and RSS-α-tocopherol) that occur in fortified foods and supplements. It does not include the *2S*-stereoisomeric forms of α-tocopherol (SRR-, SSR-, SRS-, and SSS-α-tocopherol), also found in fortified foods and supplements.

[e]As niacin equivalents (NE). 1 mg of niacin=60 mg of tryptophan; 0-6 months=preformed niacin (not NE).

[f]As dietary folate equivalents (DFE). 1 DFE=1 μg food folate=0.6 μg of folic acid from fortified food or as a supplement consumed with food=0.5 μg of a supplement taken on an empty stomach.

[g]Although AIs have been set for choline, there are few data to assess whether a dietary supply of choline is needed at all stages of the life cycle, and it may be that the choline requirement can be met by endogenous synthesis at some of these stages.

[h]Because 10 to 30 percent of older people may malabsorb food-bound $B_{12}$, it is advisable for those older than 50 years to meet their RDA mainly by consuming foods fortified with $B_{12}$ or a supplement containing $B_{12}$.

[i]In view of evidence linking folate intake with neural tube defects in the fetus, it is recommended that all women capable of becoming pregnant consume 400 μg from supplements or fortified foods in addition to intake of food folate from a varied diet.

[j]It is assumed that women will continue consuming 400 μg from supplements or fortified food until their pregnancy is confirmed and they enter prenatal care, which ordinarily occurs after the end of the periconceptional period—the critical time for formation of the neural tube.

**1–1** (Continued)

| Life Stage Group | Calcium (mg/d) | Chromium (μg/d) | Copper (μg/d) | Fluoride (mg/d) | Iodine (μg/d) | Iron (mg/d) | Magnesium (mg/d) | Manganese (mg/d) | Molybdenum (μg/d) | Phosphorus (mg/d) | Selenium (μg/d) | Zinc (mg/d) |
|---|---|---|---|---|---|---|---|---|---|---|---|---|
| Infants | | | | | | | | | | | | |
| 0-6 mo | 210* | 0.2* | 200* | 0.01* | 110* | 0.27* | 30* | 0.003* | 2* | 100* | 15* | 2* |
| 7-12 mo | 270* | 5.5* | 220* | 0.5* | 130* | **11** | 75* | 0.6* | 3* | 275* | 20* | **3** |
| Children | | | | | | | | | | | | |
| 1-3 y | 500* | 11* | **340** | 0.7* | **90** | **7** | **80** | 1.2* | **17** | **460** | **20** | **3** |
| 4-8 y | 800* | 15* | **440** | 1* | **90** | **10** | **130** | 1.5* | **22** | **500** | **30** | **5** |
| Males | | | | | | | | | | | | |
| 9-13 y | 1,300* | 25* | **700** | 2* | **120** | **8** | **240** | 1.9* | **34** | **1,250** | **40** | **8** |
| 14-18 y | 1,300* | 35* | **890** | 3* | **150** | **11** | **410** | 2.2* | **43** | **1,250** | **55** | **11** |
| 19-30 y | 1,000* | 35* | **900** | 4* | **150** | **8** | **400** | 2.3* | **45** | **700** | **55** | **11** |
| 31-50 y | 1,000* | 35* | **900** | 4* | **150** | **8** | **420** | 2.3* | **45** | **700** | **55** | **11** |
| 51-70 y | 1,200* | 30* | **900** | 4* | **150** | **8** | **420** | 2.3* | **45** | **700** | **55** | **11** |
| >70 y | 1,200* | 30* | **900** | 4* | **150** | **8** | **420** | 2.3* | **45** | **700** | **55** | **11** |
| Females | | | | | | | | | | | | |
| 9-13 y | 1,300* | 21* | **700** | 2* | **120** | **8** | **240** | 1.6* | **34** | **1,250** | **40** | **8** |
| 14-18 y | 1,300* | 24* | **890** | 3* | **150** | **15** | **360** | 1.6* | **43** | **1,250** | **55** | **9** |
| 19-30 y | 1,000* | 25* | **900** | 3* | **150** | **18** | **310** | 1.8* | **45** | **700** | **55** | **8** |
| 31-50 y | 1,000* | 25* | **900** | 3* | **150** | **18** | **320** | 1.8* | **45** | **700** | **55** | **8** |
| 51-70 y | 1,200* | 20* | **900** | 3* | **150** | **8** | **320** | 1.8* | **45** | **700** | **55** | **8** |
| >70 y | 1,200* | 20* | **900** | 3* | **150** | **8** | **320** | 1.8* | **45** | **700** | **55** | **8** |
| Pregnancy | | | | | | | | | | | | |
| ≤18 y | 1,300* | 29* | **1,000** | 3* | **220** | **27** | **400** | 2.0* | **50** | **1,250** | **60** | **12** |
| 19-30 y | 1,000* | 30* | **1,000** | 3* | **220** | **27** | **350** | 2.0* | **50** | **700** | **60** | **11** |
| 31-50 y | 1,000* | 30* | **1,000** | 3* | **220** | **27** | **360** | 2.0* | **50** | **700** | **60** | **11** |
| Lactation | | | | | | | | | | | | |
| ≤18 y | 1,300* | 44* | **1,300** | 3* | **290** | **10** | **360** | 2.6* | **50** | **1,250** | **70** | **13** |
| 19-30 y | 1,000* | 45* | **1,300** | 3* | **290** | **9** | **310** | 2.6* | **50** | **700** | **70** | **12** |
| 31-50 y | 1,000* | 45* | **1,300** | 3* | **290** | **9** | **320** | 2.6* | **50** | **700** | **70** | **12** |

NOTE: This table presents Recommended Dietary Allowances (RDAs) in **bold type** and Adequate Intakes (AIs) in ordinary type followed by an asterisk (*). RDAs and AIs may both be used as goals for individual intake. RDAs are set to meet the needs of almost all (97 to 98 percent) individuals in a group. For healthy breastfed infants, the AI is the mean intake. The AI for other life stage and gender groups is believed to cover needs of all individuals in the group, but lack of data or uncertainty in the data prevent being able to specify with confidence the percentage of individuals covered by this intake.

SOURCES: Dietary Reference Intakes for Calcium, Phosphorus, Magnesium, Vitamin D, and Fluoride (1997); Dietary Reference Intakes for Thiamin, Riboflavin, Niacin, Vitamin $B_6$, Folate, Vitamin $B_{12}$, Pantothenic Acid, Biotin, and Choline (1998); Dietary Reference Intakes for Vitamin C, Vitamin E, Selenium, and Carotenoids (2000); and Dietary Reference Intakes for Vitamin A, Vitamin K, Arsenic, Boron, Chromium, Copper, Iodine, Iron, Manganese, Molybdenum, Nickel, Silicon, Vanadium, and Zinc (2001). These reports may be accessed via www.nap.edu.

**1–2** Dietary Reference Intakes (DRIs): Recommended Intakes for Individuals, Macronutrients Food and Nutrition Board, Institute of Medicine, National Academies

| Life Stage Group | Carbohydrate (g/d) | Total Fiber (g/d) | Fat (g/d) | Linoleic Acid (g/d) | α-Linolenic Acid (g/d) | Protein[a] (g/d) |
|---|---|---|---|---|---|---|
| Infants | | | | | | |
| 0-6 mo | 60* | ND | 31* | 4.4* | 0.5* | 9.1* |
| 7-12 mo | 95* | ND | 30* | 4.6* | 0.5* | **13.5** |
| Children | | | | | | |
| 1-3 y | **130** | 19* | ND | 7* | 0.7* | **13** |
| 4-8 y | **130** | 25* | ND | 10* | 0.9* | **19** |
| Males | | | | | | |
| 9-13 y | **130** | 31* | ND | 12* | 1.2* | **34** |
| 14-18 y | **130** | 38* | ND | 16* | 1.6* | **52** |
| 19-30 y | **130** | 38* | ND | 17* | 1.6* | **56** |
| 31-50 y | **130** | 38* | ND | 17* | 1.6* | **56** |
| 51-70 y | **130** | 30* | ND | 14* | 1.6* | **56** |
| >70 y | **130** | 30* | ND | 14* | 1.6* | **56** |
| Females | | | | | | |
| 9-13 y | **130** | 26* | ND | 10* | 1.0* | **34** |
| 14-18 y | **130** | 26* | ND | 11* | 1.1* | **46** |
| 19-30 y | **130** | 25* | ND | 12* | 1.1* | **46** |
| 31-50 y | **130** | 25* | ND | 12* | 1.1* | **46** |
| 51-70 y | **130** | 21* | ND | 11* | 1.1* | **46** |
| >70 y | **130** | 21* | ND | 11* | 1.1* | **46** |
| Pregnancy | | | | | | |
| 14-18 y | **175** | 28* | ND | 13* | 1.4* | **71** |
| 19-30 y | **175** | 28* | ND | 13* | 1.4* | **71** |
| 31-50 y | **175** | 28* | ND | 13* | 1.4* | **71** |
| Lactation | | | | | | |
| 14-18 | **210** | 29* | ND | 13* | 1.3* | **71** |
| 19-30 y | **210** | 29* | ND | 13* | 1.3* | **71** |
| 31-50 y | **210** | 29* | ND | 13* | 1.3* | **71** |

NOTE: This table presents Recommended Dietary Allowances (RDAs) in **bold type** and Adequate Intakes (AIs) in ordinary type followed by an asterisk (*). RDAs and AIs may both be used as goals for individual intake. RDAs are set to meet the needs of almost all (97 to 98 percent) individuals in a group. For healthy breastfed infants, the AI is the mean intake. The AI for other life stage and gender groups is believed to cover needs of all individuals in the group, but lack of data or uncertainty in the data prevent being able to specify with confidence the percentage of individuals covered by this intake.

[a]Based on 0.8g protein/kg body weight for reference body weight.

SOURCE: Dietary Reference Intakes for Energy, Carbohydrate, Fiber, Fat, Fatty Acids, Cholesterol, Protein, and Amino Acids (2002). This report may be accessed via www.nap.edu. See also http://www.health.gov/dietaryguidelines/dga2005/report/HTML/D1_Tables.htm and Appendix 7(7-10 and 7–11, pp. 470-471).

**1–3** Dietary Reference Intakes (DRIs): Tolerable Upper Intake Levels (UL[a]), Vitamins Food and Nutrition Board, Institute of Medicine, National Academies

| Life Stage Group | Vitamin A (μg/d)[b] | Vitamin C (mg/d) | Vitamin D (μg/d) | Vitamin E (mg/d)[c,d] | Vitamin K | Thiamin | Riboflavin | Niacin (mg/d)[d] | Vitamin $B_6$ (mg/d) | Folate (μg/d)[d] | Vitamin $B_{12}$ | Pantothenic Acid | Biotin | Choline (g/d) | Carotenoids[e] |
|---|---|---|---|---|---|---|---|---|---|---|---|---|---|---|---|
| **Infants** | | | | | | | | | | | | | | | |
| 0-6 mo | 600 | ND[f] | 25 | ND | ND | ND | ND | ND | ND | ND | ND | ND | ND | ND | ND |
| 7-12 mo | 600 | ND | 25 | ND | ND | ND | ND | ND | ND | ND | ND | ND | ND | ND | ND |
| **Children** | | | | | | | | | | | | | | | |
| 1-3 y | 600 | 400 | 50 | 200 | ND | ND | ND | 10 | 30 | 300 | ND | ND | ND | 1.0 | ND |
| 4-8 y | 900 | 650 | 50 | 300 | ND | ND | ND | 15 | 40 | 400 | ND | ND | ND | 1.0 | ND |
| **Males, Females** | | | | | | | | | | | | | | | |
| 9-13 y | 1,700 | 1,200 | 50 | 600 | ND | ND | ND | 20 | 60 | 600 | ND | ND | ND | 2.0 | ND |
| 14-18 y | 2,800 | 1,800 | 50 | 800 | ND | ND | ND | 30 | 80 | 800 | ND | ND | ND | 3.0 | ND |
| 19-70 y | 3,000 | 2,000 | 50 | 1,000 | ND | ND | ND | 35 | 100 | 1,000 | ND | ND | ND | 3.5 | ND |
| >70 y | 3,000 | 2,000 | 50 | 1,000 | ND | ND | ND | 35 | 100 | 1,000 | ND | ND | ND | 3.5 | ND |
| **Pregnancy** | | | | | | | | | | | | | | | |
| ≤18 y | 2,800 | 1,800 | 50 | 800 | ND | ND | ND | 30 | 80 | 800 | ND | ND | ND | 3.0 | ND |
| 19-50 y | 3,000 | 2,000 | 50 | 1,000 | ND | ND | ND | 35 | 100 | 1,000 | ND | ND | ND | 3.5 | ND |
| **Lactation** | | | | | | | | | | | | | | | |
| ≤18 y | 2,800 | 1,800 | 50 | 800 | ND | ND | ND | 30 | 80 | 800 | ND | ND | ND | 3.0 | ND |
| 19-50 y | 3,000 | 2,000 | 50 | 1,000 | ND | ND | ND | 35 | 100 | 1,000 | ND | ND | ND | 3.5 | ND |

[a]UL=The maximum level of daily nutrient intake that is likely to pose no risk of adverse effects. Unless otherwise specified, the UL represents total intake from food, water, and supplements. Due to lack of suitable data, ULs could not be established for vitamin K, thiamin, riboflavin, vitamin $B_{12}$, pantothenic acid, biotin, or carotenoids. In the absence of ULs, extra caution may be warranted in consuming levels above recommended intakes.

[b]As preformed vitamin A only.

[c]As α-tocopherol; applies to any form of supplemental α-tocopherol.

[d]The ULs for vitamin E, niacin, and folate apply to synthetic forms obtained from supplements, fortified foods, or a combination of the two.

[e]β-Carotene supplements are advised only to serve as a provitamin A source for individuals at risk of vitamin A deficiency.

[f]ND=Not determinable due to lack of data of adverse effects in this age group and concern with regard to lack of ability to handle excess amounts. Source of intake should be from food only to prevent high levels of intake.

SOURCES: Dietary Reference Intakes for Calcium, Phosphorus, Magnesium, Vitamin D, and Fluoride (1997); Dietary Reference Intakes for Thiamin, Riboflavin, Niacin, Vitamin $B_6$, Folate, Vitamin $B_{12}$, Pantothenic Acid, Biotin, and Choline (1998); Dietary Reference Intakes for Vitamin C, Vitamin E, Selenium, and Carotenoids (2000); and Dietary Reference Intakes for Vitamin A, Vitamin K, Arsenic, Boron, Chromium, Copper, Iodine, Iron, Manganese, Molybdenum, Nickel, Silicon, Vanadium, and Zinc (2001). These reports may be accessed via www.nap.edu.

**1–3** (Continued)

| Life Stage Group | Arsenic[b] | Boron (mg/d) | Calcium (g/d) | Chromium | Copper (μg/d) | Fluoride (mg/d) | Iodine (μg/d) | Iron (mg/d) | Magnesium (mg/d)[c] | Manganese (mg/d) | Molybdenum (μg/d) | Nickel (mg/d) | Phosphorus (g/d) | Selenium (μg/d) | Silicon[d] | Vanadium (mg/d)[e] | Zinc (mg/d) |
|---|---|---|---|---|---|---|---|---|---|---|---|---|---|---|---|---|---|
| Infants | | | | | | | | | | | | | | | | | |
| 0-6 mo | ND[f] | ND | ND | ND | ND | 0.7 | ND | 40 | ND | ND | ND | ND | ND | 45 | ND | ND | 4 |
| 7-12 mo | ND | ND | ND | ND | ND | 0.9 | ND | 40 | ND | ND | ND | ND | ND | 60 | ND | ND | 5 |
| Children | | | | | | | | | | | | | | | | | |
| 1-3 y | ND | 3 | 2.5 | ND | 1,000 | 1.3 | 200 | 40 | 65 | 2 | 300 | 0.2 | 3 | 90 | ND | ND | 7 |
| 4-8 y | ND | 6 | 2.5 | ND | 3,000 | 2.2 | 300 | 40 | 110 | 3 | 600 | 0.3 | 3 | 150 | ND | ND | 12 |
| Males, Females | | | | | | | | | | | | | | | | | |
| 9-13 y | ND | 11 | 2.5 | ND | 5,000 | 10 | 600 | 40 | 350 | 6 | 1,100 | 0.6 | 4 | 280 | ND | ND | 23 |
| 14-18 y | ND | 17 | 2.5 | ND | 8,000 | 10 | 900 | 45 | 350 | 9 | 1,700 | 1.0 | 4 | 400 | ND | ND | 34 |
| 19-70 y | ND | 20 | 2.5 | ND | 10,000 | 10 | 1,100 | 45 | 350 | 11 | 2,000 | 1.0 | 4 | 400 | ND | 1.8 | 40 |
| >70 y | ND | 20 | 2.5 | ND | 10,000 | 10 | 1,100 | 45 | 350 | 11 | 2,000 | 1.0 | 3 | 400 | ND | 1.8 | 40 |
| Pregnancy | | | | | | | | | | | | | | | | | |
| ≤18 y | ND | 17 | 2.5 | ND | 8,000 | 10 | 900 | 45 | 350 | 9 | 1,700 | 1.0 | 3.5 | 400 | ND | ND | 34 |
| 19-50 y | ND | 20 | 2.5 | ND | 10,000 | 10 | 1,100 | 45 | 350 | 11 | 2,000 | 1.0 | 3.5 | 400 | ND | ND | 40 |
| Lactation | | | | | | | | | | | | | | | | | |
| ≤18 y | ND | 17 | 2.5 | ND | 8,000 | 10 | 900 | 45 | 350 | 9 | 1,700 | 1.0 | 4 | 400 | ND | ND | 34 |
| 19-50 y | ND | 20 | 2.5 | ND | 10,000 | 10 | 1,100 | 45 | 350 | 11 | 2,000 | 1.0 | 4 | 400 | ND | ND | 40 |

[a]UL=The maximum level of daily nutrient intake that is likely to pose no risk of adverse effects. Unless otherwise specified, the UL represents total intake from food, water, and supplements. Due to lack of suitable data, ULs could not be established for arsenic, chromium, and silicon. In the absence of ULs, extra caution may be warranted in consuming levels above recommended intakes.
[b]Although the UL was not determined for arsenic, there is no justification for adding arsenic to food or supplements.
[c]The ULs for magnesium represent intake from a pharmacological agent only and do not include intake from food and water.
[d]Although silicon has not been shown to cause adverse effects in humans, there is no justification for adding silicon to supplements.
[e]Although vanadium in food has not been shown to cause adverse effects in humans, there is no justification for adding vanadium to food and vanadium supplements should be used with caution. The UL is based on adverse effects in laboratory animals and this data could be used to set a UL for adults but not children and adolescents.
[f]ND=Not determinable due to lack of data of adverse effects in this age group and concern with regard to lack of ability to handle excess amounts. Source of intake should be from food only to prevent high levels of intake.
SOURCES: Dietary Reference Intakes for Calcium, Phosphorus, Magnesium, Vitamin D, and Fluoride (1997); Dietary Reference Intakes for Thiamin, Riboflavin, Niacin, Vitamin $B_6$, Folate, Vitamin $B_{12}$, Pantothenic Acid, Biotin, and Choline (1998); Dietary Reference Intakes for Vitamin C, Vitamin E, Selenium, and Carotenoids (2000); and Dietary Reference Intakes for Vitamin A, Vitamin K, Arsenic, Boron, Chromium, Copper, Iodine, Iron, Manganese, Molybdenum, Nickel, Silicon, Vanadium, and Zinc (2001). These reports may be accessed via www.nap.edu.

**1–4** Dietary Reference Intake Values for Energy: Estimated Energy Requirement (EER) Equations and Values for Active Individuals by Life Stage Group

| *Life Stage Group* | *EER Prediction Equation* | *EER for Active Physical Activity Level (kcal/day)*[a] Male | Female |
|---|---|---|---|
| 0 - 3 mo | EER = (89 x weight of infant in kg - 100) + 175 | 538 | 493 (2 mo)[c] |
| 4 - 6 mo | EER = (89 x weight of infant in kg - 100) + 56 | 606 | 543 (5 mo)[c] |
| 7 - 12 mo | EER = (89 x weight of infant in kg - 100) + 22 | 743 | 676 (9 mo)[c] |
| 1 - 2 y | EER = (89 x weight of infant in kg - 100) + 20 | 1046 | 992 (2 y)[c] |
| 3 - 9 y | | | |
| male | EER = 88.5 - (61.9 x Age in yrs) + PA[b] [26.7 x Weight in kg) + (903 x Height in m)] + 20 | 1742 (6 y)[c] | |
| female | EER = 135.3 - (30.8 x Age in yrs) + PA[b] [10.0 x Weight in kg) + (934 x Height in m)] +20 | | 1642 (6 y)[c] |
| 9 - 19 y | | | |
| male | EER = 88.5 - (61.9 x Age in yrs) + PA[b] [26.7 x Weight in kg) + (903 x Height in m)] + 25 | 2279 (11 y)[c] 3152 (16 y)[c] | |
| female | EER = 135.3 - (30.8 x Age in yrs) + PA[b] [10.0 x Weight in kg) + (934 x Height in m)] +25 | 2071 (11 y)[c] | 2368 (16 y)[c] |
| 3 - 19 y | | | |
| male overweight | TEE = −114 − 50.9 × Age (y) + PA(19.5 × Wt + 1161.4 × Ht) | | |
| female overweight | TEE = 389 − 41.2 × Age (y) + PA × (15.0 × Wt + 701 × Ht) | | |
| ≥ 19 y | | | |
| male | EER = 662 - (9.53 x Age in yrs) + PA[b] [15.91 x Weight in kg) + (539.6 x Height in m)] | 3067 (19 y)[c] | |
| female | EER = 354 - (6.91 x Age in yrs) + PA[b] [9.36 x Weight in kg) + (726 x Height in m)] | | 2403 (19 y)[c] |
| *Pregnancy* | | | |
| 14 - 19 y | | | |
| 1st trimester | Adolescent EER + 0 | | 2368 (16 y)[c] |
| 2nd trimester | Adolescent EER + 340 kcal | | 2708 (16 y)[c] |
| 3rd trimester | Adolescent EER + 452 kcal | | 2820 (16 y)[c] |
| 19 - 50 y | | | |
| 1st trimester | Adult EER + 0 | | 2403 (19 y)[c] |
| 2nd trimester | Adult EER + 340 kcal | | 2743 (19 y)[c] |
| 3rd trimester | Adult EER + 452 kcal | | 2855 (19 y)[c] |
| *Lactation* | | | |
| 14 - 18 y | | | |
| 1st 6 mo | Adolescent EER + 330 kcal | | 2698 (16 y)[c] |
| 2nd 6 mo | Adolescent EER + 400 kcal | | 2768 (16 y)[c] |
| 19 - 50 y | | | |
| 1st 6 mo | Adult EER + 330 kcal | | 2733 (19 y)[c] |
| 2nd 6 mo | Adult EER + 400 kcal | | 2803 (19 y)[c] |

[a] The intake that meets the average energy expenditure of individuals at a reference height, weight and age.
[b] See table entitled "PA Values for Different Physical Activity Levels" to determine the PA value for a specific age, gender, and activity level.
[c] Value is calculated for an individual at the age in parentheses.

**PA Values for Different Physical Activity Levels (Used to Calculate EER)**

| *Age/Gender* | *Sedentary* | | *Low-Active* | | *Active* | | *Very Active* | |
|---|---|---|---|---|---|---|---|---|
| Normal weight(NW) Over weight(OW) | N.W. | (OW) | N.W. | (OW) | N.W. | (OW) | N.W. | (OW) |
| 3 to 19 years | | | | | | | | |
| Boys | 1.00 | (1.00) | 1.13 | (1.12) | 1.26 | (1.24) | 1.42 | (1.45) |
| Girls | 1.00 | (1.00) | 1.16 | (1.18) | 1.31 | (1.35) | 1.56 | (1.60) |
| ≥ 19 years | | | | | | | | |
| Men | 1.00 | | 1.11 | | 1.25 | | 1.48 | |
| Women | 1.00 | | 1.12 | | 1.27 | | 1.45 | |

# Dietary Reference Intakes: Water, Potassium, Sodium, Chloride Sulfate

**Project:** Dietary Reference Intakes for Electrolytes and Water
**Published On:** February 11, 2004 (**Press Release)**

The Food and Nutrition Board released the sixth in a series of reports presenting dietary reference values for the intake of nutrients by Americans and Canadians. This new report establishes nutrient recommendations on water, salt and potassium to maintain health and reduce chronic disease risk. Highlights of the report include:

- The vast majority of health people adequately meet their daily hydration needs by letting thirst be their guide. The report did not specify exact requirements for water, but set general recommendations for women at approximately 2.7 liters (91 ounces) of total water – from all beverages and foods – each day, and men an average of approximately 3.7 liters (125 ounces daily) of total water. The panel did not set an upper level for water.

- About 80 percent of people's total water intake comes from drinking water and beverages – including caffeinated beverages – and the other 20 percent is derived from food.

- Prolonged physical activity and heat exposure will increase water losses and therefore may raise daily fluid needs, although it is important to note that excessive amounts can be life-threatening.

- Healthy 19-to 50-year old adults should consume 1.5 grams of sodium and 2.3 grams of chloride each day – or 3.8 grams of salt – to replace the amount lost daily on average through sweat and to achieve a diet that provides sufficient amounts of other essential nutrients.

- The tolerable upper intake level (UL) for salt is set at 5.8 grams per day. More than 95 percent of American men and 90 percent of Canadian men ages 31 to 50, and 75 percent of American women and 50 percent of Canadian women in this age range regularly consume salt in excess of the UL.

- Older individuals, African Americans, and people with chronic diseases including hypertension, diabetes, and kidney disease are especially sensitive to the blood pressure-raising effects of salt and should consume less than the UL.

- Adults should consume at least 4.7 grams of potassium per day to lower blood pressure, blunt the effects of salt, and reduce the risk of kidney stones and bone loss. However, most American women 31 to 50 years old consume no more than half of the recommended amount of potassium, and men's intake is only moderately higher.

- There is no evidence of chronic excess intakes of potassium in apparently health individuals and thus no UL was established.

1–6 Calorie Equivalent of Activities—Minutes Required at the Exercises Listed to Expend Calories in the Foods (154 lb person)

| FOOD | CALORIES | ACTIVITY | | | | |
|---|---|---|---|---|---|---|
| | | Walking<br>Minutes | Stepping<br>Minutes | Bicycling<br>Minutes | Jogging<br>Minutes | Swimming<br>Minutes |
| Apple, 1 medium | 87 | 17 | 12 | 11 | 9 | 8 |
| Banana, 1 medium | 127 | 24 | 17 | 16 | 13 | 11 |
| Beans, green, ½ cup, cooked | 15 | 3 | 2 | 2 | 2 | 1 |
| Beer, 8-ounce glass | 115 | 22 | 15 | 14 | 12 | 10 |
| Bread and butter, 1 slice | 96 | 18 | 13 | 12 | 10 | 9 |
| Cake, white layer, 1/16 of 9" cake | 250 | 48 | 33 | 31 | 25 | 22 |
| Carrot, raw, 1 large | 42 | 8 | 6 | 5 | 4 | 4 |
| Cereal, dry, 1 cup, with milk and sugar | 212 | 41 | 28 | 26 | 21 | 19 |
| Cheese, American, 1-ounce slice | 112 | 22 | 15 | 14 | 11 | 10 |
| Cheese, cottage, 1 rounded tablespoon | 30 | 6 | 4 | 4 | 3 | 3 |
| Chicken, fried, ½ breast | 232 | 45 | 31 | 28 | 23 | 21 |
| Chicken, TV dinner | 542 | 104 | 72 | 66 | 54 | 48 |
| Cola beverage, 8-ounce glass | 105 | 20 | 14 | 13 | 11 | 9 |
| Cookie, chocolate-chip, 1 average | 50 | 10 | 7 | 6 | 5 | 5 |
| Cookie, vanilla-wafer, 1 average | 15 | 3 | 2 | 2 | 2 | 1 |
| Doughnut, 1 average | 125 | 24 | 17 | 15 | 13 | 11 |
| Egg, boiled or poached, 1 medium | 78 | 15 | 10 | 10 | 8 | 7 |
| Egg, fried or scrambled, 1 medium | 108 | 21 | 14 | 13 | 11 | 10 |
| French dressing, 1 tablespoon | 57 | 11 | 8 | 7 | 6 | 5 |
| Halibut, broiled, 1 serving | 214 | 41 | 28 | 26 | 21 | 19 |
| Ham, fresh, 2 slices cooked | 254 | 49 | 34 | 31 | 25 | 23 |
| Ice cream, 2/3 cup | 186 | 36 | 25 | 23 | 19 | 17 |
| Ice milk, 2/3 cup | 137 | 26 | 18 | 17 | 14 | 12 |
| Malted milk, 8-ounce glass | 500 | 96 | 67 | 61 | 50 | 45 |
| Mayonnaise, 1 tablespoon | 100 | 19 | 13 | 12 | 10 | 9 |
| Milk, skim, 8-ounce glass | 88 | 17 | 12 | 11 | 9 | 8 |
| Milk, whole, 8-ounce glass | 160 | 36 | 21 | 20 | 16 | 14 |
| Milkshake, 8-ounce glass | 420 | 81 | 56 | 51 | 42 | 38 |
| Orange, 1 medium | 73 | 14 | 10 | 9 | 7 | 7 |
| Orange juice, 4-ounce glass | 54 | 10 | 7 | 7 | 5 | 5 |
| Pancake, 1, with 2 tablespoons syrup | 204 | 39 | 27 | 25 | 20 | 18 |
| Peach, 1 medium | 38 | 7 | 5 | 5 | 4 | 3 |
| Peach shortcake, 1 biscuit and 1 peach | 266 | 51 | 35 | 32 | 27 | 24 |
| Peas, green, ½ cup cooked | 58 | 11 | 8 | 7 | 6 | 5 |
| Pie, fruit, ½ cf of 9" pie | 400 | 77 | 53 | 49 | 40 | 36 |
| Pie, pecan, 1/6 of 9" pie | 670 | 129 | 89 | 82 | 67 | 60 |
| Pizza, cheese, 1/8 of 14" pie | 185 | 36 | 25 | 23 | 19 | 17 |
| Pork chop, 6 ounces raw | 314 | 60 | 42 | 38 | 31 | 28 |
| Potato chips, five 2" chips | 54 | 10 | 7 | 7 | 5 | 5 |
| Sandwiches: Club (bacon, chicken, tomato) | 590 | 114 | 78 | 72 | 59 | 53 |
| Hamburger | 350 | 67 | 47 | 43 | 35 | 31 |
| Roast beef with gravy | 430 | 83 | 57 | 52 | 43 | 38 |
| Tuna Salad | 278 | 54 | 37 | 34 | 28 | 25 |
| Sherbet, orange, 2/3 cup | 120 | 23 | 16 | 15 | 12 | 11 |
| Shrimp, French-fried, 3 ½ ounces | 225 | 43 | 30 | 27 | 23 | 20 |
| Spaghetti, meat sauce, 1 serving | 396 | 76 | 53 | 48 | 40 | 35 |
| Steak, T-bone, ½ pound raw | 235 | 45 | 31 | 29 | 24 | 21 |

WALKING briskly at 3.5 to 4 miles per hour on the average consumes 5.2 calories per minute. STEPPING 25 up and down steps per minute facing in the same direction consumes an average of 7.5 calories per minute. BICYLING consumes around 9.2 calories per minute. JOGGING alternated with walking (5 minutes each jogging, walking, jogging, etc.) consumes around 10 calories per minute. SWIMMING with average skill consumes approximately 11.2 calories per minute.

# PROXIMATE COMPOSITION OF GROUND SPICES, PER TEASPOON

| Spice | Wt./tsp. | Water | Food Energy | Protein | Fat | Total Carbohydrate | Fiber Carbohydrate | Ash | Calcium | Phosphorus | Sodium | Potassium | Iron | Thiamine | Riboflavin | Niacin | Ascorbic Acid | Vitamin A Activity |
|---|---|---|---|---|---|---|---|---|---|---|---|---|---|---|---|---|---|---|
| | Grams | Mg. | Cal. | Mg. | Mg. | Mg. | Mg. | Mg. | Mg. | Mg. | Mg. | Mg. | Mcg. | Mcg. | Mcg. | Mcg. | Mcg. | Int'l Units |
| Allspice | 1.7 | 150 | 6 | 102 | 112 | 1265 | 367 | 71 | 13.6 | 1.9 | 1.4 | 18.7 | 127 | 1.7 | 1.0 | 49 | 666 | 9 |
| Basil Leaves | 1.1 | 70 | 3 | 131 | 40 | 679 | 225 | 184 | 23.1 | 5.2 | 0.4 | 40.7 | 471 | 1.6 | 3.5 | 76 | 674 | 165 |
| Bay Leaves | 1.3 | 60 | 5 | 99 | 114 | 980 | 328 | 48 | 13.0 | 1.4 | 0.3 | 7.8 | 693 | 1.3 | 5.5 | 26 | 606 | 80 |
| Caraway Seed | 1.8 | 110 | 8 | 385 | 416 | 783 | 187 | 101 | 12.6 | 9.0 | 0.4 | 34.0 | 153 | 6.8 | 6.8 | 146 | N | 6 |
| Cardamom Seed | 1.8 | 150 | 6 | 176 | 52 | 1336 | 178 | 85 | 5.4 | 3.8 | 0.2 | 21.6 | 209 | 3.2 | 4.1 | 41 | N | N |
| Celery Seed | 2.4 | 120 | 11 | 434 | 547 | 1051 | 310 | 245 | 43.2 | 13.2 | 4.1 | 33.6 | 1078 | 9.8 | 11.8 | 106 | 413 | 1 |
| Cinnamon | 1.7 | 170 | 6 | 78 | 37 | 1357 | 345 | 59 | 27.2 | 0.8 | 0.2 | 6.8 | 70 | 2.4 | 3.6 | 32 | 677 | 4 |
| Cloves | 1.7 | 90 | 7 | 107 | 247 | 1170 | 189 | 85 | 1.9 | 1.9 | 4.2 | 20.4 | 161 | 1.9 | N | 5 | 1375 | 9 |
| Coriander Seed | 1.4 | 90 | 6 | 172 | 274 | 791 | 441 | 74 | 11.2 | 6.2 | 0.3 | 16.8 | 83 | 3.6 | 3.2 | 45 | N | N |
| Cumin Seed | 1.6 | 100 | 7 | 283 | 381 | 714 | 146 | 123 | 14.4 | 7.2 | 2.6 | 33.6 | 765 | 11.7 | 6.1 | 40 | 275 | 20 |
| Dill Seed | 2.1 | 140 | 9 | 275 | 376 | 1184 | 435 | 126 | 33.6 | 4.4 | 0.2 | 23.1 | 248 | 8.8 | 5.9 | 59 | N | 1 |
| Fennel Seed | 2.1 | 130 | 8 | 199 | 210 | 1277 | 388 | 281 | 27.3 | 10.1 | 1.9 | 35.7 | 233 | 8.6 | 7.6 | 126 | N | 3 |
| Garlic Powder | 1.5 | 80 | 5 | 262 | 9 | 1099 | 28 | 48 | 1.5 | 6.3 | 0.1 | 16.5 | 52 | 10.2 | 1.2 | 10 | N | N |
| Ginger | 1.6 | 110 | 6 | 138 | 102 | 1158 | 94 | 91 | 1.6 | 2.4 | 0.5 | 22.4 | 181 | 0.8 | 2.1 | 30 | N | 2 |
| Mace | 1.8 | 80 | 10 | 146 | 698 | 830 | 86 | 41 | 3.6 | 2.0 | 1.3 | 9.0 | 203 | 6.7 | 10.1 | 22 | N | 14 |
| Marjoram | 1.2 | 80 | 4 | 150 | 82 | 773 | 200 | 116 | 30.0 | 2.8 | 1.3 | 16.8 | 872 | 3.5 | 3.8 | 49 | 618 | 97 |
| Mustard Powder | 1.5 | 50 | 9 | 475 | 639 | 277 | 28 | 60 | 4.5 | 11.8 | 0.1 | 10.5 | 124 | 9.7 | 6.7 | 127 | 331 | 1 |
| Nutmeg | 1.9 | 80 | 11 | 141 | 739 | 899 | 59 | 38 | 3.8 | 3.8 | 0.2 | 7.6 | 42 | 6.8 | 4.7 | 179 | N | 2 |
| Onion Powder | 2.1 | 100 | 8 | 223 | 17 | 1690 | 134 | 73 | 6.3 | 6.1 | 0.8 | 21.0 | 46 | 8.8 | 1.3 | 12 | 309 | N |
| Oregano | 1.6 | 130 | 6 | 187 | 102 | 1038 | 176 | 144 | 27.2 | 3.2 | 0.3 | 27.2 | 853 | 5.4 | N | 99 | N | 110 |
| Paprika | 1.9 | 150 | 7 | 262 | 198 | 1146 | 365 | 144 | 3.8 | 5.7 | 0.4 | 45.6 | 439 | 11.4 | 25.8 | 291 | 1117 | 1100 |
| Parsley Flakes | 1.1 | 40 | 4 | 241 | 62 | 597 | 96 | 155 | 13.2 | 3.4 | 5.9 | 39.6 | 159 | 1.9 | 13.5 | 87 | 4312 | 256 |
| Pepper, Black | 2.3 | 190 | 9 | 239 | 235 | 1529 | 230 | 106 | 9.2 | 3.7 | 0.2 | 27.6 | 391 | 1.6 | 4.8 | 18 | N | 4 |
| Pepper, Chili | 2.1 | 140 | 9 | 294 | 296 | 1222 | 328 | 151 | 2.1 | 6.7 | 0.2 | 44.1 | 208 | 12.4 | 34.9 | 298 | 1338 | 1090 |
| Pepper, Red | 2.1 | 130 | 9 | 336 | 325 | 1140 | 546 | 168 | 2.1 | 6.7 | 0.2 | 44.1 | 208 | 10.9 | 19.5 | 286 | 617 | 659 |
| Pepper, White | 2.2 | 210 | 9 | 273 | 176 | 1518 | 99 | 22 | 4.4 | 3.3 | 0.2 | 2.2 | 152 | 0.4 | 2.9 | 4 | N | N |
| Poppy Seed | 2.5 | 90 | 13 | 577 | 887 | 755 | 217 | 187 | 40.0 | 22.0 | 0.2 | 20.0 | 247 | 17.2 | 4.5 | 22 | N | N |
| Rosemary Leaves | 1.2 | 70 | 5 | 54 | 209 | 777 | 228 | 72 | 18.0 | 0.8 | 0.5 | 12.0 | 396 | 6.1 | N | 12 | 736 | 37 |
| Sage | 1.0 | 50 | 4 | 92 | 127 | 561 | 144 | 69 | 16.2 | 0.8 | 0.1 | 9.0 | 246 | 6.7 | 3.1 | 51 | 358 | 53 |
| Savory | 1.4 | 130 | 5 | 99 | 73 | 979 | 214 | 122 | 30.8 | 2.0 | 0.3 | 15.4 | 529 | 5.2 | N | 57 | N | 71 |
| Sesame Seed | 1.9 | 60 | 9 | 450 | 426 | 895 | 716 | 68 | 1.9 | 15.0 | 0.6 | 7.6 | 118 | 15.2 | 2.5 | 108 | N | 1 |
| Tarragon | 1.4 | 60 | 5 | 339 | 102 | 721 | 95 | 172 | 18.2 | 4.3 | 1.0 | 44.8 | 500 | 3.5 | 18.8 | 125 | N | 59 |
| Thyme | 1.5 | 110 | 5 | 102 | 69 | 1024 | 364 | 198 | 31.0 | 3.0 | 1.2 | 14.1 | 2025 | 7.6 | 6.0 | 74 | N | 57 |
| Turmeric | 1.9 | 110 | 7 | 163 | 169 | 1328 | 131 | 129 | 3.8 | 4.9 | 0.2 | 47.5 | 902 | 1.7 | 3.6 | 91 | 946 | N |

Research Committee American Spice Trade Assn; 580 Slyvan Ave, Englewood Cliffs, NJ 07632.

**1–8** The Dietary Approach to Stop Hypertension (Dash) Diet—Rich in Low-Fat Foods, Fruits, Vegetables, and Dairy Foods

| **Food Group** | **Daily Servings** | **1 Serving Equals** |
|---|---|---|
| Milk and Dairy | 2-3 | 8 oz. low fat milk<br>1 cup low fat yogurt<br>1½ oz. low fat cheese |
| Fruits | 4 | 1 medium fruit<br>¼ cup dried fruit<br>½ cup fresh, frozen, or canned fruit<br>6 oz. fruit juice |
| Vegetables | 3-4 | 1 cup raw leafy vegetables<br>½ cup cooked vegetables<br>6 oz. vegetable juice |
| Grain (whole) | 6 | 1 slice ww bread<br>½ cup of dry or hot cereal<br>½ cup cooked rice or pasta |
| Meat, Fish or Poultry | 1–2 | 3 oz cooked meat, poultry or fish<br>(lean, broiled, roasted, baked, no skin) |
| Nuts, Seeds, Dried Beans | 3 week | 1/3 cup nuts<br>2 tbsp seeds<br>½ cup cooked dried beans (legumes) |

Based on 1600 calarie/day diet with two added servings of fat and oil. Reduce soduim to about 1500 mg or less/per day (e.g., limit condiments, processed foods, soy sauce, broth). Diet is rich in calcuim, magnisuim, potasuim, fiber, and protein.
From: National Institutes of Health: www.nhlbi.nib.gov/health/public/heart/hbp/dash/new_dash.pdf

**1–9** Antioxidant Scores for Common Fruits and Vegetables*

| Item | Antioxidant Score |
|---|---|
| Garlic | 23.2 |
| Kale | 24.1 |
| Spinach | 17.0 |
| Brussels sprouts | 15.8 |
| Alfalfa spouts | 14.5 |
| Broccoli flowers | 12.9 |
| Beets | 11.7 |
| Red bell pepper | 8.1 |
| Onion | 5.6 |
| Corn | 7.2 |
| Eggplant | 5.1 |
| Cauliflower | 5.1 |
| Potato | 4.6 |
| Sweet potato | 4.3 |
| Cabbage | 4.8 |
| Leaf lettuce | 4.1 |
| String beans | 3.9 |
| Carrot | 3.4 |
| Yellow squash | 2.8 |
| Iceberg lettuce | 2.3 |
| Celery | 1.1 |
| Cucumber | 1.1 |

Adapted from Cao G, Sofic E, Prior RL. Antioxidant capacity of tea and common vegetables. *J Agric Food Chem.* 1996; 44(11): 3427, Table 1.

*Other antioxidants in foods have been published by the National Institutes of Health, such as the fruits blueberries, red grapes, elderberries, red wine, green tea, and so on.

# APPENDIX 2

## Growth Grids for Special Conditions

**2–1** Down Syndrome Growth Chart, Boys, Birth–36 Months

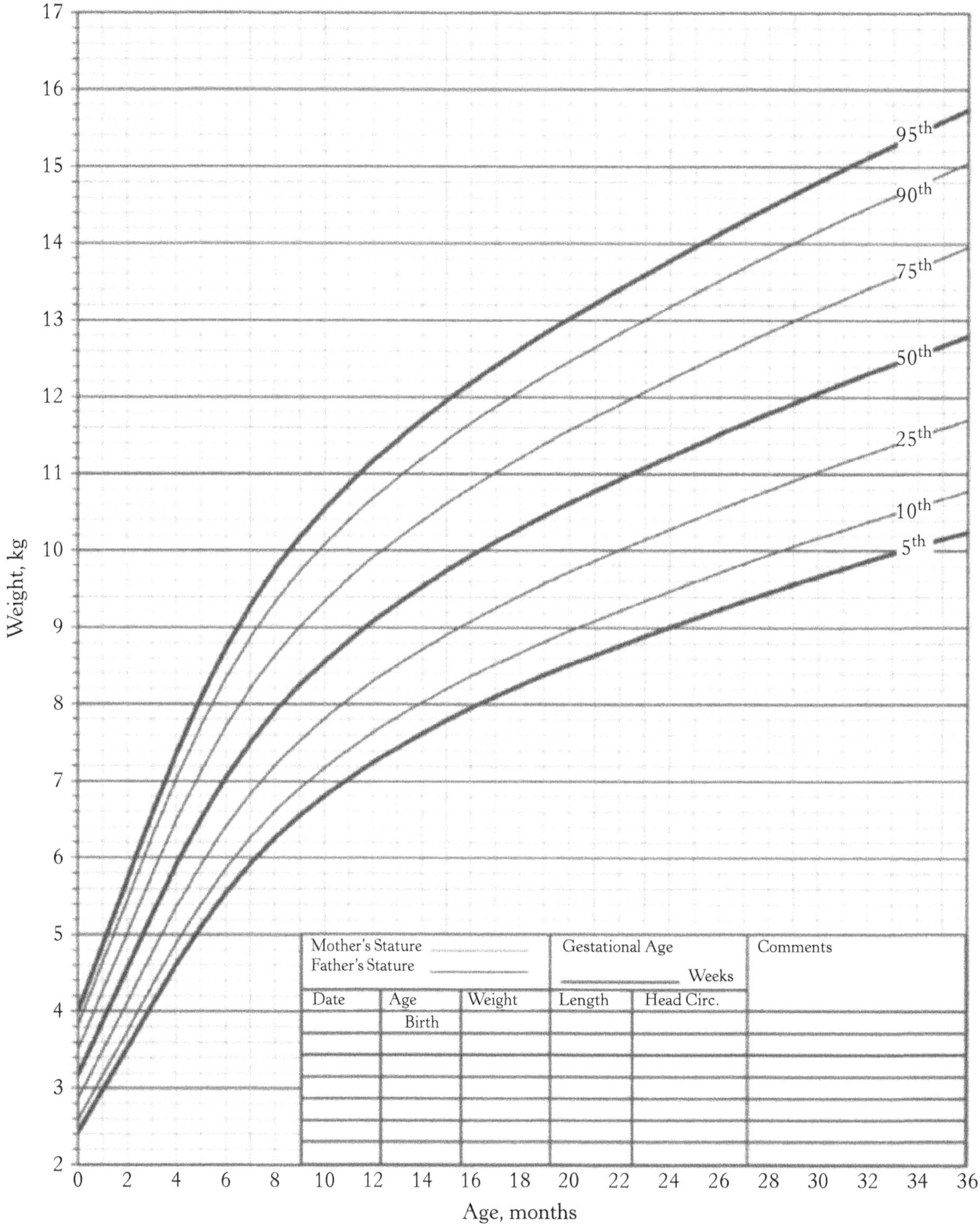


Published October 2015.
Source: Zemel BS, Pipan M, Stallings VA, Hall W, Schgadt K, Freedman DS, Thorpe P. Growth Charts for Children with Down Syndrome in the U.S. Pediatrics, 2015.

**2–2** Down Syndrome Growth Chart, Girls, Birth–36 Months

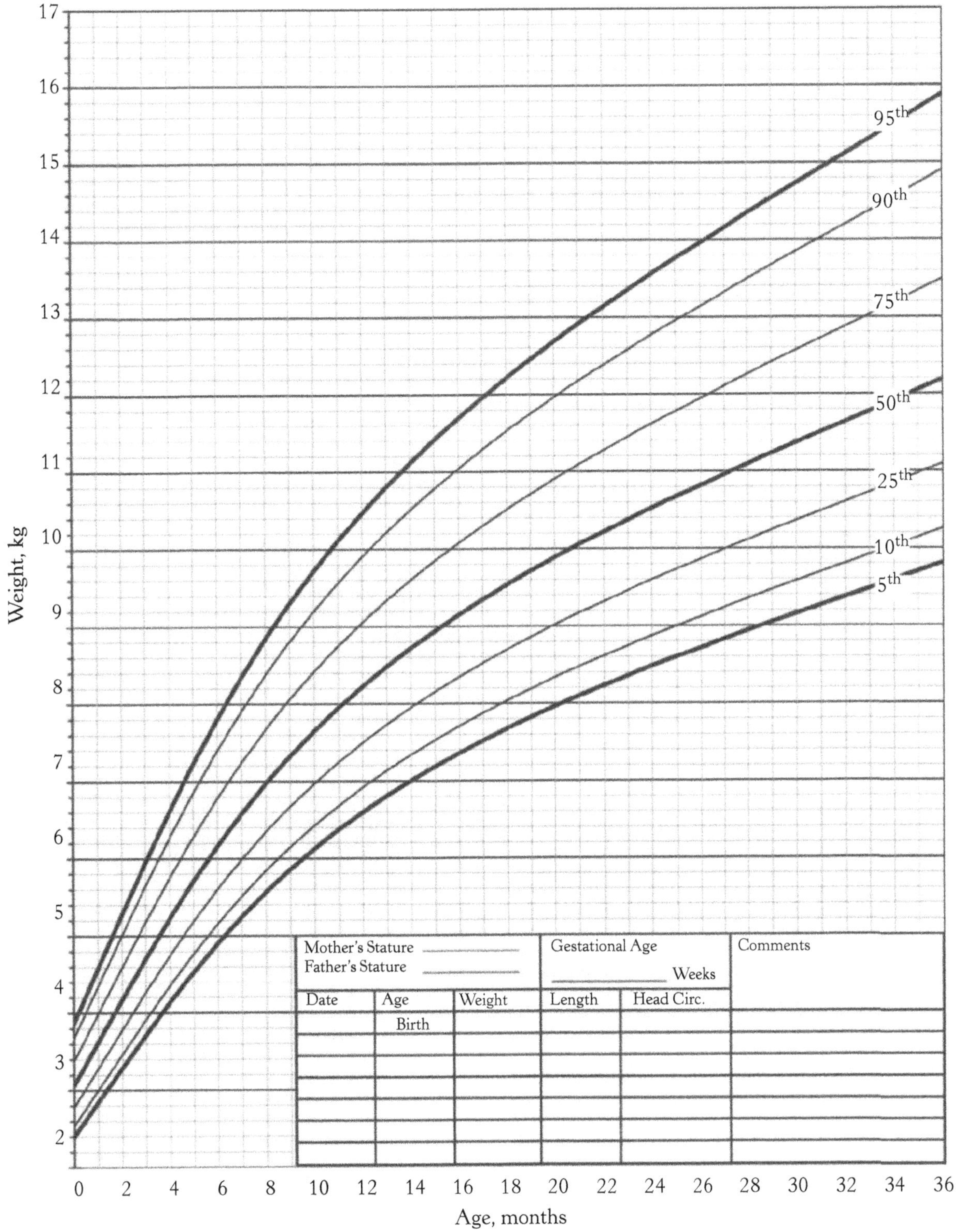


Published October 2015.
Source: Zemel BS, Pipan M, Stallings VA, Hall W, Schgadt K, Freedman DS, Thorpe P. Growth Charts for Children with Down Syndrome in the U.S. Pediatrics, 2015.

**2–3** Down Syndrome Growth Chart, Boys, 2–20 Years

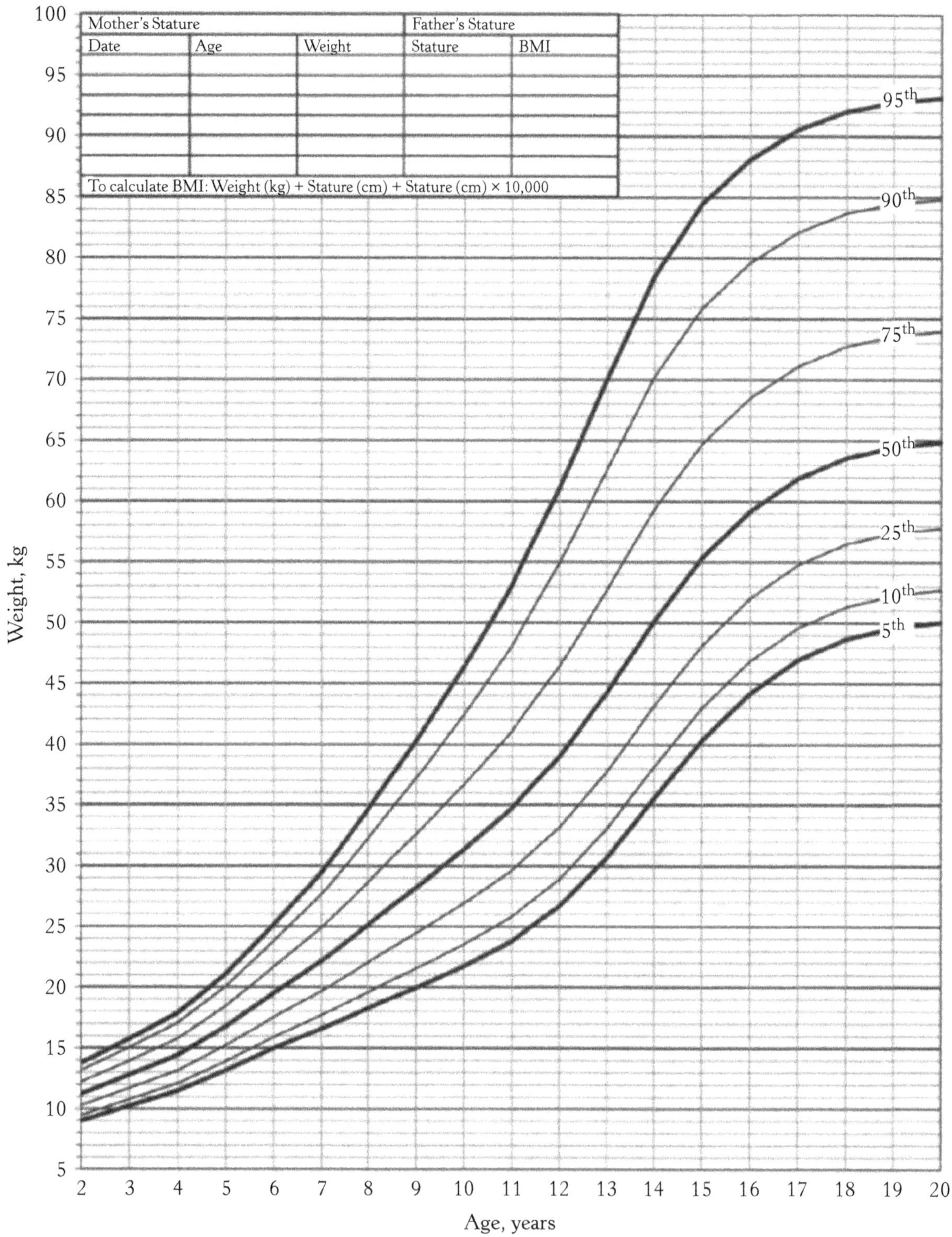


Published October 2015.
Source: Zemel BS, Pipan M, Stallings VA, Hall W, Schgadt K, Freedman DS, Thorpe P. Growth Charts for Children with Down Syndrome in the U.S. Pediatrics, 2015.

**2–4** Down Syndrome Growth Chart, Girls, 2–20 Years

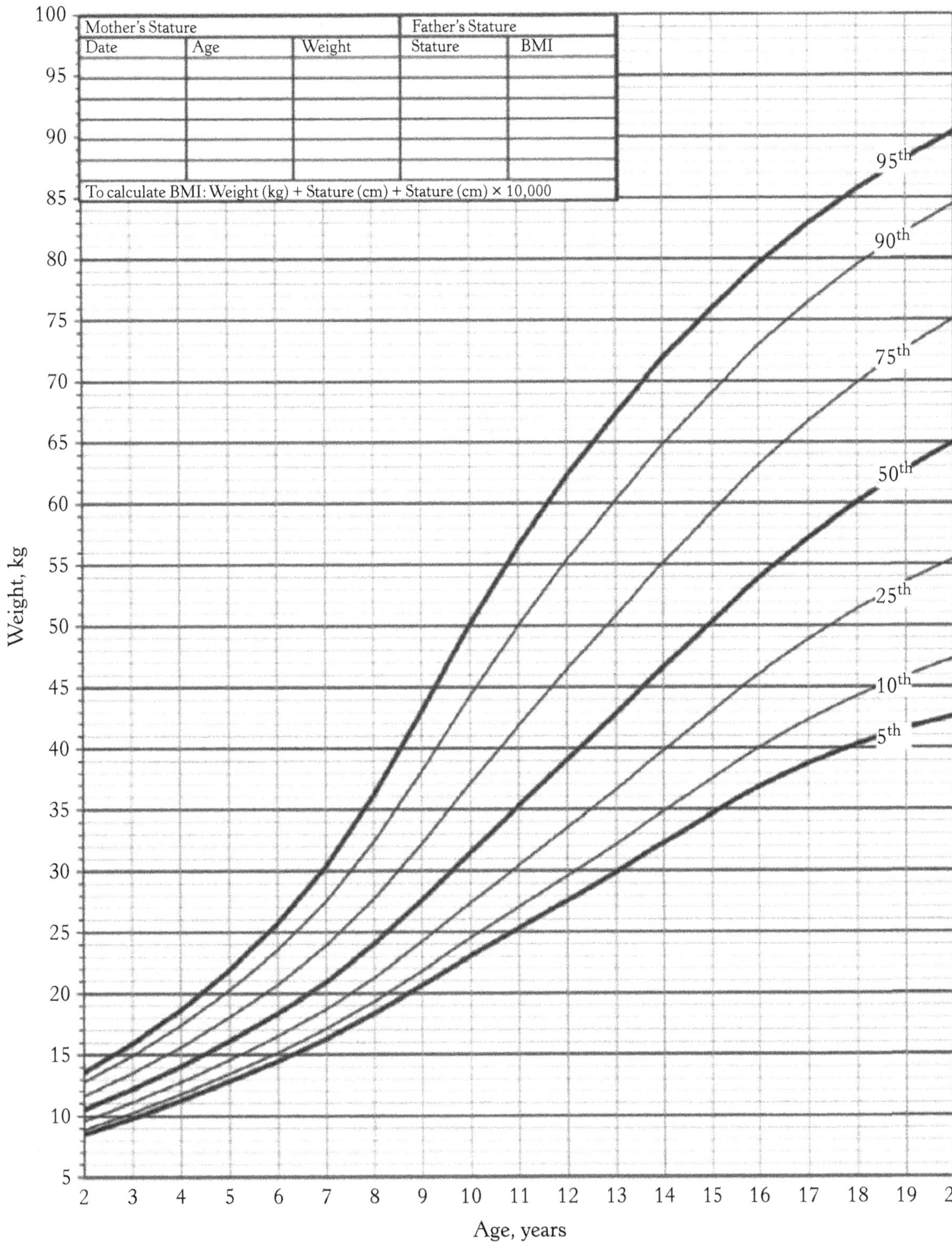


Published October 2015.
Source: Zemel BS, Pipan M, Stallings VA, Hall W, Schgadt K, Freedman DS, Thorpe P. Growth Charts for Children with Down Syndrome in the U.S. Pediatrics, 2015.

**2–5** Myelomeningocele Growth Chart, Length and Weight, 0–20 Years, Boys

## Myelomeningocele Growth Chart on Length, 0 to 20 years

**(1900 MM males)**

Myelomeningocele as ____ and CDC for normal as - - - -

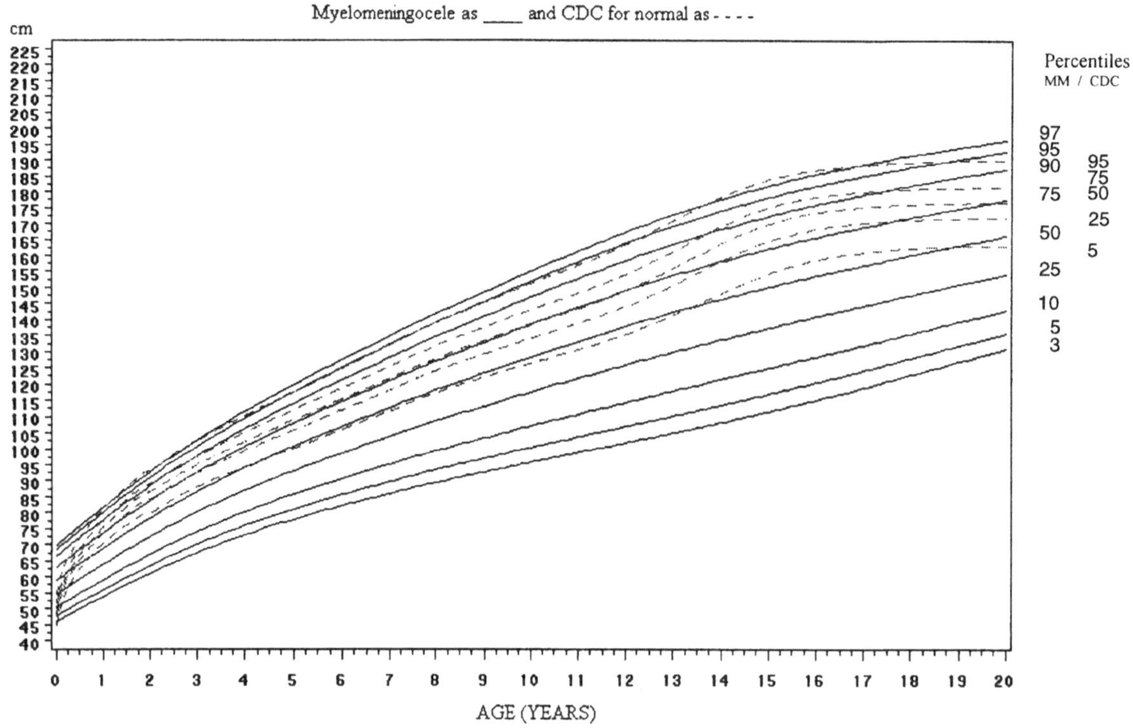


## Myelomeningocele Growth Chart on Weight, 0 to 20 years

**(1900 MM males)**

Myelomeningocele as ____ and CDC for normal as - - - -

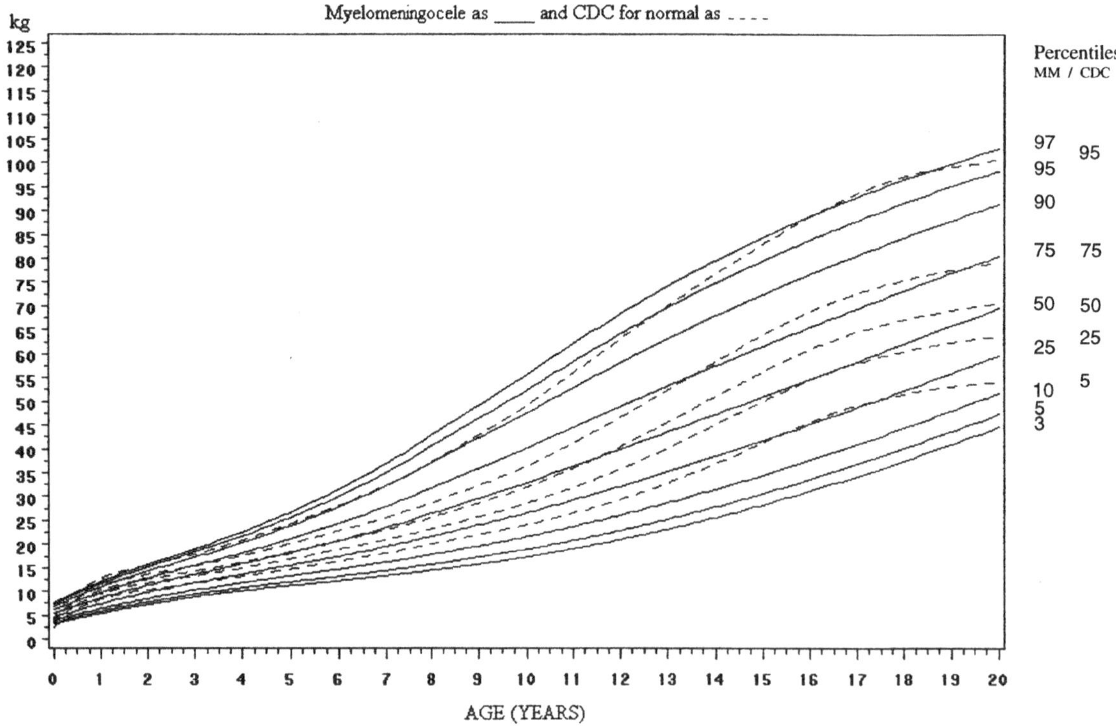


Ekvall, S., Ekvall, V., Beck, C., Leonti, G., Bigley, B., Schwiegerhat, L., Horn, P., Jiang, D. Growth charts for myelomeningocele, 2004.

**2–6** Myelomeningocele Growth Chart, Length and Weight, 0–20 Years, Girls

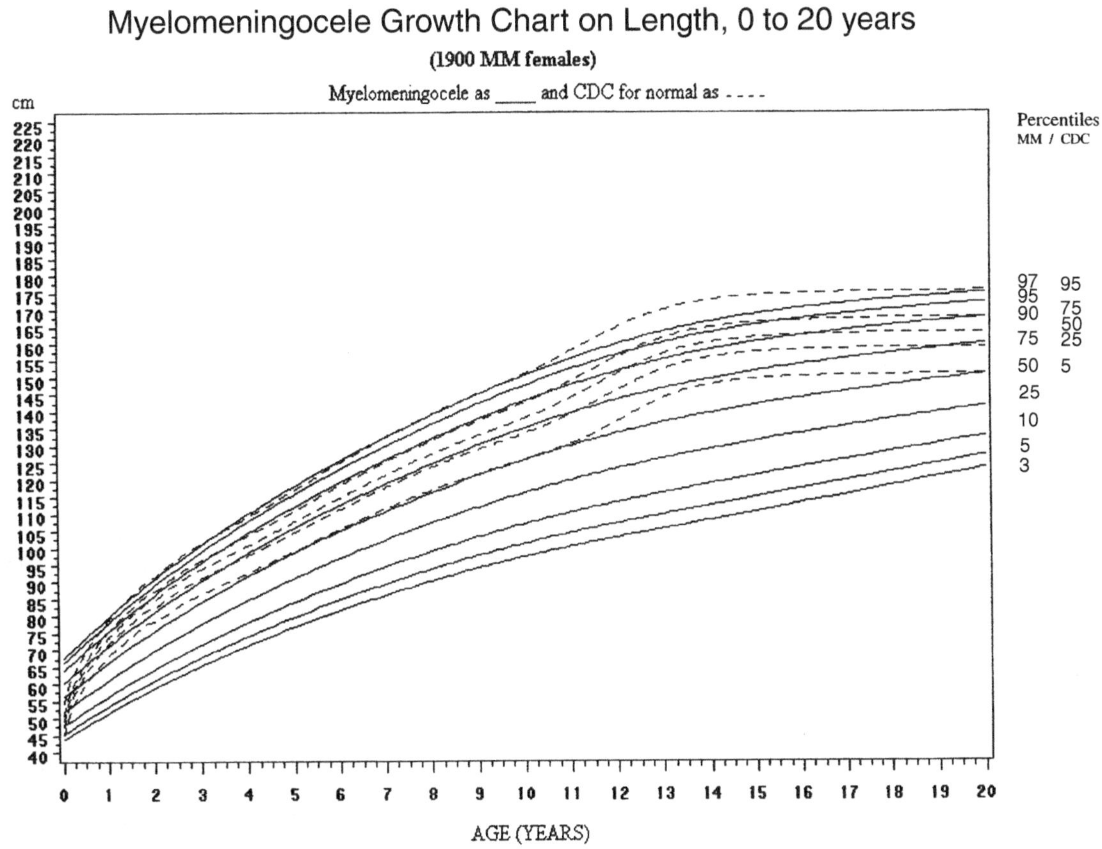


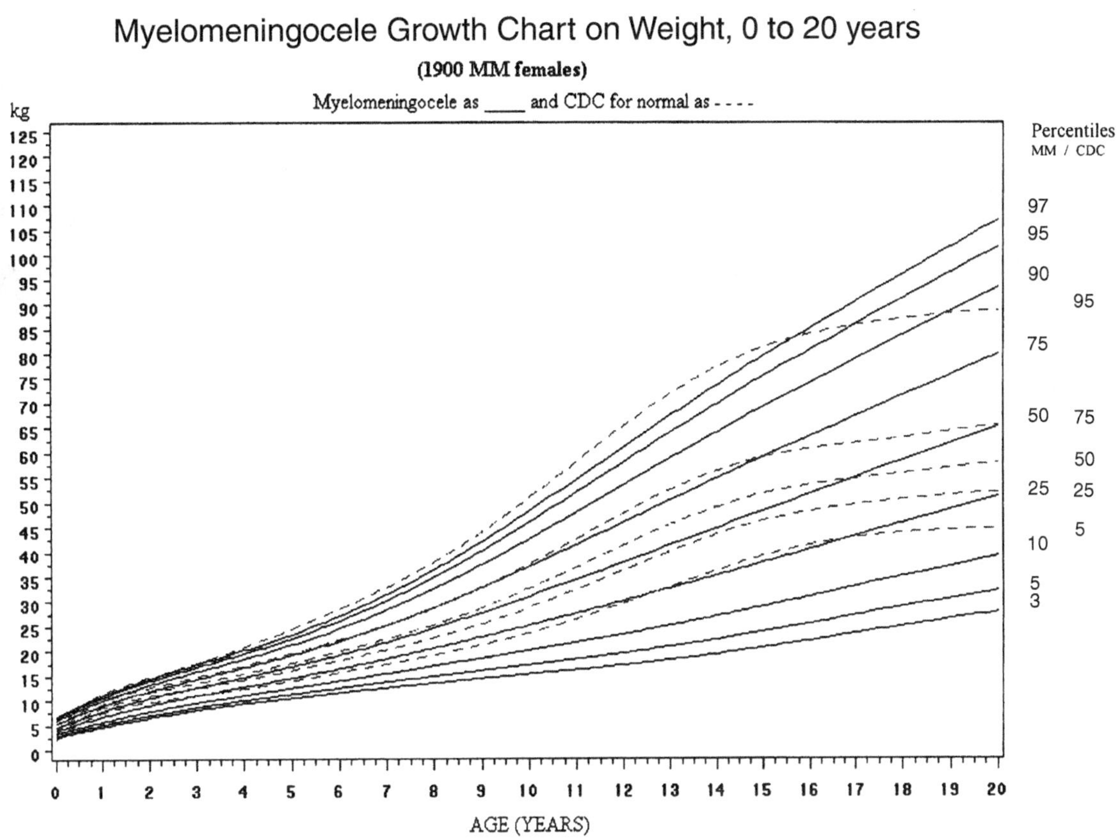


Ekvall, S., Ekvall, V., Beck, C., Leonti, G., Bigley, B., Schwiegerhat, L., Horn, P., Jiang, D. Growth charts for myelomeningocele, 2004.

## 2–7 Weight Charts for Boys with Cerebral Palsy, GMFCS Level I–V, Orally-Fed and Tube-Fed

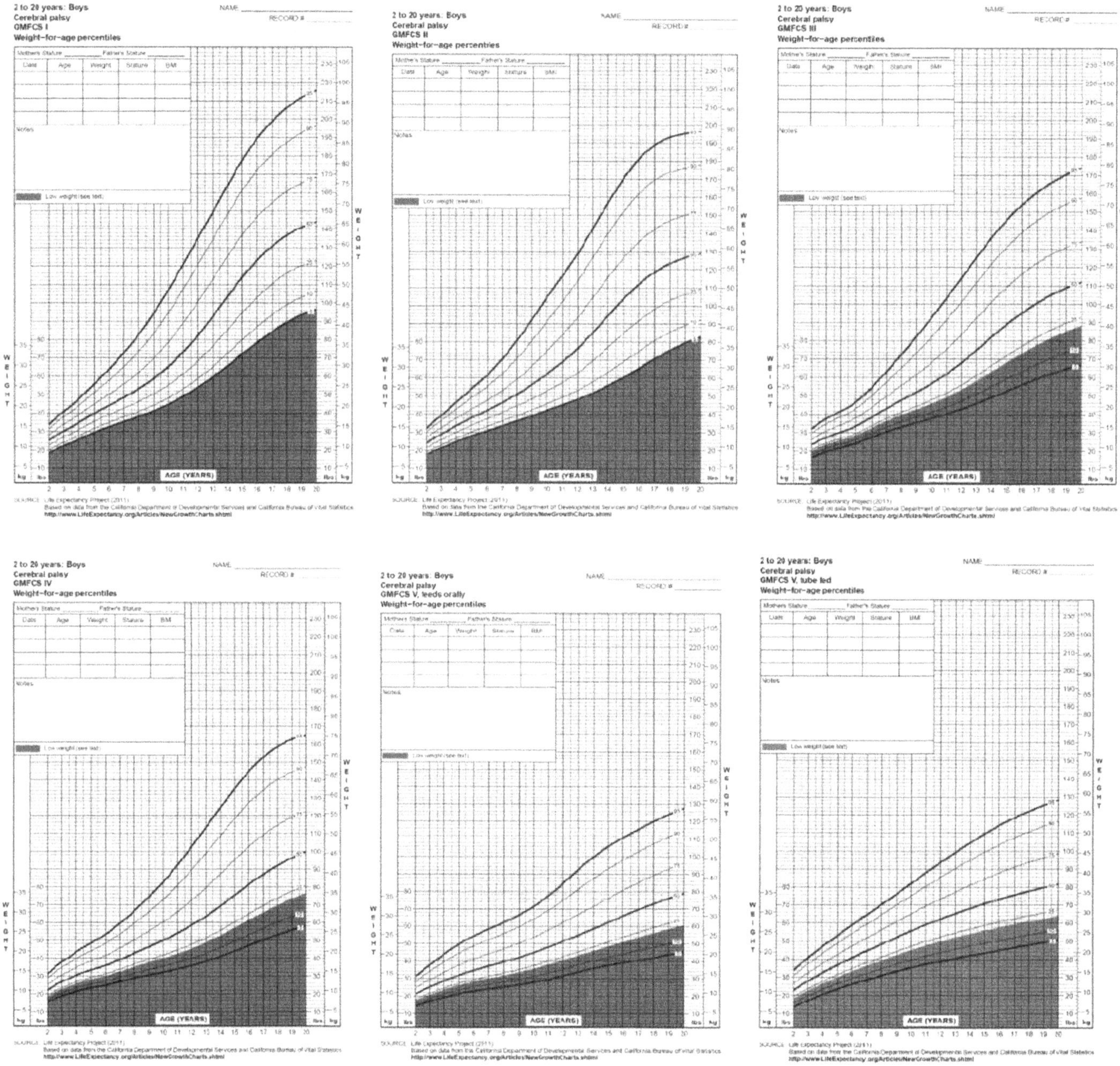


Brooks J, Day SM, Shavelle RM, Strauss DJ (2011). Low weight, morbidity, and mortality in children with cerebral palsy: New clinical growth charts. Pediatrics, 128; e299; originally published online July 18, 2011 (DOI 10.1542/peds.2010-2801).
http://www.lifeexpectancy.org/articles/NewGrowthCharts.shtml accessed May 13, 2015

**2–8** Weight Charts for Girls with Cerebral Palsy, GMFCS Level I–V, Orally-Fed and Tube-Fed

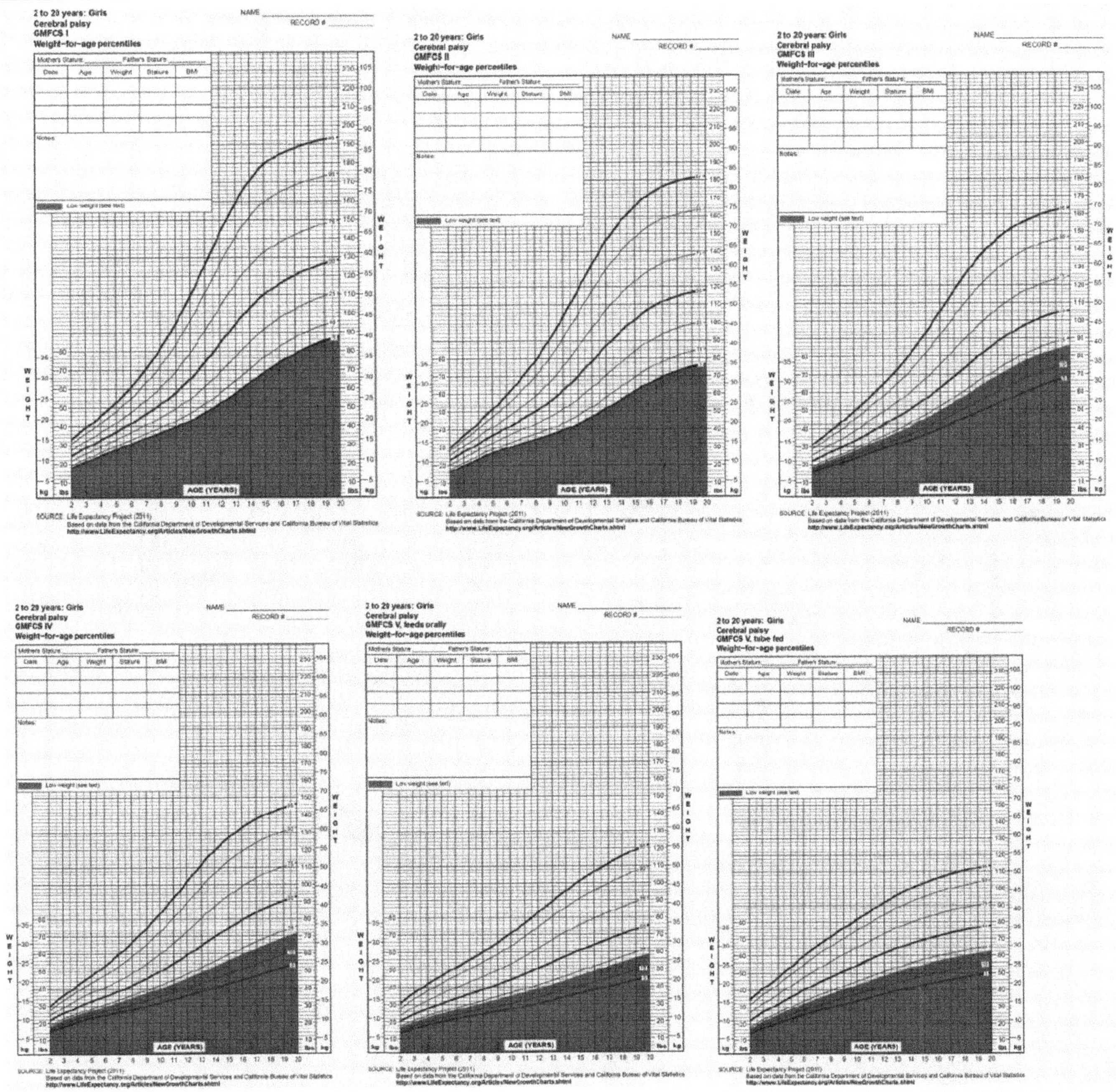


Brooks J, Day SM, Shavelle RM, Strauss DJ (2011). Low weight, morbidity, and mortality in children with cerebral palsy: New clinical growth charts. Pediatrics, 128; e299; originally published online July 18, 2011 (DOI 10.1542/peds.2010-2801).
http://www.lifeexpectancy.org/articles/NewGrowthCharts.shtml accessed May 13, 2015

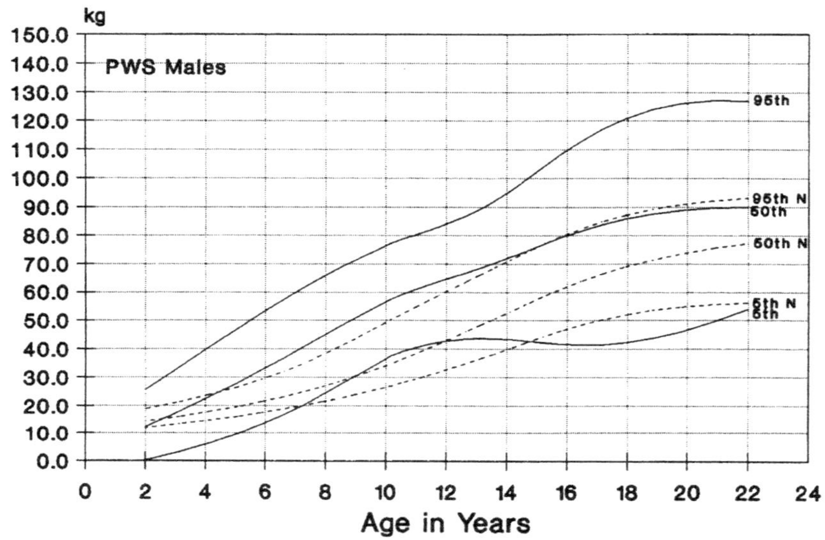


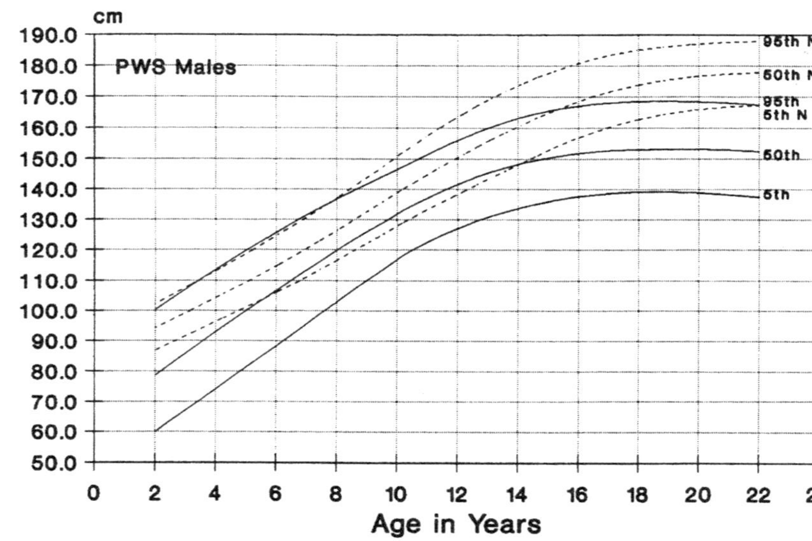


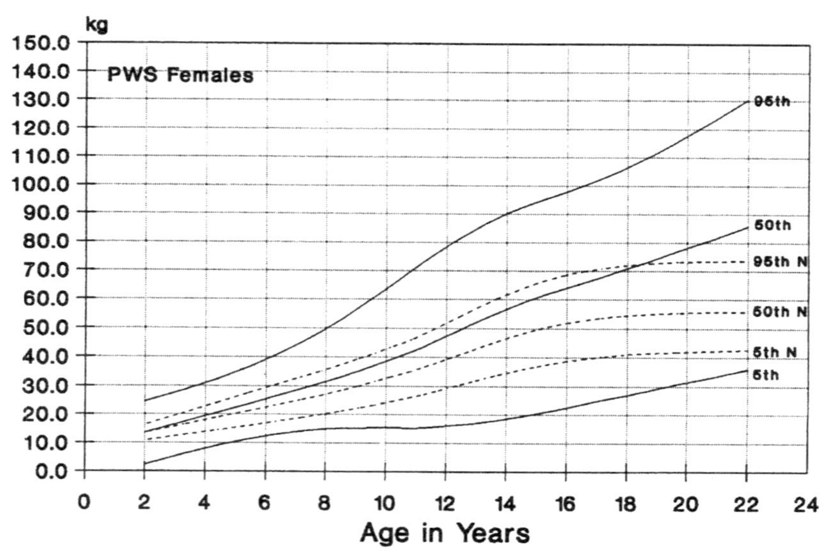


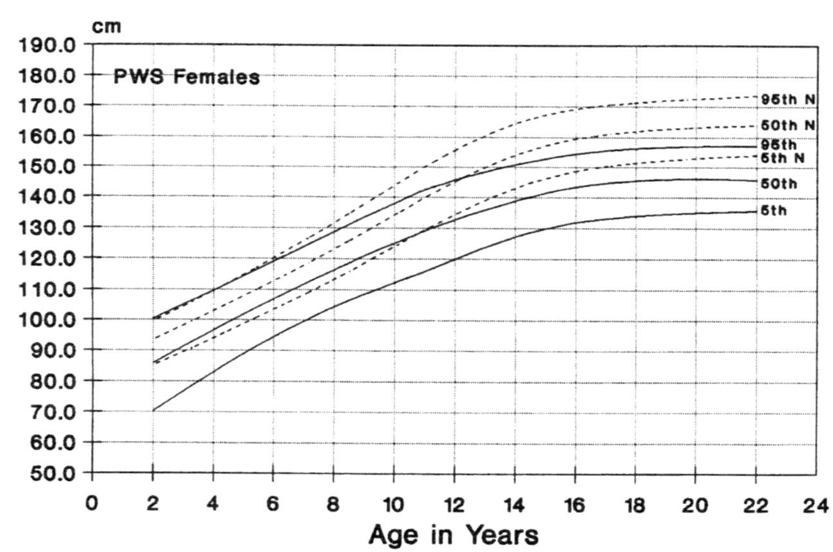


Butler, M.G., Meaney, F.J., Weight, height, sitting height, head circumference, triceps, and subscapular skinfold (plus other measures) for age 2 to 22 years. *Pediatrics* 1991;88(4):853.

**2–10** Rubinstein-Taybi Growth Chart, Boys and Girls, 2–18 Years

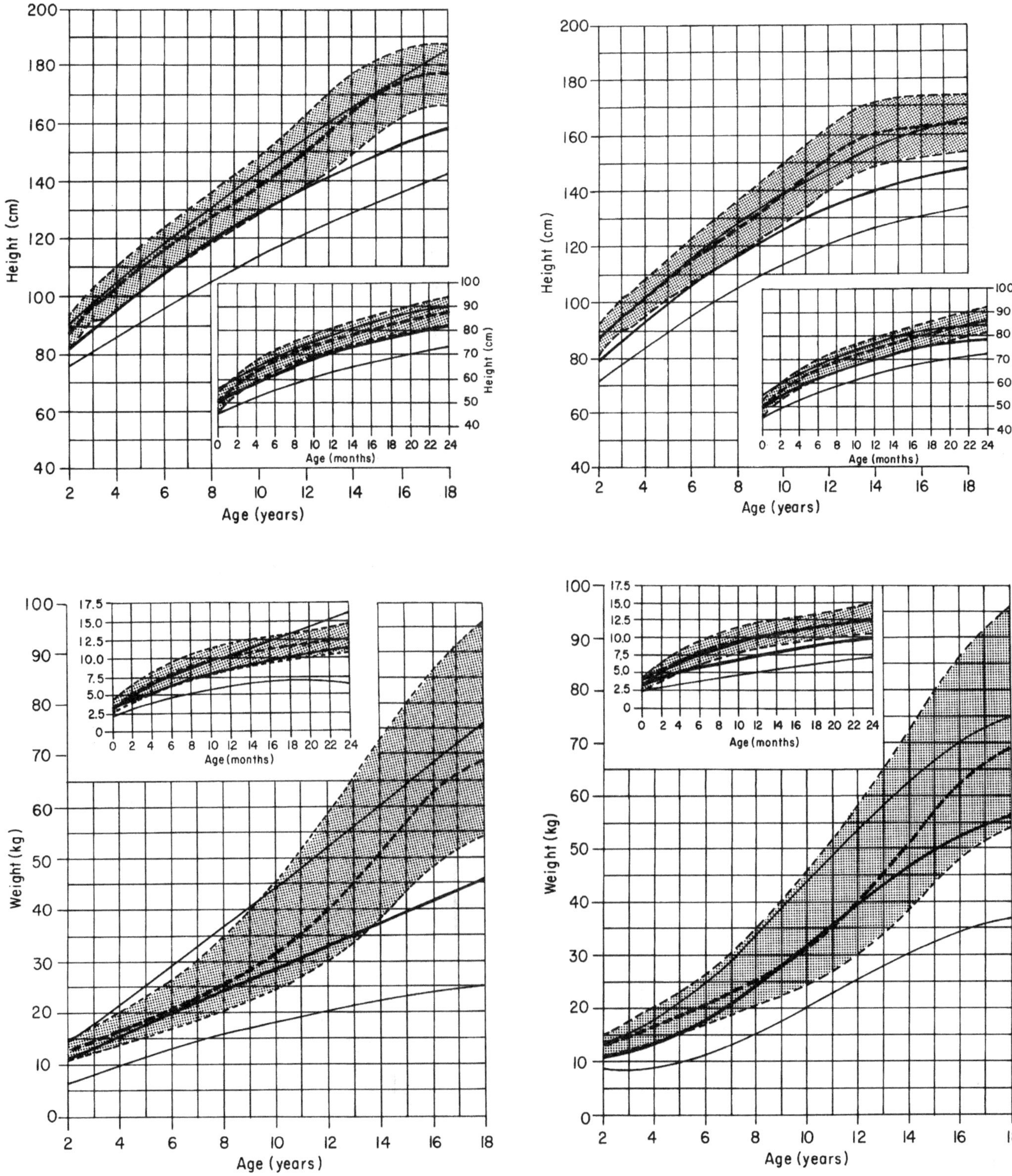


Stevens, C.A., Hennekam, R.C.M., Blackburn, B.L. Growth in the Rubinstein-Taybi syndrome. *Am. J. Med. Genet.* 1990;6:51.

**2–11** Sickle Cell Anemia Growth Chart, Boys and Girls, 2–18 Years

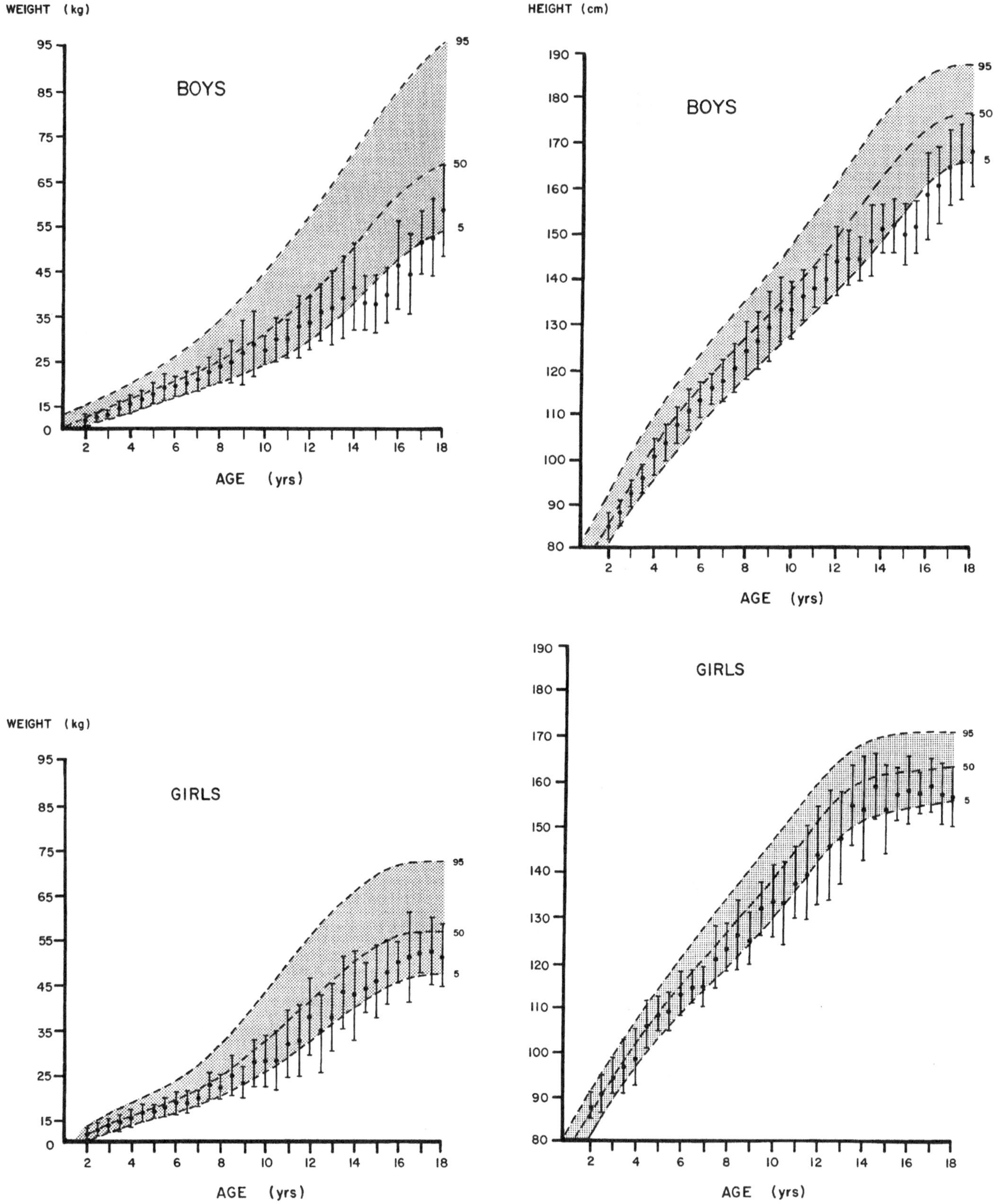


Phebus, C.K., Gloninger, M.F., Maciak, B.J. Height and weight for age birth to 18 years. *J. Pediatr.* 1985:107.

**2–12** Turner Syndrome Growth Chart, Height, Girls, 2–19 Years

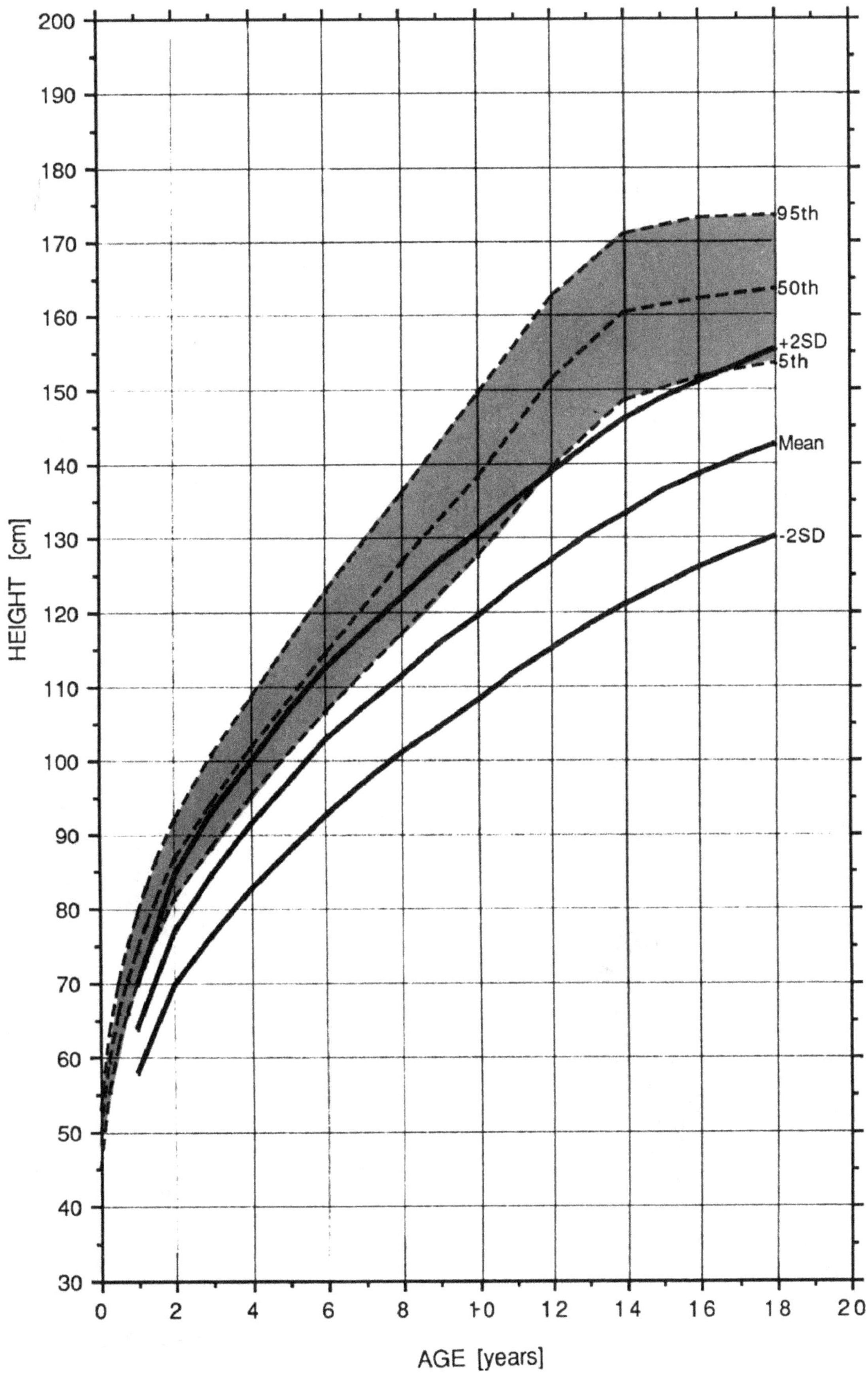


Lyon, A.J., Peece, M.A., Grant, D.B. Height for age birth to 18 years (girls). *Arch. Dis. Child.* 1985;60:932.

## 2–13 Williams Syndrome Growth Chart, Boys and Girls, 0–20 Years

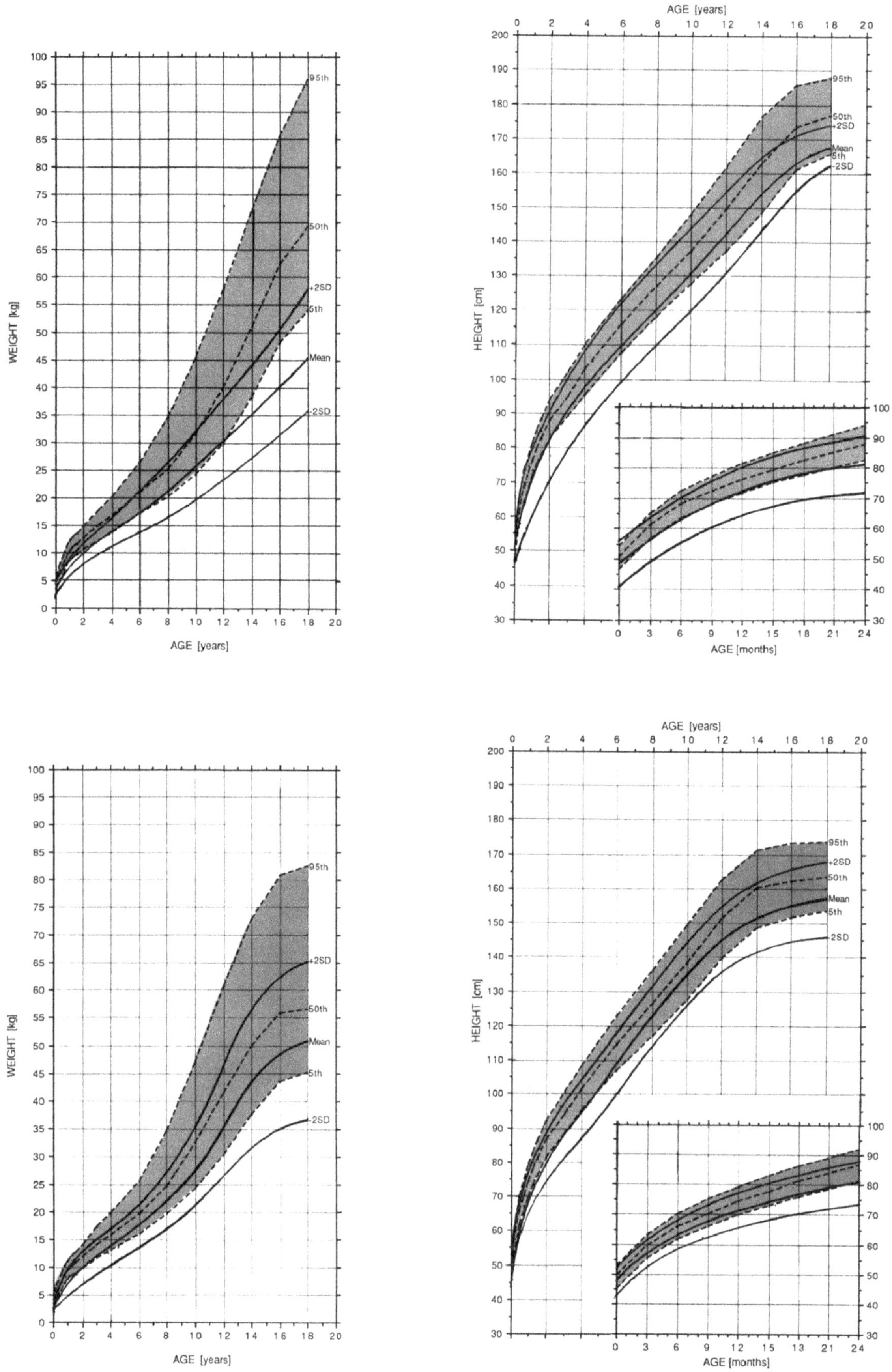


Morris, C.A., Demsey, S.A., Leonard, C.O., Dilts C., Blackburn, B.L. Stature for age birth to 24 months and birth to 18 years, weight for age birth to 18 years, and head circumference for age birth to 36 months and 2 to 18 years. *J Pediatr.* 1988;113:318.

**2–14** Noonan Syndrome Growth Chart, Boys and Girls

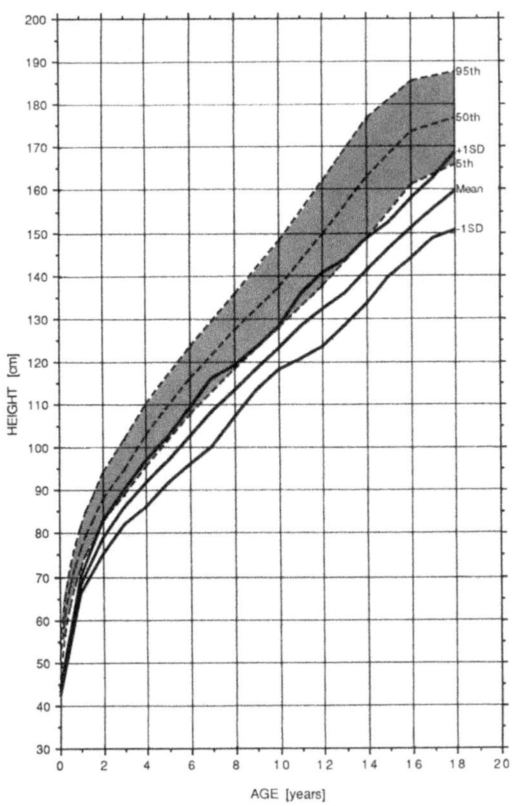


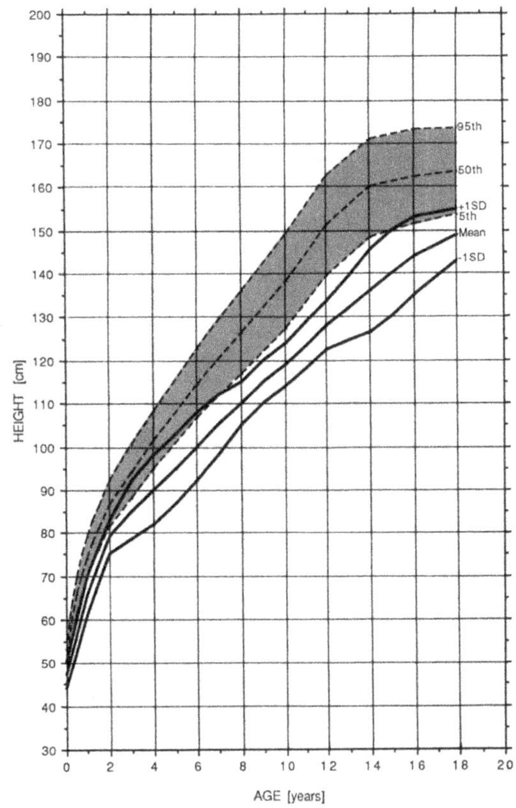


Berg, K., Oslo, J., Book, U., Mohr, J. Copenhagen: Growth curves for height in Noonan syndrome. *Clin. Genet.* 1986;30:150.

**2–15** Achondroplasia Growth Chart, Height, Boys and Girls

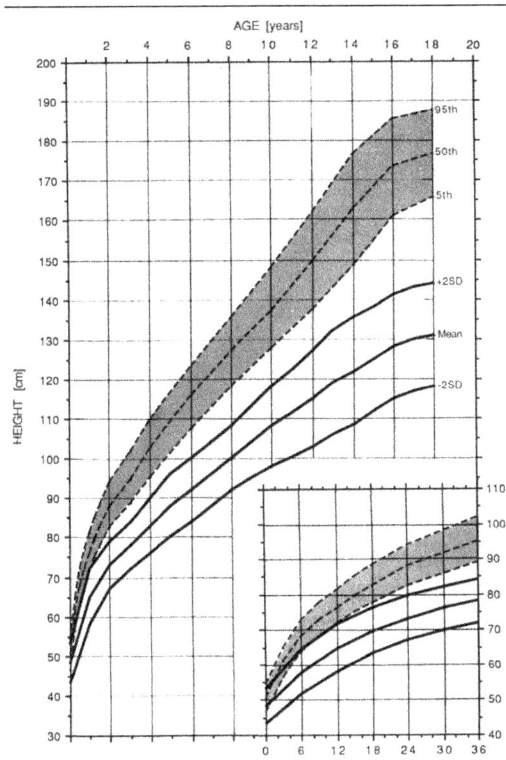


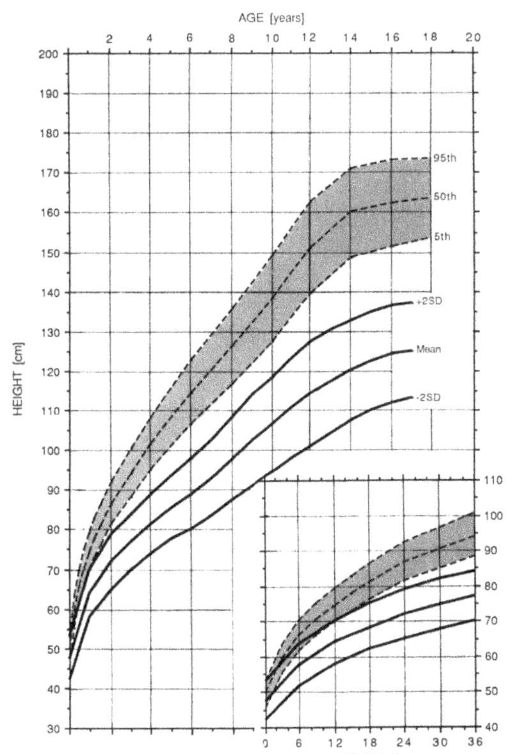


Horton, W.A., Ralter, J.L., Ramien, D.L. Standard growth curves for achondrosplasia. *J. Pediatr.* 1978;93:435.

**2–16** De Lange Syndrome Growth Chart, Weight and Height, Boys, 0–36 months and 2–18 Years

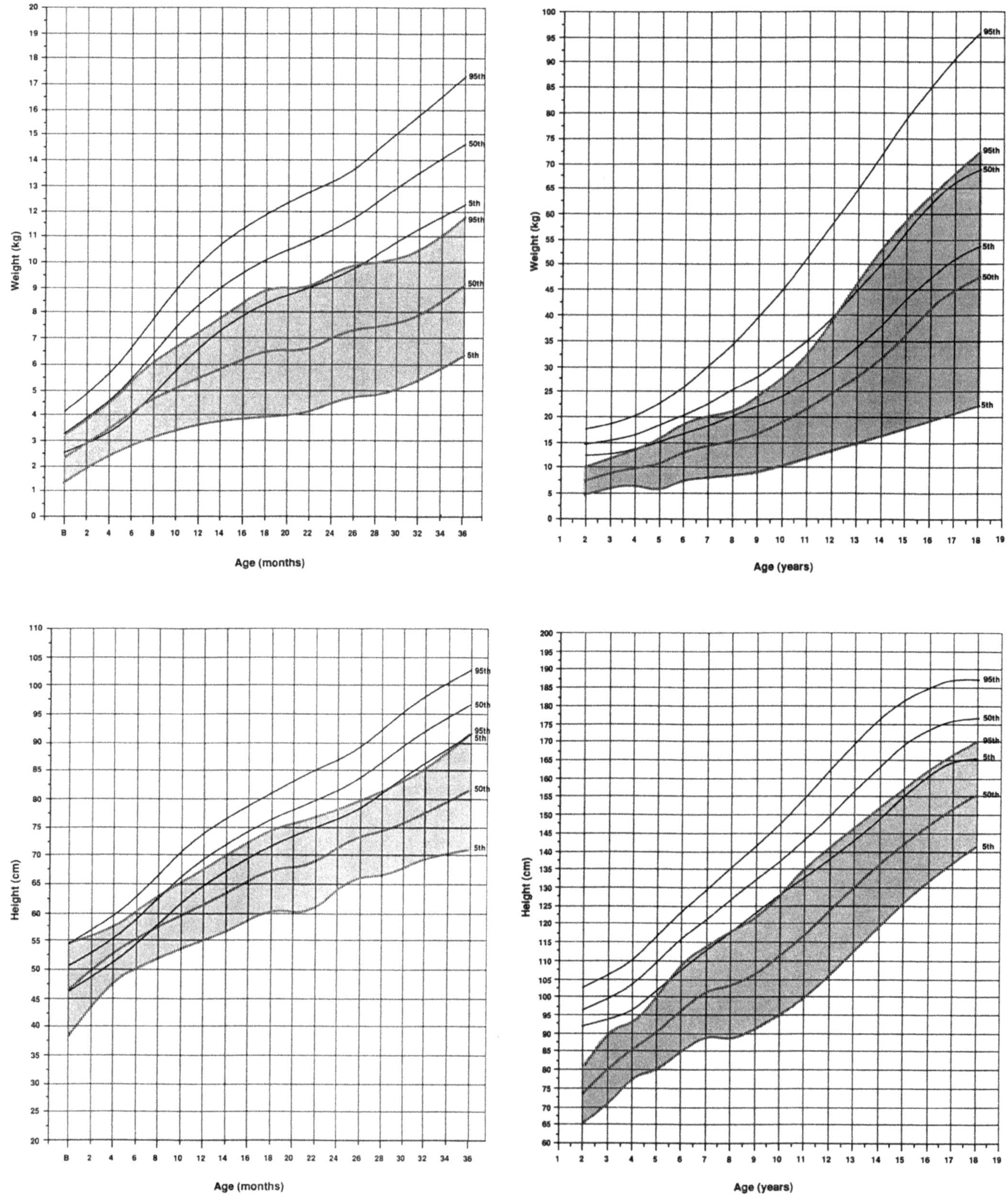


Kline, A., Barr, M., Jackson, L. Growth manifestation in Brackmann-de Lange Syndrome. *Am. J. Med. Genet.* 1993;47:1042.

**2–17** De Lange Syndrome Growth Chart, Weight and Height, 0–36 months and 2–18 Years Girls

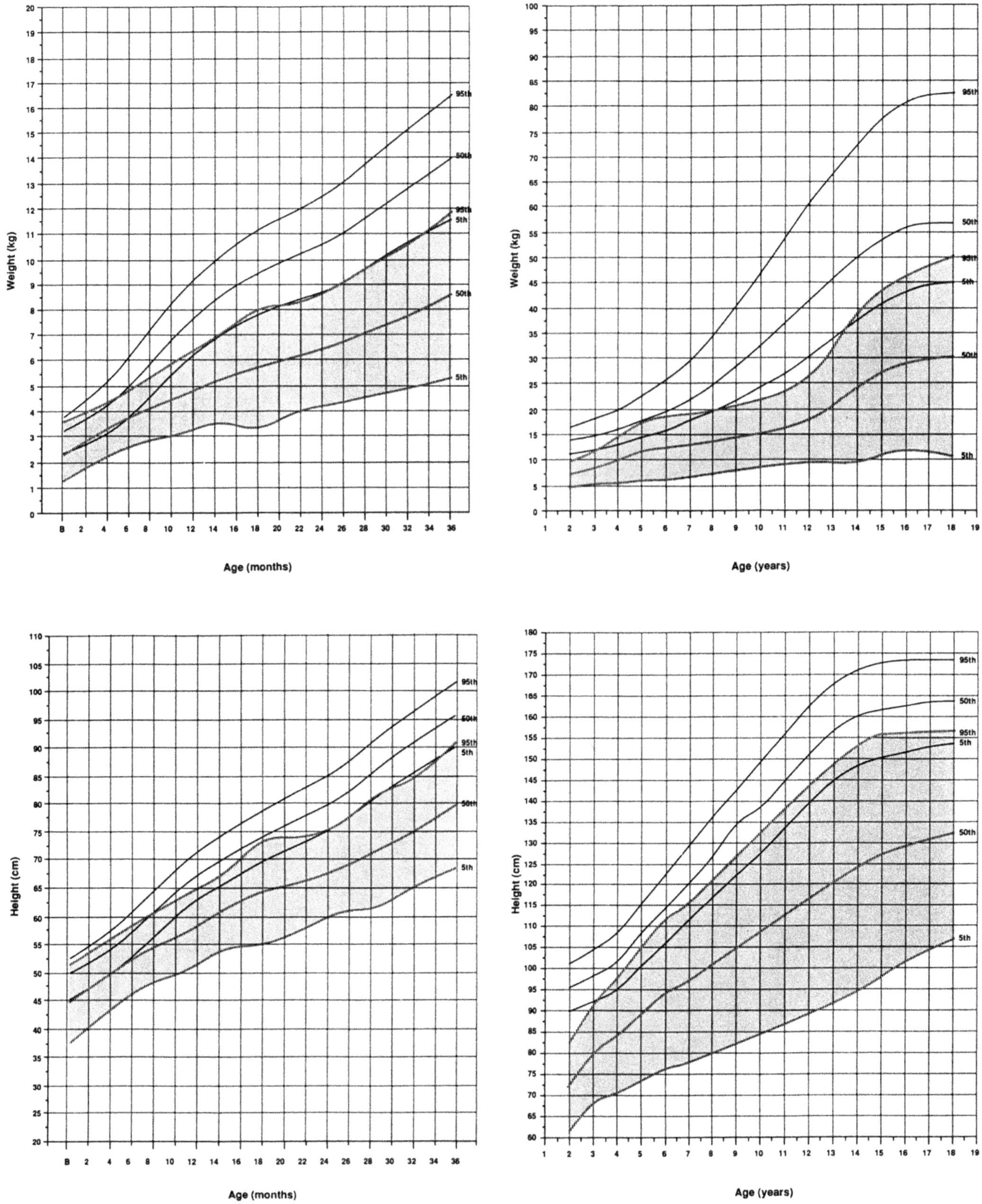

**2–18** Marfan Syndrome Growth Chart, Height and Weight, Boys and Girls, 2–24 Years

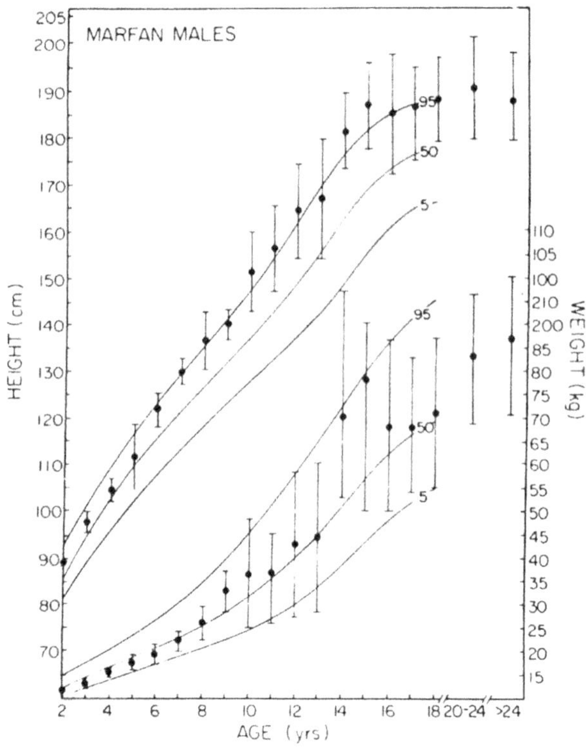


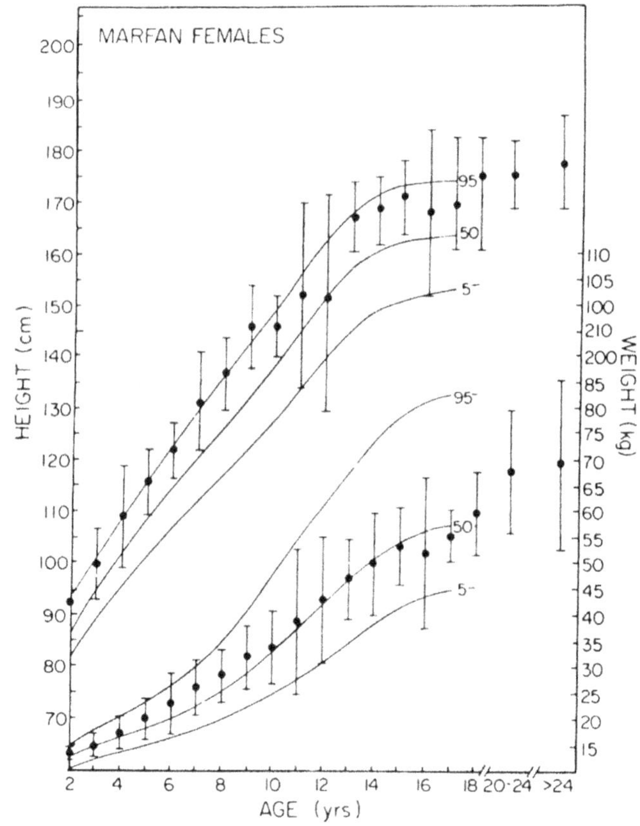


Papadatus, C.J., Bartsocoos, C.S. *Growth and Anthropometrics in Marfan Syndrome.* New York: Alan R. Liss, 1985:361.

**2–19** Fragile X Syndrome Growth Chart, Weight and Height, Boys, 0–28 Years

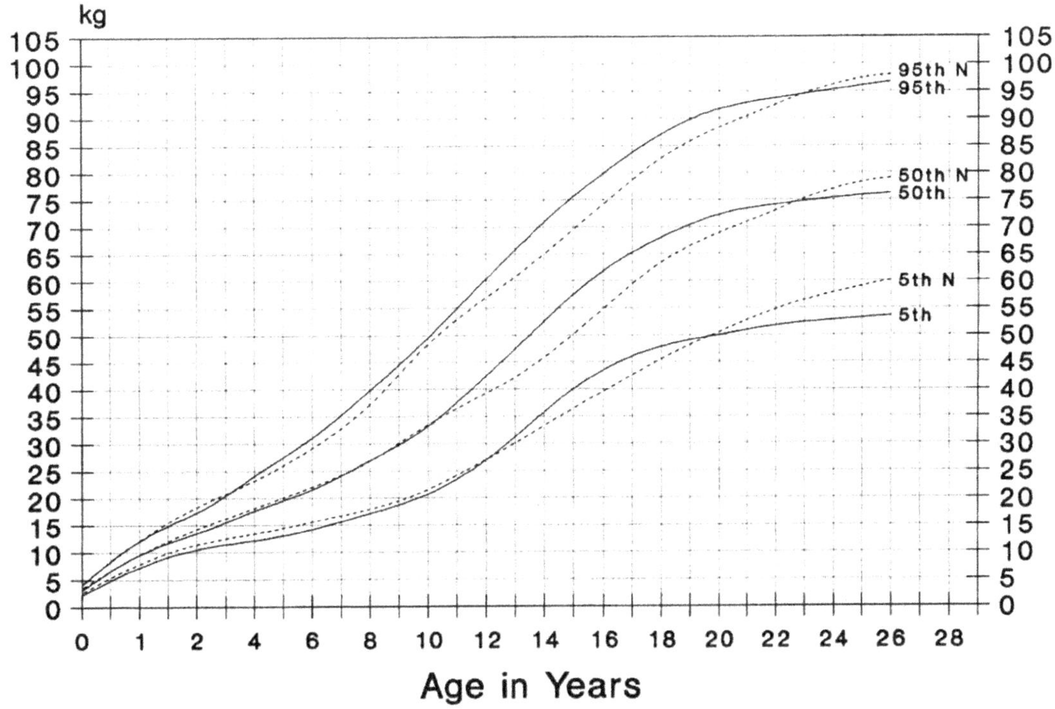


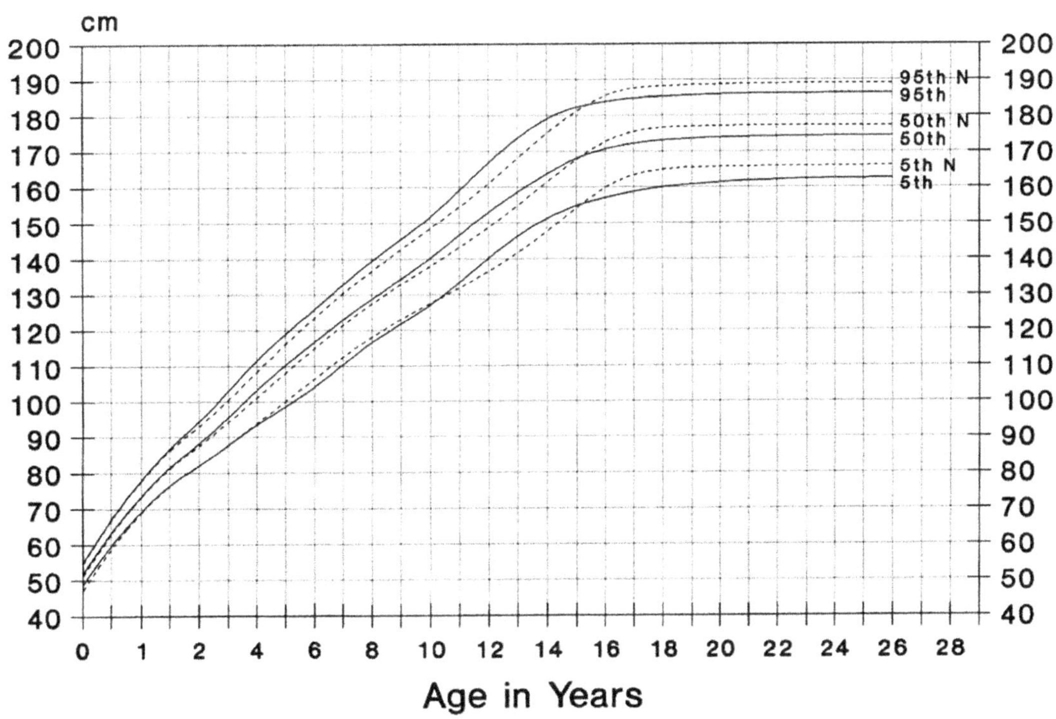


Butler, M.G., Brunschwig, A., Miller, L.K., Hagerman, R.J., *Pediatrics,* 1992:89, 1059.

# APPENDIX 3
## Growth Grids—Fenton, WHO and CDC for General Pediatric Population

**3–1** Weight and Height of Males and Females to Age 20 in the United States

**Males by Percentile**

| | *Weight, kg (lb)* | | | | | | | | | *Height, cm (in)* | | | | | | | | |
|---|---|---|---|---|---|---|---|---|---|---|---|---|---|---|---|---|---|---|
| | 3rd | 5th | 10th | 25th | 50th | 75th | 90th | 95th | 97th | 3rd | 5th | 10th | 25th | 50th | 75th | 90th | 95th | 97th |
| **Years** | | | | | | | | | | | | | | | | | | |
| 1 | 8.05 | 8.25 | 8.65 | 9.54 | 9.98 | 10.60 | 11.10 | 11.60 | 12.00 | 67.80 | 69.80 | 71.40 | 73.40 | 75.00 | 76.80 | 78.60 | 79.70 | 80.00 |
| 2 | 10.15 | 10.40 | 10.89 | 11.57 | 12.36 | 13.10 | 14.40 | 14.74 | 14.97 | 80.40 | 80.70 | 82.30 | 84.40 | 86.40 | 88.20 | 89.90 | 90.90 | 93.00 |
| 3 | 11.23 | 11.57 | 12.02 | 13.00 | 13.83 | 14.74 | 15.95 | 16.56 | 17.30 | 85.80 | 86.60 | 88.50 | 90.40 | 92.70 | 95.20 | 97.20 | 98.40 | 100.00 |
| 4 | 13.04 | 13.38 | 13.95 | 14.95 | 15.80 | 17.10 | 18.26 | 19.39 | 20.07 | 92.90 | 94.20 | 95.40 | 97.50 | 100.60 | 103.00 | 105.30 | 107.20 | 107.80 |
| 5 | 14.06 | 14.52 | 15.35 | 16.56 | 17.92 | 19.39 | 20.98 | 22.20 | 23.02 | 98.20 | 99.50 | 100.80 | 104.00 | 107.00 | 110.30 | 113.30 | 115.00 | 115.80 |
| 6 | 15.90 | 16.44 | 17.12 | 18.37 | 20.25 | 22.05 | 24.04 | 25.85 | 27.10 | 104.50 | 106.30 | 108.00 | 110.40 | 114.00 | 117.40 | 120.20 | 122.00 | 122.20 |
| 7 | 17.24 | 18.14 | 19.05 | 20.41 | 22.11 | 24.38 | 27.67 | 30.05 | 31.52 | 109.10 | 110.90 | 113.20 | 116.50 | 119.20 | 124.00 | 127.50 | 129.10 | 129.50 |
| 8 | 19.05 | 19.96 | 21.21 | 22.91 | 25.29 | 27.44 | 30.73 | 33.91 | 34.47 | 115.60 | 117.30 | 120.20 | 123.20 | 126.80 | 130.20 | 133.90 | 136.30 | 138.00 |
| 9 | 21.55 | 22.68 | 23.59 | 25.17 | 27.67 | 30.50 | 34.02 | 37.19 | 39.80 | 122.10 | 123.20 | 124.60 | 127.00 | 131.60 | 135.20 | 139.70 | 142.10 | 142.90 |
| 10 | 23.02 | 24.15 | 25.40 | 27.33 | 30.73 | 34.25 | 40.37 | 43.55 | 47.40 | 125.20 | 127.10 | 129.40 | 132.60 | 136.80 | 141.00 | 145.20 | 148.00 | 149.10 |
| 11 | 26.54 | 27.56 | 28.24 | 30.73 | 34.47 | 39.24 | 45.59 | 53.41 | 55.34 | 130.50 | 132.30 | 133.80 | 137.50 | 142.30 | 147.00 | 150.30 | 153.30 | 154.40 |
| 12 | 28.35 | 28.69 | 31.07 | 34.02 | 37.65 | 44.68 | 54.32 | 61.01 | 64.68 | 135.90 | 137.20 | 139.50 | 143.80 | 147.20 | 152.30 | 157.20 | 160.00 | 161.60 |
| 13 | 30.39 | 31.98 | 33.68 | 38.10 | 43.32 | 49.22 | 57.15 | 64.07 | 67.59 | 140.20 | 142.00 | 144.60 | 150.00 | 154.30 | 160.00 | 164.50 | 167.40 | 169.50 |
| 14 | 34.94 | 36.06 | 37.54 | 44.11 | 49.89 | 58.51 | 66.34 | 71.10 | 74.84 | 143.30 | 145.10 | 148.90 | 154.10 | 161.90 | 167.70 | 172.40 | 175.60 | 176.00 |
| 15 | 40.37 | 41.62 | 44.45 | 50.58 | 56.81 | 63.05 | 72.80 | 78.59 | 86.07 | 152.00 | 154.60 | 158.40 | 163.50 | 168.60 | 174.10 | 178.40 | 179.90 | 181.40 |
| 16 | 43.54 | 46.72 | 50.35 | 56.02 | 62.35 | 67.93 | 75.75 | 85.73 | 90.38 | 158.40 | 159.00 | 162.70 | 167.30 | 173.10 | 177.50 | 182.50 | 184.40 | 185.70 |
| 17 | 50.35 | 51.03 | 55.00 | 59.42 | 66.11 | 74.96 | 82.21 | 88.68 | 91.06 | 162.50 | 163.60 | 165.50 | 170.30 | 175.70 | 181.10 | 185.80 | 187.70 | 190.20 |
| 18 | 50.46 | 52.16 | 55.11 | 60.56 | 66.22 | 73.82 | 81.42 | 90.38 | 93.33 | 162.20 | 163.80 | 167.90 | 171.90 | 175.70 | 180.90 | 185.20 | 187.40 | 188.20 |
| 19 | 52.84 | 53.75 | 57.04 | 63.16 | 69.85 | 77.34 | 89.02 | 93.87 | 96.50 | 165.80 | 166.40 | 167.20 | 171.60 | 176.60 | 180.60 | 185.40 | 188.00 | 191.30 |
| 20 | 54.88 | 55.68 | 57.38 | 64.07 | 70.31 | 78.02 | 87.66 | 99.22 | 102.85 | 162.00 | 164.30 | 169.50 | 171.80 | 176.70 | 180.00 | 184.20 | 186.30 | 188.40 |

**Females by Percentile**

| | *Weight, kg (lb)* | | | | | | | | | *Height, cm (in)* | | | | | | | | |
|---|---|---|---|---|---|---|---|---|---|---|---|---|---|---|---|---|---|---|
| | 3rd | 5th | 10th | 25th | 50th | 75th | 90th | 95th | 97th | 3rd | 5th | 10th | 25th | 50th | 75th | 90th | 95th | 97th |
| **Years** | | | | | | | | | | | | | | | | | | |
| 1 | 7.48 | 7.48 | 7.90 | 8.62 | 9.15 | 10.05 | 10.55 | 10.85 | 11.10 | 65.80 | 68.60 | 68.80 | 71.80 | 73.50 | 74.90 | 76.70 | 78.30 | 78.80 |
| 2 | 9.45 | 9.75 | 10.09 | 10.89 | 11.79 | 12.75 | 13.49 | 13.90 | 14.17 | 79.10 | 79.20 | 80.70 | 82.40 | 84.50 | 87.00 | 88.80 | 89.90 | 90.40 |
| 3 | 11.00 | 11.23 | 11.79 | 12.47 | 13.38 | 14.52 | 15.65 | 16.44 | 17.10 | 85.00 | 85.80 | 87.00 | 89.10 | 91.90 | 94.20 | 96.80 | 97.80 | 98.80 |
| 4 | 12.40 | 12.59 | 13.27 | 14.17 | 15.31 | 16.75 | 17.92 | 18.95 | 19.63 | 92.40 | 93.20 | 94.70 | 97.00 | 99.30 | 102.40 | 104.90 | 106.30 | 107.80 |
| 5 | 13.49 | 13.95 | 14.63 | 15.76 | 17.24 | 18.80 | 20.65 | 21.89 | 24.45 | 97.40 | 97.70 | 99.70 | 102.70 | 105.60 | 109.30 | 112.20 | 113.90 | 115.00 |
| 6 | 15.65 | 16.10 | 16.85 | 17.90 | 19.80 | 22.11 | 25.25 | 28.10 | 28.92 | 103.90 | 105.20 | 107.10 | 110.50 | 113.60 | 117.00 | 120.50 | 122.80 | 125.30 |
| 7 | 16.67 | 17.12 | 17.92 | 19.62 | 21.55 | 23.81 | 27.67 | 29.48 | 30.84 | 109.30 | 110.10 | 111.80 | 115.40 | 119.00 | 122.90 | 126.50 | 128.80 | 129.90 |
| 8 | 18.94 | 19.28 | 20.18 | 21.89 | 24.27 | 26.99 | 30.39 | 32.65 | 35.15 | 114.40 | 116.20 | 117.90 | 121.20 | 125.20 | 129.40 | 113.10 | 136.50 | 138.20 |
| 9 | 21.09 | 21.77 | 22.57 | 24.38 | 27.67 | 30.73 | 36.51 | 41.05 | 42.41 | 120.30 | 122.00 | 124.60 | 127.60 | 131.80 | 135.30 | 138.70 | 140.70 | 141.30 |
| 10 | 22.79 | 23.81 | 25.40 | 27.56 | 30.84 | 35.38 | 44.45 | 47.85 | 50.35 | 124.80 | 127.00 | 128.40 | 132.60 | 136.50 | 141.00 | 145.00 | 148.40 | 149.30 |
| 11 | 25.40 | 26.31 | 27.90 | 30.62 | 34.25 | 39.01 | 45.81 | 49.33 | 53.30 | 129.40 | 130.50 | 133.80 | 138.40 | 142.50 | 147.40 | 152.20 | 155.00 | 156.80 |
| 12 | 29.03 | 29.48 | 30.62 | 34.93 | 39.92 | 47.40 | 57.15 | 63.50 | 66.34 | 135.70 | 138.70 | 140.60 | 144.20 | 149.70 | 155.20 | 159.90 | 164.50 | 165.50 |
| 13 | 32.20 | 33.45 | 36.29 | 40.60 | 46.49 | 53.75 | 61.23 | 66.00 | 70.08 | 143.00 | 144.60 | 147.50 | 151.90 | 156.50 | 160.70 | 165.00 | 166.30 | 168.40 |
| 14 | 36.17 | 36.97 | 39.01 | 44.57 | 50.12 | 56.36 | 66.22 | 72.12 | 78.70 | 147.60 | 149.50 | 150.90 | 155.50 | 169.30 | 163.20 | 167.00 | 169.90 | 172.30 |
| 15 | 40.26 | 40.94 | 43.32 | 47.51 | 52.96 | 59.99 | 69.51 | 75.07 | 78.92 | 148.40 | 150.20 | 152.80 | 156.70 | 161.60 | 166.20 | 169.90 | 172.40 | 174.10 |
| 16 | 42.86 | 44.45 | 46.27 | 49.56 | 56.25 | 60.89 | 66.79 | 76.54 | 82.78 | 151.70 | 153.10 | 155.40 | 159.20 | 164.00 | 167.80 | 171.20 | 173.90 | 175.50 |
| 17 | 43.20 | 44.11 | 45.59 | 50.69 | 55.54 | 61.80 | 71.21 | 78.70 | 88.22 | 150.10 | 151.60 | 154.40 | 158.30 | 162.50 | 166.40 | 170.90 | 173.00 | 174.20 |
| 18 | 43.77 | 45.25 | 49.33 | 52.84 | 57.61 | 63.62 | 72.69 | 84.71 | 91.29 | 150.30 | 151.80 | 154.90 | 159.30 | 163.30 | 167.00 | 171.00 | 172.80 | 175.60 |
| 19 | 42.64 | 44.00 | 47.74 | 52.73 | 56.47 | 63.16 | 69.74 | 78.02 | 79.49 | 150.30 | 152.40 | 154.90 | 159.10 | 163.70 | 167.00 | 170.70 | 173.60 | 174.20 |
| 20 | 48.99 | 49.21 | 50.80 | 54.20 | 57.95 | 64.86 | 77.00 | 80.85 | 88.68 | 151.90 | 154.20 | 155.30 | 158.60 | 163.50 | 167.40 | 171.70 | 174.00 | 175.90 |

3–2 CDC Length and Weight for Age Growth Chart, Boys, 0–24 Months

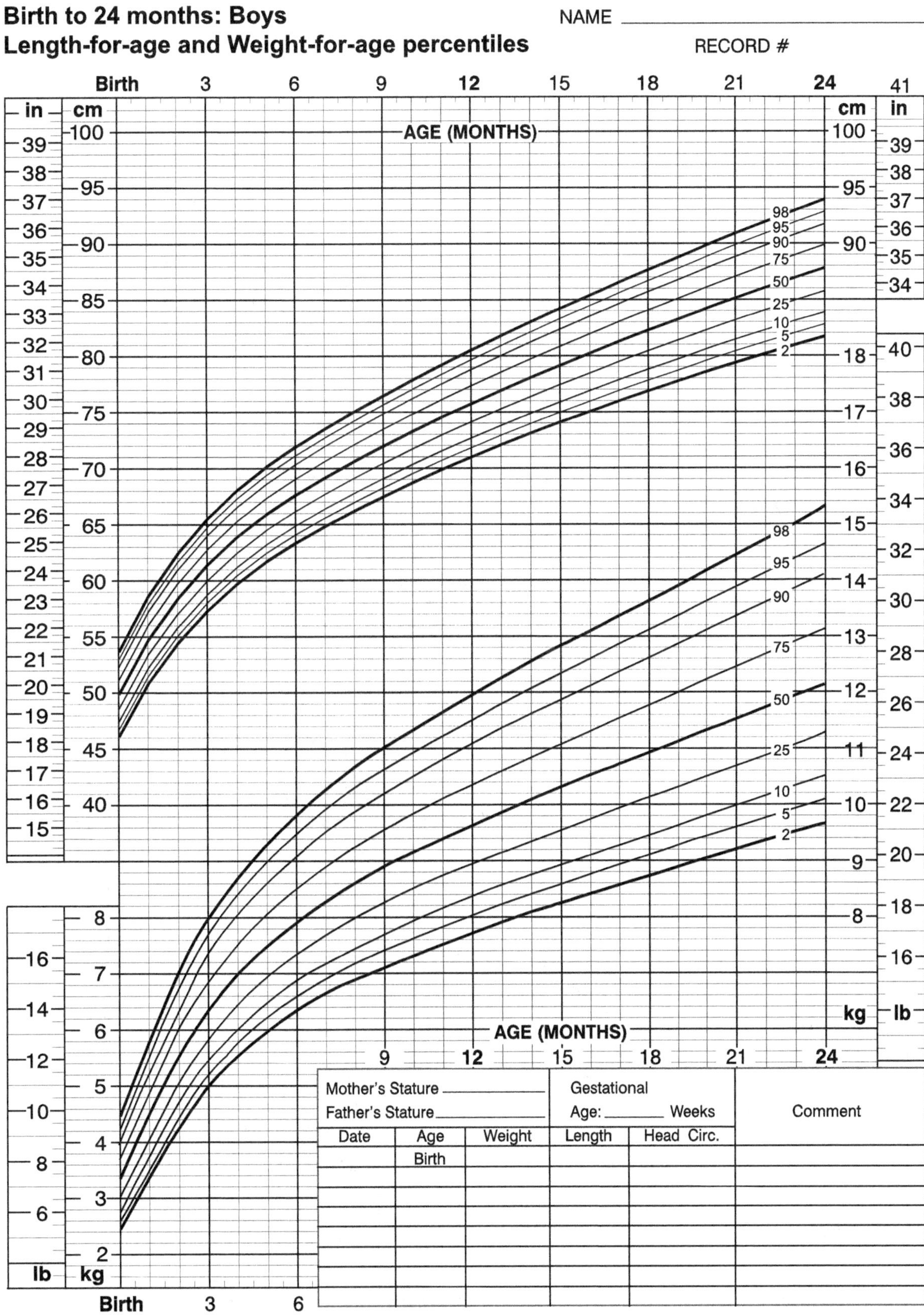


Published by the Centers for Disease Control and Prevention, November 1, 2009
SOURCE: WHO Child Growth Standards (http://www.who.int/childgrowth/en)

SAFER • HEALTHIER • PEOPLE™

**3–3** CDC Head Circumference, Weight for Length, Boys, 0–24 Months

## Birth to 24 months: Boys
## Head circumference-for-age and
## Weight-for-length percentiles

NAME ______________________

RECORD # ____________

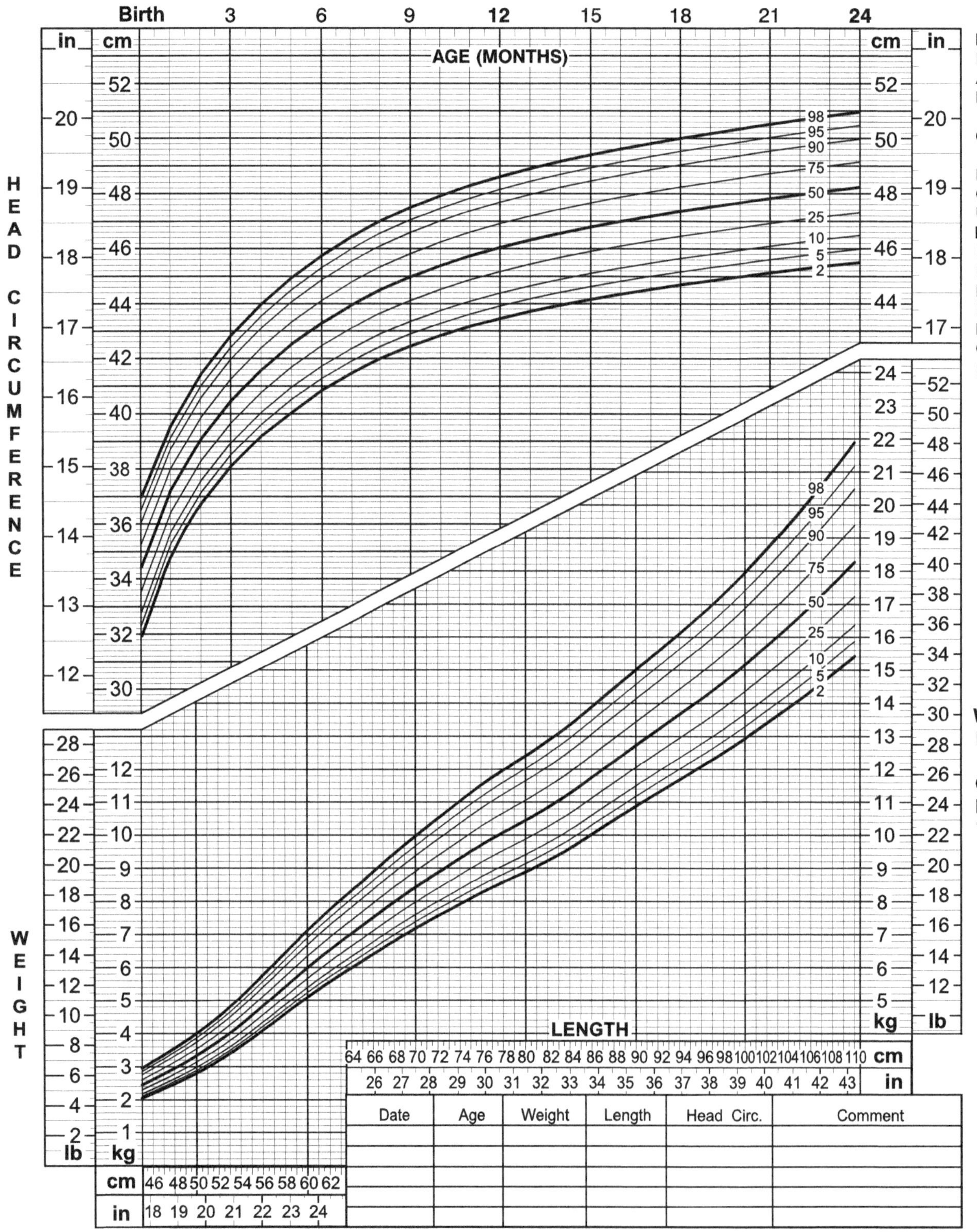


| Date | Age | Weight | Length | Head Circ. | Comment |
|---|---|---|---|---|---|
| | | | | | |
| | | | | | |
| | | | | | |
| | | | | | |

Published by the Centers for Disease Control and Prevention, November 1, 2009
SOURCE: WHO Child Growth Standards (http://www.who.int/childgrowth/en)

**3–4** CDC Length and Weight for Age Growth Chart, Girls, 0–24 Months

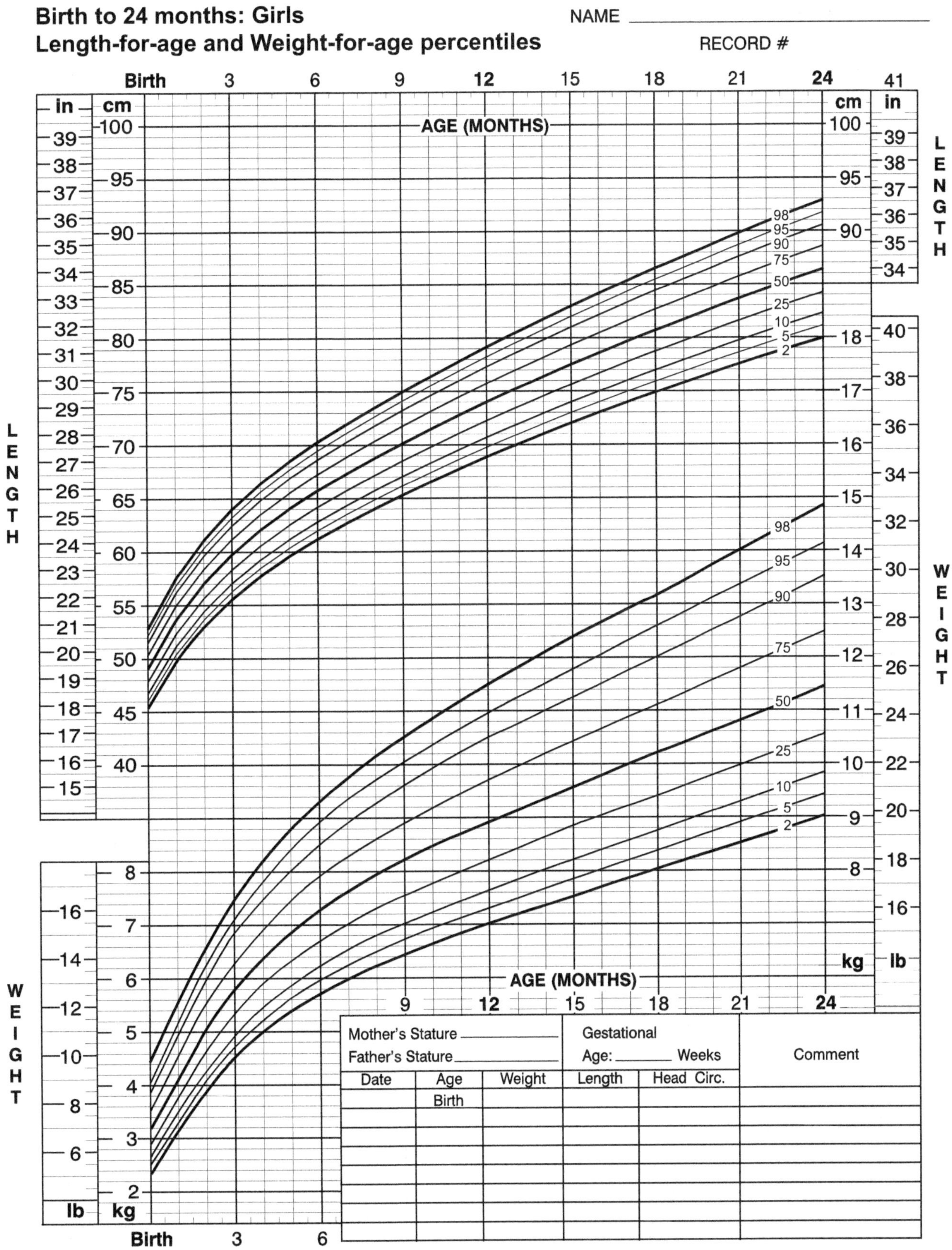


Published by the Centers for Disease Control and Prevention, November 1, 2009
SOURCE: WHO Child Growth Standards (http://www.who.int/childgrowth/en)

3–5 CDC Head Circumference, Weight for Length, Girls, 0–24 Months

## Birth to 24 months: Girls
## Head circumference-for-age and
## Weight-for-length percentiles

NAME ______________________

RECORD # ______________

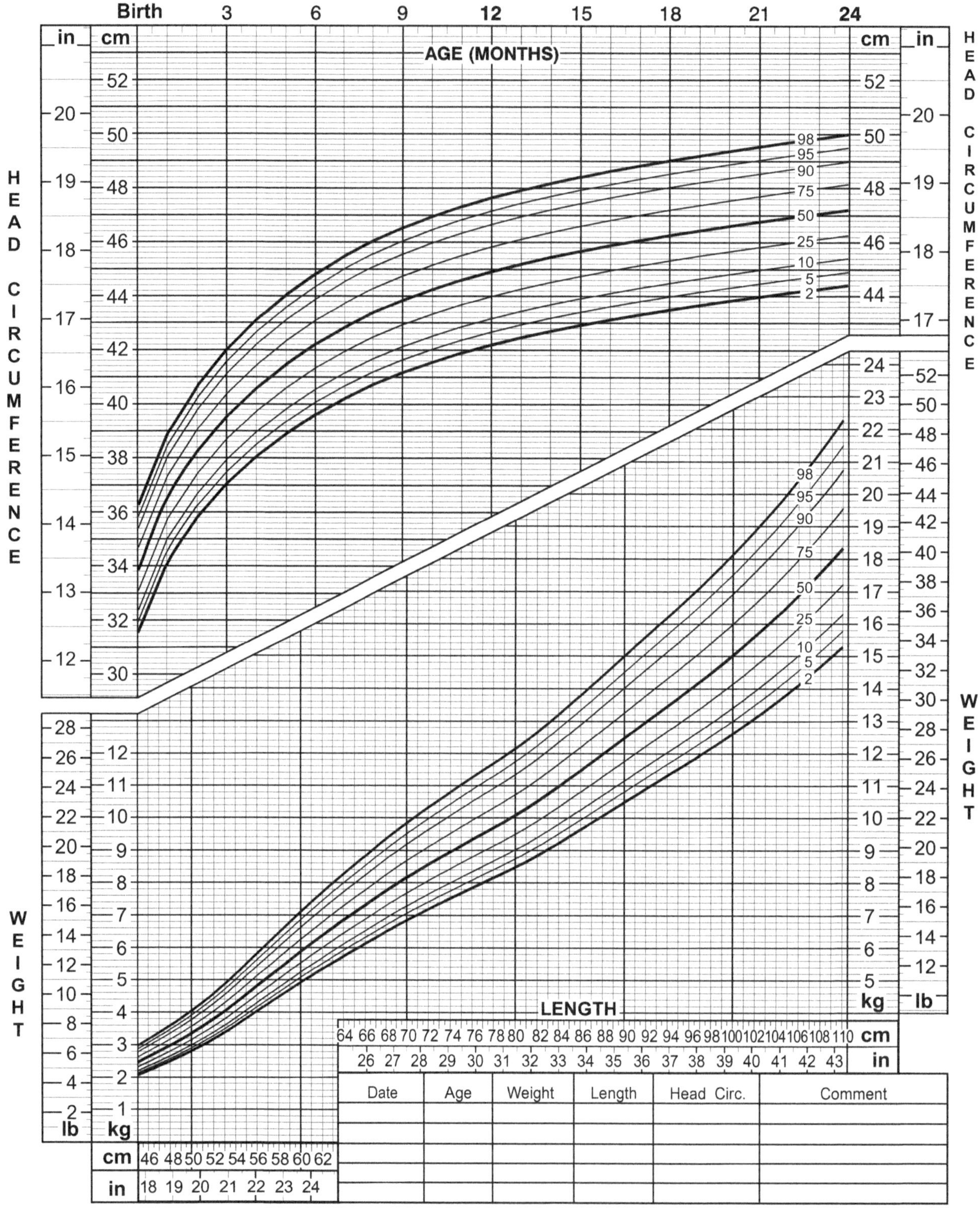


| Date | Age | Weight | Length | Head Circ. | Comment |
|---|---|---|---|---|---|
| | | | | | |
| | | | | | |
| | | | | | |
| | | | | | |

Published May 30, 2000 (modified 11/21/00).
SOURCE: Developed by the National Center for Health Statistics in collaboration with the National Center for Chronic Disease Prevention and Health Promotion (2000).
**http://www.cdc.gov/growthcharts**

**3–6** CDC Stature for Age and Weight, Boys, 2–20 Years

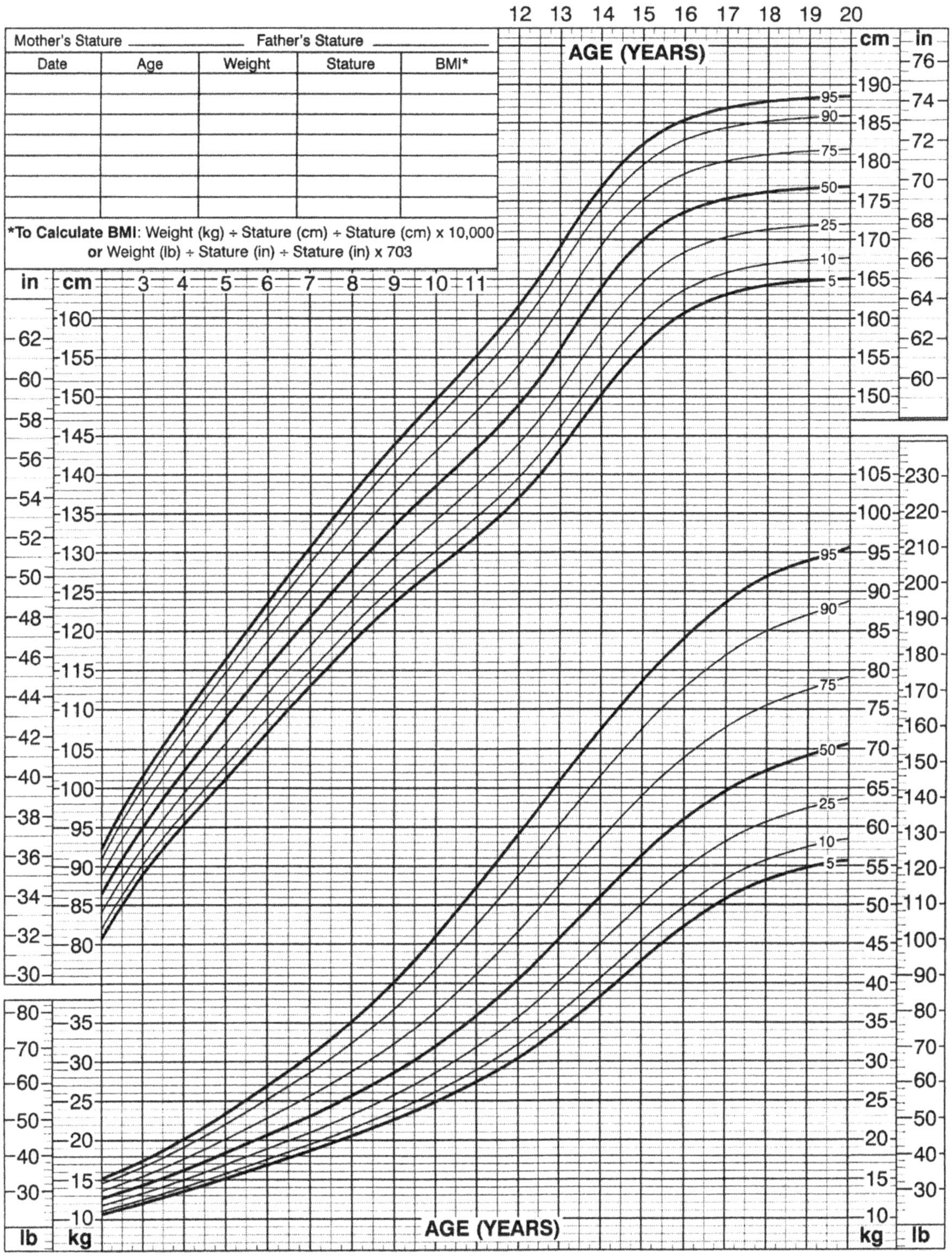


Published May 30, 2000 (modified 11/21/00).
SOURCE: Developed by the National Center for Health Statistics in collaboration with the National Center for Chronic Disease Prevention and Health Promotion (2000).
http://www.cdc.gov/growthcharts

SAFER · HEALTHIER · PEOPLE™

3–7 CDC Weight for Stature, Boys

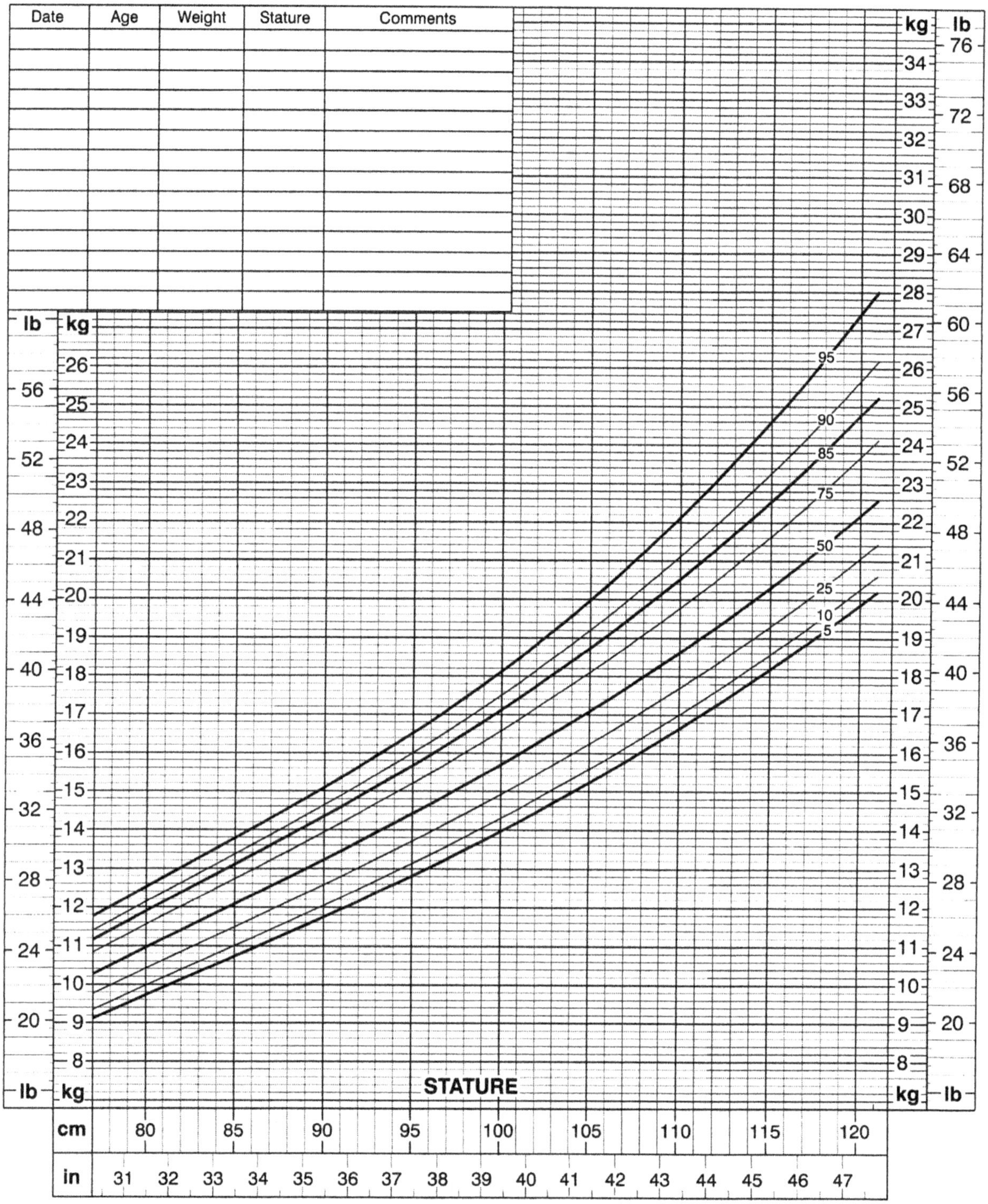


Published May 30, 2000 (modified 10/16/00).
SOURCE: Developed by the National Center for Health Statistics in collaboration with the National Center for Chronic Disease Prevention and Health Promotion (2000).
http://www.cdc.gov/growthcharts

CDC
SAFER · HEALTHIER · PEOPLE™

**3–8** CDC Stature for Age and Weight, Girls, 2–20 Years

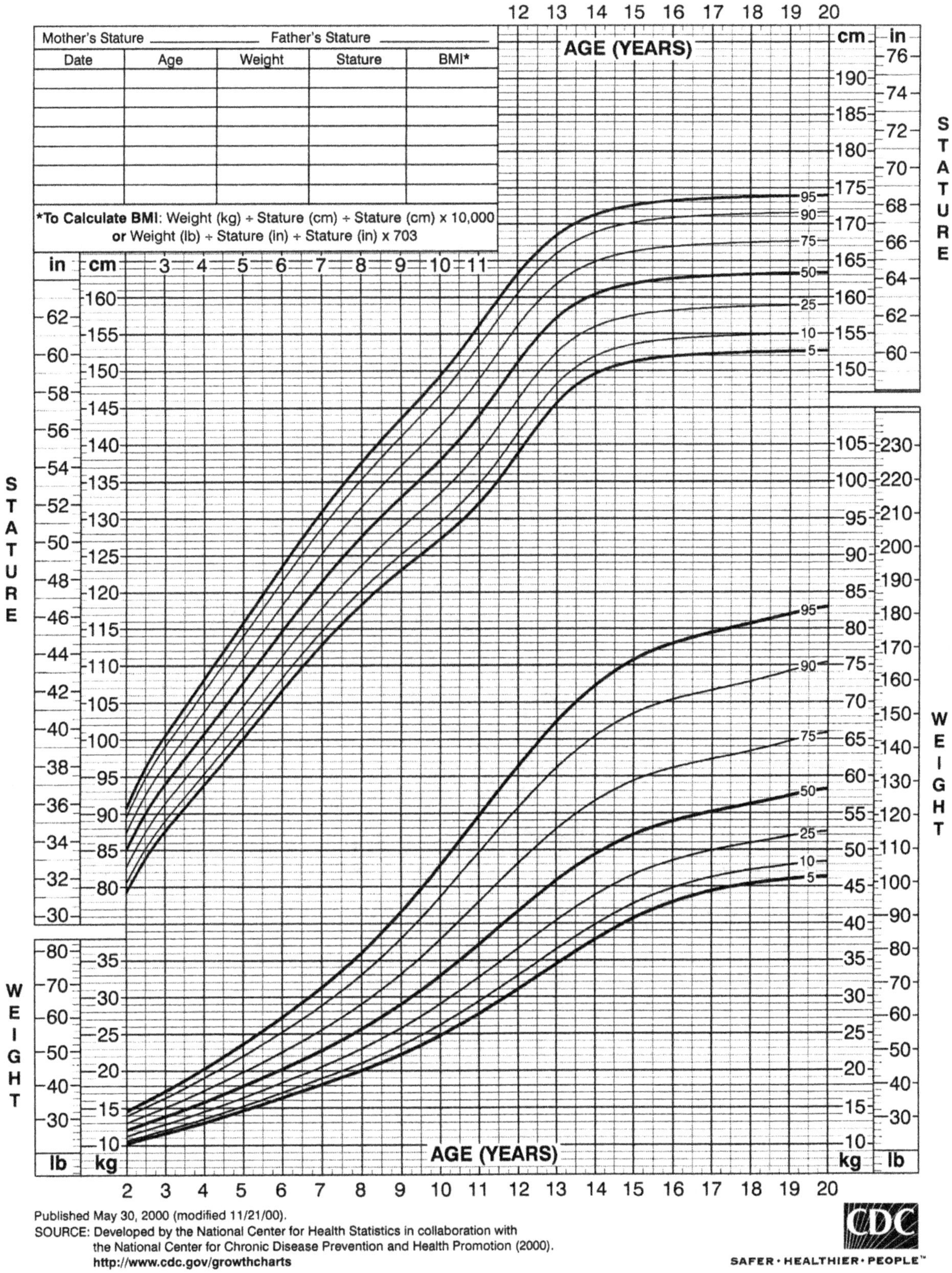

**3–9** CDC Weight for Stature, Girls

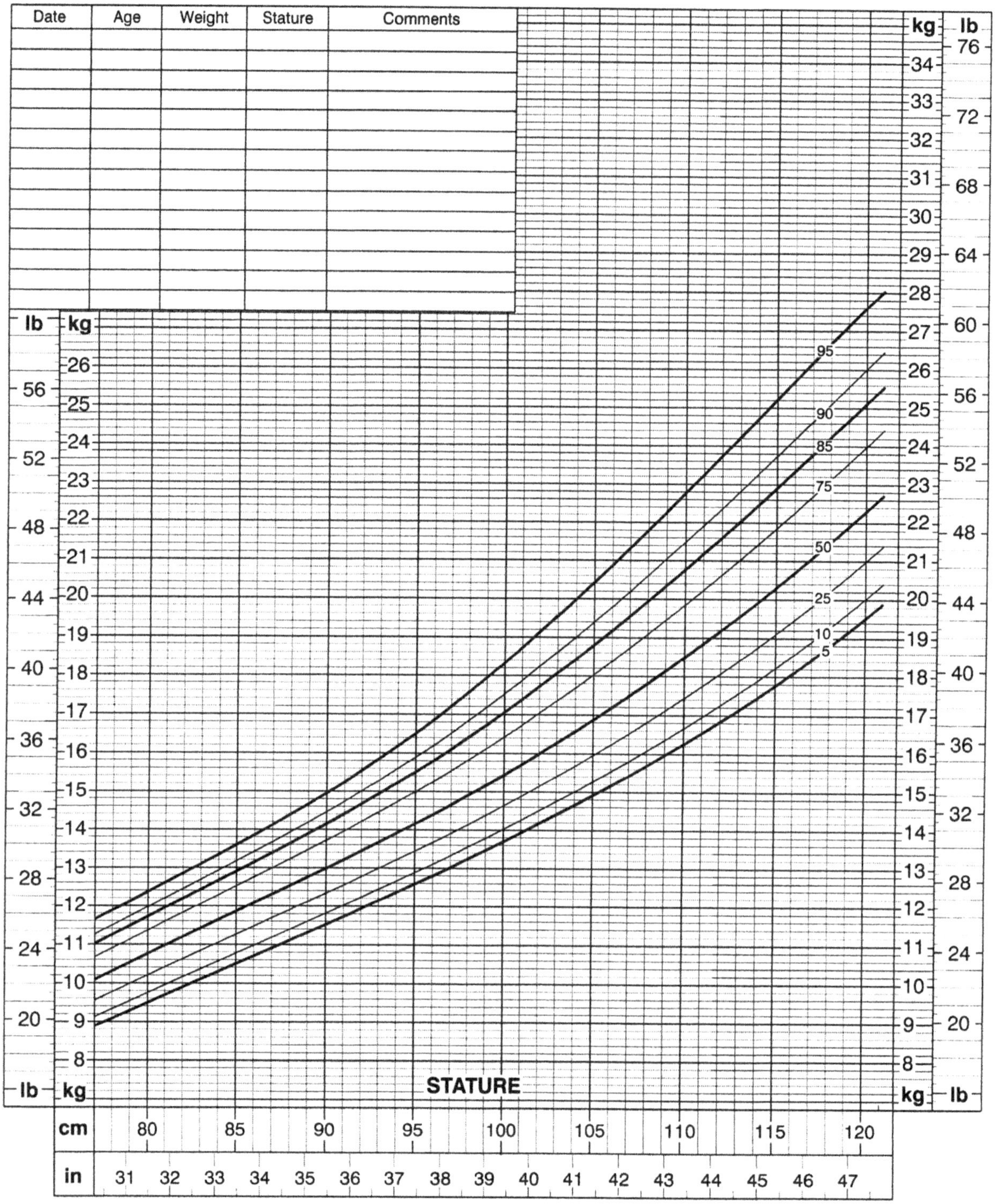


Published May 30, 2000 (modified 10/16/00).
SOURCE: Developed by the National Center for Health Statistics in collaboration with the National Center for Chronic Disease Prevention and Health Promotion (2000).
http://www.cdc.gov/growthcharts

SAFER · HEALTHIER · PEOPLE™

**3–10** CDC Body Mass Index for Age, Boys, 2–20 Years

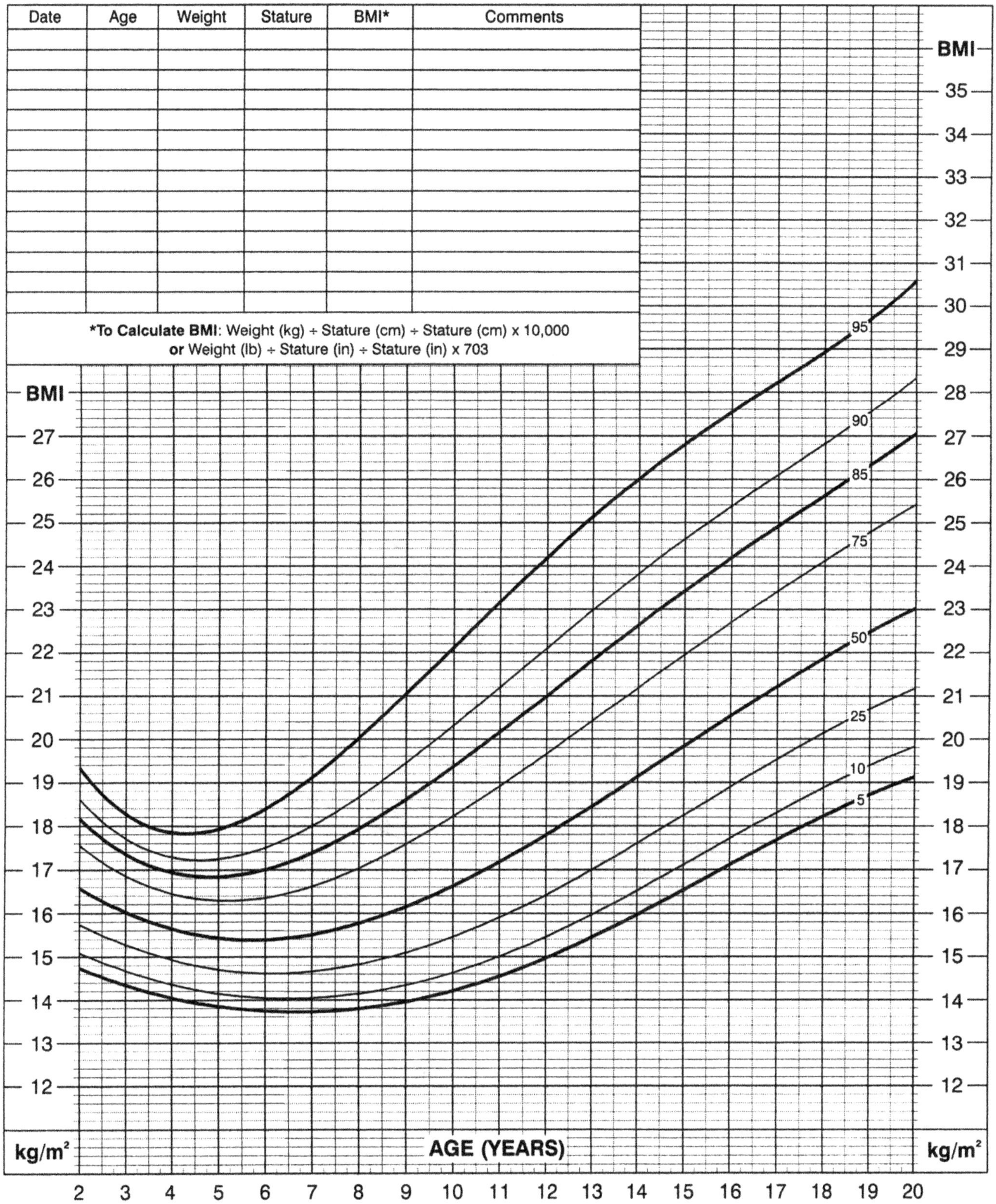


Published May 30, 2000 (modified 10/16/00).
SOURCE: Developed by the National Center for Health Statistics in collaboration with the National Center for Chronic Disease Prevention and Health Promotion (2000).
http://www.cdc.gov/growthcharts

CDC
SAFER · HEALTHIER · PEOPLE™

**3–11** CDC Body Mass Index for Age, Girls, 2–20 Years

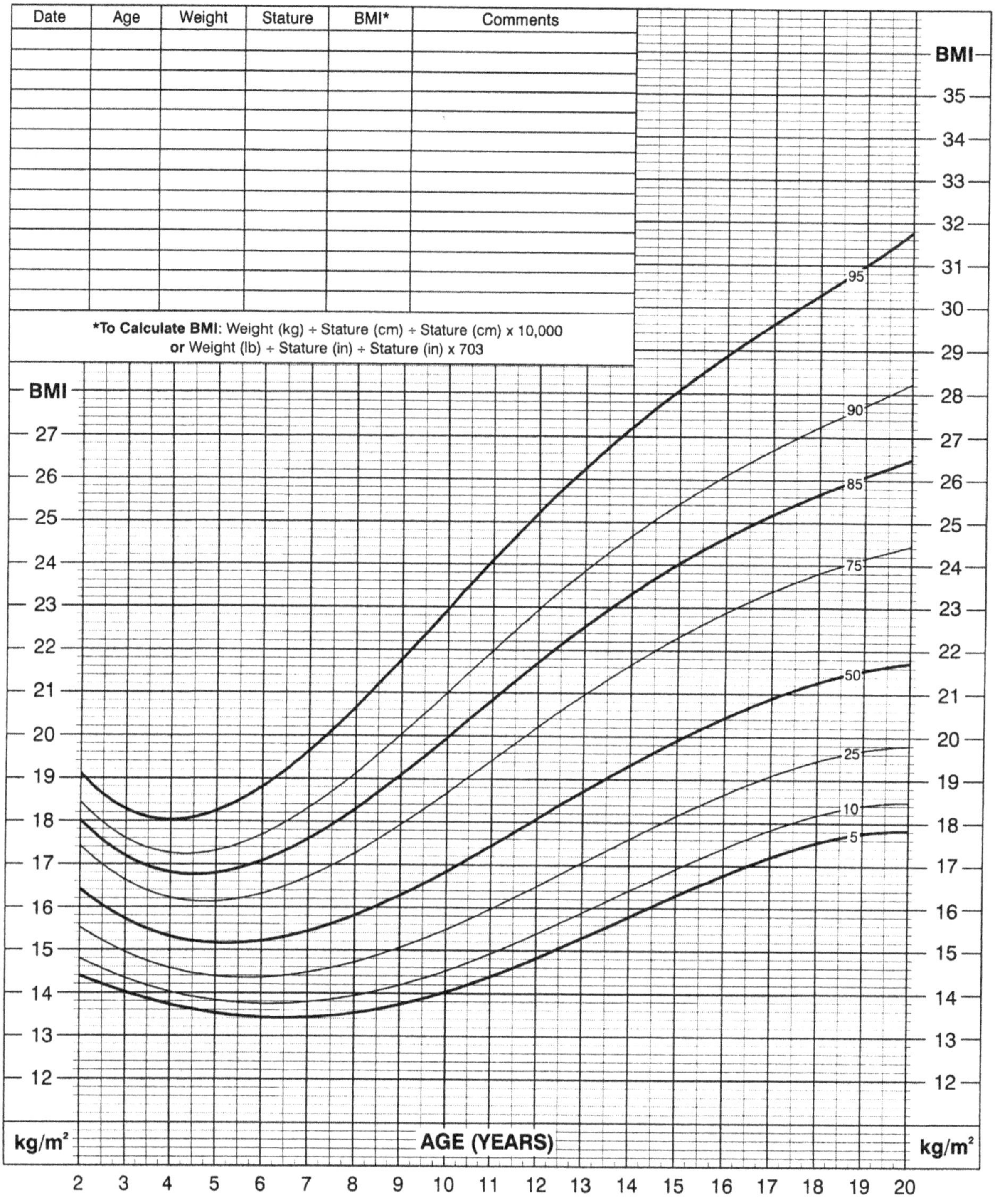


Published May 30, 2000 (modified 10/16/00).
SOURCE: Developed by the National Center for Health Statistics in collaboration with the National Center for Chronic Disease Prevention and Health Promotion (2000).
http://www.cdc.gov/growthcharts

CDC SAFER · HEALTHIER · PEOPLE™

**3–12** Fenton Revised Growth Chart, Boys

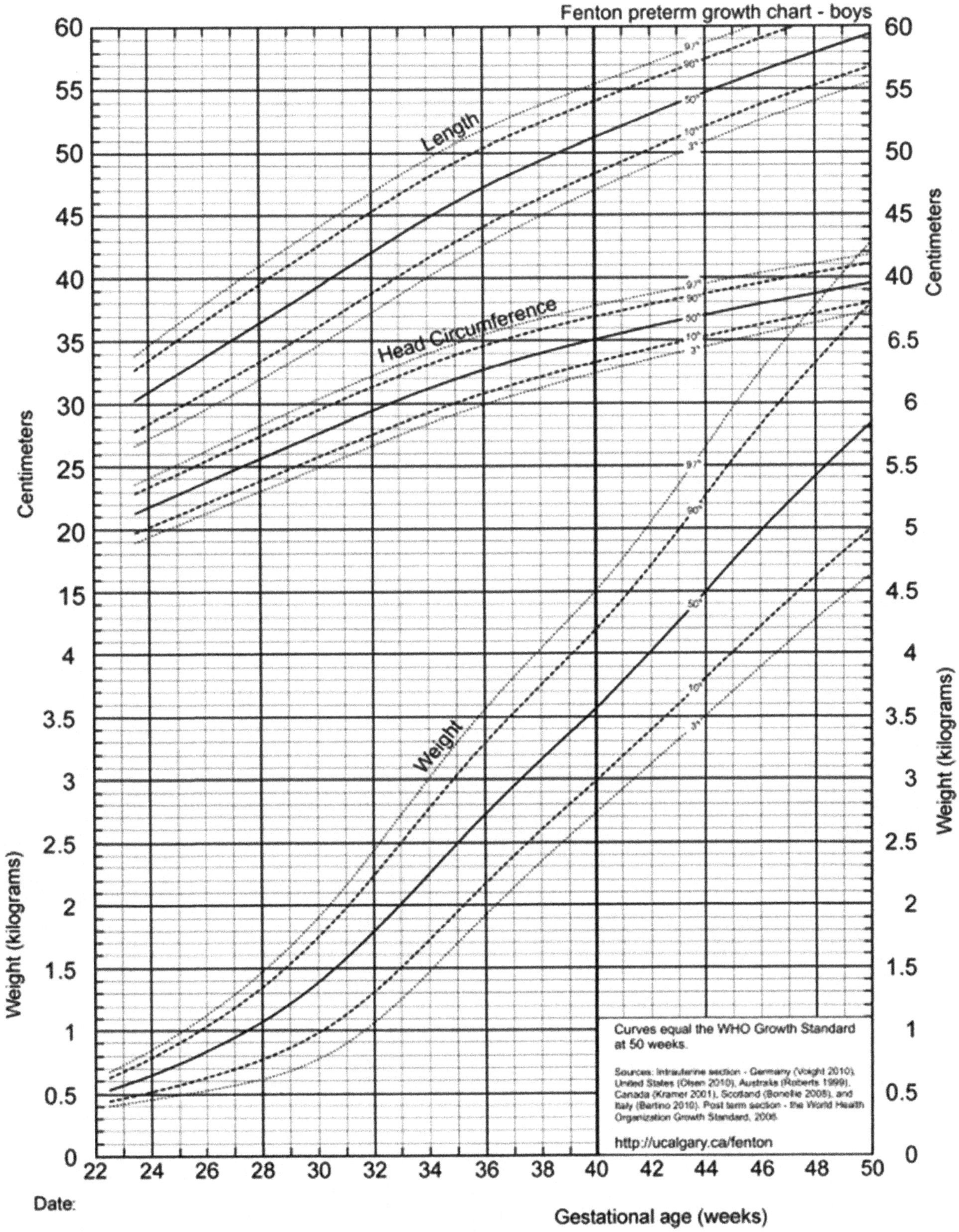

**3–13** Fenton Revised Growth Chart, Girls

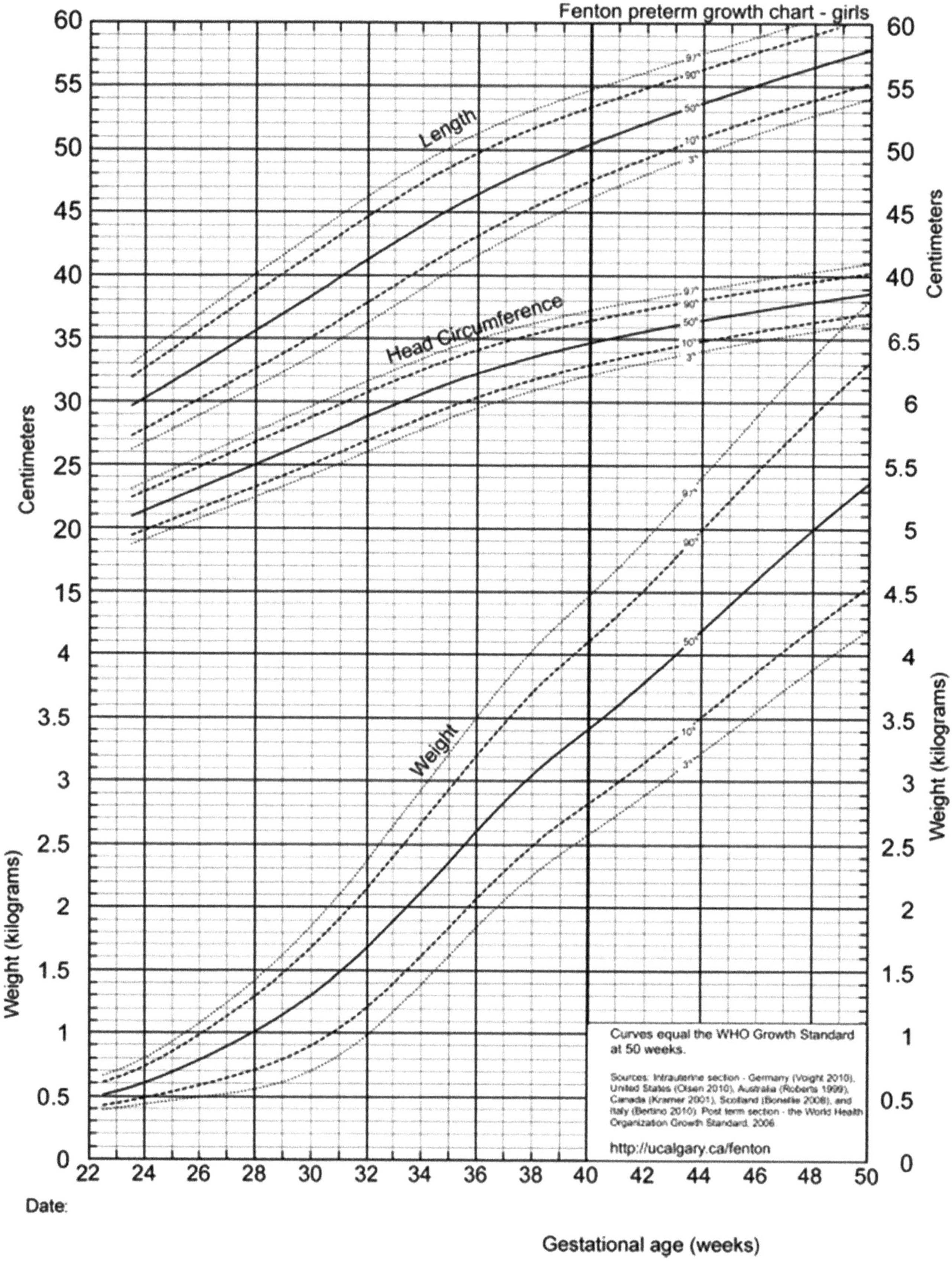

# APPENDIX 4
# Nutritional Assessment Records, Division of Developmental Disabilities, Cincinnati Children's Hospital Medical Center (CCDDD)

CINCINNATI CHILDREN'S HOSPITAL MEDICAL CENTER
DIVISION OF DEVELOPMENTAL DISABILITEIS

**NUTRITION RECORD**

**MR#**
**NAME:** ____________ **ADDRESS:** ____________
**BIRTHDATE:** ____________
**AGE:** ____ **SEX:** ____ **RACE:** ____
**BIRTH WEIGHT:** ____________ **TELEPHONE:** ____________
**DATE SEEN:** ____________ **INFORMANT:** ____________
**Case Manager:** ____________
**Interviewer:** ____________
**Pres. Nutr. Prob.** ____________

**BACKGROUND INFORMATION**

| | Mother | Father | Siblings |
|---|---|---|---|
| Height: | | | |
| Weight: | | | |
| Age: | | | |
| Parents: | | | |

**Med. Diagnosis:** ____________

**I.Q.** ____________ **A.B.** ____________

**ANTHROPOMETRIC MEASUREMENTS:**

Ht.cm ______ %ile ______
Wt.Kg ______ %ile ______
Wt/Ht Index ____ / ____ %ile
#<> Avg. ______
Calf SF ______

Upper Arm Length cm ______
Upper Arm Circum. cm ______
Fatfold Tricep mm ______
Head Circum. cm ______
Waist Circum. cm ______
Fatfold Subscapular ______

MAMC cm ______
Bone Age/Den. ______
Blood Pressure ______
MAMA $cm^2$ ______
Knee Ht. ______
%Body Fat ______

**CHEMISTRY:**
Hb. ______ Serum Fe ______
Hct. ______ Other ______
Vit/Mineral Supp. (Doctor's Orders *Y/N*)
(frequency/type) ______
Meds: ______
Nutrient/Drug Interaction Discussed Y/N
Caretaker knowledge demonstrated *Y/N*

**INTERDISCIPLINARY FINDINGS:**
Gross Motor: ______
Speech: ______

**DENTAL CARE:**
Daily Source of Fluoride? *Y/N*
Brushes teeth regularly? *Y/N*
Sees dentist regularly? *Y/N*
Caries-causing foods named ______

**SOCIO-ECONOMIC:**
Income: $ ______
Food: $ ______ *Weekly/Monthly*
No. of family members: ______
Using Food Stamp Program or Supplemental Food Program? Y/N N/A ______

**MEDICAL:**
Hx. of hospitalizations ______
Hx. Infections: ______

**PRENATAL DIETARY CARE:**

**NEONATAL FEEDING HISTORY:**
Period Breast Fed ______
Period Formula Fed ______
Type Tolerated ______
Feeding Problems: Sucking, Swallowing
Colic, Vomiting, Diarrhea,
Constipation, Weight Gain Abnormal

**ORDER OF INFANT FOOD ADDED:**

| | Age | Amts | How Taken |
|---|---|---|---|
| | | | |
| | | | |
| | | | |
| | | | |

(Solid food should not be given before four months of age)

**SUPPLEMENTS:** **AGE BEGAN:** **TIME CONTINUED:**

Age: Weaned from bottle ______ Liquid from cup ______ Unassisted ______
Age: Finger Fed ______ Used spoon ______ Unassisted ______
Bottle night feeding (other than water) Y/N

**PRESENT FEEDING ABILITIES:**

Table Foods ______ Chopped Foods ______ Jr. Foods ______ Strained ______
Normal Feeding Period ______ Behavioral Problems ______
Reward System ______

**(Circle)** Choking, Swallowing, Chewing, Tongue Thrust, Constipation, Anorexia, Pica (clay, starch, plaster, ashes, bugs, crayons – how much? ______)

**DIETARY EVALUATION**

**NAME:** ______

**FOOD INTAKE** (24 hour recall)*

| Patterns | | Amount |
|---|---|---|
| Time | ***Breakfast*** | |
| | Fruit | |
| | Meat | |
| Where | Egg | |
| | Bread | |
| With Whom | Fat | |
| | Cereal | |
| | Beverage | |
| | Other | |
| | ***Lunch*** | |
| Time | Meat | |
| | Vegetable | |
| Where | Bread | |
| | Fruit | |
| With Whom | Beverage | |
| | Other | |
| | ***Dinner*** | |
| Time | Soup | |
| | Meat/Subst. | |
| Where | Potato | |
| | Veg. cooked | |
| With Whom | Veg. raw | |
| | Salad | |
| | Bread | |
| | Fat | |
| | Dessert | |
| | Beverage | |
| | Other | |
| Time | ***Between Meals*** | |

**FOOD SUMMARY**

| GROUP | Amount Per Day | Amount Per Week | Possible Points or Daily Serv | **Actual Points |
|---|---|---|---|---|
| ***Dairy Products:*** | | | 3 | |
| Milk | | | | |
| Cheese | | | | |
| Cottage Cheese | | | | |
| Yogurt | | | | |
| Other | | | | |
| ***Meat or Alternatives: (***Fat and Ch)*** | | | 2 | |
| ***Meat, eggs | | | | |
| Fish, Poultry | | | | |
| Dr. Beans/Peas | | | | |
| Peanut Butter | | | | |
| ***Vegetables: (No Vit. A/C -½ cr.)*** | | | 3 | |
| Vit. A Veg. | | | | |
| Vit. C Veg. | | | | |
| Other | | | | |
| ***Fruits:*** | | | 2 | |
| Vit. C Fruits | | | | |
| Other Fruits | | | | |
| ***Whole Grains/Starches: (No wh/grains -½ cr.)*** | | | 6 | |
| Cereal | | | | |
| Bread | | | | |
| Pasta, Rice | | | | |
| Other/crackers | | | | |
| | | Total: | 16 | |
| ***Others:*** | | | | |
| Candy/sugar | | | If daily -1 | |
| Chips/t. salt | | | If daily -1 | |
| Soft Drinks | | | If daily -1 | |
| Desserts | | | If daily -1 | |
| Water | | | None daily -1 | |
| ***Fats, chol. | | | 3 Srv Daily -1 | |
| Fiber | | | None daily -1 | |
| | | | Total: | |

Frequency/week of eating outside of home ______
Food allergies ______
Foods regularly omitted ______
Why? ______
Favorite foods ______
Impression of diet ______
Validity of record ______
Activity score ______

Using iodized salt? Cooking ______ Table ______
Using vitamin D fortified milk? *Y / N* Caretaker knowledge of fiber and fluid? *Y / N* Can plan Basic Four Diet? *Y / N*

* If dietary recall, anthropometric measures, or clinical assessment abnormal, obtain 3-Day Food Intake Record and 3-Day Physical Activity Record for evaluation.
** When the number of servings eaten exceeds the number possible, those servings are not counted. Score below 10 requires follow-up visit, score 10-12 is borderline nutritionally.
*** Group with possibly high fat and cholesterol.

Name:________________________ Date: ____________

## PHYSICAL ACTIVITY RECORD

Estimation of Caloric Needs

Weight: kg ________ (lbs)________ %ile ______ Caloric Input__________
Height: kg. ________ (in)________ %ile ______ Caloric Input__________

RDA caloric average for ages ________ to ________ =________

RDA range for age ________- ________

**A.** Record the following activities as accurately as possible:

| Activity | Time in Hours | Calories/ lb/Hour | | Total per lb. |
|---|---|---|---|---|
| 1. Sleeping | | X 0.4 | = | |
| 2. Sitting at rest (watching TV, reading, etc.) | | X 0.7 | = | |
| 3. Sitting (hand activities, i.e., playing with toys) | | X 1.0 | = | |
| 4. Walking with crutches | | X 1.5 | = | |
| 5. Walking with crutches, total self-care | | X 2.0 | = | |
| 6. Walking doing light exercise (playground walking, sandbox playing, swinging) | | X 2.0 | = | |
| 7. Moderate exercise (active games, i.e., playing ball, stair climbing, dancing) | | X 2.7 | = | |
| 8. Strenuous exercise (running, swimming, bicycle riding, etc.) | | X 4.3 | = | |
| | | Total 24 | | TOTAL |

Caloric Output (total per lb. x weight in lbs.):______________

*Optional:*

**B.** Recommended kcal. per cm. height_______x height (cm) = _______ kcal/day

(use only for children with motor dysfunction, ages 5-12)
(ambulatory, motor dysfunction, 13.9 cal/cm.)
(Nonambulatory, severe motor dysfunction, 11.1s cal/cm.)

Caretaker demonstrates knowledge of relationship of calories to physical activity: Yes / No

## NUTRITIONAL CLINICAL EVALUATION

**Code: 0 = absent; 1 = present; 2 = does not apply**

***Hair:*** All neg. ☐

| | Code | Doubtful |
|---|---|---|
| dry | | |
| depigmented | | |
| easily pluckable | | |
| abnormal texture | | |

***Eyes:*** All neg. ☐

| | Code | Doubtful |
|---|---|---|
| cloudy | | |
| reddened | | |
| dry | | |
| | | |
| | | |

***Lips:*** All neg. ☐

| | Code | Doubtful |
|---|---|---|
| angular lesions | | |
| angular scars | | |
| | | |
| | | |

***Gums:*** All neg. ☐

| | Code | Doubtful |
|---|---|---|
| swelling | | |
| redness | | |
| hypertrophy | | |
| bleeding | | |

***Teeth:*** All neg. ☐

| | Code | Doubtful |
|---|---|---|
| visible caries | | |
| missing teeth | | |
| calculus | | |
| mottling | | |
| striated discoloration | | |
| malocclusion | | |

***Tongue:*** All neg. ☐

| | Code | Doubtful |
|---|---|---|
| glossy | | |
| fissures | | |
| magenta | | |
| geographic | | |

***Nails:*** All neg. ☐

| | Code | Doubtful |
|---|---|---|
| clubbed | | |
| ridged | | |
| spooned | | |
| blue | | |
| combinations | | |

***Face & Neck:*** All neg. ☐

| | Code | Doubtful |
|---|---|---|
| thyroid enlarged | | |
| facial stigmata of syndrome | | |
| | | |
| | | |

***Skin:*** All neg. ☐

| | Code | Doubtful |
|---|---|---|
| follicular hyperkeratosis | | |
| hyperpigmentation | | |
| dry and scaling | | |
| cold | | |
| depigmentation | | |

***Skeletal or Muscular:*** All neg. ☐

| | Code | Doubtful |
|---|---|---|
| protuberant abdomen | | |
| bowed legs | | |
| knocked-knees | | |
| beading of ribs | | |
| enlargement of wrist | | |
| winged scapula | | |
| scoliosis | | |
| muscle wasting | | |

***Lower Extremities:*** All neg. ☐

| | Code | Doubtful |
|---|---|---|
| pretibial edema | | |
| | | |
| | | |
| | | |

***General Appearance (check all that apply):***

| | |
|---|---|
| ___ Skinny | ___ Very active |
| ___ Fat | ___ Ambulatory |
| ___ Well-proportioned | ___ Nonambulatory |
| ___ Alert | ___ No speech |
| ___ Apathetic | ___ Unintelligible speech |
| ___ Irritable | ___ Intelligible speech |
| ___ Uncooperative | ___ Poor feeding behavior |

***Parent-Child Interaction (check one):***

___ Appropriate
___ Moderate
___ Slight
___ None

Name:________________ Date:__________

## FEEDING SKILL DEVELOPMENT

|  |  |
|---|---|
| *Birth* | Total body response |
| | Rooting reflex |
| | Sucking reflex |
| | Swallowing |
| | Tearless hunger cry |
| | Retrussion reflex |
| *4 Weeks* | Face brightens on saiety |
| | Looks at mother's face |
| | Tonic necks reflex position of head |
| | 2 night feedings - *8 Weeks |
| *8 Weeks* | 1 night feeding - *28 weeks |
| *12-16 Weeks* | Choking response to solids |
| *16 Weeks* | Head erect but set forward |
| | Anticipates on sight of food |
| | Arms activate at toys or food |
| | Mouth poised for nipple |
| *20 Weeks* | Pats bottle or breast - *36 weeks |
| | Closes in on bottle with both hands |
| | Scratches table top or flat surface |
| *24 Weeks* | Brings hand to mouth |
| | Sits in chair when securely supported |
| *28 Weeks* | Sits with some support |
| | Takes solids well |
| | Feet to mouth - *36 weeks |
| | Grasp spoon, nipple, cup rim |
| | Remove food quickly from spoon |
| *32 Weeks* | Bites, chews toys - *18 months |
| | Acquire sitting balance |
| | Guides mother's hand during feeding |
| *36 Weeks* | Holds feeding bottle |
| | Feeds self cracker well |
| | Prehands scissors grasp - *40 weeks |
| *40 Weeks* | Sits well, creeps |
| | Combines 2 toys, utensils |
| | Chooses pellet, finger food |
| *44 Weeks* | Treis to feed self |
| | Drinks from cup in part |
| | Tries to use spoon |
| *48 Weeks* | Net pincer grasp |
| | Cessation of drooling except when talking |
| | Scratches table top or flat surface |
| *15 Months* | Bottle discarded |
| | Grasp inhibition |
| | Uses spoon, upside down |
| | Releases finger food into cup |
| | Casts toy or finger food |
| | Grasps cup with both hands |
| | Sucks through straw |
| *18 Months* | Feeds self in part spills - *36 months |
| | Hands empty dish to mother |
| | Finger foods with pieces of food |
| *21 Months* | Handles cup well |
| | Verbalizes "eat," "all gone," asks for food |
| | Spoon to mouth right side up |
| *2 Years* | Uses spoon well |
| | Feeds doll |
| | Fond of ritual |
| *3 Years* | Spills little |
| | Pours well from small pitcher |
| | Feeds self well using utensils |

## FEEDING SKILL ASSESSMENT CHART*

Number of Observations

| | 1 | 2 | 3 | 4 | 5 | 6 | 7 | 8 | 9 | 10 |
|---|---|---|---|---|---|---|---|---|---|---|
| Breathes through mouth | | | | | | | | | | |
| Sits with good head control | | | | | | | | | | |
| Grasp response follows a tactile stimulus | | | | | | | | | | |
| Lip closure occurs | | | | | | | | | | |
| Can protrude tongue | | | | | | | | | | |
| Can lateralize tongue (moves easily from side to side) | | | | | | | | | | |
| Can elevate tongue | | | | | | | | | | |
| Removes food from spoon with lips | | | | | | | | | | |
| Control of drooling | | | | | | | | | | |
| Drinks from cup (in part) | | | | | | | | | | |
| Holds own cup (spills easily) | | | | | | | | | | |
| Holds own cup (few spills) | | | | | | | | | | |
| Holds own cup by handles, drinks well | | | | | | | | | | |
| Has hand to mouth movements | | | | | | | | | | |
| Finger feeds (cracker) | | | | | | | | | | |
| Removes food from spoon with lips, not teeth | | | | | | | | | | |
| Uses spoon (spills frequently) | | | | | | | | | | |
| Uses spoon (few spills) | | | | | | | | | | |
| Fills spoon, brings to mouth and eats | | | | | | | | | | |
| Uses fork | | | | | | | | | | |
| Uses knife | | | | | | | | | | |
| Feeds self using utensils | | | | | | | | | | |
| Shows independence in eating and talking well | | | | | | | | | | |
| Eats rapidly | | | | | | | | | | |
| Can straw suck | | | | | | | | | | |
| Pours from pitcher | | | | | | | | | | |
| Can serve self | | | | | | | | | | |
| Can set table | | | | | | | | | | |

***Key***: **X** = adequate; **/** = attempt; **+** with help; **-** unable to do; **0** = not tested

* Use Velcro on plates for stability and location of plates based on clock time, digits for consistency for the visually and hearing impaired.

**Name:**______________________ **Date:**______________

## MUELLER PRE-SPEECH AND FEEDING EVALUATION

| | *N* | *Abn* | *Nt** |
|---|---|---|---|
| 1. ***Facial Expression*** | | | |
| 2. ***Feeding Reflexes*** | | | |
| Rooting Reflex | | | |
| Suck/Swallow Reflex | | | |
| Bite Reflex | | | |
| Gag Reflex | | | |
| 3. ***Feeding Behavior*** | | | |
| Sucking/Drinking | | | |
| Swallowing | | | |
| Chewing - Rotary? | | | |
| 4. ***Response to Digital Stimulation*** | | | |
| Outside mouth | | | |
| Inside mouth | | | |
| 5. ***Dental Development*** | | | |
| Bite Reflex | | | |
| Teeth | | | |
| Gums | | | |
| 6. ***Jaws*** | | | |
| At rest | | | |
| In motion | | | |
| 7. ***Lips*** | | | |
| At rest | | | |
| In motion | | | |
| 8. ***Tongue*** | | | |
| At rest | | | |
| In motion | | | |
| 9. ***Breathing*** | | | |
| At rest | | | |
| In motion | | | |
| 10. ***Voice*** | | | |
| Pitch, range | | | |
| Loudness | | | |
| Rate | | | |
| Intonation | | | |

* Could not be tested

*SUMMARY*

*PROCEDURE RECOMMENDED*

**CINCINNATI CHILDREN'S HOSPITAL MEDICAL CENTER**
**DIVISION OF DEVELOPMENTAL DISABILITIES**

**CHILD**
Nutritional Assessment (Case Workup) Evaluation

| | Points |
|---|---|
| **I. Demographic Data – 100 Points Total** | |
| A. Chart reviewed for pertinent data from other evaluations and parental questionnaire pertaining to nutrition | 10 |
| B. Anthropometric data completed with accurate calculations and percentiles. | 10 |
| C. Prenatal, newborn and pertinent family data recorded. | 10 |
| D. Laboratory data compiled. | 10 |
| E. Twenty-four hour recall and food summary evaluated. | 20 |
| F. Physical Activity Record | 10 |
| G. Clinical Evaluation | 10 |
| H. Feeding Skill and Assessment | 20 |

| | Evaluation |
|---|---|
| **II. Nutrition Record Summary – 100 Points Total** | |
| A. Pertinent Nutritional History<br>- prenatal<br>- newborn food intake<br>- supplements<br>- feeding milestones development<br>- diet history of infancy and early childhood | 18 |
| B. Evaluation of current Nutritional Status<br>- behavior patterns during feeding/reward system<br>- present dietary pattern/fiber/fluid, caloric intake and expenditure<br>- associated problems<br>- caretaker knowledge | 12 |
| C. Anthropometric Data<br>- growth grid completed and curve plotted<br>- current measurements and percentiles/weight-height ratio and status to ideal weight and age | 8 |
| D. Biochemical Data<br>- medications<br>- drug/food interactions/caretaker knowledge<br>- laboratory values<br>- supplements | 4 |
| E. Clinical Observations<br>- physical signs and symptoms<br>- current feeding abilities – a, b and c<br>- observation of behavior during interview<br>- interaction with parents | 16 |
| F. Presenting Nutritional Problem | 6 |
| G. Impressions<br>- overall nutritional status<br>- weight/height ratio, number of pounds over or under ideal weight<br>- adequacy of diet expressed in foods and nutrients/medication interaction; % of DRI, if a 3DDD<br>- physical activity/relationship to caloric intake/expenditure<br>- feeding skills level | 20 |
| H. Recommendations: Care Plan<br>- recommendations made during interview/caretaker knowledge<br>- translate low or excessive nutrients into appropriate food sources/plus adequate fiber and fluids<br>- food budgeting, selection and preparation<br>- special techniques to improve feeding skills<br>- physical activities beneficial to client<br>- referral to other programs<br>- type of counseling, treatment needed from Nutrition Department<br>- pertinent, practical and realistic planning goals/timetable/how measured<br>- format of written report | 16 |

**CINCINNATI CHILDREN'S HOSPITAL MEDICAL CENTER**
**DIVISION OF DEVELOPMENTAL DISABILITIES**

**INFANT-TODDLER NUTRITION FORM**
(High Risk and Myelomeningocele Clinics)

Name: ______ Parents Name: ______
Birthdate: ______ Age: ______ Address: ______
Date: ______
Pediatrician: ______ Siblings: ______
Diagnosis: ______

Height______ (____cm.) ______% Hct______ low / normal
Weight______ (____kg.) ______% Hgb______ low / normal
Ht./Wt. Ratio____/____ ______% Hx of infections: Yes / No
Head Circumference______ ______% Allergies: Yes / No
Skinfold______ ______%

Growth since last clinic visits: Ht. ______ Wt.______ Plot growth curve______
Clinical Evaluation: NEG / POS (area) ______
Physical Limitations (scale 1-8, 8 high) / Dx: ______
Vitamins/Minerals: Yes / No Type: ______
Medications: Yes / No Nutrient Interaction: ______
Fluoride Source: Yes / No
WIC: Yes / No ______

Appetite: ______
Diet/Eating Concerns: ______
Feeding Problems (circle): sucking, chewing, choking, drooling, swallowing, colic, spitting, tongue thrust, pica

**DIET**

*Breast fed______
*Formula (type)______
Amount per day______
Infant foods: How taken?______
Age started:______
Yes/No: Table salt____ Table sugar____ Pop____
*Water: Amount per day______

Constipation: .......... Yes / No
Diarrhea: .......... Yes / No
*Food Allergies: .......... Yes / No
*Nursing Bottle Syndrome: .......... Yes / No
*Solid foods *should not* be given before 4 months of age.
Review quantity of food, sample menu: ...... Yes / No

Caretaker knowledge demonstrated:
Caloric expenditure .......... Yes / No
Nutrition .......... Yes / No
Fiber and fluid .......... Yes / No
Dental health .......... Yes /No
Food and drug interaction .......... Yes / No

| TIME | | 24 HOUR RECALL | Amount | Score |
|---|---|---|---|---|
| ______ | B. | Fruit______ | ______ | |
| | | Meat/Egg______ | ______ | |
| | | Bread______ | ______ | |
| | | Fat______ | ______ | |
| | | Cereal______ | ______ | |
| | | Beverage______ | ______ | ______ |
| ______ | L. | Meat______ | ______ | |
| | | Veg.______ | ______ | |
| | | Bread______ | ______ | |
| | | Fruit______ | ______ | |
| | | Beverage______ | ______ | ______ |
| ______ | D. | Meat______ | ______ | |
| | | Veg.______ | ______ | |
| | | Salad______ | ______ | |
| | | Bread______ | ______ | |
| | | Fat______ | ______ | |
| | | Dessert______ | ______ | |
| | | Beverage______ | ______ | ______ |

| TIME | BETWEEN MEALS | |
|---|---|---|
| ______ | ______ | ______ |
| ______ | ______ | ______ |
| ______ | ______ | ______ |

**INFANT-TODDLER NUTRITION FORM (Cont'd)**

**DEVELOPMENTAL ASSESSMENT:**

**FEEDING:** SPOON -- Grasps Yes / No, unable, palmer, pincer (assisted) or (unassisted)
**(fine motor)** *Control:* ______beginning ______fair ______ good

CUP -- Grasps Yes / No, both hands, one hand (assisted) or (unassisted)
*Control:* ______beginning ______fair ______ good

Bottle: .......... Yes / No
Infa-Feeder: .......... Yes / No
Finger Feeding: ...... Yes / No

**GROSS MOTOR:**
______Sitting (with or without support) ______Pullup
______Hand to mouth control ______Stand alone
______Chewing ______Cruising
______Creeping ______Walking
______Crawling ______Running

**MANNER FEED:** ______High chair ______Pumpkin seat ______Held
Transition to table foods/Reward System: ______

**OVERALL FEEDING SKILLS ASSESSMENT:** ______Age appropriate ______Delayed
Caloric intake______or______kcal/kg. ______Low ______Acceptable ______Above DRI range

*DRI range keal: 0 – 6 mos. ______kg x 115 kcal = ______(95-145)
6 mos. – 1 year ______kg x 105 kcal = ______(80-135)
1 yr – 3 yr 3000 (900-1800)

*DRI protein: 0 – 6 mos. ______kg x 2.5 gm = ______
6 mos. – 1 yr. ______kg x 2.0 gm = ______
1 yr. – 3 yr. 23 gm

Water needs______
Overall Diet Adequacy: ______Acceptable ______Not Acceptable

**ADDITIONAL COMMENTS:**

**SOAP NUTRITION CARE PLAN/RECOMMENDATIONS/FOLLOW UP**
Goals/timetable/How measured

______
Nutritionist

Prepared by J. Wessel, E. Grace, M. Schmidt and S. Ekvall 6/84, revised 10/03

**4–3** Nutrition Mid-Level Clinical Assessment Record (Above Toddler Age), CCDDD/CCHMC

**CINCINNATI CHILDREN'S HOSPITAL MEDICAL CENTER, DIVISION OF DEVELOPEMNTAL DISABILITIES**
**Myelomeningogcele Clinic and Cerebral Palsy Clinic**
Nutrition Evaluation Form
(>Toddler Age)

Today's Date:________________

MR#________________________
Name:______________________________________________
Birth Date:_____________________
Height:_______(_____cm)______%
Weight::______(_____cm)______%
Wt/Ht Ratio:_______% if under 10 years
Knee Height__________cm
Brace Weight:____________________
Head Circumference:___________________cm
Waist Circumference:________inches
Upper Arm Circumference:______(______cm)______%
Arm Muscle Area:__________cm_________%
Tricep:________mm Upper Arm length________
Thorax:________mm Abdomen___________mm
Nutrition Clinical Evaluation: Neg / Pos
Physical Limitations: Wheelchair/Braces/Walker/Self-Ambulator
Physical Activity Score (1-8):____________

Age:____________
Hct:______________low / normal Hgh__________low / normal
(from CCDDD/CCHMC record)
Hx of infections________________________ Allergies: Yes / No
Constipation Yes / No Method:____________________
Diet Restrictions: Yes / No Type:____________________
Vitamins / Minerals: Yes / No Type:____________________
Nutrients Affected:____________________
Feeding Skills Assessment: Normal / Delayed
Behavioral Problems:____________ Reward system:__________
Caretaker Knowledge Demonstrated: Yes / No
Caloric Expenditure:____________ Dental Health:____________
Nutrition:__________ Food & Drug Interaction:______________
Fiber & Fluid:______________
Food Stamps: Yes / No

Diet History: Yes / No Nutrient Deficits:________________________________________
Food Summary Score:__________________ Estimated caloric intake: ________________ Expenditure:__________________

**24-HOUR RECALL**

| ***Breakfast*** | **Amount** |
|---|---|
| Fruit______________________ | ________ |
| Meat______________________ | ________ |
| Egg______________________ | ________ |
| Bread______________________ | ________ |
| Fat______________________ | ________ |
| Cereal______________________ | ________ |
| Beverage ______________________ | ________ |
| Other______________________ | ________ |
| ***Lunch*** | |
| Meat______________________ | ________ |
| Vegetable | ________ |
| Bread______________________ | ________ |
| Fruit______________________ | ________ |
| Beverage ______________________ | ________ |
| Other______________________ | ________ |
| ***Dinner*** | |
| Soup______________________ | ________ |
| Meat/Subst.______________________ | ________ |
| Potato______________________ | ________ |
| Veg. cooked______________________ | ________ |
| Veg. raw ______________________ | ________ |
| Salad______________________ | ________ |
| Bread______________________ | ________ |
| Fat______________________ | ________ |
| Dessert______________________ | ________ |
| Beverage______________________ | ________ |
| Other______________________ | ________ |

**Time Between Meals**

______________________ ________
______________________ ________
______________________ ________

**FOOD SUMMARY**

| **GROUP** | **Day** | **Week** | **Possible Points** | ****Actual Points** |
|---|---|---|---|---|
| ***Dairy Products:*** | | | 3 | |
| Milk | ______ | ______ | ______ | ______ |
| Cheese | ______ | ______ | ______ | ______ |
| Cottage Cheese | ______ | ______ | ______ | ______ |
| Yogurt | ______ | ______ | ______ | ______ |
| Other | ______ | ______ | ______ | ______ |
| ***Meat or Alternatives: (***Fat and Ch)*** | | | 2 | |
| ***Meat, eggs | ______ | ______ | ______ | ______ |
| Fish, Poultry | ______ | ______ | ______ | ______ |
| Dr. Beans/Peas | ______ | ______ | ______ | ______ |
| Peanut Butter | | | | |
| ***Vegetables: (No Vit. A/C -½ cr.)*** | | | 3 | |
| Vit. A Veg. | ______ | ______ | ______ | ______ |
| Vit. C Veg. | ______ | ______ | ______ | ______ |
| Other | ______ | ______ | ______ | ______ |
| ***Fruits:*** | | | | |
| Vit. C Fruits | ______ | ______ | ______ | ______ |
| Other Fruits | ______ | ______ | ______ | ______ |
| ***Whole Grains/Starches: (No wh/grains -½ cr.)*** | | | 6 | |
| Cereal | ______ | ______ | ______ | ______ |
| Bread | ______ | ______ | ______ | ______ |
| Pasta, Rice | ______ | ______ | ______ | ______ |
| Other/crackers | ______ | ______ | ______ | ______ |
| | | Total: | 16 | |
| ***Others:*** | | | | |
| Candy/sugar | ______ | ______ | If daily -1 | ______ |
| Chips/t. salt | ______ | ______ | If daily -1 | ______ |
| Soft Drinks | ______ | ______ | If daily -1 | ______ |
| Desserts | ______ | ______ | If daily -1 | ______ |
| Water | ______ | ______ | None daily -1 | ______ |
| ***Fats, chol. | ______ | ______ | 3 Srv Daily -1 | ______ |
| Fiber | ______ | ______ | None daily -1 | ______ |
| | | Total: | | ______ |

(>Toddler Age) Form – Page 2
Nutrition Assessment Report and Soap Nutrition Care Plan

Recommendations/Follow-up/Goals/timetable/How Measured

______________________________
Team Nutritionist

# Nutrition Screening/Mini Evaluation

Community Outreach – Developmental Consultation Team (DCT)

*Teacher/Nurse* - Observation Checklist for Nutritional Evaluation:

| | *Yes* | *No* |
|---|---|---|
| Disproportional weight for height | ______ | ______ |
| Frequent absenteeism | ______ | ______ |
| Falls asleep in class | ______ | ______ |
| Lacks ambition | ______ | ______ |
| Behaves clumsily or falls easily | ______ | ______ |
| Delayed healing of minor injuries | ______ | ______ |
| Bites nails | ______ | ______ |
| Signs of hyperactivity | ______ | ______ |
| Many food dislikes (if known) | ______ | ______ |
| Balanced lunch including protein, fruit and milk | ______ | ______ |
| Frequent colds or respiratory infections | ______ | ______ |
| Good appetite | ______ | ______ |
| Frequent headaches | ______ | ______ |
| Frequent digestive disturbances | ______ | ______ |
| Allergies (if known) | ______ | ______ |

Additional health of nutritional information of importance not included in above______________________

________________________________________________________________________

________________________________________________________________________

Checklist for screening to be complete by *Nutritionist*:

Height________________________________ Percentile__________

Weight________________________________ Percentile__________

Head Circumference____________________ Percentile__________

*Physical Appearances:*

| | Satisfactory | If Unsatisfactory-describe |
|---|---|---|
| Hair | __________ | ____________________ |
| Skin | __________ | ____________________ |
| Nails | __________ | ____________________ |
| Eyes | __________ | ____________________ |
| Teeth | __________ | ____________________ |
| Gums | __________ | ____________________ |
| Tongue | __________ | ____________________ |
| Posture | __________ | ____________________ |
| Abdomen | __________ | ____________________ |
| Skeletal development | __________ | ____________________ |

Other Comments ________________________________________________________

The *Social Worker* Interview with parents:

Questions on family food practices, such as feeding history (feeding difficulties) and dietary history (food purchasing, food preparation, eating habits)_______________________________________

________________________________________________________________________

*Prepared by Catherine Grogan, M.Ed., RD, and Patricia Lierman, M.Ed, RD; DCT Staff Nutritionists
From *Clinical Instruction Techniques in an Interdisciplinary Setting*, S. Ekvall

NAME:____________________ AGE:__________

WT:________ HT:__________ Dates: *from* ____________ *to*________

## Instruction Sheet for Recording of Dietary Intake

1. Record what the child has eaten immediately after each meal or snack. (Do not trust your memory at the end of the day)

2. Date each sheet – have consecutive days (unless illness intervenes).

3. Be exact as to amounts, i.e., report in terms of level tablespoons, cups, dimensions of slices of meat, size of fruit, etc. (*Bowlfuls*, *glasses* and *servings* do not indicate accurate measures of food contained therein).

4. Describe *accurately* the kind of food recorded:
   a. State brand name whenever possible
   b. Type of milk used, i.e., *whole, powdered, evaporated*, etc. Mention whenever butter, milk, sugar are used in cream sauce, etc.
   c. Differentiate between ice milk and ice cream.
   d. Type of bread/cereal used, i.e., *whole wheat, white, rye, cornflakes, oatmeal*, etc.
   e. Method of cooking, i.e, *boiled, fried, creamed, roasted*, etc. and give entire recipes (list of ingredients) of mixed dishes.
   f. State whether canned, dried, fresh or frozen product.

5. Be sure to record *everything* eaten:
   a. Vitamin preparations and medicines.
   b. "Hidden foods," i.e., *sugar* on cereal or fruit; *butter, oleo or mayonnaise* on bread, vegetables, or popcorn; *crumb or cheese topping*, etc.
   c. Candy, pop, potato chips – state kind and amount.

6. At the end of this period, please complete the following:
   g. Was this a typical week – does the child usually eat these foods and these amounts?____________________
   b. If not, how was it different?____________________
   c. Was there any illness during this period?____________________

Day

| Meal Pattern | Kind of Food Calories | Amount | |
|---|---|---|---|
| ***Breakfast***<br>Time:<br>Where:<br>With Whom: | | | |
| ***Mid-Morning***<br>Snacks | | | |
| ***Lunch***<br>Time:<br>Where:<br>With Whom: | | | |
| ***Afternoon***<br>Snacks | | | |
| ***Dinner***<br>Time:<br>Where:<br>With Whom: | | | |
| ***Afternoon***<br>Snack | | | |
| ***Evening***<br>Snacks | | | |
| **Water** | | | |
| **Vitamins and Minerals** | | | |
| **Appetite** | | | |

*Total Calories:*____________

### Physical Activity Record

Record below all activities during the day from time of waking up until going to bed in the evening and falling asleep.

*Example:*

| Time From | Time Until | Kind of Activity | Where |
|---|---|---|---|
| 11:00 | 11:30 | Played ball | Outdoors |

# APPENDIX 5
## Nutritional Assessment Records, Developmental Evaluation Center, Boston Children's Hospital Medical Center, and Other Nutritional Assessment Forms

**5–1** In-Depth Nutrition Assessment Record, Developmental Evaluation Center, Boston Children's Hospital Medical Center

Child's Name Date

Child's Birth Date Age

Person Completing Form

Relationship to child

What are your child's feeding problems?

1.

2.

3.

4.

5.

How much did your child weigh at birth?

What was your child's length at birth?

Was your child a full term baby?

How long did your child stay in hospital at birth?

Has your child had any hospitalizations since birth?

Has your child ever been treated with a special diet?

Circle the answer that applies

Weight gain from birth has been: satisfactory slow fluctuating

Weight gain recently has been: satisfactory slow fluctuating

How does this child compare to siblings at the same age? larger same smaller

How much does mother weigh?

How tall is mother?

How much does father weigh?

How tall is father?

Has your child ever been treated with a special diet?

Early Feeding Problems

| | Never | 0-6 Months | 6-12 Months | 1-3 Years | 3-6 Years |
|---|---|---|---|---|---|
| Sucking | | | | | |
| Swallowing | | | | | |
| Chewing | | | | | |
| Tongue Control | | | | | |
| Lip Control | | | | | |
| Color Change with Feeding | | | | | |
| Gagging | | | | | |
| Colic | | | | | |
| Spitting-up | | | | | |
| Vomiting | | | | | |
| Appetite | | | | | |
| Food Intolerances | | | | | |
| Diarrhea | | | | | |
| Constipation | | | | | |
| Anemia | | | | | |
| Dehydration | | | | | |
| Underweight | | | | | |
| Overweight | | | | | |
| Poor Growth | | | | | |
| Gastrostomy | | | | | |
| Nasogastric | | | | | |
| Hyperalimentation | | | | | |
| Intravenous | | | | | |

How Often Does Your Child Eat These Foods?

| | Daily | Occasionally | Seldom |
|---|---|---|---|
| Milk | | | |
| Cheese, ice cream | | | |
| Cold or hot cereal | | | |
| Sweet rolls or donuts | | | |
| Sandwiches | | | |
| Soup | | | |
| Fruit or fruit juice | | | |
| Peanut butter or nuts | | | |
| Dried peas or beans | | | |
| Meat in casseroles | | | |
| Red meat, fish or poultry | | | |
| Cooked or raw vegetable | | | |
| Potato, rice or noodles | | | |
| Cookies or crackers | | | |
| Pie, cake or brownies | | | |
| Potato chips or corn chips | | | |
| Candy | | | |
| Soft drinks or kool-aid | | | |

Feeding Development

| | 0-3 Months | 4-6 Months | 7-9 Months | 10-12 Months | 13-15 Months | 16-18 Months | 19-21 Months | 22-24 Months | 2-2½ Years | 2½-3 Years | Not Yet |
|---|---|---|---|---|---|---|---|---|---|---|---|
| Baby Food Introduction | | | | | | | | | | | |
| Junior Foods | | | | | | | | | | | |
| Finger Feeding | | | | | | | | | | | |
| Cup Drinking | | | | | | | | | | | |
| Weaning | | | | | | | | | | | |
| Whole Table Foods | | | | | | | | | | | |
| Use of Spoon | | | | | | | | | | | |
| Independent Feeding | | | | | | | | | | | |
| Self Preparation of Food | | | | | | | | | | | |

Present Feeding

What is the hungriest time of the day for your child? a.m. noon p.m.

Does your child ever crave or eat non-food items? yes no

Please Record the Usual Daily Food Intake:

| Time of meal or snack | Food eaten | Amount |
|---|---|---|
| | | |

Is your child on a vitamin-mineral supplement? yes name no

List the medications taken by your child

Past____________________

Now____________________

What is your child's position during feeding? held in seat sits independently

How long does a feeding take? 15 minutes or less ½ hour ½ hour or more

Who usually feeds your child? mother father other

Describe the texture of your child's food. strained ground cut regular

How is your child fed? bottle cup spoon gastrostomy nasogastric

Describe your child's appetite: excellent fair poor

Does your child bring toys or fingers to his or her mouth? yes no

Describe your child's level of independece. totally independent partially dependent

Does your child close his or hands around a bottle? yes no

Does your child finger feed? yes no

Does your child attempt to grasp the spoon as you feed? yes no

Is your child sipping from a cup? yes no

Does your child: Drink independently from a cup?

raises cup
drinks
replaces

Does your child eat independently with a spoon?

- grasps spoon
- dips in dish
- fills spoon
- brings spoon to mouth
- replaces spoon

Does your child use a fork? yes no

DEVELOPMENTAL EVALUATION CLINIC

NAME:-------------------- PARENTS:------------------------
D.O.B.:--------- AGE:------ ADDRESS:--------------------------
D.O.E.:-------
EVALUATOR:----------------- TELEPHONE:------------------------
DIAGNOSIS:---------------------------------------------------

ANTHROPOMETRICS

HEIGHT:--------/--------IN./CM ------% ------%(DS)
WEIGHT:--------/--------LBS./KG------% ------%(DS)
WT/HT RELATIONSHIP:--------% HEAD CIRCUMFERENCE:------IN/CM----%
HEIGHT AGE:------ WEIGHT AGE:------- IDEAL BODY WEIGHT:--------
SKIN FOLD:------MM/------% ARM CIRCUMFERENCE:--------MM/------%
MAMC:---------CM/---------%

ACTIVITY LEVEL AND MUSCLE TONE

-----AMBULATORY -----WHEELCHAIR BOUND ------INVOLUNTARY MOVEMENTS -----NORMAL TONE -----HYPERTONIA -----HYPOTONIA
-----VARIABLE TONE -----SIT WITH /WITHOUT SUPPORT
-----STAND WITH/WITHOUT SUPPORT.

PRENATAL AND INFANT HISTORY:

GESTATIONAL LENGTH:------------- PRENATAL WEIGHT GAIN:-----------
BIRTH COMPLICATIONS:-------------------------------------------
BIRTH WEIGHT:---------------- BIRTH LENGTH:-------------------
BREAST FED:------- BOTTLE FED:----------- FORMULA:---------------
AGE SOLID FOODS WERE STARTED:----------------------------------
DIFFICULTIES:--------------------------------------------------

BIOCHEMICAL DATA:

SERUM ALBUMIN:-------(GM/DL) SERUM TOTAL PROTEIN:------(GM/DL)
HEMOGLOBIN:-------(GM/DL) HCT:------(%) SERUM TRANSFERRIN(MG/DL) ------- OTHER:-----------------------------------------------

NUTRITIONAL HISTORY:

FEEDING SKILLS:
------NO SELF-FEEDING SKILLS -----ABLE TO FEED SELF WITH ASSISTANCE -----HOLDS BOTTLE -----FINGER FEEDS -----WEANED FROM BOTTLE
INDEPENDENT WITH -----SPOON ------FORK ------STRAW
DIET TEXTURE:
------STRAINED BABY FOODS ------JUNIOR BABY FOODS
------BLENDERIZED/MASHED TABLE FOODS ------GROUND ------CHOPPED FINE -------REGULAR

24-HOUR RECALL(TYPICAL DAY):

| BREAKFAST | LUNCH | DINNER | SNACKS |
|---|---|---|---|
| -------------- | ------------- | ------------- | ------------- |
| -------------- | ------------- | ------------- | ------------- |
| -------------- | ------------- | ------------- | ------------- |
| -------------- | ------------- | ------------- | ------------- |
| -------------- | ------------- | ------------- | ------------- |
| -------------- | ------------- | ------------- | ------------- |
| -------------- | ------------- | ------------- | ------------- |
| -------------- | ------------- | ------------- | ------------- |

TOTAL CALORIES:------------- KCAL/KG:---------
PROTEIN(GMS)/KG:------------ FLUID INTAKE:--------(OZ/CC)
ESTIMATED NEEDS:
CALORIES:---------- KCAL/DAY, ----------KCAL/KG
PROTEIN:----------- GM/DAY, -----------GM/KG
FLUID: -----------CC/DAY

NUTRITIONAL RELATED CONCERNS:

ORAL MOTOR--------- BEHAVIORAL--------- POSITIONING------------
FOOD TOLERANCES----------------- VOMITING/GAGGING-------------
CONSTIPATION/DIARRHEA-------------- DENTAL PROBLEMS:-------------
MEDICATIONS:--------------------------------------------------
VITAMIN/MINERAL SUPPLEMENTS:-----------------------------------
OTHER CONCERNS:-----------------------------------------------

NUTRITIONAL IMPRESSIONS:--------------------------------------

RECOMMENDATIONS:

1.--------------------------------------------------------

2.--------------------------------------------------------

3.--------------------------------------------------------

4.--------------------------------------------------------

8/88

## 5–2 WIC Nutrition Education/Care Plan, Ohio

Date ____________

Participant's Name ____________

Participant's Age ____________

Location of Program Application:

____________

Circle type of encounter: Initial

Recert

Follow-up: Date ____________

Ind Grp HR Tel

Minimum Requirements for Nutrition Education

Required at initial certification. Restate needed thereafter.

( ) Information Covered.

___ 1. Explanation of nutritional need condition.
___ 2. Explanation that foods are for recipient and not entire family.
___ 3. Information regarding what constitutes an adequate diet for the participant.
___ 4. Explanation that the WIC foods are supplemental.
___ 5. Information regarding possible uses of the WIC foods.
___ 6. Information regarding the nutritional value of the WIC foods.
___ 7. Explanation of the importance of health care.
___ 8. Explanation of breastfeeding (pregnant women only).

**SUBJECTIVE**

Participant comments/statements:

Health professional comments/observations:

Language Barrier? Yes No

**OBJECTIVE**

Ht:___in___%ile
Wt:___lb___oz___%ile
Hct/Hgb: ______
See: ___ Growth chart
___ Certification form
Location of medical chart ______
Other clinical/medical data:

Parental heights: Mother ______ Father ______
Weight gain/loss: _____lb at ____ weeks gestation
Wrist Measurement: ____ in Frame size ______
EDC (Date) ____________

**ASSESSMENT**

| | WIC CODE | PRIORITY | COMMENTS |
|---|---|---|---|
| Anthropometric | | | |
| Weight/Growth: WNL O U | 11, 12, 13, 14, 15 | 1,6 | |
| Height: WNL Low Stature | 51, 52, 53, 54 | 1,3 | |
| Hematological | | | |
| WNL LOW N/A | 20 | 1, 3, 6 | |
| Nutritional | | | |
| 24 hour recall: | | | |
| WNL Inadequate | | | |
| Food Frequency: | 30, 62 | 4, 5, 6 | |
| WNL Inadequate | | | |
| Other Risk Assessments | | | |
| Age | 40, 41 | 1, 3 | |
| Breastfeeding | 70, 71, 72 | 1, 2, 4 | |
| Infants | 61, 64 | 2 | |
| Medical Condition | 44 | 1, 3 | |
| Previous/Current OB History | 42, 43, 45 | 1, 4 | |
| Prevention of Regression | 63 | 1, 3, 6 | |
| Substance Abuse | 46, 47, 48 | 1 | |
| Transfers | 80, 81 | 1, 2, 3, 4, 6 | |

Other Assessment Information

Receptive to counseling? Yes No
Objectives met? Yes No

High risk ____ Reason:
Ineligible ____ Reason:

**PLAN**

| COUNSELING | HANDOUTS |
|---|---|
| ___ Basic Nutrition | ___ Daily Food Guide |
| ___ Breastfeeding | ___ Breastfeeding: Baby's Best Start |
| ___ Dental/Baby Bottle Tooth Decay | ___ Food For the Preschooler: I II III |
| ___ Infant Feeding/Solids | ___ Feeding Your Baby |
| ___ Iron | ___ Eating Right For Your Baby |
| ___ Postpartum Nutrition | ___ Relief From Common Problems |
| ___ Prenatal Nutrition | ___ ABC's of Smart Snacking |
| ___ Snacking | ___ Food For Red Blood |
| ___ Vitamins/Minerals | ___ Counting Your Calories |
| ___ Weight Control | ___ Your Baby's Weight |
| ___ Other: | ___ Your Child's Weight |
| | ___ Other: |

Objectives set:

____________
Health Professional's Signature

Follow-up Contact (Date):

High Risk Plan:

Referrals:

| | |
|---|---|
| ___ Well Child CLinic | ___ Headstart |
| ___ Immunizations | ___ Physician |
| ___ HEALTHCHEK | ___ Dentist |
| ___ Prenatal Clinic | ___ Food Stamps |
| ___ Family Planning | ___ Childbirth Class |
| ___ Breastfeeding Support | ___ Other: |
| ___ Human Services/Medicaid | |

## FOOD FREQUENCY FOR WOMEN

Name: ______________ Today's Date: ______________

DIRECTIONS: For each GROUP of foods, write in the number of times PER DAY or WEEK the woman eats any of them and CIRCLE the serving size that is closest to what she USUALLY eats.

| Foods | Frequency | Your Usual Serving Size 1/2 | 1 | 2 | Tally + or - |
|---|---|---|---|---|---|
| Milk, Yogurt, Pudding, Custard, Creamed Soup | | 4 oz or 1/2 C | 8 oz or 1 C | 12-16 oz or 1-1/2 C | |
| Cheese | | 1/2-1 slice | 1-1/2 slices | 2-3 slices | |
| Cottage Cheese, Ice Cream, Milk Shake | | 1/2-1 C | 2 C | 3-4 C | |
| Meat, Poultry, Fish, Eggs | | 1 oz or 1 egg | 2 oz or 1 egg | 4 oz or 1 egg | |
| Dried Beans (Pinto, Kidney, etc.), Dried Peas (Split Peas) | | 1/4 C cooked | 3/4 C cooked | 1-1/2 C cooked | |
| Nuts, Seeds, Peanut Butter | | 1/2 oz or 1 T | 1 oz or 2 T | 2 oz or 4 T | |
| Vit C - Citrus Fruit or Juice, Tomato, Broccoli, Brussels Sprouts, Strawberries enriched Apple Juice, Green Peppers, Greens | | 1/4 C cooked or juice or 1/2 C raw | 1/2 C cooked or juice or 1 C raw | 1 C cooked or juice or 1-1/2 C raw | |
| Vit A - Spinach, Cantaloupe, Apricots Peaches, Sweet Potato, Yams, Carrots | | 1/4 C fresh 1/2 piece | 1/2 C fresh 1 piece | 1 C fresh 2 pieces | |
| White Potato, Peas, Corn, Lettuce, Zucchini, Green or Yellow Beans, Beets, Celery, Cucumber | | 1/4 C cooked or 1/2 C raw | 1/2 C cooked or 1 C raw | 1 C cooked or 2 C raw | |
| Apples, Banana, Plums, Pears, Grapes | | 1/4 C or 1/2 piece | 1/2 C or 1 piece | 1 C or 2 pieces | |
| Enriched or Whole Grain Breads, Muffins, Biscuits, Pancakes, Waffles, Crackers | | 1/2 slice | 1 slice | 2 slices | |
| Cereal (hot) and Rice, Pasta, Grits | | 1/4 C | 1/2-3/4 C | 1-1 1/2 C | |
| Cereals, Ready-to-Eat | | 1/2 C | 1 C | 2 C | |
| Sweet Roll, Donut, Cake, Pie, Cookies | | 1/2 piece | 1 piece | 2 pieces | |
| French Fries, Potato Chips, Corn Chips Cheese Curls, Pretzels, etc. | | 1 oz bag | 1 C | 2 C | |
| Pot Pies, TV Dinners, Canned or Packaged Spaghetti, Ravioli, Macaroni and Cheese, Beefaroni, or Canned Soup | | 1/2 C | 1 C | 2 C | |
| Coffee (regular), Tea | | 1/2 C | 1 C | 2 C | |
| Soda Pop, Hi-C, Kool-Aid, Cocoa, Fruit Drinks | | 6 oz | 12 oz | 16 oz | |
| Sugar, Honey, Maple Syrup | | 1 T | 2 T | 4 T | |

List any other foods you usually eat and how often: ______________

Name: ______________ Date: ______________

| What did you eat for: | HOW MUCH? (Amount of each food) | Milk | Meat & Alternatives | Fruit & Vegetables | Grain | Other |
|---|---|---|---|---|---|---|
| Morning | | | | | | |
| Between Meals | | | | | | |
| Noon | | | | | | |
| Between Meals | | | | | | |
| Evening | | | | | | |
| In Evening Before Bedtime | | | | | | |
| | Totals | | | | | |

From: Ohio Dept. of Health, Division of WIC. Used with permission.

5–3 Nutrition Assessment, Perinatal, California

## Perinatal *

Name: ______ Date of HV: ______

Address: ______ City: ______

Birth Date: ______ Age: ______ Phone #: ______

Race: ☐ White ☐ Asian ☐ Indochinese ☐ Phillipino Language Spoken ______

☐ Black ☐ Amer. Indian ☐ Pacific Islander ☐ Hispanic Head of Household, Family Name ______

Evaluator ______

Program ☐☐☐ Signature ______

### I. ANTHROPOMETRIC

| | DATA | A | AG/I |
|---|---|---|---|
| 0 Height | | | |
| 1 Current Weight | | | |
| Post Partum (PP) | | | |
| 2 Recommended Body Weight (RBW) | | | |
| ◇ 3 Percent RBW | | | |
| ◇ 4 Weight Change | | | |
| Ante Partum (AP) | | | |
| 6 Pregravid Weight | | | |
| 7 Pregravid RBW | | | |
| 8 Pregravid Percent RBW | | | |
| 9 Prenatal Weight Change | | | |

GOAL O

PP - Client at RBW ☐

AP - Adequate weight gain rate ☐

### III. DIETARY

| | DATA | A | AG/I |
|---|---|---|---|
| 30 Adequate Food Groups | | | |
| ◇ 31 Vitamin-mineral supplements | | | |
| | | | |
| ◇ 33 Fad Diet | | | |
| ◇ 34 Pica | | | |
| ◇ 35 Food allergy/intolerance/dislikes | | | |
| | | | |
| | | | |
| 36 Change in appetite | | | |
| 38 Fat intake | | | |
| 39 Sugar intake | | | |
| 40 Alcohol intake | | | |
| 41 Salt intake | | | |
| 42 Caffeine intake | | | |
| 43 Fluid intake | | | |
| 44 Exercise | | | |
| 45 Financial resources | | | |
| 46 Food preparation/storage facilities | | | |
| 47 Food preparation ability | | | |
| 48 Breastfeeding | | | |
| ◇ 49 Special diet | | | |

GOAL O

59 DIETARY is WNL ☐

### II. BIOCHEMICAL

| | DATA | A | AG/I |
|---|---|---|---|
| ◇ 20 Hemoglobin | | | |
| ◇ 21 Hematocrit | | | |
| ◇ 22 Blood glucose | | | |
| 23 Urinalysis -- protein | | | |
| 24 glucose | | | |
| 25 ketones | | | |

GOAL O

29 BIOCHEM is WNL ☐

### IV. MEDICAL

| | DATA | A | AG/I |
|---|---|---|---|
| ◇ 60 Blood pressure | | | |
| ◇ 61 Days of hospitalization | | | |
| 62 Chewing ability | | | |
| ◇ 64 Malnutrition | | | |
| ◇ 65 Nutrient-drug interactions | | | |
| | | | |
| | | | |
| ◇ 66 Nausea/vomiting | | | |
| ◇ 67 Heartburn | | | |
| ◇ 68 Constipation | | | |
| ◇ 69 Diarrhea | | | |
| ◇ 70 Frequent conception | | | |
| ◇ 71 Age | | | |
| 72 Gravida/Para | | | |
| 73 Multiple births | | | |
| 74 Smoking | | | |
| ◇ 76 Dental caries | | | |

### HYPERMETABOLIC CONDITIONS

| | * | AG/I |
|---|---|---|
| ◇ 80 Major surgery | | |
| 81 Minor surgery | | |
| 82 Burns | | |
| 83 Long bone fracture | | |
| 84 Other | | |

### PREVIOUS OBSTETRICAL COMPLICATIONS

| | | AG/I |
|---|---|---|
| ◇ 90 Birthweight < 5 lbs 8 oz or > 8 lbs 13 oz | | |
| ◇ 91 Glucose intolerance in pregnancy | | |
| 92 Congenital anomalies | | |
| 93 Fetal or neonatal deaths | | |
| ◇ 94 Pre-eclampsia/Toxemia | | |
| ◇ 95 Anemia | | |
| ◇ 96 Weight gain < 20 or > 40 lbs | | |

### CHRONIC DISEASE

| | | AG/I |
|---|---|---|
| 101 Cardiovascular disease | | |
| ◇ 102 —anemia | | |
| ◇ 105 —G6PD | | |
| ◇ 106 —hyperlipidemia | | |
| ◇ 107 —hypertension | | |
| ◇ 108 —sickle cell | | |
| 109 Endocrine disorder | | |
| ◇ 110 —diabetes | | |
| 112 Gastrointestinal disease | | |
| 118 Infectious disease | | |
| 120 Kidney disease | | |
| 125 Liver and Biliary disease | | |
| ◇ 127 —cholecystitis | | |
| 129 Metabolic disease | | |
| 132 Neurological disease | | |
| 138 Orthopedic disease | | |
| 142 Psychological dysfunction | | |
| ◇ 143 —alcoholism | | |
| ◇ 144 —depression | | |
| ◇ 145 —eating disorder | | |
| ◇ 146 —substance abuse | | |
| 147 Respiratory disease | | |
| 149 Other | | |
| | | |

GOAL O

150 MEDICAL is WNL ☐

**LEGEND**

AG = Anticipatory Guidance
- T = Teach
- D = Demonstrate
- L = Literature
- R = Refer
- S = Supervise
- C = Contract
- K = Counsel

◇ = Refer to nutritionist/RD

A = Assessment
- ✓ = WNL
- P = Problem
- + = Optimal Problem Management
- — = Not appropriate

Y = Yes, condition is present

N = No, condition is not present

I = Intervention

0 = Outcome
- 1 = Goal Met
- = Goal Not Met
- 2a = Still working towards goal
- 2b = Lost to follow up
- 2c = Refused
- 2d = Client failed to follow through
- 2e = Referred to another District or Co.
- 3 = Continue on appropriate flow sheet

*page 2 - weight grid, summary and referral

County of San Bernardino — Department of Public Health

341.003.H41

Clay, G., Bouchard, C., and Hemphill, K.: A comprehensive nutrition case management system. *J. Am Diet Assoc* 88 (2):197, 1988. Used with permission.

| Living Area/Ward | Sex | Age | Height | Weight | Ideal Weight |
|---|---|---|---|---|---|
| Weight History | Mid Arm Circ. | | Triceps Skinfold | | Mid Arm Musc. Circ. |

Admitting Diagnosis

Pertinent Medical History

Diet Order

Medications

Pertinent Lab Values (date and result)

| HGB | HCT | Alb | FBS |
|---|---|---|---|
| BUN | Chol | Other | |

Motor Development (dexterity, coordination)

Sensory Skills

| Speech/Communication | Vision | Hearing |
|---|---|---|

**Habits Related to Foods**

Occupation/Daily Activity

Sleep Patterns
Total Hours: ☐ Continuous ☐ Interrupted

Exercise
☐ Restrictive ☐ Inactive ☐ Moderate ☐ Excessive

| Tobacco (kind, amount) | Alcohol (kind, amount) | Drugs (kind, amount) |
|---|---|---|

Elimination
☐ Regular ☐ Diarrhea ☐ Constipation ☐ Laxatives

Appetite
☐ Excessive ☐ Good ☐ Fair ☐ Poor

| Food Likes | Food Dislikes |
|---|---|

Allergies, Intolerances, Religious Restrictions

Special Problems Affecting Eating

Dentition
☐ Own Teeth ☐ Dentures ☐ No Teeth ☐ Swallowing

Feeding
☐ Feeds Self ☐ Needs Assistance ☐ Adaptive Equipment (specify)

Ambulation
☐ Ambulatory ☐ Mobil Nonambulatory ☐ Nonambulatory

Comments:

DMH-0021

**DIETARY HISTORY**
Rev. 8/82 DMH-MedR-1017

Amount of Foods Eaten Daily

| Milk | Meat | Eggs | Vegetables | Fruit Juices | Desserts |
|---|---|---|---|---|---|
| Bread | Cereal | Potato, Pasta | Fats | Sugar, Candy | Snack Foods |

Family History (diabetes, mental deficiency, obesity, etc.)

Assessment

**Nutritional Care Plan**

Goals

| Objectives | Strategies |
|---|---|
| | |

Source of Information (if other than patient)

| Signature of Interviewer (if other than Dietitian) | Date | Signature of Dietitian | Date |
|---|---|---|---|

DMH-MedR-1017

From: Department of Mental Health, Ohio. Used with permission.

5–5 Nutrition Screening Questionnaire, Health Department, New Mexico

CHILD__________________ BIRTHDATE__________ TODAY'S DATE__________

HOME PHONE__________

**HOW IS YOUR CHILD EATING AND GROWING?**

(Please circle yes or no in response to the following questions)

(7) yes no 1. Is it easy to tell when your child is hungry or thirsty?
(10) yes no 2. Do you have any concerns about his/her eating or growing?
(5B) yes no 3. Is your child on a special diet? If yes, what? __________
(5D) yes no 4. Does he/she take vitamins and minerals? If yes, what? __________
(5E) yes no 5. Does he/she take medications? If yes, what? __________
(5C) yes no 6. Does your child eat anything that is not food, such as paint or dirt?
(5A) yes no 7. Do you have trouble buying or making your child's food?
yes no 8. Does your child participate in the WIC Program? If yes, where? __________

**WHAT DOES YOUR CHILD EAT AND DRINK?**

(5A) 9. How many meals and snacks does he/she eat most days? _____Meals _____Snacks

(8E) 10. How long does it take him/her to finish a meal or feeding? _____ Minutes

(6) 11. Please check the choice(s) that best describe(s) what your child eats.

| | | |
|---|---|---|
| ___Breastmilk | ___Baby Cereal | ___Ground Meats/Finely Ground Table Foods |
| ___Formula | ___Strained Baby Foods | ___Cut Up Meats/Soft Table Foods |
| ___Cow's Milk | ___Junior Foods | ___Finger Foods |

(5A) 12. Circle any of the following food groups that you feel your child is not eating enough of.

1. Milk & Milk Products 2. Meat, Beans, Eggs 3. Fruits & Vegetables 4. Breads & Cereals

(5A) 13. Fill in the amount (cups or ounces) your child usually drinks in one day (24 hours).

Water_____ Sweet Drinks_____ Juice_____ Cow's Milk_____

Baby Formula_____ What kind of formula?__________

How do you make formula? __________

**(8) ARE ANY OF THESE A PROBLEM FOR YOUR CHILD? IF YES, PLEASE CHECK.**

| | | |
|---|---|---|
| ___Vomiting | ___Eating too slowly | ___Holding up his/her head |
| ___Diarrhea | ___Refusing to eat | ___Sitting up alone |
| ___Constipation | ___Spitting out food | ___Sucking on nipple |
| ___Food Allergies | ___Gagging & Choking | ___Chewing |
| ___Bad Teeth/Sore Mouth | ___Getting upset at meals | ___Swallowing |
| | | ___Drooling |

**STAFF USE ONLY**

(9) DX__________

(1,2) Height_____ Weight_____ %tiles : Ht/Age_____ Wt/Age_____ Wt/Ht_____

(3)(4) Birthweight (birth to 2 years) _____ Hematocrit _____% Hemoglobin _____gm/dl

Comments:__________

Name__________ Agency__________ Phone__________

Nutrition Bureau, Public Health Division, New Mexico Health & Environment Department
Adapted from Child Nutrition Questionnaire, Colorado Department of Health
Used with permission.

**5–6 Early Intervention Nutrition Screening—Peach Survey**

**Agency:**______________________ **Date:**______________
**Child's Name:**______________________ **Date of Birth:**______________
**Address:**______________________ **Phone#:**______________
______________________

**Please circle YES or NO for each question as it applies to your child.**

| Question | | Points |
|---|---|---|
| Does your child have a health problem (do not include colds or flu)? If yes, what is it? | YES NO | 1 |
| Is your child: small for age______ , too thin_______, too heavy_______ (If you checked any of the above, please circle YES) | YES NO | 3 |
| Does your child have feeding problems? If yes, what are they? | YES NO | 3 |
| Is you child's appetite a problem? If yes, describe: | YES NO | 1 |
| Is your child on a special diet? If yes, what type of diet? | YES NO | 2 |
| Does your child take medicine for a health problem (do not include vitamins, iron or fluoride)? | YES NO | 1 |
| Does your child have food allergies? If yes, to what foods? | YES NO | 1 |
| Does your child use a feeding tube or other special feeding method? If yes, explain | YES NO | 4 |
| Circle *YES* if your child does not eat any of these foods: Milk____ Meats____ Vegetables____ Fruits____ (Check all that apply) | YES NO | 1 |
| Circle *YES* if your child has problems with: Sucking____ Swallowing____ Chewing____ Gagging____ (Check all that apply) | YES NO | 3 |
| Circle *YES* if your child has problems with: Loose stools____ Hard stools____ Throwing up____ Spitting up____ (Check all that apply) | YES NO | 3 |
| Does your child eat clay, paint chips, dirt, or other things that are no food? If yes, what? | YES NO | 2 |
| Does your child refuse to eat, throws food or do other things that upset you at mealtime? If yes, explain. | YES NO | 2 |
| For infants *under* 12 months who are bottle-feed: Does your child drink less than 3 (8 oz.) bottles of milk per day? | YES NO | 1 |
| For children *over* 12 months: Is your child not using a cup____ Is your child not finger feeding____ (check if applies and circle YES) | YES NO | 1 |
| For children *over* 18 months: Does your child still take liquids from a bottle? | YES NO | 2 |
| Circle yes if your child is not using a spoon. | YES NO | 2 |
| | **Total** = | |

Score *under* 4 points: re-screen in six months or whenever there is a concern.
Score 4 points and above: refer to Registered Dietitian at a Children's Hospital for a complete nutrition assessment.

Referred to:______________________ Date:______________
Feedback:______________________

*Parent Eating and Nutrition Assessment for children with Special Health Care Needs. 

**5–7** Surface Area Assessment

| Males: Age at Last Birthday | Males: Mean (cal/m²/hr) | Females: Age at Last Birthday | Females: Mean (cal/m²/hr) |
|---|---|---|---|
| 6 | 53.00 | 6 | 50.62 |
| 7 | 52.45 | 6½ | 50.23 |
| 8 | 51.78 | 7 | 49.12 |
| 8½ | 51.20 | 7½ | 47.84 |
| 9 | 50.54 | 8 | 47.00 |
| 9½ | 49.42 | 8½ | 46.50 |
| 10 | 48.50 | 9–10 | 45.90 |
| 10½ | 47.71 | 11 | 45.26 |
| 11 | 47.18 | 11½ | 44.80 |
| 12 | 46.75 | 12 | 44.28 |
| 13–15 | 46.35 | 12½ | 43.58 |
| 16 | 45.72 | 13 | 42.90 |
| 16½ | 45.30 | 13½ | 42.10 |
| 17 | 44.80 | 14 | 41.45 |
| 17½ | 44.03 | 14½ | 40.74 |
| 18 | 43.25 | 15 | 40.10 |
| 18½ | 42.70 | 15½ | 39.40 |
| 19 | 42.32 | 16 | 38.85 |
| 19½ | 42.00 | 16½ | 38.30 |
| 20–21 | 41.43 | 17 | 37.82 |
| 22–23 | 40.82 | 17½ | 37.40 |
| 24–27 | 40.24 | 18–19 | 36.74 |
| 28–29 | 39.81 | 20–24 | 36.18 |
| 30–34 | 39.34 | 25–44 | 35.70 |
| 35–39 | 38.68 | 45–49 | 34.94 |
| 40–44 | 38.00 | 50–54 | 33.96 |
| 45–49 | 37.37 | 55–59 | 33.18 |
| 50–54 | 36.73 | 60–64 | 32.61 |
| 55–59 | 36.10 | 65–69 | 32.30 |
| 60–64 | 35.48 | * | |
| 65–69 | 34.80 | | |

*Obtain numbers beyond 69 by extrapolation. From Pike & Brown, *Nutrition: An Integrated Approach,* 2nd ed. New York, Wiley and Sons.

**5–8** Spice and Herb Nutrient Composition

## PROXIMATE COMPOSITION OF GROUND SPICES, 100 GRAMS, EDIBLE PORTION†

| Spice | Water | Food Energy | Protein | Fat | Total Carbohydrate | Fiber Carbohydrate | Ash | Calcium | Phosphorus | Sodium | Potassium | Iron | Thiamine | Riboflavin | Niacin | Ascorbic Acid | Vitamin A Activity |
|---|---|---|---|---|---|---|---|---|---|---|---|---|---|---|---|---|---|
| | Grams | Cal. | Grams | Grams | Grams | Grams | Grams | Grams | Mg. | Mg. | Grams | Mg. | Mcg. | Mcg. | Mg. | Mg. | Int'l Units |
| Allspice | 9.0 | 380 | 6.0 | 6.6 | 74.4 | 21.6 | 4.2 | 0.8 | 110 | 80 | 1.1 | 7.5 | 100 | 60 | 2.9 | 39 | 540 |
| Basil Leaves | 6.0 | 325 | 12.0 | 3.6 | 61.7 | 20.5 | 16.7 | 2.1 | 470 | 40 | 3.7 | 42.8 | 150 | 320 | 6.9 | 61 | 15000 |
| Bay Leaves | 4.5 | 410 | 7.5 | 8.8 | 75.4 | 25.2 | 3.7 | 1.0 | 110 | 20 | 0.6 | 53.3 | 100 | 420 | 2.0 | 47 | 6180 |
| Caraway Seed | 6.0 | 465 | 21.0 | 23.1 | 43.5 | 10.4 | 5.6 | 0.7 | 500 | 20 | 1.9 | 8.5 | 380 | 380 | 8.1 | N | 360 |
| Cardamom Seed | 8.0 | 360 | 10.0 | 2.9 | 74.2 | 9.9 | 4.7 | 0.3 | 210 | 10 | 1.2 | 11.6 | 180 | 230 | 2.3 | N | N |
| Celery Seed | 5.0 | 450 | 18.0 | 22.8 | 43.8 | 12.9 | 10.2 | 1.8 | 550 | 170 | 1.4 | 44.9 | 410 | 490 | 4.4 | 17 | 50 |
| Cinnamon | 10.0 | 355 | 4.5 | 2.2 | 79.8 | 20.3 | 3.5 | 1.6 | 50 | 10 | 0.4 | 4.1 | 140 | 210 | 1.9 | 40 | 260 |
| Cloves | 5.0 | 430 | 6.0 | 14.5 | 68.8 | 11.1 | 5.0 | 0.7 | 110 | 250 | 1.2 | 9.5 | 110 | N | 1.5 | 81 | 530 |
| Coriander Seed | 6.0 | 450 | 12.0 | 19.6 | 56.5 | 31.5 | 5.3 | 0.8 | 440 | 20 | 1.2 | 5.9 | 260 | 230 | 3.2 | N | N |
| Cumin Seed | 6.0 | 460 | 18.0 | 23.8 | 44.6 | 9.1 | 7.7 | 0.9 | 450 | 160 | 2.1 | 47.8 | 730 | 380 | 2.5 | 17 | 1270 |
| Dill Seed | 6.5 | 435 | 13.0 | 17.9 | 56.4 | 20.7 | 6.0 | 1.6 | 210 | 10 | 1.1 | 11.8 | 420 | 280 | 2.8 | N | 50 |
| Fennel Seed | 6.0 | 370 | 9.5 | 10.0 | 60.8 | 18.5 | 13.4 | 1.3 | 480 | 90 | 1.7 | 11.1 | 410 | 360 | 6.0 | N | 135 |
| Garlic Powder | 5.0 | 365 | 17.5 | 0.6 | 73.3 | 1.9 | 3.2 | 0.1 | 420 | 10 | 1.1 | 3.5 | 680 | 80 | 0.7 | N | N |
| Ginger | 7.0 | 380 | 8.5 | 6.4 | 72.4 | 5.9 | 5.7 | 0.1 | 150 | 30 | 1.4 | 11.3 | 50 | 130 | 1.9 | N | 150 |
| Mace | 4.5 | 565 | 8.0 | 38.8 | 46.1 | 4.8 | 2.3 | 0.2 | 110 | 70 | 0.5 | 11.3 | 370 | 560 | 1.2 | N | 800 |
| Marjoram | 6.5 | 365 | 12.5 | 6.8 | 64.4 | 16.7 | 9.7 | 2.5 | 230 | 110 | 1.4 | 72.7 | 290 | 320 | 4.1 | 51 | 8070 |
| Mustard Powder | 3.0 | 580 | 32.0 | 42.6 | 18.5 | 1.9 | 4.0 | 0.3 | 790 | 10 | 0.7 | 8.3 | 650 | 450 | 8.5 | 22 | 60 |
| Nutmeg | 4.0 | 565 | 7.0 | 38.9 | 47.3 | 3.1 | 2.0 | 0.2 | 200 | 10 | 0.4 | 2.2 | 360 | 250 | 9.4 | N | 100 |
| Onion Powder | 4.5 | 370 | 10.5 | 0.8 | 80.5 | 6.4 | 3.5 | 0.3 | 290 | 40 | 1.0 | 2.2 | 420 | 60 | 0.6 | 15 | N |
| Oregano | 8.0 | 360 | 12.0 | 6.4 | 64.9 | 11.0 | 9.0 | 1.7 | 200 | 20 | 1.7 | 53.3 | 340 | N | 6.2 | N | 6900 |
| Paprika | 7.0 | 390 | 14.0 | 10.4 | 60.3 | 19.2 | 8.6 | 0.2 | 300 | 20 | 2.4 | 23.1 | 600 | 1360 | 15.3 | 59 | 58000 |
| Parsley Flakes | 4.0 | 355 | 22.0 | 5.6 | 54.3 | 8.7 | 14.1 | 1.2 | 310 | 540 | 3.6 | 14.5 | 170 | 1230 | 7.9 | 392 | 23300 |
| Pepper, Black | 8.0 | 400 | 10.0 | 10.2 | 66.5 | 10.0 | 4.6 | 0.4 | 160 | 10 | 1.2 | 17.0 | 70 | 210 | 0.8 | N | 190 |
| Pepper, Chili | 6.5 | 415 | 14.0 | 14.1 | 58.2 | 15.6 | 7.2 | 0.1 | 320 | 10 | 2.1 | 9.9 | 590 | 1660 | 14.2 | 64 | 51800 |
| Pepper, Red | 6.0 | 420 | 16.0 | 15.5 | 54.3 | 26.0 | 8.0 | 0.1 | 320 | 10 | 2.1 | 9.9 | 520 | 930 | 13.6 | 29 | 31400 |
| Pepper, White | 9.5 | 395 | 12.0 | 8.0 | 69.0 | 4.5 | 1.0 | 0.2 | 150 | 10 | 0.1 | 6.9 | 20 | 130 | 0.2 | N | N |
| Poppy Seed | 3.5 | 530 | 23.0 | 35.5 | 30.2 | 8.7 | 7.5 | 1.6 | 880 | 10 | 0.8 | 9.9 | 690 | 180 | 0.9 | N | N |
| Rosemary Leaves | 5.5 | 440 | 4.5 | 17.4 | 66.4 | 19.0 | 6.0 | 1.5 | 70 | 40 | 1.0 | 33.0 | 510 | N | 1.0 | 61 | 3100 |
| Sage | 5.5 | 415 | 10.0 | 14.1 | 62.3 | 16.0 | 7.7 | 1.8 | 90 | 10 | 1.0 | 27.3 | 750 | 340 | 5.7 | 40 | 5900 |
| Savory | 9.0 | 355 | 7.0 | 5.2 | 69.9 | 15.3 | 8.7 | 2.2 | 140 | 20 | 1.1 | 37.8 | 370 | N | 4.1 | N | 5100 |
| Sesame Seed | 3.0 | 480 | 24.0 | 22.4 | 47.1 | 37.7 | 3.6 | 0.1 | 790 | 30 | 0.4 | 6.2 | 800 | 130 | 5.7 | N | 65 |
| Tarragon | 4.5 | 365 | 24.0 | 7.3 | 51.5 | 6.8 | 12.3 | 1.3 | 310 | 70 | 3.2 | 35.7 | 250 | 1340 | 8.9 | N | 4200 |
| Thyme | 7.0 | 340 | 7.0 | 4.6 | 68.3 | 24.3 | 13.2 | 2.1 | 200 | 80 | 0.9 | 135.0 | 510 | 400 | 4.9 | N | 3800 |
| Turmeric | 6.0 | 390 | 8.5 | 8.9 | 69.9 | 6.9 | 6.8 | 0.2 | 260 | 10 | 2.5 | 47.5 | 90 | 190 | 4.8 | 50 | N |

Research Committee, American Spice Trade Association, 580 Sylvan Avenue, Englewood Cliffs, NJ 07632.

APPENDIX 6

# Intensive Care Nursery Protocol Formula Composition and Preventive Nutrition

**6–1** Specialty Pediatrics Medical Nutrition Products: Composition and Features

| Product | Ages | Standard Dilution | Per 100 Calories | | | Indications | Unique Features | Manufacturer and Website |
|---|---|---|---|---|---|---|---|---|
| | | | Protein, g(% Total kcal)Source(s) | Carbohydrate, g(% Total kcal)Sources | Fat, g(% Total kcal)Sources | | | |
| [1]Neocate Infant DHA/ARA, [2]Neocate Junior, unflavored | [1]0–12 mo, [2]1+ yr | [1]20 kcal/fl oz, [2]30 kcal/fl oz[1,2] (1 kcal/mL) | [1]2.8 g (11.2%),[2] 3.3 g (13%) free amino acids | [1]10.8 g (43.1%), [2]10.4 g (42%) corn syrup solids | [1]5.1 g (45.7%) MCT (modified coconut and/or palm kernel), sunflower, canola, *M. alpina* & *C. cohnii* (DHA & ARA), [2]5.0 g (45%) MCT (modified palm kernel and/or coconut), canola, high-oleic safflower | CMA, EoE, GER, MFPI, SBS | CMA, EoE, GER, MFPI, SBS [1]Nucleotides, free of soy oil, osmolality = 340 mOsm/kg[2], [2]Hypoallergenic, nutritionally complete | Nutricia www. nutricia-na.com |
| Neocate Junior with prebiotics: unflavored, vanilla, strawberry, tropical & chocolate | 1+ years | 30 kcal/fl oz (1.0 kcal/mL) | 3.3 - 3.5 g (13%) free amino acids | 10.4 - 11.3 g (42 - 45%) corn syrup solids, fructo-oligosaccharide, inulin | 4.6 - 5.0 g (41 - 45%) MCT (modified palm kernel and/or coconut), canola, high-oleic safflower | CMA, EoE, GER, MFPI, SBS | Only hypoallergenic formula with prebiotics | Nutricia www. nutricia-na.com |
| Neocate Splash unflavored | 1+ yr | 30 kcal/fl oz (1.0 kcal/mL) | 3.0 g (12%) free amino acids | 10.5 g (42%) maltodextrin (corn), sugar | 5.1 g (46%) high-oleic sunflower, MCT (modified palm kernel and/or coconut), canola | CMA, EoE, GER, MFPI, SBS | Hypoallergenic, nutritionally-complete; RTF tetrapak, easy to decant | Nutricia www. nutricia-na.com |
| E028 Splash: grape, tropical fruit, & orange-pineapple | 1+ yr | 30 kcal/fl oz (1.0 kcal/mL) | 2.5 g (10%) free amino acids | 14.6 g (58%) maltodextrin (corn), sugar (orange-pineapple also contains corn syrup solids) | 3.5 g (32%) MCT (modified palm kernel and/or coconut), canola, high-oleic sunflower | CMA, EoE, GER, MFPI, SBS | Hypoallergenic, RTF tetrapack | Nutricia www. nutricia-na.com |
| Neocate Nutra | 6+ mo | — | 1.7 g (7%) free amino acids | 14.3 g (57%) corn syrup solids, rice starch, sugar | 4.0 g (36%) coconut, high-oleic sunflower, canola, sunflower | CMA, EoE, GER, MFPI, SBS | Hypoallergenic semi-solid medical food | Nutricia www. nutricia-na.com |
| Phenex[1,2] | [1]Infant-toddler [2]Child-adult | [1]20, [2]30 kcal/fl oz | [1]3.1 g (12.4%), [2]7.3 g (29.2%) L-amino acids | [1]11.0 g (44%), [2]8.5 g (34.0%) corn syrup solids | [1]4.5 g (40.5%), [2]3.4 g (30.6%) high-oleic safflower oil, coconut oil, soy oil | PKU | Phenylalanine free, contains L-tyrosine | Abbott www. abbottnutrition.com |
| Ketonex[1,2] | [1]Infant-toddler [2]Child-adult | [1]20, [2]30 kcal/fl oz | [1]3.1 g (12.4%), [2]7.3 g (29.2%) L-amino acids | [1]11.0 g (44.0%), [2]8.5 g (34.0%) corn syrup solids | [1]4.5 g (40.5%),[2] 3.4 g (30.6%) high-oleic safflower oil, coconut oil, soy oil | MSUD | Branched-chain amino acid free | Abbott www. abbottnutrition.com |

| | | | | | | | | |
|---|---|---|---|---|---|---|---|---|
| Cyclinex[1,2] | [1]Infant-Toddler [2]Child-Adult | [1]20, [2]30 kcal/fl oz | [1]1.5 g (6.0%), [2]3.4 g (13.6%) L-amino acids | [1]11.2 g (44.8%), [2]10.2 g (40.8%) corn syrup solids | [1]4.9 g (44.1%), [2]3.9 g (35.1%) high-oleic safflower oil, coconut oil, soy oil | Urea cycle disorder, gyrate atrophy, of HHH syndrome | Nonessential amino acid free | Abbott www.abbottnutrition.com |
| Propimex[1,2] | [1]Infant-toddler [2]Child-adult | [1]20, [2]30 kcal/fl oz | [1]3.1 g (12.4%) L-amino acids [2]7.3 g (29.2%) L-amino acids | [1]11.0 g (44%) [2]8.5 g (34.0%) corn syrup solids | [1]4.5 g (40.5%) [2]3.2 g (28.8%) high-oleic safflower oil, coconut oil, soy oil | Propionic or methylmalonic acidemia | Methionine and valine free; low in isoleucine and threonine | Abbott www.abbottnutrition.com |
| Nutramigen with Enflora LGG | 0–12 mo | 20 kcal/fl oz (0.68 kcal/mL) | 2.8 (11%) casein hydrolysate and amino acids | 10.3 (41%) corn syrup solids, modified corn starch | 5.3 (48%) palm olein, soy, coconut, high oleic sunflower oils, and single cell oils (DHA & ARA) | CMA, MFPI | *Lactobacillus rhamnosus* LGG 1 × $10^6$ CFUs LGG/g of powder formula | Mead Johnson Nutrition www.meadjohnson.com/pediatrics |
| PurAmino | 0–24 mo | 20 kcal/fl oz (0.68 kcal/mL) | 2.8 (11%) free amino acids | 10.6 (42%) Corn syrup solids, modified tapioca starch | 5.3 (47%) high-oleic sunflower, MCT, soy, single cell oils (DHA & ARA) | CMA, EoE, MFPI, SBS | 33% of fat from MCT oil | Mead Johnson Nutrition www.meadjohnson.com/pediatrics |
| | | | | Per 100 g Powder | | | | |
| Phenyl-Free 1 | 0–36 mo | Varies, 5 kcal/g powder | 16.2 g protein equivalents (13%), free amino acids | 51 g (40%), corn syrup solids, modified corn starch, sugar | 26 g (47%), Palm olein, soy, coconut, high oleic sunflower, single cell oils (DHA & ARA) | PKU | DHA (0.34% of total fatty acids), ARA (0.67% of total fatty acids) | Mead Johnson Nutrition www.meadjohnson.com/pediatrics |
| Phenyl-Free 2 | 3 yr + | Varies, 4.1 kcal/g powder | 22 g protein equivalents (22%), free amino acids | 60 g (59%), sugar, corn syrup solids, modified corn starch | 8.6 g (19%), soy oil | PKU | Phenyl-Free 2 HP has 40 g protein equivalents per 100 g powder | Mead Johnson Nutrition www.meadjohnson.com/pediatrics |

## 6–2 Neonatal Intensive Care Unit Protocol, Baylor University, Texas[1]

**Milk Selection**

1. Infants < 34 weeks and < 2000 grams should receive human milk or premature infant formula. When 100 cc/kg/day of human milk is achieved, 2 packets of human milk fortifier are added to the 100 cc of milk for 1 day. The next day, the fortifier addition is increased to 4 packets per 100 cc of milk. The following day, milk volume is advanced.

2. Infant ≥ 34 weeks and ≥ 2000 grams should receive human milk or term, infant formula.

**Vitamin and Iron Supplementation**

**A. Preterm Infants**

1. Vitamin Supplementation: Not indicated. Preterm infants will meet needs when human milk fortifiers are added to human milk or when infant formulas designed for preterm infants are provided.

2. Iron Supplementation: 2 mg/kg/day is recommended. Human milk fortifiers that contain iron or iron fortified formulas will meet needs. Infants receiving human milk with a fortifier, which does not contain iron, should receive 2 mg/kg at 1 month of age. This level of intake should continue through the first year of life.

**B. Term Infants**

1. Vitamin Supplementation: The exclusively breastfed infant should receive 200 IU/day of vitamin D supplementation by 2 months of age. Triple vitamin supplements are recommended at 0.5 ml/day. Vitamin supplementation is not indicated for formula fed infants.

2. Iron Supplementation: Iron should be provided at 6 months of age for the exclusively breast fed infant. Iron fortified foods and/or iron drops can meet needs. Infants who have had significant blood loss will require iron supplementation while in the nursery and supplementation should continue through the first year of life. Iron fortified formulas will meet needs. Low iron infant formulas are not recommended.

**Intake Guidelines**

1. Volume intake is provided to support growth and fluid needs. Weekly weight gains should be 10 – 20 g/kg/day for infants who weigh ≤ 2000 g and 20 – 30 g/day for infants who weight > 2000 g. Milk volumes to meet needs are listed below.
   - 150 – 160 ml/kg/day of preterm formula
   - 160 –180 ml/kg/day of fortified human milk or premature transitional formula
   - 180 – 200 ml/kg/day of unfortified human milk or term formula

2. Infants requiring fluid restriction will often need formula powder added to fortified human milk or ready to feed premature infant formula to meet nutrient needs for growth. Formulas available in powder or liquid concentrate form; can be concentrated to a more nutrient dense product.

**Feeds Initiation, Advancement and Tolerance**

**A. Trophic Feedings**

1. On day of life 2 to 4, trophic feedings should be introduced for infants who weight < 1250 grams. Feeding volumes of 10 to 20 cc/kg/day of human milk or premature infant formula should be provided for 7 to 10 days at a volume of 10 to 20 cc/kg/day. Post trophic feeding period advance feedings should be advanced by 10 to 20 cc/kg/day. Trophic feedings can lead to improved gastrointestinal development and feeding tolerance.

2. Infants who weigh 1250 – 1500 grams may be considered for trophic feedings.

**B. Volume Advancement**

1. Infants < 1500 grams advance volume by 10 – 20 cc/kg/day.

2. Healthy infants ≥ 1500 grams and ≥ 32 weeks gestation may tolerate up to 35 cc/kg/day

3. Relatively, healthy term infants may tolerate 50 cc/kg/day to ab lib feeding.

**C. Feeding Method for Tube Feeding**

1. Intermittent bolus gastric feedings are preferred for improved feeding tolerance and growth

2. Continuous infusions are recommended for infants with short guts.

3. Transpyloric feedings are suggested for infants who do not tolerate bolus gastric feeding as demonstrated by delayed gastric emptying. Feedings should be provided continuously.

**D. Tolerance**

Feeding intolerance and illness are common occurrence for infants in the NICU. Infants must be assessed as to the readiness to advance feedings. Signs of illness such as temperature instability, apnea and bradycardia, gastric distension and or large gastric residuals require physical examination and further medical evaluation. In the absence of illness, a gastric residual volume of ≤ 50% of a 3 hour feeding volume is acceptable. When trophic feedings are began, residuals equal to the feeding volumes may be seen, and trophic feedings can continue.

[1]Nutrition, Metabolic Management, and Gastroenterology Review Committee. Nutrition Support. In Adams JM, Adcock L, Anderson DM, Garcia-Prats JA, Haney PM, Speer ME, Weisman LE, editors. Guidelines for the acute care of the neonate. 12th edition. Houston: Newborn Section, Department of Pediatrics, Baylor College of Medicine. 2004

6–3 Naturally Occurring Toxins and Syndromes They Produce in Humans

| TYPE OF TOXIN | EFFECTS IN HUMANS |
|---|---|
| Protease inhibitors* | IgE antibodies to the Kunitz soybean trypsin inhibitor produce angioedema and anaphylaxis |
| Hemagglutinins/lectins | Diarrhea and poor growth |
| Glucosinolates/thioglucosides | Goitrogenic syndromes of theoretical concern only |
| Cyanogens* | Tropical ataxic syndrome from chronic ingestion. Acute poisoning is similar to that from inorganic cyanide |
| Saponins/glycosides | No obvious effects |
| Gossypol polyphenolic pigments | Anorexia, cachexia, and infertility |
| Lathyrogens* | Neurolathyrism (osteolathyrism does not occur in humans) |
| Pyrimidine analogues* | Favism-acute hemolytic anemia in patients with deficiency of glucose 6 phosphate dehydrogenase |
| Non-physiologic amino acids* | L-canavanine can induce or exacerbate the lupus syndrome |
| Allergens* | Target of allergies may be the skin, lungs, gastrointestinal tract, musculoskeletal or nervous system |
| Carcinogens and mutagens* | Aflatoxins are probably etiologic in the pathogenesis of some malignancies |
| Anti-vitamin factors* | Pellagra is endemic in India because of an antiniacin factor on jowar, a plant with a high content of leucine (which interferes with the metabolism of tryptophan and nicotinic acid) |
| Estrogenic products of plants | None described |
| Hallucinogens* | Acute or chronic hallucinosis, drug dependence, or both |
| Pressor amines* | High levels in some fruits, cheeses, beans, and nuts increase blood pressure |
| Hypoglycemic agents* | Intake of unripe ackee fruit in Jamaica and Nigeria has been associated with hypoglycemia and depression of the central nervous system |
| Antienzymes* | Solanine, an anticholinestrase present in sprouts and skin of "night-shade plants," can act as a poison |
| Other toxins | Purple mint plant has a ketone substitutedfuran and can cause pulmonary emphysema in several species of animals. Rose in humans is unknown |

*Clinically significant.

From: Corman, L.C. The relationship between nutrition, infection and immunity. *Med Clin N Am*, 69(3):519, 1985. Used with permission.

## 6–4 Food Classifications

### *PLANT SOURCES*

**Grain Family**
Corn
- corn starch
- corn oil
- corn sugar
- corn syrup
- cerulose
- dextrose
- glucose

Barley
- malt

Oats
Rice
Rye
Sorghum
Wheat
- graham flour
- gluten flour
- bran
- wheat germ

Wild rice

**Arrow Root Family**
Taro
- poi

Cane
- cane sugar
- molasses

**Sprurge Family**
Tapioca

**Buckwheat Family**
Buckwheat
Rhubarb

**Composite Family**
Leaf lettuce
Head lettuce
Endive
Escarole
Artichoke
Dandelion
Oyster plant
Chicory

**Goosefoot Family**
Beet
- beet sugar

Spinach
Swiss chard

**Gourd Family**
Pumpkin
Squash
Cucumber
Cantaloupe
Muskmelon
Honeydew
Casaba
Watermelon

**Legume Family**
Navy bean
Kidney bean
Lima bean
String bean
Soybean
- soybean oil

Lentil
Black-eyed pea
Peanut
- peanut oil

Licorice
Anacia
Senna

**Lily Family**
Asparagus
Onion
Garlic
Leek
Chive
Aloes

**Morning Glory Family**
Sweet Potato
Yam

**Mustard Family**
Mustard
Cabbage
Cauliflower
Broccoli
Brussel Sprouts
Turnip
Rutabaga
Kale
Collard
Celery cabbage
Kohlrabi
Radish
Horseradish
Watercress

**Parsley Family**
Parsley
Parsnip
Carrot
Celery
Caraway
Anise
Dill
Coriander
Fennel

**Pomegranate Family**
Pomegranate

**Potato Family**
Potato
Tomato
Eggplant
Red Pepper
- cayenne

Green Pepper
Chili

**Sunflower Family**
Jerusalem artichoke
Sunflower seed oil

**Apple Family**
Apple
- cider
- vinegar
- apple pectin

Pear
Quince
- quince seed

**Banana Family**
Banana
Plantain

**Citrus Family**
Orange
Grapefruit
Lemon
Lime
Tangerine
Kumquat

**Ebony Family**
Persimmon

**Gooseberry Family**
Gooseberry
Currant

**Grape Family**
Grape
- raisin
- cream of tartar

**Heath Family**
Cranberry
Bluebarry

**Honeysuckle Family**
Elderberry

**Laurel Family**
Avocado
Cinnamon
Bay leaves

**Olive Family**
Green Olive
Ripe Olive
- olive oil

**Pawpaw Family**
Papaya

**Pineapple Family**
Pineapple

**Plum Family**
Plum
- prune

Cherry
Peach
Apricot
Nectarine
Almond

**Rose Family**
Raspberry
Blackberry
Loganberry
Youngberry
Dewberry
Strawberry

**Beech Family**
Beechnut
Chestnut

**Birch Family**
Filbert
Hazelnut
Oil of birch (wintergreen)

**Cashew Family**
Cashew
Pistachio
Mango

**Fungi Family**
Mushroom
Yeast

**Ginger Family**
Ginger
Tumeric
Cadamon

**Legythis Family**
Brazil nut

**Madder Family**
Coffee

**Mellow Family**
Okra (gumbo)
Cottonseed

**Maple Family**
Maple syrup
- maple sugar

**Mint Family**
Mint
Peppermint
Spearmint
Thyme
Sage
Majoram
Savory

**Miscellaneous**
Honey
Mulberry
Fig
Hop
Breadfruit

**Myrtle Family**
Allspice
Cloves
Pimento
Guava

**Nutmeg Family**
Nutmeg

**Orchid Family**
Vanilla

**Palm Family**
Coconut
Date
Sago

**Pedalium Family**
Sesame oil

**Pepper Family**
Black pepper

**Pine Family**
Juniper

**Poppy Family**
Poppy seed

**Stercula Family**
Cocoa
- chocolate

Tea Family
Tea

**Walnut Family**
English walnut
Black walnut
Butternut
Hickory Nut
Pecan

### *ANIMAL SOURCES*

**Amphibians**
Frog

**Crustaceans**
Crab
Lobster
Shrimp
Squid

**Fish**
Sturgeon
caviar
Anchovy
Sardine
Herring
Smelt
Trout
Salmon
Whitefish
Chub
Shad
Eel
Carp
Sucker
Buffalo
Catfish
Bullhead
Pike
Pickerel
Muskellunge
Mullet
Barracuda
Mackerel
Tuna
Pompano
Bluefish
Butterfish
harverstfish
Swordfish
Sunfish
Bass
Perch
Snapper
Croaker
Weakfish
Drum
Scup
Porgy
Flounder
Sole
Halibut
Rosefish
Codfish
Scrod
haddock
Hake
Pollack
Cusk

**Mollusks**
Abalone
Mussell
Oyster
Scallop
Clam

**Reptiles**
Turtles

**Birds**
Chicken
- chicken eggs

Duck
- duck eggs

Goose
- goose eggs

Turkey
Guinea hen
Pheasant
Partridge
Grouse

**Mammals**
Beef
- veal
- cow's milk
- butter
- cheese

Goat
- goat's milk
- cheese

Mutton
- lamb

Pork
- ham
- bacon

Venison
Horse meat
Rabbit
Squirrel

---

*Sometimes placed in composite family. Modified from Sheldon, J.M., Lovell, R.G. and Mathews, K.P. (Eds.):Food and Gastrointestinal Allergy. In a manual of Clinical Allergy, Philadelphia, Saunders, 1967. Used with permission.

**6–5** Factors in Cancer Causation and Prevention

| Disease | Risk factors | Mechanism | Protective elements | Mechanism |
|---|---|---|---|---|
| Lung cancer | Cigarette smoking | Complex mixture of genotoxic carcinogens, polycyclic aromatic hydrocarbons and tobacco specific nitrosamines and risk-determining enhancing, promoting agents. Asbestos, air pollutants have strong cocarcinogenic effect | Yellow-green vegetables | Retinoids, $\beta$-carotene inhibit development of early lesions through strengthening patency of gap junctions |
| | Occupational | Polycyclic hydrocarbons coal gas work, bis(chloromethyl)ether, bis(chloroethyl)sulfide, arsenic, nickel, and chromate ores | | |
| Oral cancer | Smoking: tobacco chewing; betel chewing; smoking and alcohol | Carcinogens in tobacco (mainly tobacco-specific nitrosamines), betel nut; hydroxy radicals | Yellow-green vegetables | Retinoids, $\beta$-carotene |
| Kidney cancer | Smoking; other factors unknown | Carcinogens from tobacco, unknown mechanisms | ? | ? |
| | Obesity | Endocrines: fat cells produce estrogens acting as carcinogens? | Weight control/loss | Lowers excessive nonphysiologic estrogen levels |
| Nasopharyngeal cancer | Salted, pickled fish | Contains specific nitrosamine? | ? | ? |
| | Viral factors | Can increase cell cycling | Vaccination? | |
| | Occupational | Wood and leather workers | | |
| Esophageal cancer | Salted, pickled food? | Specific nitrosamine | Yellow-green vegetables | Role of vegetables unknown if risk factor present in food |
| | Alcohol intake + smoking | Alcohol modifies esophageal metabolism of tobacco-specific carcinogens | Yellow-green vegetables | ($\beta$-carotene, protective element) |
| | Tobacco chewing | Tobacco-specific carcinogens and promoters? | Vegetables | $\beta$-Carotene, retinoids |
| Gastric cancer (intestinal) | Salted, pickled food | Nitrosoindoles, phenolic diazotates | Green-yellow vegetables | Role of vegetables unknown if risk factor present in food, but may assist in differentiation |
| | Geochemical nitrate and salt | Formation of gastric carcinogens, above, in stomach | Green-yellow vegetables, fruits, vitamins C and E | Prevent formation of carcinogen: cellular tissue defenses |
| Bladder cancer | Bilharzia: schistosomiasis | Carcinogens unknown; increased cell proliferation enhances risk | Yellow-green vegetables | ? |
| | Smoking | Unknown | Yellow-green vegetables | Retinoids |
| | Occupational | Arylamines | — | — |

**6–5** (Continued)

| | | | | |
|---|---|---|---|---|
| Endocrine-related cancers; prostate, breast, ovary | Total dietary fat (saturated + ω-6 polyunsaturated lipids) | Complex multieffector elements; hormonal balances, membrane and intracellular effectors | Monounsaturated oil (olive); ω-3 polyunsaturated oils | Neutral or protective action on hormone metabolism |
| | | | Medium-chain triglycerides | Caloric equivalent to carbohydrate |
| | | | Cereal fiber and pectin; yellow-green vegetables | Affects enteroheptic cycling of hormones |
| Endometrium | Same as above; excessive body weight | Same as above; fat cells generate estrogen | Same as above; weight control/loss | Same as above; lowers excessive nonphysiologic estrogen levels |
| Pancreas | Same as endocrine; | Fat affects physiology | Low-fat diets | Protects function |
| | Cigarette smoking | Tobacco-specific nitrosamines | ? | ? |
| Colon cancer | | | | |
| Proximal | ? | ? | ? | ? |
| Distal | Same as endocrine related cancers | Biosynthesis of cholesterol, thence bile acids, and colon cancer promotion including higher cell cycling | Cereal fiber | Increases stool bulk; dilutes promoters; lower intestinal pH |
| Rectal cancer | Alcoholic beverages, especially beer | Increases cell cycling in rectum | Cereal fiber? | Dilutes effectors by increasing stool bulk |
| Liver cancer | Mold contaminated foods | Mycotoxins | Avoid moldy, pickled foods, improve nutrition, more protein, fruits and vegetables | Lower carcinogen intake |
| | Some plants | Pyrrolizidine alkaloids | | |
| | Pickled foods | Nitrosamines | | |
| | Chronic virus | Hepatitis B | Vaccination | |
| | High level of specific alcoholic beverages | Damages liver, risk of cirrhosis potentiates effect of carcinogens | Decrease intake of alcohol | May lower cell duplication rates |
| | Occupational | Vinyl chloride | Lower exposure | |
| | Iatrogenic | Some oral contraceptives (infrequent occurrence) | | |

From: Weisburger, J.H.: Nutrtional approach to cancer prevention with emphasis on vitamins, antioxidants and carotenoids. *Am J Clin Nut*, 53(1):227S, 19991. Used with permission.

6–6 Color Your Daily Diet with Fruits and Vegetables (*Fresh, Frozen, Dried and Canned Varieties all count)

| | Phytonutrient | Benefits | Found In |
|---|---|---|---|
| GREEN | Lutein (Yellow-Green and Leafy Greens) | Helps Maintain Good Vision; Decreases the Risk of Cataracts or Macular Degeneration | Spinach, Kale, Leafy Greens (Turnip, Collard, Mustard), Romaine Lettuce, Broccoli, Green Peas, Kiwifruit, Honeydew Melon. |
| | Indoles (Cruciferous Vegetables) | Decreases the Risk of Cancer (Particularly Breast and Prostate Cancers); Reduce the Risk of Tumor Growth in Cancer Patients. | Brussels Sprouts, Broccoli, Cabbage, Bok Choy, Arugala, Swiss Chard, Turnips, Rutabaga, Watercress, Cauliflower, Kale. |
| ORANGE | Beta-Carotene (Dark Orange) | Powerful Antioxidant; Boosts Immunity; Reduces the Risk for Cancer; Reduces the Risk of Heart Attacks; Helps Maintain Good Vision. | Sweet Potatoes, Carrots, Pumpkin, Butternut Squash, Cantaloupe; Mangos, Apricots, Peaches |
| | Bioflavonoids (Yellow-Orange) | Powerful Antioxidants; Works with Vitamin C to Reduce the Risk of Heart Attacks, Reduce the Risk of Cancer, and to Help Maintain Strong Bones/Teeth, Healthy Skin, and Good Vision | Lemons, Oranges, Grapefruit, Tangerines, Clementines, Peaches, Papaya, Apricots, Nectarines, Pears, Pineapple, Yellow Raisins, Yellow Pepper. |
| RED | Lycopene | Reduces the Risk of Prostate, Breast and Skin Cancer; Reduces the Risk of heart Attacks. | Fresh Tomato, Tomato-based Products (Tomato Juice, Spaghetti Sauce, Tomato Soup, Tomato Paste), Watermelon, Pink Grapefruit, Guava. |
| | Anthocyanins | Decreases the Risk of Cancer; Powerful Antioxidants; Helps Control High Blood Pressure, Reduce the Risk of Diabetes Complications; Reduce the Risk of heart Attacks; Reduce the Risk of Alzheimer's Disease. | Sweet Cherries, Red Raspberries, Strawberries, Cranberries, Beets, Red Apples (with skin), Red Cabbage, Red Onion, Kidney Beans, Red Beans. |
| BLUE/PURPLE | Anthocyanins | Decreases the Risk of Cancer; Powerful Antioxidants; Reduce the Risk of Age-Related memory Loss; help control High Blood Pressure; Reduce the Risk of Diabetes Complications; Reduce the Risk of Heart Attacks; Reduce the Risk of Alzheimer's Disease. | Blackberries, Blueberries, Purple Grapes, Black Currants, Elderberries. |
| | Phenolics | Powerful Antioxidants; May Slow Some of the Effects of Aging. | Plums, Dried Plums (Prunes), Raisins, Eggplant |
| WHITE | Allicin | Increases Immunity; Helps Lower High Cholesterol; Helps Control High Blood Pressure; Reduces the Risk of Heart Attacks; Reduces the Risk for Spread of Cancer (particularly stomach and color cancer). | Onions, Garlic, Leeks, Scallions, Chives |

6–7 Calorie Control

| 800 CALORIES | 1000 CALORIES | 1200 CALORIES | 1500 CALORIES | 1800 CALORIES |
|---|---|---|---|---|
| P-60 grams | P-65 grams | P-70 grams | P-75 grams | P-85 grams |
| F-25 grams | P-30 grams | F-40 grams | F-65 grams | F-70 grams |
| C-85 grams | C-120 grams | C-135 grams | C-150 grams | C-180 grams |
| **BREAKFAST** | **BREAKFAST** | **BREAKFAST** | **BREAKFAST** | **BREAKFAST** |
| 1 x egg or cereal | 1 x cereal or egg | 1 x egg or cereal | 1 x cereal or egg | 1 x egg or cereal |
| ½ x bread | ½ x bread | 1 x bread | 1 x bread | 1 x bread |
| 1 x fruit (citrus) | 1 x fruit (citrus) | 1 x fruit (citrus) | 1 x fruit (citrus) | 2 x fruit (citrus) |
| 1 x skim milk | 1 x skim milk | 1 x skim milk | 1 x milk 2% | 1 x milk 2% |
| | ¼ x fat | ½ x fat | 1 x fat | 1 x fat |
| **LUNCH** | **LUNCH** | **LUNCH** | **LUNCH** | **LUNCH** |
| 2 x meat | 2 x meat | 2 x meat | 2 x meat | 3 x meat |
| 2 x vegetable A | 1 x vegetable A | 1 x vegetable A | 1 x vegetable A | 1 x vegetable A |
| 1 x fruit | 1 x fruit | 1 x fruit | 1 x fruit | 2 x fruit |
| 1 x bread | 2 x bread | 2 x bread | 2 x bread | 2 x bread |
| 1 x skim milk | ¼ x fat | ½ x fat | 1 x fat | 1 x fat |
| | 1 x skim milk | 1 x skim milk | 1 x milk 2% | 1 x milk 2% |
| **SUPPER** | **SUPPER** | **SUPPER** | **SUPPER** | **SUPPER** |
| 2 x meat | 2 x meat | 2 x meat | 3 x meat | 3 x meat |
| 1 x vegetable A | 1 x vegetable A | 1 x vegetable A | 1 x vegetable A | 1 x vegetable A |
| 1 x vegetable B | 1 x vegetable B | 1 x vegetable B | 1 x vegetable B | 1 x vegetable B |
| 1 x fruit | 1 x fruit | 1 x fruit | 1 x fruit | 2 x fruit |
| 1 x skim milk | ½ x bread | 1 x bread | 2 x bread | 2 x bread |
| | ½ x fat | 2 x fat | 2 x fat | 2 x fat |
| | 1 x skim milk | 1 x skim milk | 1 x milk 2% | 1 x milk 2% |

To insure nutritional adequacy:

1. Serve citrus fruit at least once per day (cranberry with Vitamin C added is okay).
2. Serve a yellow or deep green leafy vegetable every day.
3. Serve eggs three (3) days per week, cooked cereal two days, and dry cereal two days.
4. Use a skim milk or 2% milk which is fortified with vitamin A and D.
5. Use enriched or whole wheat bread and cereal products.
6. Use lite or iodized salt only – (not needed if using seafood 2x/week).
7. Make liver your choice of meat once per week, unless on a low cholesterol diet.
8. Make lean pork your choice at least twice per week (if diet is 800 calories).
9. Make puddings, custard, etc. with skim milk or non-fat dried milk.

This diet is adequate in protein, minerals and vitamins and should not need supplementation in any form.

**ADA Exchange lists – Meal Planning**

| Conversion to Glucose | C (100%) | P (58%) | F (10%) |
|---|---|---|---|
| Meat Group, lean | - | 7 | 5 |
| Vegetable Group | 5 | 2 | - |
| Fruit Group | 15 | - | - |
| Bread/Starch Group | 15 | 3 | - |
| Milk Group, 2% | 12 | 8 | 5 |
| Fat Group | - | - | 5 |

6–7 (Continued)

**VEGETABLES – A**

*One serving equals 1 cup cooked, 25 calories (raw as desired)*

| | |
|---|---|
| Asparagus | Lettuce |
| Broccoli | Mushrooms |
| Brussel Sprouts | Okra |
| Cabbage | Pepper |
| Cauliflower | Radishes |
| Celery | Sauerkraut |
| Chicory | String Beans |
| Cucumbers | Summer Squash |
| Escarole | Tomato (limit one to a meal) |
| Eggplant | Tomato Juice (limit ½ cup at a meal) |
| Greens: | Zucchini |
| Beet Greens | |
| Chard | |
| Dandelion Greens | |
| Mustard Greens | |
| Spinach | |
| Turnip Greens | |

**VEGETABLES – B**

*One serving equals ½ cup, 35 calories*

| | |
|---|---|
| Beets | Pumpkin |
| Carrots | Rutabagas |
| Onions | Winter squash |
| Green Peas | Turnips |

**MEATS**

*Equals 1 oz. of any lean meat 75 calories*

| | |
|---|---|
| Beef, veal, lamb, pork, ham, Chicken (trim off all fat) | 1 ounce |
| Cold Cuts – low fat | |
| Salami, Minced Ham, Bologna, Liverwurst, Luncheon Loaf | 1 slice |
| Frankfurters (8-9 per lb.) low fat | 1 |
| Egg | 1 |
| Fish | 1 ounce |
| Salmon, Tuna, Crab, Lobster | ¼ cup |
| Shrimp, Clams, Oysters | 5 small |
| Sardines | 3 medium |
| Cheese, cheddar type | 1 ounce |
| Cottage Cheese | ¼ cup |
| Peanut Butter | 2 Tbsp. |
| Dried Peas or Beans (measure cooked) | ½ cup |
| Baked Beans (no pork) | ¼ cup |

**FATS**

*One serving equals 45 calories*

| | |
|---|---|
| Butter or Fortified Margarine | 1 tsp. |
| Bacon, crisp | 1 slice |
| Cream, light (sweet or sour) | 2 Tbsp. |
| Cream, heavy | 1 Tbsp. |
| Cream cheese | 1 Tbsp. |
| Avocado | 1/8 |
| French Dressing | 1 Tbsp. |
| Mayonnaise | 1 tsp. |
| Oil | 1 tsp. |
| Cooking Fat | 1 tsp. |
| Nuts | 6 small |
| Olives | 5 small |

**BREAD**

*Equals 1 slice bread or toast, 70 calories*

| | |
|---|---|
| Biscuit or Roll (2 inches diameter) | 1 |
| Muffin (2 inches diameter) | 1 |
| Cornbread (1½ inches diameter) | 1 |
| Cereals, cooked | ½ cup |
| Dry, flake and puff types | ¾ cup |
| Rice, Noodles, Macaroni, or Spaghetti (measure cooked) | ½ cup |
| Crackers, graham | 2 |
| Oyster crackers | 20 or ½ cup |
| Saltines | 5 |
| Uneeda | 3 |
| Ritz | 5 |
| Corn (1 small ear) | 1/3 cup |
| Parsnips | 1/3 cup |
| Pop Corn (plain) | 2/3 cup |
| Potatoes, white ½ cup mashed or 1 small (Use fat allowance) | 1 |
| Sweet Potato | ¼ cup |
| Sponge Cake (plain) 1 ½ inch cube | 1 |
| Ice Milk or Sherbet | ½ cup |
| Ice Cream (Omit 2 teaspoons fat) | ½ cup |

**FRUITS**

*One serving equals 40 calories*

| | |
|---|---|
| Apple | 1 small |
| Applesauce | ½ cup |
| Apricots, fresh | 2 medium |
| Apricots, dried | 4 halves |
| Banana | ½ small |
| Blackberries | 1 cup |
| Raspberries | 1 cup |
| * Strawberries | 1 cup |
| Blueberries | 2/3 cup |
| Cantaloupe | ¼ medium |
| Cherries | 10 large |
| Cranberry juice | ½ cup |
| Dates | 2 |
| Figs, fresh | 2 large |
| * Grapefruit | ½ |
| * Grapefruit juice | ½ cup |
| Grapes | 12 |
| Grape juice | ¼ cup |
| Honeydew Melon | 1/8 medium |
| Mango | ½ small |
| * Orange | 1 small |
| * Orange juice | ½ cup |
| Peach | 1 medium |
| Pear | 1 small |
| Pineapple | ½ cup |
| Pineapple juice | 1/3 cup |
| Plums | 2 medium |
| Prunes, dried | 2 medium |
| Raisins | 2 Tbsp. |
| * Tangerine | 1 large |
| * Tomato juice | 1 cup |
| Watermelon | ½ slice (1" thick) or 1 cup |

* Vitamin C Source

# APPENDIX 7
# Quality Assurance Standards, Choose My Plate and Selected Pyramids

7–1 Nutrition Quality Assurance Criteria, Developmental Disorders

**Target Population:** Patients With Developmental Disabilities (Generic)
**Variables:** Age 0 to 18 Years, Ambulatory Care, Nonacute

| Criteria* | Critical time | Accepted level of performance | Exceptions | References | Audit data source |
|---|---|---|---|---|---|
| (P) 1. Nutrition screening completed, including the following minimal elements:<br>a. Diagnosis<br>b. Review of health history†<br>c. Weight/height (or length)<br>d. Rate of growth<br>e. Dietary intake<br>f. Ambulation | Each clinic visit | | Clinic visit for nutrition assessment or routine therapy | | Medical record |
| (P) 2. Nutrition assessment completed, including the following minimal elements:<br>a. Height (or length) and weight<br>b. Triceps and subscapular skin-fold measurements<br>c. Iron status<br>d. Dietary<br>e. Clinical/dental<br>f. Feeding skills/behaviors<br>g. Elimination patterns<br>h. Nutrient-drug interaction<br>i. Nutrient supplementation<br>j. Frequent infections<br>k. Physical activity/ambulation<br>l. Maturation | Initial evaluation period and as indicated in nutrition care plan<br>Nutrient-drug interactions evaluated with each medication change<br>Maturation evaluated during preadolescence and adolescence | | | 1, 2 | Medical record |
| (P) 3. Nutrition care plan developed jointly by patient/caregiver and nutritionist according to established guidelines for documentation. | At or within 2 wk of completion of nutrition assessment | | | | Medical record |
| (P) 4. Nutrition care plan implemented as written or revised. | Duration of treatment or according to timetable identified in nutrition care plan | | | | Medical record |
| (P) 5. Patient/caregiver given food and fluid information appropriate to patient's age, development, and condition. | Initial clinic visit and as indicated in nutrition care plan | | | 3, 4 | Medical record |
| (O) 6. Patient/caregiver reports patient consumes (or progresses toward) diet as specified in nutrition care plan. | Following initial instruction and with each change in diet | | | | Medical record |
| (O) 7. Solid or supplemental foods introduced no earlier than age 4 mo. | First 4 mo of life | | Solid or supplemental foods introduced to patient prior to initial clinic visit | 5 | Medical record |
| (O) 8. Patient's texture progression of food appropriate for developmental status. | Until mature eating pattern achieved | | Team assessment identifies that patient's maximum potential achieved but is below mature eating pattern | 3, 6 | Medical record |
| (O) 9. Patient progresses toward or achieves mature feeding skills. | Until mature feeding skills achieved | | Team assessment identifies that patient's maximum potential achieved but is below mature feeding skills | 6 | Medical record |
| (O) 10. Patient with prescribed diet modification and/or caregiver can devise 1-day meal plan with number of servings, portion sizes, and kinds of foods specified in diet pattern agreed upon with nutritionist. | Clinic visit following initial counseling, or as specified in nutrition care plan | | Precluded by functioning level of patient and/or caregiver | | Medical record |
| (O) 11. Patient/caregiver can identify diet and activity as factors contributing to patient's weight status. | Clinic visit following initial counseling, or as specified in nutrition care plan | | Precluded by functioning level of patient and/or caregiver; patient's weight is appropriate and unlikely to be affected adversely by condition | 7, 8 | Medical record |
| (O) 12. Patient/caregiver can identify fluid and dietary fiber intake and exercise as important factors in prevention of constipation. | Clinic visit following initial counseling, or as specified in nutrition care plan | | Precluded by functioning level of patient and/or caregiver; constipation not usual manifestation of clinical condition | 9, 10 | Medical record |

**7–1** (Continued)

| | | | | |
|---|---|---|---|---|
| (O) 13. Patient/caregiver reports appropriate use of rewards (reinforcers). | Clinic visit following initial counseling, or as specified in nutrition care plan | | 3, 8 | Medical record |
| (P) 14. Patient/caregiver counseled on relationship between diet and dental/oral health. | Initial evaluation period and/or as indicated in nutrition care plan | | 8, 11 | Medical record |
| (O) 15. Patient/caregiver can identify inappropriate bottle feeding. | Clinic visit following initial counseling, or as indicated in nutrition care plan | Patient no longer using bottle | 11 | Medical record |
| (O) 16. Patient maintains, progresses toward, or achieves weight/height between the 10th and 90th percentiles according to National Center for Health Statistics (NCHS) growth chart, and/or triceps and subscapular skin-fold measurements between 10th and 90th percentiles of most appropriate reference data available.‡ | Each clinic visit following initial visit, or as indicated in nutrition care plan | Growth potential compromised by nonnutritional factors | 12–15 | Medical record |
| (O) 17. Patient/caregiver can identify nutrition risk related to nutrient-drug interactions. | Clinic visit following initial counseling, or as indicated in nutrition care plan | Precluded by functioning level of patient and/or caregiver; patient is not receiving drugs that affect nutrition | 16, 17 | Medical record |

§

* P, process; O, outcome.

‡ These percentiles are used because of the importance of detecting a potential growth problem early, as growth problems are often found in this population.

§ This criteria set was one of the first to be developed. It does not include a specific criterion regarding referral of the client to food and/or nutrition resources. Practitioners are encouraged to add such a criterion when using this criteria set.

† Iron status, feeding skills/behaviors, elimination patterns, nutrient supplementation, nutrient-drug interaction, frequent infections.

## References


1. Smith MAH, et al: Developmental feeding tool, in: *Feeding Management of a Child With a Handicap: A Guide for Professionals.* Memphis, University of Tennessee Center for the Health Sciences Child Development Center, 1982.
2. Smith MAH (ed): *Guides for Nutritional Assessment of the Mentally Retarded and Developmentally Disabled.* Memphis, University of Tennessee Center for the Health Sciences Child Development Center, 1976.
3. Pipes PL, Carmen P: Nutrition and feeding of children with developmental delays and related problems, in Pipes PL and Carman P (eds): *Nutrition in Infancy and Childhood.* St. Louis, Times Mirror/Mosby Co, 1985.
4. Rickard K, Brady MS, Gresham EL: Nutrition in the chronically ill child. Congenital heart disease and myelomeningocele. *Pediatr Clin North Am* 24:157, 1977.
5. American Academy of Pediatrics Committee on Nutrition: On the feeding of supplemental foods to infants. *Pediatrics* 65:1178, 1980.
6. Smith MAH, et al: Normal feeding development chart, in: *Feeding Management of a Child With a Handicap: A Guide for Professionals.* Memphis, University of Tennessee Center for the Health Sciences Child Development Center, 1982.
7. Heins JN: Obesity in children, in Palmer S, Ekvall S (eds): *Pediatric Nutrition Developmental Disorders.* Springfield, IL, Charles C Thomas, 1978.
8. Howard RB, Harbold NH: *Nutrition in Clinical Care.* New York, McGraw-Hill, 1982.
9. Infant and child nutrition: Concerns regarding the developmentally disabled. *J Am Diet Assoc* 78:443, 1981.
10. Frequently reported nutrition problems and factors contributing to high nutritional risk of children with handicapping conditions, in Baer MT (ed): *Nutrition Services for Children With Handicaps. A Manual for State Title V Programs.* Los Angeles, University Affiliated Training Program, Center for Child Developmental Disorders, 1982.
11. Nizel AE: Nutritional support for optimizing children's dental health, in Suskind R (ed): *Textbook of Pediatric Nutrition.* New York, Raven Press, 1981.
12. National Center for Health Statistics: *NCHS Growth Curves for Children 0-18 Years, US.* Vital and Health Statistics, series 11, no. 165. Health Resources Administration, US Government Printing Office, 1977.
13. National Center for Health Statistics: *Height and Weight of Youths 12-17 Years, US.* Vital and Health Statistics, series 11, no. 124. Health Services and Mental Health Administration, US Government Printing Office, 1973.
14. National Center for Health Statistics: *Basic Data on Anthropometric Measurements and Angular Measurement of the Hip and Knee Joints for Selected Age Groups, 1-74 Years of Age, US 1971-1975.* Vital and Health Statistics, series 11, no. 219. US Government Printing Office, 1981.
15. Cronk CE: Growth of children with Down's syndrome: Birth to age 3 years. *Pediatrics* 61:564, 1978.
16. Springer NS, Fricke NL: Endogenous malnutrition following drug therapy, in Palmer S, Ekvall S (eds): *Pediatric Nutrition in Developmental Disorders.* Springfield, IL, Charles C Thomas, 1978.
17. Springer NS: Drug-nutrient interactions, in: *Nutrition Casebook on Developmental Disabilities.* Syracuse, NY, Syracuse University Press, 1982.


## Developmental Disabilities Quality Assurance Committee

Among those involved in the development and/or field testing of these criteria were:

Mariel Caldwell, MS, MPH, RD, chairperson
Marion Baer, PhD, RD
Elaine Blyler, MS, RD
Harriet Cloud, MS, RD
Sandra Eardley, PhD, RD
Shirley M. Ekvall, PhD, RD
Sheila Farnan, MPH, RD
Barbara Free, MS, RD
Kate Hohenbrink, MS, RD
Betty Kozlowski, PhD
Jackie Krick, MS, RD
Judith Oliver, MS, RD
Peggy Pipes, MPH, RD

**Field-test Sites:**

Southern Illinois University School of Medicine
Springfield, Illinois

Sparks Center for Developmental and Learning Disorders
University of Alabama at Birmingham
Birmingham, Alabama

University Affiliated Cincinnati Center for Developmental Disorders
University of Cincinnati
Cincinnati, Ohio

7–2 Nutrition Quality Assurance Criteria, Myelomeningocele

**Target Population:** Patients With Myelodysplasia
**Variables:** Age 0-18 Years, Ambulatory Care, Nonacute

| Criteria* | Critical time | Accepted level of performance | Exceptions | References | Audit data source |
|---|---|---|---|---|---|
| (P) 1. Nutrition screening completed, including the following minimal elements:<br>a. Review of health history†<br>b. Weight/height (or length) and/or skin-fold | Each clinic visit or as indicated in nutrition care plan | | Clinic visit for nutrition assessment | | Medical record |
| (P) 2. Nutrition assessment completed, including the following minimal elements:<br>a. Height (or length)<br>b. Weight and/or skin-fold<br>c. Iron status<br>d. Dietary intake<br>e. Clinical/medical history<br>f. Feeding skills | Initial clinic visit and as indicated in nutrition care plan | | | 1 | Medical record |
| (P) 3. Nutrition care plan developed jointly by patient/caregiver and nutritionist according to established guidelines for documentation. | At or within 2 wk of completion of nutrition assessment | | | | Medical record |
| (P) 4. Nutrition care plan implemented as written or revised. | According to timetable identified in nutrition care plan | | | | Medical record |
| (P) 5. Patient maintains, progresses toward, or achieves: | Duration of treatment | | | 2-5 | Medical record |
| a. Body weight/height between the 10th and 75th percentiles according to National Center for Health Statistics (NCHS) growth chart (for patients aged 2-10 yr) and/or | | | Patient is not aged 2-10 yr | | |
| b. Body weight/height between the 10th and 90th percentiles according to Health and Nutrition Examination Survey (HANES) data (for patients aged 12-17 yr) and/or | | | Patient is not aged 12-17 yr | | |
| c. A triceps or subscapular skin-fold between the 10th and 90th percentiles for age and sex according to HANES data (for patients aged 1-18 yr)‡ | | | Patient is not aged 1-18 yr | | |
| (O) 6. Patient/caregiver given the following information related to patient's age, development, and condition (each element evaluated separately):<br>a. Appropriate food and fluid intake<br>b. Avoidance of high-calorie, low-nutrient foods | Each clinic visit or as indicated in nutrition care plan | | | 2 | Medical record |
| c. Nursing bottle syndrome | | | Patient is no longer using bottle | | |
| (O) 7. Patient/caregiver reports patient consumes or progresses toward diet as specified in nutrition care plan. | Following initial diet instruction and as indicated by nutrition care plan | | | | Medical record |
| (O) 8. Solid or supplemental foods introduced no earlier than age 4 mo. | First 4 mo of life | | Solid or supplemental foods introduced to patient prior to intial clinic visit | 6 | Medical record |
| (O) 9. Patient/caregiver reports texture progression of food appropriate for developmental readiness. | Until mature feeding skills achieved | | Team assessment identifies that patient's maximum potential is achieved, but is below mature eating pattern | 7 | Medical record |
| (O) 10. Patient progresses toward or achieves mature feeding skills appropriate for developmental or chronologic age. | Until mature feeding skills achieved | | Team assessment identifies that patient's maximum potential is achieved, but is below mature feeding skills | 8 | Medical record |
| (O) 11. Patient/caregiver correctly identifies low-nutrient, high-calorie foods in patient's diet history. | Clinic visit following initial counseling, or as specified in nutrition care plan | | Patient has diagnosis of failure to thrive; patient is below 5th percentile as measured in criterion 5 | 2, 9 | Medical record |

**7–2** (Continued)

| | | | | |
|---|---|---|---|---|
| (O) 12. Patient with prescribed diet modification and/or caregiver can devise 1-day meal with recommended number of servings, portion sizes, and kinds of foods consistent with those specified in diet pattern agreed upon with nutrition counselor. | Clinic visit following initial instruciton or as specified in nutrition care plan | Patient does not have prescribed diet modification | | Medical record |
| (O) 13. Patient/caregiver can identify that patient's specific diet and activity factors contribute to weight control. | Clinic visit following initial instruction or as specified in nutrition care plan | | 10 | Medical record |
| (O) 14. Patient/caregiver can identify fluid and dietary fiber intake and exercise as important factors in prevention of constipation. | Clinic visit following initial instruction or as specified in nutrition care plan | | 11 | Medical record |
| (O) 15. Patient/caregiver reports use of only nonfood items as rewards. | Clinic visit following initial instruction or as specified in nutrition care plan | | | Medical record |
| (O) 16. Patient's drug/medical intake evaluated for effect on nutrient utilization. | At initial clinic visit and following each drug/medication change | | 12 | Medical record |

§

* P, process; O, outcome.

§ This criteria set was one of the first to be developed. It does not include a specific criterion regarding referral of the client to food and/or nutrition resources. Practitioners are encouraged to add such a criterion when using this criteria set.

‡ These percentiles are used because of the importance of detecting a potential growth problem early, as growth problems are often found in this population.

## References


1. Christakis G (ed): Nutrition assessment in health programs. *Am J Public Health* 63:38, 1973.
2. Rickard K, Brady MS, Gresham EL: Nutritional management of the chronically ill child: Congenital heart disease and myelomeningocele, in Neumann CG, Jelliffe DB (eds): *Pediatric Clinics of North America*. Philadelphia, W.B. Saunders Co, 1977.
3. National Center for Health Statistics: *NCHS Growth Curves for Children 0-18 Years, US*. Vital and Health Statistics, series 11, no. 165. Health Resources Administration, US Government Printing Office, 1977.
4. National Center for Health Statistics: *Height and Weight of Youths 12-17 Years, US*. Vital and Health Statistics, series 11, no. 124. Health Services and Mental Health Administration, US Government Printing Office, 1973.
5. National Center for Health Statistics: *Basic Data on Anthropometric Measurements and Angular Measurement of the Hip and Knee Joints for Selected Age Groups, 1-74 Years of Age, US, 1971-1975*. Vital and Health Statistics, series 11, no. 219. US Government Printing Office, 1981.
6. American Academy of Pediatrics Committee on Nutrition: On the feeding of supplemental foods to infants. *Pediatrics* 65:1178, 1980.
7. Pipes PL (ed): *Nutrition in Infancy and Childhood*. St. Louis, C.V. Mosby, 1981.
8. Smith MAH, et al: Normal feeding development chart, in: *Feeding Management of a Child With a Handicap: A Guide for Professionals*. Memphis, University of Tennessee Center for the Health Sciences Child Development Center, 1982.
9. *Nutritive Value of Foods*. Home and Garden Bulletin no. 72. Department of Agriculture, 1981.
10. Heins JN: Obesity in children, in Palmer S, Ekvall S (eds): *Pediatric Nutrition in Developmental Disorders*. Springfield, IL, Charles C Thomas, 1978.
11. Infant and child nutrition: Concerns regarding the developmentally disabled. *J Am Diet Assoc* 78:443, 1981.
12. Springer NS, Fricke NL: Endogenous malnutrition following drug therapy, in Palmer S, Ekvall S (eds): *Pediatric Nutrition in Developmental Disorders*. Springfield, IL, Charles C. Thomas, 1978.


## Myelodysplasia Quality Assurance Committee

Among those involved in the development and/or field testing of these criteria were:

Mariel Caldwell, MS, MPH, RD, chairperson
Mary Sue Brady, RD, DMSc
Shirley M. Ekvall, PhD, RD
Sheila Farnan, MPH, RD
Barbara Free, MS, RD
Betty Krauss, RD
Anne Nalepp, RD
Jill Reynolds, MPH, RD
Karyl Rickard, RD, PhD
Alice Smith, MS, RD

**Field-test Sites**

Children's Hospital of Michigan
Detroit, Michigan

Children's Memorial Hospital
Chicago, Illinois

James Whitcomb Riley Hospital for Children
Indiana University Medical Center
Indianapolis, Indiana

Mary Freebed Hospital
Grand Rapids, Michigan

University Affiliated Cincinnati Center for Developmental Disorders
University of Cincinnati
Cincinnati, Ohio

7–3 Medical Nutrition Therapy Protocol, Cystic Fibrosis

Setting: Ambulatory Care or adapted for other health care settings (Diagnosis through Adulthood)
Number of encounters: 1-4 per year

| No. of encounters | Length of contact | Time between encounters |
|---|---|---|
| 1 | 45-60 minutes | Determined by physician |
| 2 | 20-30 minutes | Determined by physician |
| 3 | 20-30 minutes | Determined by physician |
| 4 | 20-30 minutes | Determined by physician |

**Expected Outcomes of Medical Nutrition Therapy**

| Outcome Assessment Factors | Baseline | Evaluation of Intervention | | | Expected Outcomes | Ideal/goal value |
|---|---|---|---|---|---|---|
| | Interventions | | | | | |
| | 1 | 2 | 3 | 4 | | |
| **Clinical Assessment**[1] | | | | | | |
| **Laboratory parameters** | | | | | | • Maintain normal values for age, no indication of anemia or uncontrolled hyperglycemia |
| • Prealbumin, albumin | ✓ | | ✓ | | • Improve or maintain values for age | |
| • CBC: HgB, Hct, MCV | ✓ | | ✓ | | | |
| • Glucose, OGTT per need | ✓ | | | | | |
| • Glycated HgB with diabetes | ✓ | | ✓ | | | |
| • Electrolytes, BUN, creatinine | ✓ | | ✓ | | | |
| **Nutrition Physical** | | | | | | • Appropriate weight gain and growth velocity for age and gender |
| • Length (<2 yr), Height (>2 yr) | ✓ | ✓ | ✓ | ✓ | | |
| • Length/height-for-age plotted | ✓ | ✓ | ✓ | ✓ | | • >5th %tile for length or height |
| • Weight-for-age plotted | ✓ | ✓ | ✓ | ✓ | • CDC:US[2] growth charts reflect appropriate growth patterns for age and gender (for clients < 20 years of age) | |
| • Body Mass Index (BMI) (> 2 yr) | ✓ | ✓ | ✓ | ✓ | | • 90% IBW/height |
| • Weight-for-stature or IBW | ✓ | ✓ | ✓ | ✓ | | • BMI in normal range for age |
| • Weight-for-length (<3 yr) | ✓ | ✓ | ✓ | ✓ | • Calculate BMI | |
| • Head circumference (HC) (<3 yr) | | ✓ | ✓ | ✓ | | • HC normal for age |
| • TSF, MAMC, AMA[3] | | ✓ | ✓ | | • Normal fat area and muscle for height age | • Maintain normal fat area and muscle mass |
| **Clinical Signs and Symptoms** | | | | | | |
| • Symptoms of CF Malabsorption | ✓ | ✓ | ✓ | ✓ | • GI symptoms, eg, malabsorption minimized | • GI symptoms controlled<br>• Fecal fat results indicate 85-90% absorption |
| **Nutrition and Behavior Education*** | | | | | | **MNT Goals** |
| • Food and meal planning | ✓ | ✓ | ✓ | ✓ | • Consumes appropriate foods, fluids, and snacks | • Consumes adequate calories, protein, salt and fluids. |
| • Pancreatic enzymes, vitamin and mineral supplements or other dietary supplements as prescribed | ✓ | ✓ | ✓ | ✓ | • Adheres to prescribed pancreatic enzyme and vitamin/mineral therapies | • Adheres to appropriate diet, pancreatic enzyme and vitamin/mineral therapies to maintain normal growth velocity, normal weight–for-height (stature) and laboratory values. |
| • High-calorie/nutrient-dense foods and adequate salt intake | | ✓ | ✓ | ✓ | • Identifies & provides high-calorie & -protein foods, diet adequate in salt | |
| • Recipe modification | | ✓ | ✓ | ✓ | • Capable of modifying recipes | |
| • Feeding and eating behaviors | ✓ | ✓ | ✓ | ✓ | • Appropriate eating & behavioral skills and meals | |
| • Potential food/drug interaction | ✓ | ✓ | ✓ | ✓ | • Verbalizes potential food/drug interactions | |
| • Exercise and physical activity | ✓ | ✓ | ✓ | ✓ | • Participates in regular exercise for age | • Understands CF in relation to nutrition health, diet, growth, infection and disease process. |
| • Tube feeding or oral food supplements, dietary supplements as needed | ✓ | ✓ | ✓ | ✓ | • Follows tube-feeding prescription or consumes dietary supplements as needed | |

[1] Additional labs or tests may include liver function test (eg, AST, ALT, alkaline phosphatase), calcium, phosphorus, magnesium, vitamin A, vitamin E, PT, 25, OH vitamin D, bone mineral status (Dual Emission Xenon Absorpiometry (DEXA)).
[2] Center for Disease Control (CDC): United States (US) growth charts, June 2000.
[3] Tricep Skinfold (TSF), Mid-Arm Muscle Circumference (MAMC), Arm Muscle Area (AMA)
* Encounter in which behavioral topics are covered may vary according to client and caregiver's readiness, skills, resources, and need for lifestyle changes.

7–4 Medical Nutrition Therapy Protocol for General High-Risk Premature Infants (Children)

**Setting: Ambulatory Care** (Children ≤ 3 years corrected age) **Number of encounters:** 5

| No. of encounters | Length of contact | Goal age at encounters * |
|---|---|---|
| 1 | 45-60 minutes | 2-4 weeks after NICU discharge |
| 2 | 30-45 minutes | at approximately 3 months corrected age |
| 3 | 30-45 minutes | at approximately 7 months corrected age |
| 4 | 30-45 minutes | at approximately 18 months corrected age |
| 5 | 30-45 minutes | at approximately 36 months corrected age |

* Coordinate with routine medical visits.

**Expected Outcomes of Medical Nutrition Therapy**

| Outcome assessment factors | Baseline<br>Interventions 1 | Evaluation of Intervention<br>2 | 3 | 4 | 5 | Expected outcome | Ideal/goal value |
|---|---|---|---|---|---|---|---|
| **Clinical Assessment** [1] | | | | | | | |
| **Nutrition Physical**<br>• Weight<br>• Length/height (stature)<br>• Head circumference (≤ 36 mo)<br>• Weight-for-age, %tile<br>• Length/height-for-age, %tile<br>• Head circumference-for-age, %tile<br>• Weight-for-length/height, %tile | ✓<br>✓<br>✓<br>✓<br>✓<br>✓<br>✓ | ✓<br>✓<br>✓<br>✓<br>✓<br>✓<br>✓ | ✓<br>✓<br>✓<br>✓<br>✓<br>✓<br>✓ | ✓<br>✓<br>✓<br>✓<br>✓<br>✓<br>✓ | ✓<br>✓<br>✓<br>✓<br>✓<br>✓<br>✓ | Growth is appropriate. CDC:US[2] growth charts reflect appropriate growth for **corrected age** and gender. However, comparing actual with reference incremental[3] gains in weight (g/d) and length (mm/d) for **corrected age** is a more sensitive assessment of growth. | Achieves/maintains incremental growth[3] at a minimum of 25-75th %tile for **corrected age** during the first 2 years of life. Over time, achieves/maintains growth on the CDC:US[2] growth charts at 25-75th %tile for **corrected age**. |
| **Clinical signs and symptoms**<br>• Feeding issues<br>• Voiding & stool pattern | ✓ | ✓ | ✓ | ✓ | ✓ | Appetite and feeding cues expressed. Tolerates feedings. Ad libitum and fluid intakes adequate. Stools and voiding patterns normal. | Appetite is good. Optimum dietary intake achieved and corresponds to observed growth. No nutrient deficiencies observed. |
| **Functional/Feeding Assessment** | | | | | | | |
| • Breast-feeding skills | ✓ | ✓ | ✓ | ✓ | ✓ | Breast-fed infants: transition to breast completed and support in place. | Achieves/maintains effective breast feeding at frequency and duration mother/infant desire. |
| • General feeding skills | ✓ | ✓ | ✓ | ✓ | ✓ | All infants: feeding progression and behavior appropriate. | Enjoys eating, takes feedings easily, uses developmentally appropriate skills and utensils. |
| **Nutrition and Behavior Education*** | | | | | | | **MNT Goals** |
| • Food and meal planning<br>• Food preparation and food safety<br>• Dietary intake and mealtime management | ✓<br>✓<br>✓ | ✓<br>✓<br>✓ | ✓<br>✓<br>✓ | ✓<br>✓<br>✓ | ✓<br>✓<br>✓ | Parent or caregiver:<br>• Has access to food and other appropriate resources.<br>• Prepares and stores infant or pediatric formula recipe and foods appropriately and safely.<br>• Includes vitamin and mineral supplements appropriately.<br>• Delays solids until 4-6 months corrected age or until developmentally appropriate.<br>• Offers developmentally appropriate amounts at appropriate times. | • Utilizes resources appropriately.<br>• Minimizes risks of inappropriate formula dilution, food preparation, and food borne illness.<br>• Maintains optimum dietary intake and adheres to appropriate feeding treatment plan set by Registered dietitian to promote growth. Achieves developmentally appropriate feeding skills. |

[1]Recheck in 1 month if abnormal. Change to the MNT protocol for Complex High -Risk Premature if clinical outcomes remain abnormal.
[2]Centers for Disease Control (CDC:US) growth charts provide reasonable standards for monitoring the growth of premature infants when corrected age is used. [3]Guo, Roche, Fomon, et al. (1991) provide reasonable reference data for increments in size during the first two years of life when corrected age is used (*refer to pages 32-33*).
*Encounter in which behavioral topics are covered may vary according to caregiver's readiness, skills, resources, and need for lifestyle changes.

7–5 Medical Nutrition Therapy Protocol, Complex High-Risk Premature Infants (Children)

**Setting: Ambulatory Care:** (Children ≤ 5 years old) **Number of encounters:** 5

| No. of encounters | Length of contact | Time between encounters |
|---|---|---|
| 1 | 45-60 minutes | 1-2 weeks |
| 2 | 30-45 minutes | 2-4 weeks |
| 3 | 30-45 minutes | 1-2 months |
| 4 , 5 and beyond | 30-45 minutes | 1-2 months |

**Expected Outcomes of Medical Nutrition Therapy**

| Outcome assessment factors | Baseline: Interventions 1 | Evaluation of Intervention: 2 | 3 | 4 | 5 | Expected outcome | Ideal/goal value |
|---|---|---|---|---|---|---|---|
| **Clinical Assessment** [1] | | | | | | | |
| **Laboratory Values**[2] | | | | | | | |
| • Albumin, BUN, creatinine<br>• Electrolytes, calcium,<br>• Phosphorus, alkaline phosphatase | ✓ | ✓ | ✓ | ✓ | ✓ | Achieves and maintains normal levels. | Maintains laboratory values within normal range based on institution standards. |
| **Nutrition Physical**<br>• Weight<br>• Length/height (stature)<br>• Head circumference (≤ 36 mo)<br>• Weight-for-age, %tile<br>• Length-for-age, %tile<br>• Head circumference-for-age, %tile<br>• Weight-for-length/height, %tile (< 5 yrs)<br>• Clinical signs and symptoms | ✓ | ✓ | ✓ | ✓ | ✓ | Growth is appropriate. CDC:US[3] growth charts reflect appropriate growth for **corrected age**. However, comparing actual with reference incremental[4] gains in weight (g/d) and length (mm/d) for **corrected age** is a more sensitive assessment of growth. Appetite/ feeding cues expressed. Tolerates feedings, in appropriate time interval and volume.<br>Fluid intakes adequate; stools normal. | Achieves/maintains incremental growth[4] at a minimum of 25-75th %tile for **corrected age** during the first 2 years of life. Over time, achieves/maintains growth on the CDC:US[3] growth charts at 25-75th %tile for **correct age** and for weight-for-length-height.<br>Appetite is good. Optimum dietary intake achieved and corresponds to observed growth. No nutrient deficiencies observed. |
| **Functional Assessment** | | | | | | | |
| • Feeding skills | ✓ | ✓ | ✓ | ✓ | ✓ | Develops oral feeding skills whether breast or bottle fed. Feeding progression and behavior appropriate. | Maintains/advances oral eating.<br>Enjoys eating, takes feedings easily, uses developmentally appropriate skills and utensils. |
| **Nutrition and Behavior Education*** | | | | | | **Parent or caregiver:** | **MNT Goals:** |
| • Food and meal planning | ✓ | ✓ | ✓ | ✓ | ✓ | • Has access to food and other appropriate resources. | • Utilizes resources appropriately. |
| • Food preparation and food safety | ✓ | ✓ | ✓ | ✓ | ✓ | • Prepares and stores infant or pediatric formula recipe and foods appropriately and safely.<br>• Includes vitamin and mineral supplements appropriately. | • Minimizes risks of inappropriate formula dilution, food preparation, and food borne illness. |
| • Dietary intake and mealtime management | ✓ | ✓ | ✓ | ✓ | ✓ | • Delays solids until 4-6 months corrected age or until developmentally appropriate.<br>• Offers developmentally appropriate amounts at appropriate times.<br>• Is able to identify and resolve feeding problems.<br>• Keeps accurate food records.[5] | • Maintains optimum dietary intake and adheres to appropriate feeding treatment plan set by registered dietitian to promote growth. Achieves developmentally appropriate feeding skills. Contacts registered dietitian for help with significant feeding problems. |

[1]Recheck in 1 month if abnormal. If outcomes are consistently within normal limits and complex problems appear resolved, consider a change to the MNT protocol for General High-Risk Premature Infants. [2] As appropriate, general labs suggested for complex premature infants would include hematocrit, albumin, BUN, and creatinine. (For infants receiving diuretics consider electrolytes. For infants with osteopathy of prematurity consider calcium, phosphorus, and alkaline phosphatase.) [3]Centers for Disease Control (CDC: US) growth charts provide reasonable standards for monitoring the growth of premature infants when corrected age is used. [4]Guo, Roche, Fomon, et al. provide reasonable reference data for increments in size during the first two years of life when corrected age is used (see *pages 32-33)*. [5] Food records requested as needed.
*Encounter in which behavioral topics are covered may vary according to caregiver's readiness, skills, resources, and need for lifestyle changes. [5]Food records requested as needed.

7–6 Medical Nutrition Therapy Protocol, Pediatric Failure to Thrive

**Setting: Ambulatory Care or adapted for other health care settings** (Birth through 7 years)
**Number of encounters**: 5

| No. of encounters | Length of contact | Time between encounters |
|---|---|---|
| 1 | 60-90 minutes | 1-2 weeks |
| 2 | 30-45 minutes | determined by need |
| 3 | 30 minutes | determined by need |
| 4 | 30 minutes | determined by need |
| 5 | 30 minutes | determined by need |

**Expected Outcomes of Medical Nutrition Therapy**

| | Base-Line | Evaluation of Intervention | | | | | |
|---|---|---|---|---|---|---|---|
| **Outcome Assessment Factors** | **Interventions** 1 | 2 | 3 | 4 | 5 | **Expected Outcome** | **Ideal/goal value** |
| **Clinical Assessment** [1] | | | | | | | |
| **Laboratory parameters** [2] | | | | | | | |
| • HgB | ✓ | | ✓ | | | ↑ HgB | HgB 10.5-12.5 g/dL (6m–6yr) |
| • Hct | ✓ | | ✓ | | | ↑ Hct | Hct 33-37 g/dL/ 6m-6yr) |
| Other Labs (specific to needs of child) | ✓ | | ✓ | | | Progress towards normal levels | Within normal ranges for age |
| **Nutrition Physical** | | | | | | | |
| • Weight | ✓ | ✓ | ✓ | ✓ | ✓ | CDC:US growth charts[3] reflect progress towards appropriate growth velocity for age, gender | Accelerated growth velocity of 150% >average wt gain/age/day<br>Preemie 22-45 g/day |
| • Length/height (stature) | ✓ | ✓ | ✓ | ✓ | ✓ | | 0-3m 30-45 g/day |
| • Length/stature-for-age (%tile) | ✓ | ✓ | ✓ | ✓ | ✓ | | 3-6m 22-32 g/day |
| • Weight-for-age (%tile) | ✓ | ✓ | ✓ | ✓ | ✓ | | 6-12m 15-20 g/day |
| • Weight %tile for stature (length < 3 years) | ✓ | ✓ | ✓ | ✓ | ✓ | | 1-6yr 8-12 g/day |
| • Z scores, if available [4] | ✓ | ✓ | ✓ | ✓ | ✓ | Improvement in Z scores | |
| • Head circumference (HC) (<3 years) | ✓ | ✓ | ✓ | ✓ | ✓ | | HC > 5th %tile |
| • TSF, MAC | ✓ | ✓ | ✓ | ✓ | ✓ | Progress towards ideal goal | TSF, MAC > 5th %tile |
| **Clinical signs and symptoms**<br>• Elimination & reflux patterns (if applicable) | ✓ | ✓ | ✓ | ✓ | ✓ | Improvement in reflux or elimination patterns | Normal elimination and resolved reflux |
| **Functional Assessment** | | | | | | | |
| • Self-feeding skills | ✓ | ✓ | ✓ | ✓ | ✓ | Advancement in feeding skills | Achieves age-appropriate feeding skills |
| **Nutrition and Behavioral Education** [•] | | | | | | | **MNT Goals** |
| • Mealtime management | ✓ | ✓ | ✓ | ✓ | ✓ | • Improvement in mealtime management skills | • Consistently provides appropriate foods, liquids, supplements, modular additives, and appropriate mealtime management skills in order to promote growth within goals set by practitioner |
| • Appropriate texture for age | ✓ | ✓ | ✓ | ✓ | ✓ | • Consumes or progresses towards age-appropriate foods | |
| • Appropriate supplements/modular nutrients | | ✓ | ✓ | ✓ | ✓ | • Consumes appropriate supplements/modular nutrients | |
| • Resources utilized | ✓ | ✓ | ✓ | ✓ | ✓ | • Utilizes resources appropriately | |
| • Food records [5] | ✓ | ✓ | | ✓ | ✓ | • Caregiver records accurate food records | • Appropriate utilization of resources |
| • Knowledge of high-calorie/nutrient-dense foods or other nutrition care plan | ✓ | ✓ | | ✓ | | • Caregiver identifies and provides appropriate or high calorie and high quality foods | |
| • Food labels | ✓ | ✓ | ✓ | ✓ | | • Caregiver understands food labels | |
| • Recipe modification | | ✓ | | ✓ | | • Caregiver is capable of modifying recipes | |

[1] Recheck in 1 month if normal. [2] Additional lab or tests may include lead, zinc, ferritin, serum Fe+, bone age, thyroid function tests, prealbumin, albumin, growth hormone. (HC should be monitored until 36th month.) [3] Center for Disease Control (CDC: US) Growth Charts [4] Refer to reference Waterlow et al, 1977, and Dibley et al, 1987. [•] Encounters in which behavioral topics are covered may vary according to caregiver's readiness, skills, resources, and need for lifestyle changes. [5] Additional food records only if poor growth.

**7–7** My Vegetarian Plate

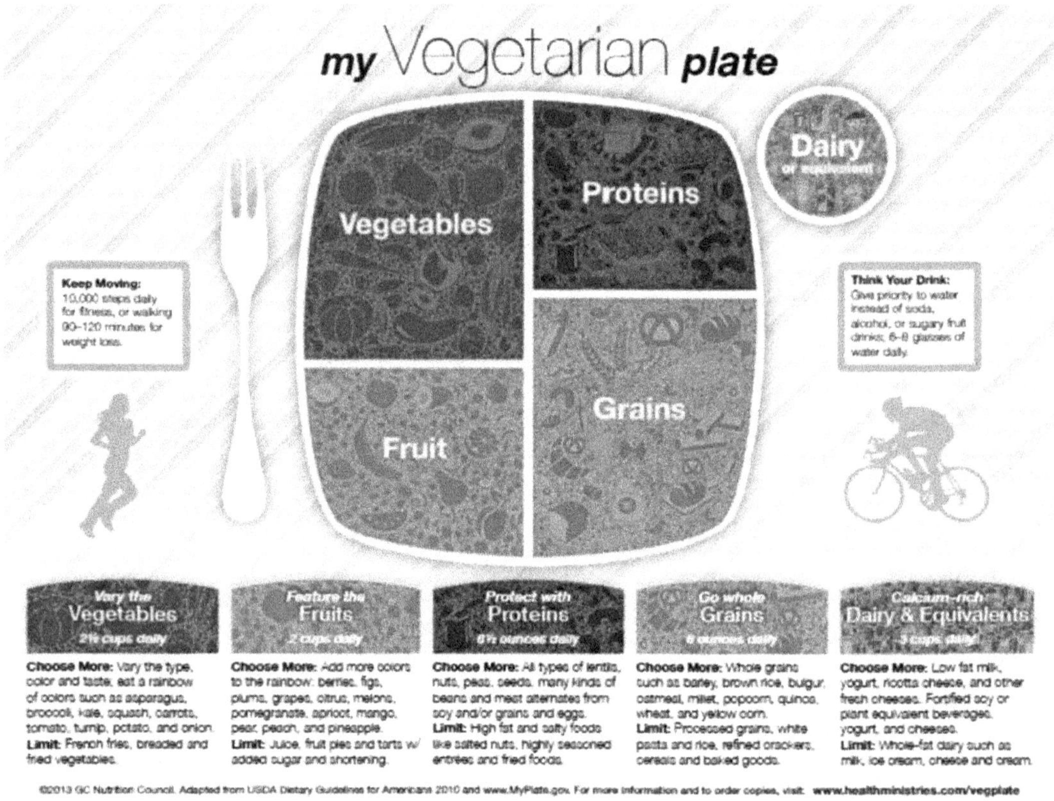

**7–8** My Vegetarian Plate Food Guide

# My Vegetarian Plate Food Guide

| Food Groups | Many Women & Older Adults<br>1600 Calories Daily | Children, Active Girls and Women<br>2000 Calories Daily | Boys and Active Men<br>2400 Calories Daily | Sample Serving Sizes<br>g=grams / ml=milliliters / 1oz=28g | Best Foods from Each Food Group | Nutrients Contributed by Each Group |
|---|---|---|---|---|---|---|
| Go Whole Grains | Servings: 5 | Servings: 6 | Servings: 8 | ½ bagel, ½ English muffin<br>¼ [4 oz] muffin, 1 slice [30g] bread<br>¾ cup [40g] dry unsweetened cereal<br>¼ cup granola, ½ cup [100g] hot cereal<br>3–4 [30g] crackers, 1 [30g] chapati<br>6" tortilla, ½ cup rice or pasta | Amaranth, barley, brown rice, buckwheat, bulgur, kamut, maize, millet, multigrain, oats, popcorn, quinoa, rye, sorghum, teff, triticale, wheat, wild rice, yellow corn | Carbohydrates (complex and simple), B vitamins (thiamine, riboflavin, niacin, folate), iron, protein, fiber, and trace minerals |
| Vary the Vegetables | Servings: 4 | Servings: 5 | Servings: 6 | 1 cup [50g] raw leafy vegetable salad<br>½ cup [50g] chopped raw vegetables<br>½ cup [80g] cooked vegetables<br>¾ cup [100g] vegetable juice<br>Unlimited: basil, cilantro, dill, ginger, oregano, parsley, rosemary, turmeric, etc. | **Green:** Asparagus, bok choy, broccoli, cabbage, collards, kale, mustard greens, okra, romaine, spinach, turnip greens<br>**Orange:** Carrot, pumpkin, rutabaga, sweet potato, squash<br>**Red:** Beet, eggplant, radish, red cabbage and pepper, tomato<br>**White:** Cauliflower, garlic, onion, potato, turnip | Carotenoids, vitamin C, fiber, protein, potassium, folate, magnesium, vitamin K, phytochemicals |
| Focus on Fruits | Servings: 3 | Servings: 4 | Servings: 4 | 1 medium [100g or 1 cup] whole fruit<br>1 cup [100g] berries<br>½ cup [125g] lite or unsweetened canned or frozen fruit<br>½ cup [100g] lite or unsweetened fruit juice<br>¼ cup [35g] dried fruit | **Blue-Red-Purple:** Blueberries, blackberries, boysenberries, cranberries, cherries, grapes, plums, prunes, raspberries, pomegranate, strawberries, watermelon<br>**Citrus:** Grapefruit, kumquat, lemon, lime, orange, tangerine<br>**Orange:** Apricot, cantaloupe, papaya, persimmon<br>**Yellow:** Banana, durian, mango, peach, pear, pineapple<br>**Green:** Honeydew, kiwi **Dry:** Dates, figs, raisins, prunes | Vitamin C, carotenoids, fiber, potassium, folate, magnesium, flavonoids |
| Delight in Dairy / Equivalents | Servings: 3 | Servings: 3 | Servings: 4 | 1 cup [240ml] non-fat or low fat milk<br>1 cup [240ml] full fat, fortified soy milk<br>1 cup [240ml] low fat or non-fat yogurt<br>1½ cup [290g] low fat cottage cheese<br>½ cup [125g] non-fat ricotta cheese<br>¾ cup [165g] soy cheese | **Dairy Products:** Low fat milk, yogurt, ricotta cheese, other fresh cheeses<br>**Fortified Dairy Equivalents** with vitamins D & $B_{12}$ and calcium: soy beverages, soy yogurt, soy cheese | Protein, calcium, vitamins A, $B_2$, $B_{12}$, D, soy, riboflavins |
| Protect with Proteins | Servings: 3 | Servings: 5½ | Servings: 6 | **Protein g**<br>[100g] cooked beans 7<br>½ cup [100g] cooked lentils 9<br>½ cup [100g] tofu 6<br>1 egg or 2 egg whites 7<br>¼ cup [35g] seeds, whole 7<br>¼ cup [28g] nuts 7<br>2 tbsp [32g] nut butter 8 | **Beans:** adzuki, black, fava, kidney, lima, navy, pinto, soy<br>**Peas:** Blackeyed, chick, lentil, pigeon, purple hull, split<br>**Meat Alternates:** Grains with legumes, soymeats, tofu, edamame, meat substitutes<br>**Nuts:** Almonds, hazelnuts, pecans, pistachios, walnuts<br>**Seeds:** Pumpkin, sunflower | Protein, iron, zinc, vitamins $B_{12}$, $B_6$, E, niacin, complex carbohydrate, fiber, linoleic acid, linolenic acid |
| Find Healthy Fats | Servings: 5 | Servings: 6 | Servings: 7 | **Fat g**<br>⅛ cup [36g] avocado 5<br>2 tbsp [16g] flax seed, ground 5<br>1 tbsp [8g] nuts, chopped 5<br>1½ tsp [15g] nut butter 5<br>1 tsp [5g] margarine, oil, mayo 5 | **Nuts & Seeds:** Brazil nuts, cashews, hazelnuts, flax seeds, macadamias, pecans, sesame seeds, walnuts<br>**Oils:** Canola, olive, soy and walnut oils, flax seed spreads made from healthy oils<br>**Other:** Avocado & olives | Vitamin E, linoleic acid, linolenic acid |
| Discern Desserts | Limit intake of refined sugar/high-fat desserts to occasional small servings. | | | ⅛ fruit pie [270 to 486 calories]<br>1 tbsp fruit preserves [50 calories]<br>½ cup ice cream [111 to 377 calories]<br>1.5 oz chocolate bar [200 calories] | **Fruits:** Dried or fresh fruit, fruit cobbler, fruit crisp<br>**Other Desserts:** Low in fat, sugar and calories | Fat, refined sugars are empty calories containing no nutrients |

***To calculate your own nutrition profile, visit: https://www.supertracker.usda.gov***

**7–9** Ethnic Diet Pyramids: Asian, Mediterranean, Latin American, and African American

The Traditional Healthy
Asian Diet Pyramid

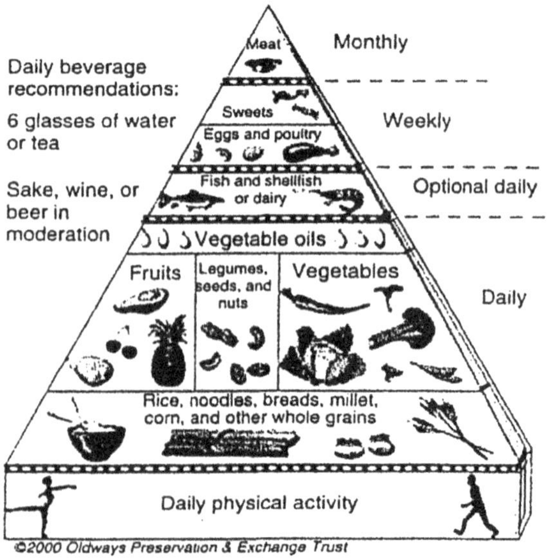




The Traditional Healthy
Mediterranean Diet Pyramid

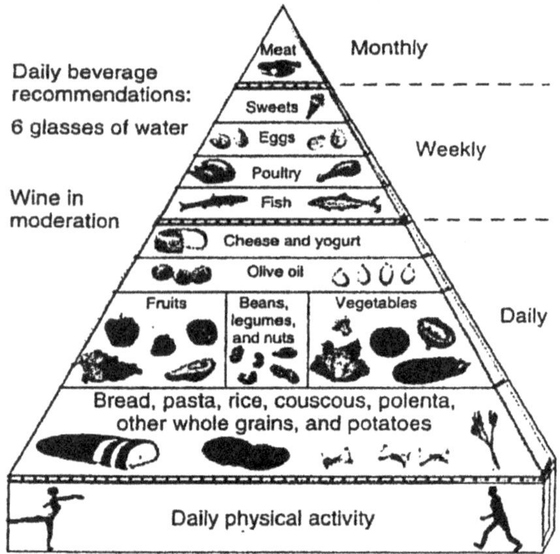




The Traditional Healthy
Latin American Diet Pyramid

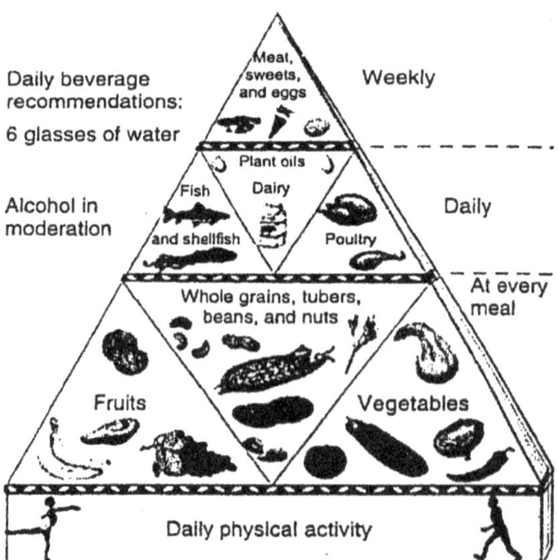




The *Soul* Food Diet Pyramid

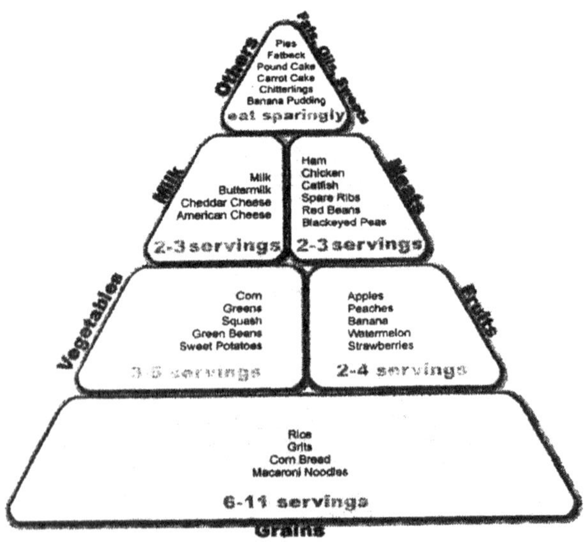

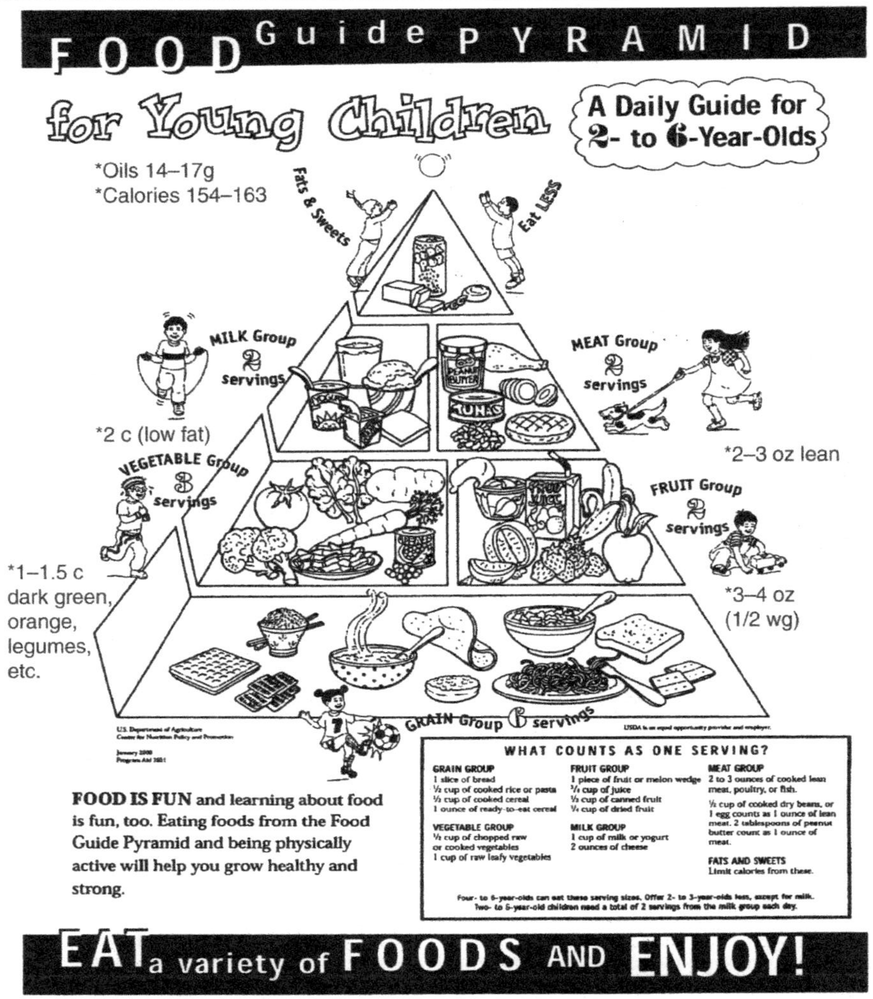


* Food Guide Pyramid 2005, adapted from U.S. Department of Agriculture, Center for Nutrition Promotion, 6th edition, 2005 text, Tables D1–13 and D1–14. See Appendix 7 ( 7–10 and 7–11, pp. 470–471) and http://www.health.gov/dietaryguidelines/dga2005/report/HTML/D1_Tables.htm. Based on calories from 1000–2000.

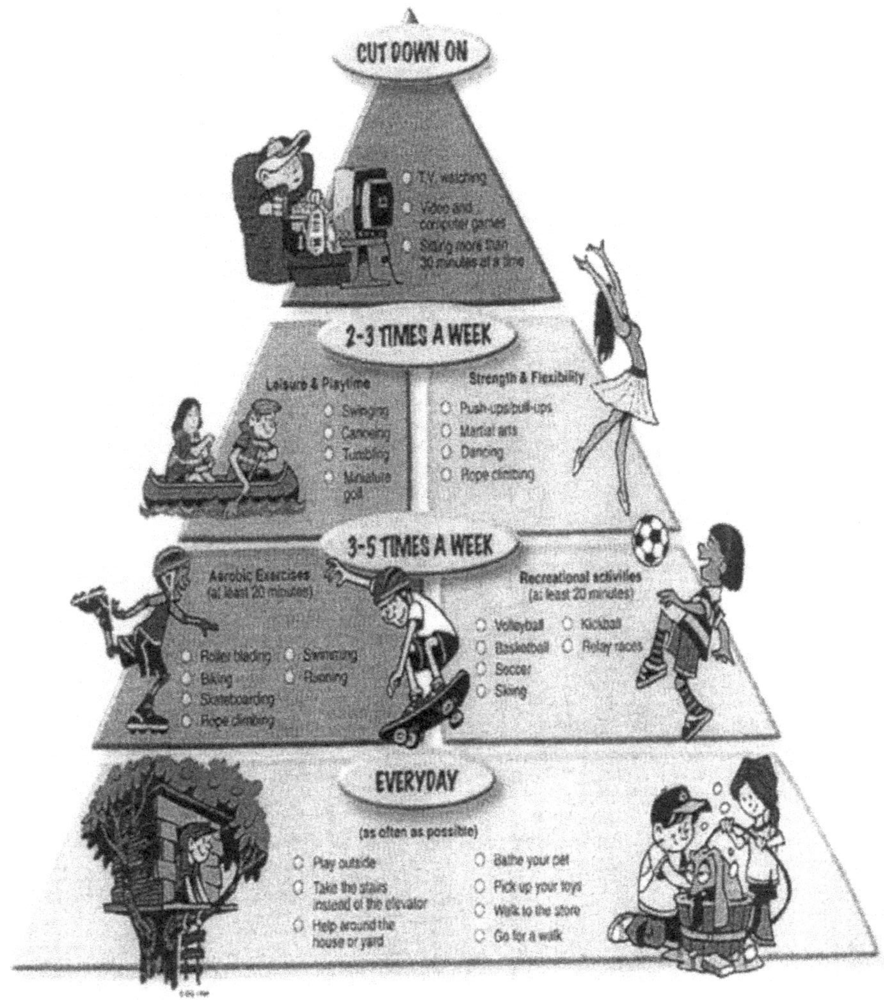


From: Family Nutrition Education Programs. University of Missouri Entension. Used with permission.

**7–11** Revised USDA Food Intake Patterns for Meeting Recommended Nutrient Intakes (for 2005 Pyramid)

This table shows the suggested amounts of food to consume from the basic food groups, subgroups, and oils to meet recommended nutrient intakes at 12 different calorie levels. Nutrient and engergy contributions from each group are calculated based on nutrient dense forms of foods in each group (e.g., lean meats, fat-free milk). The table also shows the amount of discretionary calories that can be accommodated within each calorie level in addition to the suggested amounts of nutrient dense forms of foods in each group.

**Daily Amount of Food from Each Group in Pattern (Vegetable subgroup amounts are per week)**

| Calorie Level | 1,000 | 1,200 | 1,400 | 1,600 | 1,800 | 2,000 | 2,200 | 2,400 | 2,600 | 2,800 | 3,000 | 3,200 |
|---|---|---|---|---|---|---|---|---|---|---|---|---|
| **FOOD GROUP**[1] | **Food group amounts shown in cup (c) or ounce equivalents (oz eq) with number of servings (srv) in parentheses when it differs from the other units. See note for quantity equivalents for foods in each group.[2] Oils are shown in grams (g).** | | | | | | | | | | | |
| **FRUITS** | 1 c(2 srv) | 1 c(2 srv) | 1.5 c(3 srv) | 1.5 c(3 srv) | 1.5 c(3 srv) | 2 c(4 srv) | 2 c(4 srv) | 2 c(4 srv) | 2 c(4 srv) | 2.5 c(5 srv) | 2.5 c(5 srv) | 2.5 c(5 srv) |
| **VEGETABLES**[3] | 1 c(2 srv) | 1.5 c(3 srv) | 1.5 c(3 srv) | 2 c(4 srv) | 2.5 c(5 srv) | 2.5 c(5 srv) | 3 c(6 srv) | 3 c(6 srv) | 3.5 c(7 srv) | 3.5 c(7 srv) | 4 c(8 srv) | 4 c(8 srv) |
| **Dark-green veg.** | 1 c/wk | 1 1/2 c/wk | 1 1/2 c/wk | 2 c/wk | 3 c/wk | 3 c/wk | 3 c/wk | 3 c/wk | 3 c/wk | 3 c/wk | 3 c/wk | 3 c/wk |
| **Orange veg.** | 1/2 c/wk | 1 c/wk | 1 c/wk | 1 1/2 c/wk | 2 c/wk | 2 c/wk | 2 c/wk | 2 c/wk | 2 1/2 c/wk | 2 1/2 c/wk | 2 1/2 c/wk | 2 1/2 c/wk |
| **Legumes** | 1/2 c/wk | 1 c/wk | 1 c/wk | 2 1/2 c/wk | 3 c/wk | 3 c/wk | 3 c/wk | 3 c/wk | 3 1/2 c/wk | 3 1/2 c/wk | 3 1/2 c/wk | 3 1/2 c/wk |
| **Starchy veg.** | 1 1/2 c/wk | 2 1/2 c/wk | 2 1/2 c/wk | 2 1/2 c/wk | 3 c/wk | 3 c/wk | 6 c/wk | 6 c/wk | 7 c/wk | 7 c/wk | 9 c/wk | 9 c/wk |
| **Other veg.** | 4 c/wk | 4 1/2 c/wk | 4 1/2 c/wk | 5 1/2 c/wk | 6 1/2 c/wk | 6 1/2 c/wk | 7 c/wk | 7 c/wk | 8 1/2 c/wk | 8 1/2 c/wk | 10 c/wk | 10 c/wk |
| **GRAINS**[4] | 3 oz eq | 4 oz eq | 5 oz eq | 5 oz eq | 6 oz eq | 6 oz eq | 7 oz eq | 8 oz eq | 9 oz eq | 10 oz eq | 10 oz eq | 10 oz eq |
| **Whole grains** | 1.5 | 2 | 2.5 | 3 | 3 | 3 | 3.5 | 4 | 4.5 | 5 | 5 | 5 |
| **Other grains** | 1.5 | 2 | 2.5 | 2 | 3 | 3 | 3.5 | 4 | 4.5 | 5 | 5 | 5 |
| **MEAT AND BEANS** | 2 oz eq | 3 oz eq | 4 oz eq | 5 oz eq | 5 oz eq | 5 1/2 oz eq | 6 oz eq | 6 1/2 oz eq | 6 1/2 oz eq | 7 oz eq | 7 oz eq | 7 oz eq |
| **MILK** | 2 c | 2 c | 2 c | 3 c | 3 c | 3 c | 3 c | 3 c | 3 c | 3 c | 3 c | 3 c |
| **Oils**[5] | 14 g | 17 g | 18 g | 20 g | 22 g | 24 g | 27 g | 27 g | 30 g | 34 g | 40 g | 46 g |
| **Discretionary calories**[6] | 154 | 163 | 173 | 181 | 190 | 208 | 235 | 235 | 244 | 262 | 298 | 334 |

Notes:
1. Food items included in each group and subgroup:

| | |
|---|---|
| **Fruits** | All fresh, frozen, canned, and dried fruits and fruit juices: for example, oranges and orange juice, apples and apple juice, bananas, grapes, melons, berries, raisins. In developing the food patterns, only fruits and juice with no added sugars or fats were used. **See note 6 on discretionary calories if products with added sugars or fats are consumed.** |
| **Vegetables** | In developing the food patterns, only vegetables with no added fats or sugars were used. **See note 6 on discretionary calories if products with added sugars or fats are consumed.** |
| Dark-green vegetables | All fresh, frozen, and canned dark-green vegetables, cooked or raw: for example, broccoli; spinach; romaine; collard, turnip, and mustard greens. |
| Orange vegetables | All fresh, frozen, and canned orange and deep-yellow vegetables, cooked or raw: for example, carrots, sweet potatoes, winter squash, pumpkin. |
| Legumes (dry beans and peas) | All cooked dry beans and peas and soybean products: for example, pinto beans, kidney beans, lentils, chickpeas, tofu. (See comment under meat and beans group about counting legumes in the vegetable or the meat and beans group.) |
| Starchy vegetable | All fresh, frozen, and canned starchy vegetables: for example, white potatoes, corn, green peas. |
| Other vegetables | All fresh, frozen, and canned other vegetables, cooked or raw: for example, tomatoes, tomato juice, lettuce, green beans, onions. |
| **Grains** | In developing the food patterns, only grains in low-fat and low sugars forms were used. **See note 6 on discretionary calories if products that are higher in fat and/or added sugars are consumed.** |
| Whole grains | All whole grain products and whole grains used as ingredients: for example, whole wheat and rye breads, whole grain cereals and crackers, oatmeal, brown rice. |
| Other grains | All refined grain products and refined grains used as ingredients: for example, white breads, enriched grain cereals and crackers, enriched pasta, white rice. |
| **Meat, poultry, fish, dry beans, eggs, and nuts (Meat & beans)** | All meat, poultry, fish, dry beans and peas, eggs, nuts, seeds. Most choices should be lean or low fat. **See note 6 on discretionary calories if higher fat products are consumed.** Drbeans and peas and soybean products are considered part of this group as well as the vegetable group, but should be counted in one group only. |
| **Milk, yogurt, and cheese (Milk)** | All milks, yogurts, frozen yogurts, dairy desserts, cheese (except cream cheese), including lactose-free and lactose-reduced products. Most choices should be fat-free or low-fat. In developing the food patterns, only fat-free milk was used. **See note 6 on discretionary calories if one consumes low-fat, reduced fat, or whole milk or milk products—or milk products that contain added sugars.** Calcium-fortified soy beverages are an option for those who want a non-dairy calcium source. |

2. Quantity **equivalents for each food group:**
**Grains** The following each count as 1 ounce equivalent (1 serving) of grains: 1/2 cup cooked rice, pasta, or cooked cereal; 1 ounce dry pasta or rice; 1 slice bread; 1 small muffin (1 oz); 1 cup ready-to-eat cereal flakes.
**Fruits and vegetables** The following each count as 1 cup (2 servings) of fruits or vegetables: 1 cup cut-up raw or cooked fruit or vegetable, 1 cup fruit or vegetable, 1 cup fruit or vegetable juice, 2 cups leafy salad greens.
**Meat and beans** The following each count as 1 ounce equivalent: 1 ounce lean meat, poultry, or fish; 1 egg; 1/4 cup cooked dry beans or tofu; 1 Tbsp peanut butter; 1/2 ounce nuts or seeds.
**Milk** The following each count as 1 cup (1 serving) of milk: 1 cup milk or yogurt, 1 1/2 ounces natural cheese such as cheddar cheese, or 2 ounces process cheese. Discretionary calories must be counted for all choices except nonfat milk.

3. **Explanation of vegetable subgroup amounts:**
Vegetable subgroup amounts are shown in this table as weekly amounts, because it would be difficult for consumers to select foods from each subgroup daily. A daily amount that is one-seventh of the weekly amount listed is used in calculations of nutrient and energy levels in each pattern.

4. **Explanation of grain subgroup amounts:**
The whole grain subgroup amounts shown in this table represent at least 3 one-ounce servings, and one-half of the total amount as whole grains for all calorie levels of 1600 and above. This is the minimum suggested amount of whole grains to consume as part of the food patterns. More whole grains up to all of the grains recommended may be selected, with offsetting decreases in the amount of other (enriched) grains. In patterns designed for younger children (1,000, 1,200, and 1,400 calories), one-half of the total amount of grains is shown as whole grains.

5. **Explanation of oils:**
Oils (including *trans*-free soft margarine) shown in this table represent the amounts that are added to foods during processing, cooking, or at the table. Oils and soft margarines include vegetable oils and soft vegetable oil table spreads that are trans-free. The amounts of oils listed in this table are not considered to be part of discretionary calories because they are a major source of the vitamin E and polyunsaturated fatty acids, including the essential fatty acids, in the food pattern. In contrast, solid fats are listed separately in the discretionary calorie table (Table D1-14) because, compared with oils, they are higher in saturated fatty acids and lower in vitamin E and mono- and polyunsaturated fatty acids, including essential fatty acids. The amounts of each type of fat in the food intake pattern were based on 60% oils and/or trans-free soft margarines and 40% solid fat. The amounts in typical American diets are about 42% oils or soft margarines and about 58% solid fats.

6. **Discretionary calories** are the remaining amount of calories in each food pattern after selecting the specified number of nutrient dense forms of foods in each food group. The number of discretionary calories assumes that food items in each food group are selected in nutrient dense forms (that is, forms that are fat-free or low-fat and that contain no added sugars). Solid fat and sugar calories always need to be counted as discretionary calories, as in the following examples:
The fat in low-fat, reduced fat, or whole milk or milk products or cheese and the sugar and fat in chocolate milk, ice cream, pudding, etc.
The fat in higher fat meats (e.g., ground beef with more than 5% fat by weight, poultry with skin, higher fat luncheon meats, sausages)
The sugars added to fruits and fruit juices with added sugars or fruits canned in syrup
The added fats and/or sugars in vegetables prepared with added fat or sugars
The added fats and/or sugars in grain products containing higher levels of fats and/or sugars (e.g., sweetened cereals, higher fat crackers, pies and other pastries, cakes, cookies)

Total discretionary calories should be limited to the amounts shown in the table at each calorie level. Additional information about discretionary calories, including an example of the division of these calories between solid fats and added sugars, is provided in Table D1-14. See http:www.health.gov/dietaryguidelines/dga2005/report/HTML/D1_Tables.htm

**7–12** Discretionary Calories in Revised USDA Food Intake Patterns

Discretionary calories are the remaining amount of calories in each food pattern after nutrient dense forms of foods in each food group are selected. This table shows the number of discretionary calories remaining in each food intake pattern if nutrient dense foods are selected. Those trying to lose weight may choose not to use discretionary calories. For those wanting to maintain their weight, discretionary calories may be used to increase the amount of food selected from each food group; to consume foods that are not in the lowest fat form (such as 2% milk or medium fat meat) or that contain added sugars; to add oil, fat, or sugars to foods; or to consume alcohol. The table shows an example of how these calories may be divided between solid fats and added sugars.

**Discretionary calories that remain in food patterns at each calorie level**

| FOOD PATTERN CALORIE LEVEL | 1,000 | 1,200 | 1,400 | 1,600 | 1,800 | 2,000 | 2,200 | 2,400 | 2,600 | 2,800 | 3,000 | 3,200 |
|---|---|---|---|---|---|---|---|---|---|---|---|---|
| **Discretionary calories**[1] | 154 | 163 | 172 | 181 | 190 | 208 | 235 | 235 | 244 | 262 | 298 | 334 |
| **Example of division of discretionary calories:** | | | | | | | | | | | | |
| Solid fats are shown in grams (g); added sugars in grams (g) and teaspoons (tsp). | | | | | | | | | | | | |
| **Solid fats**[2] | 10 g | 11 g | 12 g | 13 g | 14 g | 16 g | 19 g | 19 g | 20 g | 22 g | 26 g | 30 g |
| **Added sugars**[3] | 16 g (4tsp) | 20 g (5tsp) | 20 g (5tsp) | 24 g (6tsp) | 32 g (8tsp) | 40 g (10tsp) | 48 g (12tsp) | 56 g (14tsp) | 64 g (16tsp) | 72 g (18tsp) | 80 g (20tsp) | 112 g (28tsp) |

Adults most deficient nutrients are vitamins A, C, E, folate, calcium, magnesium, potassium, and fiber. Children's most deficient nutrients are vitamin E, folate, calcium, magnesium, potassium and fiber. See http://www.health.gov/dietaryguidelines/dga2005/report/HTML/D1_Tables.htm

# APPENDIX 8

## Skinfold Grids—Children Other Anthropometry Standards/ Laboratory Data

| Age (yrs) | Percentiles | | | | | | | | |
|---|---|---|---|---|---|---|---|---|---|
| | 5 | 10 | 15 | 25 | 50 | 75 | 85 | 90 | 95 |
| **Males** | | | | | | | | | |
| 1.0–1.9 | 14.2 | 14.7 | 14.9 | 15.2 | 16.0 | 16.9 | 17.4 | 17.7 | 18.2 |
| 2.0–2.9 | 14.3 | 14.8 | 15.1 | 15.5 | 16.3 | 17.1 | 17.6 | 17.9 | 18.6 |
| 3.0–3.9 | 15.0 | 15.3 | 15.5 | 16.0 | 16.8 | 17.6 | 18.1 | 18.4 | 19.0 |
| 4.0–4.9 | 15.1 | 15.5 | 15.8 | 16.2 | 17.1 | 18.0 | 18.5 | 18.7 | 19.3 |
| 5.0–5.9 | 15.5 | 16.0 | 16.1 | 16.6 | 17.5 | 18.5 | 19.1 | 19.5 | 20.5 |
| 6.0–6.9 | 15.8 | 16.1 | 16.5 | 17.0 | 18.0 | 19.1 | 19.8 | 20.7 | 22.8 |
| 7.0–7.9 | 16.1 | 16.8 | 17.0 | 17.6 | 18.7 | 20.0 | 21.0 | 21.8 | 22.9 |
| 8.0–8.9 | 16.5 | 17.2 | 17.5 | 18.1 | 19.2 | 20.5 | 21.6 | 22.6 | 24.0 |
| 9.0–9.9 | 17.5 | 18.0 | 18.4 | 19.0 | 20.1 | 21.8 | 23.2 | 24.5 | 26.0 |
| 10.0–10.9 | 18.1 | 18.6 | 19.1 | 19.7 | 21.1 | 23.1 | 24.8 | 26.0 | 27.9 |
| 11.0–11.9 | 18.5 | 19.3 | 19.8 | 20.6 | 22.1 | 24.5 | 26.1 | 27.6 | 29.4 |
| 12.0–12.9 | 19.3 | 20.1 | 20.7 | 21.5 | 23.1 | 25.4 | 27.1 | 28.5 | 30.3 |
| 13.0–13.9 | 20.0 | 20.8 | 21.6 | 22.5 | 24.5 | 26.6 | 28.2 | 29.0 | 30.8 |
| 14.0–14.9 | 21.6 | 22.5 | 23.2 | 23.8 | 25.7 | 28.1 | 29.1 | 30.0 | 32.3 |
| 15.0–15.9 | 22.5 | 23.4 | 24.0 | 25.1 | 27.2 | 29.0 | 30.3 | 31.2 | 32.7 |
| 16.0–16.9 | 24.1 | 25.0 | 25.7 | 26.7 | 28.3 | 30.6 | 32.1 | 32.7 | 34.7 |
| 17.0–17.9 | 24.3 | 25.1 | 25.9 | 26.8 | 28.6 | 30.8 | 32.2 | 33.3 | 34.7 |
| 18.0–24.9 | 26.0 | 27.1 | 27.7 | 28.7 | 30.7 | 33.0 | 34.4 | 35.4 | 37.2 |
| 25.0–29.9 | 27.0 | 28.0 | 28.7 | 29.8 | 31.8 | 34.2 | 35.5 | 36.6 | 38.3 |
| 30.0–34.9 | 27.7 | 28.7 | 29.3 | 30.5 | 32.5 | 34.9 | 35.9 | 36.7 | 38.2 |
| 35.0–39.9 | 27.4 | 28.6 | 29.5 | 30.7 | 32.9 | 35.1 | 36.2 | 36.9 | 38.2 |
| 40.0–44.9 | 27.8 | 28.9 | 29.7 | 31.0 | 32.8 | 34.9 | 36.1 | 36.9 | 38.1 |
| 45.0–49.9 | 27.2 | 28.6 | 29.4 | 30.6 | 32.6 | 34.9 | 36.1 | 36.9 | 38.2 |
| 50.0–54.9 | 27.1 | 28.3 | 29.1 | 30.2 | 32.3 | 34.5 | 35.8 | 36.8 | 38.3 |
| 55.0–59.9 | 26.8 | 28.1 | 29.2 | 30.4 | 32.3 | 34.3 | 35.5 | 36.6 | 37.8 |
| 60.0–64.9 | 26.6 | 27.8 | 28.6 | 29.7 | 32.0 | 34.0 | 35.1 | 36.0 | 37.5 |
| 65.0–69.9 | 25.4 | 26.7 | 27.7 | 29.0 | 31.1 | 33.2 | 34.5 | 35.3 | 36.6 |
| 70.0–74.9 | 25.1 | 26.2 | 27.1 | 28.5 | 30.7 | 32.6 | 33.7 | 34.8 | 36.0 |
| **Females** | | | | | | | | | |
| 1.0–1.9 | 13.6 | 14.1 | 14.4 | 14.8 | 15.7 | 16.4 | 17.0 | 17.2 | 17.8 |
| 2.0–2.9 | 14.2 | 14.6 | 15.0 | 15.4 | 16.1 | 17.0 | 17.4 | 18.0 | 18.5 |
| 3.0–3.9 | 14.4 | 15.0 | 15.2 | 15.7 | 16.6 | 17.4 | 18.0 | 18.4 | 19.0 |
| 4.0–4.9 | 14.8 | 15.3 | 15.7 | 16.1 | 17.0 | 18.0 | 18.5 | 19.0 | 19.5 |
| 5.0–5.9 | 15.2 | 15.7 | 16.1 | 16.5 | 17.5 | 18.5 | 19.4 | 20.0 | 21.0 |
| 6.0–6.9 | 15.7 | 16.2 | 16.5 | 17.0 | 17.8 | 19.0 | 19.9 | 20.5 | 22.0 |
| 7.0–7.9 | 16.4 | 16.7 | 17.0 | 17.5 | 18.6 | 20.1 | 20.9 | 21.6 | 23.3 |
| 8.0–8.9 | 16.7 | 17.2 | 17.6 | 18.2 | 19.5 | 21.2 | 22.2 | 23.2 | 25.1 |
| 9.0–9.9 | 17.6 | 18.1 | 18.6 | 19.1 | 20.6 | 22.2 | 23.8 | 25.0 | 26.7 |
| 10.0–10.9 | 17.8 | 18.4 | 18.9 | 19.5 | 21.2 | 23.4 | 25.0 | 26.1 | 27.3 |
| 11.0–11.9 | 18.8 | 19.6 | 20.0 | 20.6 | 22.2 | 25.1 | 26.5 | 27.9 | 30.0 |
| 12.0–12.9 | 19.2 | 20.0 | 20.5 | 21.5 | 23.7 | 25.8 | 27.6 | 28.3 | 30.2 |
| 13.0–13.9 | 20.1 | 21.0 | 21.5 | 22.5 | 24.3 | 26.7 | 28.3 | 30.1 | 32.7 |
| 14.0–14.9 | 21.2 | 21.8 | 22.5 | 23.5 | 25.1 | 27.4 | 29.5 | 30.9 | 32.9 |
| 15.0–15.9 | 21.6 | 22.2 | 22.9 | 23.5 | 25.2 | 27.7 | 28.8 | 30.0 | 32.2 |
| 16.0–16.9 | 22.3 | 23.2 | 23.5 | 24.4 | 26.1 | 28.5 | 29.9 | 31.6 | 33.5 |
| 17.0–17.9 | 22.0 | 23.1 | 23.6 | 24.5 | 26.6 | 29.0 | 30.7 | 32.8 | 35.4 |
| 18.0–24.9 | 22.4 | 23.3 | 24.0 | 24.8 | 26.8 | 29.2 | 31.2 | 32.4 | 35.2 |
| 25.0–29.9 | 23.1 | 24.0 | 24.5 | 25.5 | 27.6 | 30.6 | 32.5 | 34.3 | 37.1 |
| 30.0–34.9 | 23.8 | 24.7 | 25.4 | 26.4 | 28.6 | 32.0 | 34.1 | 36.0 | 38.5 |
| 35.0–39.9 | 24.1 | 25.2 | 25.8 | 26.8 | 29.4 | 32.6 | 35.0 | 36.8 | 39.0 |
| 40.0–44.9 | 24.3 | 25.4 | 26.2 | 27.2 | 29.7 | 33.2 | 35.5 | 37.2 | 38.8 |
| 45.0–49.9 | 24.2 | 25.5 | 26.3 | 27.4 | 30.1 | 33.5 | 35.6 | 37.2 | 40.0 |
| 50.0–54.9 | 24.8 | 26.0 | 26.8 | 28.0 | 30.6 | 33.8 | 35.9 | 37.5 | 39.3 |
| 55.0–59.9 | 24.8 | 26.1 | 27.0 | 28.2 | 30.9 | 34.3 | 36.7 | 38.0 | 40.0 |
| 60.0–64.9 | 25.0 | 26.1 | 27.1 | 28.4 | 30.8 | 34.0 | 35.7 | 37.3 | 39.6 |
| 65.0–69.9 | 24.3 | 25.7 | 26.7 | 28.0 | 30.5 | 33.4 | 35.2 | 36.5 | 38.5 |
| 70.0–74.9 | 23.8 | 25.3 | 26.3 | 27.6 | 30.3 | 33.1 | 34.7 | 35.8 | 37.5 |

| Age (yrs) | Percentiles | | | | | | | | |
|---|---|---|---|---|---|---|---|---|---|
| | 5 | 10 | 15 | 25 | 50 | 75 | 85 | 90 | 95 |
| **Males** | | | | | | | | | |
| 1.0–1.9 | 9.7 | 10.4 | 10.8 | 11.6 | 13.0 | 14.6 | 15.4 | 16.3 | 17.2 |
| 2.0–2.9 | 10.1 | 10.9 | 11.3 | 12.4 | 13.9 | 15.6 | 16.4 | 16.9 | 18.4 |
| 3.0–3.9 | 11.2 | 12.0 | 12.6 | 13.5 | 15.0 | 16.4 | 17.4 | 18.3 | 19.5 |
| 4.0–4.9 | 12.0 | 12.9 | 13.5 | 14.5 | 16.2 | 17.9 | 18.8 | 19.8 | 20.9 |
| 5.0–5.9 | 13.2 | 14.2 | 14.7 | 15.7 | 17.6 | 19.5 | 20.7 | 21.7 | 23.2 |
| 6.0–6.9 | 14.4 | 15.3 | 15.8 | 16.8 | 18.7 | 21.3 | 22.9 | 23.8 | 25.7 |
| 7.0–7.9 | 15.1 | 16.2 | 17.0 | 18.5 | 20.6 | 22.6 | 24.5 | 25.2 | 28.6 |
| 8.0–8.9 | 16.3 | 17.8 | 18.5 | 19.5 | 21.6 | 24.0 | 25.5 | 26.6 | 29.0 |
| 9.0–9.9 | 18.2 | 19.3 | 20.3 | 21.7 | 23.5 | 26.7 | 28.7 | 30.4 | 32.9 |
| 10.0–10.9 | 19.6 | 20.7 | 21.6 | 23.0 | 25.7 | 29.0 | 32.2 | 34.0 | 37.1 |
| 11.0–11.9 | 21.0 | 22.0 | 23.0 | 24.8 | 27.7 | 31.6 | 33.6 | 36.1 | 40.3 |
| 12.0–12.9 | 22.6 | 24.1 | 25.3 | 26.9 | 30.4 | 35.9 | 39.3 | 40.9 | 44.9 |
| 13.0–13.9 | 24.5 | 26.7 | 28.1 | 30.4 | 35.7 | 41.3 | 45.3 | 48.1 | 52.5 |
| 14.0–14.9 | 28.3 | 31.3 | 33.1 | 36.1 | 41.9 | 47.4 | 51.3 | 54.0 | 57.5 |
| 15.0–15.9 | 31.9 | 34.9 | 36.9 | 40.3 | 46.3 | 53.1 | 56.3 | 57.7 | 63.0 |
| 16.0–16.9 | 37.0 | 40.9 | 42.4 | 45.9 | 51.9 | 57.8 | 63.6 | 66.2 | 70.5 |
| 17.0–17.9 | 39.6 | 42.6 | 44.8 | 48.0 | 53.4 | 60.4 | 64.3 | 67.9 | 73.1 |
| 18.0–24.9 | 34.2 | 37.3 | 39.6 | 42.7 | 49.4 | 57.1 | 61.8 | 65.0 | 72.0 |
| 25.0–29.9 | 36.6 | 39.9 | 42.4 | 46.0 | 53.0 | 61.4 | 66.1 | 68.9 | 74.5 |
| 30.0–34.9 | 37.9 | 40.9 | 43.4 | 47.3 | 54.4 | 63.2 | 67.6 | 70.8 | 76.1 |
| 35.0–39.9 | 38.5 | 42.6 | 44.6 | 47.9 | 55.3 | 64.0 | 69.1 | 72.7 | 77.6 |
| 40.0–44.9 | 38.4 | 42.1 | 45.1 | 48.7 | 56.0 | 64.0 | 68.5 | 71.6 | 77.0 |
| 45.0–49.9 | 37.7 | 41.3 | 43.7 | 47.9 | 55.2 | 63.3 | 68.4 | 72.2 | 76.2 |
| 50.0–54.9 | 36.0 | 40.0 | 42.7 | 46.6 | 54.0 | 62.7 | 67.0 | 70.4 | 77.4 |
| 55.0–59.9 | 36.5 | 40.8 | 42.7 | 46.7 | 54.3 | 61.9 | 66.4 | 69.6 | 75.1 |
| 60.0–64.9 | 34.5 | 38.7 | 41.2 | 44.9 | 52.1 | 60.0 | 64.8 | 67.5 | 71.6 |
| 65.0–69.9 | 31.4 | 35.8 | 38.4 | 42.3 | 49.1 | 57.3 | 61.2 | 64.3 | 69.4 |
| 70.0–74.9 | 29.7 | 33.8 | 36.1 | 40.2 | 47.0 | 54.6 | 59.1 | 62.1 | 67.3 |
| **Females** | | | | | | | | | |
| 1.0–1.9 | 8.9 | 9.7 | 10.1 | 10.8 | 12.3 | 13.8 | 14.6 | 15.3 | 16.2 |
| 2.0–2.9 | 10.1 | 10.6 | 10.9 | 11.8 | 13.2 | 14.7 | 15.6 | 16.4 | 17.3 |
| 3.0–3.9 | 10.8 | 11.4 | 11.8 | 12.6 | 14.3 | 15.8 | 16.7 | 17.4 | 18.8 |
| 4.0–4.9 | 11.2 | 12.2 | 12.7 | 13.6 | 15.3 | 17.0 | 18.0 | 18.6 | 19.8 |
| 5.0–5.9 | 12.4 | 13.2 | 13.9 | 14.8 | 16.4 | 18.3 | 19.4 | 20.6 | 22.1 |
| 6.0–6.9 | 13.5 | 14.1 | 14.6 | 15.6 | 17.4 | 19.5 | 21.0 | 22.0 | 24.2 |
| 7.0–7.9 | 14.4 | 15.2 | 15.8 | 16.7 | 18.9 | 21.2 | 22.6 | 23.9 | 25.3 |
| 8.0–8.9 | 15.2 | 16.0 | 16.8 | 18.2 | 20.8 | 23.2 | 24.6 | 26.5 | 28.0 |
| 9.0–9.9 | 17.0 | 17.9 | 18.7 | 19.8 | 21.9 | 25.4 | 27.2 | 28.3 | 31.1 |
| 10.0–10.9 | 17.6 | 18.5 | 19.3 | 20.9 | 23.8 | 27.0 | 29.1 | 31.0 | 33.1 |
| 11.0–11.9 | 19.5 | 21.0 | 21.7 | 23.2 | 26.4 | 30.7 | 33.5 | 35.7 | 39.2 |
| 12.0–12.9 | 20.4 | 21.8 | 23.1 | 25.5 | 29.0 | 33.2 | 36.3 | 37.8 | 40.5 |
| 13.0–13.9 | 22.8 | 24.5 | 25.4 | 27.1 | 30.8 | 35.3 | 38.1 | 39.6 | 43.7 |
| 14.0–14.9 | 24.0 | 26.2 | 27.1 | 29.0 | 32.8 | 36.9 | 39.8 | 42.3 | 47.5 |
| 15.0–15.9 | 24.4 | 25.8 | 27.5 | 29.2 | 33.0 | 37.3 | 40.2 | 41.7 | 45.9 |
| 16.0–16.9 | 25.2 | 26.8 | 28.2 | 30.0 | 33.6 | 38.0 | 40.2 | 43.7 | 48.3 |
| 17.0–17.9 | 25.9 | 27.5 | 28.9 | 30.7 | 34.3 | 39.6 | 43.4 | 46.2 | 50.8 |
| 18.0–24.9 | 19.5 | 21.5 | 22.8 | 24.5 | 28.3 | 33.1 | 36.4 | 39.0 | 44.2 |
| 25.0–29.9 | 20.5 | 21.9 | 23.1 | 25.2 | 29.4 | 34.9 | 38.5 | 41.9 | 47.8 |
| 30.0–34.9 | 21.1 | 23.0 | 24.2 | 26.3 | 30.9 | 36.8 | 41.2 | 44.7 | 51.3 |
| 35.0–39.9 | 21.1 | 23.4 | 24.7 | 27.3 | 31.8 | 36.7 | 43.1 | 46.1 | 54.2 |
| 40.0–44.9 | 21.3 | 23.4 | 25.5 | 27.5 | 32.3 | 39.8 | 45.8 | 49.5 | 55.8 |
| 45.0–49.9 | 21.6 | 23.1 | 24.8 | 27.4 | 32.5 | 39.5 | 44.7 | 48.4 | 56.1 |
| 50.0–54.9 | 22.2 | 24.6 | 25.7 | 28.3 | 33.4 | 40.4 | 46.1 | 49.6 | 55.6 |
| 55.0–59.9 | 22.8 | 24.8 | 26.5 | 28.7 | 34.7 | 42.3 | 47.3 | 52.1 | 58.8 |
| 60.0–64.9 | 22.4 | 24.5 | 26.3 | 29.2 | 34.5 | 41.1 | 45.6 | 49.1 | 55.1 |
| 65.0–69.9 | 21.9 | 24.5 | 26.2 | 28.9 | 34.6 | 41.6 | 46.3 | 49.6 | 56.5 |
| 70.0–74.9 | 22.2 | 24.4 | 26.0 | 28.8 | 34.3 | 41.8 | 46.4 | 49.2 | 54.6 |

Modified from Fisancho, A.R.: *Anthropometric Standards for the Assessment of Growth and Nutritional Status*, Ann Arbor, The University of Michigan Press, 1990.

| Age (yrs) | Percentiles | | | | | | | | |
|---|---|---|---|---|---|---|---|---|---|
| | 5 | 10 | 15 | 25 | 50 | 75 | 85 | 90 | 95 |
| **Males** | | | | | | | | | |
| 1.0–1.9 | 6.5 | 7.0 | 7.5 | 8.0 | 10.0 | 12.0 | 13.0 | 14.0 | 15.5 |
| 2.0–2.9 | 6.0 | 6.5 | 7.0 | 8.0 | 10.0 | 12.0 | 13.0 | 14.0 | 15.0 |
| 3.0–3.9 | 6.0 | 7.0 | 7.0 | 8.0 | 9.5 | 11.5 | 12.5 | 13.5 | 15.0 |
| 4.0–4.9 | 5.5 | 6.5 | 7.0 | 7.5 | 9.0 | 11.0 | 12.0 | 12.5 | 14.0 |
| 5.0–5.9 | 5.0 | 6.0 | 6.0 | 7.0 | 8.0 | 10.0 | 11.5 | 13.0 | 14.5 |
| 6.0–6.9 | 5.0 | 5.5 | 6.0 | 6.5 | 8.0 | 10.0 | 12.0 | 13.0 | 16.0 |
| 7.0–7.9 | 4.5 | 5.0 | 6.0 | 6.0 | 8.0 | 10.5 | 12.5 | 14.0 | 16.0 |
| 8.0–8.9 | 5.0 | 5.5 | 6.0 | 7.0 | 8.5 | 11.0 | 13.0 | 16.0 | 19.0 |
| 9.0–9.9 | 5.0 | 5.5 | 6.0 | 6.5 | 9.0 | 12.5 | 15.5 | 17.0 | 20.0 |
| 10.0–10.9 | 5.0 | 6.0 | 6.0 | 7.5 | 10.0 | 14.0 | 17.0 | 20.0 | 24.0 |
| 11.0–11.9 | 5.0 | 6.0 | 6.5 | 7.5 | 10.0 | 16.0 | 19.5 | 23.0 | 27.0 |
| 12.0–12.9 | 4.5 | 6.0 | 6.0 | 7.5 | 10.5 | 14.5 | 18.0 | 22.5 | 27.5 |
| 13.0–13.9 | 4.5 | 5.0 | 5.5 | 7.0 | 9.0 | 13.0 | 17.0 | 20.5 | 25.0 |
| 14.0–14.9 | 4.0 | 5.0 | 5.0 | 6.0 | 8.5 | 12.5 | 15.0 | 18.0 | 23.5 |
| 15.0–15.9 | 5.0 | 5.0 | 5.0 | 6.0 | 7.5 | 11.0 | 15.0 | 18.0 | 23.5 |
| 16.0–16.9 | 4.0 | 5.0 | 5.1 | 6.0 | 8.0 | 12.0 | 14.0 | 17.0 | 23.0 |
| 17.0–17.9 | 4.0 | 5.0 | 5.0 | 6.0 | 7.0 | 11.0 | 13.5 | 16.0 | 19.5 |
| 18.0–24.9 | 4.0 | 5.0 | 5.5 | 6.5 | 10.0 | 14.5 | 17.5 | 20.0 | 23.5 |
| 25.0–29.9 | 4.0 | 5.0 | 6.0 | 7.0 | 11.0 | 15.5 | 19.0 | 21.5 | 25.0 |
| 30.0–34.9 | 4.5 | 6.0 | 6.5 | 8.0 | 12.0 | 16.5 | 20.0 | 22.0 | 25.0 |
| 35.0–39.9 | 4.5 | 6.0 | 7.0 | 8.5 | 12.0 | 16.0 | 18.5 | 20.5 | 24.5 |
| 40.0–44.9 | 5.0 | 6.0 | 6.9 | 8.0 | 12.0 | 16.0 | 19.0 | 21.5 | 26.0 |
| 45.0–49.9 | 5.0 | 6.0 | 7.0 | 8.0 | 12.0 | 16.0 | 19.0 | 21.0 | 25.0 |
| 50.0–54.9 | 5.0 | 6.0 | 7.0 | 8.0 | 11.5 | 15.0 | 18.5 | 20.8 | 25.0 |
| 55.0–59.9 | 5.0 | 6.0 | 6.5 | 8.0 | 11.5 | 15.0 | 18.0 | 20.5 | 25.0 |
| 60.0–64.9 | 5.0 | 6.0 | 7.0 | 8.0 | 11.5 | 15.5 | 18.5 | 20.5 | 24.0 |
| 65.0–69.9 | 4.5 | 5.0 | 6.5 | 8.0 | 11.0 | 15.0 | 18.0 | 20.0 | 23.5 |
| 70.0–74.9 | 4.5 | 6.0 | 6.5 | 8.0 | 11.0 | 15.0 | 17.0 | 19.0 | 23.0 |
| **Females** | | | | | | | | | |
| 1.0–1.9 | 6.0 | 7.0 | 7.0 | 8.0 | 10.0 | 12.0 | 13.0 | 14.0 | 16.0 |
| 2.0–2.9 | 6.0 | 7.0 | 7.5 | 8.5 | 10.0 | 12.0 | 13.5 | 14.5 | 16.0 |
| 3.0–3.9 | 6.0 | 7.0 | 7.5 | 8.5 | 10.0 | 12.0 | 13.0 | 14.0 | 16.0 |
| 4.0–4.9 | 6.0 | 7.0 | 7.5 | 8.0 | 10.0 | 12.0 | 13.0 | 14.0 | 15.5 |
| 5.0–5.9 | 5.5 | 7.0 | 7.0 | 8.0 | 10.0 | 12.0 | 13.5 | 15.0 | 17.0 |
| 6.0–6.9 | 6.0 | 6.5 | 7.0 | 8.0 | 10.0 | 12.0 | 13.0 | 15.0 | 17.0 |
| 7.0–7.9 | 6.0 | 7.0 | 7.0 | 8.0 | 10.5 | 12.5 | 15.0 | 16.0 | 19.0 |
| 8.0–8.9 | 6.0 | 7.0 | 7.5 | 8.5 | 11.0 | 14.5 | 17.0 | 18.0 | 22.5 |
| 9.0–9.9 | 6.5 | 7.0 | 8.0 | 9.0 | 12.0 | 16.0 | 19.0 | 21.0 | 25.0 |
| 10.0–10.9 | 7.0 | 8.0 | 8.0 | 9.0 | 12.5 | 17.5 | 20.0 | 22.5 | 27.0 |
| 11.0–11.9 | 7.0 | 8.0 | 8.5 | 10.0 | 13.0 | 18.0 | 21.5 | 24.0 | 29.0 |
| 12.0–12.9 | 7.0 | 8.0 | 9.0 | 11.0 | 14.0 | 18.5 | 21.5 | 24.0 | 27.5 |
| 13.0–13.9 | 7.0 | 8.0 | 9.0 | 11.0 | 15.0 | 20.0 | 24.0 | 25.0 | 30.0 |
| 14.0–14.9 | 8.0 | 9.0 | 10.0 | 11.5 | 16.0 | 21.0 | 23.5 | 26.5 | 32.0 |
| 15.0–15.9 | 8.0 | 9.5 | 10.5 | 12.0 | 16.5 | 20.5 | 23.0 | 26.0 | 32.5 |
| 16.0–16.9 | 10.5 | 11.5 | 12.0 | 14.0 | 18.0 | 23.0 | 26.0 | 29.0 | 32.5 |
| 17.0–17.9 | 9.0 | 10.0 | 12.0 | 13.0 | 18.0 | 24.0 | 26.5 | 29.0 | 34.5 |
| 18.0–24.9 | 9.0 | 11.0 | 12.0 | 14.0 | 18.5 | 24.5 | 28.5 | 31.0 | 36.0 |
| 25.0–29.9 | 10.0 | 12.0 | 13.0 | 15.0 | 20.0 | 26.5 | 31.0 | 34.0 | 38.0 |
| 30.0–34.9 | 10.5 | 13.0 | 15.0 | 17.0 | 22.5 | 29.5 | 33.0 | 35.5 | 41.5 |
| 35.0–39.9 | 11.0 | 13.0 | 15.5 | 18.0 | 23.5 | 30.0 | 35.0 | 37.0 | 41.0 |
| 40.0–44.9 | 12.0 | 14.0 | 16.0 | 19.0 | 24.5 | 30.5 | 35.0 | 37.0 | 41.0 |
| 45.0–49.9 | 12.0 | 14.5 | 16.5 | 19.5 | 25.5 | 32.0 | 35.5 | 38.0 | 42.5 |
| 50.0–54.9 | 12.0 | 15.0 | 17.5 | 20.5 | 25.5 | 32.0 | 36.0 | 38.5 | 42.0 |
| 55.0–59.9 | 12.0 | 15.0 | 17.0 | 20.5 | 26.0 | 32.0 | 36.0 | 39.0 | 42.5 |
| 60.0–64.9 | 12.5 | 16.0 | 17.5 | 20.5 | 26.0 | 32.0 | 35.5 | 38.0 | 42.5 |
| 65.0–69.9 | 12.0 | 14.5 | 16.0 | 19.0 | 25.0 | 30.0 | 33.5 | 36.0 | 40.0 |
| 70.0–74.9 | 11.0 | 13.5 | 15.5 | 18.0 | 24.0 | 29.5 | 32.0 | 35.0 | 38.5 |

| Age (yrs) | Percentiles | | | | | | | | |
|---|---|---|---|---|---|---|---|---|---|
| | 5 | 10 | 15 | 25 | 50 | 75 | 85 | 90 | 95 |
| **Males** | | | | | | | | | |
| 1.0–1.9 | 4.0 | 4.0 | 4.5 | 5.0 | 6.0 | 7.0 | 8.0 | 8.5 | 10.0 |
| 2.0–2.9 | 3.5 | 4.0 | 4.0 | 4.5 | 5.5 | 7.0 | 7.5 | 8.5 | 10.0 |
| 3.0–3.9 | 3.5 | 4.0 | 4.0 | 4.5 | 5.0 | 6.0 | 7.0 | 7.0 | 9.0 |
| 4.0–4.9 | 3.0 | 3.5 | 4.0 | 4.0 | 5.0 | 6.0 | 6.5 | 7.0 | 8.0 |
| 5.0–5.9 | 3.0 | 3.5 | 4.0 | 4.0 | 5.0 | 5.5 | 6.5 | 7.0 | 8.0 |
| 6.0–6.9 | 3.0 | 3.5 | 3.5 | 4.0 | 4.5 | 5.5 | 6.5 | 8.0 | 13.0 |
| 7.0–7.9 | 3.0 | 3.5 | 4.0 | 4.0 | 5.0 | 6.0 | 7.0 | 8.0 | 12.0 |
| 8.0–8.9 | 3.0 | 3.5 | 4.0 | 4.0 | 5.0 | 6.0 | 7.5 | 9.0 | 12.5 |
| 9.0–9.9 | 3.0 | 3.5 | 4.0 | 4.0 | 5.0 | 7.0 | 9.5 | 12.0 | 14.5 |
| 10.0–10.9 | 3.5 | 4.0 | 4.0 | 4.5 | 6.0 | 8.0 | 11.0 | 14.0 | 19.5 |
| 11.0–11.9 | 4.0 | 4.0 | 4.0 | 5.0 | 6.0 | 9.0 | 15.0 | 18.5 | 26.0 |
| 12.0–12.9 | 4.0 | 4.0 | 4.5 | 5.0 | 6.0 | 9.5 | 15.0 | 19.0 | 24.0 |
| 13.0–13.9 | 4.0 | 4.0 | 5.0 | 5.0 | 6.5 | 9.0 | 13.0 | 17.0 | 25.0 |
| 14.0–14.9 | 4.0 | 5.0 | 5.0 | 5.5 | 7.0 | 9.0 | 12.0 | 15.5 | 22.5 |
| 15.0–15.9 | 5.0 | 5.0 | 5.5 | 6.0 | 7.0 | 10.0 | 13.0 | 16.0 | 22.0 |
| 16.0–16.9 | 5.0 | 6.0 | 6.0 | 7.0 | 8.0 | 11.0 | 14.0 | 16.0 | 22.0 |
| 17.0–17.9 | 5.0 | 6.0 | 6.0 | 7.0 | 8.0 | 11.0 | 14.0 | 17.0 | 21.5 |
| 18.0–24.9 | 6.0 | 7.0 | 7.0 | 8.0 | 11.0 | 16.0 | 20.0 | 24.0 | 30.0 |
| 25.0–29.9 | 7.0 | 7.0 | 8.0 | 9.0 | 13.0 | 20.0 | 24.5 | 26.5 | 31.0 |
| 30.0–34.9 | 7.0 | 8.0 | 9.0 | 11.0 | 15.5 | 22.0 | 25.5 | 29.0 | 33.0 |
| 35.0–39.9 | 7.0 | 8.0 | 9.5 | 11.0 | 16.0 | 22.5 | 25.5 | 28.0 | 33.0 |
| 40.0–44.9 | 7.0 | 8.0 | 9.0 | 11.5 | 16.0 | 22.0 | 25.5 | 29.5 | 33.0 |
| 45.0–49.9 | 7.0 | 8.0 | 9.5 | 11.5 | 17.0 | 23.5 | 27.0 | 30.0 | 34.5 |
| 50.0–54.9 | 7.0 | 8.0 | 9.0 | 11.5 | 16.0 | 22.5 | 26.5 | 29.5 | 34.0 |
| 55.0–59.9 | 6.5 | 8.0 | 9.5 | 11.5 | 16.5 | 23.0 | 26.0 | 28.5 | 32.0 |
| 60.0–64.9 | 7.0 | 8.0 | 10.0 | 12.0 | 17.0 | 23.0 | 26.0 | 29.0 | 34.0 |
| 65.0–69.9 | 6.0 | 7.5 | 8.5 | 10.5 | 15.0 | 21.5 | 25.0 | 28.0 | 32.5 |
| 70.0–74.9 | 6.5 | 7.0 | 8.0 | 10.3 | 15.0 | 21.0 | 25.0 | 27.5 | 31.0 |
| **Females** | | | | | | | | | |
| 1.0–1.9 | 4.0 | 4.0 | 4.5 | 5.0 | 6.0 | 7.5 | 8.5 | 9.0 | 10.0 |
| 2.0–2.9 | 4.0 | 4.0 | 4.5 | 5.0 | 6.0 | 7.0 | 8.0 | 9.0 | 10.5 |
| 3.0–3.9 | 3.5 | 4.0 | 4.0 | 5.0 | 5.5 | 7.0 | 7.5 | 8.5 | 10.0 |
| 4.0–4.9 | 3.5 | 4.0 | 4.0 | 4.5 | 5.5 | 7.0 | 8.0 | 9.0 | 10.5 |
| 5.0–5.9 | 3.5 | 4.0 | 4.0 | 4.5 | 5.0 | 7.0 | 8.0 | 9.0 | 12.0 |
| 6.0–6.9 | 3.5 | 4.0 | 4.0 | 4.5 | 5.5 | 7.0 | 8.0 | 10.0 | 11.5 |
| 7.0–7.9 | 3.5 | 4.0 | 4.0 | 4.5 | 6.0 | 7.5 | 9.5 | 11.0 | 13.0 |
| 8.0–8.9 | 3.5 | 4.0 | 4.0 | 5.0 | 6.0 | 8.0 | 11.5 | 14.5 | 21.0 |
| 9.0–9.9 | 4.0 | 4.5 | 5.0 | 5.0 | 6.5 | 9.5 | 13.0 | 18.0 | 24.0 |
| 10.0–10.9 | 4.0 | 4.5 | 5.0 | 5.5 | 7.0 | 11.5 | 16.0 | 19.5 | 24.0 |
| 11.0–11.9 | 4.5 | 5.0 | 5.0 | 6.0 | 8.0 | 12.0 | 16.0 | 20.0 | 28.5 |
| 12.0–12.9 | 5.0 | 5.5 | 6.0 | 6.5 | 9.0 | 13.0 | 17.0 | 22.0 | 30.0 |
| 13.0–13.9 | 5.0 | 6.0 | 6.0 | 7.0 | 10.0 | 15.5 | 19.0 | 23.0 | 26.5 |
| 14.0–14.9 | 6.0 | 6.0 | 7.0 | 7.5 | 10.0 | 16.0 | 20.5 | 25.0 | 30.0 |
| 15.0–15.9 | 6.0 | 7.0 | 7.5 | 8.0 | 10.0 | 15.0 | 20.0 | 23.0 | 28.0 |
| 16.0–16.9 | 7.0 | 7.5 | 8.0 | 9.0 | 11.5 | 16.5 | 24.0 | 26.0 | 34.0 |
| 17.0–17.9 | 6.0 | 7.0 | 7.5 | 9.0 | 12.5 | 19.0 | 24.5 | 28.0 | 34.0 |
| 18.0–24.9 | 6.5 | 7.0 | 8.0 | 9.5 | 13.0 | 20.0 | 25.5 | 29.0 | 36.0 |
| 25.0–29.9 | 6.5 | 7.0 | 8.0 | 10.0 | 14.0 | 23.0 | 29.0 | 33.0 | 38.5 |
| 30.0–34.9 | 6.5 | 7.5 | 8.5 | 10.5 | 16.0 | 26.5 | 32.5 | 37.0 | 43.0 |
| 35.0–39.9 | 7.0 | 8.0 | 9.0 | 11.0 | 18.0 | 28.5 | 34.0 | 36.5 | 43.0 |
| 40.0–44.9 | 6.5 | 8.0 | 9.0 | 11.5 | 19.0 | 28.5 | 34.0 | 37.0 | 42.0 |
| 45.0–49.9 | 7.0 | 8.5 | 10.0 | 12.5 | 20.0 | 29.5 | 34.0 | 37.5 | 43.5 |
| 50.0–54.9 | 7.0 | 9.0 | 11.0 | 14.0 | 21.9 | 30.0 | 35.0 | 39.0 | 43.5 |
| 55.0–59.9 | 7.0 | 9.0 | 11.0 | 13.5 | 22.0 | 31.0 | 35.0 | 38.0 | 45.0 |
| 60.0–64.9 | 7.5 | 9.0 | 11.0 | 14.0 | 21.5 | 30.5 | 35.0 | 38.0 | 43.0 |
| 65.0–69.9 | 7.0 | 8.0 | 10.0 | 13.0 | 20.0 | 28.0 | 33.0 | 36.0 | 41.0 |
| 70.0–74.9 | 6.5 | 8.5 | 10.0 | 12.0 | 19.5 | 27.0 | 32.0 | 35.0 | 38.5 |

Modified from Fisancho, A.R.: *Anthropometric Standards for the Assessment of Growth and Nutritional Status,* Ann Arbor, The University of Michigan Press, 1990.

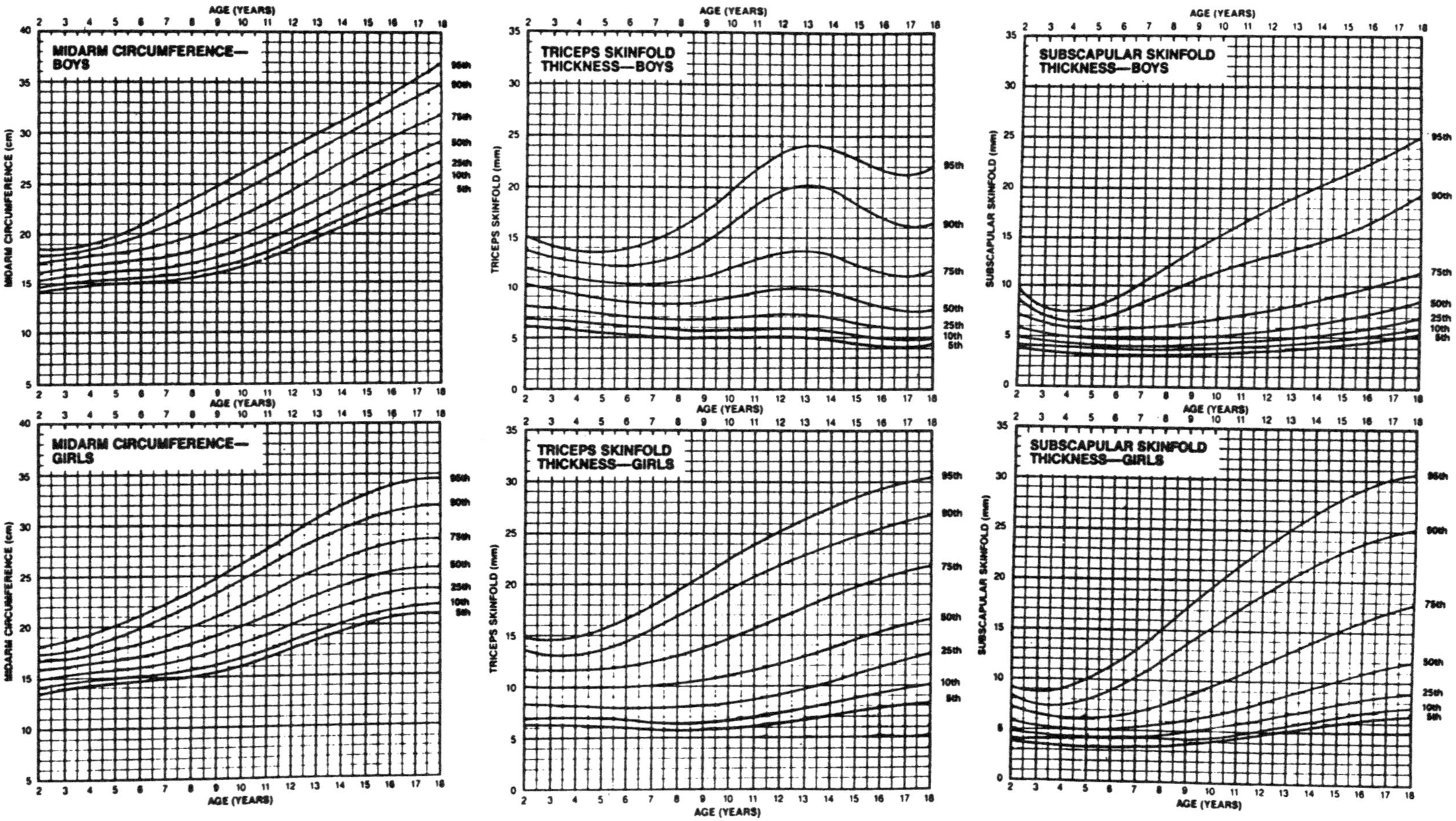


Figures adapted from Johnson, C.L., Fullwood, R., Abraham, S., et al: Basic data on anthropometric measuements and angular measurements of the hip and knee joints for selected age groups, 1–74 years of age, United States, 1971–1975. Vital and Health Statistics Series 11, No. 219. DHHS Publication No. (PHS) 81-1669, 1981.

## 8–4 Acromial Radiale (Upper Arm) Length and Knee Height Growth Chart, 2–18 Years

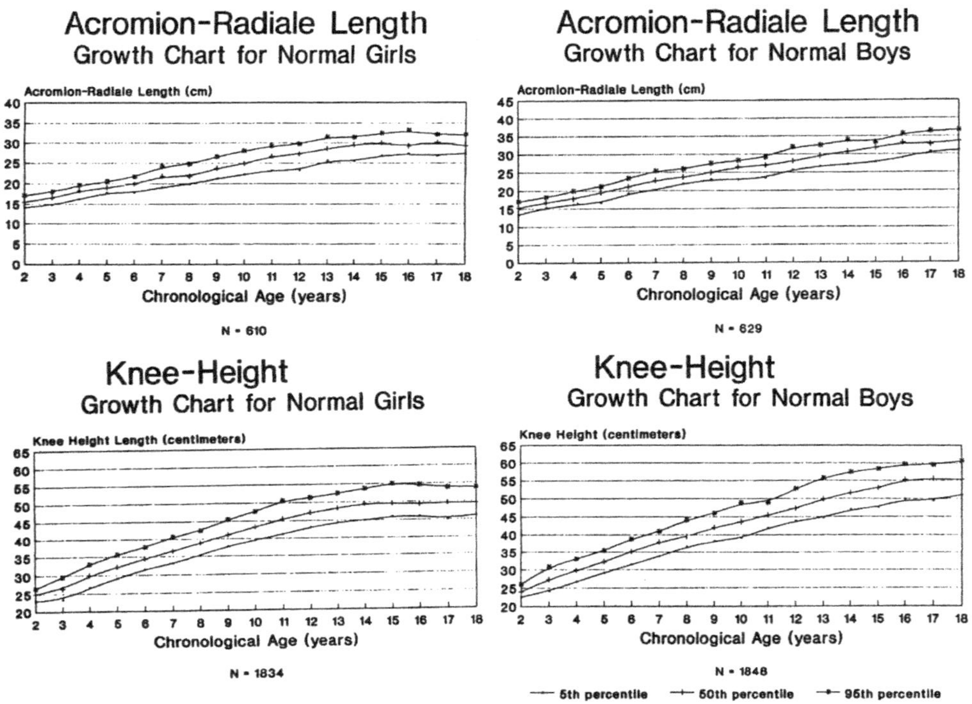


**From charts developed by T. K. White and S. W. Ekvall, 1992 as adapted from data by Snyder, R. G., Highway Safety Research Institute, University of Michigan, 1977.**

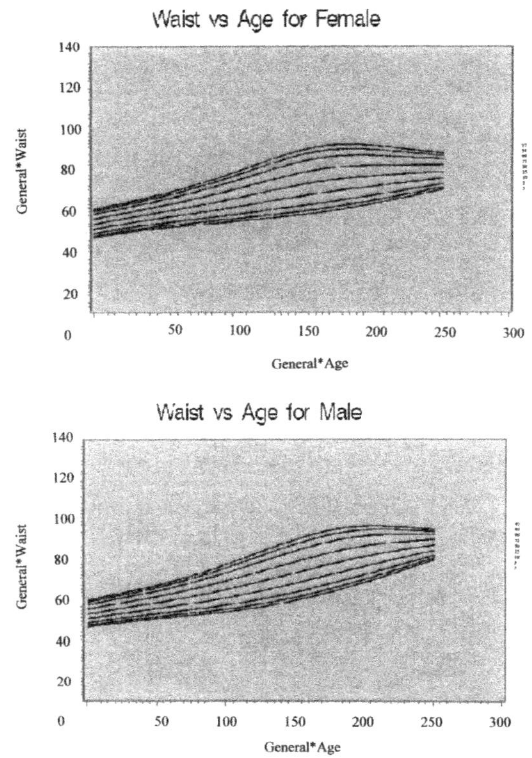


Waist circumference in centimeters for age in months—1006 normal girls and 986 normal boys. From charts developed by Ekvall, S., Sexton, T., Jaeger, L., Flaig, V., Laffert, V., Frondorf, J., Rittmeyer, K., Ekvall, V., Janecko, T., and Johnston, S. 2004.

8–5 Directions for Ross Knee Height Caliper Measurement

# DIRECTIONS FOR THE ROSS KNEE HEIGHT CALIPER

Stature can be estimated from knee height when standing height cannot be measured. Estimated stature can be used in nutritional assessment parameters, including reference weights for height, energy expenditure equations, body surface area equations, and the creatinine-height and body mass indices. Knee height may also be used with midarm circumference to predict weight in individuals who cannot be weighed by conventional methods.

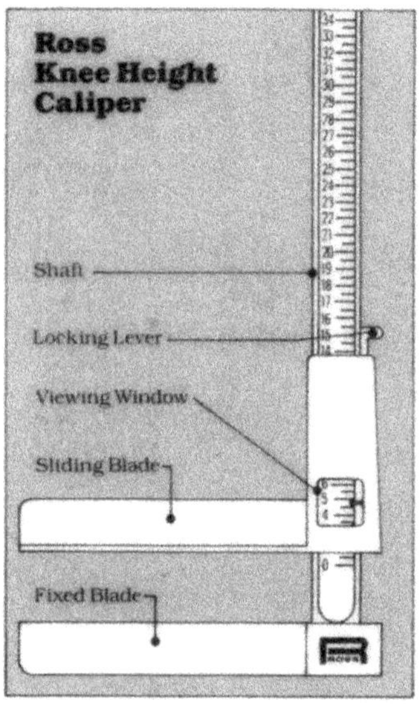


## KNEE HEIGHT MEASUREMENTS

**1.** With the subject lying on his or her back, bend both the left knee and left ankle to a 90° angle (Fig 1). Check the angles using the triangle (Fig 2).

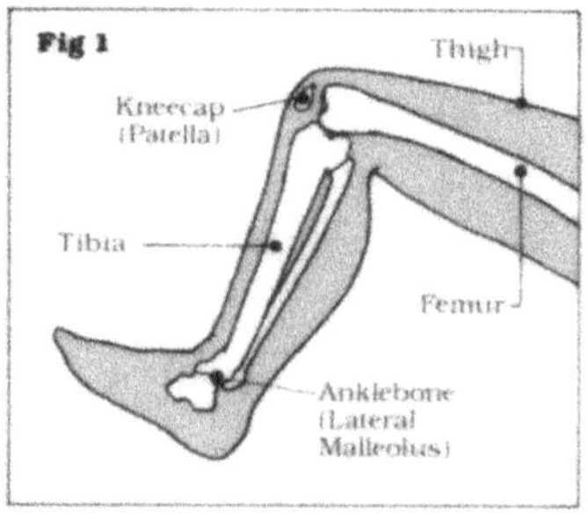

Fig 1

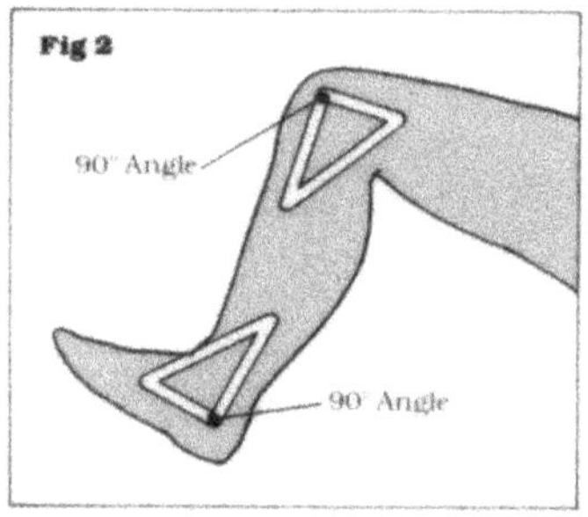

Fig 2

**2.** Open the caliper and place the fixed blade under the heel. Press the sliding blade down against the thigh about 2 in. behind the kneecap (patella) (Fig 3). The shaft of the caliper should be in line with the large bone in the lower leg (tibia) and be over the ankle bone (lateral malleolus) (Fig 4).

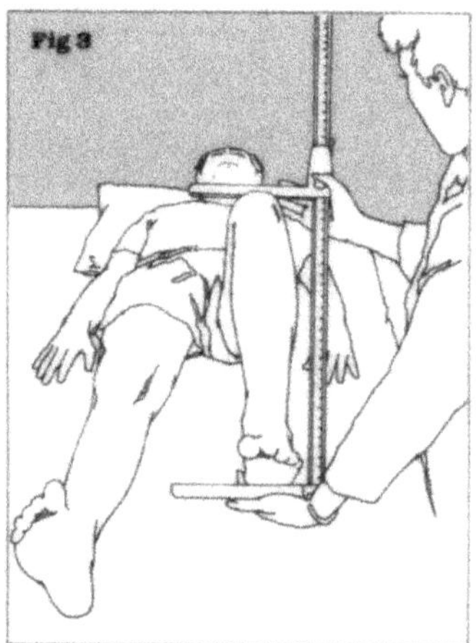
Fig 3

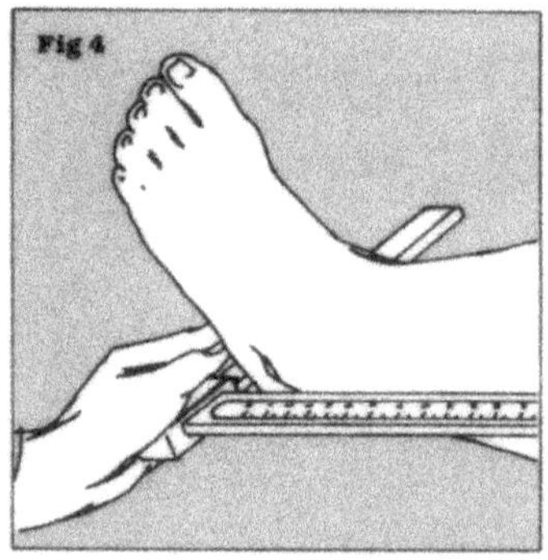
Fig 4

**3.** To hold the measurement, push the locking lever away from the blades (Fig 5). Read the measurement through the viewing window to the nearest 0.1 cm (Fig 6).

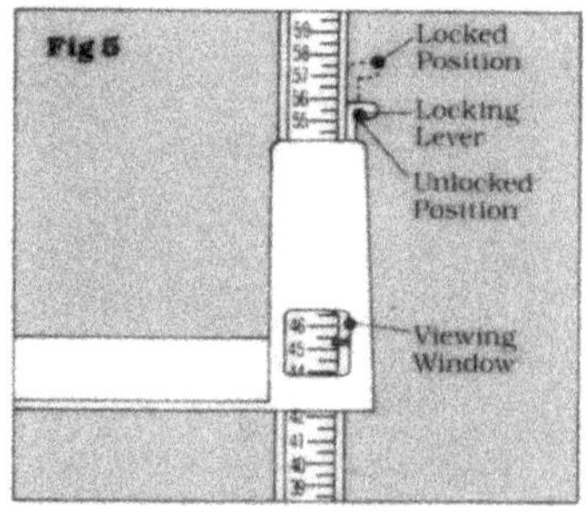

Fig 5

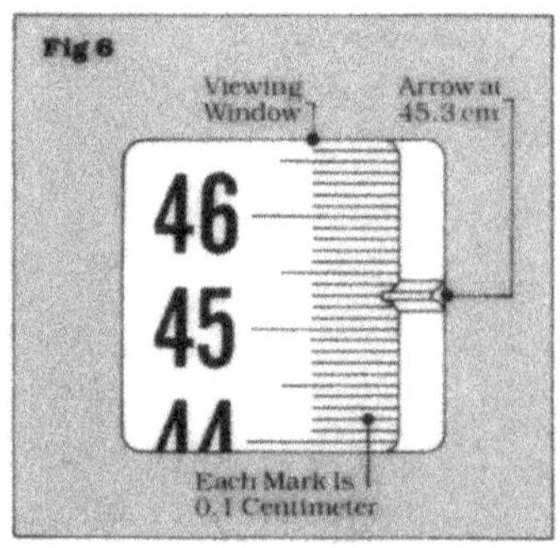

Fig 6

**4.** Release the locking lever by pushing it toward the caliper blades. Repeat the process to take a second measurement. Both measurements should be within 0.5 cm of each other.

**8–6** Estimations of Stature and Weight from Knee Height

Stature may be estimated from knee height for children, adults, and the elderly using age-, gender-, and race-specific equations. Equations have been developed from national surveys of healthy, normal individuals and reflect normal patterns of growth and development.

1. Average the two knee height measurements, rounding the result to the nearest 0.1 cm.
2. Use the appropriate equation to determine height.
3. To convert the estimated stature from centimeters to inches, use the following:

$$\textbf{Stature in inches} = \frac{\textbf{Stature in cm}}{\textbf{2.54}}$$

| MALES 6 TO 18 YEARS | | NOTE: Estimated stature should be within... |
|---|---|---|
| White Males | Stature (cm) = [Knee Height (cm) × 2.22] + 40.54 | ± 8.42 cm of actual stature for 95% of white boys. |
| Black Males | Stature (cm) = [Knee Height (cm) × 2.18] + 39.60 | ± 9.16 cm of actual stature for 95% of black boys. |
| **MALES 19 TO 59 YEARS** | | |
| White Males | Stature (cm) = [Knee Height (cm) × 1.88] + 71.85 | ± 7.94 cm of actual stature for 95% of white men. |
| Black Males | Stature (cm) = [Knee Height (cm) × 1.79] + 73.42 | ± 7.20 cm of actual stature for 95% of black men. |
| **MALES 60 TO 80 YEARS** | | |
| White Males | Stature (cm) = [Knee Height (cm) × 2.08] + 59.01 | ± 7.84 cm of actual stature for 95% of white men. |
| Black Males | Stature (cm) = [Knee Height (cm) × 1.37] + 95.79 | ± 8.44 cm of actual stature for 95% of black men. |
| **FEMALES 6 TO 18 YEARS** | | |
| White Females | Stature (cm) = [Knee Height (cm) × 2.15] + 43.21 | ± 7.79 cm of actual stature for 95% of white girls. |
| Black Females | Stature (cm) = [Knee Height (cm) × 2.02] + 46.59 | ± 8.77 cm of actual stature for 95% of black girls. |
| **FEMALES 19 TO 59 YEARS** | | |
| White Females | Stature (cm) = [Knee Height (cm) × 1.86] − [Age (years) × 0.05] + 70.25 | ± 7.20 cm of actual stature for 95% of white women. |
| Black Females | Stature (cm) = [Knee Height (cm) × 1.86] − [Age (years) × 0.06] + 68.10 | ± 7.60 cm of actual stature for 95% of black women. |
| **FEMALES 60 TO 80 YEARS** | | |
| White Females | Stature (cm) = [Knee Height (cm) × 1.91] − [Age (years) × 0.17] + 75.00 | ± 8.82 cm of actual stature for 95% of white women. |
| Black Females | Stature (cm) = [Knee Height (cm) × 1.96] + 58.72 | ± 8.26 cm of actual stature for 95% of black women. |

# ESTIMATING WEIGHT FROM KNEE HEIGHT

Weight can be estimated using age-, gender-, and race-specific equations. Measurements of midarm circumference (MAC) are also needed. Equations have been developed from national surveys of healthy, normal individuals and reflect normal patterns of growth and development.

1. Average the two knee height and midarm circumference measurements, rounding the results to the nearest 0.1 cm.
2. Use the appropriate equation to determine weight.
3. To convert weight in kilograms to pounds, use the following:

**Weight (lbs) = [Weight (kg) × 2.2]**

| MALES 6 TO 18 YEARS | | NOTE: Estimated weight should be within... |
|---|---|---|
| White Males | Weight (kg) = [Knee Height (cm) × 0.68] + [MAC (cm) × 2.64] − 50.08 | ± 7.82 kg of actual weight for 95% of white boys. |
| Black Males | Weight (kg) = [Knee Height (cm) × 0.59] + [MAC (cm) × 2.73] − 48.32 | ± 7.50 kg of actual weight for 95% of black boys. |
| **MALES 19 TO 59 YEARS** | | |
| White Males | Weight (kg) = [Knee Height (cm) × 1.19] + [MAC (cm) × 3.21] − 86.82 | ± 11.42 kg of actual weight for 95% of white men. |
| Black Males | Weight (kg) = [Knee Height (cm) × 1.09] + [MAC (cm) × 3.14] − 83.72 | ± 11.30 kg of actual weight for 95% of black men. |
| **MALES 60 TO 80 YEARS** | | |
| White Males | Weight (kg) = [Knee Height (cm) × 1.10] + [MAC (cm) × 3.07] − 75.81 | ± 11.46 kg of actual weight for 95% of white men. |
| Black Males | Weight (kg) = [Knee Height (cm) × 0.44] + [MAC (cm) × 2.86] − 39.21 | ± 7.04 kg of actual weight for 95% of black men. |
| **FEMALES 6 TO 18 YEARS** | | |
| White Females | Weight (kg) = [Knee Height (cm) × 0.77] + [MAC (cm) × 2.47] − 50.16 | ± 7.20 kg of actual weight for 95% of white girls. |
| Black Females | Weight (kg) = [Knee Height (cm) × 0.71] + [MAC (cm) × 2.59] − 50.43 | ± 7.65 kg of actual weight for 95% of black girls. |
| **FEMALES 19 TO 59 YEARS** | | |
| White Females | Weight (kg) = [Knee Height (cm) × 1.01] + [MAC (cm) × 2.81] − 66.04 | ± 10.60 kg of actual weight for 95% of white women. |
| Black Females | Weight (kg) = [Knee Height (cm) × 1.24] + [MAC (cm) × 2.97] − 82.48 | ± 11.98 kg of actual weight for 95% of black women. |
| **FEMALES 60 TO 80 YEARS** | | |
| White Females | Weight (kg) = [Knee Height (cm) × 1.09] + [MAC (cm) × 2.68] − 65.51 | ± 11.42 kg of actual weight for 95% of white women. |
| Black Females | Weight (kg) = [Knee Height (cm) × 1.50] + [MAC (cm) × 2.58] − 84.22 | ± 14.52 kg of actual weight for 95% of black women. |

| Age (yrs) | Percentiles 5 | 10 | 15 | 25 | 50 | 75 | 85 | 90 | 95 |
|---|---|---|---|---|---|---|---|---|---|
| **Males** | | | | | | | | | |
| 2.0–2.9 | 50.0 | 51.0 | 51.3 | 52.0 | 54.0 | 56.0 | 57.0 | 57.0 | 58.0 |
| 3.0–3.9 | 52.1 | 54.0 | 54.0 | 55.0 | 57.0 | 58.8 | 59.6 | 60.0 | 61.0 |
| 4.0–4.9 | 55.0 | 56.0 | 57.0 | 58.0 | 60.0 | 61.7 | 63.0 | 63.0 | 64.3 |
| 5.0–5.9 | 57.9 | 59.0 | 59.3 | 60.0 | 62.3 | 64.0 | 65.0 | 66.0 | 67.0 |
| 6.0–6.9 | 59.5 | 61.0 | 62.0 | 63.0 | 65.0 | 67.0 | 68.0 | 69.0 | 69.4 |
| 7.0–7.9 | 62.0 | 63.2 | 64.0 | 65.3 | 67.2 | 69.2 | 70.0 | 71.0 | 72.0 |
| 8.0–8.9 | 64.1 | 65.4 | 66.0 | 67.5 | 69.0 | 71.4 | 72.6 | 73.0 | 74.6 |
| 9.0–9.9 | 66.0 | 67.5 | 68.0 | 69.0 | 71.4 | 74.0 | 75.0 | 75.6 | 76.7 |
| 10.0–10.9 | 68.0 | 69.0 | 70.0 | 71.6 | 73.8 | 76.0 | 77.0 | 78.0 | 79.4 |
| 11.0–11.9 | 69.3 | 71.0 | 71.9 | 73.0 | 76.0 | 78.0 | 79.6 | 80.4 | 82.0 |
| 12.0–12.9 | 71.7 | 72.9 | 74.0 | 75.1 | 78.0 | 81.0 | 82.3 | 84.2 | 86.0 |
| 13.0–13.9 | 74.0 | 75.0 | 76.0 | 78.0 | 81.7 | 85.3 | 87.2 | 88.5 | 90.5 |
| 14.0–14.9 | 76.7 | 79.3 | 80.5 | 82.5 | 86.0 | 88.9 | 90.5 | 91.5 | 92.9 |
| 15.0–15.9 | 80.4 | 82.0 | 83.5 | 85.4 | 88.1 | 91.1 | 92.6 | 93.8 | 95.0 |
| 16.0–16.9 | 84.1 | 85.2 | 86.1 | 87.6 | 90.5 | 93.4 | 94.5 | 95.1 | 96.5 |
| 17.0–17.9 | 84.3 | 86.0 | 87.0 | 88.4 | 91.1 | 93.5 | 94.7 | 95.9 | 97.3 |
| 18.0–24.9 | 86.2 | 87.6 | 88.5 | 90.0 | 92.4 | 94.7 | 96.3 | 97.2 | 98.5 |
| 25.0–29.9 | 86.5 | 88.0 | 89.0 | 90.3 | 92.9 | 95.2 | 96.7 | 97.6 | 98.8 |
| 30.0–34.9 | 86.7 | 87.9 | 88.8 | 90.3 | 92.7 | 95.1 | 96.4 | 97.4 | 98.7 |
| 35.0–39.9 | 86.4 | 87.6 | 88.6 | 90.0 | 92.5 | 95.1 | 96.4 | 97.0 | 98.3 |
| 40.0–44.9 | 86.3 | 87.8 | 88.8 | 90.1 | 92.4 | 94.5 | 96.0 | 96.9 | 98.2 |
| 45.0–49.9 | 85.5 | 87.2 | 88.3 | 89.6 | 92.1 | 94.2 | 95.6 | 96.4 | 97.8 |
| 50.0–54.9 | 85.3 | 86.8 | 87.6 | 89.2 | 91.6 | 93.8 | 95.1 | 96.0 | 97.3 |
| 55.0–59.9 | 84.9 | 86.2 | 87.3 | 88.6 | 91.1 | 93.5 | 94.6 | 95.4 | 96.6 |
| 60.0–64.9 | 84.8 | 86.1 | 86.8 | 88.0 | 90.5 | 92.9 | 94.1 | 94.8 | 96.1 |
| 65.0–69.9 | 83.3 | 84.5 | 85.5 | 86.7 | 89.4 | 91.7 | 93.3 | 94.1 | 95.2 |
| 70.0–74.9 | 81.9 | 83.6 | 84.8 | 86.2 | 88.7 | 91.0 | 92.4 | 93.5 | 94.4 |
| **Females** | | | | | | | | | |
| 2.0–2.9 | 49.0 | 49.8 | 50.0 | 51.0 | 53.0 | 54.4 | 55.0 | 56.0 | 56.7 |
| 3.0–3.9 | 51.0 | 52.3 | 53.0 | 54.0 | 55.7 | 57.2 | 58.3 | 59.0 | 60.0 |
| 4.0–4.9 | 54.0 | 55.0 | 56.0 | 57.0 | 58.8 | 60.7 | 61.3 | 62.0 | 63.0 |
| 5.0–5.9 | 56.6 | 58.0 | 58.9 | 60.0 | 61.6 | 63.1 | 64.2 | 65.0 | 66.0 |
| 6.0–6.9 | 59.2 | 60.0 | 61.0 | 62.0 | 64.0 | 66.0 | 67.0 | 68.0 | 69.0 |
| 7.0–7.9 | 62.0 | 62.8 | 63.1 | 64.5 | 66.1 | 68.4 | 69.8 | 70.2 | 71.8 |
| 8.0–8.9 | 64.0 | 64.7 | 65.9 | 67.0 | 69.0 | 71.0 | 72.0 | 73.0 | 74.1 |
| 9.0–9.9 | 65.5 | 66.7 | 67.8 | 69.0 | 71.0 | 73.5 | 75.0 | 76.0 | 77.2 |
| 10.0–10.9 | 68.0 | 69.2 | 70.1 | 71.4 | 73.5 | 75.8 | 77.3 | 78.9 | 81.0 |
| 11.0–11.9 | 70.0 | 71.6 | 72.2 | 74.0 | 76.6 | 80.0 | 81.2 | 82.3 | 83.9 |
| 12.0–12.9 | 73.0 | 74.0 | 75.1 | 77.2 | 80.5 | 83.1 | 84.6 | 85.5 | 86.4 |
| 13.0–13.9 | 76.2 | 77.7 | 76.7 | 80.1 | 82.7 | 85.0 | 86.3 | 86.9 | 87.8 |
| 14.0–14.9 | 78.1 | 79.1 | 80.4 | 81.7 | 84.3 | 86.9 | 87.8 | 88.6 | 89.5 |
| 15.0–15.9 | 79.8 | 81.1 | 82.2 | 83.3 | 85.3 | 87.5 | 88.5 | 89.9 | 91.5 |
| 16.0–16.9 | 79.3 | 81.0 | 81.9 | 83.5 | 85.8 | 88.0 | 88.8 | 89.8 | 91.5 |
| 17.0–17.9 | 80.0 | 81.1 | 82.4 | 83.8 | 86.0 | 88.1 | 89.4 | 90.3 | 92.0 |
| 18.0–24.9 | 80.4 | 81.9 | 82.8 | 84.0 | 86.4 | 88.5 | 89.8 | 90.6 | 91.9 |
| 25.0–29.9 | 80.9 | 82.2 | 83.1 | 84.4 | 86.5 | 88.7 | 89.9 | 90.6 | 92.0 |
| 30.0–34.9 | 81.0 | 82.3 | 83.1 | 84.4 | 86.5 | 89.0 | 90.1 | 91.1 | 92.3 |
| 35.0–39.9 | 81.0 | 82.1 | 83.1 | 84.5 | 86.7 | 88.8 | 90.2 | 91.0 | 92.0 |
| 40.0–44.9 | 80.6 | 82.0 | 82.8 | 84.1 | 86.3 | 88.4 | 89.7 | 90.5 | 91.7 |
| 45.0–49.9 | 80.5 | 82.0 | 83.0 | 84.2 | 86.4 | 88.3 | 89.4 | 90.3 | 91.6 |
| 50.0–54.9 | 80.5 | 81.6 | 82.4 | 83.4 | 85.5 | 87.7 | 88.8 | 89.7 | 90.7 |
| 55.0–59.9 | 78.9 | 80.5 | 81.5 | 82.6 | 85.0 | 87.1 | 88.3 | 89.1 | 90.0 |
| 60.0–64.9 | 78.6 | 80.0 | 80.9 | 82.1 | 84.4 | 86.5 | 87.7 | 88.4 | 89.7 |
| 65.0–69.9 | 77.4 | 78.8 | 79.7 | 81.0 | 83.3 | 85.5 | 86.7 | 87.4 | 88.6 |
| 70.0–74.9 | 76.5 | 77.9 | 78.7 | 80.0 | 82.4 | 84.4 | 85.7 | 86.5 | 87.6 |

| Age, years | BMI 50th M | 50th F | 85th M | 85th F | 95th M | 95th F | Sum of Two Skinfolds 50th M | 50th F | 85th M | 85th F | 95th M | 95th F |
|---|---|---|---|---|---|---|---|---|---|---|---|---|
| 6 | 15.4 | 15.2 | 16.8 | 17.1 | 18.2 | 18.5 | 12 | 14 | 16 | 19 | 20 | 27 |
| 7 | 15.6 | 15.4 | 17.1 | 17.6 | 18.9 | 19.6 | 12 | 15 | 17 | 22 | 24 | 28 |
| 8 | 16.0 | 15.9 | 18.1 | 18.6 | 20.2 | 21.1 | 13 | 16 | 19 | 25 | 28 | 36 |
| 9 | 16.2 | 16.3 | 19.0 | 19.5 | 22.4 | 22.9 | 14 | 17 | 23 | 29 | 34 | 41 |
| 10 | 16.5 | 16.9 | 19.2 | 20.6 | 21.8 | 23.6 | 14 | 18 | 24 | 32 | 33 | 43 |
| 11 | 17.2 | 17.5 | 20.9 | 21.7 | 24.2 | 24.8 | 15 | 19 | 28 | 31 | 39 | 43 |
| 12 | 17.8 | 18.6 | 21.4 | 22.6 | 24.1 | 26.2 | 15 | 20 | 24 | 34 | 44 | 47 |
| 13 | 18.7 | 19.4 | 22.6 | 23.4 | 26.6 | 26.8 | 15 | 21 | 28 | 39 | 46 | 52 |
| 14 | 19.6 | 20.2 | 23.2 | 24.1 | 26.7 | 26.5 | 14 | 24 | 27 | 37 | 39 | 53 |
| 15 | 20.4 | 20.7 | 24.0 | 24.7 | 27.8 | 29.4 | 14 | 25 | 25 | 41 | 40 | 56 |
| 16 | 20.8 | 20.9 | 24.0 | 24.9 | 26.9 | 29.6 | 14 | 26 | 24 | 42 | 39 | 58 |
| 17 | 21.5 | 21.0 | 24.9 | 24.3 | 28.5 | 29.3 | 15 | 27 | 26 | 42 | 41 | 59 |

From Lohman, T: Advances in Body Composition Assessment. Champaign, Human Kinetics, 1992.

| Characteristics | Computation | Variable |
|---|---|---|
| Child's stature (CS) | N.A. | 123.0 cm |
| Father's stature | N.A. | 187.0 cm |
| Mother's stature | N.A. | 165.0 cm |
| Midparent stature (MPS) | (187 + 165)/2 | 176.0 cm |
| Adjusted for midparent stature | 123 - 4.27 | 118.7 cm |
| Weight | N.A. | 31.0 kg |
| Sitting Height | N.A. | 69.0 cm |
| Sitting Height Index | (69/123) x 100 | 56.0% |
| Triceps Skinfold | 11/10 = 1.1 cm | 11.0 mm |
| Subscapular Skinfold | N.A. | 5.0 mm |
| Sum of Skinfold Thicknesses | N.A. | 16.0 mm |
| Upper Arm Circumference | N.A. | 22.0 cm |
| Total Upper Arm Fat Area (TUA) | $22^2/12.57$ | 38.5 $cm^2$ |
| Upper Arm Muscle Area (UMA) | $[(22.0 - 1.1) \times 3.1416]^2/12.57$ | 27.4 $cm^2$ |
| Upper Arm Fat Area (UFA) | 38.5 - 27.4 | 11.1 $cm^2$ |
| Arm Fat Index (AFI) | (11.1/38.5) x 100 | 28.8% |

**Growth and Nutritional Status Evaluation**

| Reference | Z-score | Category | Percentile | Category |
|---|---|---|---|---|
| Stature by Age | -1.08 | Below Ave. | >5th but <15 | Below Ave. |
| Adj. midparent stature | -1.87 | Short | < 5th | Short |
| Wt. by Age | N.A. | N.A. | >15th but <85th | Average |
| Wt. by Ht. | N.A. | N.A. | >95th | High Wt. |
| Sitting Ht. Index | 0.76 | Average | >95th | Large Trunk |
| UMA by Age | 1.26 | Above Ave. | >85th but <95th | Above Ave. |
| UMA by Ht. | 2.19 | Above Ave. | >85th but <95th | Above Ave. |
| Sum of Skinfolds | N.A. | N.A. | >15th but <85th | Average |
| Arm Fat Index | N.A. | N.A. | >15th but <85th | Average |

Interpretation. The subject is short for his age and, considering his parents' height, he should have been taller than he is now. In other words, he seems to be below his genetic potential as far as his height is concerned. However, the subject is heavy for his age. As judged by the measurements of body composition, the excess weight is not due to an excess of fat but to the subjects' high muscularity and short legs (which is indicated by the high sitting height index).

Modified from Fisancho, A.R.: *Anthropometric Standards for the Assessment of Growth and Nutritional Status,* Ann Arbor, The University of Michigan Press, 1990.

**8–8** Percentage Body Fat from Triceps plus Subscapular Skinfolds, Equations and Chart, Children

<u>For Triceps and Subscapular</u>

Prepubescent White Males: $PFDWB = 1.21\,(triceps + subscapular) - .008\,(triceps + subscapular)^2 - 1.7$

Prepubescent Black Males: $PFDWB = 1.21\,(triceps + subscapular) - .008\,(triceps + subscapular)^2 - 3.2$

Pubescent White Males: $PFDWB = 1.21\,(triceps + subscapular) - .008\,(triceps + subscapular)^2 - 3.4$

Pubescent Black Males: $PFDWB = 1.21\,(triceps + subscapular) - .008\,(triceps + subscapular)^2 - 5.2$

Postpubescent White Males: $PFDWB = 1.21\,(triceps + subscapular) - .008\,(triceps + subscapular)^2 - 5.5$

Postpubescent Black Males: $PFDWB = 1.21\,(triceps + subscapular) - .008\,(triceps + subscapular)^2 - 6.8$

All Females: $PFDWB = 1.33\,(triceps + subscapular) - .013\,(triceps + subscapular)^2 - 2.5$

For a sum of tricep and subscapular greater than 35 mm, the following equation should be applied.

All Males $PFDWB = .783\,(triceps + subscapular) + 1.6$

All Females $PFDWB = .546\,(triceps + subscapular) + 9.7$

From Slaughter, M.H. Lohman, T.G., Boileau, R.A., Horswill, C.A., Stillman, R.J., Van Loan, M.D. and Bemben, D.A.: Skinfold equations for estimation of body fatness in children and youth. *Human Biol*, 60:709, 1988. Used with permission.

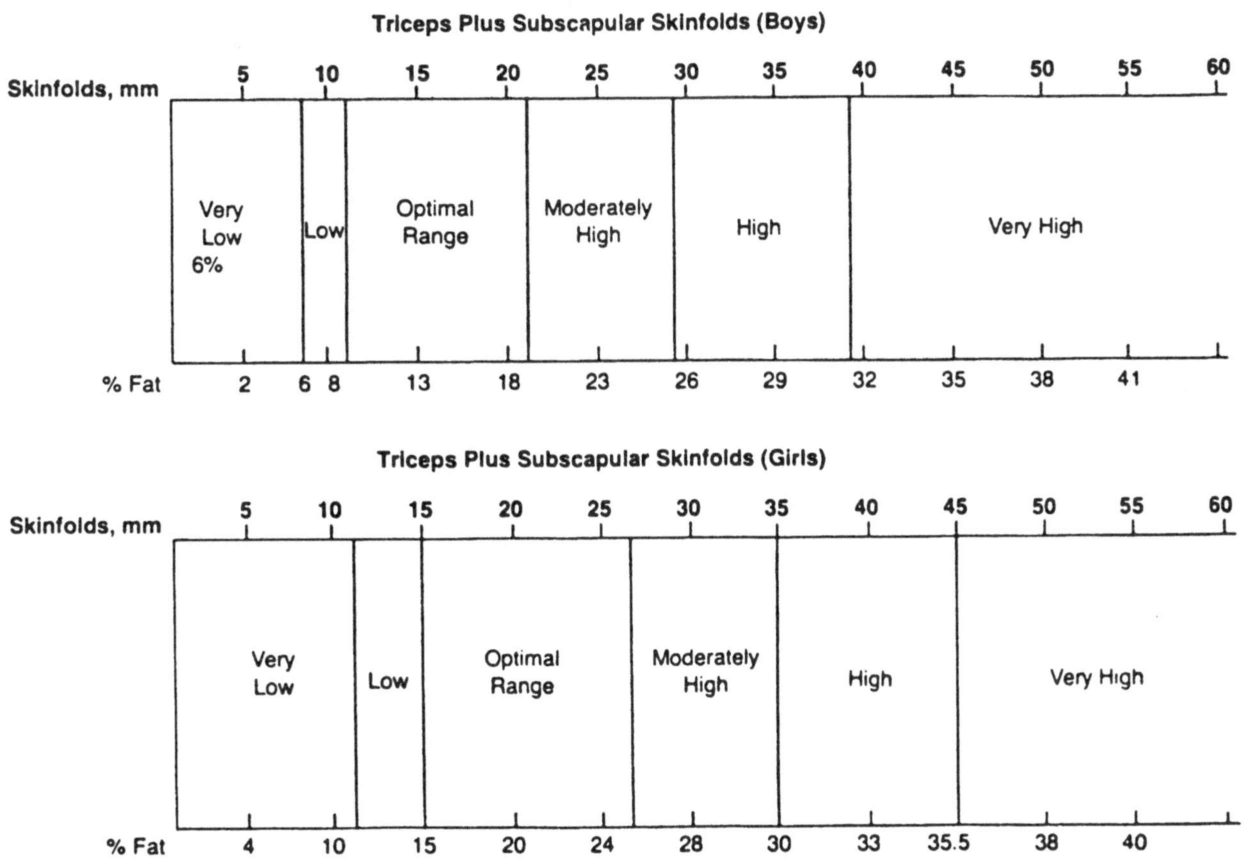


**Figure 1.**

Lohman, T.G.: The use of skinfold to estimate body fatness on children and youth. *J Phy Ed Rec,* 58:98, 1987.

**8–9** Percentage Body Fat from Triceps plus Calf Skinfolds, Equations and Chart, Children

For Triceps and Calf
Males:PFDWB = .735 (triceps + calf) + 1.0
Females:PFDWB = .610 (triceps + calf) + 5.1

From Slaughter, M. H. Lohman, T. G., Boileau, R. A., Horswill, C. A., Stillman, R. J., Van Loan, M.D. and Bemben, D. A.: Skinfold equations for estimation of body fatness in children and youth. Human Biol, 60:709, 1988. Used with permission.

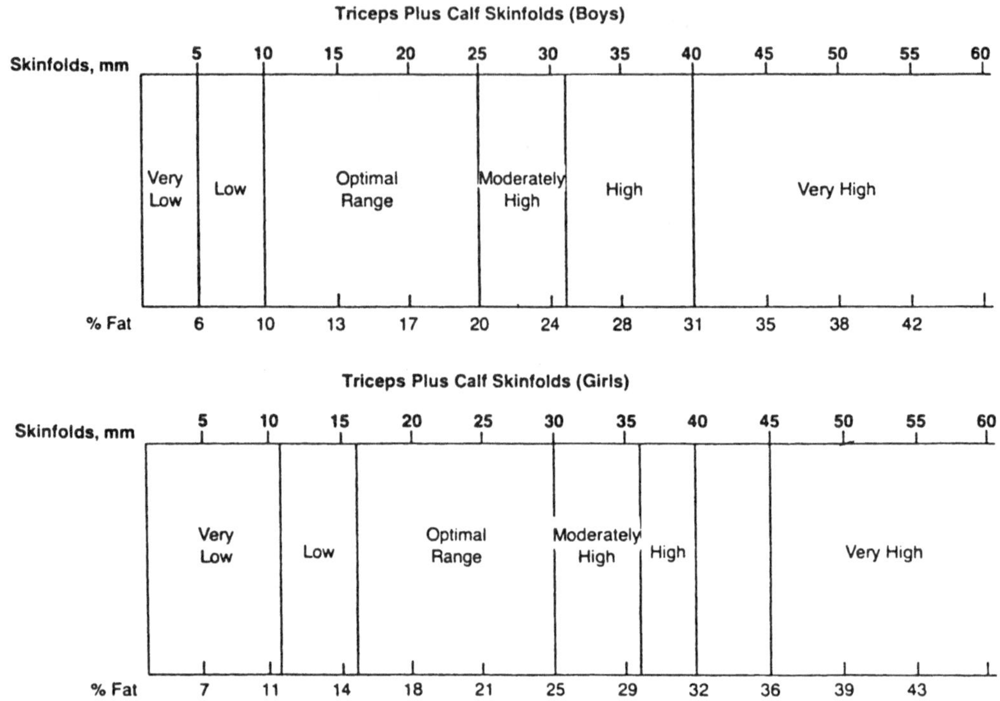


Figure 1.

Lohman, T.G.: The use of skinfold to estimate body fatness on children and youth. *J Phy Ed Rec,* 58:98, 1987.

## 8–10 Free Amino Acids in Serum

| | micromol per liter | | |
|---|---|---|---|
| | Children Birth–6 yrs | Normal Adults Mean (S.D) | |
| | | MALE | FEMALE |
| Taurine | 110 (40) | 86 (28) | 80 (25) |
| Aspartic Acid | 33 (14) | 28 (11) | 21 (10) |
| Hydroxyproline | 31 (14) | 15 ( 6) | 13 ( 5) |
| Threonine | 157 (47) | 150 (26) | 147 (47) |
| Serine | 194 (54) | 192 (45) | 177 (58) |
| Asparagine | 71 (18) | 63 (21) | 60 (21) |
| Glutamic Acid | 113 (43) | 103 (41) | 88 (32) |
| Glutamine | 647 (116) | 599 (61) | 562 (98) |
| Proline | 223 (58) | 210 (64) | 173 (58) |
| Glycine | 367 (95) | 298 (52) | 303 (84) |
| Alanine | 417 (107) | 376 (96) | 354 (99) |
| Citrulline | 22 (8) | 34 ( 8) | 31 ( 8) |
| Aminobutyric Acid | 10) 6) | 21 (12) | 17 (11) |
| Valine | 213 (53) | 271 (48) | 214 (36) |
| Cystine | 36 (10) | 44 (18) | 39 (12) |
| Methionine | 34 (11) | 24 ( 4) | 20 ( 4) |
| Isoleucine | 66 (21) | 70 (14) | 54 (12) |
| Leucine | 122 (32) | 143 (24) | 112 (20) |
| Tyrosine | 81 (28) | 61 (15) | 57 (17) |
| Phenylalanine | 72 (17) | 76 (18) | 61 (15) |
| Tryptophan | 40 (13) | 42 (12) | 40 (13) |
| Ornithine | 95 (38) | 115 (23) | 103 (33) |
| Lysine | 169 (41) | 199 (37) | 172 (38) |
| Histidine | 90 (16) | 98 (18) | 90 (18) |
| Arginine | 95 (29) | 54 ( 9) | 54 (22) |

From the Metabolic Disease Center, Children's Hospital Medical Center, Cincinnati, OH, 45229 (unpublished data). Data for children represent the 10th to 90th percentiles of values from 440 consecutive amino acid analyses on a Beckman 6300 Amino Acid Analyzer (Beckman Instruments, Fullerton, CA) using operating settings and reagents recommended by the manufacturer for analysis of physiological fluids. Adult values represent two specimens each from 10 men and 18 women.

## 8–10A Estimates of Daily Amino Acid Requirements

| | Requirements, by age group | | | |
|---|---|---|---|---|
| | Infants 3–4 mo* | Children under 2 yr† | Children 10–12 yr‡ | Adults§ |
| Amino acid | (mg/kg/day) | | | |
| Histidine | 28 | ? | ? | 8-12 |
| Isoleucine | 70 | 31 | 28 | 10 |
| Leucine | 161 | 73 | 42 | 14 |
| Lysine | 103 | 64 | 44 | 12 |
| Methionine plus cystine | 58 | 27 | 22 | 13 |
| Phenylalinine plus tyrosine | 125 | 69 | 22 | 14 |
| Threonine | 87 | 37 | 28 | 7 |
| Tryptophan | 17 | 12.5 | 3.3 | 3.5 |
| Valine | 93 | 38 | 25 | 10 |
| Total without histidine | 714 | 352 | 214 | 84 |

*Based on amounts of amino acids in human milk or cow's milk formulas fed at levels that supported good growth. Data from Formon, S.J., Filer, L.J., Jr. Amino acid requirements for normal growth. In: Nyhan, W.L., ed. *Amino Acid Metabolism and Genetic Variation*. New York: McGraw-Hill; 1967.

†Based on achievement of nitrogen balance sufficient to support adequate lean tissue gain (16 mg N/kg per day). Data from Pineda, O., Torun, B., Viteri, F.E., Arroyave, G. Protein quality in relation to estimates of essential amino acids requirements. In: Bodwell, C.E., Adkins, J.S. Hopkins, D.T., eds. *Protein Quality in Humans: Assessment and In Vitro Estimation*. Westport, CT: AVI Publishing; 1981.

‡Based on upper range of requirement for positive nitrogen balance. Recalculated by Williams, H.H., Harper, A.E., Hegsted, D.M., Arroyave, G., Holt, I.E., Jr. Nitrogen and amino acid requirements. In: Food and Nutrition Board. *Improvement of Protein Nutriture. Report of the Committee on Amino Acids*. Washington, DC: National Academy of Sciences; 1974.

§Based on highest estimate of requirement to achieve nitrogen balance. Data from several investigators (reviewed by) FAO/WHO (Food and Agriculture Organization/World Health Organization). *Energy and Protein Requirements. Report of a Joint FAO/WHO Ad Hoc Expert Committee*. Technical Report Series No. 552; FAO Nutrition Meetings Report Series 52. Rome: World Health Organization; 1973.

From National Research Council[16] with permission.

| Nutrient & Units | Age of Subject (years) | Criteria of Status: Deficient | Marginal | Acceptable |
|---|---|---|---|---|
| Hemoglobin (g/dl) | 1 week | | | 13–20 |
| | 1 month | | | > 14 |
| | 6–23 months | < 9.0 | 9.0–9.9 | 10.0+ |
| | 2–5 | < 10.0 | 10.0–10.9 | 11.0+ |
| | 6–12 | < 10.0 | 10.0–11.4 | 11.5+ |
| | 13–16M | < 12.0 | 12.0–12.9 | 13.0+ |
| | 13–16F | < 10.0 | 10.0–11.4 | 11.5+ |
| | 16+M | < 12.0 | 12.0–13.9 | 14.0+ |
| | 16+F | < 10.0 | 10.0–11.9 | 12.0+ |
| | Pregnant | | | |
| | 2nd trimester | < 9.5 | 9.5–10.9 | 11.0+ |
| | 3rd trimester | < 9.0 | 9.0–10.5 | 10.5+ |
| Hematocrit (packed cell volume in %) | 1 week | | | 43–66 |
| | 1 month | | | > 50 |
| | 3 months | | | > 35 |
| | 6 months–5 years | | | > 38 |
| | 6–12 | < 30 | 30–35 | 36+ |
| | 13–16M | < 37 | 37–39 | 40+ |
| | 13–16F | < 31 | 31–35 | 36+ |
| | 16+M | < 37 | 37–43 | 44+ |
| | 16+F | < 31 | 31–37 | 33+ |
| | Pregnant | < 30 | 30–32 | 33+ |
| Mean corpuscular volume ($\mu m^3$) | All ages | | | 80–94 |
| Mean corpuscular hemoglobin (μg) | All ages | | | 27–35 |
| Mean corpuscular hemoglobin concentration (%) | All ages | | | 32–36 |
| Serum iron (μg/dl) | < 2 | < 30 | | 30+ |
| | 2–5 | < 40 | | 40+ |
| | 6–12 | < 50 | | 50+ |
| | 12+M | < 60 | | 60+ |
| | 12+F or pregnant | < 40 | 40 | 40+ |
| Transferrin saturation (%) | < 2 | < 15.0 | | 15.0+ |
| | 2–12 | < 20.0 | | 20.0+ |
| | 12+M | < 20.0 | | 20.0+ |
| | 12+F or pregnant | < 15.0 | 15 | 15.0+ |
| Serum ascorbic acid (mg/dl) | All ages | < 0.1 | 0.1–0.19 | 0.2+ |
| Plasma vitamin A (μg/dl) | All ages | < 10 | 10–19 | 20+ |
| Plasma carotene (μ/dl) | All ages | < 20 | 20–39 | 40+ |
| | pregnant | | 40–79 | 80+ |

| Nutrient & Units | Age of Subject (years) | Criteria of Status: Deficient | Marginal | Acceptable |
|---|---|---|---|---|
| Serum folic acid (ng/ml) | All ages; pregnant | < 2.0 | 2.1–5.9 | 6.0+ |
| Serum vitamin $B_{12}$ (pg/ml) | All ages; pregnant | < 100 | 100 | 100+ |
| Thiamine in urine (μg/g of creatinine) | 1–3 | < 120 | 120–175 | 175+ |
| | 4–5 | < 85 | 85–120 | 120+ |
| | 6–9 | < 70 | 70–180 | 180+ |
| | 10–15 | < 55 | 55–150 | 150+ |
| | 16+ | < 27 | 27–65 | 65+ |
| | Pregnant | < 21 | 21–49 | 50+ |
| Riboflavin in urine (μg/g of creatinine) | 1–3 | < 150 | 150–499 | 500+ |
| | 4–5 | < 100 | 100–299 | 300+ |
| | 6–9 | < 85 | 85–269 | 270+ |
| | 10–16 | < 80 | 70–199 | 200+ |
| | 16+ | < 27 | 27–79 | 80+ |
| | Pregnant | < 30 | 30–89 | 90+ |
| Tryptophan load (mg xanthurenic acid excreted) | Adults (Dose: 100 mg/kg body weight) | 6 hr 25+ | | < 25 |
| | | 24 hr 75+ | | < 75 |
| Urinary pyridoxine (μg/g of creatinine) | 1–3 | < 90 | | 90+ |
| | 4–6 | < 80 | | 80+ |
| | 7–9 | < 60 | | 60+ |
| | 10–12 | < 40 | | 40+ |
| | 13–15 | < 30 | | 30+ |
| | 16+ | < 20 | | 20+ |
| Urinary N'methyl nicotinamide (mg/g of creatinine) | All ages | < 0.2 | 0.2–5.59 | 0.6+ |
| | Pregnant | < 0.8 | 0.8–2.49 | 2.5+ |
| Urinary pantothenic acid (μg) | All ages | < 200 | | 200+ |
| Vitamine E (serum tocopherol) (mg/dl) | Birth | | | 0.22 |
| | 2 mos. | | | 0.33 |
| | 2–12 yr. | | | 0.72 |
| | Adults | | | 0.85 |
| Transaminase index (ratio) | | | | |
| EGOT | Adult | 2.0+ | | < 2.0 |
| EGPT | Adult | 1.25+ | | < 1.25 |

Modified from: Zeman, F.J.: *Clinical Nutrition and Dietetics*. New York, Macmillan, 1991. M=male subjects; F=female subjects; EGOT=erythrocyte glutamic oxaloacetic transaminase; EGPT=erythrocyte glutamic pyruvic transaminase.

**8–12** Depletion of Body Iron, Increases in Urinary Nitrogen Excretion, and Changes in Resting Metabolism Over Time

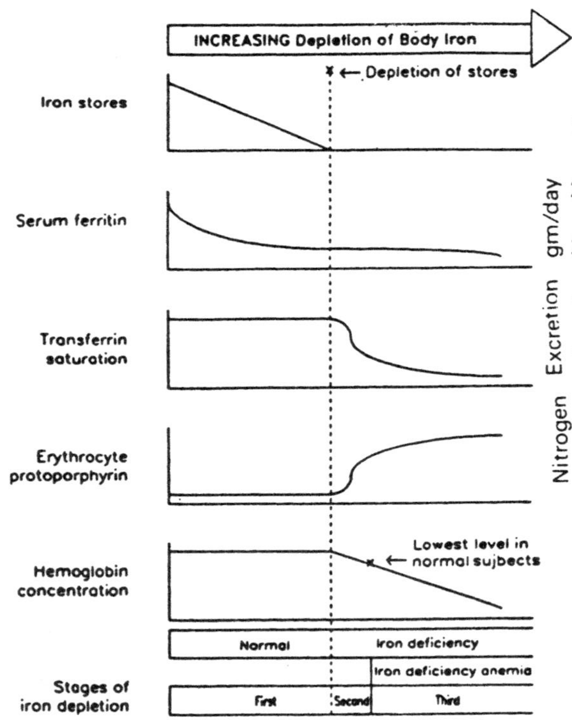


From: LSRO, FASEB. 1989. Nutrition Monitoring in the United States: An Update Report on Nutrition Monitoring Washington, D.C.: U.S. Government Printing Office, Figure 6.1, page 131.

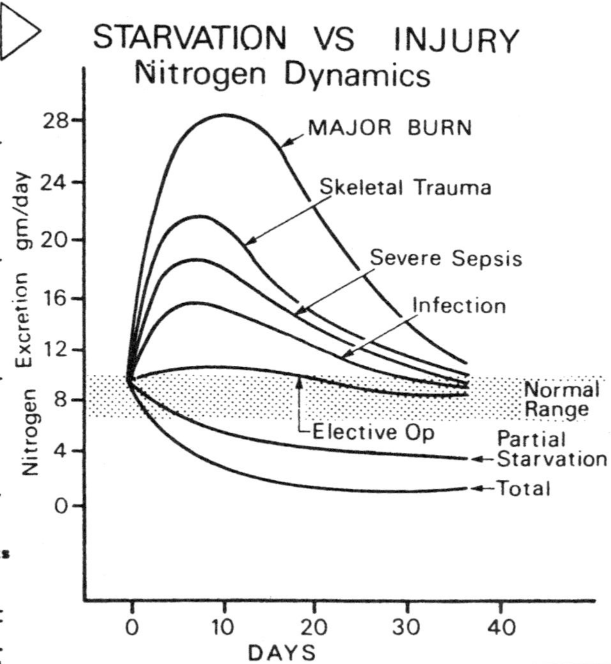


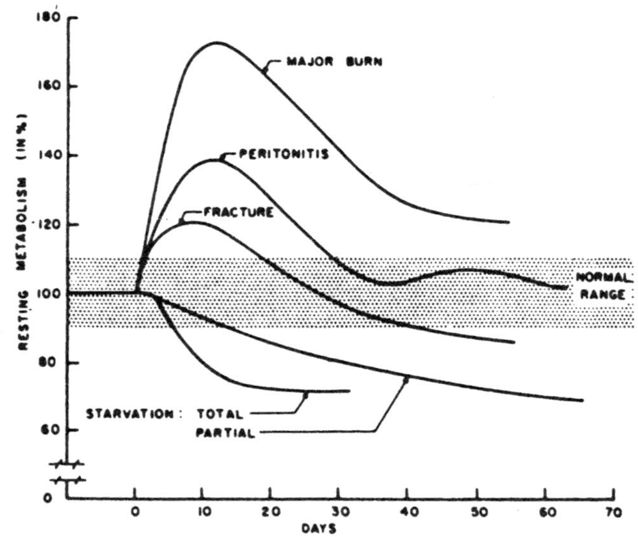


Long, C.L., Schaffel, N., Geiger, J.W., Schiller, W.R., and Blakemore, W.S.: Metabolic Response to Injury and Illness: Estimation of Energy and Protein Needs from Indirect Calorimetry and Nitrogen Balance. *JPEN*, Vol 3 (6): 452:1979. Used with permission.

**8–13** Other Anthropometric Measurement Procedures

**Anthropometric Measurement Procedures**

*Biceps skinfold thickness:* 1) place child in sitting position with right arm relaxed and flexed 90 degrees at the elbow; 2) use midpoint mark as in the triceps skinfold measure; 3) grasp the skin and the subcutaneous tissue on the bicep of the relaxed arm, which is flexed 90 degrees at the elbow; 4) place the calipers 1 cm below the fingers to the fatfold; and 5) read the biceps skinfold measurement with arm hanging freely and not compressed.

*Abdominal skinfold:* 1) place child in standing position breathing quietly; 2) grasp skin and subcutaneous tissues 3 cm to the right and 1 cm below the umbilical cord; and 3) apply the calipers horizontally to the abdominal skinfold.

*Thorax or midaxillary skinfold:* 1) place child in standing position with arms extended to shoulder line; 2) grasp skin and subcutaneous tissue parallel over the tenth rib or xiphi-sternal junction in the axillary line; and 3) place the calipers on a horizontal fold adjacent to the grasping fingers.

*Anterior thigh skinfold:* 1) extend child's leg flat on the bed; 2) measure the anterior upper thigh with a flexible tape from the lower pelvis to the upper knee cap, and mark the midpoint as for measuring thigh circumference; and 3) grasp the skin and subcutaneous fat at the mark, and apply the calipers 1 cm distal to the marked level.

*Anterior chest skinfold:* 1) place the child in standing position with the arm hanging relaxed at the side; 2) grasp the anterior axillary skinfold as high as possible. The long axis of the fold should slant medially and inferior; and 3) place the caliper perpendicular to the length of the fold about 1 cm below the fingers.

*Superilliac skinfold:* 1) place child in standing position; 2) select site in midaxillary line, superior to the illiac crest; and 3) apply the calipers parallel to the cleavage line of the skin, not quite horizontal.

*Thigh skinfold:* 1) use the thigh circumference marked area; 2) grasp a double fold of skin and subcutaneous tissue 1 cm distal to marked level; and 3) apply calipers perpendicular to fold at marked level.

*Chest circumference:* 1) place child in a sitting position with arms at side; and 2) apply the tape to the chest so as to encompass the areolae for boys and the axillae above the area of breast fullness for girls.

*Wrist circumference:* 1) place the child in a standing position, arm flexed at the elbow, palm side up (useful for frame size); and 2) apply tape perpendicular to long axis of the forearm, just distal to the styloid processes of the radius and ulna.

*Elbow breadth:* 1) elbow breadth is a good indicator of skeletal dimensions (frame size) because it is not affected by percent fat weight; 2) use sliding caliper on frameter (distributed by Health Products, 2126 Ridge, Ann Arbor, Michigan, 48104); 3) place child in a sitting position facing the examiner; 4) extend the right arm and bend the forearm toward the shoulder at a 90 degree angle, turning the palm of the hand toward the body and place the elbow on a table or board containing calipers; 5) slide the caliper jaws against the side the child's elbow; and 6) measure the greatest bony width across the elbow.

*Ankle breadth:* 1) place child in an erect, standing position with feet apart and weight evenly distributed; 2) use a sliding caliper; 3) with paddle blades of the sliding caliper, measure the minimum horizontal breadth of the right ankle (narrowest part) above the malleous (ankle bone).

# APPENDIX 9
# Adolescent Maturation Charts and Psychological Tests

**9–1** Male Pubertal Development, Tanner

## Pubertal development in size of male genitalia.

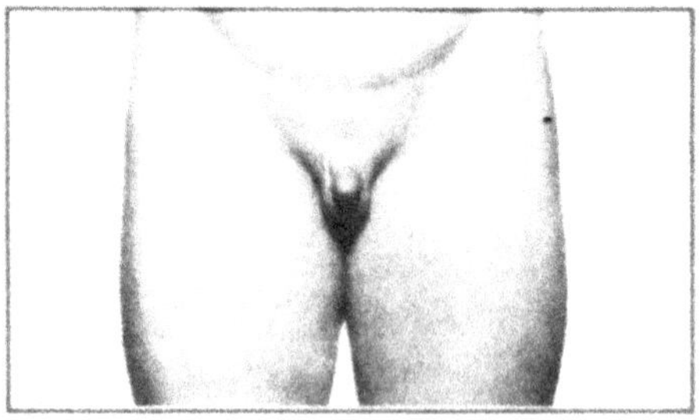

**Stage 1.** The penis, testes, and scrotum are of childhood size.

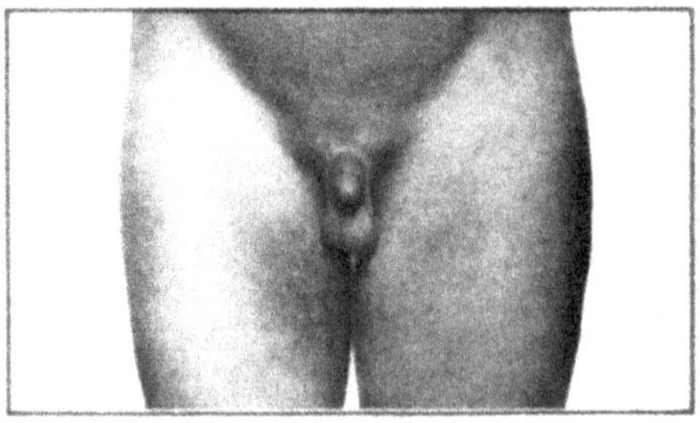

**Stage 2.** There is enlargement of the scrotum and testes, but the penis usually does not enlarge. The scrotal skin reddens.

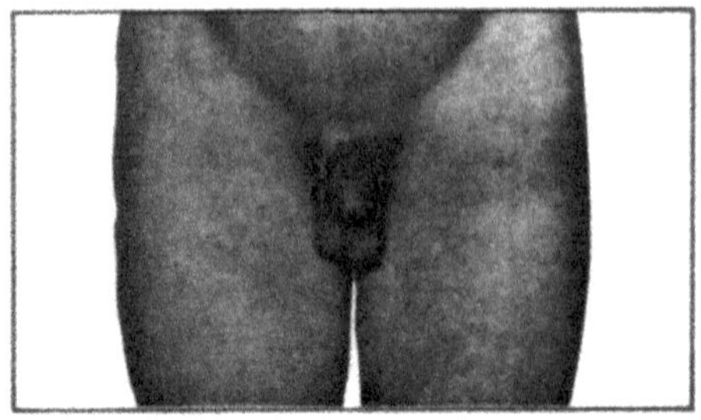

**Stage 3.** There is further growth of the testes and scotum and enlargement of the penis, mainly in length.

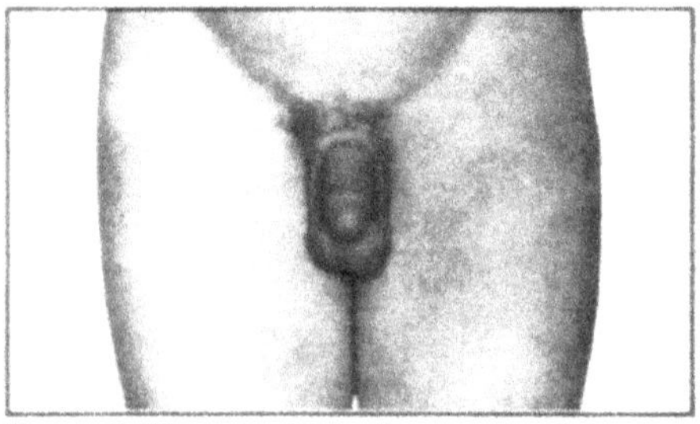

**Stage 4.** There is still further growth of the testes and scrotum and increased size of the penis, especially in breadth.

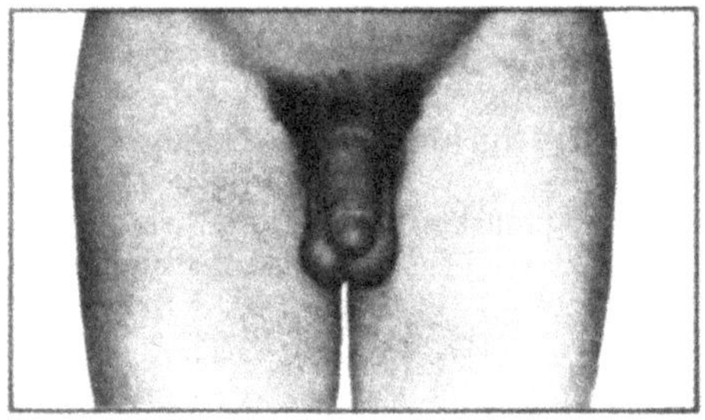

**Stage 5.** The genitalia are adult in size and shape.

## Pubertal development of male pubic hair.

**Stage 1.** There is no pubic hair.

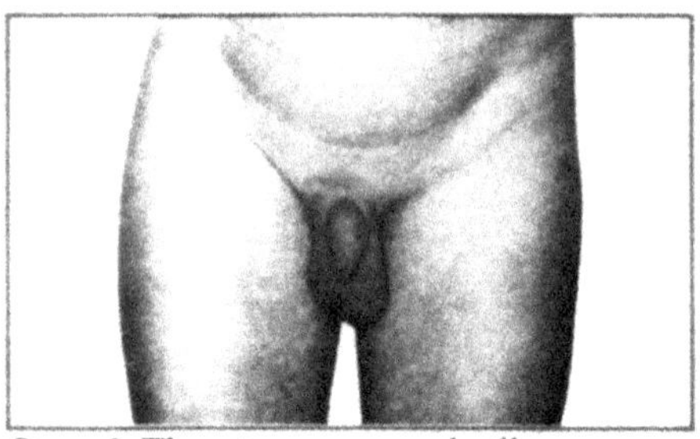

**Stage 2.** There is sparse growth of long, slightly pigmented, downy hair, straight or only slightly curled, primarily at the base of the penis.

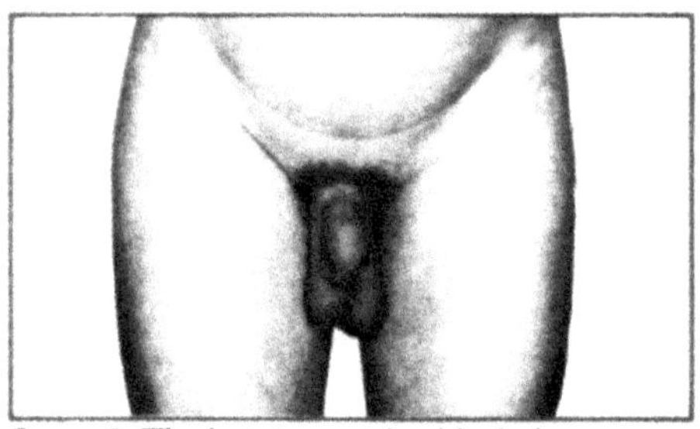

**Stage 3.** The hair is considerably darker, coarser, and more curled. The hair spreads sparsely over the junction of the pubes.

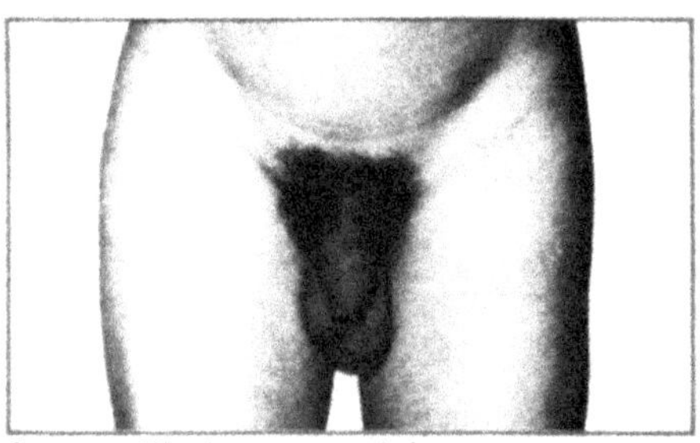

**Stage 4.** The hair, now adult in type, covers a smaller area than in the adult and does not extend onto the thighs.

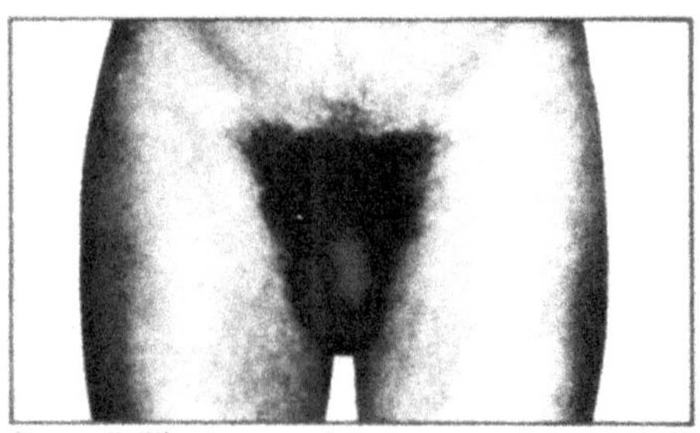

**Stage 5.** The hair is adult in quantity and type, with extension onto the thighs.

**9–2** Female Pubertal Development, Tanner

## Pubertal development in size of female breasts.

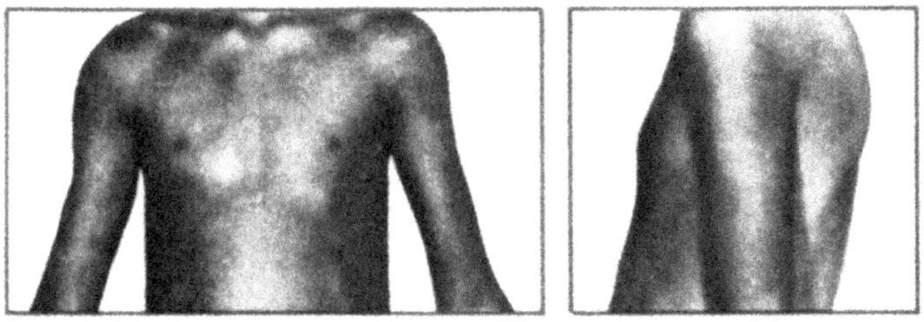

**Stage 1.** The breasts are preadolescent. There is elevation of the papilla only.

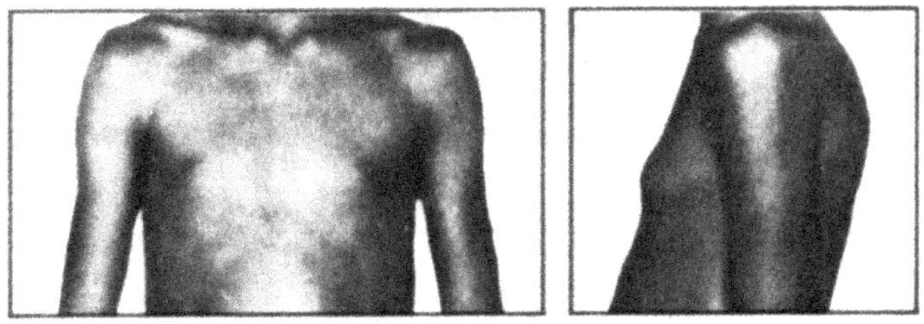

**Stage 2.** Breast bud stage. A small mound is formed by the elevation of the breast and papilla. The areolar diameter enlarges.

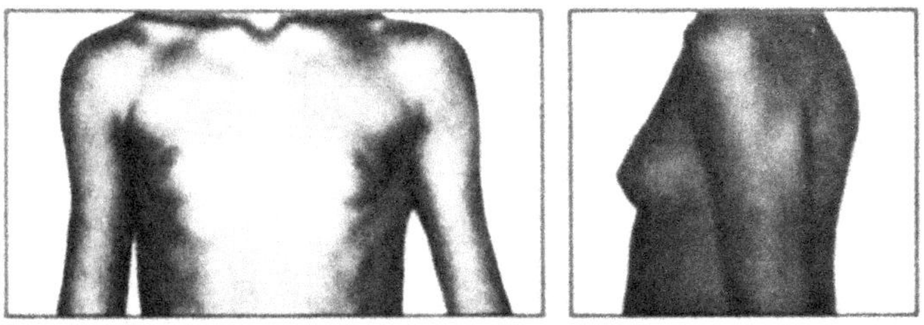

**Stage 3.** There is further enlargement of breasts and areola with no separation of their contours.

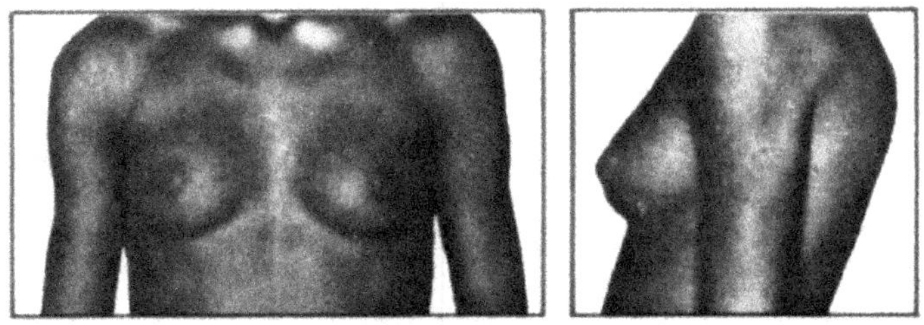

**Stage 4.** There is a projection of the areola and papilla to form a secondary mound above the level of the breast.

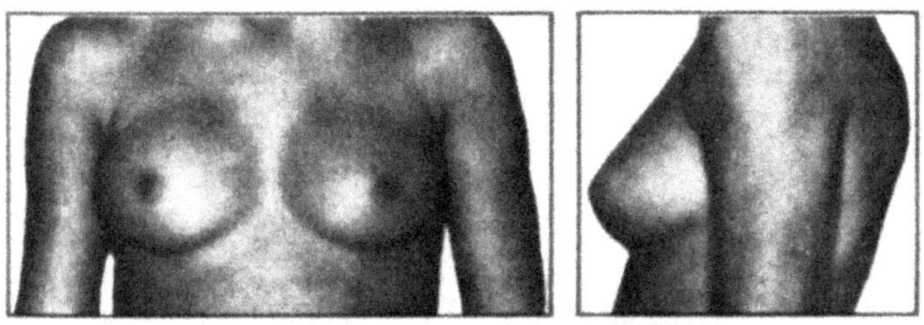

**Stage 5.** The breasts resemble those of a mature female as the areola has recessed to the general contour of the breast.

---

## Pubertal development of female pubic hair.

**Stage 1.** There is no pubic hair.

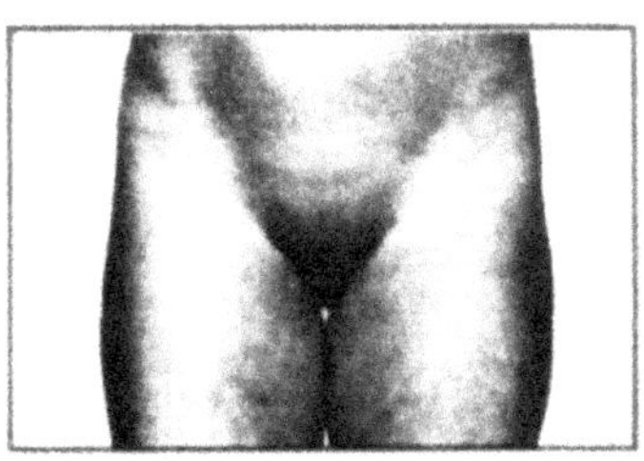

**Stage 2.** There is sparse growth of long, slightly pigmented, downy hair, straight or only slightly curled, primarily along the labia.

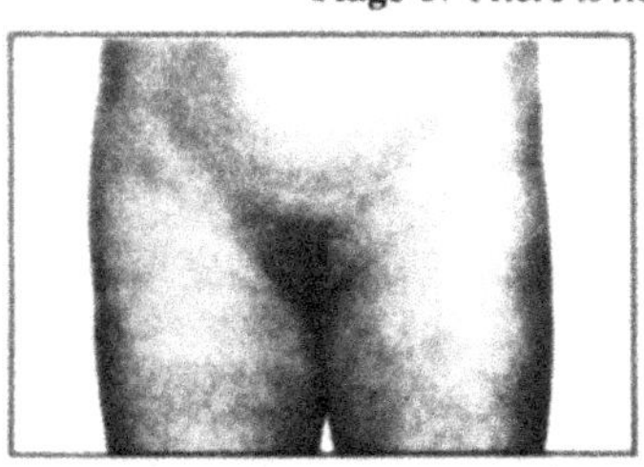

**Stage 3.** The hair is considerably darker, coarser, and more curled. The hair spreads sparsely over the junction of the pubes.

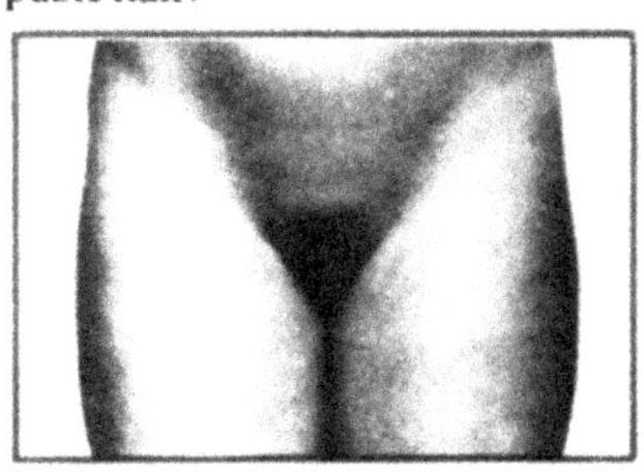

**Stage 4.** The hair, now adult in type, covers a smaller area than in the adult and does not extend onto the thighs.

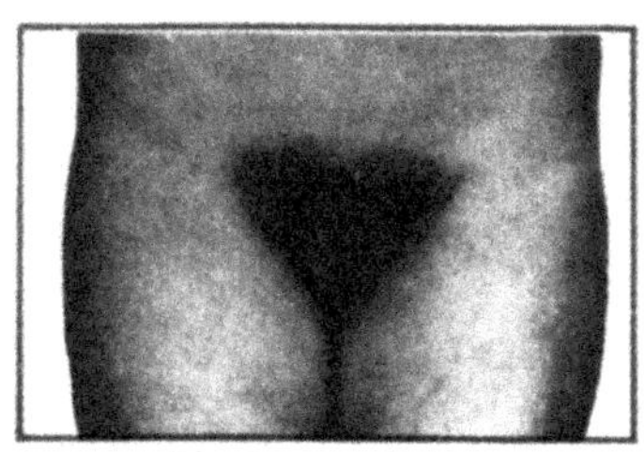

**Stage 5.** The hair is adult in quantity and type, with extension onto the thighs.

**9–3** Male and Female Sequence of Pubertal Events

## Sequence of Pubertal Events—Average American Male

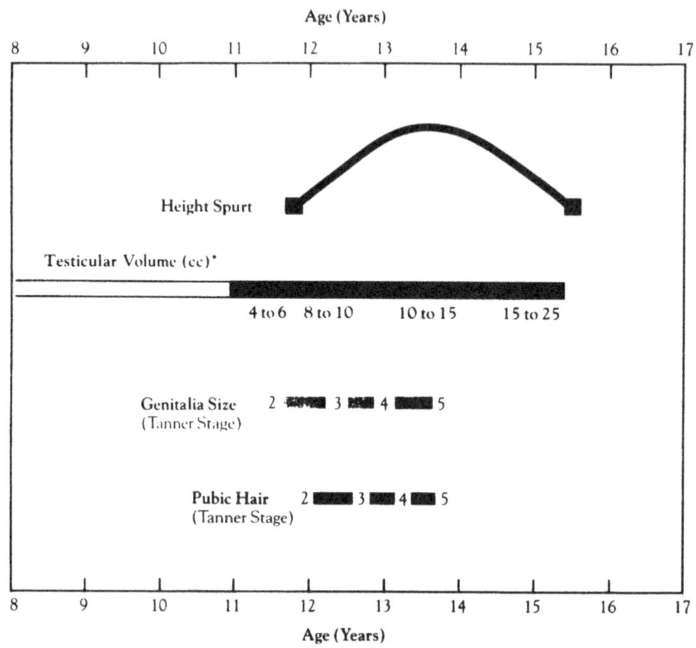


Adapted from Brookman RR, Rauh JL, Morrison JA, et al: The Princeton Maturation Study, 1976, unpublished data for adolescents in Cincinnati, Ohio.

*Testicular volume less than 4 cc using orchidometer (Prader Beads) represents prepubertal stage.

Prader Beads may be obtained from M. Benesch, Secretary to Professor Prader, Universitats-Kinderklinik, Steinwiesstrasse 75, CH-8032, Zurich, Switzerland. Enclose check for 70 Swiss francs and allow 4 to 5 months for delivery.

**9–3** (Continued)

# Sequence of Pubertal Events— Average American Female

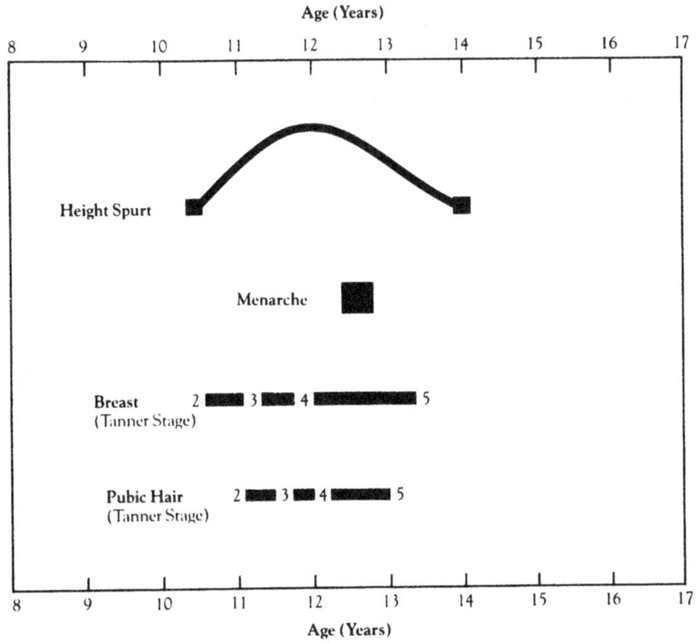


Adapted from Brookman RR, Rauh JL, Morrison JA, et al: The Princeton Maturation Study, 1976, unpublished data for adolescents in Cincinnati, Ohio.

**9–4** Hormonal Correlates of Physical Maturation, Males and Females

| | MATURATIONAL STAGE | | | | | |
|---|---|---|---|---|---|---|
| | I | II | III | IV | V | Adult |
| Follicle-stimulating hormone (mIU/ml)* | | | | | | |
| Male mean - 21 Range 16–21 | 4.5 | 5.9 | 8.1 | 8.5 | 8.0 | range 5.0–20.0 |
| Female mean - 21 | 4.2 | 5.5 | 8.0 | 8.0 | 12.3 | range 4.0–20.0 |
| Luteinizing hormone (mIU/ml)* | | | | | | |
| Male mean - 21 Range 16–21 | 3.9 | 6.8 | 8.5 | 9.5 | 11.5 | range 5.0–20.0 |
| Female mean - 21 | 2.9 | 3.9 | 8.4 | 11.3 | 18.9 | range 4.0–25.0 |
| Follicle-stimulating hormone (mIU/ml)** | | | | | | |
| Male mean - 24 | 3.8 | 3.9 | 6.8 | 7.4 | 6.4 | |
| Luteinzing hormone (mIU/ml)** | | | | | | |
| Male mean - 24 | 5.4 | 5.6 | 7.5 | 9.1 | 9.3 | |
| Follicle stimulating hormone (IU)++ | | | | | | |
| Male mean - 22 | 1.6 | 3.2 | 3.7 | 4.7 | 2.8 | |
| Female mean - 22 | 1.5 | 4.0 | 6.0 | 3.8 | 2.3 | |
| Luteinizing hormone (IU)++ | | | | | | |
| Male mean - 22 | 2.0 | 5.9 | 13.5 | 17.0 | 21.6 | |
| Female mean - 22 | 1.9 | 5.0 | 13.7 | 14.9 | 16.6 | |
| Prolactin (mIU/ml)** | | | | | | |
| Male mean - | 3.6–10.3 | 2.4–18.9 | 3.0–15.2 | 4.3–18.1 | 3.1–15.7 | |
| Female mean - 20 | 3.8–13.5 | 3.1–11.7 | 3.8–19.2 | 4.2–16.8 | 5.0–18.0 | |
| Estrone (ng/dl)* | | | | | | |
| Male mean - 16 | 2.0 | 3.0 | 3.0 | 4.0 | 3.0 | range 2.0– 6.0 |
| Female mean - 16 | 4.0 | 5.0 | 7.0 | 12.0 | 3.0 | range 2.0–18.2 |
| Estradiol (ng/dl)* | | | | | | |
| Male mean - 16 | 2.0 | 1.0 | 2.0 | 4.0 | 3.0 | range 1.5– 5.0 |
| Female mean - 16 | 2.0 | 3.0 | 13.0 | 16.0 | 8.0 | range 1.5–40.0 |
| Progesterone (ng/dl)* | | | | | | |
| Male mean - 21 | 30.0 | 36.0 | 40.0 | 40.0 | 35.0 | range 16– 60 |
| Female mean - 21 | 10–13 | 16.0 | 16–23 | 30–161 | 29–75 (follicular) | range 20–2000 |
| 17-hydroxyprogesterone (ng/dl)* | | | | | | |
| Male mean - 21 | 30–60 | 34–40 | 52–62 | 78–93 | 97.0 | range 38–200 |
| Female mean - 21 | 32–38 | 38–52 | 55–69 | 101–127 | 11–80 | range |
| Testosterone (ng/dl)* | | | | | | |
| Male mean - 16 | 10 | 18 | 52 | 170 | 350 | range 300–800 |
| Female mean - 16 | 11 | 19 | 28 | 48 | 38 | range 15– 85 |
| Dehydrotestosterone (ng/dl)* | | | | | | |
| Male mean - 16 | 3 | 4 | 13 | 26 | 16 | range 30–80 |
| Female mean - 21 | 2–16 | 3–24 | 9–25 | 9–32 | | range 10–32 |
| Androstenedione (nd/dl)* | | | | | | |
| Male mean - 16 | 54 | 49 | 85 | 69 | 90 | range 100–180 |
| Female mean - 16 | 35 | 72 | 103 | 176 | 141 | range 40–300 |
| Dehydroepiandrosterone (ng/dl)* | | | | | | |
| Male mean - 16 | 192 | 300 | 396 | 396 | 450 | range 200–700 |
| Female mean - 16 | 133 | 326 | 427 | 498 | 741 | range 200–1500 |
| Dehydroepiandrosterone sulfate (mg/dl)* | | | | | | |
| Male mean - 33 | 42 | 63 | 73 | 103 | 123 | range 125–300 |
| Female mean - 33 | 43 | 49 | 71 | 86 | 120 | range 125–300 |
| Testosterone (ng/dl)* | | | | | | |
| Male mean - 24 | 31 | 132 | 368 | 423 | 490 | |

* plasma ** serum ++ 24 hour urine collection

9–5 Body Composition of Reference Adolescents

| Age (years) | Height (cm) | Weight (kg) | Fat (kg) | Fat (%) | FFBM (kg) | Components of Fat-Free Body Mass (FFBM) (% of body weight) Protein | Water Total Body | Water Extracellular | Water Cellular | Minerals OM | Minerals NOM | Carbohydrate | FFBM Density (g/cm$^{-3}$) |
|---|---|---|---|---|---|---|---|---|---|---|---|---|---|
| Males | | | | | | | | | | | | | |
| 10.5 | 140.3 | 33.30 | 5.34 | 16.0 | 27.96 | 16.2 | 63.1 | 27.2 | 36.0 | 3.3 | 0.9 | 0.6 | 1.086 |
| 11.5 | 146.4 | 37.46 | 6.46 | 17.2 | 31.00 | 16.1 | 62.2 | 26.5 | 35.7 | 3.2 | 0.8 | 0.6 | 1.086 |
| 12.5 | 153.0 | 42.27 | 6.90 | 16.3 | 35.37 | 16.4 | 62.7 | 26.4 | 36.4 | 3.2 | 0.9 | 0.6 | 1.086 |
| 13.5 | 159.9 | 47.81 | 7.05 | 14.8 | 40.76 | 16.8 | 63.7 | 26.4 | 37.3 | 3.4 | 0.9 | 0.6 | 1.087 |
| 14.5 | 166.2 | 53.76 | 7.32 | 13.6 | 46.44 | 17.1 | 64.4 | 26.2 | 38.2 | 3.5 | 0.9 | 0.6 | 1.088 |
| 15.5 | 171.5 | 59.51 | 7.73 | 13.0 | 51.78 | 17.4 | 64.6 | 25.8 | 38.8 | 3.6 | 0.9 | 0.6 | 1.090 |
| 16.5 | 175.2 | 64.39 | 8.22 | 12.8 | 56.17 | 17.6 | 64.5 | 25.4 | 39.1 | 3.8 | 0.9 | 0.6 | 1.091 |
| 17.5 | 176.7 | 67.78 | 8.61 | 12.7 | 59.17 | 17.7 | 64.4 | 25.0 | 39.4 | 3.8 | 0.9 | 0.7 | 1.092 |
| 18.5 | 177.0 | 69.88 | 9.01 | 12.9 | 60.87 | 17.7 | 64.1 | 24.7 | 39.4 | 3.9 | 0.9 | 0.7 | 1.093 |
| Females | | | | | | | | | | | | | |
| 10.5 | 141.5 | 34.72 | 8.14 | 23.5 | 26.58 | 15.0 | 57.3 | 25.3 | 32.0 | 3.0 | 0.8 | 0.5 | 1.087 |
| 11.5 | 148.2 | 39.23 | 8.90 | 22.7 | 30.33 | 15.2 | 57.7 | 25.4 | 32.3 | 3.2 | 0.8 | 0.5 | 1.088 |
| 12.5 | 154.6 | 43.84 | 9.41 | 21.5 | 34.43 | 15.4 | 58.5 | 25.6 | 32.9 | 3.4 | 0.8 | 0.5 | 1.090 |
| 13.5 | 159.0 | 48.26 | 10.53 | 21.8 | 37.73 | 15.4 | 58.0 | 25.2 | 32.8 | 3.6 | 0.8 | 0.5 | 1.092 |
| 14.5 | 161.2 | 52.10 | 12.09 | 23.2 | 40.01 | 15.1 | 56.8 | 24.4 | 32.4 | 3.6 | 0.8 | 0.5 | 1.093 |
| 15.5 | 162.1 | 54.96 | 13.59 | 24.7 | 41.37 | 14.9 | 55.5 | 23.7 | 31.8 | 3.7 | 0.8 | 0.5 | 1.094 |
| 16.5 | 162.7 | 56.44 | 14.34 | 25.4 | 42.10 | 14.8 | 54.9 | 23.4 | 31.6 | 3.7 | 0.7 | 0.4 | 1.095 |
| 17.5 | 163.4 | 56.71 | 14.28 | 25.2 | 42.43 | 14.8 | 55.1 | 23.4 | 31.7 | 3.7 | 0.7 | 0.4 | 1.095 |
| 18.5 | 164.0 | 56.97 | 14.24 | 25.0 | 42.77 | 14.9 | 55.2 | 23.5 | 31.7 | 3.7 | 0.7 | 0.4 | 1.096 |

OM = osseous minerals, NOM = nonosseous minerals

From Haschke, F.: Body Composition During Adolescence. In Klish, W.J. and Kretchmer, N. (Eds.): Body Composition Measurements in Infants and Children, Report of the Ninety-Eighth Ross Conference on Pediatric Research, Columbus, Ohio, Ross Laboratories, 1989, p. 78. Used with permission.

DRIVE FOR THINNESS: Subscale Items
I eat sweets and carbohydrates without feeling nervous.
I think about dieting.
I feel extremely guilty after overeating.
I am terrified of gaining weight
I exaggerate or magnify the importance of weight.
I am preoccupied with the desire to be thinner.
If I gain a pound, I worry that I will keep gaining.

INTEROCEPTIVE AWARENESS: Subscale Items
I get frightened when my feelings are too strong.
I get confused about what emotion I am feeling.
I can clearly identify what emotion I am feeling.
I don't know what's going on inside me.
I get confused as to whether or not I am hungry.
I worry that my feelings will get out of control.
I feel bloated after eating a small meal.
When I am upset, I don't know if I am sad, frightened or angry.
I have feelings I can't quite identify.
When I am upset, I worry that I will start eating.

BULIMIA: Subscale Items
I eat when I am upset.
I stuff myself with food.
I have gone on eating binges where I have felt that I could not stop.
I thing about binging (overeating).
I eat moderately in front of others and stuff myself when they're gone.
I have the thought of trying to vomit in order to lose weight.
I eat or drink in secrecy.

BODY DISSATISFACTION: Subscale Item
I think that my stomach is too big.
I think that my thighs are too large.
I think that my stomach is just the right size.
I feel satisfied with the shape of my body.
I like the shape of my buttocks.
I think my hips are too big.
I think that my thighs are just the right size.
I think my buttocks are too large.
I think that my hips are just the right size.

INEFFECTIVENESS: Subscale Items
I feel ineffective as a person.
I feel alone in the world.
I feel generally in control of things in my life.
I wish I were someone else.
I feel inadequate.
I feel secure about myself.
I have a low opinion of myself.
I feel that I can achieve my standards.
I feel that I am a worthwhile person.
I feel empty inside (emotionally).

MATURITY FEARS: Subscale Items
I wish that I could return to the security of childhood.
I wish that I could be younger.
The happiest time in life is when you are a child.
I would rather be an adult than a child.
The demands of adulthood are too great.
I feel happy that I am not a child anymore.
I feel that people are happiest when they are children.
The best years of your life are when you become an adult.

PERFECTIONISM: Subscale Items
Only outstanding performance is good enough in my family.
As a child, I tried very hard to avoid disappointing my parents and teachers.
I hate being less than best at things.
My parents have expected excellence of me.
I feel that I must do things perfectly or not do them at all.
I have extremely high goals.

INTERPERSONAL DISTRUST: Subscale Items
I am open about my feelings.
I trust others.
I can communicate with others easily.
I have close relationships.
I have trouble expressing my emotions to others.
I need to keep people at a certain distance (feel uncomfortable if someone tries to get too close).
I can talk about personal thoughts or feelings.

Adapted from: Garner, D.M., Olmstead, M.P., and Polivy, J.: Development and validation of a multidimensional eating disorder inventory for anorexia nervosa and bulimia. *Int'l J Eating Disorders,* 2(2):15, 1989.

SELF

1. Am terrified about being overweight.
2. Avoid eating when I am hungry.
3. Find myself preoccupied with food.
4. Have gone on eating binges where I feel that I may not be able to stop.
5. Cut my food into small pieces.
6. Am aware of the calorie content of foods that I eat.
7. Particularly avoid foods with a high carbohydrate content (e.g. bread, rice, potatoes, etc.).
8. Feel that others would prefer if I ate more.
9. Vomit after I eat.
10. Feel extremely guilty after eating.
11. Am preoccupied with a desire to be thinner.
12. Think about burning calories when I exercise.
13. Other people think that I am too thin.
14. Am preoccupied with the thought of having fat on my body.
15. Take longer than others to eat my meals.
16. Avoid foods with sugar in them.
17. Eat diet foods.
18. Feel that food controls my life.
19. Display self-control around food.
20. Feel that others pressure me to eat.
21. Give too much time and thought to food.
22. Feel uncomfortable after eating sweets.
23. Engage in dieting behavior.
24. Like my stomach to be empty.
25. Enjoy trying new rich foods.
26. Have the impulse to vomit after meals.
27. Exercise to prevent weight gain.
28. Use laxatives or diuretics to prevent weight gain.

PARENT

1. Is terrified about being overweight.
2. Avoids eating when she is hungry.
3. Is preoccupied with food.
4. Has gone on eating binges where she is not able to stop.
5. Cuts her food into small pieces.
6. Is aware of the calorie content of foods that she eats.
7. Particularly avoids foods with a high carbohydrate content (e.g. bread, rice, potatoes, etc).
8. Feels that others would prefer if she ate more.
9. Vomits after she eats.
10. Feels extremely guilty after eating.
11. Is preoccupied with a desire to be thinner.
12. Thinks about burning up calories when she exercises.
13. Feels other epople think she is too thin.
14. Is preoccupied with the thought of having fat on her body.
15. Takes longer than others to eat her meals.
16. Avoids foods with sugar in them.
17. Eats diet foods.
18. Feels that food controls her life.
19. Displays self-control around food.
20. Feels that others pressure her to eat.
21. Gives too much time and thought to food.
22. Feels uncomfortable after eating sweets.
23. Engages in dieting behavior.
24. Likes her stomach to be empty.
25. Enjoys trying new rich foods.
26. Has the impulse to vomit after meals.
27. Exercises to prevent weight gain.
28. Uses laxatives or diuretics to prevent weight gain.

0 = Never  1 = Rarelv  2 = Sometimes  3 = Often  4 = Usuallv  5 = Always

Adapted from: Kagan, D.M. and Squires, R.L.: Eating disorders among adolescents: patterns and prevalence. *Adolesc*, 19(73):15, 1984. Kagan, D.M. and Squires, R.L.: Dieting, compulsive eating and feelings of failure among adolescents. *Int'l J Eating Disorders*, 3(1):15, 1983.

## 9–8 Depression Inventory (Symptoms, Attitude, Categories)

A (Mood)
0 I do not feel sad
1 I feel blue or sad
2a I am blue or sad all the time and I can't snap out of it
2b I am so sad or unhappy that it is very painful
3 I am so sad or unhappy that I can't stand it

B (Pessimism)
0 I am not particularly pessimistic or discouraged about the future
1a I feel discouraged about the future
2a I feel I have nothing to look forward to
2b I feel that I won't ever get over my troubles
3 I feel that the future is hopeless and that things cannot improve

C (Sense of Failure)
0 I do not feel like a failure
1 I feel I have failed more than the average person
2a I feel I have accomplished very little that is worthwhile or that means anything
2b As I look back on my life all I can see is a lot of failures
3 I feel I am a complete failure as a person (parent, husband, wife)

D (Lack of Satisfaction)
0 I am not particularly dissatisfied
1a I feel bored most of the time
1b I don't enjoy things the way I used to
2 I don't get satisfaction out of anything any more
3 I am dissatisfied with everything

E (Guilty Feeling)
0 I don't feel particularly guilty
1 I feel bad or unworthy a good part of the time
2a I feel quite guilty
2b I feel bad or unworthy practically all the time now
3 I feel as though I am very bad or worthless

*Scoring: None, mild, moderate, severe

F (Sense of Punishment)
0 I don't feel I am being punished
1 I feel that something bad may happen to me
2 I feel I am being punished or will be punished
3a I feel I deserve to be punished
3b I want to be punished

G (Self Hate)
0 I don't feel disappointed in myself
1a I am disappointed in myself
1b I don't like myself
2 I am disgusted with myself
3 I hate myself

H (Self Accusations)
0 I don't feel I am any worse than anybody else
1 I am very critical of myself for my weaknesses or mistakes
2a I blame myself for everything that goes wrong

I (Self-Punitive Thoughts)
0 I don't have any thought of harming myself
1 I have thoughts of harming myself but I would not carry them out
2a I feel I would be better off dead
2b I have definite plans about committing suicide
2c I feel my family would be better off if I were dead
3 I would kill myself if I could

J (Crying Spells)
0 I don't cry any more than usual
1 I cry more now than I used to
2 I cry all the time now. I can't stop it
3 I used to be able to cry but now I can't cry at all even though I want to

K (Irratability)
0 I am no more irritated now that I ever am
1 I get annoyed or irritated more easily than I used to
2 I feel irritated all the time now
3 I don't get irritated at all the things that used to irritate me

L (Social Withdrawal)
0 I have not lost interest in other people
1 I am less interested in other people now than I used to be
2 I have lost all my interest in other people and have little feeling for them
3 I have lost all my interest in other poeple and don't care about them at all

M (Indecisiveness)
0 I make decisions about as well as ever
1 I am less sure of myself now try to put off making decisions
2 I can't make decisions at all without help
3 I can't make any decisions at all any more

N (Body Image)
0 I don't feel I look any worse than I used to
1 I am worried that I am looking old or unattractive
2 I feel that there are permanent changes in my appearance and they make me look unattractive
3 I feel that I am ugly or repulsive looking

O (Work Inhibition)
0 I can work about as well as before
1a It takes extra effort to get started at doing something
1b I don't work as well as I used to
2 I have to push myself very hard to do anything
3 I can't do any work at all

P (Sleep Disturbance)
0 I can sleep as well as usual
1 I wake up more tired in the morning than I used to
2 I wake up 1-2 hours earlier than usual and find it hard to get back to sleep
3 I wake up early every day and can't get more than 5 hours sleep

Q (Fatigability)
0 I don't get any more tired than usual
1 I get tired more easily than I used to
2 I get tired from doing anything
3 I get too tired to do anything

R (Loss of Appetite)
0 My appetite is no worse than usual
1 My appetite is not as good as it used to be
2 My appetite is much worse now
3 I have no appetite at all any more

S (Weight Loss)
0 I haven't lost much weight, if any, lately
1 I have lost more than 5 pounds
2 I have lost more than 10 pounds
3 I have lost more than 15 pounds

T (Somatic Preoccupation)
0 I am no more concerned about my health than usual
1 I am concerned about aches and pains or upset stomach or constipation or other upleasant feelings in my body
2 I am so concerned with how I feel or what I feel that it's hard to think of much else
3 I am completely absorbed in what I feel

U (Loss of Libido)
0 I have not noticed any recent change in my interest in sex
1 I am less interested in sex than I used to be
2 I am much less interested in sex now
3 I have lost interest in sex completely

Adapted from Kagan, D.M., Squires, R.L. Eating disorders among adolescents: patterns and prevalence. *Adolescence* 1984;19(73):15. Kagan, D.M., Squires, R.L. Dieting, compulsive eating and feelings of failure among adolescents. *Int. J. Eat. Disord.* 1983;3(1):15.
Van der Ster Wallin, G., Hambraeus, L. An anthropometric and biochemical assessment of nutritional status in eating disordered patients: is there a problem of interpretation? *Nutr. Res.* 1996;16(7):1095.

**9–9** Twelve Step Approach for Eating Disorders and Questionnaire on Health and Nutrition for the Homeless

1. Admit being powerless over food
2. Request power within self to restore self to sanity.
3. Make decisions to turn life over to God.
4. Make searching and fearless inventory of self.
5. Confess to God, self, and another person that eating habits are bad.
6. Be entirely ready to ask God to remove all defects of character.
7. Humbly ask God to remove all shortcomings.
8. Make a list of all people harmed and make willing amends.
9. Make direct amends.
10. Continue to take personal inventory, and admit any wrong doings.
11. Seek through prayer and meditation a conscience which is content with God.
12. Having had a spiritual awakening, try to carry this message to other people with eating disorders and practice these principles in all affairs.

From: Devlin, C. L., Twelve Step Approach Intervention in Compulsive Eating. *J Am Diet Assoc*, 1991:A186.

Percentage of 96 homeless persons answering "yes" to questions on a health and nutrition questionnaire.

| Question | Yes % |
|---|---|
| 1. Do you have enough to eat? | 90 |
| 2. Do you have a good appetite? | 73 |
| 3. Are there cooking facilities available to you? | 43 |
| 4. How many meals do you prepare for yourself per day? | |
| 0 meals | 57 |
| 1 meal | 16 |
| 2–3 meals | 27 |
| 5. Do you have any money to buy food? How much per week? | |
| 0 dollars | 15 |
| 20 dollars | 31 |
| 21–50 dollars | 38 |
| 51 dollars or more | 16 |
| 6. Have you been told by an M.D. that you should or should not eat particular foods? | 52 |
| 7. If yes, are you able to follow this diet? | 48 |
| 8. Do you smoke cigarettes? | 65 |
| 9. Do you drink alcohol? | 32 |
| 10. Do you use street drugs? | 5 |
| 11. Do you use vitamin supplements? | 47 |
| 12. Has your weight changed over the past year? | 58 |
| If yes, did it go up? | 47 |
| Or, did it go down? | 53 |
| 13. Do you have any medical conditions? | 89 |
| If yes, are you taking medications for these conditions? | 98 |

From: Luder, E., Cupens-Okado, E., Karen-Roth, A., Martinez-Weber, C. Health and nutrition survey in a group of urban homeless adults. *J Am Diet Assoc*, 1990, 90:1387.

**9–10** Attention Deficit Hyperactivity Disorder (ADHD) Assessment Scale

Today's Date: ___________ Child's Name: ______________________________ Date of Birth: ______________

Parent's Name: ______________________________ Parent's Phone Number: ______________________

**Directions: Each rating should be considered in the context of what is appropriate for the age of your child. When completing this form, please think about your child's behaviors in the past 6 months.**

**Is this evaluation based on a time when the child ☐ was on medication ☐ was not on medication ☐ not sure?**

| Symptoms | Never | Occasionally | Often | Very Often |
|---|---|---|---|---|
| 1. Does not pay attention to details or makes careless mistakes with, for example, homework | 0 | 1 | 2 | 3 |
| 2. Has difficulty keeping attention to what needs to be done | 0 | 1 | 2 | 3 |
| 3. Does not seem to listen when spoken to directly | 0 | 1 | 2 | 3 |
| 4. Does not follow through when given directions and fails to finish activities (not due to refusal or failure to understand) | 0 | 1 | 2 | 3 |
| 5. Has difficulty organizing tasks and activities | 0 | 1 | 2 | 3 |
| 6. Avoids, dislikes, or does not want to start tasks that require ongoing mental effort | 0 | 1 | 2 | 3 |
| 7. Loses things necessary for tasks or activities (toys, assignments, pencils, or books) | 0 | 1 | 2 | 3 |
| 8. Is easily distracted by noises or other stimuli | 0 | 1 | 2 | 3 |
| 9. Is forgetful in daily activities | 0 | 1 | 2 | 3 |
| 10. Fidgets with hands or feet or squirms in seat | 0 | 1 | 2 | 3 |
| 11. Leaves seat when remaining seated is expected | 0 | 1 | 2 | 3 |
| 12. Runs about or climbs too much when remaining seated is expected | 0 | 1 | 2 | 3 |
| 13. Has difficulty playing or beginning quiet play activities | 0 | 1 | 2 | 3 |
| 14. Is "on the go" or often acts as if "driven by a motor" | 0 | 1 | 2 | 3 |
| 15. Talks too much | 0 | 1 | 2 | 3 |
| 16. Blurts out answers before questions have been completed | 0 | 1 | 2 | 3 |
| 17. Has difficulty waiting his or her turn | 0 | 1 | 2 | 3 |
| 18. Interrupts or intrudes in on others' conversations and/or activities | 0 | 1 | 2 | 3 |
| 19. Argues with adults | 0 | 1 | 2 | 3 |
| 20. Loses temper | 0 | 1 | 2 | 3 |
| 21. Actively defies or refuses to go along with adults' requests or rules | 0 | 1 | 2 | 3 |
| 22. Deliberately annoys people | 0 | 1 | 2 | 3 |
| 23. Blames others for his or her mistakes or misbehaviors | 0 | 1 | 2 | 3 |
| 24. Is touchy or easily annoyed by others | 0 | 1 | 2 | 3 |
| 25. Is angry or resentful | 0 | 1 | 2 | 3 |
| 26. Is spiteful and wants to get even | 0 | 1 | 2 | 3 |
| 27. Bullies, threatens, or intimidates others | 0 | 1 | 2 | 3 |
| 28. Starts physical fights | 0 | 1 | 2 | 3 |
| 29. Lies to get out of trouble or to avoid obligations (ie, "cons" others) | 0 | 1 | 2 | 3 |
| 30. Is truant from school (skips school) without permission | 0 | 1 | 2 | 3 |
| 31. Is physically cruel to people | 0 | 1 | 2 | 3 |
| 32. Has stolen things that have value | 0 | 1 | 2 | 3 |

The information contained in this publication should not be used as a substitute for the medical care and advice of your pediatrician. There may be variations in treatment that your pediatrician may recommend based on individual facts and circumstances.



Adapted from the Vanderbilt Rating Scales developed by Mark L. Wolraich, MD.

Revised - 1102

American Academy of Pediatrics

DEDICATED TO THE HEALTH OF ALL CHILDREN™

NICHQ

National Initiative for Children's Healthcare Quality

McNeil

Consumer & Specialty Pharmaceuticals

HE0350

**9–10** (Continued)

Today's Date: ___________ Child's Name: ______________________________ Date of Birth: ____________

Parent's Name: ______________________________ Parent's Phone Number: ____________________

| Symptoms (continued) | Never | Occasionally | Often | Very Often |
|---|---|---|---|---|
| 33. Deliberately destroys others' property | 0 | 1 | 2 | 3 |
| 34. Has used a weapon that can cause serious harm (bat, knife, brick, gun) | 0 | 1 | 2 | 3 |
| 35. Is physically cruel to animals | 0 | 1 | 2 | 3 |
| 36. Has deliberately set fires to cause damage | 0 | 1 | 2 | 3 |
| 37. Has broken into someone else's home, business, or car | 0 | 1 | 2 | 3 |
| 38. Has stayed out at night without permission | 0 | 1 | 2 | 3 |
| 39. Has run away from home overnight | 0 | 1 | 2 | 3 |
| 40. Has forced someone into sexual activity | 0 | 1 | 2 | 3 |
| 41. Is fearful, anxious, or worried | 0 | 1 | 2 | 3 |
| 42. Is afraid to try new things for fear of making mistakes | 0 | 1 | 2 | 3 |
| 43. Feels worthless or inferior | 0 | 1 | 2 | 3 |
| 44. Blames self for problems, feels guilty | 0 | 1 | 2 | 3 |
| 45. Feels lonely, unwanted, or unloved; complains that "no one loves him or her" | 0 | 1 | 2 | 3 |
| 46. Is sad, unhappy, or depressed | 0 | 1 | 2 | 3 |
| 47. Is self-conscious or easily embarrassed | 0 | 1 | 2 | 3 |

| Performance | Excellent | Above Average | Average | Somewhat of a Problem | Problematic |
|---|---|---|---|---|---|
| 48. Overall school performance | 1 | 2 | 3 | 4 | 5 |
| 49. Reading | 1 | 2 | 3 | 4 | 5 |
| 50. Writing | 1 | 2 | 3 | 4 | 5 |
| 51. Mathematics | 1 | 2 | 3 | 4 | 5 |
| 52. Relationship with parents | 1 | 2 | 3 | 4 | 5 |
| 53. Relationship with siblings | 1 | 2 | 3 | 4 | 5 |
| 54. Relationship with peers | 1 | 2 | 3 | 4 | 5 |
| 55. Participation in organized activities (eg, teams) | 1 | 2 | 3 | 4 | 5 |

**Comments:**

**For Office Use Only**

Total number of questions scored 2 or 3 in questions 1–9: ____________

Total number of questions scored 2 or 3 in questions 10–18: ____________

Total Symptom Score for questions 1–18: ____________

Total number of questions scored 2 or 3 in questions 19–26: ____________

Total number of questions scored 2 or 3 in questions 27–40: ____________

Total number of questions scored 2 or 3 in questions 41–47: ____________

Total number of questions scored 4 or 5 in questions 48–55: ____________

Average Performance Score: ____________

American Academy of Pediatrics

DEDICATED TO THE HEALTH OF ALL CHILDREN™

NICHQ

National Initiative for Children's Healthcare Quality

McNeil Consumer & Specialty Pharmaceuticals

11-19/rev1102

**9–11** Pediatric Behavior Scale—ADHD

This checklist asks you to provide some information about your child's behavior. Below is a list of items that describe common behavior problems in children. Some of the items may be true of your child and some may not. Similar items are listed together. Please read each statement and decide how well it describes your child during the past two months.

1. Disobedient; won't mind or follow rules
2. Argues or quarrels
3. Uncooperative; won't help or work together with others
4. Defies authority or talks back
5. Mean or cruel to others
6. Threatens, bullies, or picks on other children
7. Starts fights
8. Hits, bites, or throws things at people
9. Destructive; breaks or smashes things on purpose
10. Lies or cheats
11. Steals
12. Hangs around with "bad" friends who often get into trouble
13. Explosive, unpredictable, or violent outbursts
14. Irritable; gets angry or annoyed easily
15. Overreacts to minor problems; "flies off the handle"
16. Loses temper; has temper tantrums
17. Shouts or screams a lot
18. Excitable; gets "wound up" easily
19. Can't concentrate or pay attention for long; short attention span
20. Easily distracted
21. Shifts frequently from one activity to another
22. Doesn't listen to directions
23. Fails to finish things he or she starts
24. Impulsive; acts without stopping to think
25. Can't stand waiting, wants things right away
26. Interrupts, talks out of turn, or blurts things out
27. Grabs for things; gets "into" everything
28. Rushes into danger without thinking about getting hurt
29. Hyperactive; always "on the go"
30. Restless; can't sit still
31. Squirms or fidgets
32. Constantly in motion; rarely slows down
33. Always running about or climbing on things
34. Tense, can't seem to relax
35. Nervous, "jumpy," or jittery; seems "on edge"
36. Nervous movements, shaking, or twitching
37. Picks at things (such as skin, clothes, or hair)
38. Fearful, anxious, or worried
39. Shy or timid
40. Self-conscious or easily embarrassed
41. Afraid to try new things for fear of making mistakes
42. Makes self "sick" with worry
43. Clings to adults or is too dependent on others
44. Panic attacks, gets so worried or upset that he/she can't be easily comforted
45. Feelings are easily hurt; sensitive to criticism
46. Lacks self-confidence; has low self-esteem
47. Feels worthless or inferior
48. Blames self for problems; feels guilty
49. Feels lonely, unwanted, or unloved; complains that no one loves him/her
50. Lacks motivation; gives up easily or doesn't try
51. Sad, unhappy, or depressed
52. Cries a lot; cries easily for no good reason
53. Show little interest or pleasure in activities; apathetic, doesn't seem to care about anything
54. Thinks too much about death or dying; preoccupied with death
55. Talks about harming or killing self
56. Deliberately harms self or attempts suicide
57. Doesn't get along with other children
58. Has a hard time making friends
59. Ignored or rejected by others
60. Gets teased or picked on by other children
61. Withdrawn, doesn't get involved with others; spends a lot of time alone
62. Doesn't take part in normal social activities
63. Acts too young for his or her age, "childish" or immature
64. Acts silly or giggles too much
65. Pesters or nags, is demanding, won't take "no" for an answer
66. Asks personal or embarrassing questions
67. Loud
68. Talks too much
69. Hums or makes odd noises in public
70. Poor social judgment; not sensitive to other people's feelings or reactions
71. Careless about how he/she looks or dresses
72. Talks or thinks about sex too much
73. Plays with own sex parts too much
74. Bites or hits self, bangs head, or repeats other acts causing self-injury
75. Odd movements or unusual posturing (such as hand-flapping or toe-walking)
76. Needs close or constant supervision
77. Talks or thinks about the same things over and over
78. Repeats certain actions over and over (please explain)
79. Once he/she gets an idea, it's hard to get it out of his/her mind
80. Repeats or "echoes" words or phrases said by others
81. Upset by changes in routine; insists on doing things the same way every time
82. Sudden changes in mood or feelings; moody
83. Rapid shifts between sadness and excitement
84. Inconsistent; behavior or learning varies greatly from day to day
85. Shows changes in personality; is not always his/her "same old self"
86. Sees or hears things that aren't really there
87. Confuses reality and fantasy; unable to tell the difference between real and imaginary things
88. Says strange things that don't make sense; has odd or peculiar ideas (please explain)
89. Strange, unusual, or bizarre behavior (please explain)
90. Very suspicious of others; thinks people are out to get him or her
91. Drowsy or sleepy; not alert or wide awake
92. Sluggish or slow-moving; lacks energy
93. Stares into space; seems preoccupied or "in a world of his/her own"
94. Confused or disoriented; seems to be in a fog
95. Unresponsive; doesn't show feelings or emotions
96. Clumsy, awkward, or poorly coordinated
97. Bumps into things or falls a lot
98. Speech is slurred or hard to understand
99. Shaky movements or tremor; hands tremble or shake
100. Draws or writes poorly
101. Has trouble hitting, kicking, or throwing a ball
102. Eats too much
103. Overweight or gains too much weight
104. Poor appetite; doesn't eat much
105. Underweight or loses too much weight
106. Eats things that are not food (please explain)
107. Goes on eating binges; eats large amounts of food all at once
108. Vomits after eating (not due to illness or medication)
109. Sleeps more than most other children
110. Sleeps less than most other children
111. Has trouble falling asleep
112. Sleep is restless or disturbed; often tosses and turns in sleep
113. Wakes up often in the night
114. Has nightmares or bad dreams
115. Talks, walks, or cries out in sleep

**9–11** (Continued)

116. Wakes up too early in the morning
117. Headaches
118. Stomach aches
119. Aches or pains in muscles, limbs, chest, or back
120. Complains of feeling "sick"
121. Complains of dizziness of feeling faint
122. Nausea or vomiting when nervous or emotionally upset
123. Nausea or vomiting due to illness or medication
124. Diarrhea or loose bowels
125. Fever or high temperatures
126. Complains of hot or cold spells (without having a fever)
127. Hearing problems (please explain)
128. Problems with eyes or vision (other than needing eyeglasses) (please explain)
129. Rashes or other skin problems
130. Asthma, wheezing, or trouble breathing
131. Seizures that cause falling and loss of consciousness
132. Seizures that are brief and do not cause complete loss of consciousness
133. Tires easily; lacks stamina or physical endurance
134. Constipated; doesn't have regular bowel movements
135. Has bowel movements outside of the toilet; soils pants
136. Wets the bed at night
137. Wets self during the day
138. Accident-prone; gets frequent cuts, scrapes, or bruises
139. Illness requiring emergency room treatment or a stay in the hospital (please explain)
140. Other physical problems (please explain)
141. Doesn't follow doctor's orders for health problems
142. Refuses or "forgets" to take pills or medicine he/she is supposed to take
143. Refuses or "forgets" to complete special exercises or physical activities he/she is supposed to do
144. If on a restricted diet, he/she sneaks food or eats foods he/she is not supposed to eat
145. Worries about or is fearful of medical procedures (shots, blood tests, etc.)
146. Physically resists or combats medical procedures (shots, blood tests, etc.)
147. Careless or irresponsible about his/her health
148. Has trouble expressing self; "can't get the words out"
149. Quiet; doesn't talk very much
150. Speech or articulation problems (please explain)
151. Gets mixed up when telling a story or explaining how something happened
152. Has trouble remembering names for things or thinking of the right words to say
153. Makes up words or substitutes words with similar meanings (such as "door" for "window")
154. Thinks and works slowly
155. Unable to think clearly and logically; has trouble figuring out how to solve problems
156. Comprehension problems; difficulty in understanding directions or discussions
157. Has trouble remembering things; forgets easily
158. Thoughts are rambling or disorganized
159. Has difficulty learning, even when he or she tries hard
160. Underachieving; not working up to potential
161. Has trouble with reading, writing, or arithmetic
162. Fails to complete schoolwork or homework
163. Schoolwork is sloppy, careless, or disorganized
164. Gets low grades on school papers or tests
165. Does not like school; doesn't want to go to school

From Lindgren, S. D. *Pediatric Behavior Scale.* Solon, IA: Linden Press; 1985.
Used with Permission. Note: Items 19–33 comprise the attention deficits subscale.

**9–12** Quality of Life Index Scoring Form

*Score each heading 2, 1 or 0 according to your most recent assessment of the patient.*

ACTIVITY *During the last week, the patient*
- has been working or studying full-time, or nearly so, in usual occupation, or managing own household, or participating in unpaid or voluntary activities, whether retired or not .......... 2
- has been working or studying in usual occupation or managing own household or participating in unpaid or voluntary activities; but requiring major assistance or a significant reduction in hours worked or a sheltered situation or was on sick leave .......... 1
- has not been working or studying in any capacity and not managing own household .......... 0

DAILY LIVING *During the last week, the patient*
- has been self-reliant in eating, washing, toileting and dressing; using public transport or driving own car .......... 2
- has been requiring assistance (another person or special equipment) for daily activities and transport but performing light tasks .......... 1
- has not been managing personal care nor light tasks and/or not leaving own home or institution at all .......... 0

HEALTH *During the last week, the patient*
- has been appearing to feel well or reporting feeling "great" most of the time .......... 2
- has been lacking energy or not feeling entirely "up to par" more than just occasionally .......... 1
- has been feeling very ill or "lousy", seeming weak and washed out most of the time or was unconscious .......... 0

SUPPORT *During the last week,*
- the patient has been having good relationships with others and receiving strong support from *at least one* family member and/or friend .......... 2
- support received or perceived has been limited from family and friends and/or by the patient's condition .......... 1
- support from family and friends occurred infrequently or only when absolutely necessary or patient was unconscious .......... 0

OUTLOOK *During the last week, the patient*
- has usually been appearing calm and positive in outlook, accepting and in control of personal circumstances, including surroundings .......... 2
- has sometimes been troubled because not fully in control of personal circumstances or has been having periods of obvious anxiety or depression .......... 1
- has been seriously or very frightened or consistently anxious and depressed or unconscious .......... 0

QL INDEX TOTAL

How confident are you that your scoring of the preceding dimensions is accurate? Please ring the appropriate category.

| Absolutely Confident | Very Confident | Quite Confident | Not Very Confident | Very Doubtful | Not at all Confident |
|---|---|---|---|---|---|
| 1 | 2 | 3 | 4 | 5 | 6 |

Adapted from Spitzer, W.O., Dobson, A.J., Hall, J., et al. Measuring the quality of life of cancer patients: a concise QL-Index for use by physicians. *J. Chronic Dis.* 1981;34:585.

# APPENDIX 10

## Adult Nutrition Records and Nutrition Values

**NAME:** ____________ **ADDRESS:** ____________
**BIRTHDATE:** ____________
**AGE:** ____________ **TELEPHONE:** ____________
**MARITAL STATUS:** ____________ **WORK HOURS:** ____________
**OCCUPATION:** ____________ **DATE SEEN:** ____________

**BACKGROUND INFORMATION:**

| PARENTS: | DIED FROM | AT AGE |
|---|---|---|
| Mother | ____ | ____ |
| Father | ____ | ____ |
| SIBLINGS: | | |
| Brother/s | ____ | ____ |
| Sister/s | ____ | ____ |

Current Diagnosis: ____________
Sex: _____ Race: ____________
Interviewer: ____________

**ANTHROPOMETRIC MEASUREMENTS:**

| | Present | Ideal |
|---|---|---|
| Ht. cm | ____ | ____ |
| Wt. kg | ____ | ____ |

Wt. loss or gain (circle one) in 6 mo.
Amt. (kg.) ____________
Usual weight–Current Weight x 100= ____ %
Usual Weight wt. loss

Upper arm circ. cm__ Pulse rate___
Fatfold tricep mm__ B.P. ________
Muscle mass cm__
Bone Age ______ Bone density ______

**CHEMISTRY:**
Hb. ______ Hct. ______ CBC ______
Transferin ____ Urinalysis ______
TG ______ Serum Albumin ______
Chol. _____ Blood Sugar ______
Kidney ___ Chest ___ Stomach ___
Eyes _______ Hearing _______

**INTERDISCIPLINARY FINDINGS:**
Dental: ____________
Gross Motor: ____________
Speech: ____________
Hx. Infections: ____________

**CLINICAL/PHYSICAL DATA** (check if appropriate)

Chronic Diseases
- Cancer _____
- Chronic Liver Disease _____
- Chronic Renal Disease _____
- Coronary Artery Disease _____
- Diabetes Mellitus _____
- Hypertension _____

Recent Major Surgery or Illness
Type of Surgery Performed
Increased Metabolic Needs:
- burns _____
- fever _____
- infection _____
- trauma _____

Gastrointestinal Function:
- Dysgeusian _____ Dysphasia _____
- Enteric Fistula _____
- Head/neck cancer-radiation or trauma___
- Inflammatory bowel disease _____
- Mechanical Obstruction of GI tract___
- Persistent diarrhea___ or vomiting___

Increased Losses:
- burns _____
- draining abscesses _____
- draining fistulas _____
- open wounds _____

**PRESENT FEEDING ABILITIES:**
Table foods _____ Chpd. foods _____ Jr. Foods _____ Strained _____
Length of Normal Feeding Period ____________
Circle: Choking, Swallowing, Chewing, Tongue Thrust, Constipation, Anorexia

**Name:** ____________

**DIETARY EVALUATION**

**FOOD INTAKE** (24 Hr. Recall)

| Patterns: | | Breakfast | Amt. |
|---|---|---|---|
| Time | Fruit | ____ | ____ |
| | Meat | ____ | ____ |
| ____ | Egg | ____ | ____ |
| Where | Bread | ____ | ____ |
| ____ | Fat | ____ | ____ |
| With Whom | Cereal | ____ | ____ |
| ____ | Beverage | ____ | ____ |
| Who Prepared | Other | ____ | ____ |
| | | **Lunch** | |
| Time | Meat | ____ | ____ |
| ____ | Veg. | ____ | ____ |
| Where | Bread | ____ | ____ |
| ____ | Fruit | ____ | ____ |
| With Whom | Beverage | ____ | ____ |
| ____ | Other | ____ | ____ |
| Who Prepared | | | |
| | | **Dinner** | |
| Time | Soup | ____ | ____ |
| ____ | Meat or subst. | ____ | ____ |
| Where | | | |
| ____ | Potato | ____ | ____ |
| With Whom | Vegetable: | | |
| | Cooked | ____ | ____ |
| Who Prepared | Raw | ____ | ____ |
| | Salad | ____ | ____ |
| | Bread | ____ | ____ |
| | Fat | ____ | ____ |
| | Dessert | ____ | ____ |
| | Beverage | ____ | ____ |
| | Other | ____ | ____ |
| Time: | | **Between Meals** | |
| ____ | | ____ | ____ |
| ____ | | ____ | ____ |
| ____ | | ____ | ____ |

Alcohol ____________ Smoking ______
How much salt is used at each meal ______
Vit. & Mineral Supp. ____________
Drugs: ____________
Income ______ Spent on Food ______/wk.mo.

**FOOD SUMMARY**

| GROUP | Amt. per day | Amt. per week | Possible points or daily serv. | **Actual Points |
|---|---|---|---|---|
| Dairy Products: | | | 3 | |
| Milk | ___ | ___ | ___ | ___ |
| Cheese | ___ | ___ | ___ | ___ |
| Cottage Cheese | ___ | ___ | ___ | ___ |
| Yogurt | ___ | ___ | ___ | ___ |
| Other | ___ | ___ | ___ | ___ |
| Meat or Alternates:*** Fat & Chol. | | | 2 | |
| ***Meat, Eggs | ___ | ___ | ___ | ___ |
| Fish, Poultry | ___ | ___ | ___ | ___ |
| Dr. Beans/peas | ___ | ___ | ___ | ___ |
| Peanut Butter | ___ | ___ | ___ | ___ |
| Vegetables: (No Vit. A/C-1/2 cr) | | | 3 | |
| Vit A Veg. | ___ | ___ | ___ | ___ |
| Vit C Veg. | ___ | ___ | ___ | ___ |
| Other | ___ | ___ | ___ | ___ |
| Fruits: | | | 2 | |
| Vit C Fruit | ___ | ___ | ___ | ___ |
| Other Fruits | ___ | ___ | ___ | ___ |
| Whole Grains/Starches: (No w/grains-1/2 cr) | | | 6 | |
| Cereal | ___ | ___ | ___ | ___ |
| Bread | ___ | ___ | ___ | ___ |
| Pasta, Rice | ___ | ___ | ___ | ___ |
| Other | ___ | ___ | ___ | ___ |
| | | TOTAL | 16 | ___ |
| Others: | | | | |
| Candy/Sugar | ___ | ___ | If daily-1 | ___ |
| Chips/t. salt | ___ | ___ | If daily-1 | ___ |
| Soft Drinks | ___ | ___ | If daily-1 | ___ |
| Desserts | ___ | ___ | If daily-1 | ___ |
| Water | ___ | ___ | None daily-1 | ___ |
| ***Fats & Chol. | ___ | ___ | 3 ser. d.-1 | ___ |
| Fiber | ___ | ___ | None daily-1 | ___ |
| | | TOTAL | | |

Frequency/wk. of eating outside the home: ______
Food allergies: ____________
Foods regularly ommitted: ____________
____________ Why: ____________
Favorite Foods: ____________
Impression of diet: ____________
Validity of record: ____________
Activity Score: ____________

Are you using iodized salt? ______ Are you using vitamin D fortified milk? ______ Are you on food stamp or supplemental food program? ______
Favorite Foods ____________ What foods do you believe are good for you? ____________ Are other factors (religion, region, nationality, illness, special diet, allergies, etc.) affecting the diet? ____________ Foods regularly omitted ____________

**10–1** (Continued)

**PHYSICAL ACTIVITY RECORDS**
**Estimation of Caloric Needs**

WEIGHT: kg.________(lbs.)____%ile____ Caloric Input____________

HEIGHT: cm.________(in.)____%ile____ Caloric Output____________

RDA calorie average for ages ____ to ____ = ________

RDA range for age ______-______

A. Record the following activities as accurately as possible:

| Activity | Time in Hours | Calories/ lb/hr. | Total per lb. |
|---|---|---|---|
| 1. Sleeping | | x 0.4 | = |
| 2. Sitting at rest (watching TV, reading, etc.) | | x 0.7 | = |
| 3. Sitting (Hand activities, i.e., playing with toys) | | x 1.0 | = |
| 4. Walking with crutches | | x 1.5 | = |
| 5. Walking with crutches, total self care | | x 2.0 | = |
| 6. Walking doing light exercise (playground walking, sandbox playing, swinging) | | x 2.0 | = |
| 7. Moderate exercise (active games, i.e., playing ball, stair climbing dancing) | | x 2.7 | = |
| 8. Strenuous exercise (running, swimming, bicycle riding, etc.) | | x 4.3 | = |
| | Total 24 | | TOTAL |

Calorie Output (total per lb. x weight in lbs.):________________

Optional:

B. Recommended kcal. per cm. height:____ x height (cm) = ____kcal/day (use only for children with motor dysfunction, ages 5-12.) (ambulatory, motor dysfunction, 13.9 cal/cm.) (nonambulatory, severe motor dysfunction, 11.1 cal/cm.)

Caretaker demonstrates knowledge of relationship of calories to physical activity: YES/NO

**NUTRITIONAL CLINICAL EVALUATION**

Code: 0 = absent; 1 = present; 2 = does not apply

| Code | Doubtful |
|---|---|
| **Hair:** | |
| all | dry ______ |
| neg. | dispigmented ______ |
| | easily pluckable ______ |
| ___ | abnormal texture ______ |
| **Eyes:** | |
| all | cloudy ______ |
| neg. | reddened ______ |
| ___ | dry ______ |
| **Lips:** | |
| all | angular lesions ______ |
| neg. | angular scars ______ |
| ___ | |
| **Gums:** | |
| all | swelling ______ |
| neg. | redness ______ |
| ___ | hypertrophy ______ |
| | bleeding ______ |
| **Teeth:** | |
| all | visible caries ______ |
| neg. | missing teeth ______ |
| ___ | calculus ______ |
| | mottling ______ |
| | striated discoloration ______ |
| | malocclusion ______ |
| **Tongue:** | |
| all | glossy ______ |
| neg. | fissures ______ |
| ___ | magenta ______ |
| | geographic ______ |
| **Nails:** | |
| all | clubbed ______ |
| neg. | ridged ______ |
| ___ | spooned ______ |
| | blue ______ |
| | combinations ______ |

| Code | Doubtful |
|---|---|
| **Face & Neck:** | |
| all | thyroid enlarged ______ |
| neg. | facial stigmata of syndrome ______ |
| ___ | |
| **Skin:** | |
| all | follicular hyperkeratosis ______ |
| neg. | hyperpigmentation ______ |
| ___ | dry and scaling ______ |
| | cold ______ |
| | dispigmentation ______ |
| **Skeletal or Muscular:** | |
| all | protuberant abdomen ______ |
| neg. | bowed legs ______ |
| ___ | knocked-knees ______ |
| | beading of ribs ______ |
| | enlargement of wrist ______ |
| | winged scapula ______ |
| | scoliosis ______ |
| | muscle wasting ______ |
| **Lower Extremities:** | |
| all | pretibial edema ______ |
| neg. | |
| ___ | |

General Appearance: Circle if appropriate

| | |
|---|---|
| skinny | ambulatory |
| fat | nonambulatory |
| well proportioned | no speech |
| alert | unintelligible speech |
| apathetic | intelligible speech |
| irritable | poor feeding behavior |
| uncooperative | very active |

Parent-Child Interaction

___ Appropriate ___ Slight

___ Moderate ___ None

**10–1** (Continued)

| | Evaluation |
|---|---|
| **Demographic Data**<br>anthropometric data<br>family data<br>lab data | 9 |
| **Pertinent Nutritional History**<br>medication and disease history<br>diet history | 6 |
| **Current Nutritional and Feeding Status**<br>present dietary pattern<br>any neurological impairment that affects feeding<br>physical activity<br>socioeconomic problems<br>presenting nutrition problem<br>anthropometric - height, weight, skinfold, circumference | 27 |
| **Biochemical**<br>medications, drug interaction, nutrition supplements lab data | 16 |
| **Clinical Observations**<br>physical signs and symptoms/overt signs of poor nutrition<br>feeding skill evaluation<br>behavioral problems<br>interaction with people | 12 |
| **Impressions**<br>1. Height and weight, percentiles and statements to reflect nutritional status such as thin or overweight, etc.<br>2. Adequacy of diet expressed in nutrients.<br>3. Feeding skills level. | 12 |
| **Recommendations**<br>1. Good nutrition-translation of low or excessive nutrients into appropriate food sources.<br>2. Food planning, purchasing and preparation suggestions.<br>3. Social interaction - suggestions in eating or techniques in feeding.<br>4. Physical activity suggestions.<br>5. Follow up or disposition of case. | 18 |

A nutritional assessment for this population includes these five steps:

**Step 1.** Anthropometric evaluation
- Height
- Actual weight
- Body frame size
- Expected weight range -% expected body weight
- Usual weight - % usual body weight
- Body composition
- % body fat (sum of four skinfolds) - kg body fat and kg lean body mass
- Midarm muscle circumference
- Triceps skinfold
- Upper arm muscle area
- Upper arm fat area

**Step 2.** Biochemical evaluation
- Visceral proteins
- Serum albumin
- Serum transferrin
- Immunocompetence
- Total lymphocyte count
- Delayed cutaneous hyperse3nsitivity

**Step 3.** Nutritional diagnosis
- Adequate
- Marasmus (starvation)
- Visceral protein depletion (kwashiorkor)
- Maramus with visceral protein depletion (maramuskwashiorkor mix)

**Step 4.** Energy and protein requirements
- Harris-Benedict equations basal energy expenditure (BEE)
- Maintenance
  - Oral: BEE x 1.2
  - Parenteral: BEE x 1.5
  - Anabolic
    - Oral: BEE x 1.5
  - Parenteral: BEE x 1.75
  - Protein requirement = 1.0 to 1.4 g/kg body weight
    - Use expected weight if normal weight or obese
    - Use actual weight if underweight

**Step 5.** Evaluation of nutritional therapy
- Daily weights
- Anthropometric measurements
- Laboratory tests
- Indirect calorimetry
- Nitrogen balance"

An Individual Nutrition Assessment form for this age group is found in Appendix 10.

**10–2** Nutrition Assessment Summary, Adult

# NUTRITION TODAY

**Individual Patient**

**Nutritional Assessment Summary © ***

PATIENT ________

INSTITUTION ________

By ________

DATE ________

| | | |
|---|---|---|
| Triceps Skin-fold | % of standard | ___ |
| Mid Upper Arm Circum. | % of standard | ___ |
| Mid Upper Arm Muscle Circumference (Mid Arm Circum. cm-πx Triceps Skinfold cm) (N adult male 25.3, female 23.2 cm) | % of standard | ___ |
| Albumin | % of standard | ___ |

**Height/Creatinine mg/24 hrs/cm Height**
(See tables on reverse side for normal values for males and females of ideal weight for their height, of urinary creatinine/cm body height.)

**Height/Creatinine** % of standard ___

**Total Lymphocyte Count**
(Should be 1,500/mm$^3$) ___ /mm$^3$

**Total Lymphocyte Count** % of standard ___

**Transferrin**
(or TIBC level) % of standard ___

**Cellular Immunity Skin Testing**

| | Reactive | Unre-active |
|---|---|---|
| PPD (0.1 mg, 5 Tuberculin units) | ___ | ___ |
| Candida (Hollister-Stier) | ___ | ___ |
| DNCB | ___ | ___ |

Assessment of CMI—adequate ........ Impaired ........

**SUMMARY** (CHECK)

| STANDARD PARAMETERS | >90% | 60-90% | <60% |
|---|---|---|---|
| Weight/Height | | | |
| Triceps Skinfold | | | |
| Mid Arm Circumference | | | |
| Mid Arm Muscle Circum. | | | |
| Albumin | | | |
| Height/Creatinine | | | |
| Lymphocyte Count | | | |
| Transferrin | | | |
| Cellular Immunity | | | |

| **Other Risk Factors:** | **Absent** | **Present** |
|---|---|---|
| Vitamin Deficiency | | |
| a. Clinical Signs | | |
| b. Laboratory Evidence | | |
| Mineral or Electrolyte Imbalance | | |
| a. Clinical Signs | | |
| b. Laboratory Evidence | | |
| Drug-Nutrient-Hormone Interaction | | |
| General Assessment (Socio-Economic, Habits, Behavior, Underlying Diagnosis, etc.) | | |

**Types of Protein-Calorie Malnutrition (Check):**

**Acute Visceral Attrition ("Kwashiorkor-like")**
(Wt/Ht, TSF, MUAC, MUAMC, Ht/Creat, Preserved; alb and transferrin acutely depressed) ☐

**Chronic Depletion of Parietal Muscle & Fat**
("Adult Marasmus")
(Wt/Ht, TSF, MUAC, MUAMC, Ht/Creat, depressed; Alb and Transferrin preserved until late) ☐

**Acute Visceral Attrition Superimposed on Chronic Depletion of Muscle & Fat**
(Advanced PCM:)
(Wt/Ht, TSF, MUAC, MUAMC, Ht/Creat, Alb, Transferrin, Lymphocytes, Immunity, all depressed) ☐

**Other Nutritional Disorders (Check):**

Vitamin Deficiency ☐
Specify Predominant Syndromes,
Or if multiple, so state

Mineral or Electrolyte Imbalance ☐
(e.g. Iron, Calcium, Magnesium, Phosphorus, Zinc, Sodium, Potassium, etc.)
Specify

**PRIMARY DIAGNOSIS**

*From "Hospital Malnutrition and Nutritional Assessment," Nutrition Today 10:8 (March/April) '75. This form is copyrighted by Nutrition Today, Inc., 101 Ridgely Ave., Annapolis, Md. 21404. Available in pads of 100 sheets each at $4.00 a pad, postpaid. Nutrition Today Society members entitled to 10 percent discount. Payment must accompany order.

From Hospital malnutrition and nutritional assessment. *Nutr. Today* 1975; 10:8. Jones, J.M. The methodology of nutritional screening and assessment tools. *J. Hum. Nutr. Diet.* 2002; 15(1):59. Defining nutritional status. Galveston College Library, E-Reserves, Health Occupations. Available at: www.gc.edu/library/e_reserves/team-nursing/rnsg1115_SP04/

**10–3** Weight for Height–Males and Females, 18–74 Years

| Height in inches | Percentile | Age group in years 18-24 | 25-34 | 35-44 | 45-54 | 55-64 | 65-74 |
|---|---|---|---|---|---|---|---|
| 62 inches | 50 | 130 | 141 | 143 | 147 | 143 | 143 |
| | 15 | 102 | 109 | 115 | 118 | 113 | 116 |
| | 5 | 85 | 91 | 98 | 100 | 96 | 100 |
| 63 inches | 50 | 135 | 145 | 148 | 152 | 147 | 147 |
| | 15 | 107 | 113 | 120 | 123 | 117 | 120 |
| | 5 | 90 | 95 | 103 | 105 | 100 | 104 |
| 64 inches | 50 | 140 | 150 | 153 | 156 | 153 | 151 |
| | 15 | 112 | 118 | 125 | 127 | 123 | 124 |
| | 5 | 95 | 100 | 108 | 109 | 106 | 108 |
| 65 inches | 50 | 145 | 156 | 158 | 160 | 158 | 156 |
| | 15 | 117 | 124 | 130 | 131 | 128 | 129 |
| | 5 | 100 | 106 | 113 | 113 | 111 | 113 |
| 66 inches | 50 | 150 | 160 | 163 | 164 | 163 | 160 |
| | 15 | 122 | 128 | 135 | 135 | 133 | 133 |
| | 5 | 105 | 110 | 118 | 117 | 116 | 117 |
| 67 inches | 50 | 154 | 165 | 169 | 169 | 168 | 164 |
| | 15 | 126 | 133 | 141 | 140 | 138 | 137 |
| | 5 | 109 | 115 | 124 | 122 | 121 | 121 |
| 68 inches | 50 | 159 | 170 | 174 | 173 | 173 | 169 |
| | 15 | 131 | 138 | 146 | 144 | 143 | 142 |
| | 5 | 114 | 120 | 129 | 126 | 126 | 126 |
| 69 inches | 50 | 164 | 174 | 179 | 177 | 178 | 173 |
| | 15 | 136 | 142 | 151 | 148 | 148 | 146 |
| | 5 | 119 | 124 | 134 | 130 | 131 | 130 |
| 70 inches | 50 | 168 | 179 | 184 | 182 | 183 | 177 |
| | 15 | 140 | 147 | 156 | 153 | 153 | 150 |
| | 5 | 123 | 129 | 139 | 135 | 136 | 134 |
| 71 inches | 50 | 173 | 184 | 190 | 187 | 189 | 182 |
| | 15 | 145 | 152 | 162 | 158 | 159 | 155 |
| | 5 | 128 | 134 | 145 | 140 | 142 | 139 |
| 72 inches | 50 | 178 | 189 | 194 | 191 | 193 | 186 |
| | 15 | 150 | 157 | 166 | 162 | 163 | 159 |
| | 5 | 133 | 139 | 149 | 144 | 146 | 143 |
| 73 inches | 50 | 183 | 194 | 200 | 196 | 197 | 190 |
| | 15 | 155 | 162 | 172 | 167 | 167 | 163 |
| | 5 | 138 | 144 | 155 | 149 | 150 | 147 |
| 74 inches | 50 | 188 | 199 | 205 | 200 | 203 | 194 |
| | 15 | 160 | 167 | 177 | 171 | 173 | 167 |
| | 5 | 143 | 149 | 160 | 153 | 156 | 150 |

| Height in inches | Percentile | Age group in years 18-24 | 25-34 | 35-44 | 45-54 | 55-64 | 65-74 |
|---|---|---|---|---|---|---|---|
| 57 inches | 50 | 114 | 118 | 125 | 129 | 132 | 130 |
| | 15 | 85 | 85 | 89 | 94 | 97 | 100 |
| | 5 | 68 | 65 | 67 | 73 | 77 | 82 |
| 58 inches | 50 | 117 | 121 | 129 | 133 | 136 | 134 |
| | 15 | 88 | 88 | 93 | 98 | 101 | 104 |
| | 5 | 71 | 68 | 71 | 77 | 81 | 86 |
| 59 inches | 50 | 120 | 125 | 133 | 136 | 140 | 137 |
| | 15 | 91 | 92 | 97 | 101 | 105 | 107 |
| | 5 | 74 | 72 | 75 | 80 | 85 | 89 |
| 60 inches | 50 | 123 | 128 | 137 | 140 | 143 | 140 |
| | 15 | 94 | 95 | 101 | 105 | 108 | 110 |
| | 5 | 77 | 75 | 79 | 84 | 88 | 92 |
| 61 inches | 50 | 126 | 132 | 141 | 143 | 147 | 144 |
| | 15 | 97 | 99 | 105 | 108 | 112 | 114 |
| | 5 | 80 | 79 | 83 | 87 | 92 | 96 |
| 62 inches | 50 | 129 | 136 | 144 | 147 | 150 | 147 |
| | 15 | 100 | 103 | 108 | 112 | 115 | 117 |
| | 5 | 83 | 83 | 86 | 91 | 95 | 99 |
| 53 inches | 50 | 132 | 139 | 148 | 150 | 153 | 151 |
| | 15 | 103 | 106 | 112 | 115 | 118 | 121 |
| | 5 | 86 | 86 | 90 | 94 | 98 | 103 |
| 64 inches | 50 | 135 | 142 | 152 | 154 | 157 | 154 |
| | 15 | 106 | 109 | 116 | 119 | 122 | 124 |
| | 5 | 89 | 89 | 94 | 98 | 102 | 106 |
| 65 inches | 50 | 138 | 146 | 156 | 158 | 160 | 158 |
| | 15 | 109 | 113 | 120 | 123 | 125 | 128 |
| | 5 | 92 | 93 | 98 | 102 | 105 | 110 |
| 66 inches | 50 | 141 | 150 | 159 | 161 | 164 | 161 |
| | 15 | 112 | 117 | 123 | 126 | 129 | 131 |
| | 5 | 95 | 97 | 101 | 105 | 109 | 113 |
| 67 inches | 50 | 144 | 153 | 163 | 165 | 167 | 165 |
| | 15 | 115 | 120 | 127 | 130 | 132 | 135 |
| | 5 | 98 | 100 | 105 | 109 | 112 | 117 |
| 68 inches | 50 | 147 | 157 | 167 | 168 | 171 | 169 |
| | 15 | 118 | 124 | 131 | 133 | 136 | 139 |
| | 5 | 101 | 104 | 109 | 112 | 116 | 121 |

From: Weight by Height and Age for Adults 18–74 Years: U.S. 1971–74, National Health Survey. Vital Health Statisitcs Series 11, No. 208. U.S. Dept. Health, Education, and Welfare, P.H.S., 1979 and 15th percentile Bishop, C.W., Bowen, P.E., Ritchey, S.J.: Norms for nutritional anthropometery of Americans and adults by upper arm anthropometry. *Am J Clin Nutr,* 34:2530, 1981. Used with permission.

## 10–4 Elbow Breadth/Percentiles, 1–75 Years, and Elbow Breadth/Stature Index for Frame Size, 18–75 Years

| Age (yrs) | Percentiles 5 | 10 | 15 | 25 | 50 | 75 | 85 | 90 | 95 |
|---|---|---|---|---|---|---|---|---|---|
| **Males** | | | | | | | | | |
| 1.0–1.9 | 36.0 | 37.0 | 37.0 | 39.0 | 40.0 | 42.0 | 43.0 | 44.0 | 45.0 |
| 2.0–2.9 | 38.0 | 39.0 | 40.0 | 41.0 | 42.0 | 44.0 | 45.0 | 46.0 | 47.0 |
| 3.0–3.9 | 40.0 | 41.0 | 42.0 | 43.0 | 44.0 | 46.0 | 47.0 | 48.0 | 50.0 |
| 4.0–4.9 | 42.0 | 43.0 | 43.0 | 44.0 | 46.0 | 48.0 | 49.0 | 50.0 | 52.0 |
| 5.0–5.9 | 43.0 | 44.0 | 45.0 | 46.0 | 48.0 | 50.0 | 51.0 | 52.0 | 53.0 |
| 6.0–6.9 | 45.0 | 46.0 | 47.0 | 48.0 | 50.0 | 52.0 | 54.0 | 55.0 | 56.0 |
| 7.0–7.9 | 47.0 | 48.0 | 49.0 | 49.0 | 52.0 | 54.0 | 55.0 | 56.0 | 57.0 |
| 8.0–8.9 | 48.0 | 49.0 | 50.0 | 51.0 | 54.0 | 56.0 | 57.0 | 58.0 | 60.0 |
| 9.0–9.9 | 50.0 | 51.0 | 52.0 | 53.0 | 56.0 | 58.0 | 60.0 | 61.0 | 63.0 |
| 10.0–10.9 | 51.0 | 53.0 | 54.0 | 56.0 | 58.0 | 60.0 | 62.0 | 63.0 | 65.0 |
| 11.0–11.9 | 53.0 | 54.0 | 56.0 | 57.0 | 60.0 | 62.0 | 64.0 | 65.0 | 67.0 |
| 12.0–12.9 | 55.0 | 57.0 | 58.0 | 60.0 | 63.0 | 66.0 | 68.0 | 68.0 | 72.0 |
| 13.0–13.9 | 59.0 | 61.0 | 61.0 | 63.0 | 66.0 | 69.0 | 71.0 | 72.0 | 74.0 |
| 14.0–14.9 | 62.0 | 64.0 | 64.0 | 66.0 | 69.0 | 71.0 | 73.0 | 74.0 | 75.0 |
| 15.0–15.9 | 63.0 | 64.0 | 65.0 | 67.0 | 70.0 | 72.0 | 74.0 | 75.0 | 77.0 |
| 16.0–16.9 | 64.0 | 66.0 | 66.0 | 68.0 | 70.0 | 73.0 | 74.0 | 76.0 | 77.0 |
| 17.0–17.9 | 64.0 | 66.0 | 67.0 | 68.0 | 71.0 | 73.0 | 75.0 | 76.0 | 77.0 |
| 18.0–24.9 | 65.0 | 66.0 | 67.0 | 69.0 | 71.0 | 74.0 | 75.0 | 76.0 | 78.0 |
| 25.0–29.9 | 65.0 | 67.0 | 68.0 | 69.0 | 72.0 | 74.0 | 76.0 | 77.0 | 78.0 |
| 30.0–34.9 | 65.0 | 67.0 | 68.0 | 69.0 | 72.0 | 74.0 | 76.0 | 77.0 | 79.0 |
| 35.0–39.9 | 66.0 | 67.0 | 69.0 | 70.0 | 72.0 | 75.0 | 77.0 | 77.0 | 79.0 |
| 40.0–44.9 | 67.0 | 68.0 | 69.0 | 70.0 | 73.0 | 75.0 | 77.0 | 78.0 | 80.0 |
| 45.0–49.9 | 66.0 | 68.0 | 69.0 | 70.0 | 73.0 | 76.0 | 78.0 | 78.0 | 80.0 |
| 50.0–54.9 | 67.0 | 68.0 | 70.0 | 71.0 | 73.0 | 76.0 | 77.0 | 78.0 | 80.0 |
| 55.0–59.9 | 67.0 | 68.0 | 69.0 | 71.0 | 73.0 | 77.0 | 78.0 | 80.0 | 81.0 |
| 60.0–64.9 | 67.0 | 68.0 | 69.0 | 71.0 | 73.0 | 76.0 | 78.0 | 79.0 | 81.0 |
| 65.0–69.9 | 66.0 | 68.0 | 69.0 | 71.0 | 73.0 | 76.0 | 78.0 | 79.0 | 81.0 |
| 70.0–74.9 | 67.0 | 68.0 | 69.0 | 71.0 | 73.0 | 76.0 | 78.0 | 79.0 | 81.0 |
| **Females** | | | | | | | | | |
| 1.0–1.9 | 34.0 | 35.0 | 36.0 | 37.0 | 39.0 | 41.0 | 42.0 | 42.0 | 43.0 |
| 2.0–2.9 | 36.0 | 37.0 | 38.0 | 39.0 | 41.0 | 42.0 | 44.0 | 44.0 | 45.0 |
| 3.0–3.9 | 38.0 | 39.0 | 40.0 | 41.0 | 43.0 | 44.0 | 45.0 | 46.0 | 47.0 |
| 4.0–4.9 | 40.0 | 41.0 | 41.0 | 42.0 | 44.0 | 46.0 | 47.0 | 48.0 | 49.0 |
| 5.0–5.9 | 42.0 | 43.0 | 43.0 | 44.0 | 46.0 | 48.0 | 49.0 | 50.0 | 51.0 |
| 6.0–6.9 | 43.0 | 44.0 | 45.0 | 46.0 | 48.0 | 50.0 | 51.0 | 52.0 | 53.0 |
| 7.0–7.9 | 44.0 | 45.0 | 46.0 | 48.0 | 50.0 | 52.0 | 53.0 | 54.0 | 55.0 |
| 8.0–8.9 | 46.0 | 47.0 | 48.0 | 49.0 | 51.0 | 54.0 | 55.0 | 56.0 | 58.0 |
| 9.0–9.9 | 48.0 | 50.0 | 50.0 | 51.0 | 54.0 | 56.0 | 57.0 | 59.0 | 60.0 |
| 10.0–10.9 | 50.0 | 51.0 | 51.0 | 53.0 | 55.0 | 58.0 | 60.0 | 61.0 | 62.0 |
| 11.0–11.9 | 52.0 | 53.0 | 53.0 | 55.0 | 58.0 | 61.0 | 63.0 | 63.0 | 64.0 |
| 12.0–12.9 | 54.0 | 55.0 | 55.0 | 57.0 | 59.0 | 61.0 | 62.0 | 64.0 | 65.0 |
| 13.0–13.9 | 54.0 | 55.0 | 56.0 | 57.0 | 60.0 | 62.0 | 63.0 | 64.0 | 66.0 |
| 14.0–14.9 | 55.0 | 56.0 | 57.0 | 58.0 | 60.0 | 62.0 | 64.0 | 65.0 | 66.0 |
| 15.0–15.9 | 54.0 | 56.0 | 57.0 | 58.0 | 61.0 | 63.0 | 65.0 | 66.0 | 66.0 |
| 16.0–16.9 | 55.0 | 56.0 | 57.0 | 58.0 | 61.0 | 63.0 | 65.0 | 66.0 | 67.0 |
| 17.0–17.9 | 54.0 | 56.0 | 57.0 | 58.0 | 61.0 | 64.0 | 65.0 | 66.0 | 67.0 |
| 18.0–24.9 | 55.0 | 56.0 | 57.0 | 59.0 | 61.0 | 63.0 | 64.0 | 66.0 | 67.0 |
| 25.0–29.9 | 55.0 | 57.0 | 57.0 | 59.0 | 61.0 | 63.0 | 65.0 | 66.0 | 68.0 |
| 30.0–34.9 | 56.0 | 57.0 | 58.0 | 59.0 | 62.0 | 64.0 | 66.0 | 67.0 | 69.0 |
| 35.0–39.9 | 56.0 | 58.0 | 59.0 | 60.0 | 62.0 | 65.0 | 66.0 | 67.0 | 69.0 |
| 40.0–44.9 | 57.0 | 58.0 | 59.0 | 60.0 | 62.0 | 65.0 | 67.0 | 68.0 | 70.0 |
| 45.0–49.9 | 57.0 | 59.0 | 59.0 | 61.0 | 63.0 | 66.0 | 68.0 | 69.0 | 71.0 |
| 50.0–54.9 | 57.0 | 59.0 | 60.0 | 61.0 | 63.0 | 67.0 | 68.0 | 69.0 | 71.0 |
| 55.0–59.9 | 58.0 | 59.0 | 60.0 | 61.0 | 64.0 | 67.0 | 69.0 | 70.0 | 73.0 |
| 60.0–64.9 | 58.0 | 60.0 | 61.0 | 62.0 | 64.0 | 67.0 | 69.0 | 70.0 | 72.0 |
| 65.0–69.9 | 58.0 | 59.0 | 60.0 | 61.0 | 64.0 | 67.0 | 69.0 | 70.0 | 72.0 |
| 70.0–74.9 | 58.0 | 60.0 | 60.0 | 62.0 | 64.0 | 67.0 | 69.0 | 71.0 | 72.0 |

Categories of frame size derived with reference to Frame Index 2 {[elbow breadth (mm) / stature (cm)] x 100}, by age and by height

| Frame Index 2 = [elbow breadth (mm) / stature (cm)] x 100 | | | | | | |
|---|---|---|---|---|---|---|
| | Male | | | Female | | |
| | Small | Medium | Large | Small | Medium | Large |
| Age (yrs.) | Frame Index 1: elbow breadth (mm) | | | | | |
| 18.0–24.9 | <38.4 | 38.4 to 41.6 | >41.6 | <35.2 | 35.2 to 38.6 | >38.6 |
| 25.0–29.9 | <38.6 | 38.6 to 41.8 | >41.8 | <35.7 | 35.7 to 38.7 | >38.7 |
| 30.0–34.9 | <38.6 | 38.6 to 42.1 | >42.1 | <35.7 | 35.7 to 39.0 | >39.0 |
| 35.0–39.9 | <39.1 | 39.1 to 42.4 | >42.4 | <36.2 | 36.2 to 39.8 | >39.8 |
| 40.0–44.9 | <39.3 | 39.3 to 42.5 | >42.5 | <36.7 | 36.7 to 40.2 | >40.2 |
| 45.0–45.9 | <39.6 | 39.6 to 43.0 | >43.0 | <36.7 | 37.2 to 40.7 | >40.7 |
| 50.0–54.9 | <39.9 | 39.9 to 43.3 | >43.3 | <37.2 | 37.2 to 41.6 | >41.6 |
| 55.0–59.9 | <40.2 | 40.2 to 43.8 | >43.8 | <37.8 | 37.8 to 41.9 | >41.9 |
| 60.0–64.9 | <40.2 | 40.2 to 43.6 | >43.6 | <38.2 | 38.2 to 41.8 | >41.8 |
| 65.0–69.9 | <40.2 | 40.2 to 43.6 | >43.6 | <38.2 | 38.2 to 41.8 | >41.8 |
| 70.0–74.9 | <40.2 | 40.2 to 43.6 | >43.6 | <38.2 | 38.2 to 41.8 | >41.8 |

| Frame Index 2: Elbow breadth by height | | | | | | |
|---|---|---|---|---|---|---|
| | Male | | | Female | | |
| | Small | Medium | Large | Small | Medium | Large |
| Height (cm) | Elbow breadth (mm) | | | | | |
| 141–146 | — | — | — | <56 | 56 to 61 | >61 |
| 147–152 | — | — | — | <57 | 57 to 62 | >62 |
| 153–158 | <66 | 66 to 70 | >70 | <60 | 60 to 63 | >63 |
| 159–164 | <66 | 66 to 71 | >71 | <61 | 61 to 65 | >65 |
| 165–170 | <68 | 68 to 72 | >72 | <61 | 61 to 65 | >65 |
| 171–176 | <70 | 70 to 73 | >73 | <62 | 62 to 65 | >65 |
| 177–182 | <71 | 71 to 75 | >75 | <62 | 62 to 66 | >66 |
| 183–188 | <71 | 71 to 76 | >76 | — | — | — |
| 189–194 | <73 | 73 to 76 | >76 | — | — | — |

Modified from Fisancho, A.R. *Anthropometric Standards for the Assessment of Growth and Nutritional Status,* Ann Arbor: University of Michigan Press, 1990. Chumlea, W.C., Wisemandle, W., Guo, S.S., Siervogel, R.M. Relations between frame size and body composition and bone mineral status. *Am. J. Clin. Nutr.* 2002; 75:1012.

## 10–5 Percentile Weight by Frame Size, Adults

| Age (yrs) | Percentiles | | | | | | | | |
|---|---|---|---|---|---|---|---|---|---|
| | 5 | 10 | 15 | 25 | 50 | 75 | 85 | 90 | 95 |
| **Males with small frames** | | | | | | | | | |
| 18.0–24.9 | 54.5 | 57.4 | 59.8 | 63.2 | 69.3 | 76.4 | 81.0 | 83.9 | 89.6 |
| 25.0–29.9 | 57.9 | 60.9 | 62.1 | 66.1 | 73.1 | 81.6 | 85.8 | 88.3 | 97.9 |
| 30.0–34.9 | 59.6 | 63.0 | 65.1 | 68.4 | 75.4 | 83.3 | 87.0 | 91.5 | 97.6 |
| 35.0–39.9 | 56.6 | 61.7 | 63.3 | 67.9 | 76.5 | 83.9 | 88.6 | 91.6 | 96.0 |
| 40.0–44.9 | 62.3 | 64.6 | 68.8 | 71.9 | 77.6 | 87.4 | 93.0 | 96.8 | 101.3 |
| 45.0–49.9 | 58.8 | 62.3 | 63.8 | 68.3 | 76.8 | 84.1 | 89.4 | 92.6 | 96.4 |
| 50.0–54.9 | 57.3 | 62.8 | 65.2 | 67.5 | 75.4 | 83.0 | 88.2 | 90.5 | 99.4 |
| 55.0–59.9 | 54.0 | 58.2 | 61.8 | 66.4 | 75.1 | 81.5 | 87.2 | 90.9 | 94.7 |
| 60.0–64.9 | 56.4 | 60.2 | 62.5 | 65.8 | 73.6 | 80.8 | 85.7 | 88.4 | 93.3 |
| 65.0–69.9 | 51.1 | 56.0 | 59.0 | 62.9 | 71.4 | 79.9 | 84.1 | 86.8 | 91.8 |
| 70.0–74.9 | 50.1 | 54.5 | 58.7 | 62.6 | 70.5 | 78.1 | 82.6 | 84.9 | 92.2 |
| **Males with medium frames** | | | | | | | | | |
| 18.0–24.9 | 57.9 | 60.8 | 62.4 | 65.9 | 72.3 | 81.0 | 87.0 | 93.1 | 100.5 |
| 25.0–29.9 | 59.5 | 63.0 | 65.2 | 69.3 | 76.7 | 84.6 | 88.9 | 93.2 | 100.7 |
| 30.0–34.9 | 60.0 | 63.4 | 66.2 | 69.7 | 78.1 | 85.7 | 91.6 | 94.0 | 99.1 |
| 35.0–39.9 | 60.9 | 66.3 | 69.8 | 73.7 | 80.6 | 87.1 | 91.5 | 94.6 | 101.6 |
| 40.0–44.9 | 61.2 | 65.3 | 68.4 | 72.5 | 79.9 | 88.4 | 93.4 | 97.8 | 102.6 |
| 45.0–49.9 | 60.1 | 65.2 | 67.3 | 72.1 | 79.8 | 88.6 | 93.3 | 96.7 | 101.3 |
| 50.0–54.9 | 58.6 | 63.4 | 66.4 | 70.9 | 78.5 | 86.4 | 91.7 | 96.7 | 102.2 |
| 55.0–59.9 | 60.2 | 65.8 | 67.1 | 71.2 | 78.0 | 85.4 | 91.1 | 95.4 | 100.9 |
| 60.0–64.9 | 58.4 | 61.8 | 65.3 | 69.2 | 76.9 | 84.5 | 88.6 | 91.5 | 97.8 |
| 65.0–69.9 | 56.7 | 60.7 | 63.4 | 67.9 | 75.1 | 83.2 | 87.0 | 90.8 | 96.7 |
| 70.0–74.9 | 55.2 | 59.1 | 62.9 | 66.6 | 73.7 | 81.8 | 86.6 | 90.3 | 93.9 |
| **Males with large frames** | | | | | | | | | |
| 18.0–24.9 | 58.4 | 61.5 | 62.7 | 67.6 | 75.0 | 85.4 | 91.2 | 95.0 | 103.3 |
| 25.0–29.9 | 61.2 | 66.0 | 68.3 | 72.8 | 82.0 | 90.9 | 99.3 | 102.1 | 113.5 |
| 30.0–34.9 | 64.6 | 69.1 | 70.9 | 76.3 | 86.0 | 94.0 | 101.0 | 104.3 | 115.5 |
| 35.0–39.9 | 59.6 | 67.4 | 71.4 | 75.4 | 83.6 | 92.6 | 98.4 | 104.1 | 115.3 |
| 40.0–44.9 | 63.6 | 67.4 | 68.7 | 73.4 | 81.8 | 92.2 | 100.3 | 107.4 | 113.8 |
| 45.0–49.9 | 64.2 | 67.3 | 69.4 | 75.3 | 83.9 | 92.5 | 97.9 | 103.2 | 113.2 |
| 50.0–54.9 | 64.3 | 66.6 | 68.8 | 73.0 | 82.4 | 92.5 | 100.9 | 102.8 | 110.2 |
| 55.0–59.9 | 64.8 | 68.1 | 71.5 | 75.1 | 84.5 | 92.8 | 100.0 | 102.6 | 116.3 |
| 60.0–64.9 | 62.7 | 66.7 | 69.5 | 73.1 | 80.1 | 89.4 | 94.5 | 98.9 | 107.3 |
| 65.0–69.9 | 58.2 | 62.0 | 66.3 | 71.0 | 78.9 | 87.5 | 92.2 | 95.7 | 103.9 |
| 70.0–74.9 | 55.8 | 61.6 | 64.8 | 68.4 | 76.9 | 83.2 | 90.5 | 94.7 | 99.6 |

| Age (yrs) | Percentiles | | | | | | | | |
|---|---|---|---|---|---|---|---|---|---|
| | 5 | 10 | 15 | 25 | 50 | 75 | 85 | 90 | 95 |
| **Females with small frames** | | | | | | | | | |
| 18.0–24.9 | 44.0 | 46.7 | 48.5 | 50.6 | 54.9 | 60.9 | 64.5 | 66.9 | 71.5 |
| 25.0–29.9 | 44.4 | 47.3 | 48.5 | 51.3 | 55.9 | 60.9 | 63.7 | 66.1 | 72.6 |
| 30.0–34.9 | 46.1 | 48.3 | 50.0 | 52.6 | 57.0 | 62.5 | 66.8 | 68.8 | 77.1 |
| 35.0–39.9 | 45.9 | 48.2 | 50.8 | 53.4 | 59.4 | 66.2 | 71.0 | 74.7 | 78.4 |
| 40.0–44.9 | 48.0 | 50.3 | 51.8 | 54.5 | 58.8 | 65.2 | 69.3 | 72.5 | 78.1 |
| 45.0–49.9 | 46.5 | 48.8 | 50.9 | 53.5 | 60.1 | 66.3 | 70.5 | 73.1 | 79.7 |
| 50.0–54.9 | 46.8 | 49.3 | 51.5 | 54.4 | 60.1 | 66.7 | 70.4 | 72.9 | 76.5 |
| 55.0–59.9 | 45.4 | 49.3 | 51.6 | 54.4 | 59.2 | 64.9 | 69.6 | 72.3 | 79.1 |
| 60.0–64.9 | 46.6 | 48.5 | 50.6 | 54.2 | 60.7 | 67.9 | 71.4 | 73.9 | 79.8 |
| 65.0–69.9 | 45.1 | 48.4 | 51.1 | 53.5 | 60.0 | 67.3 | 70.8 | 73.5 | 79.0 |
| 70.0–74.9 | 42.6 | 45.9 | 48.5 | 51.5 | 59.6 | 66.4 | 72.0 | 74.2 | 79.3 |
| **Females with medium frames** | | | | | | | | | |
| 18.0–24.9 | 46.6 | 48.8 | 50.2 | 52.6 | 57.9 | 64.1 | 68.1 | 71.9 | 77.8 |
| 25.0–29.9 | 46.9 | 49.1 | 50.2 | 52.7 | 58.1 | 66.1 | 72.2 | 76.0 | 81.6 |
| 30.0–34.9 | 47.2 | 50.0 | 51.7 | 54.2 | 60.1 | 66.3 | 73.7 | 78.6 | 83.6 |
| 35.0–39.9 | 49.2 | 51.7 | 53.0 | 55.9 | 60.8 | 67.6 | 72.8 | 76.7 | 83.5 |
| 40.0–44.9 | 49.0 | 51.0 | 53.2 | 56.1 | 61.6 | 68.8 | 75.4 | 80.1 | 90.6 |
| 45.0–49.9 | 47.7 | 50.9 | 53.0 | 55.9 | 62.8 | 71.2 | 76.9 | 81.9 | 89.0 |
| 50.0–54.9 | 48.8 | 52.4 | 54.5 | 57.3 | 63.6 | 72.3 | 78.0 | 81.6 | 89.6 |
| 55.0–59.9 | 48.2 | 50.6 | 53.6 | 57.3 | 64.5 | 73.3 | 78.4 | 84.1 | 89.2 |
| 60.0–64.9 | 49.1 | 51.7 | 53.3 | 57.3 | 64.2 | 72.7 | 77.6 | 81.1 | 87.2 |
| 65.0–69.9 | 48.5 | 51.3 | 53.3 | 56.3 | 64.4 | 72.7 | 78.1 | 81.1 | 87.8 |
| 70.0–74.9 | 47.1 | 50.6 | 52.5 | 56.6 | 62.5 | 70.2 | 75.9 | 79.1 | 83.9 |
| **Females with large frames** | | | | | | | | | |
| 18.0–24.9 | 48.6 | 50.8 | 52.7 | 55.3 | 62.1 | 74.3 | 81.9 | 86.4 | 102.1 |
| 25.0–29.9 | 49.8 | 52.7 | 55.1 | 57.8 | 66.0 | 79.7 | 87.7 | 96.3 | 104.0 |
| 30.0–34.9 | 50.5 | 53.6 | 56.8 | 60.1 | 69.3 | 87.2 | 95.6 | 101.3 | 109.4 |
| 35.0–39.9 | 52.3 | 55.0 | 56.7 | 61.5 | 71.8 | 86.1 | 94.5 | 98.9 | 108.9 |
| 40.0–44.9 | 52.3 | 56.8 | 59.9 | 64.0 | 73.5 | 86.8 | 94.9 | 100.6 | 110.8 |
| 45.0–49.9 | 56.0 | 60.3 | 63.2 | 65.8 | 76.0 | 86.1 | 97.6 | 102.2 | 112.5 |
| 50.0–54.9 | 50.6 | 58.7 | 61.2 | 65.5 | 73.0 | 85.5 | 93.1 | 98.5 | 106.7 |
| 55.0–59.9 | 55.9 | 59.8 | 61.9 | 66.1 | 76.4 | 88.2 | 92.9 | 99.1 | 105.6 |
| 60.0–64.9 | 56.0 | 58.5 | 61.3 | 65.7 | 75.8 | 84.7 | 91.3 | 98.8 | 104.2 |
| 65.0–69.9 | 54.8 | 58.4 | 60.8 | 63.8 | 73.8 | 82.5 | 90.8 | 97.2 | 105.7 |
| 70.0–74.9 | 53.9 | 57.6 | 60.7 | 65.7 | 74.4 | 81.9 | 87.0 | 90.0 | 93.9 |

Modified from Fisancho, A.R.: *Anthropometric Standards for the Assessment of Growth and Nutritional Status*, Ann Arbor, The University of Michigan Press, 1990.

## 10–6 Percentiles of Percent Body Fat by Age, and Nonograms for Conversion of Skinfolds to Percent Body Fat, Adults

| Age (yrs) | Percentiles | | | | | | | | |
|---|---|---|---|---|---|---|---|---|---|
| | 5 | 10 | 15 | 25 | 50 | 75 | 85 | 90 | 95 |
| **Males** | | | | | | | | | |
| 18.0–24.9 | 8.0 | 9.0 | 10.0 | 12.0 | 16.0 | 20.0 | 23.0 | 25.0 | 28.0 |
| 25.0–29.9 | 9.0 | 10.0 | 11.0 | 13.0 | 18.0 | 23.0 | 25.0 | 26.0 | 29.0 |
| 30.0–34.9 | 16.0 | 17.0 | 18.0 | 20.0 | 23.0 | 26.0 | 27.0 | 28.0 | 30.0 |
| 35.0–39.9 | 15.0 | 17.0 | 18.0 | 20.0 | 23.0 | 25.0 | 27.0 | 27.0 | 29.0 |
| 40.0–44.9 | 14.0 | 16.0 | 18.0 | 21.0 | 26.0 | 30.0 | 32.0 | 34.0 | 36.0 |
| 45.0–49.9 | 15.0 | 17.0 | 19.0 | 21.0 | 26.0 | 30.0 | 32.0 | 34.0 | 36.0 |
| 50.0–54.9 | 15.0 | 17.0 | 19.0 | 22.0 | 27.0 | 31.0 | 33.0 | 35.0 | 37.0 |
| 55.0–59.9 | 15.0 | 18.0 | 20.0 | 22.0 | 27.0 | 31.0 | 33.0 | 35.0 | 37.0 |
| 60.0–64.9 | 16.0 | 18.0 | 20.0 | 22.0 | 27.0 | 31.0 | 33.0 | 35.0 | 37.0 |
| 65.0–69.9 | 13.0 | 16.0 | 18.0 | 21.0 | 26.0 | 30.0 | 33.0 | 35.0 | 37.0 |
| 70.0–74.9 | 13.0 | 16.0 | 18.0 | 21.0 | 26.0 | 30.0 | 33.0 | 34.0 | 36.0 |
| **Females** | | | | | | | | | |
| 18.0–24.9 | 17.0 | 19.0 | 21.0 | 23.0 | 27.0 | 33.0 | 35.0 | 37.0 | 40.0 |
| 25.0–29.9 | 18.0 | 20.0 | 21.0 | 24.0 | 29.0 | 34.0 | 37.0 | 39.0 | 41.0 |
| 30.0–34.9 | 21.0 | 23.0 | 25.0 | 27.0 | 31.0 | 36.0 | 38.0 | 40.0 | 42.0 |
| 35.0–39.9 | 22.0 | 24.0 | 25.0 | 28.0 | 32.0 | 37.0 | 39.0 | 40.0 | 42.0 |
| 40.0–44.9 | 25.0 | 28.0 | 29.0 | 31.0 | 35.0 | 39.0 | 41.0 | 42.0 | 43.0 |
| 45.0–49.9 | 26.0 | 28.0 | 29.0 | 32.0 | 36.0 | 39.0 | 41.0 | 42.0 | 44.0 |
| 50.0–54.9 | 27.0 | 30.0 | 32.0 | 35.0 | 39.0 | 43.0 | 46.0 | 47.0 | 48.0 |
| 55.0–59.9 | 27.0 | 30.0 | 32.0 | 35.0 | 39.0 | 44.0 | 45.0 | 47.0 | 49.0 |
| 60.0–64.9 | 28.0 | 31.0 | 32.0 | 35.0 | 40.0 | 43.0 | 45.0 | 46.0 | 48.0 |
| 65.0–69.9 | 27.0 | 30.0 | 32.0 | 34.0 | 38.0 | 42.0 | 44.0 | 46.0 | 47.0 |
| 70.0–74.9 | 26.0 | 29.0 | 31.0 | 34.0 | 38.0 | 42.0 | 44.0 | 45.0 | 47.0 |

Modified from Frisancho, A.R.: *Anthropometric Standards for the Assessment of Growth and Nutritional Status,* Ann Arbor, The University of Michigan Press, 1990.

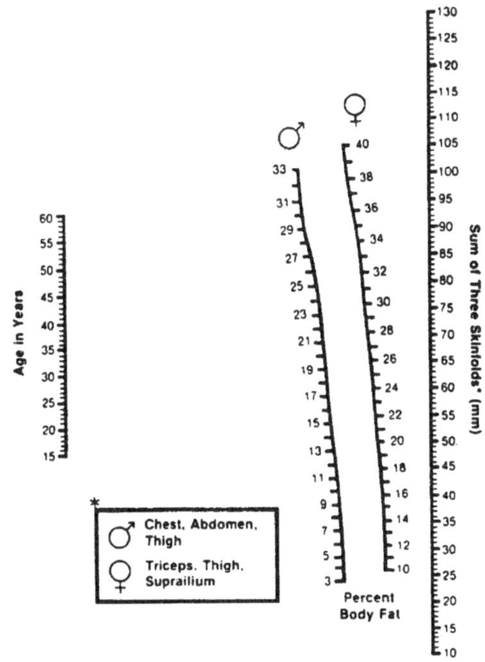


From: *The Research Quarterly for Exercise and Sport,* 1981, 52:380. Used with permission.

## 10–6A Lutein and Zeaxanthin Content of Selected Foods (Beneficial for Vision)

**Fresh Vegetables**

| Vegetable, 1 cup | Lutein/ Zeaxanthin, mcg |
|---|---|
| Mushroom | 0 |
| Onion | 16 |
| Cabbage-red | 44 |
| Iceberg lettuce | 194 |
| Tomato | 234 |
| Celery | 278 |
| Sweet Red Peppers | 325 |
| Carrots-1 cup sliced | 437 |
| Okra | 516 |
| Green Olives | 750 |
| Pea Pods | 816 |
| Black Olives | 831 |
| Cucumber-with peel | 856 |
| Green Peppers | 891 |
| Asparagus | 920 |
| Seaweed-dehydrated | 1,044 |
| Sweet Yellow Pepper | 1,147 |
| Romaine lettuce | 1,476 |
| Broccoli | 2,152 |
| Watercress | 2,546 |
| Swiss Chard | 2,906 |
| Collards | 3,381 |
| Spinach | 3,581 |
| Turnip Greens | 4,642 |
| Mustard Greens | 4,726 |
| Kelp | 16,822 |

**Cooked Vegetables**

| Vegetable, 1 cup | Lutein/ Zeaxanthin, mcg |
|---|---|
| Onion | 15 |
| Acorn Squash | 162 |
| Leeks | 515 |
| Sweet Red Peper | 541 |
| Frozen Okra | 718 |
| Green Beans | 875 |
| Frozen Lima Beans | 1,190 |
| Green Pepper | 1,288 |
| Asparagus | 1,328 |
| Sweet Yellow Pepper | 1,476 |
| Fresh Brussels Sprouts | 2,012 |
| Pea Pods | 2,160 |
| Green Peas | 2,648 |
| Broccoli | 2,928 |
| Corn | 2,952 |
| Fresh Zucchini | 4,500 |
| Frozen Zucchini | 5,575 |
| Watercress | 10,260 |
| Turnip Greens | 12,154 |
| Fresh Spinach | 12,677 |
| Frozen Spinach | 13,382 |
| Fresh Collards | 15,373 |
| Swiss Chard | 17,225 |
| Kale | 20,537 |

**Fruit Juices**

| Juice, 1 cup | Lutein/ Zeaxanthin, mcg |
|---|---|
| Pineapple juice | 4 |
| Cranberry juice | 23 |
| Grapefruit juice | 25 |
| Grape juice | 65 |
| Apple juice | 121 |
| Tomato juice | 146 |
| Orange juice | 217 |

**Cereals/Grains**

| Cereal, 1 cup | Lutein/ Zeaxanthin, mcg |
|---|---|
| Corn Chex | 301 |
| Cornflakes | 300 |
| Cornbread-3" × 3" piece | 240 |
| Corn tortilla 2-six inch | 390 |

**Fruit**

| Fruit, 1 cup | Lutein/ Zeaxanthin, mcg |
|---|---|
| Banana | 0 |
| Pineapple-canned | 0 |
| 1/2 Grapefruit | 13 |
| Cranberries-fresh | 27 |
| Strawberries | 35 |
| Cranberries-dried | 40 |
| Apple | 78 |
| Pears-canned | 83 |
| Cherries-fresh | 104 |
| Papaya-fresh | 105 |
| Peaches-canned | 149 |
| Raspberries | 182 |
| Rhubarb-fresh | 216 |
| Blueberries | 290 |
| Rhubarb-frozen | 242 |
| Plum | 282 |
| Orange | 337 |
| Mandarin Oranges | 474 |
| Kiwi | 526 |
| Blackberries | 936 |

Analyzed using Nutrition Data System for Research software versions 5.0_35 (8-3-04) developed by the Nutrition Coordinating Center (NCC), University of Minnesota, Minneapolis, MN.

**10–7** Sum of Skinfold to Determine Body Fat in Adults by Jackson and Pollack, Three Sites

**Percent Fat: Men, Sum of three sites:**

1. Abdomen
2. Ilium
3. Tricep

Percent fat $= .39287\ (\Sigma 3) - .00105\ (\Sigma 3^2) + .15772\ (AGE) + 5.18845$

R = .893 SE = 3.63% fat

Percent Fat Estimates for Three Sites - Men

| Sum of 3 skin-folds | Age to Last Year 18-22 | 23-27 | 28-32 | 33-37 | 38-42 | 43-47 | 48-52 | 53-57 | >58 |
|---|---|---|---|---|---|---|---|---|---|
| 8-12 | 1.8 | 2.6 | 3.4 | 4.2 | 4.9 | 5.7 | 6.5 | 7.3 | 8.1 |
| 13-17 | 3.6 | 4.4 | 5.2 | 6.0 | 6.8 | 7.6 | 8.4 | 9.1 | 9.9 |
| 18-22 | 5.4 | 6.2 | 7.0 | 7.8 | 8.6 | 9.3 | 10.1 | 10.9 | 11.7 |
| 23-27 | 7.1 | 7.9 | 8.7 | 9.5 | 10.3 | 11.1 | 11.9 | 12.6 | 13.4 |
| 28-32 | 8.8 | 9.6 | 10.4 | 11.2 | 12.0 | 12.8 | 13.5 | 14.3 | 15.1 |
| 33-37 | 10.4 | 11.2 | 12.0 | 12.8 | 13.6 | 14.4 | 15.2 | 15.9 | 16.7 |
| 38-42 | 12.0 | 12.8 | 13.6 | 14.4 | 15.2 | 15.9 | 16.7 | 17.5 | 18.3 |
| 43-47 | 13.5 | 14.3 | 15.1 | 15.9 | 16.7 | 17.5 | 18.3 | 19.0 | 19.8 |
| 48-52 | 15.0 | 15.8 | 16.6 | 17.4 | 18.1 | 18.9 | 19.7 | 20.5 | 21.3 |
| 53-57 | 16.4 | 17.2 | 18.0 | 18.8 | 19.6 | 20.3 | 21.1 | 21.9 | 22.7 |
| 58-62 | 17.8 | 18.5 | 19.3 | 20.1 | 20.9 | 21.7 | 22.5 | 23.3 | 24.1 |
| 63-67 | 19.1 | 19.9 | 20.6 | 21.4 | 22.2 | 23.0 | 23.8 | 24.6 | 25.4 |
| 68-72 | 20.3 | 21.1 | 21.9 | 22.7 | 23.5 | 24.3 | 25.1 | 25.8 | 26.6 |
| 73-77 | 21.5 | 22.3 | 23.1 | 23.9 | 24.7 | 25.5 | 26.3 | 27.0 | 27.8 |
| 78-82 | 22.7 | 23.5 | 24.3 | 25.0 | 25.8 | 26.6 | 27.4 | 28.2 | 29.0 |
| 83-87 | 23.8 | 24.6 | 25.3 | 26.1 | 26.9 | 27.7 | 28.5 | 29.3 | 30.1 |
| 88-92 | 24.8 | 25.6 | 26.4 | 27.2 | 28.0 | 28.8 | 29.6 | 30.3 | 31.1 |
| 93-97 | 25.8 | 26.6 | 27.4 | 28.2 | 29.0 | 29.8 | 30.5 | 31.3 | 32.1 |
| 98-102 | 26.7 | 27.5 | 28.3 | 29.1 | 29.9 | 30.7 | 31.5 | 32.3 | 33.1 |
| 103-107 | 27.6 | 28.4 | 29.2 | 30.0 | 30.8 | 31.6 | 32.4 | 33.2 | 33.9 |
| 108-112 | 28.5 | 29.3 | 30.1 | 30.8 | 31.6 | 32.4 | 33.2 | 34.0 | 34.8 |
| 113-117 | 29.3 | 30.0 | 30.8 | 31.6 | 32.4 | 33.2 | 34.0 | 34.8 | 35.6 |
| 118-122 | 30.0 | 30.8 | 31.6 | 32.4 | 33.1 | 33.9 | 34.7 | 35.5 | 36.3 |
| 123-127 | 30.7 | 31.5 | 32.2 | 33.0 | 33.8 | 34.6 | 35.4 | 36.2 | 37.0 |
| 128-132 | 31.3 | 32.1 | 32.9 | 33.7 | 34.4 | 35.2 | 36.0 | 36.8 | 37.6 |
| 133-137 | 31.9 | 32.7 | 33.4 | 34.2 | 35.0 | 35.8 | 36.6 | 37.4 | 38.2 |
| 138-142 | 32.4 | 33.2 | 34.0 | 34.8 | 35.5 | 36.3 | 37.1 | 37.9 | 38.7 |
| 143-147 | 32.9 | 33.6 | 34.4 | 35.2 | 36.0 | 36.8 | 37.6 | 38.4 | 39.2 |
| 148-152 | 33.3 | 34.1 | 34.8 | 35.6 | 36.4 | 37.2 | 38.0 | 38.8 | 39.6 |
| 153-157 | 33.6 | 34.4 | 35.2 | 36.0 | 36.8 | 37.6 | 38.4 | 39.2 | 39.9 |
| 158-162 | 33.9 | 34.7 | 35.5 | 36.3 | 37.1 | 37.9 | 38.7 | 39.5 | 40.3 |
| 163-167 | 34.2 | 35.0 | 35.8 | 36.6 | 37.4 | 38.1 | 38.9 | 39.7 | 40.5 |
| 168-172 | 34.4 | 35.2 | 36.0 | 36.8 | 37.6 | 38.4 | 39.1 | 39.9 | 40.7 |
| 173-177 | 34.6 | 35.3 | 36.1 | 36.9 | 37.7 | 38.5 | 39.3 | 40.1 | 40.9 |
| 178-182 | 34.7 | 35.4 | 36.2 | 37.0 | 37.8 | 38.6 | 39.4 | 40.2 | 41.0 |

**Percent Fat: Women, Sum of three sites:**

1. Abdomen
2. Ilium
3. Tricep

Percent fat $= .41563\ (\Sigma 3) - .00112\ (\Sigma 3^2) + .03661\ (AGE) + 4.03653$

R = .825 SE = 3.98% fat

Percent Fat Estimates for Three Sites - Women

| Sum of 3 skin-folds | Age to Last Year 18-22 | 23-27 | 28-32 | 33-37 | 38-42 | 43-47 | 48-52 | 53-57 | >58 |
|---|---|---|---|---|---|---|---|---|---|
| 8-12 | 8.8 | 9.0 | 9.2 | 9.4 | 9.5 | 9.7 | 9.9 | 10.1 | 10.3 |
| 13-17 | 10.8 | 10.9 | 11.1 | 11.3 | 11.5 | 11.7 | 11.8 | 12.0 | 12.2 |
| 18-22 | 12.6 | 12.8 | 13.0 | 13.2 | 13.4 | 13.5 | 13.7 | 13.9 | 14.1 |
| 23-27 | 14.5 | 14.6 | 14.8 | 15.0 | 15.2 | 15.4 | 15.6 | 15.7 | 15.9 |
| 28-32 | 16.2 | 16.4 | 16.6 | 16.8 | 17.0 | 17.1 | 17.3 | 17.5 | 17.7 |
| 33-37 | 17.9 | 18.1 | 18.3 | 18.5 | 18.7 | 18.9 | 19.0 | 19.2 | 19.4 |
| 38-42 | 19.6 | 19.8 | 20.0 | 20.2 | 20.3 | 20.5 | 20.7 | 20.9 | 21.1 |
| 43-47 | 21.2 | 21.4 | 21.6 | 21.8 | 21.9 | 22.1 | 22.3 | 22.5 | 22.7 |
| 48-52 | 22.8 | 22.9 | 23.1 | 23.3 | 23.5 | 23.7 | 23.8 | 24.0 | 24.2 |
| 53-57 | 24.2 | 24.4 | 24.6 | 24.8 | 25.0 | 25.2 | 25.3 | 25.5 | 25.7 |
| 58-62 | 25.7 | 25.9 | 26.0 | 26.2 | 26.4 | 26.6 | 26.8 | 27.0 | 27.1 |
| 63-67 | 27.1 | 27.2 | 27.4 | 27.6 | 27.8 | 28.0 | 28.2 | 28.3 | 28.5 |
| 68-72 | 28.4 | 28.6 | 28.7 | 28.9 | 29.1 | 29.3 | 29.5 | 29.7 | 29.8 |
| 73-77 | 29.6 | 29.8 | 30.0 | 30.2 | 30.4 | 30.6 | 30.7 | 30.9 | 31.1 |
| 78-82 | 30.9 | 31.0 | 31.2 | 31.4 | 31.6 | 31.8 | 31.9 | 32.1 | 32.3 |
| 83-87 | 32.0 | 32.2 | 32.4 | 32.6 | 32.7 | 32.9 | 33.1 | 33.3 | 33.5 |
| 88-92 | 33.1 | 33.3 | 33.5 | 33.7 | 33.8 | 34.0 | 34.2 | 34.4 | 34.6 |
| 93-97 | 34.1 | 34.3 | 34.5 | 34.7 | 34.9 | 35.1 | 35.2 | 35.4 | 35.6 |
| 98-102 | 35.1 | 35.3 | 35.5 | 35.7 | 35.9 | 36.0 | 36.2 | 36.4 | 36.6 |
| 103-107 | 36.1 | 36.2 | 36.4 | 36.6 | 36.8 | 37.0 | 37.2 | 37.3 | 37.5 |
| 108-112 | 36.9 | 37.1 | 37.3 | 37.5 | 37.7 | 37.9 | 38.0 | 38.2 | 38.4 |
| 113-117 | 37.8 | 37.9 | 38.1 | 38.3 | 39.2 | 39.4 | 39.6 | 39.8 | 39.5 |
| 118-122 | 38.5 | 38.7 | 38.9 | 39.1 | 39.4 | 39.6 | 39.8 | 40.0 | 40.0 |
| 123-127 | 39.2 | 39.4 | 39.6 | 39.8 | 40.0 | 40.1 | 40.3 | 40.5 | 40.7 |
| 128-132 | 39.9 | 40.1 | 40.2 | 40.4 | 40.6 | 40.8 | 41.0 | 41.2 | 41.3 |
| 133-137 | 40.5 | 40.7 | 40.8 | 41.0 | 41.2 | 41.4 | 41.6 | 41.7 | 41.9 |
| 138-142 | 41.0 | 41.2 | 41.4 | 41.6 | 41.7 | 41.9 | 42.1 | 42.3 | 42.5 |
| 143-147 | 41.5 | 41.7 | 41.9 | 42.0 | 42.2 | 42.4 | 42.6 | 42.8 | 43.0 |
| 148-152 | 41.9 | 42.1 | 42.3 | 42.8 | 42.6 | 42.8 | 43.0 | 43.2 | 43.4 |
| 153-157 | 42.3 | 42.5 | 42.6 | 52.8 | 43.0 | 43.2 | 43.4 | 43.6 | 43.7 |
| 158-162 | 42.6 | 42.8 | 42.0 | 43.1 | 43.3 | 43.5 | 43.7 | 43.9 | 44.1 |
| 163-167 | 42.9 | 43.0 | 43.2 | 43.4 | 43.6 | 43.8 | 44.0 | 44.1 | 44.3 |
| 168-172 | 43.1 | 43.2 | 43.4 | 43.6 | 43.8 | 44.0 | 44.2 | 44.3 | 44.5 |
| 173-177 | 43.2 | 43.4 | 43.6 | 43.8 | 43.9 | 44.1 | 44.3 | 44.5 | 44.7 |
| 178-182 | 43.3 | 43.5 | 43.7 | 43.8 | 44.0 | 44.2 | 44.4 | 44.6 | 44.8 |

Equations and tables based on Jackson, A.S. and Pollock, M.L.: Generalized equations for predicting body density of man. *Br J Nutr,* 40:497, 1978. From Golding, L.A., Myers, C.R., and Sinning, W.E.: *Y's Way to Physical Fitness,* Champaign, IL., Human Kinetics, 1989. Used with permission.

## 10–8 Sum of Skinfold to Determine Body Fat in Adults by Jackson and Pollock, Four Sites

Percent Fat: Men - Sum of four sites:
1. Abdomen
2. Ilium
3. Tricep
4. Thigh

Percent fat $= .29288\ (\Sigma 4) - .0005\ (\Sigma 4^2) + .15845\ (\text{AGE}) - 5.76377$

R = .901 SE = 3.49% fat

### Percent Fat Estimates for Four Sites - Men

| Sum of 4 skin-folds | Age to Last Year | | | | | | | | |
|---|---|---|---|---|---|---|---|---|---|
| | 18-22 | 23-27 | 28-32 | 33-37 | 38-42 | 43-47 | 48-52 | 53-57 | >58 |
| 13-17 | 1.7 | 2.5 | 3.3 | 4.1 | 4.9 | 5.6 | 6.4 | 7.2 | 8.0 |
| 18-22 | 3.1 | 3.9 | 4.6 | 5.4 | 6.2 | 7.0 | 7.8 | 8.6 | 9.4 |
| 23-27 | 4.4 | 5.2 | 6.0 | 6.8 | 7.6 | 8.4 | 9.2 | 10.0 | 10.7 |
| 28-32 | 5.7 | 6.5 | 7.3 | 8.1 | 8.9 | 9.7 | 10.5 | 11.3 | 12.1 |
| 33-37 | 7.0 | 7.8 | 8.6 | 9.4 | 10.2 | 11.0 | 11.8 | 12.6 | 13.4 |
| 38-42 | 8.3 | 9.1 | 9.9 | 10.7 | 11.5 | 12.3 | 13.1 | 13.9 | 14.6 |
| 43-47 | 9.6 | 10.3 | 11.1 | 11.9 | 12.7 | 13.5 | 14.3 | 15.1 | 15.9 |
| 48-52 | 10.8 | 11.6 | 12.4 | 13.2 | 13.9 | 14.7 | 15.5 | 16.3 | 17.1 |
| 53-57 | 12.0 | 12.8 | 13.6 | 14.4 | 15.1 | 15.9 | 16.7 | 17.5 | 18.3 |
| 58-62 | 13.1 | 13.9 | 14.7 | 15.5 | 16.3 | 17.1 | 17.9 | 18.7 | 19.5 |
| 63-67 | 14.3 | 15.1 | 15.9 | 16.7 | 17.5 | 18.2 | 19.0 | 19.8 | 20.6 |
| 68-72 | 15.4 | 16.2 | 17.0 | 17.8 | 18.6 | 19.4 | 20.2 | 21.0 | 21.8 |
| 73-77 | 16.5 | 17.3 | 18.1 | 18.9 | 19.7 | 20.5 | 21.3 | 22.1 | 22.8 |
| 78-82 | 17.6 | 18.4 | 19.2 | 20.0 | 20.7 | 21.5 | 22.3 | 23.1 | 23.9 |
| 83-87 | 18.6 | 19.4 | 20.2 | 21.0 | 21.8 | 22.6 | 23.4 | 24.2 | 25.0 |
| 88-92 | 19.6 | 20.4 | 21.2 | 22.0 | 22.8 | 23.6 | 24.4 | 25.2 | 26.0 |
| 93-97 | 20.6 | 21.4 | 22.2 | 23.0 | 23.8 | 24.6 | 25.4 | 26.2 | 27.0 |
| 98-102 | 21.6 | 22.4 | 23.2 | 24.0 | 24.8 | 25.6 | 26.4 | 27.1 | 27.9 |
| 103-107 | 22.5 | 23.3 | 24.1 | 24.9 | 25.7 | 26.5 | 27.3 | 28.1 | 28.9 |
| 108-112 | 23.5 | 24.2 | 25.0 | 25.8 | 26.6 | 27.4 | 28.2 | 29.0 | 29.8 |
| 113-117 | 24.3 | 25.1 | 25.9 | 26.7 | 27.5 | 28.3 | 29.1 | 29.9 | 30.7 |
| 118-122 | 25.2 | 26.0 | 26.8 | 27.6 | 28.4 | 29.2 | 30.0 | 30.8 | 31.6 |
| 123-127 | 26.0 | 26.8 | 27.6 | 28.4 | 29.2 | 30.0 | 30.8 | 31.6 | 32.4 |
| 128-132 | 26.9 | 27.7 | 28.4 | 29.2 | 30.0 | 30.8 | 31.6 | 32.4 | 33.2 |
| 133-137 | 27.7 | 28.4 | 29.2 | 30.0 | 30.8 | 31.6 | 32.4 | 33.2 | 34.0 |
| 138-142 | 28.4 | 29.2 | 30.0 | 30.8 | 31.6 | 32.4 | 33.2 | 34.0 | 34.8 |
| 143-147 | 29.2 | 29.9 | 30.7 | 31.5 | 32.3 | 33.1 | 33.9 | 34.7 | 35.5 |
| 148-152 | 29.9 | 30.7 | 31.5 | 32.2 | 33.0 | 33.8 | 34.6 | 35.4 | 36.2 |
| 153-157 | 30.6 | 31.3 | 32.1 | 32.9 | 33.7 | 34.5 | 35.3 | 36.1 | 36.9 |
| 158-162 | 31.2 | 32.0 | 32.8 | 33.6 | 34.4 | 35.2 | 36.0 | 36.8 | 37.6 |
| 163-167 | 31.8 | 32.6 | 33.4 | 34.2 | 35.0 | 35.8 | 36.6 | 37.4 | 38.2 |
| 168-172 | 32.5 | 33.3 | 34.0 | 34.8 | 35.6 | 36.4 | 37.2 | 38.0 | 38.8 |
| 173-177 | 33.0 | 33.8 | 34.6 | 35.4 | 36.2 | 37.0 | 37.8 | 38.6 | 39.4 |
| 178-182 | 33.6 | 34.4 | 35.2 | 36.0 | 36.8 | 37.6 | 38.4 | 39.2 | 39.9 |
| 183-187 | 34.1 | 34.9 | 35.7 | 36.5 | 37.3 | 38.1 | 38.9 | 39.7 | 40.5 |

Percent Fat: Women, Sum of four sites:
1. Abdomen
2. Ilium
3. Tricep
4. Thigh

Percent fat $= .29669\ (\Sigma 4) - .00043\ (\Sigma 4^2) + .02963\ (\text{AGE}) + 1.4072$

R = .846 SE = 3.89% fat

### Percent Fat Estimates for Four Sites - Women

| Sum of 4 skin-folds | Age to Last Year | | | | | | | | |
|---|---|---|---|---|---|---|---|---|---|
| | 18-22 | 23-27 | 28-32 | 33-37 | 38-42 | 43-47 | 48-52 | 53-57 | >58 |
| 23-27 | 8.6 | 9.3 | 9.4 | 9.6 | 9.7 | 9.9 | 10.0 | 10.2 | 10.3 |
| 28-32 | 10.0 | 10.7 | 10.8 | 11.0 | 11.0 | 11.3 | 11.4 | 11.6 | 11.7 |
| 33-37 | 11.3 | 12.0 | 12.2 | 12.3 | 12.4 | 12.6 | 12.7 | 12.9 | 13.0 |
| 38-42 | 12.6 | 13.3 | 13.5 | 13.6 | 13.7 | 13.9 | 14.1 | 14.2 | 14.4 |
| 43-47 | 13.9 | 14.6 | 14.8 | 14.9 | 15.0 | 15.2 | 15.4 | 15.5 | 15.7 |
| 48-52 | 15.2 | 15.9 | 16.1 | 16.2 | 16.3 | 16.5 | 16.7 | 16.8 | 17.0 |
| 53-57 | 16.5 | 17.2 | 17.3 | 17.5 | 17.5 | 17.8 | 17.9 | 18.1 | 18.2 |
| 58-62 | 17.7 | 18.4 | 18.6 | 18.7 | 18.8 | 19.0 | 19.1 | 19.3 | 19.4 |
| 63-67 | 18.9 | 19.6 | 19.8 | 19.9 | 20.0 | 20.2 | 20.4 | 20.5 | 20.7 |
| 68-72 | 20.1 | 20.8 | 21.0 | 21.1 | 21.2 | 21.4 | 21.6 | 21.7 | 21.9 |
| 73-77 | 21.3 | 22.0 | 22.1 | 22.3 | 22.3 | 22.6 | 22.7 | 22.9 | 23.0 |
| 78-82 | 22.5 | 23.1 | 23.3 | 23.4 | 23.5 | 23.7 | 23.9 | 24.0 | 24.2 |
| 83-87 | 23.6 | 24.3 | 24.4 | 24.6 | 24.6 | 24.9 | 25.0 | 25.2 | 25.3 |
| 88-92 | 24.7 | 25.4 | 25.5 | 25.7 | 25.7 | 26.0 | 26.1 | 26.3 | 26.4 |
| 93-97 | 25.8 | 26.5 | 26.6 | 26.8 | 26.8 | 27.1 | 27.2 | 27.4 | 27.5 |
| 98-102 | 26.8 | 27.5 | 27.7 | 27.8 | 27.9 | 28.1 | 28.3 | 28.4 | 28.6 |
| 103-107 | 27.9 | 28.6 | 28.7 | 28.9 | 28.9 | 29.2 | 29.3 | 29.5 | 29.6 |
| 108-112 | 28.9 | 29.6 | 29.7 | 29.9 | 30.0 | 30.2 | 30.3 | 30.5 | 30.6 |
| 113-117 | 29.9 | 30.6 | 30.7 | 30.9 | 31.0 | 31.2 | 31.3 | 31.5 | 31.6 |
| 118-122 | 30.9 | 31.6 | 31.7 | 31.9 | 31.9 | 32.2 | 32.3 | 32.5 | 32.6 |
| 123-127 | 31.9 | 32.5 | 32.7 | 32.8 | 32.9 | 33.1 | 33.3 | 33.4 | 33.6 |
| 128-132 | 32.8 | 33.5 | 33.6 | 33.8 | 33.8 | 34.1 | 34.2 | 34.4 | 34.5 |
| 133-137 | 33.7 | 34.4 | 34.5 | 34.7 | 34.7 | 35.0 | 35.1 | 35.3 | 35.4 |
| 138-142 | 34.6 | 35.3 | 35.4 | 35.6 | 35.6 | 35.9 | 36.0 | 36.2 | 36.3 |
| 143-147 | 35.5 | 36.2 | 36.3 | 36.5 | 36.5 | 36.7 | 36.9 | 37.0 | 37.2 |
| 148-152 | 36.3 | 37.0 | 37.2 | 37.3 | 37.4 | 37.6 | 37.8 | 37.9 | 38.0 |
| 153-157 | 37.2 | 37.8 | 38.0 | 38.1 | 38.2 | 38.4 | 38.6 | 38.7 | 38.9 |
| 158-162 | 38.0 | 38.6 | 38.8 | 38.9 | 39.0 | 39.2 | 39.4 | 39.5 | 39.7 |
| 163-167 | 38.8 | 39.4 | 39.6 | 39.7 | 39.8 | 40.0 | 40.2 | 40.3 | 40.5 |
| 168-172 | 39.5 | 40.2 | 40.3 | 40.5 | 40.6 | 40.8 | 40.9 | 41.1 | 41.2 |
| 173-177 | 40.3 | 40.9 | 41.1 | 41.2 | 41.3 | 41.5 | 41.7 | 41.8 | 42.0 |
| 178-182 | 41.0 | 41.7 | 41.8 | 42.0 | 42.0 | 42.3 | 42.4 | 42.6 | 42.7 |
| 183-187 | 41.7 | 42.4 | 42.5 | 42.7 | 42.7 | 43.0 | 43.1 | 43.3 | 43.4 |
| 188-192 | 42.4 | 43.0 | 43.2 | 43.3 | 43.4 | 43.6 | 43.8 | 43.9 | 44.1 |
| 193-197 | 43.0 | 43.7 | 43.9 | 44.0 | 44.1 | 44.3 | 44.4 | 44.6 | 44.7 |
| 198-202 | 43.7 | 44.3 | 44.5 | 44.6 | 44.7 | 44.9 | 45.1 | 45.2 | 45.4 |

Equations and tables based on Jackson, A.S. and Pollock, M.L.: Generalized equations for predicting body density of man. *Br J Nutr*, 40:497, 1978. From Golding, L.A., Myers, C.R., and Sinning, W.E.: *Y's Way to Physical Fitness*, Champaign, IL., Human Kinetics, 1989. Used with permission.

**10–9** Sample Adult Body Composition and Body Fat Classifications for Athletes and Non-Athletes

| Men | | Women | |
|---|---|---|---|
| Age | = 20-24 | Age | = 20-24 |
| Height | = 68.5 in. | Height | = 64.5 in. |
| Weight | = 154 lb. | Weight | = 125 lb. |
| Total fat | = 23.1 lb. (15.0%) | Total fat | = 3.8 lb. (27.0%) |
| Storage fat | = 18.5 lb. (12.0%) | Storage fat | = 18.8 lb. (15.0%) |
| Essential fat | = 4.6 lb. (3.0%) | Essential fat | = 15.0 lb. (12.0%) |
| Muscle | = 69 lb. (44.8%) | Muscle | = 45 lb. (36.0%) |
| Bone | = 23 lb. (14.9%) | Bone | = 15 lb. (12.0%) |
| Remainder | = 38.9 lb. (25.3%) | Remainder | = 31.2 lb. (25.0%) |
| Lean body weight | = 136 lb. | Minimal weight | = 107 lb. |

**Gross body composition of a reference man and woman.**

Adapted from McArdle, W.D., Katch, F.I., and Katch, V.L.: *Exercise Physiology,* Lea & Febiger, 1983.

**BODY FAT VALUES in ATHLETES and $VO_2$ max**

| Athletic Group or Sport | MALE %fat | MALE $VO_2$ max ml/kg/min | FEMALE %fat | FEMALE $VO_2$max ml/kg/min |
|---|---|---|---|---|
| Baseball | 12-15 | 48-56 | | |
| Basketball | 7-12 | 45-55 | 18-27 | 40-44 |
| Canoeing | 10-14 | 55-67 | | |
| Football: | | | | |
| Defensive backs | 9-12 | 48-55 | | |
| Offensive backs | 9-12 | 48-55 | | |
| Linebackers | 13 | 48-55 | | |
| Offensive linemen | 19 | 46-52 | | |
| Defensive linemen | 19 | 42-48 | | |
| Quarterback, kickers | 14 | 48-55 | | |
| Gymnastics | 3-6 | 52-58 | 8-18 | 37-44 |
| Ice hockey | 12-16 | 50-63 | | |
| Jockeys | 6-14 | 50-60 | | |
| Skiing: | | | | |
| Alpine | 10-17 | 57-68 | 20-28 | 48-60 |
| Cross-country | 7-13 | 65-90 | 18-24 | 60-75 |
| Ski jumping | 12-16 | 58-63 | | |
| Soccer | 7-12 | 54-64 | 16-22 | 45-55 |
| Swimming | 4-10 | 50-70 | 14-25 | 40-55 |
| Track and field: | | | | |
| Runners | | | | |
| Distance, elite | 5-12 | 60-80 | 10-18 | 60-75 |
| Distance | | | 15-20 | 50-60 |
| Sprint | 5-12 | 55-65 | 15-20 | 50-60 |
| Discus | 12-18 | 42-52 | 22-28 | |
| Jumpers and hurdlers | 6-13 | 50-60 | 12-22 | 48-60 |
| Shot put | 14-20 | 40-46 | 23-30 | 35-42 |
| Tennis | 12-16 | | 15-22 | |
| Volleyball | 10-15 | | 20-23 | |
| Weight lifting | 6-16 | | | |
| Wrestling | 6-12 | | | |

**BODY FAT CLASSIFICATIONS for NON-ATHLETES**

| | | Male | Female |
|---|---|---|---|
| Very low fat | skinny | 7 - 9.9 | 14 -16.9 |
| Low fat | trim | 10 -12.9 | 17 -19.9 |
| Average fat | normal | 13 -16.9 | 20 - 26.9 |
| Above normal | plump | 17 - 24.9 | 27 - 30.9 |
| Very high fat | fat | 25+ | 31+ |

From: Tufts University and United States Department of Agriculture, Human Nutrition Research Center on Aging.

# 10–10 Pathophysiology of Obesity, Waist to Hip Ratio, and Blood Pressure Classifications, Male and Female, Adult

**PATHOPHYSIOLOGY OF OBESITY**

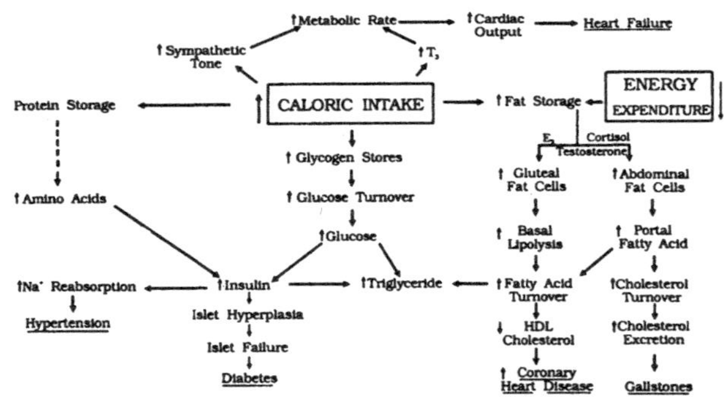


**Waist Hip Ratio by Age and Sex***

| Risk | 20–29 | 30–39 | 40–49 | 50–59 | 60–69 |
|---|---|---|---|---|---|
| Very High | 0.95(0.82) | 0.96(0.85) | 1.00(0.87) | 1.20(0.88) | 1.39(0.91) |
| Moderate | 0.87(0.78) | 0.92(0.79) | 0.94(0.80) | 0.95(0.82) | 0.97(0.85) |
| Low | 0.83(0.71) | 0.84(0.73) | 0.88(0.75) | 0.90(0.76) | 0.91(0.78) |

*Female values in parenthesis.

Adapted from: Bray, G., Pathophysiology of obesity. *Am J Clin Nutr,* 1992: 55, 4885.

**CLASSIFICATION OF BLOOD PRESSURE# IN ADULTS AGE 18 YEARS OR OLDER**

| Range, mm Hg | Category* |
|---|---|
| Diastolic | |
| < 85 | Normal Blood Pressure |
| 85–89 | High normal blood pressure |
| 90–104 | Mild Hypertension |
| 105–114 | Moderate hypertension |
| ≥ 115 | Severe Hypertension |

Systolic, when diastolic blood pressure is <90

| | |
|---|---|
| < 140 | Normal blood pressure |
| 140–159 | Borderline isolated systolic hypertension |
| ≥ 160 | Isolated systolic hypertension |

#Classification based on the average of two or more readings on two or more occasions.

*A classification of borderline isolated systolic hypertension (SBP 140 to 159 mm Hg) or isolated systolic hypertension (SBP ≥ 160 mm Hg) takes precedence over high normal blood pressure (diastolic blood pressure, 85 to 89 mm Hg) when both occur in the same person. High normal blood pressure (DBP 85 to 39 mm Hg) take precedence over a classification of normal blood pressure (SBP < 140 mm Hg) when both occur in the same person.

From: The 1988 Report of the Joint National Committee on *Detection, Evaluation, and Treatment of High Blood Pressure,* U.S. Dept. of Health and Human Services, Public Health Services, National Institute of Health.

**10–11** Nomograms to Determine Body Fat by Body Mass Index, and Nomograms to Determine Body Fat by Abdominal (Waist) and Hip Circumstances, Adults

BODY MASS INDEX NOMOGRAM

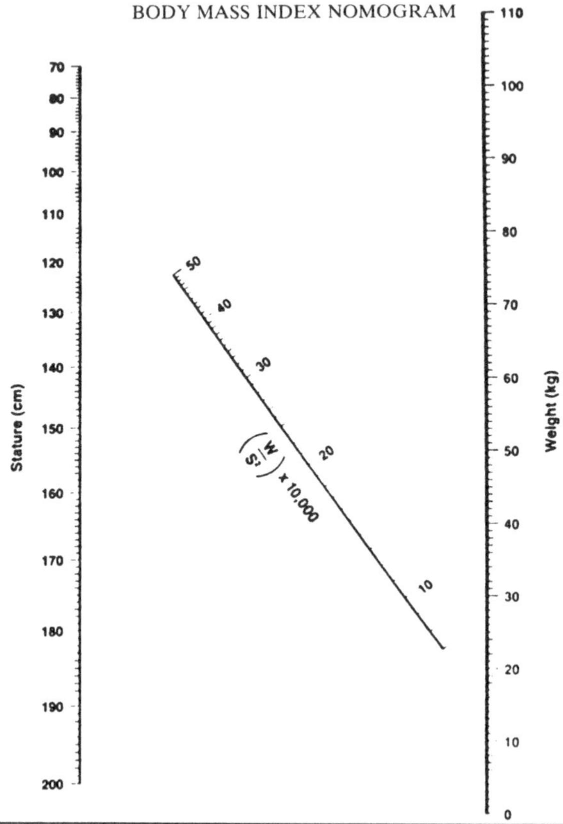


From: *Am J Clin Nutr*, 34, 2831, 1981. © *Am J Clin Nutr*, American Society for Clinical Nutrition. Used with permission.

BODY FAT NOMOGRAM

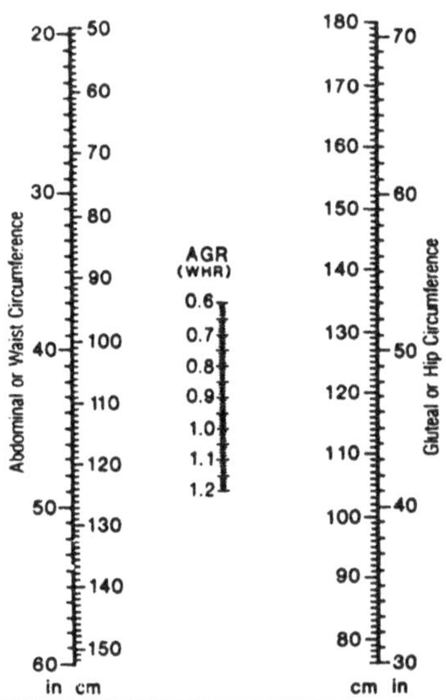


From: Bray, G. A., and D. S. Gray. Obesity. Part I: pathogenesis. *Western Medical Journal*, 1988, 149:429. Used with permission.

## 10–12 Nomograms for Adults and Upper Arm Anthropometry

**Triceps Skinfold (mm), Males**

| Age (years) | Percentile | | |
|---|---|---|---|
| | *50th* | *15th* | *5th* |
| 18-24 | 9.5 | 6.0 | 4.0 |
| 25-34 | 12.0 | 6.0 | 4.5 |
| 35-44 | 12.0 | 7.0 | 5.0 |
| 45-54 | 11.0 | 7.0 | 5.0 |
| 55-64 | 11.0 | 6.5 | 5.0 |
| 65-74 | 11.0 | 6.5 | 4.5 |

**Triceps Skinfold (mm), Females**

| Age (years) | Percentile | | |
|---|---|---|---|
| | *50th* | *15th* | *5th* |
| 18-24 | 18.0 | 12.0 | 9.4 |
| 25-34 | 21.0 | 13.5 | 10.5 |
| 35-44 | 23.0 | 16.0 | 12.0 |
| 45-54 | 25.0 | 17.0 | 13.0 |
| 55-64 | 25.0 | 16.0 | 11.0 |
| 65-74 | 23.0 | 16.0 | 11.5 |

**Midarm Muscle Circumference (cm), Males**

| Age (years) | Percentile | | |
|---|---|---|---|
| | *50th* | *15th** | *5th* |
| 18-24 | 27.2 | 25.0 | 23.5 |
| 25-34 | 28.0 | 25.8 | 24.2 |
| 35-44 | 28.7 | 26.2 | 25.0 |
| 45-54 | 28.1 | 25.6 | 24.0 |
| 55-64 | 27.9 | 25.4 | 22.8 |
| 65-74 | 26.9 | 24.3 | 22.5 |

**Midarm Muscle Circumference (cm), Females**

| Age (years) | Percentile | | |
|---|---|---|---|
| | *50th* | *15th** | *5th* |
| 18-24 | 20.6 | 18.8 | 17.7 |
| 25-34 | 21.4 | 19.3 | 18.3 |
| 35-44 | 22.0 | 19.7 | 18.5 |
| 45-54 | 22.2 | 19.9 | 18.8 |
| 55-64 | 22.6 | 20.1 | 18.6 |
| 65-74 | 22.5 | 20.0 | 18.6 |

**Midarm Circumference (cm), Males**

| Age (years) | Percentile | | |
|---|---|---|---|
| | *50th* | *15th* | *5th* |
| 18-24 | 30.7 | 27.6 | 25.7 |
| 25-34 | 32.0 | 28.9 | 27.0 |
| 35-44 | 32.7 | 29.5 | 27.8 |
| 45-54 | 32.0 | 28.9 | 26.7 |
| 55-64 | 31.7 | 28.2 | 25.6 |
| 65-74 | 30.7 | 27.3 | 25.3 |

**Midarm Circumference (cm), Females**

| Age (years) | Percentile | | |
|---|---|---|---|
| | *50th* | *15th* | *5th* |
| 18-24 | 26.4 | 23.5 | 22.1 |
| 25-34 | 27.8 | 24.8 | 23.3 |
| 35-44 | 29.2 | 25.8 | 24.1 |
| 45-54 | 30.3 | 26.6 | 24.3 |
| 55-64 | 30.2 | 26.1 | 23.9 |
| 65-74 | 29.9 | 26.2 | 23.8 |

*Values provided by investigator, Charles W. Bishop, PhD, University of Wisconsin From Bishop, C.W., Bowen P.D., Ritchey, S.J.: Norms for nutritional assessment of American adults by upper arm anthropometry, *Am J Clin Nutr* 34:2530, 1981. Used with permission..

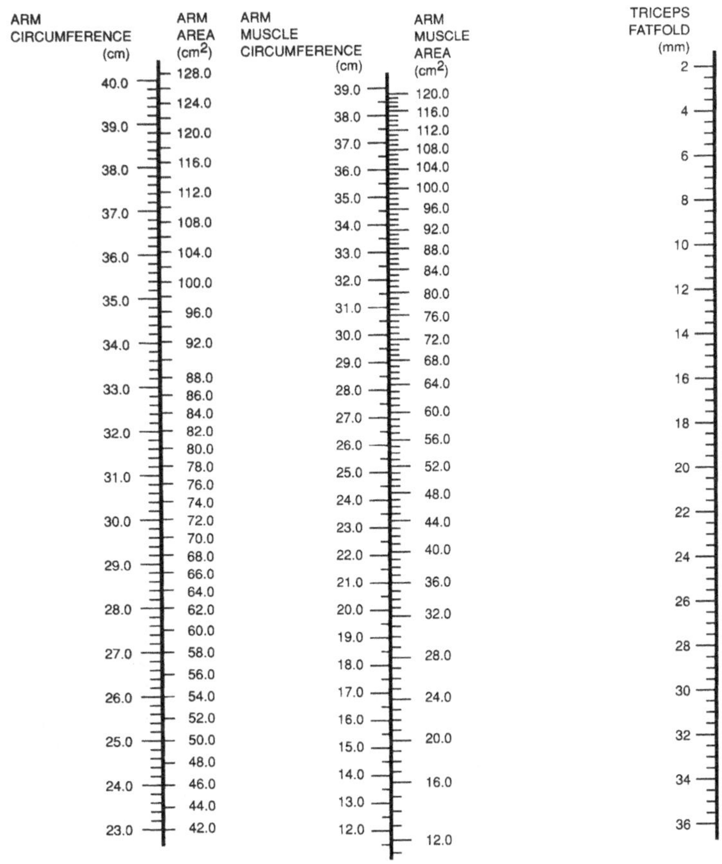


ARM ANTHROPOMETRY NOMOGRAM FOR ADULTS

*Reproduced with permission from: Gurney, J. and Jellife, D.: Arm anthropometry in nutritional assessments: nomogram for rapid calculation of muscle circumference and cross-sectional muscle and fat areas. *Am J Clin Nutr*, 26:912, 1973.

**10–13** Target Weight by Percent Body Fat, Women and Men

**Target Weight - Women (23% Fat)**

| | Body Weight (lb) | | | | | | | | | | | | | | | | | | |
|---|---|---|---|---|---|---|---|---|---|---|---|---|---|---|---|---|---|---|---|
| %fat | 105 | 110 | 115 | 120 | 125 | 130 | 135 | 140 | 145 | 150 | 155 | 160 | 165 | 170 | 175 | 180 | 185 | 190 | 195 |
| 24 | 104 | 109 | 114 | 118 | 123 | 128 | 133 | 138 | 143 | 148 | 153 | 158 | 163 | 168 | 173 | 178 | 183 | 188 | 192 |
| 25 | 102 | 107 | 112 | 117 | 122 | 127 | 131 | 136 | 141 | 146 | 151 | 156 | 161 | 166 | 170 | 175 | 180 | 185 | 190 |
| 26 | 101 | 106 | 111 | 115 | 120 | 125 | 130 | 135 | 139 | 144 | 149 | 154 | 159 | 163 | 168 | 173 | 178 | 183 | 187 |
| 27 | 100 | 104 | 109 | 114 | 119 | 123 | 128 | 133 | 137 | 142 | 147 | 152 | 156 | 161 | 166 | 171 | 175 | 180 | 185 |
| 28 | 98 | 103 | 108 | 112 | 117 | 122 | 126 | 131 | 136 | 140 | 145 | 150 | 154 | 159 | 164 | 168 | 173 | 178 | 182 |
| 29 | 97 | 101 | 106 | 111 | 115 | 120 | 124 | 129 | 134 | 138 | 143 | 148 | 152 | 157 | 161 | 166 | 171 | 175 | 180 |
| 30 | 95 | 100 | 105 | 109 | 114 | 118 | 123 | 127 | 132 | 136 | 141 | 145 | 150 | 155 | 159 | 164 | 168 | 173 | 177 |
| 31 | 94 | 99 | 103 | 108 | 112 | 116 | 121 | 125 | 130 | 134 | 139 | 144 | 149 | 152 | 157 | 161 | 166 | 170 | 175 |
| 32 | 93 | 97 | 102 | 106 | 110 | 115 | 119 | 124 | 129 | 132 | 137 | 141 | 146 | 150 | 155 | 159 | 163 | 168 | 172 |
| 33 | 91 | 96 | 100 | 104 | 109 | 113 | 117 | 122 | 126 | 131 | 135 | 139 | 144 | 148 | 152 | 157 | 161 | 165 | 170 |
| 34 | 90 | 94 | 99 | 103 | 107 | 111 | 116 | 120 | 124 | 129 | 133 | 137 | 141 | 146 | 150 | 154 | 159 | 163 | 167 |
| 35 | 89 | 93 | 97 | 101 | 106 | 110 | 114 | 118 | 122 | 127 | 131 | 135 | 139 | 144 | 148 | 152 | 156 | 160 | 165 |
| 36 | 87 | 91 | 96 | 100 | 104 | 108 | 112 | 116 | 121 | 125 | 129 | 133 | 137 | 141 | 145 | 150 | 154 | 158 | 162 |
| 37 | 86 | 90 | 94 | 98 | 102 | 106 | 110 | 115 | 119 | 123 | 127 | 131 | 135 | 139 | 143 | 147 | 151 | 155 | 160 |
| 38 | 85 | 89 | 93 | 97 | 101 | 105 | 109 | 113 | 117 | 121 | 125 | 129 | 133 | 137 | 141 | 145 | 149 | 153 | 157 |
| 39 | 83 | 87 | 91 | 95 | 99 | 103 | 107 | 111 | 115 | 119 | 123 | 127 | 131 | 135 | 139 | 143 | 147 | 151 | 154 |
| 40 | 82 | 86 | 90 | 94 | 97 | 101 | 105 | 109 | 113 | 117 | 121 | 125 | 129 | 132 | 136 | 140 | 144 | 148 | 152 |

**Target Weight - Men (16% Fat)**

| | Body Weight (lb) | | | | | | | | | | | | | | | | | | | | | | | | |
|---|---|---|---|---|---|---|---|---|---|---|---|---|---|---|---|---|---|---|---|---|---|---|---|---|---|
| %Fat | 120 | 125 | 130 | 135 | 140 | 145 | 150 | 155 | 160 | 165 | 170 | 175 | 180 | 185 | 190 | 195 | 200 | 205 | 210 | 215 | 220 | 225 | 230 | 235 | 240 |
| 17 | 119 | 123 | 129 | 133 | 138 | 143 | 148 | 153 | 158 | 163 | 168 | 173 | 179 | 183 | 188 | 193 | 198 | 203 | 208 | 212 | 217 | 222 | 227 | 232 | 237 |
| 18 | 117 | 122 | 127 | 132 | 137 | 142 | 146 | 151 | 156 | 161 | 166 | 171 | 176 | 181 | 186 | 190 | 195 | 200 | 205 | 210 | 215 | 220 | 225 | 229 | 234 |
| 19 | 116 | 121 | 125 | 130 | 135 | 140 | 145 | 149 | 154 | 159 | 164 | 169 | 174 | 178 | 183 | 188 | 193 | 198 | 203 | 207 | 212 | 217 | 222 | 225 | 231 |
| 20 | 114 | 119 | 124 | 129 | 133 | 138 | 143 | 148 | 152 | 157 | 162 | 167 | 171 | 176 | 181 | 186 | 190 | 195 | 200 | 205 | 210 | 214 | 219 | 224 | 229 |
| 21 | 113 | 118 | 122 | 127 | 132 | 136 | 141 | 146 | 150 | 155 | 160 | 165 | 169 | 174 | 179 | 183 | 188 | 193 | 198 | 202 | 207 | 212 | 216 | 221 | 226 |
| 22 | 111 | 116 | 121 | 125 | 130 | 135 | 139 | 144 | 149 | 153 | 158 | 162 | 167 | 172 | 176 | 181 | 186 | 190 | 195 | 200 | 204 | 209 | 214 | 218 | 223 |
| 23 | 110 | 115 | 119 | 123 | 128 | 133 | 138 | 142 | 147 | 151 | 156 | 160 | 165 | 170 | 174 | 179 | 183 | 188 | 193 | 197 | 202 | 206 | 211 | 215 | 220 |
| 24 | 109 | 113 | 118 | 122 | 127 | 131 | 136 | 140 | 145 | 149 | 154 | 158 | 163 | 167 | 172 | 176 | 181 | 186 | 190 | 195 | 199 | 204 | 208 | 213 | 217 |
| 25 | 107 | 112 | 116 | 121 | 125 | 129 | 134 | 138 | 143 | 147 | 152 | 156 | 161 | 165 | 170 | 174 | 179 | 183 | 188 | 192 | 196 | 201 | 205 | 210 | 214 |
| 26 | 106 | 110 | 115 | 119 | 123 | 128 | 132 | 137 | 141 | 145 | 150 | 154 | 159 | 163 | 167 | 172 | 176 | 181 | 185 | 189 | 194 | 198 | 203 | 207 | 211 |
| 27 | 104 | 109 | 113 | 117 | 122 | 126 | 130 | 135 | 139 | 143 | 148 | 152 | 156 | 161 | 165 | 169 | 174 | 178 | 183 | 187 | 191 | 196 | 200 | 204 | 209 |
| 28 | 103 | 107 | 111 | 116 | 120 | 124 | 129 | 133 | 137 | 141 | 146 | 150 | 154 | 159 | 163 | 167 | 171 | 176 | 180 | 184 | 189 | 193 | 197 | 201 | 208 |
| 29 | 102 | 106 | 110 | 114 | 118 | 123 | 127 | 131 | 135 | 139 | 144 | 148 | 152 | 156 | 161 | 165 | 169 | 173 | 178 | 182 | 186 | 190 | 194 | 199 | 203 |
| 30 | 100 | 104 | 108 | 113 | 117 | 121 | 125 | 129 | 133 | 137 | 142 | 146 | 150 | 154 | 158 | 162 | 167 | 171 | 175 | 179 | 183 | 188 | 192 | 196 | 200 |
| 31 | 99 | 103 | 107 | 111 | 115 | 119 | 123 | 127 | 131 | 136 | 140 | 144 | 149 | 152 | 156 | 160 | 164 | 168 | 173 | 177 | 181 | 185 | 189 | 193 | 197 |
| 32 | 97 | 101 | 105 | 109 | 113 | 117 | 121 | 125 | 130 | 134 | 138 | 142 | 146 | 150 | 154 | 158 | 162 | 166 | 170 | 174 | 178 | 182 | 186 | 190 | 194 |
| 33 | 96 | 100 | 104 | 108 | 112 | 116 | 120 | 124 | 128 | 132 | 136 | 140 | 144 | 148 | 152 | 156 | 160 | 164 | 168 | 171 | 175 | 179 | 183 | 187 | 191 |
| 34 | 94 | 98 | 102 | 106 | 110 | 114 | 118 | 122 | 126 | 130 | 134 | 137 | 141 | 145 | 149 | 153 | 157 | 161 | 165 | 169 | 173 | 177 | 181 | 185 | 189 |
| 35 | 93 | 97 | 101 | 104 | 108 | 112 | 116 | 120 | 124 | 128 | 132 | 135 | 139 | 143 | 147 | 151 | 155 | 159 | 163 | 166 | 170 | 174 | 178 | 182 | 186 |
| 36 | 91 | 95 | 99 | 103 | 107 | 110 | 114 | 118 | 122 | 126 | 130 | 133 | 137 | 141 | 145 | 149 | 152 | 156 | 160 | 164 | 168 | 171 | 175 | 179 | 183 |
| 37 | 90 | 94 | 98 | 101 | 105 | 109 | 113 | 116 | 120 | 124 | 128 | 131 | 135 | 139 | 143 | 146 | 150 | 154 | 158 | 161 | 165 | 169 | 173 | 176 | 180 |
| 38 | 89 | 92 | 96 | 100 | 103 | 107 | 111 | 114 | 118 | 122 | 125 | 129 | 133 | 137 | 140 | 144 | 148 | 151 | 155 | 159 | 162 | 166 | 170 | 174 | 177 |
| 39 | 87 | 91 | 94 | 98 | 102 | 105 | 109 | 112 | 116 | 120 | 123 | 127 | 131 | 134 | 138 | 142 | 145 | 149 | 153 | 156 | 160 | 163 | 167 | 171 | 174 |
| 40 | 86 | 89 | 93 | 96 | 100 | 104 | 107 | 111 | 114 | 118 | 121 | 125 | 129 | 132 | 136 | 139 | 143 | 146 | 150 | 154 | 157 | 161 | 164 | 168 | 173 |

NOTE: To use, find the subject's present weight at the top of the table, then descend vertically to the horizontal row corresponding to the estimated percent fat. From Golding, L.A., Myers, C.R., and Sinning, W.E.: *Y's Way to Fitness,* Champaign, IL., Human Kinetics, 1989. Used with permission.

**10–14** Coronary Heart Disease and Stroke Risk Factor Prediction Charts

## Stroke Risk Factor Prediction Chart

American Heart Association

**1. Find Points For Each Risk Factor**

**Men**

| Age | SBP | HYP RX | Diabetes | Cigs | CVD | AF | LVH |
|---|---|---|---|---|---|---|---|
| 54–56 = 0 | 95–105 = 0 | No = 0 | No = 0 | No = 0 | No = 0 | No = 0 | No = 0 |
| 57–59 = 1 | 106–116 = 1 | Yes = 2 | Yes = 2 | Yes = 3 | Yes = 3 | Yes = 4 | Yes = 6 |
| 60–62 = 2 | 117–126 = 2 | | | | | | |
| 63–65 = 3 | 127–137 = 3 | | | | | | |
| 66–68 = 4 | 138–148 = 4 | | | | | | |
| 69–71 = 5 | 149–159 = 5 | | | | | | |
| 72–74 = 6 | 160–170 = 6 | | | | | | |
| 75–77 = 7 | 171–181 = 7 | | | | | | |
| 78–80 = 8 | 182–191 = 8 | | | | | | |
| 81–83 = 9 | 192–202 = 9 | | | | | | |
| 84–86 = 10 | 203–213 = 10 | | | | | | |

**Women**

| Age | SBP | HYP RX | Diabetes | Cigs | CVD | AF | LVH |
|---|---|---|---|---|---|---|---|
| 54–56 = 0 | 95–104 = 0 | No = 0 | No = 0 | No = 0 | No = 0 | No = 0 | No = 0 |
| 57–59 = 1 | 105–114 = 1 | If Yes see below | Yes = 3 | Yes = 3 | Yes = 2 | Yes = 6 | Yes = 4 |
| 60–62 = 2 | 115–124 = 2 | | | | | | |
| 63–65 = 3 | 125–134 = 3 | | | | | | |
| 66–68 = 4 | 135–144 = 4 | | | | | | |
| 69–71 = 5 | 145–154 = 5 | | | | | | |
| 72–74 = 6 | 155–164 = 6 | | | | | | |
| 75–77 = 7 | 165–174 = 7 | | | | | | |
| 78–80 = 8 | 175–184 = 8 | | | | | | |
| 81–83 = 9 | 185–194 = 9 | | | | | | |
| 84–86 = 10 | 196–204 = 10 | | | | | | |

If Currently Under Anti-Hypertensive Therapy Add The Following Points Depending On SBP Level

| SBP | 95–104 | 105–114 | 115–124 | 125–134 | 135–144 | 145–154 |
|---|---|---|---|---|---|---|
| Points | 6 | 5 | 5 | 4 | 3 | 3 |

| SBP | 155–164 | 165–174 | 175–184 | 185–194 | 195–204 |
|---|---|---|---|---|---|
| Points | 2 | 1 | 1 | 0 | 0 |

**2. Sum Points For All Risk Factors**

_____ Age + _____ SBP + _____ HYP RX + _____ Diabetes + _____ CIGS + _____ CVD + _____ AF + _____ LVH = _____ Point Total

**3. Look Up Risk Corresponding To Point Total**

**Men 10 Yr.**

| Pts. | Prob. | Pts. | Prob. | Pts. | Prob. |
|---|---|---|---|---|---|
| 1 | 2.6% | 11 | 11.2% | 21 | 41.7% |
| 2 | 3.0% | 12 | 12.9% | 22 | 46.6% |
| 3 | 3.5% | 13 | 14.8% | 23 | 51.8% |
| 4 | 4.0% | 14 | 17.0% | 24 | 57.3% |
| 5 | 4.7% | 15 | 19.5% | 25 | 62.8% |
| 6 | 5.4% | 16 | 22.4% | 26 | 68.4% |
| 7 | 6.3% | 17 | 25.5% | 27 | 73.8% |
| 8 | 7.3% | 18 | 29.0% | 28 | 79.0% |
| 9 | 8.4% | 19 | 32.9% | 29 | 83.7% |
| 10 | 9.7% | 20 | 37.1% | 30 | 87.9% |

**Women 10 Yr.**

| Pts. | Prob. | Pts. | Prob. | Pts. | Prob. |
|---|---|---|---|---|---|
| 1 | 1.1% | 11 | 7.6% | 21 | 43.4% |
| 2 | 1.3% | 12 | 9.2% | 22 | 50.0% |
| 3 | 1.6% | 13 | 11.1% | 23 | 57.0% |
| 4 | 2.0% | 14 | 13.3% | 24 | 64.2% |
| 5 | 2.4% | 15 | 16.0% | 25 | 71.4% |
| 6 | 2.9% | 16 | 19.1% | 26 | 78.2% |
| 7 | 3.5% | 17 | 22.8% | 27 | 84.4% |
| 8 | 4.3% | 18 | 27.0% | | |
| 9 | 5.2% | 19 | 31.9% | | |
| 10 | 6.3% | 20 | 37.3% | | |

**4. Compare To Average 10-Year Risk**

Avg. 10 Yr. Prob. By Age

| Men | | Women | |
|---|---|---|---|
| 55–59 | 5.9% | 55–59 | 3.0% |
| 60–64 | 7.8% | 60–64 | 4.7% |
| 65–69 | 11.0% | 65–69 | 7.2% |
| 70–74 | 13.7% | 70–74 | 10.9% |
| 75–79 | 18.0% | 75–79 | 15.5% |
| 80–84 | 22.3% | 80–84 | 23.9% |

Key For Symbols:

**SBP** — Systolic blood pressure
**HYP RX** — Under anti-hypertensive therapy?
**DIABETES** — History of diabetes?
**CIGS** — Smokes cigarettes?
**CVD** — History of myocardial infarction, angina pectoris, coronary insuffiency, intermittent claudication or congestive heart failure?
**AF** — History of atrial fibrillation?
**LVH** — Left ventricular hypertrophy on ECG?

## Coronary Heart Disease Risk Factor Prediction Chart

**1. Find Points For Each Risk Factor**

| Age (If Female) Age | Pts. | Age | Pts. | Age (If Male) Age | Pts. | Age | Pts. | HDL-Cholesterol HDL-C | Pts. | Total-Cholesterol Total-C | Pts. | Systolic Blood Pressure SBP | Pts. | Other | Pts. |
|---|---|---|---|---|---|---|---|---|---|---|---|---|---|---|---|
| 30 | −12 | 47–48 | 5 | 30 | −2 | 57–59 | 13 | 25–26 | 7 | 139–151 | −3 | 98–104 | −2 | Cigarettes | 4 |
| 31 | −11 | 49–50 | 6 | 31 | −1 | 60–61 | 14 | 27–29 | 6 | 152–166 | −2 | 105–112 | −1 | Diabetic-male | 3 |
| 32 | −9 | 51–52 | 7 | 32–33 | 0 | 62–64 | 15 | 30–32 | 5 | 167–182 | −1 | 113–120 | 0 | Diabetic-female | 6 |
| 33 | −8 | 53–55 | 8 | 34 | 1 | 65–67 | 16 | 33–35 | 4 | 183–199 | 0 | 121–129 | 1 | ECG-LVH | 9 |
| 34 | −6 | 56–60 | 9 | 35–36 | 2 | 68–70 | 17 | 36–38 | 3 | 200–219 | 1 | 130–139 | 2 | | |
| 35 | −5 | 61–67 | 10 | 37–38 | 3 | 71–73 | 18 | 39–42 | 2 | 220–239 | 2 | 140–149 | 3 | 0 pts for each NO | |
| 36 | −4 | 68–74 | 11 | 39 | 4 | 74 | 19 | 43–46 | 1 | 240–262 | 3 | 150–160 | 4 | | |
| 37 | −3 | | | 40–41 | 5 | | | 47–50 | 0 | 263–288 | 4 | 161–172 | 5 | | |
| 38 | −2 | | | 42–43 | 6 | | | 51–55 | −1 | 289–315 | 5 | 173–185 | 6 | | |
| 39 | −1 | | | 44–45 | 7 | | | 56–60 | −2 | 316–330 | 6 | | | | |
| 40 | 0 | | | 46–47 | 8 | | | 61–66 | −3 | | | | | | |
| 41 | 1 | | | 48–49 | 9 | | | 67–73 | −4 | | | | | | |
| 42–43 | 2 | | | 50–51 | 10 | | | 74–80 | −5 | | | | | | |
| 44 | 3 | | | 52–54 | 11 | | | 81–87 | −6 | | | | | | |
| 45–46 | 4 | | | 55–56 | 12 | | | 88–96 | −7 | | | | | | |

**2. Sum Points For All Risk Factors**

_____ Age + _____ HDL-C + _____ Total-C + _____ SBP + _____ Smoker + _____ Diabetes + _____ ECG-LVH = _____ Point Total

NOTE: *Minus Points Subtract From Total.*

**3. Look Up Risk Corresponding To Point Total**

| Pts. | Probability 5 Yr. | 10 Yr. | Pts. | Probability 5 Yr. | 10 Yr. | Pts. | Probability 5 Yr. | 10 Yr. | Pts. | Probability 5 Yr. | 10 Yr. |
|---|---|---|---|---|---|---|---|---|---|---|---|
| ≤1 | <1% | <2% | 10 | 2% | 6% | 19 | 8% | 16% | 28 | 19% | 33% |
| 2 | 1% | 2% | 11 | 3% | 6% | 20 | 8% | 18% | 29 | 20% | 36% |
| 3 | 1% | 2% | 12 | 3% | 7% | 21 | 9% | 19% | 30 | 22% | 38% |
| 4 | 1% | 2% | 13 | 3% | 8% | 22 | 11% | 21% | 31 | 24% | 40% |
| 5 | 1% | 3% | 14 | 4% | 9% | 23 | 12% | 23% | 32 | 25% | 42% |
| 6 | 1% | 3% | 15 | 5% | 10% | 24 | 13% | 25% | | | |
| 7 | 1% | 4% | 16 | 5% | 12% | 25 | 14% | 27% | | | |
| 8 | 2% | 4% | 17 | 6% | 13% | 26 | 16% | 29% | | | |
| 9 | 2% | 5% | 18 | 7% | 14% | 27 | 17% | 31% | | | |

**4. Compare To Average 10 Year Risk**

| Age | Probability Women | Men |
|---|---|---|
| 30–34 | <1% | 3% |
| 35–39 | <1% | 5% |
| 40–44 | 2% | 6% |
| 45–49 | 5% | 10% |
| 50–54 | 8% | 14% |
| 55–59 | 12% | 16% |
| 60–64 | 13% | 21% |
| 65–69 | 9% | 30% |
| 70–74 | 12% | 24% |

These charts were prepared with the help of William B. Kannel, M.D., Professor of Medicine and Public Health and Ralph D'Agostino, Ph.D., Head, Department of Mathematics, both at Boston University; Keaven Anderson, Ph.D., Statistician, NHLBI, Framingham Study; Daniel McGee, Ph.D., Associate Professor, University of Arizona.

Framingham Heart Study

## 10–15 Percentiles of Anthropometry, Older Adults

### Subscapular Skinfold Thickness

| Age (years) | Men 95% | Men 50% | Men 5% | Age (years) | Women 95% | Women 50% | Women 5% |
|---|---|---|---|---|---|---|---|
| 65 | 35.7 | 20.0 | 11.2 | 65 | 33.1 | 16.4 | 8.5 |
| 70 | 34.0 | 18.2 | 9.4 | 70 | 32.5 | 15.8 | 7.9 |
| 75 | 32.2 | 16.4 | 7.7 | 75 | 31.9 | 15.2 | 7.3 |
| 80 | 30.4 | 14.7 | 5.9 | 80 | 31.3 | 14.6 | 6.7 |
| 85 | 28.7 | 12.9 | 4.1 | 85 | 30.7 | 14.0 | 6.1 |
| 90 | 26.9 | 11.2 | 2.4 | 90 | 30.1 | 13.5 | 5.5 |

### Midarm Muscle Area

| Age (years) | Men 95% | Men 50% | Men 5% | Age (years) | Women 95% | Women 50% | Women 5% |
|---|---|---|---|---|---|---|---|
| 65 | 77.1 | 59.4 | 43.2 | 65 | 66.4 | 44.5 | 33.5 |
| 70 | 75.3 | 57.7 | 41.4 | 70 | 65.9 | 44.1 | 33.0 |
| 75 | 73.5 | 55.9 | 39.6 | 75 | 65.5 | 43.6 | 32.6 |
| 80 | 71.7 | 54.1 | 37.8 | 80 | 65.1 | 43.2 | 32.2 |
| 85 | 69.9 | 52.3 | 36.0 | 85 | 64.7 | 42.8 | 31.8 |
| 90 | 68.2 | 50.5 | 34.3 | 90 | 64.2 | 42.4 | 31.3 |

### Midarm Circumference

| Age (years) | Men 95% | Men 50% | Men 5% | Age (years) | Women 95% | Women 50% | Women 5% |
|---|---|---|---|---|---|---|---|
| 65 | 37.8 | 31.9 | 26.7 | 65 | 37.0 | 30.5 | 25.3 |
| 70 | 37.2 | 31.3 | 26.0 | 70 | 36.6 | 30.2 | 24.9 |
| 75 | 36.6 | 30.7 | 25.4 | 75 | 36.3 | 29.8 | 24.6 |
| 80 | 36.0 | 30.1 | 24.8 | 80 | 35.9 | 29.5 | 24.2 |
| 85 | 35.3 | 29.4 | 24.2 | 85 | 35.6 | 29.1 | 23.9 |
| 90 | 34.7 | 28.8 | 23.5 | 90 | 35.2 | 28.9 | 23.5 |

### Weight

| Age (years) | Men 95% | Men 50% | Men 5% | Age (years) | Women 95% | Women 50% | Women 5% |
|---|---|---|---|---|---|---|---|
| 65 | 102.0 (224.9) | 79.5 (175.0) | 62.6 (138.0) | 65 | 87.1 (192.0) | 66.8 (147.3) | 51.2 (112.9) |
| 70 | 99.1 (218.5) | 76.5 (168.7) | 59.7 (131.6) | 70 | 84.9 (187.2) | 64.6 (142.4) | 49.0 (108.0) |
| 75 | 96.3 (212.3) | 73.6 (162.3) | 56.8 (125.2) | 75 | 82.8 (182.5) | 62.4 (137.6) | 46.8 (103.2) |
| 80 | 93.4 (205.9) | 70.7 (155.9) | 53.9 (118.8) | 80 | 80.6 (177.7) | 60.2 (132.7) | 44.7 ( 98.5) |
| 85 | 90.5 (199.5) | 67.8 (149.5) | 51.0 (112.4) | 85 | 78.4 (172.8) | 58.0 (127.9) | 42.5 ( 93.7) |
| 90 | 87.6 (193.1) | 64.9 (142.8) | 48.1 (106.0) | 90 | 76.2 (168.0) | 55.9 (123.2) | 40.3 ( 88.8) |

### Stature

| Age (years) | Men 95% | Men 50% | Men 5% | Age (years) | Women 95% | Women 50% | Women 5% |
|---|---|---|---|---|---|---|---|
| 65 | 181.6 (71.5) | 170.3 (67.0) | 159.1 (62.6) | 65 | 171.6 (67.6) | 161.0 (63.4) | 153.1 (60.3) |
| 70 | 181.6 (71.5) | 169.9 (66.9) | 158.7 (62.5) | 70 | 169.8 (66.9) | 159.1 (62.6) | 151.3 (59.6) |
| 75 | 181.2 (71.3) | 169.5 (66.7) | 158.4 (62.4) | 75 | 167.9 (66.1) | 157.3 (61.9) | 149.4 (58.8) |
| 80 | 180.9 (71.2) | 169.1 (66.6) | 158.0 (62.2) | 80 | 166.1 (65.4) | 155.4 (61.2) | 147.6 (58.1) |
| 85 | 180.5 (71.1) | 168.8 (66.5) | 157.7 (62.1) | 85 | 164.2 (64.6) | 153.6 (60.5) | 145.7 (57.4) |
| 90 | 180.2 (70.9) | 168.5 (66.3) | 157.3 (61.9) | 90 | 162.4 (63.9) | 151.7 (59.7) | 143.9 (56.6) |

### Triceps Skinfold Thickness

| Age (years) | Men 95% | Men 50% | Men 5% | Age (years) | Women 95% | Women 50% | Women 5% |
|---|---|---|---|---|---|---|---|
| 65 | 27.0 | 13.8 | 8.6 | 65 | 33.0 | 21.6 | 13.5 |
| 70 | 26.1 | 12.9 | 7.7 | 70 | 32.0 | 20.6 | 12.5 |
| 75 | 25.2 | 12.0 | 6.8 | 75 | 31.0 | 19.6 | 11.5 |
| 80 | 24.3 | 11.2 | 6.0 | 80 | 30.0 | 18.6 | 10.5 |
| 85 | 23.4 | 10.3 | 5.1 | 85 | 29.0 | 17.6 | 9.5 |
| 90 | 22.6 | 9.4 | 4.2 | 90 | 28.0 | 16.6 | 8.5 |

From: *Nutritional Assessment of the Elderly through Anthropometry,* Chumlea, W.C., Roches, A.F., and Mukherjee, D., Fels Research Institute, Yellow Springs Ross Laboratories, Columbus, Ohio. Used with permission.

**10–16** Triceps Skinfold Thickness, Body Mass Index, Whites and Blacks, Women

| Body Mass Index (kg/m²) | Total | Age Group 65-74 | 75-84 | 85+ | Disability Level Moderate[3] | ADL Difficulty Receives No Help | Receives Help |
|---|---|---|---|---|---|---|---|
| Total | (N=924) | (N=358) | (N=287) | (N=279) | (N=333) | (N=455) | (N=136) |
| Mean | 28.9 | 31.1 | 27.6 | 26.1 | 27.9 | 29.6 | 29.4 |
| Median | 27.4 | 29.5 | 27.1 | 25.6 | 27.0 | 27.9 | 27.0 |
| Percent underweight (≤21.44)[4] | 11.7 | 5.9 | 15.3 | 19.1 | 12.7 | 10.0 | 15.5 |
| Percent overweight (≥31.58)[5] | 28.5 | 39.1 | 23.1 | 12.5 | 24.0 | 31.1 | 31.8 |
| Whites | (N=667) | (N=235) | (N=208) | (N=224) | (N=221) | (N=352) | (N=94) |
| Mean | 28.0 | 29.8 | 27.2 | 25.9 | 27.0 | 28.6 | 28.7 |
| Median | 26.9 | 28.8 | 27.0 | 25.4 | 26.5 | 27.7 | 26.3 |
| Percent underweight (≤21.44)[4] | 12.5 | 5.6 | 15.7 | 20.9 | 12.1 | 10.8 | 20.4 |
| Percent overweight (≥31.58)[5] | 24.9 | 33.7 | 21.6 | 12.1 | 17.8 | 28.0 | 31.4 |
| Blacks | (N=254) | (N=120) | (N=79) | (N=55) | (N=111) | (N=101) | (N=42) |
| Mean | 31.3 | 33.8 | 28.8 | 26.9 | 29.7 | 33.1 | 30.9 |
| Median | 28.9 | 31.5 | 28.0 | 27.0 | 29.0 | 29.4 | 28.2 |
| Percent underweight (≤21.44)[4] | 9.9 | 6.6 | 13.9 | 12.0 | 14.1 | 7.2 | 4.6 |
| Percent overweight (≥31.58)[5] | 37.5 | 49.2 | 27.5 | 14.0 | 35.8 | 41.2 | 32.6 |

(Women's Health and Aging Study, physical assessment, 1992-1995)

[1] Weight(kg)/height(m)². If a participant's height was not measured, it was estimated from the average of two knee height measurements. The estimated height in cm = 84.88 + 1.83 (knee height) - 0.24(age). Chumlea WC, Roche AF, Steinbaugh ML. Estimating stature from knee height for persons 60 to 90 years of age. J Am Geriatr Soc 1958, 33: 116-120.
[2] Descriptive statistics are based on weighted data.
[3] No ADL difficulty; disabled in two or more domains (see Chapter 1).
[4] 15th percentile or below, based on data from NHANES I for females age 70 to 74 years in Must A, Dallal GE, Dietz WH. (1991). Reference data for obesity: 85th and 95th percentiles of body mass index (wt/ht²) and triceps skinfold thickness. Am J Clin Nutr 53:839-846.
[5] 85th percentile or above, based on previous reference.

| Triceps Skinfold Thickness (mm) | Total | Age Group 65-74 | 75-84 | 85+ | Disability Level Moderate[3] | ADL Difficulty Receives No Help | Receives Help |
|---|---|---|---|---|---|---|---|
| Total | (N=995) | (N=384) | (N=309) | (N=302) | (N=342) | (N=473) | (N=180) |
| Mean | 21.9 | 24.4 | 20.8 | 17.4 | 21.8 | 22.0 | 21.7 |
| Median | 20.7 | 24.0 | 19.8 | 17.4 | 21.0 | 20.4 | 19.9 |
| Percent low (≤16.3)[4] | 25.6 | 14.6 | 29.9 | 45.9 | 24.4 | 24.5 | 31.3 |
| Percent high (≥30.8)[5] | 15.2 | 22.1 | 11.6 | 5.2 | 14.3 | 14.9 | 17.9 |
| Whites | (N=709) | (N=248) | (N=219) | (N=242) | (N=228) | (N=361) | (N=120) |
| Mean | 21.4 | 24.2 | 20.4 | 17.1 | 21.2 | 21.6 | 21.0 |
| Median | 20.2 | 23.3 | 20.2 | 17.3 | 20.8 | 20.2 | 19.6 |
| Percent low (≤16.3)[4] | 25.3 | 13.4 | 28.0 | 47.1 | 24.0 | 24.2 | 32.0 |
| Percent high (≥30.8)[5] | 12.2 | 20.3 | 7.6 | 3.9 | 10.3 | 12.7 | 14.3 |
| Blacks | (N=281) | (N=131) | (N=90) | (N=60) | (N=113) | (N=109) | (N=59) |
| Mean | 23.1 | 25.0 | 21.9 | 18.4 | 23.1 | 23.3 | 23.0 |
| Median | 21.1 | 24.8 | 19.5 | 18.7 | 22.2 | 20.9 | 20.7 |
| Percent low (≤16.3)[4] | 26.9 | 17.8 | 35.5 | 40.9 | 25.4 | 26.3 | 31.1 |
| Percent high (≥30.8)[5] | 23.4 | 26.4 | 22.8 | 10.6 | 23.0 | 22.6 | 25.6 |

(Women's Health and Aging Study, physical assessment, 1992-1995)

[1] Skinfold thickness was usually computed by averaging the first two measures. A third measure was taken if the difference between the first two exceeded 2 mm. If the third measure was within 2 mm of just one of the earlier measures then the average of the two close measures was computed. Otherwise, the average of three measures was used. When a single measure was taken then it was used for the thickness.
[2] Descriptive statistics are based on weighted data.
[3] No ADL difficulty; disabled in two or more domains (see Chapter 1).
[4] 15th percentile or below, based on data from NHANES I for females age 70 to 74 years in Must A, Dallal GE, Dietz WH. (1991). Reference data for obesity: 85th and 95th percentiles of body mass index (wt/ht²) and triceps skinfold thickness. Am J Clin Nutr 53:839-846.
[5] 85th percentile or above, based on previous reference.

# APPENDIX 11
## Helpful Resources

### APPENDIX 11–1

Helpful Resources
http://health.gov/dietaryguidelines/2015/guidelines/
http://www.choosemyplate.gov/

# Index

Page references for figures are indicated by *f,* for tables by *t,* and for boxes by *b.*